Essentials of
Oral and Maxillofacial Radiology

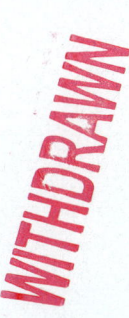

Essentials of
Oral and Maxillofacial Radiology

Freny R Karjodkar MDS (Mumbai University)

Professor and Head
Department of Oral Medicine and Radiology
Nair Hospital Dental College
Mumbai, Maharashtra, India

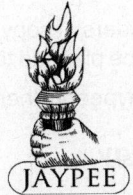

JAYPEE BROTHERS Medical Publishers (P) Ltd

New Delhi • London • Philadelphia • Panama

Jaypee Brothers Medical Publishers (P) Ltd.

Headquarters
Jaypee Brothers Medical Publishers (P) Ltd.
4838/24, Ansari Road, Daryaganj
New Delhi 110 002, India
Phone: +91-11-43574357
Fax: +91-11-43574314
Email: jaypee@jaypeebrothers.com

Overseas Offices

J.P. Medical Ltd.
83, Victoria Street, London
SW1H 0HW (UK)
Phone: +44-2031708910
Fax: +02-03-0086180
Email: info@jpmedpub.com

Jaypee-Highlights Medical Publishers Inc.
City of Knowledge, Bld. 237, Clayton
Panama City, Panama
Phone: +1 507-301-0496
Fax: +1 507-301-0499
Email: cservice@jphmedical.com

Jaypee Medical Inc.
The Bourse
111, South Independence Mall East
Suite 835, Philadelphia, PA 19106, USA
Phone: +1 267-519-9789
Email: jpmed.us@gmail.com

Jaypee Brothers Medical Publishers (P) Ltd.
17/1-B, Babar Road, Block-B, Shaymali
Mohammadpur, Dhaka-1207
Bangladesh
Mobile: +08801912003485
Email: jaypeedhaka@gmail.com

Jaypee Brothers Medical Publishers (P) Ltd.
Bhotahity, Kathmandu, Nepal
Phone: +977-9741283608
Email: kathmandu@jaypeebrothers.com

Website: www.jaypeebrothers.com
Website: www.jaypeedigital.com

© 2014, Jaypee Brothers Medical Publishers

Inquiries for bulk sales may be solicited at: jaypee@jaypeebrothers.com

Essentials of Oral and Maxillofacial Radiology

First Edition: **2014**
ISBN: 978-93-5152-229-4
Printed at Replika Press Pvt. Ltd.

Dedicated to

You discern how it is.
You choose a book, open to the dedication page, and find that, once again,
the book is dedicated to someone else and not to you.
Here is the change.
It could be that we have not yet met, may have met or may never meet,
I trust despite that you will remember...
This one's for you.
To all the readers of this book...

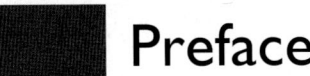# Preface

"You can teach a student a lesson for a day; but if you can teach him to learn by creating curiosity, he will continue the learning process as long as he lives."

—*Clay P Bedford*

"Any fool can know. The point is to understand."

—*Albert Einstein*

There are already plenty of good books out there on dental radiology, then why did I write this book on *Essentials of Oral and Maxillofacial Radiology*?

When the dental surgeon starts out looking at a film, he often has no idea what the diagnosis is. Experienced dental radiologists usually have no trouble generating an appropriate differential diagnosis. But what do you do if you are just starting out in dental radiology? The dental surgeon has the additional responsibility of interpreting his own radiographs.

Besides, in the recent decade, dental radiography has witnessed a radical change with advances in diagnostic imaging which has made dental diagnosis and treatment planning much more precise and accurate, but only if the interpreter is well versed with his basic radiology knowledge.

The dominant vision was to satisfy a need that is not currently addressed by any radiology textbook presently in the market. We wanted to create a single volume textbook that has all its information presented in a standardized way. We wished to avoid long descriptive sentence constructions that would make information retrieval inefficient. We tried to cover the basics of dental radiology, how and when to take dental radiographs and most important how to read and interpret, recognizing the fact that while there are hundreds of potential diagnosis lurking out there for the dental radiologist, in real life, one keeps bumping into the same old stuff over and over, and only rarely finds cases of the unusual disorders.

I wish to express my gratitude to all the persons who have directly or indirectly helped in the realization of this book, our dean Dr SJ Nagda, my colleagues Dr K Sansare and Dr S Sontakke, and all my postgraduate students with a special thanks to Dr Nimish Prakash and Dr Shahnaz Tambawala. My association with M/s Jaypee Brothers Medical Publishers (P) Ltd, New Delhi, and the editorial and production staff in Mumbai and Delhi branches goes a long way and I truly appreciate their unstinted support and co-operation. The love, affection and patience of my family, my mother, aunt, husband Rashmiraj and children Mohnish and Raveena who have incited me to complete this book. I offer my intense thanks to the Almighty, for giving me the courage and confidence to realize my endeavor.

Finally my sincere submission to all my students and readers of this book in the words of Elie Wiesel, "There is a divine beauty in learning... To learn means to accept the postulate that life did not begin at birth. Others have been here before me and I walk in their footsteps..."

Freny R Karjodkar

Contents

Section VII   Role of Radiology in Specialized Dental Fields

Plate 1

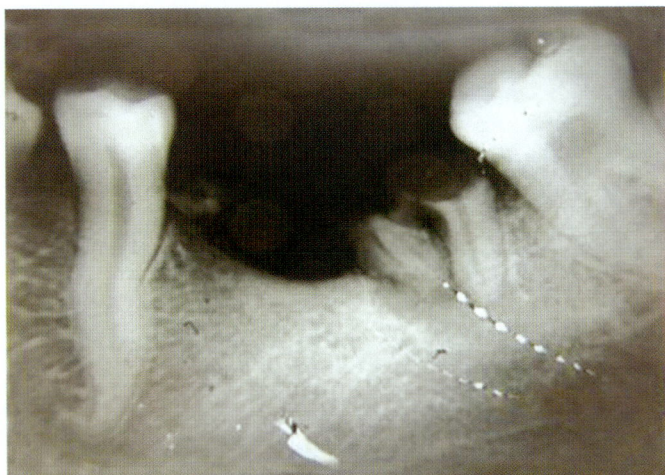

Figure 8.25 Yellow or brown stains

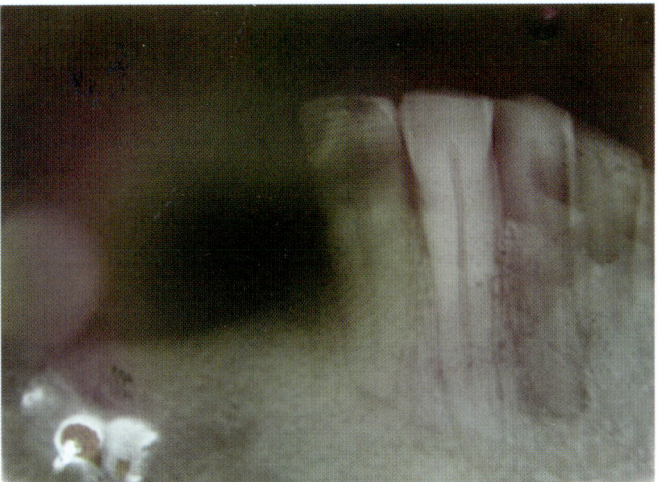

Figure 8.26 Dichroic (showing two colors)

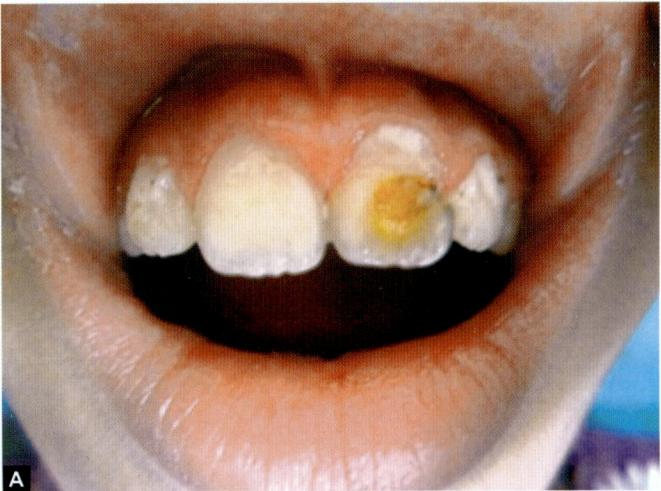

Figure 17.7 Facial caries on the labial aspect of the central incisor seen as a circular radiolucency overlapping the pulp chamber in the radiograph. The central also shows proximal caries on mesial and distal surface involving the enamel and dentine

Section I

Introduction

History of Dental Radiography

Prologue to discovery

Nothing materializes as if by magic overnight. Even Roentgen's discovery depended upon the development and application of three converging thoughts; Electricity, Vacuum and Magnetism.

DISCOVERY OF X-RAYS

Sir William Morgan (1785) (**Fig. 1.1**), unknowingly was the *first man to produce X-rays* while conducting one of his experiments, where he was investigating the discharge of high tension current using 100% vacuum, the glass of the tube cracked and there was an amazing display of colors, beginning with yellow-green and followed by red, violet and blue.

Wilhelm Hittorf (1870) (**Fig. 1.2**) improved vacuum pumps. He observed that fluorescent discharge increased in size as the tube was evacuated and identified the source of the phenomenon as cathode and termed it as 'cathode rays'. He found that these rays traveled in straight lines, produced heat and triggered fluorescence on glass; cast shadow of the object placed in their way and were deflected by a magnet. His work was subsequently verified by Eugen Goldstein (1879).

In 1880s, Sir William Crookes (**Fig. 1.3**) described additional changes that took place in fluorescence. He considered 'radiant matter' to be the 'ultra gaseous state'. He established that recently opened photographic plates were peculiarly fogged and blackened. He also mentioned a 'molecular' and 'emissive' ray which was emitted from his tube which could only be perceived when a fluorescent screen was placed in the path of the ray. He had unintentionally and accidentally generated X-rays.

Philip Lenard (**Fig. 1.4**) demonstrated that cathode rays on passing through a special aluminium window built into the wall of a discharge tube; reserved sufficient energy outside the tube to cause a glow on the fluorescent screen. The emitted glow spread in all directions for about five centimeters in air and he named it as 'Lenard's Ray'. Lenard may have discovered X-rays, had he used barium platinocyanide instead of a less sensitive fluorescent material, keton (pentadecyl paratolylketon).

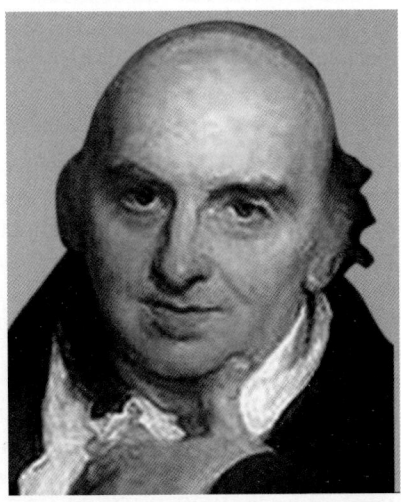

Figure 1.1 Sir William Morgan (1785)

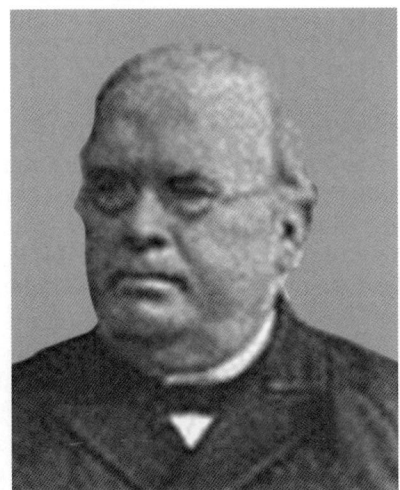

Figure 1.2 Wilhelm Hittorf (1870)

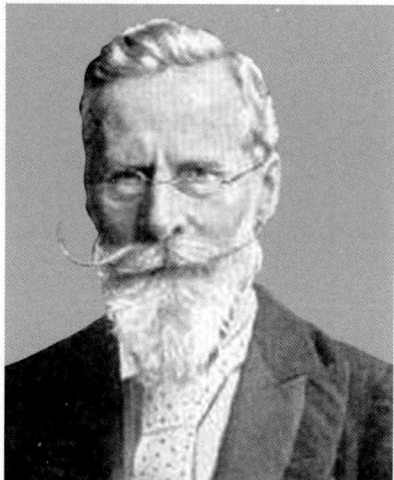

Figure 1.3 Sir William Crookes

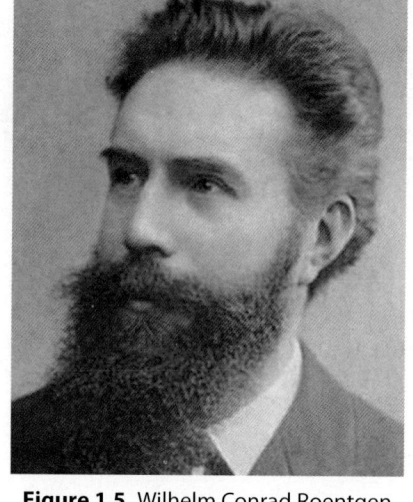

Figure 1.5 Wilhelm Conrad Roentgen

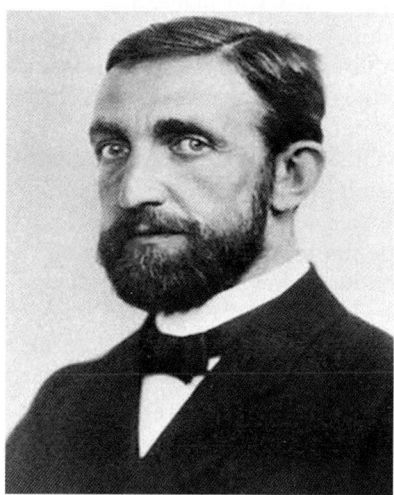

Figure 1.4 Philip Lenard

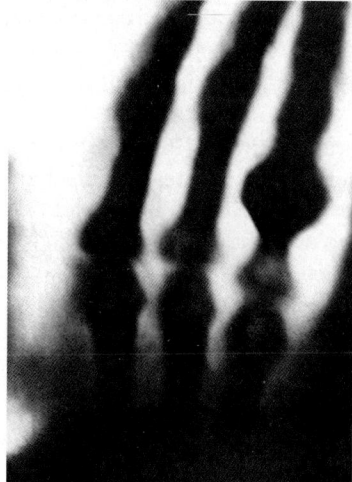

Figure 1.6 First radiograph, which was the hand of Roentgen's wife Bertha Roentgen. Note images of soft tissue, bones and two rings

We owe honor and gratitude for discovering the most striking and outstanding property of cathode rays to Professor Wilhelm Conrad Roentgen of Wurzberg, Bavaria (1895) (**Fig. 1.5**). He termed these rays 'X-rays' after the mathematical symbol for the unknown—'X' which were ultimately, called 'Roentgen Rays'.

Roentgen was the first person to radiograph the human body; by placing his wife's hand on a photographic plate and exposing it to the 'unknown rays' for 15 minutes (**Fig. 1.6**).

It is uncertain who took the first dental radiograph, but the honors are fairly shared between the Germans, Koenig and Walkhoff, (**Fig. 1.7**) Frank Harrison in Britain and C. Edmund Kells (**Fig. 1.8**) in New Jersey, all of whom were producing crude but recognizable dental 'skiagrams' (**Fig. 1.9**) in 1896.

Dr C Edmund Kells (1880), (**Fig. 1.8**) known as the *Father of Dental Radiology*, was the first dentist to practice radiography in root canal therapy on May 10, 1899.

Eight weeks after, Roentgen announced his discovery, on March 23, 1896, Dr. John Daniel, a physicist from Vanderbilt University, Nashville, reported to the editor of Science stating about his observation of hair loss from the head of his colleague in the region that was exposed to radiation.

The real breakthrough in the tube design, which actually ushered in the 'golden age of radiology' was the development of the hot cathode tube by William David Coolidge, (1913) (**Fig. 1.10**).

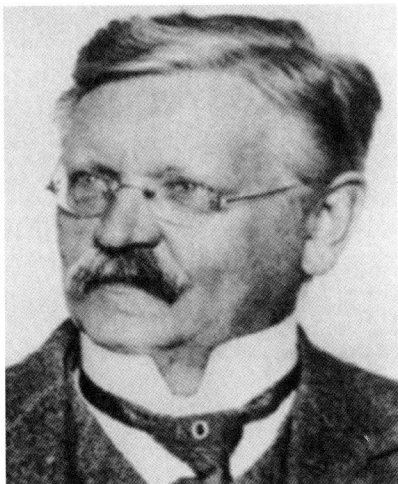

Figure 1.7 Friedrich Otto Walkhoff

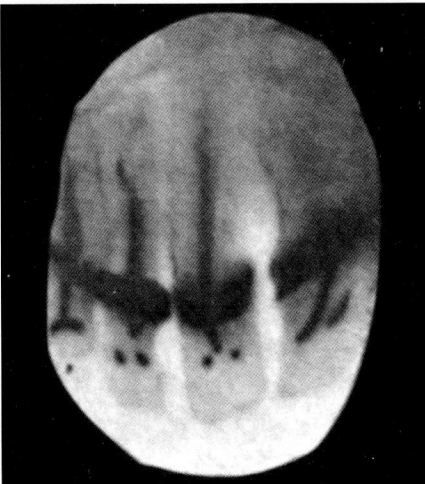

Figure 1.9 Skiagram, the upper right central and lateral incisors; fitted with 'Downie' crowns. Ten minutes exposure

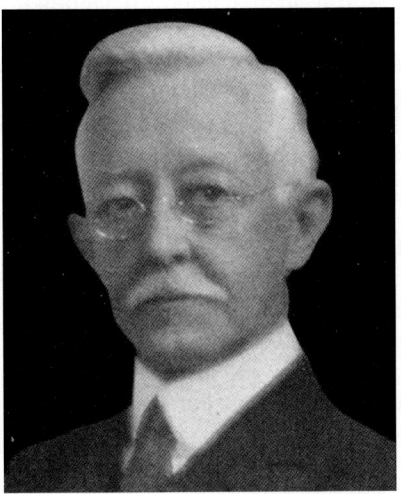

Figure 1.8 C Edmund Kells

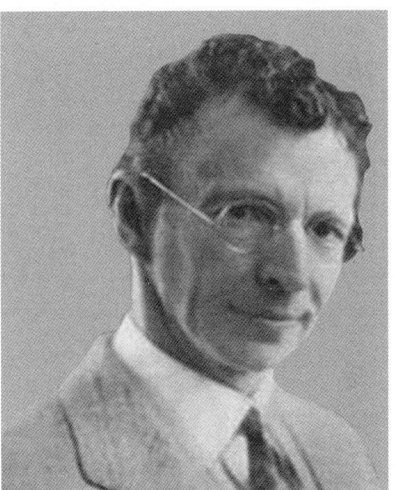

Figure 1.10 William David Coolidge

The X-ray tube stand initially had limited mobility, as it was suspended between two clamps, one on either side of the bulb or from the ceiling.

Dr William Rollins (1896) designed an exclusive X-ray apparatus for the dental surgeon, which also had a protective screen and an adaptable diaphragm to prevent excessive radiation to the patient. He was the first person to report the harmful effects of X-rays and designed a protective tube housing to shield the X-ray tube.

X-ray Films

The first dental radiographs were taken on small glass plates so that they would not distort during development.

Kells and Rollins initiated the use of photographic films because of their flexibility to adapt to the tissues and reduced chances of breakage. Initially the films were hand-made from glass plates or roll films, customized in size and wrapped in black paper and rubber dam to avoid moisture contamination. However they lacked emulsion sensitivity.

The first machine wrapped dental X-ray film packet, called Regular film (Kodak), and became commercially available in 1919. It was a single emulsion, relatively slow but produced sharp images. The Ekta speed film (Kodak), introduced in 1980s has again reduced the exposure by 50 percent.

GROWTH OF DENTAL RADIOLOGY

William Herbert Rollins (1852–1929) (**Fig. 1.11**) '*Dentistry's Forgotten Man*' was an introvert, he is also known as the '*Father of Radiation Protection*'. He experimented with guinea pigs (1901) and inferred that the adverse physiological effects related with X-ray exposure were a result of the X-ray beams themselves and he suggested three protective measures to dental and medical X-ray users:

1. Use radiopaque (leaded) glasses to protect the eyes.
2. Encompass the X-ray tube in a leaded housing.
3. Expose only the area of interest of the patient and cover all neighboring areas with radiopaque materials.

He suggested the use of the collimator to reduce the beam size and proposed a long target film distance to improve image quality and patient safety. In 1903, he was the first to use selective filtration of the X-ray beam which helped to remove the dangerous low energy X-rays.

Dr Weston A Price in 1904 (**Fig. 1.12**), introduced two techniques for film positioning in the oral cavity—the paralleling and the bisecting angle technique. He was instrumental in proposing an X-ray projection technique based on the 'rule of isometry', which is today known as 'bisection of the angle' technique. Price also used opaque (leaded) gloves to protect his hands when he held the film in the patient's mouth.

In 1909, Howard Riley Raper (1887–1978) (**Fig. 1.13**), created a new discipline and a new name for it—*Radiodontia*. In 1925 Dr. Raper introduced the idea of bite-wing films and approached George Eastman of the Eastman Kodak Company.

Franklin W McCormack a medical X-ray technician from San Francisco, California, was the first to use the paralleling principles in intraoral dental radiography.

In 1940, Dr Gordon Fitzgerald (1907–1981) designed a long cone for the dental X-ray machine, based on McCormack's tabletop long-distance (36-inch FFD) technique and adapted it to the dental chair.

In 1949, the American Academy of Oral Roentgenology, (now known as American Academy of Dental Radiology) was formed.

The '*Rotational Panoramic Radiography*' method is by far the most popular method of panoramic radiography. Dr H Numata (**Fig. 1.14**) was the first to propose (1933) and experiment (1934) with this method of panoramic radiography. Numata placed a curved film in the mouth lingual to the teeth and used a slit or narrow X-ray beam that rotated around the patient's jaws to expose the film. Twelve years later, in 1946 Y.V. Paatero (**Fig. 1.15**) of the Institute of Dentistry, Finland, proposed (1946), experimented (1948) and demonstrated a slit beam method of panoramic radiography for the dental arches (1949). In 1960s, SS White and Company marketed the first Panoramic machine (Panorex).

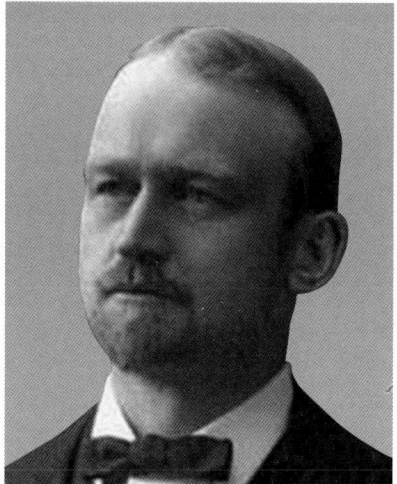

Figure 1.11 Dr William Herbert Rollins

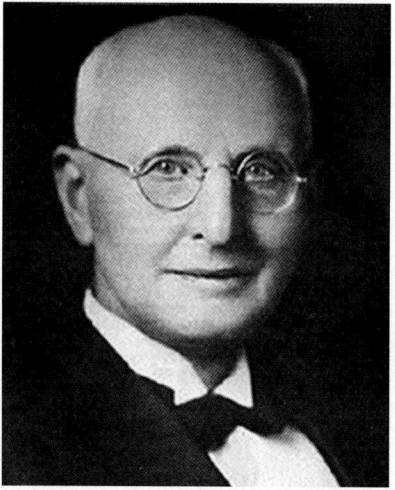

Figure 1.12 Dr Weston A Price

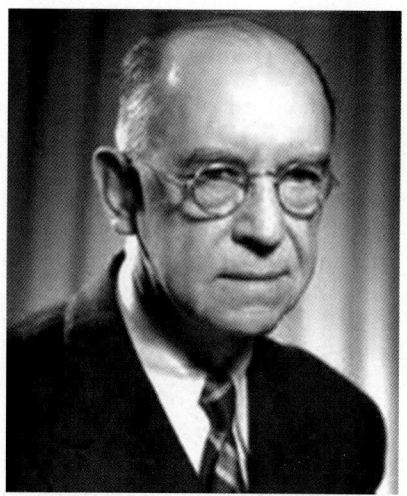

Figure 1.13 Howard Riley Raper

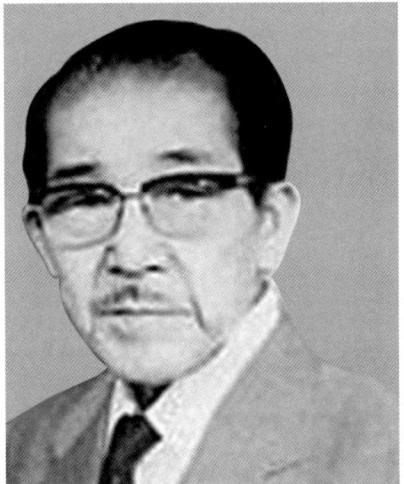

Figure 1.14 Dr H Numata

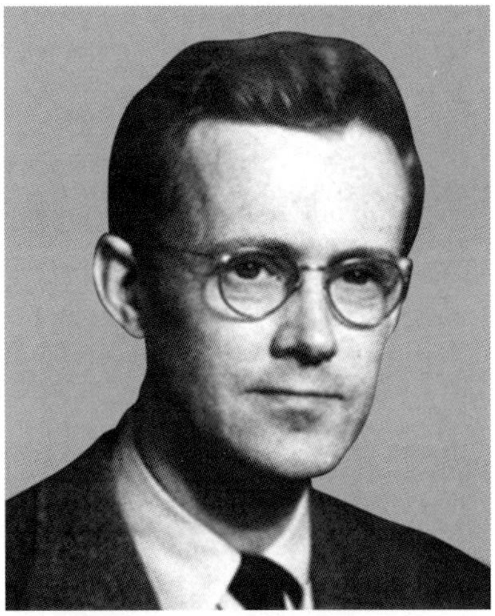

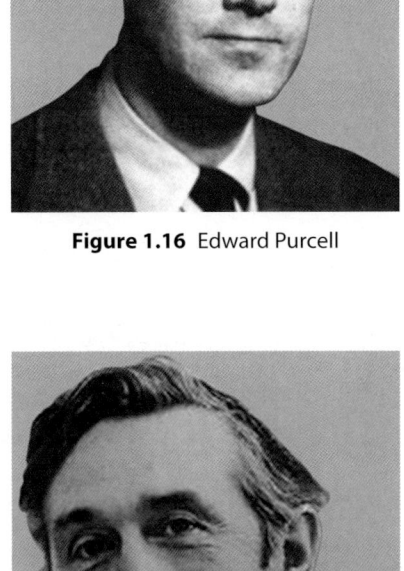

Figure 1.16 Edward Purcell

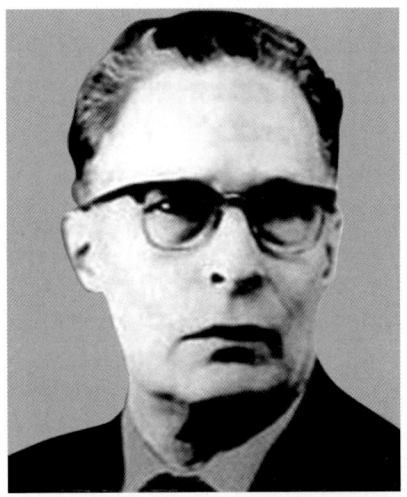

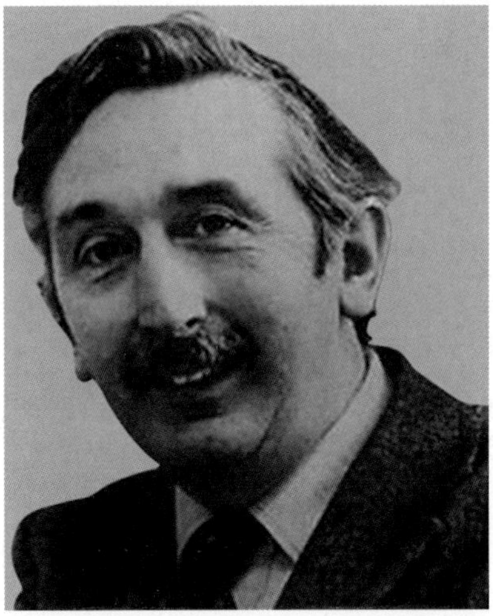

Figure 1.15 YV Paatero

Figure 1.17 Godfrey Hounsfield

In 1968, the International Association of Dento-Maxillofacial Radiology was established.

Magnetic resonance imaging (MRI) is a relatively new medical imaging technology, with its roots dating back in the year 1946. Felix Bloch and Edward Purcell (**Fig. 1.16**) individually discovered the magnetic resonance phenomena. Till 1970s MRI was used for chemical and physical analysis. In 1971 Raymond Damadian established that nuclear magnetic relaxation times of tissues and tumors differed, inspiring scientists to practice MRI to study disease. With the dawn of *Computed Tomography* (using computer techniques to develop images from MRI information) in 1973 by Godfrey Hounsfield (**Fig. 1.17**), and echo-planar imaging (a rapid imaging technique) in 1977 by Mansfield, MRI and CT Imaging techniques evolved over the next 20 years.

Cone beam computed tomography (CBCT) technology was first introduced in the European market in 1998 and into the US market in 2001. This is a specific technology which has created an uprising in maxillofacial imaging enabling the advancement of dental imaging from 2D to 3D images and increasing the role of imaging from diagnosis to image guidance for operative and surgical procedures via third party application softwares.

Highlights in the history of dental radiology

Years	Concepts	Persons associated with
1895	Discovery of X-rays	WC Roentgen
1896	First dental radiograph	O Walkhoff
1896	First dental radiograph in US (skull)	WJ Morton
1896	First dental radiograph in US (live)	CE Kells
1901	First paper on dangers of X-radiation	WH Rollins
1904	Introduction of bisecting technique	WA Price
1913	First dental text	HR Raper
1913	First prewrapped dental films	Eastman Kodak Company
1913	First X-ray tube	WD Coolidge
1920	Concept of paralleling technique	F McCormack
1920	First machine-made film packets	Eastman Kodak Company
1923	First dental X-ray machine	Victor X-ray Corporation of Chicago
1925	Introduction of bite-wing technique	HR Raper
1933	Concept of rotational panoramics proposed	Dr Hisatugu Numata
1947	Introduction of long cone paralleling technique	FG Fitzgerald
1948	Introduction of panaromic radiography	Dr Yrjo Veli Paatero
1955	Introduction of D-speed film	
1957	First variable kilovoltage dental X-ray machine	General electric
1960	First panoramic X-ray machine	Marketed SS White and Co.
1969	Prototype scanner developed	Godfrey Hounsfield
1978	Introduction of dental xeroradiography	
1981	Introduction of E-speed film	
1987	Introduction of intraoral digital radiography	
1987	Denta scan designed	
1998	CBCT	European market
2000	Introduction of 'F' Speed Films	
2001	CBCT	US market

BIBLIOGRAPHY

1. Gibbs SJ. Nashville, Tenn. Radiology Chasing a Century, Opening a Millennium, Oral Surg, Oral Med, Oral Pathol, Oral Radiol. Endod. 1996;81:603-6.
2. Goaz DW, White SC. Oral Radiology, Principles and Interpretation. 2nd, CV Mosby; 1987.pp.1-17.
3. JW Preece. Roentgen Alchemy Part I, American Academy of Dental Radiology. 1969;28(5):680-91.
4. JW Preece. Roentgen Alchemy Part II, American Academy of Dental Radiology. 1969;28(6):830-43.
5. Langland OE, Langlas RP. Early Pioneers of Oral and Maxillofacial Radiology, Oral Surg, Oral Med, Oral Pathol, Oral Radiol, Endod. 1995;80:496-511.
6. Mc Call JO, Wald SS. Clinical Dental Roentgenology. WB Saunders Co. Philadelphia; 1947.
7. Mc Coy JD. Dental and Oral Radiology. St. Louis, The CV Mosby Co. 1919.
8. Taylor JA. History of Dentistry. Philadelphia: Lea and Febiger; 1522.

Section II

Physics of Ionizing Radiation

Radiation Physics | 2

BASIC CONSIDERATIONS

The world is composed of matter and energy.

Matter is the substance of which all physical things are composed, it occupies space, has inertia, mass, can exert force and can be acted upon by force. It occurs in three states, solid, liquid and gaseous and may be divided into elements and compounds, which are essentially made of molecules and atoms. When matter is altered it results in the production of *energy*.

An *atom* is the fundamental unit of any particular element, which cannot be subdivided by ordinary chemical methods, but may be broken down into subatomic particles by special high energy techniques.

A *molecule* is defined as a sufficiently stable, electrically neutral group of at least two atoms in a definite arrangement held together by strong chemical bonds.

The atom consists of two parts, a central nucleus and orbiting electrons. The identity of an atom is determined by the composition of its nucleus and the arrangement of its orbiting electrons.

The *nucleus*, or the dense core of the atom is composed of particles known as protons and neutrons (nucleons); protons carry the positive electrical charges, whereas neutrons carry no electrical charge. The nucleus of the atom occupies very little space. Atoms differ from one another based on their nuclear composition. The number of protons and neutrons in the nucleus of an atom determines its *mass number* or *atomic weight*. The number of protons inside the nucleus equals the number of electrons outside the nucleus and determines the atomic number of the atom. Each atom has an atomic number ranging from that of Hydrogen, the simplest atom, which has an atomic number of 1, to that of Hahnium, the most complex atom, which has an atomic number of 105.

Electrons are tiny negatively charged particles that have very little mass; an electron weighs approximately 1/1800 as much as a proton or neutron. The arrangement of the electrons and neutrons in an atom resemble that of a miniature solar system. Just as the planets revolve around the sun, electrons travel around the nucleus in well defined paths known as orbits or shells.

An atom contains a maximum of seven shells, each located at a specific distance from the nucleus and representing different energy levels. The shells are designated with the letters K, L, M, N, O, P, and Q. Each shell has a maximum number of electrons it can hold, which is determined by the formula, $(2n^2)$, where n is the quantum number.

Electrons are maintained in their orbits by the electrostatic force, or attraction, between the positive nucleus and the negative electrons, and it also balances the centrifugal force of the rapidly moving electrons. This is known as the binding energy or binding force of an electron. The binding energies of orbital electrons are measured in electron volts (eV) or kiloelectron volts (keV). (1 keV = 1000 eV).

Atoms can exist in a neutral or an electrically unbalanced state. Atoms that gain or lose an electron and become electrically unbalanced are called ions.

Ionization (**Fig. 2.1**) is the production of ions, or the process of converting an atom into ions. When an electron is removed from an atom; in the process of ionization; an ion pair results.

Just as an electron has to receive energy to escape from its orbit, so when it transfers from one orbit to another closer to the nucleus it must surrender some energy. It has to in fact, give up the difference between the binding energy of the two orbits and this energy is emitted in the form of *electromagnetic radiation*.

The binding energy of different orbits depends on the nuclear charge and therefore will be different for different elements, furthermore, the difference between the binding

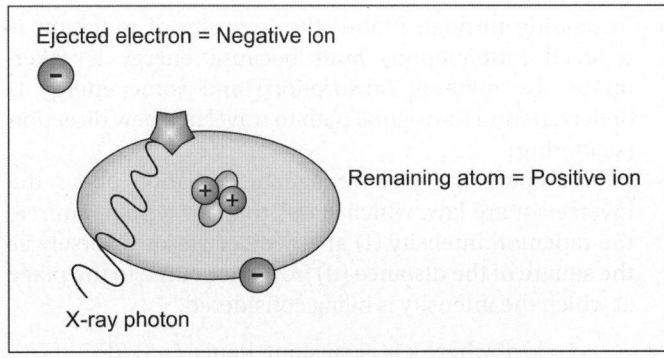

Figure 2.1 An ion pair is formed when an electron is removed from an atom; the atom is the positive ion and the ejected electron is the negative ion

energy will vary from element to element and so will the energy of the radiation emitted following ionization. The energy level values and their difference are characteristic of the element and thus the radiation emitted constitutes a *line spectrum* and are usually called the *characteristic radiation* of the element.

The process of raising an electron to a higher level is called excitation. When the atom is in an 'excited' state it is often more chemically reactive than normal, thus excitation may enable it to take part in a chemical process into which in a normal state it would not enter. *Excitation in biological material is an important cause of biological damage caused by radiation.*

ELECTROMAGNETIC SPECTRUM

Electromagnetic radiation can be defined as the propagation of wave like energy (without mass) through space or matter. Electromagnetic radiations are arranged according to their energies in what is termed *electromagnetic spectrum*.

Electromagnetic radiations are believed to move through space as both a particle and a wave; hence an explanation of the characteristics of electromagnetic radiation requires a *dualistic theory*:
- Wave theory
- Quantum theory.

Properties of Electromagnetic Radiations

- They travel through space in a wave motion along a straight line.
- They have neither mass nor weight nor electrical charge.
- They travel at the speed of light, in a vacuum, i.e. 3×10^8 m/sec or 186,000 miles/second.
- As they travel through space they give off an electric field at right angles to the path of propagation and a magnetic field at right angles to both (the path of propagation and electric field) (**Fig. 2.2**).
- They transfer energy from place to place in quanta (photons).
- In passing through matter the intensity of radiation is reduced (attenuation) both because energy is taken up by the material (absorption) and some energy is deflected from its original path to travel in a new direction (scattering).
- In free space the electromagnetic radiation obeys the inverse square law, which states that, for a point source, the radiation intensity (I) at any place varies inversely as the square of the distance (d) from the source to the place at which the intensity is being considered.

  $I = k/d^2$ where k is a constant, hence $I \propto 1/d^2$

- All electromagnetic radiations have a measureable frequency and wavelength but different temperature and energy.

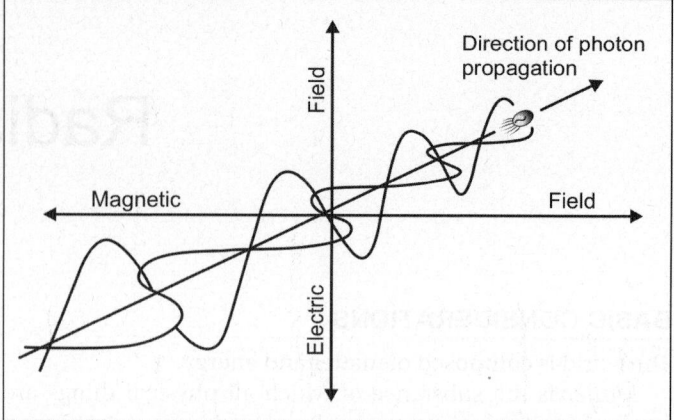

Figure 2.2 Line diagram of electromagnetic radiation illustrating electric and magnetic fields associated with a photon

- All electromagnetic radiations are invisible to the naked eye, with the exception of those falling within the range of the visible spectrum.

Main Types of Radiations Comprising the Electromagnetic Spectrum (Fig. 2.3)

- *Electric waves*: These have the longest wavelength, 10^{15} Å.
- *Hertzian waves*: These waves are used by high altitude transmission satellites, and have a wavelength of 10^{16} Å to 10^{13} Å.
- *Communication waves or radiowaves*: These waves can pass through most materials except that of great bulk. The wavelength varies from 10^{13} Å to 10^8 Å.
- *Short wave diathermy or microwaves*: These have wave lengths from 3×10^{-2} m to 3×10^{-4} m, these overlap the wave lengths of the communication waves on one end and infra red waves on the other end.
- *Infrared waves*: Infrared means 'below the red'. These have wavelengths ranging from 40,000 Å to 1,00,000 Å. These occupy the part of the spectrum with a frequency less than that of visible light and greater than that of radio waves.
- *Visible light*: This ranges from 4,000 Å to 7,700 Å. The range of color is often called VIBGYOR, with red having the longest wavelength and violet having the shortest wavelength. R-red, O-orange, Y-yellow, G-green, B-blue, I-indigo, V-violet.
- *Ultraviolet light*: This ranges from 1,000 Å to 2,000 Å. These rays have a slight penetrating power (up to density of quartz) and can penetrate living tissues for a depth of a few millimeters and cause biological effects like:
  - Photo erythema (sun burn).
  - Photo pigmentation (sun tan).
  - Photo chemical cornification of skin and skin carcinoma (malignant dermal changes).
  - Bactericidal effect.

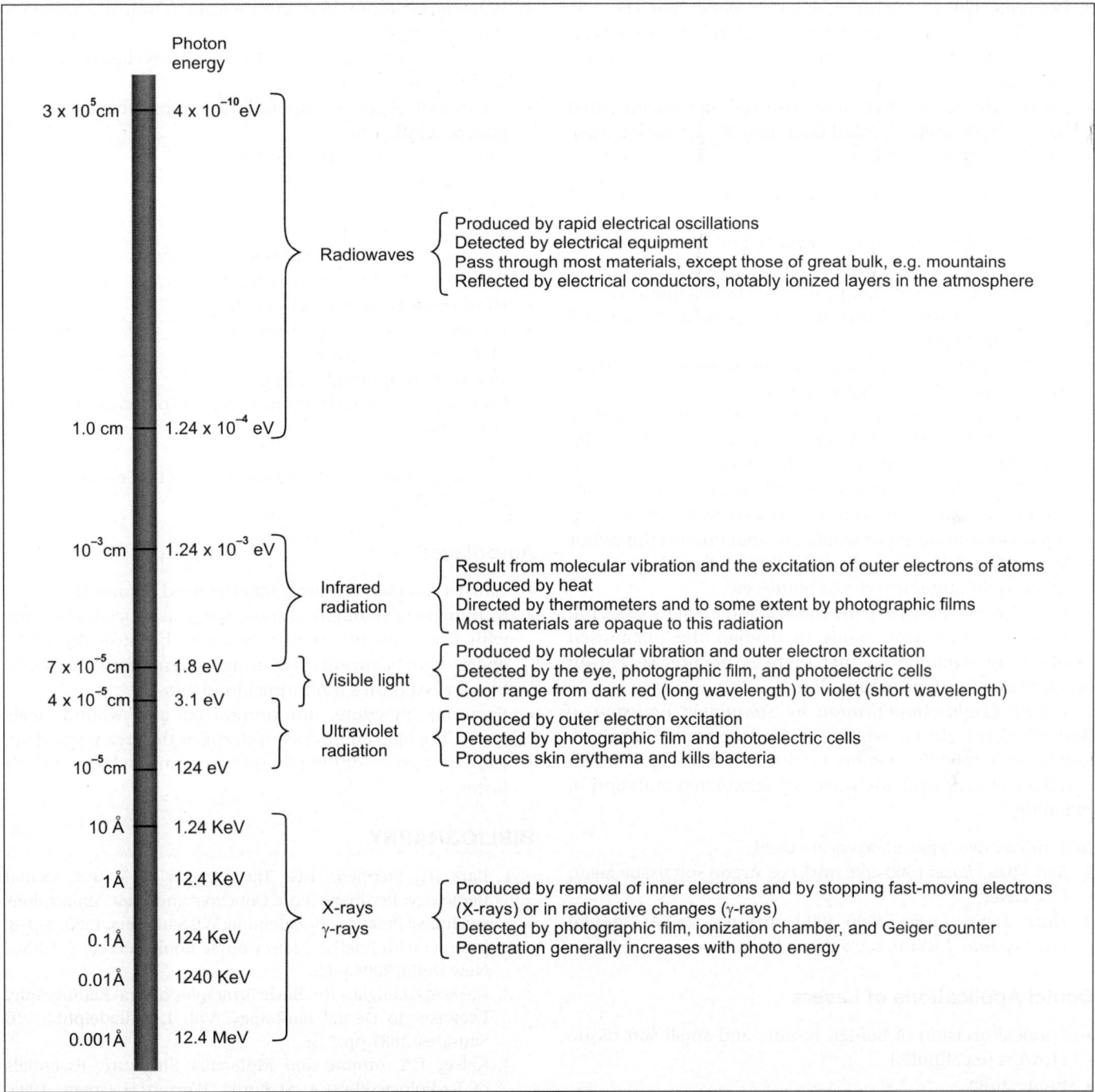

Figure 2.3 Diagrammatic representation of the Electromagnetic Spectrum (EMS)

– Aging of skin.
– Eyes are sensitive to UV rays which can cause cataract or keratitis.
– Is an agent in the production of vitamin D.

The ultraviolet spectrum can be divided into three groups based on the wave lengths:

1. Between 200 and 290 nm, *short or germicidal UV rays* (UVC), these can cause genetic mutations, altered reproductive cycles and cell death.
2. Between 290 and 320 nm, *middle or erythemal UV rays* (UVB), these can cause skin erythema and are commercially available as sun or mercury vapor lamps.

3. Between 320 and 380 nm, *long or black light UV rays* (UVA), on its own it is not damaging but when used with sensitizing chemicals, it can cause extensive biological damage.

- *X-rays*: The X-rays were first observed and documented in 1895 by Wilhelm Conard Roentgen. X-rays have a wave length from 1Å to 0.001 Å.

X-rays are divided into four types depending on their wave lengths:

1. 1–2 Å—*Grenz or Super Soft X-rays*, mainly used to treat superficial lesions and in crystalogy.
2. 1–0.5 Å—*Soft X-rays*, mainly used in contact therapy.
3. 0.5–0.1 Å—*Medium X-rays*, mainly used in diagnostic and superficial therapy.
4. 0.1 Å—*Hard X-rays*, mainly used for deep X-ray therapy and for industrial roentgenography.

- *Gamma rays*: These are high powered X-rays, having a wave-length of 0.001 Å. These are electromagnetic radiations, but their source is from the radioactive decay process. They have shorter wave length and greater penetrating power and are used in the treatment of tumors, e.g. Radon needles or seeds which are implanted at the tumor site, radioactive iridium in nylon threaded seeds, percutaneous radiotantalum wire implants, etc.
- *Cosmic rays*: These have the shortest wave length, 0.0001 Å.

Each radiation type tends to overlap the juxtaposed neighboring radiation so that there is no precise cut-off boundary for any type of radiation.

LASER (Light Amplification by Stimulated Emission of Radiation) is a device which can operate in the infra-red, visible or ultraviolet region of the spectrum and which amplifies electromagnetic waves by stimulated emission of radiation.

In dentistry two types of lasers are used:

1. *Soft Tissue Laser* (800–990 nm), e.g. Argon soft tissue laser, CO_2 Laser.
2. *Hard Tissue Laser* (2500–3000 nm), e.g. Er:YAG dental laser system, Erbium hard tissue laser.

Dental Applications of Lasers

- Surgical excision of benign tumors and small soft tissue growths (e.g. Epulis)
- Frenectomy
- Nerve regeneration
- Sleep apnea (LAUP—Laser Assisted Uvula Palatoplasty).
- Cavity detection

- Viewing of tooth and gum tissue (Optical coherence tomography)
- Treatment of cold sores—low intensity lasers used to reduce pain
- Treatment of temporomandibular joint for reduction of pain and inflammation
- Treatment of ulcerative lesions
- Oral biopsies
- Treatment of gummy smile
- Treatment of tooth sensitivity
- Treatment of melanin pigmented gingiva
- Local anesthesia free cavity preparation
- Hard tissue roughening or etching
- Enameloplasty, excavation of pits and fissures for placement of sealants
- Osseous crown lengthening
- Cutting, shaving and contouring of oral osseous structures.
- Ostectomy
- Apicectomy
- For early detection of dysplastic cells (Optical coherence tomography).

Advantages

- Causes less pain thereby reducing need for anesthesia.
- Minimizes bleeding and most surgical procedures done with lasers do not require sutures, because the high-energy light beam aids in clotting (coagulation) of exposed blood vessels thus inhibiting blood loss.
- Bacterial infections are minimized and wound heals faster. The high energy beam sterilizes the area worked on.
- Damage to surrounding tissue is minimized. Wound heals faster.

BIBLIOGRAPHY

1. Barr JH, Stephens RG. The Physics of X-rays. Dental Radiology: Pertinent Basic Concepts and their Applications in Clinical Practice. Philadelphia: WB Saunders; 1980.pp.1-8.
2. Interact with English Main Course Book. Secretary, CBSC, New Delhi; 2004.p.52.
3. Kasle MJ, Langlais RP. Basic Principles of Oral Radiography Exercises in Dental Radiology. Vol. 4. Philadelphia: WB Saundes; 1981.pp.2-36.
4. Kelsey CA. Atomic and Molecular Structure. Essentials of Radiology Physics. St Louis, Warren H Green; 1985. pp.34-42.
5. WJ Merdith, JB Massey. Fundamental Physics of Radiology. Second edition, Bristol: John Wright and Sons; 1972.

Properties of X-rays | 3

DEFINITION

X-rays are defined as weightless packages of pure energy (photons) that are without electrical charge and that travel in waves along a straight line with a specific frequency and speed.

The properties of X-rays may be classified into four broad categories:
1. Physical
2. Chemical
3. Biological
4. Physiochemical.

PHYSICAL PROPERTIES

- X-rays belong to a family of electromagnetic radiations having a wavelength between 10 Å and 0.01 Å.
- They travel through space in a wave motion.
- In free space they travel in a straight line.
- They travel with the same speed as that of visible light (i.e. 1,86,000 miles per second).
- As they travel through space, they can produce an electrical field at right angles to their path of propagation and a magnetic field at right angles to the electric field.
- They are invisible to the eye and cannot be seen; heard or smelt (they remain undetected by the human senses).
- They cannot be focused by a lens.
- They cannot be reflected, refracted or deflected by a magnet or electric field as they do not possess any charge.
- They show the properties of interference, diffraction and polarization, similar to that of visible light.
- They do not require a medium for propagation.
- X-rays are pure energy, no mass and they transfer energy from place to place in the form of quanta (photons). ($E = h\nu$).
- In free space they obey the inverse square law, which states that for a point source of radiation the intensity (I) at any given place varies inversely as the square of the distance (d) from the source to the place at which the intensity is being considered.
  $I \propto 1/d^2$ or $I = k/d^2$, where k is a constant.
  Intensity is determined by the number or quantity of X-ray photons in a beam.
- X-rays are produced by the collision of electrons with tungsten atoms. The collisions which occur are of two types, thus giving rise to two types of spectra:

– *Continuous spectra (General radiation, Bremsstrahlung radiation or braking radiation) (Fig. 3.1)*: The incoming electron penetrates the outer electron shell and passes close to the nucleus of the tungsten atom. The incoming electron is dramatically slowed down and deflected by the nucleus with a large loss of energy, which is emitted in the form of X-rays. The amount of deceleration and the degree of deflection determines the amount of energy lost by the bombarding electron and hence the energy of the resultant emitted photon has a wide range or spectrum of energies and therefore called continuous spectrum.
– *Characteristic spectrum or line spectrum (Fig. 3.2)*: The incoming electron collides with an inner shell tungsten electron, displacing it to an outer shell (excitation), or displacing it from the atom (ionization), with a large loss of energy and subsequently the orbiting tungsten electrons rearrange themselves to return the atom to neutral or ground state. This involves electron 'jumps' which results in the emission of X-ray photons with a specific energy called characteristic spectrum.

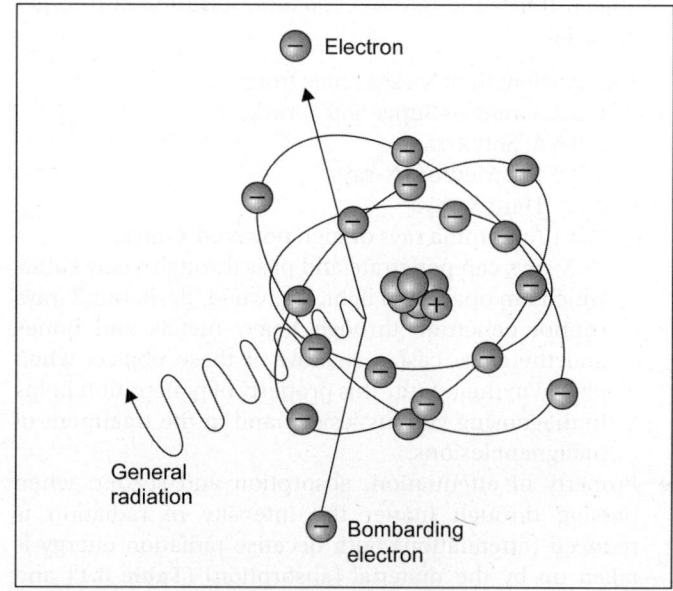

Figure 3.1 When an electron comes close to the nucleus of a tungsten atom, it is slowed down and deflected, an X-ray photon of lower energy known as general radiation results

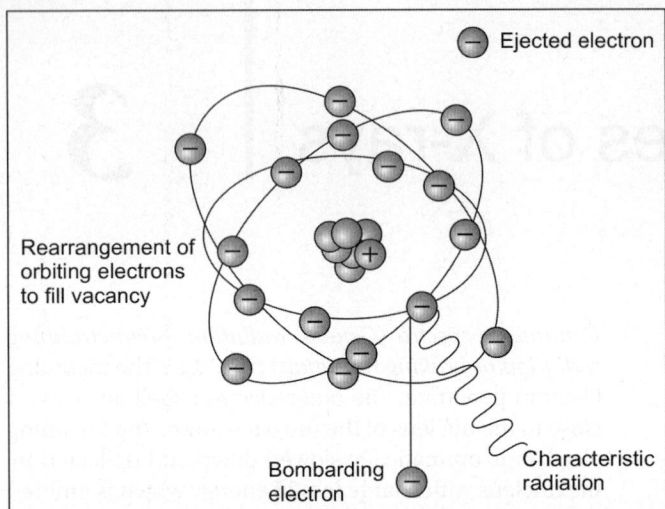

Figure 3.2 An electron that dislodges an inner shell electron from the tungsten atom results in the rearrangement of the remaining orbiting electrons and the production of an X-ray photon known as characteristic radiation

Table 3.1 Components of the body arranged in order of their power to absorb X-rays, starting from the lowest value to the highest value

- Air
- Fat
- Soft tissues, blood, body fluids
- Medullary bone
- Cancellous bone
- Cortical bone
- Dentin and cementum
- Enamel

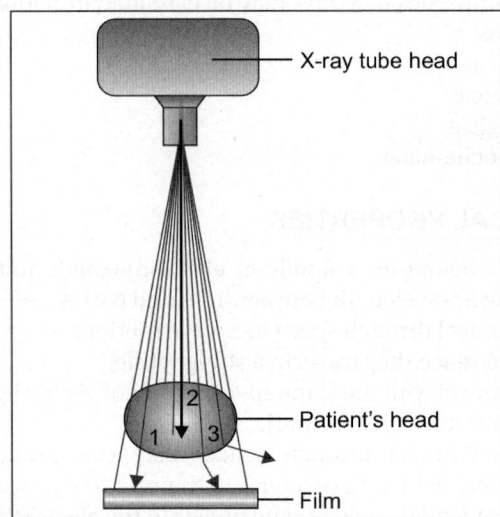

Figure 3.3 Three types of radiation interactions with the patient, may occur: 1. The X-ray photon may pass through the patient without interaction and reach the film; 2. Photon may be totally absorbed; 3. The photon may be scattered onto the film or away from the film

- X-rays can penetrate various objects and the degree of penetration depends upon the quality of the X-ray beam, and also on the intensity and wavelength of the X-ray beam.

  Quality (penetrating power of X-ray beam) is defined as the energy carried by the X-ray beam. The quality of the X-ray beam is determined by the kilo voltage, milli amperage, distance between the target and the object, time or length of exposure, filtration and target material.

  The wavelength of X-rays range from:
  - 1–2 Å: Grenz or Super Soft X-rays
  - 1–0.5 Å: Soft X-rays
  - 0.5–0.1 Å: Medium X-rays
  - 0.1 Å: Hard X-rays
  - 0.001 Å: Gamma rays or high powered X-rays.

    X-rays can penetrate and pass through many solids which are opaque to light, e.g. wood, flesh, but X-rays cannot penetrate through heavy metals and bones and therefore cast a shadow of these objects when placed in their path. This property of penetration helps in diagnosing various lesions and in the treatment of malignant lesions.
- Property of attenuation, absorption and scatter; when passing through matter the intensity of radiation is reduced (attenuation) both because radiation energy is taken up by the material (absorption) (**Table 3.1**) and some is deflected from the original path, to travel in a new direction (scattering) (**Fig. 3.3**).

Effect of Interaction of X-rays with Matter (**Fig. 3.4**): In the case of the diagnostic X-ray beam there are three mechanisms by which these processes take place:
1. Coherent scattering (**Fig. 3.5**)
2. Photoelectric effect (**Fig. 3.6**)
3. Compton scattering (**Fig. 3.7**).
- Due to their energy X-rays can release photoelectrons from the metals, when allowed to fall on them.
- *Heating effect*: The production of heat is one of the initial results of the slowing down of the primary electrons, it also arises as an end product of the chemical reactions induced by radiations. This change in temperature is very small and can only be detected by very sensitive instruments.

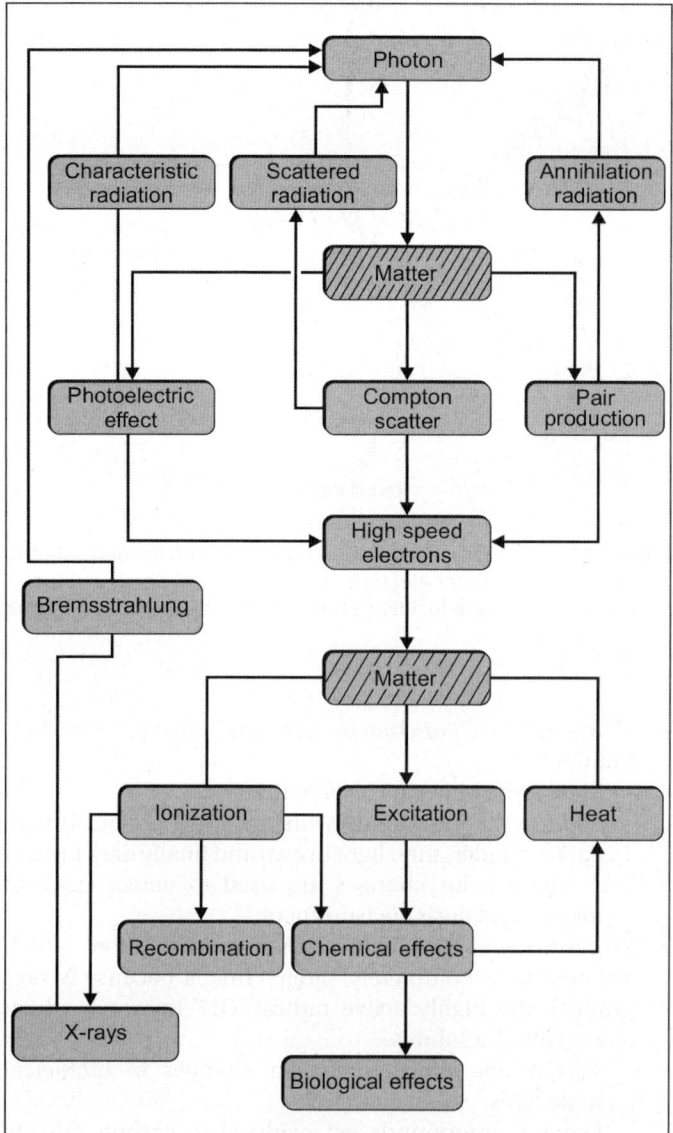

Figure 3.4 The effect of interaction of X-rays with matter

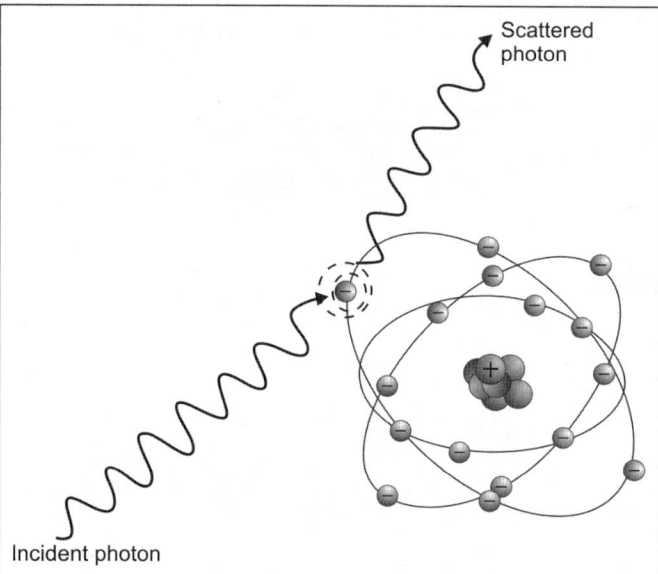

Figure 3.5 Coherent scattering results from the interaction of low energy incident photon with outer electron, causing it to vibrate momentarily. After this interaction, scattered photon of the same energy is emitted at a different angle to the path of incident photon

- *Fluorescence*: When X-rays fall upon certain materials, visible light is emitted called fluorescence, and it was this very property which led to the discovery of X-rays.

  There are different ways in which materials may emit light (luminescence) when X-rays are incident upon them.
  - *Phosphorescent materials*: These materials continue to emit light for a period of time after the X-ray absorption has taken place. This is called 'after glow' and it is used in the advertisement hoardings and lightings.
  - *Fluorescent materials*: Here the emission of light is instantaneous, quickly completed following X-ray irradiation. This property is used in intensifying screens and mass miniature radiography (photo fluorography).

  - *Thermoluminescent materials*: These emit visible radiations during or after irradiation of X-rays but only if heated to a few 100 degrees centigrade. This is used in comparative dosimetry and TLD badges.
- *Ionization*: This is a process of converting atoms into ions (refer **Fig. 2.1**).
  - X-rays can ionize gases and thus increase the electro conductivity of a gas through which it passes. Ionized air is accepted as the basis for X-ray measurement and for the definition of unit of X-ray quantity (Roentgen).

    Various devices that work on the principle of ionization are:
    - Ionization chamber
    - Thimble chamber
    - Condenser chamber
    - Geiger Muller counter
    - Scintillation counter.
  - Ionization also takes place whenever an X-ray photon strikes matter producing secondary radiation, and the effects of X-rays is largely due to this process.
  - X-ray radiation by virtue of its intrinsic ionizing potential can activate and dissociate silver ions in silver halide. This property is used in diagnostic radiology.

CHEMICAL PROPERTIES

The outer electrons of the atoms play an important role in chemical combinations and therefore any disturbance in the outer electron configuration of an atom brings about a chemical change.

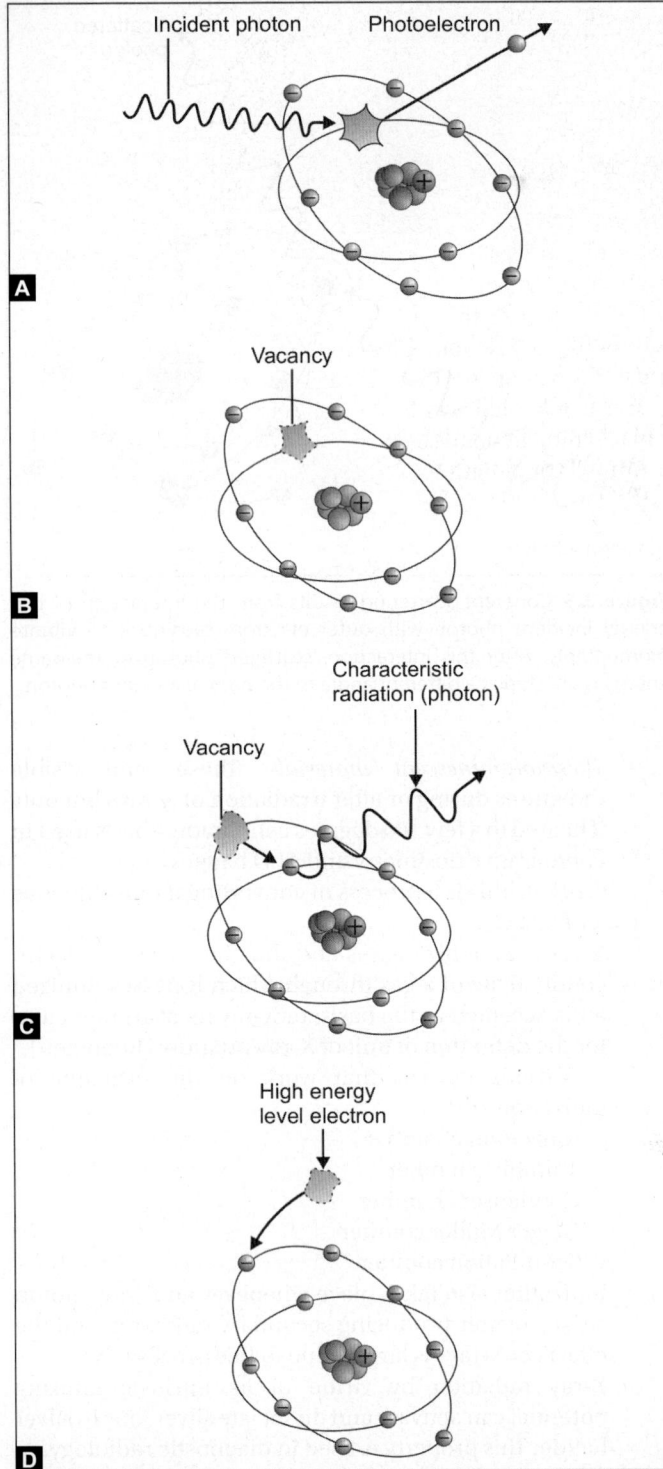

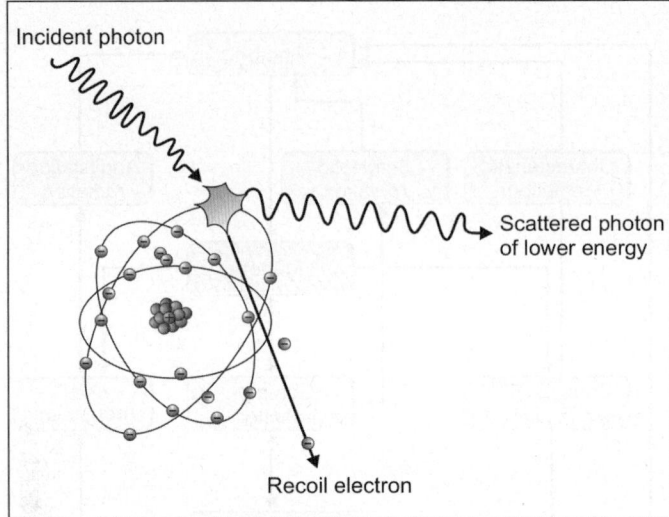

Figure 3.7 Compton absorption occurs when the incident photon interacts with the outer electron, resulting in a scattered photon of lower energy than the incident photon and a recoil electron ejected from target atom

- X-rays induce color changes of several substances or their solutions.
    - Methylene blue gets bleached.
    - Sodium platinocyanide which is apple green turns to darker shades, then light brown and finally dark brown.
        These color changes are used to detect cases of forgery and dose measurement.
- X-rays bring about chemical changes in solutions which are otherwise completely stable. This is because X-rays produce the highly active radical 'OH' in water, which reacts with the solutes.
    - This brings about molecular changes in biological molecules.
    - Organic compounds get oxidized to carbon dioxide with release of hydrogen when exposed to radiation, because water in organic substances undergoes oxidation and reduction reactions when irradiated.
    - X-rays can cause oxidation of ferrous sulfate to ferric sulfate and this is used as a method of measuring X-ray dosage (Frickle Dosimeter).
- X-rays can cause destruction of the fermenting power of enzymes, which are vital substances for the metabolism of cells of all living materials.

BIOLOGICAL PROPERTIES

When X-rays are incident on an atom, one of the reaction it produces is 'excitation'. These state of 'excitation' in biological materials enable it to take part in a chemical process into which in the normal state it would not enter. This is an important cause of biological damage produced by radiation.

Figures 3.6A to D (A) Photoelectric absorption occurs when the incident photon gives up all its energy to inner electron, ejected from atom as photoelectron; (B) An electron vacancy in the inner orbit results in ionization of the atom; (C) An electron from a higher energy level fills the vacancy and emits characteristics radiation; (D) All orbits are subsequently filled, completing energy exchange

- This property of excitation is used in the treatment of malignant lesions
- X-rays also have a germicidal or bactericidal effect and are used for sterilization and preservation of food.

The biological effects of X-rays may be classified into two types:

1. *Somatic effect*: This ranges from a simple sun burn to severe dermatitis, to changes in the blood supply and/or malignancy. The effect is cumulative and depends upon the type of tissues and intensity of the radiation.

Diagnostic properties of X-rays

- X-rays travel in a straight line.
- *Penetration*: X-rays can penetrate liquids, solids and gases. The composition of the substance determines whether the X-rays penetrate or are absorbed.
- *Absorption*: X-rays are absorbed by matter, the absorption depends on the atomic structure of the matter and the wavelength of the X-ray.
- *Ionizing capability*: X-rays interact with materials they penetrate and cause ionization, dissociate silver ions in film emulsions.
- *Fluorescence*: X-rays can cause substances to fluorescence or emit light radiation in longer wavelengths. (e.g. visible light or ultra-violet light).
- *Effect on films*: X-rays can produce an image on a photographic film.
- *Effect on living tissues*: X-rays cause biological changes in living cells.

2. *Genetic effect*: This effect is due to radiation induced mutation of genes and chromosomes. These effects are usually seen in the off-springs of the irradiated parents. The fetus is more sensitive to radiation in the early stage of development.

PHYSIOCHEMICAL PROPERTIES

The photographic effect: Photographic paper or film when exposed to X-ray radiation and then developed will be found blackened. The irradiation affects the silver salts in the emulsion, so that after the chemical process called developing, the radiograph metallic silver is released and the film or paper appears blackened.

This blackening is known as 'film density' and the degree of blackening depends upon:

- Amount of radiation
- Quality of radiation
- Characteristic of a film
- Concentration and age of developing solution
- Length of developing time
- Use of intensifying screens.

The difference between the degrees of density is known as 'film contrast'.

BIBLIOGRAPHY

1. Curry TS, Dowdy JE, Marry RC. Christensen's Introduction to the Physics of Diagnostic Radiology, 3rd edition, Philadelphia: Lea and Febiger; 1984.
2. John HE, Cunningham JR. The Physics of Radiology, (4th edition), Springfield, Charles C Thomas, Publisher, 1985.
3. Merdith WJ, Massey JB. Fundamental Physics of Radiology, 2nd edition, Bristol: John Wright and Sons; 1972.

Production of X-rays | 4

X-rays are produced by the sudden deceleration or stoppage of a rapidly moving stream of electrons at a metal target in a high vacuum tube. The X-ray tube is an important part of any X-ray machine. Dental X-ray machines can be used to expose intraoral as well as extra oral films. Some machines are used only for intraoral films whereas others are for extraoral films. Now, digital radiography units are also available.

DENTAL X-RAY MACHINE

The dental X-ray machine is made up of three parts or components (**Fig. 4.1**):
1. Control panel.
2. Extension arm.
3. Tube head.

- *Control panel*: The control panel of the dental X-ray machine contains:
  - An on and off switch and an indicator light
  - An exposure button and indicator light
  - Control devices (time, kilo voltage, milli amperage selectors) to regulate the X-ray beam.
  The control panel is plugged into an electrical outlet.
- *Extension arm*: The extension arm suspends the X-ray tube head and houses the electrical wires that extend from the control panel to the tube head. The extension arm also allows the movement and positioning of the tube head.

- *Tube head*: It is a tightly sealed, heavy metal housing that contains the X-ray tube that produces dental X-rays. The component parts of the X-ray tube include the following (**Fig. 4.2**):
  - *Metal housing*: This is the metal body of the tube head that surrounds the X-ray tube and transformer and is filled with oil, it protects the X-ray tube and grounds the high voltage component.
  - *Insulating oil*: It is that which surrounds the X-ray tube and transformer inside the tube head, it prevents over heating by absorbing the heat created by the production of X-rays. The surrounding oil both maintains the insulation properties of the glass envelope and also insulates the tube from the metal shield.
    With rise in temperature the oil expands and occupies a greater volume. It is essential in any such tube that there should be no air bubbles within the space surrounding the glass. The problem therefore, is how to provide for expansion of oil without having any bubbles in the tube case when cold. This is solved by inserting *metal bellows*, which extends as the heated oil expands, simultaneous acting as a safety device. If the bellows expand beyond a certain point then they operate a micro switch which prevents operation of the tube until the oil has cooled sufficiently.

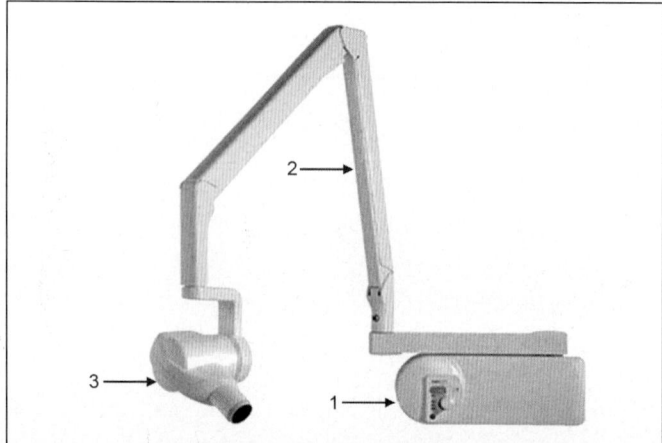

Figure 4.1 Three component parts of the dental X-ray machine: 1. Control panel; 2. Extension arm; 3. Tube head

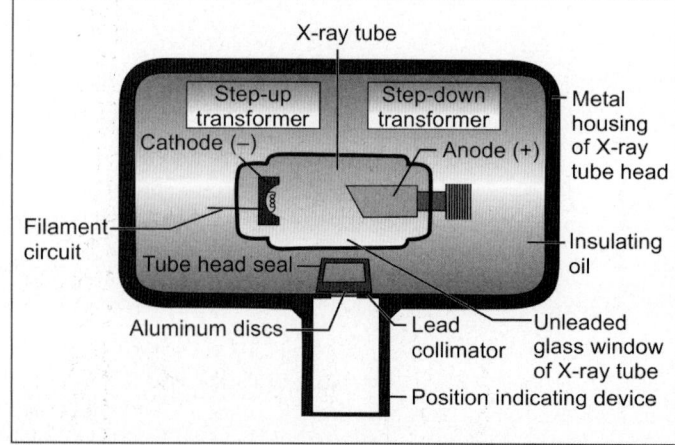

Figure 4.2 Schematic diagram of the dental X-ray tube head

– *Tube head seal*: Aluminum or leaded glass of the tube head that permits the exit of X-rays from the tube head, it seals the oil in the tube head and acts as a filter to the X-ray beam.

– *X-ray tube (Fig. 4.3)*: It is the main X-ray generating system.

• *Aluminum discs (Fig. 4.4)*: The sheets of 0.5 mm thick aluminum are placed in the path of the X-ray beam. They filter out the nonpenetrating, longer wave-length X-rays, resulting in a higher energy and more penetrating useful beam, which is less harmful to the patient (decreased skin dose). In the dental X-ray tube head there are two types of filtration:

– *Inherent filtration* takes place when the primary beam passes through the glass window of the X-ray tube, the insulating oil and the tube head seal. In the dental X-ray machines the inherent filtration is approximately equivalent to 0.5 to 1 mm of aluminum.

– *Added filtration* refers to the placement of aluminum discs in the path of the X-ray beam between the collimator and the tube head seal in the dental X-ray tube head. Aluminum discs may be added in 0.5 mm increments.

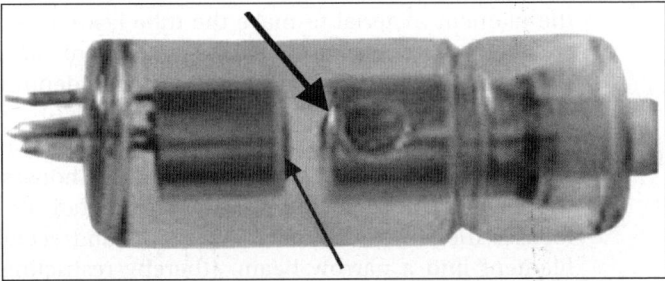

Figure 4.3 X-ray tube showing focusing cup (thin arrow cathode) and focal spot area (thick arrow anode)

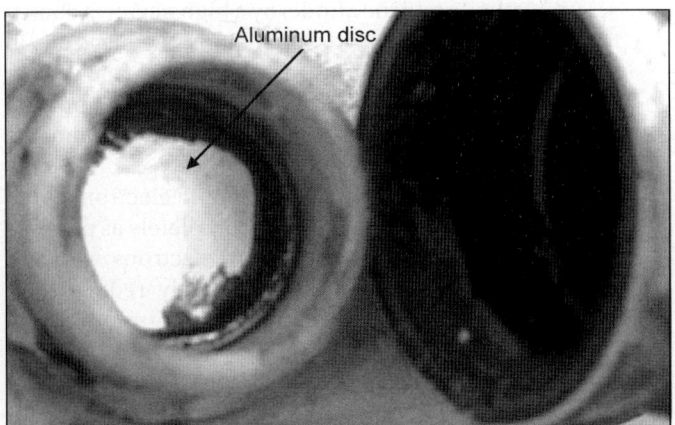

Figure 4.4 X-ray tube head with aluminum disc seen when the PID is removed

Total filtration (inherent + added filtration) is regulated by the state and federal law (in USA). Dental machines operating:

i. At or below 70 kVp require a minimum total filtration of 1.5 mm of aluminum thickness.

ii. Above 70 kVp require a minimum total filtration of 2.5 mm of aluminum thickness.

• *Lead collimator*: It is a lead plate with a central hole that fits directly over the opening of the metal housing where the X-rays exit.

Collimation is used to restrict the size and shape of the X-ray beam and thus reduce exposure to the patient.

Collimators are of two types:

1. Fixed
2. Adjustable

– In the dental X-ray machine usually the fixed collimators are used, they may either have a round or rectangular opening.

– A rectangular collimator restricts the size of the X-ray beam to an area slightly larger than a size 2 intraoral (normal adult intraoral periapical films) and thus significantly reduces the patient exposure.

– A circular collimator produces a cone shaped beam that is 2.75 inches in diameter and is considerably larger than the size of two intraoral periapical films, and thus leads to an increased skin dose to the patient.

• *Position indicating device (Fig. 4.5)*: Position indicating device (PID) or open ended lead cylinder, that extends from the opening of the metal housing of the tube head also called the 'cone'.

The PID appears as an extension of the tube head and it aims and shapes the X-ray beam. There are three types of PIDs:

1. Conical
2. Rectangular
3. Round.

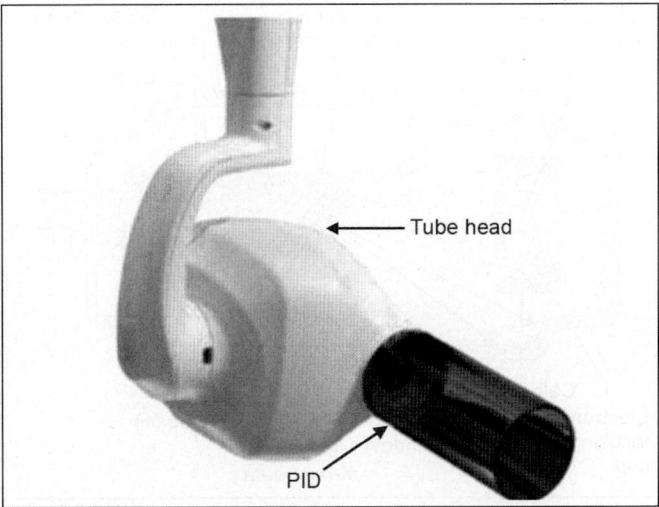

Figure 4.5 The position indicating device (PID) or cone

The conical PID appears as a closed, pointed plastic cone and when X-rays exit they penetrate the plastic and produce scattered radiation (see **Fig. 6.7**).

Nowadays lead lined rectangular or round PIDs are preferred as they do not produce scattered radiation.

Both rectangular and round PIDs are available in two lengths:
1. Short (8 inches)
2. Long (16 inches).

The long PID is preferred because less divergence of X-ray beam occurs. The rectangular type is most effective in reducing patient exposure.

- *The X-ray tube (Fig. 4.6)*: It is the heart of the X-ray generating system. This consists of a glass vacuum tube from which all of the air has been removed. The X-ray tube used in dentistry measures approximately several inches long by one inch in diameter. The component parts of the X-ray tube consist of:
    - *Leaded glass housing*: It is a leaded glass vacuum tube that prevents X-rays from escaping in all directions (radiation leakage). One central area of the leaded glass tube has a 'window' that permits the X-ray beam to exit the tube and directs the X-ray beam towards the aluminum disc, lead collimator and PID. This is also used for earthing.
    - *Negative cathode*: It is principally composed of two parts:
        i. Filament
        ii. Focussing cup.
    - The filament is the source of electrons in the tube; it is made up of a coil of tungsten wire (atomic number 74, melting point 3380°C), approximately 0.2 cm in diameter, 1–2 mm wide, 0.1–0.2 mm thick and 7 to 15 mm in length. It is mounted on two strong stiff wires that support it and carry the electric current. These two mounted wires lead through the glass envelope to serve as a connection to the low and high voltage electrical source.

The filament is heated to incandescence through a range of temperatures by varying voltage (10 V), across the filament from a step down transformer in a low voltage circuit. The hot filament emits electrons that are separated from the outer orbits of tungsten atoms at a rate proportional to its temperature by a process called 'Thermionic emission'. The electrons lost by the filament form a cloud or space charge around the filament. (These are replaced from the negative side from the high voltage circuit which is connected to one of the filament mounting wire).

A milli ampere control provides for fine adjustment of voltage across the filament and in turn the flow of heating current through it. The milli ampere control, thereby controls the quantity of electrons the filament emits, which in turn controls tube current.

Vaporization of the filament occurs over a period of time. When the particles vaporize (turn into gaseous form) they solidify on the glass of the X-ray tube, which is called 'sun-burning' or 'sun-tanning' of the tube. This reduces the output of the X-ray tube, destruction of the vacuum and integrity of the tube, resulting in 'arcing' and ultimate tube failure. Thorium (a radioactive metallic element) is added to the filament material to make the tube last longer.

Other materials used for the filament are; Rhenium (melting point—3,186°C), Molybdenum (melting point—2,623°C).

The *focussing cup* is a negatively charged concave reflector cup of molybdenum or nickel and houses the filament. The focussing cup electrostatically focuses the electrons emitted by the incandescent filament into a narrow beam, (thereby restricting the size of the electron cloud) directed at a small rectangular area in the anode—the focal spot.

The electrons are caused to move in this direction because of a strong electric field interposed between the cathode and the anode, by a high negative charge placed on the cathode which repels the electrons in the electron cloud towards the anode which has a high positive charge. This is achieved by applying a high voltage circuit between the anode and the cathode.

To facilitate the movement of the electron cloud, the X-ray tube is evacuated as completely as possible to prelude collision of moving electrons with gas molecules, which could significantly reduce their speed. It also prevents oxidation or 'burn out' of the filament.

- *Grid controlled focusing cups*: Some X-ray procedures (for example; portable capacitor discharge units, digital subtraction angiography, digital radiography, cineradiography) require exposures to be taken at regular

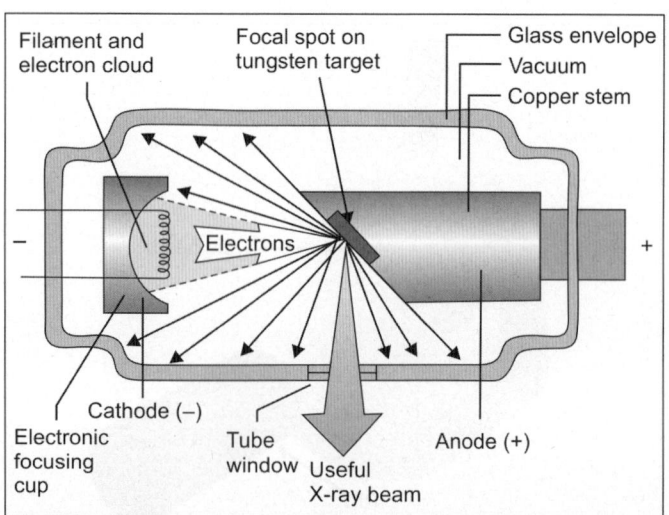

Figure 4.6 X-ray tube with the major components labeled

intervals. In grid controlled focusing cups, they have a variable charge applied to the focusing cup that acts as an exposure switch. When the tube is activated, the charge increases or decreases rapidly. Short bursts of electrons flow to the target.

- *Positive anode or the positive electrode*: It consists of a wafer thin tungsten plate (target) embedded in a solid copper stem. The purpose of the target is to convert the kinetic energy of the electrons generated from the filament into X-ray photons. The position of the anode is indicated externally as a depression, usually a red dot on the tube head by the manufacturer.

Tungsten is usually selected as the target material because it represents an effective compromise between the features of an ideal target material, namely:

- *High atomic number*: This is desired for more efficient production of X-rays. High atomic number indicates high charge on the nucleus (more protons) and high binding energy of orbital electrons. This high charge on the nucleus causes greater deceleration of bombarding electrons which approach the nucleus and of incoming electrons that collide with the inner shell electrons producing higher energy radiation. In brief, high atomic number gives rise to increased interaction between electrons and atoms, thereby increasing X-ray photons.
- *High melting point*: 3380°C, so that even if the temperature rises the target will not melt.
- *Low vapour pressure*: So that at high temperatures, it does not evaporate.
- *High specific heat* (conduction of heat) to facilitate dissipation of heat, but tungsten is a poor conductor of heat.

Therefore, the tungsten target is embedded in a copper block which is a good thermal conductor.

The methods of heat dissipation are:
- *Conduction*: Through the copper stem.
- *Convection*: Through the oil surrounding the tube.
- *Radiation*: Through the radiator device attached to the copper stem.
- Rotating anode.

There are two types of anodes:
1. Stationary or fixed anode.
2. *Rotating anode*: This type of anode is used to help dissipate heat from a small focal spot. The tungsten target is in the form of a small bevelled disc that rotates when the tube is in operation. As a result electrons strike successive areas of the target as it rotates. This widens the focal spot to an amount corresponding to the circumference of the bevelled disc and distributes heat over an expanded area. As a result of using rapidly rotating bevelled disc target, fractional millimeter focal spots can be used with currents up to 100 mA to 500 mA, that is ten to fifty times that of stationary anode.

The target and the rotor (armature) of the motor are located within the X-ray tube whereas the coils which drive the rotor at about 3000 rpm are situated outside the tube. Such rotating anodes are not used in conventional dental X-ray machines, but may be used in cephalometric or extra oral X-ray machines.

Target size: The radiographic image quality is dependent upon the geometry of the target. Sharpness of the radiographic image increases as the size of the radiographic source (that is focal spot) decreases.

The focal spot is the area on the target onto which the focussing cup directs the electrons from the filament.

As the focal spot becomes smaller, heat generated per unit target area becomes greater. Thus in order to derive benefit from a small focal spot and yet to effectively distribute the bombarding electrons over a greater surface of a large target, the target is placed at an angle to the electron beam. (The effective focal spot will be smaller than the actual size of the focal spot that is projected, perpendicular to the target).

In practice the target is inclined at an angle of 20° to the central ray of electrons. This causes the *effective focal spot* to be 1 mm × 1 mm, in contrast to 1 mm × 3 mm of the actual focal spot size. This results in a smaller source of X-rays and sharper image with a larger actual focal spot for effective heat dissipation. This is known as 'line focus principle' and the twenty degree angle is called as 'the angle of truncation' (**Fig. 4.7**).

Rectification: It is the conversion of alternating current to direct current.

The dental X-ray tube acts as a self rectifier, in that it changes AC to DC while producing X-rays.

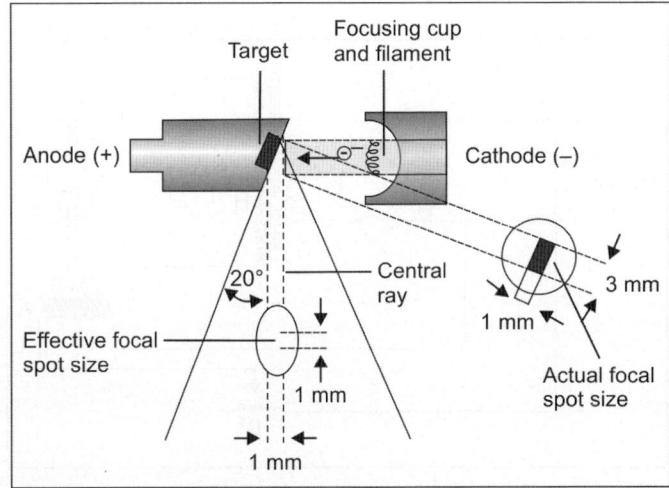

Figure 4.7 The angle of the target to the central ray of the X-ray beam has a strong influence on the apparent size of the focal spot. The projected effective focal spot is much smaller than the actual focal spot size

During the first phase, the cathode is negatively charged and the anode is positively charged, the electrons flow from the cathode and hit the anode and X-rays are produced. But when the current changes direction, the cathode becomes positively charged and therefore the electrons present at the anode will travel backwards and hit the filament, this occurs in general X-ray machines where very high voltage is used. In the dental X-ray machine, however, the amount of heat produced at the anode does not give rise to excessive electrons as a result, when the current changes its direction, there are no electrons at the anode to travel back to the cathode, this half of the cycle is called inverse voltage or reverse bias, hence the dental X-ray tube is called *self rectifying* or *half wave rectifying*.

The newer consistent potential X-ray machines produce a homogeneous beam of consistent wavelengths during exposure and this helps to reduce patient exposure to radiation by 20 percent.

Amperage: It is the measurement of the number of electrons moving through a conductor.

Current is measured in amperes (A) or milliamperes (mA). If the milli amperes (mA) increase, the number of electrons passing through the cathode filament increases.

Voltage: It is the measurement of electric force that causes electron to move from a negative pole to a positive one. It is measured in volts (V) or kilovolts (kV). If there is increase in kilovoltage wavelength is decreased, penetration will increase.

Circuit: It is a path of electrical current.

In the production of X-ray, two circuits are used (**Fig. 4.8**):
1. *Filament circuit:* It is low voltage (3–5 volts) and regulates the flow of electrical current to the filament of the X-ray

tube. It is controlled by the mA setting in the Control Panel.
2. *High voltage circuit:* It uses 65,000–1,00,000 volts, providing a high voltage required to accelerate electrons to generate X-rays in the X-ray tube. It is controlled by the kVp setting in the control panel.
   • *Transformer (Fig. 4.9):* It is a device that is used to either increase or decrease the voltage in an electrical circuit. It alters the voltage of the incoming electrical current and then routes the electrical energy to the X-ray tube.

In the production of X-rays three transformers are used:
1. *Step down transformer:* It is used to decrease the voltage from the incoming 110–220 line voltage to 3–4 V as required for the filament circuit. (This transformer has more coils in the primary coil than in the secondary coil).
2. *Step up transformer:* It is used to increase the voltage from the incoming 110–220 line voltage to 65,000–1,00,000 volts as required by the high voltage circuit.
3. *Auto transformer:* This serves as a voltage compensator that corrects the minor fluctuations in the current.

Timer: A timing control device, used to control X-ray exposure time. It is included in the primary high voltage supply. The timer completes the circuit with the high voltage transformer thereby controlling the time that the high voltage is applied to the tube and thus the time during which the tube current flows and X-rays are produced.

The timing circuit first sends a current through the filament to get it to the proper operating temperature. Once the filament is heated, a time delay switch applies power to the high voltage circuit.

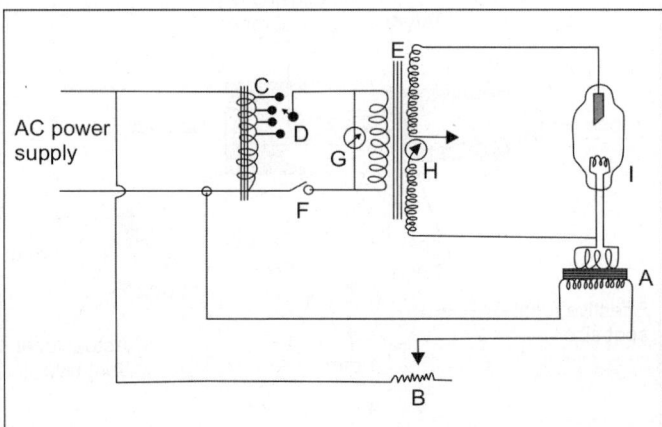

Figure 4.8 Dental X-ray machine circuit, with the major components labeled: A. Filament step down transformer, B. Filament current control (mA switch), C. Auto transformer; D. kVp selector dial (switch); E. High voltage transformer; F. X-ray timer (switch); G. Tube voltage indicator (volt meter); H. Tube current indicator (Ammeter); I. X-ray tube

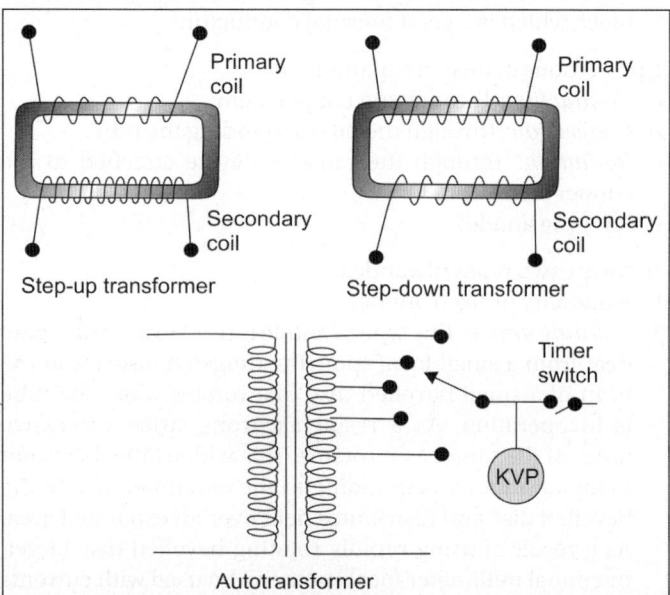

Figure 4.9 Three different transformers used in the production of X-rays

Tube rating and duty cycle: Each tube has a rating specification that describes the operating limits of the tube. These specifications are on the tube rating charts that describe in a graph like representation the maximum safe intervals (seconds) the tube may be energized at a given range of voltage (kVp) and the tube current (mA) values.

The duty cycle refers to how frequently successive exposures can be made. The heat build up at the anode is calculated as Heat Unit (Hu).

$$Hu = kVp \times mA \times sec \text{ (watt sec)}$$

PRODUCTION OF DENTAL X-RAYS (FIG. 4.10)

- Electricity from the wall outlet supplies the power to generate X-rays. When the X-ray machine is turned on, the electric current enters the control panel, via the plugged in cord and from there to the tube head via electrical wires in the extension arm.
- The current is directed to the filament circuit through the step down transformer, which reduces the 110–220 voltage to 3–5 volts.
- The filament circuit uses the 3–5 volts to heat the tungsten filament. Thermionic emission occurs, which results in the release of electrons from the tungsten filament, which forms an 'electron cloud'. This cloud remains around the filament till the high voltage circuit is activated.

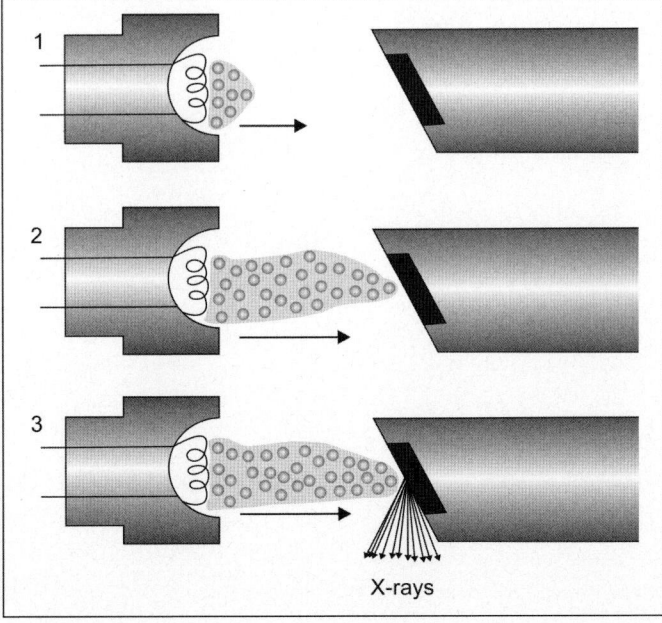

Figure 4.10 The production of dental X-ray occurs in the X-ray tube: 1. When the filament circuit is activated, the filament heats up and thermionic emission occurs; 2. When the exposure button is activated, the electrons are accelerated from the cathode to the anode; 3. The electrons strike the tungsten target, and their kinetic energy is converted to X-rays and heat

- When the exposure button is pushed the high voltage circuit is activated. The electron cloud produced at the cathode is accelerated across the X-ray tube to the anode. The molybdenum cup of the cathode directs the electrons to the tungsten target in the anode.
- The electrons travel from the cathode to the anode. When the electrons strike the tungsten target, their energy motion (kinetic energy) is converted to X-ray energy and heat. Less than 1 percent of the energy is converted to X-rays, the remaining 99 percent is lost as heat.
- The heat produced is carried away by the copper stem and absorbed by the insulating oil in the tube head. The X-rays produced are emitted from the target in all directions. However, the leaded glass housing prevents the X-rays from escaping from the X-ray tube in any direction. Only a small number of X-rays are able to exit from the X-ray tube via the unleaded glass window portion of the tube.
- The X-rays travel through the unleaded glass window, the tube head seal, the aluminum discs, which filter the long wave X-rays from the beam.
- The size and shape of the X-ray beam is controlled by the lead collimator. The X-ray beam then travels down the lead lined PID and exits the tube head at the opening of the PID.

TYPES OF X-RAYS PRODUCED

The X-rays produced in the X-ray tube vary in energy and wavelength, depending on how the electrons interacted with the tungsten atoms in the anode. The kinetic energy of the electrons is converted to X-ray photons via one of the following mechanism:

- *General (Bremsstrahlung radiation or braking radiation) radiation (refer Fig. 3.1)*: The term refers to the sudden 'braking' of high speed electrons when they hit the tungsten target in the anode. The 70 percent of the X-rays are produced in this manner.
  - If the electron hits the nucleus of the tungsten atom all its kinetic energy is converted into 'High Energy X-ray Photon'. But most of the time, instead of hitting the nucleus, most electrons just miss the nucleus of the tungsten atom. When the electron comes close to the nucleus, it is attracted to the nucleus and slows down, consequently an X-ray photon is released (due to the decrease in the kinetic energy of the photon).
  - The electron that misses the nucleus continues to penetrate many such tungsten atoms producing many lower energy X-ray photons before it imparts all its kinetic energy. As a result general radiation consists of X-rays of many different energies and wavelengths. It is also called continuous spectrum.
- *Characteristic radiation (refer Fig. 3.2)*: It is produced when a high speed electron dislodges an inner shell electron from the tungsten atom and causes ionization of

the atom. Once the electron is dislodged the remaining orbiting electrons are rearranged to fill the vacancy. This rearrangement produces a loss of energy that results in the X-ray photon, with the energy equal to the difference in the two orbital energy states. The X-ray thus produced is called *characteristic radiation*.

- Characteristic radiation accounts for a very small part of X-rays produced in the dental X-ray machine and occur only at 70 kVp and above, because the binding energy of 'K' shell electron is approximately 70 kVp.
- The difference between the binding energy of the electrons will vary from element to element and thus, so will the energies of the photons emitted following ionization. The energy level values and their differences are characteristic of the element and the radiation emitted constitutes the 'Line Spectrum', and is usually called the characteristic radiation of that elements.

BIBLIOGRAPHY

1. O'Brien RC. The Nature and Generation of X-rays. Dental Radiography: An introduction for Dental Hygienists and Assistants, 4th edition. Philadelphia: WB Saunders; 1982. pp.1-12.
2. WJ Merdith, JB Massey. Fundamental Physics of Radiology, 2nd edition, Bristol: John Wright and Sons; 1972.

Section III

Radiation and Health Physics

Radiation Biology | 5

RADIATION EFFECTS

Radiation biology is defined as the study of the effects of ionizing radiation on living systems (**Flow chart 5.1**).

DETERMINISTIC EFFECT (FLOW CHART 5.2)

It is an effect in which the severity of the response is proportional to the dose. These effects have a dose threshold below which the response is not seen. For example, oral changes after radiation therapy. This effects usually in cell killing, and may occur in all people when the dose is large enough.

STOCHASTIC EFFECT

It is that effect for which the probability of the occurrence of a change, rather than its severity is dose dependent. These effects do not have a dose threshold. For example, radiation induced cancer, because the greater exposure of a person or population to radiation increases the probability of the cancer but not its severity.

ACTION THEORY OF BIOLOGICAL TISSUES

Direct or Target Action Theory (Fig. 5.1)

Direct or target action theory is that effect which occurs when the energy of a photon or secondary electron ionizes biological macromolecules.

Indirect Action or Poison Chemical Theory (Figs 5.2 and 5.3)

Water is a predominant molecule of the biological system. When the photon is absorbed by the water molecule, it is ionized and releases free radicals which further interact and produce changes in the biologic molecule, this effect is termed 'indirect'.

Flow chart 5.1 Sequence of events which occur when an X-ray photon strikes matter

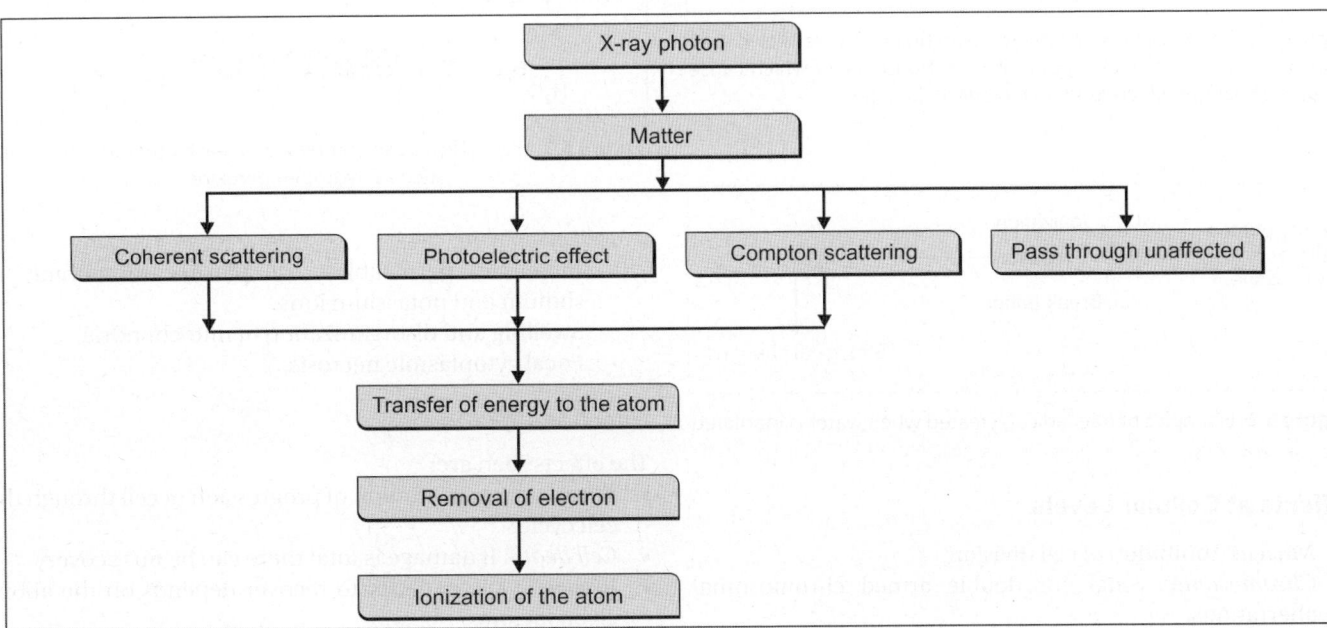

Flow chart 5.2 Effect of radiation on the biological tissues

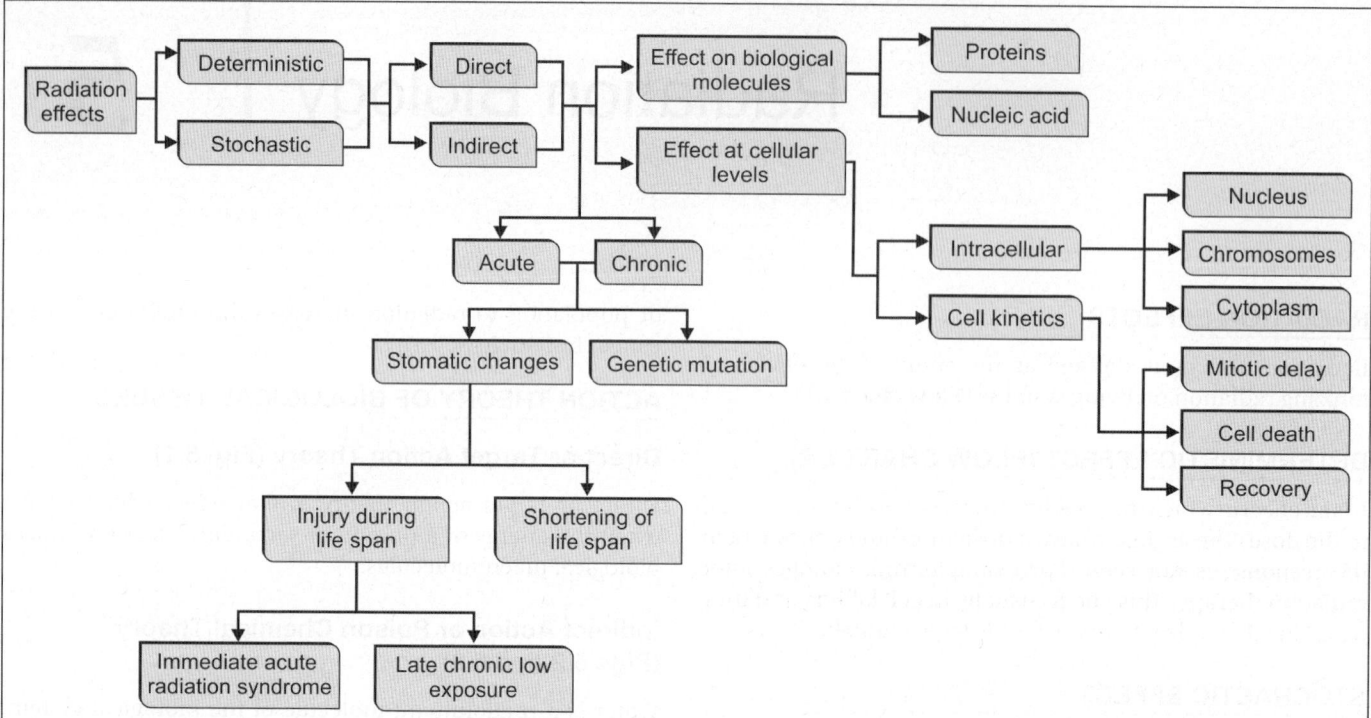

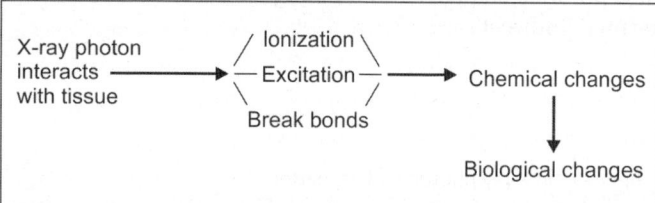

Figure 5.1 The X-ray photon interacts with tissues and results in ionization, excitation or breaking of molecular bonds, all of which cause chemical changes which result in biological damage

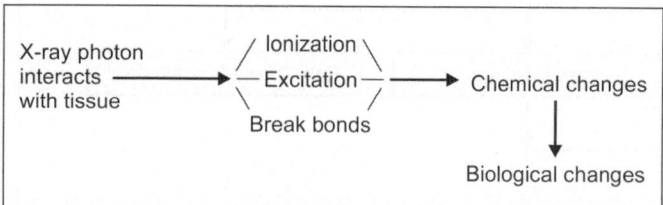

Figure 5.2 Examples of free radicals created when water is irradiated

Effects at Cellular Levels

- *Nucleus*: Inhibition of cell division.
- *Chromosomes*: Single or double armed chromosomal aberrations.

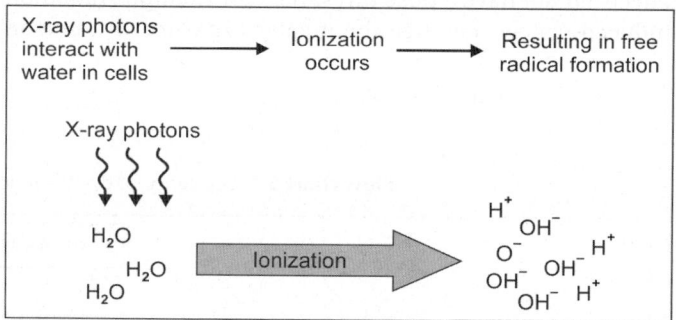

Figure 5.3 Free radicals can combine with each other to form toxins such as hydrogen peroxide

- *Cell cytoplasm*:
  - Increased permeability of plasma membrane to sodium and potassium ions.
  - Swelling and disorganization of mitochondria.
  - Focal cytoplasmic necrosis.

Effect on Cell Kinetics

The effects seen are:
- *Mitotic delay*: Inhibition of progression of cell through the cell cycle.
- *Cell death*: If damage is total there can be no recovery.
- *Recovery*: The capacity to recover depends on the above given factors.

Acute Exposure

This occurs when a large dose of radiation is absorbed in a short period of time, e.g. nuclear accident.

The radiation damage caused by acute radiation is much more than that caused by chronic exposure to radiation.

This type of exposure is not seen when using *dental diagnostic radiations.*

Chronic Exposure

This occurs when small amounts of radiations are absorbed repeatedly over a long period of time.

Stomatic Damage

This damage occurs in the living cell/organism and is not carried forward once the cell/organism dies. This can be observed as:

- Injuries during the life span
  - The most important are the radiation induced cancers. It is believed that radiation causes cancer by modifying the DNA, still the exact mechanism of induction of cancer by ionizing radiation is not well understood. The most commonly found cancers are:
    - Thyroid cancer.
    - Esophageal cancer.
    - Brain and nervous system cancers.
    - *Salivary gland cancers*: The incidence is increased in patients treated for diseases of the head and neck. It was believed that the risk of salivary gland tumors may be highest in patients receiving full mouth examinations before the age of 20 years but it has been seen that this may be true only in individuals who have received a cumulative parotid dose of 500 mGy or more.
    - Cancer of other organs, like skin, paranasal sinuses and bone marrow also shows excess neoplasia after exposure.
    - Leukemia.
  - *Other late somatic changes*:
    - Growth and development is retarded subject to the age and amount of radiation the individual was exposed to.
    - *Mental retardation*: As estimated 4 percent chance of mental retardation per 100 mSv exists at 8 to 15 weeks of gestation age.

      The exposure to the embryo from a full set of dental radiographs, using lead apron, is less than 3 mSv.
    - *Cataracts*: The threshold for induction of cataracts is from 2 Gy to more than 5 Gy.
  - *Shortening the life span*: There is an acceleration of the aging process resulting in a shortened life span.

Genetic Damage

Genetic cells are the germ cells found in the reproductive organs. These contain chromosomes which have genes which are made up of DNA. Any damage will lead to loss or rearrangement of the genetic material, which results in genetic mutations. These changes are more commonly seen in the next and subsequent generations.

Short-term Effects

These effects of radiation on a tissue are determined primarily by the sensitivity of its parenchymal cells.

If continuously proliferating cells are irradiated (bone marrow, oral mucous membrane), the effect of irradiation becomes apparent relatively quickly, (highly radiosensive). Tissues composed of cells that rarely or never divide (muscle) demonstrate little or no radiation induced hypoplasia (low radiosensitivity) over a short-term.

Long-term Effects

The long-term deterministic effects of radiation on tissues and organs depend primarily on the extent of damage to the fine vasculature. The relative radiosensitivity of capillaries and connective tissue is intermediate. Irradiation of capillaries causes swelling, degeneration and necrosis, which increase capillary permeability and initiate progressive fibrosis around the vessels, leading to deposition of fibrous scar tissue and premature narrowing of vascular lumens. This impairs transport of oxygen, nutrients and waste products resulting in cell death, leading to progressive fibroatrophy of the irradiated tissue, and loss of cell function with a reduced resistance of the irradiated tissue to infection and trauma.

In India, around 40 percent of all cancers are detected as oral cancers. In addition for patients with cancer of the nose, nasopharynx, paranasal sinuses and oropharynx, radiotherapy is one of the modality of treatment used.

Radiotherapy is frequently used as an adjuvant form of treatment in the management of head and neck cancer. This radiotherapy may produce an oral sequelae that causes considerable misery to the patient.

Radiocurability is defined as the ability of radiations to reduce the number of malignant cells below a critical level such that no further clinical manifestation of their presence will occur during the remaining life time of the host.

Radiosensitivity is defined as the ability of radiations to biologically change, (i.e. cell killing or a destruction of reproduction integrity) cells comprising a tumor or other tissue.

Radioresponsiveness refers to the time required for any changes to occur and can be measured in terms of the rate at which the clinical manifestations of radiation induced biological change take place.

Different cells of the same individual may respond differently to the same irradiation. Casarett has divided mammalian cells into five categories of radiosensitivity on the basis of histologic observations of early cell death.

- *Vegetative intermitotic cells* are the most radiosensitive. These cells divide regularly, have long mitotic potentials and do not undergo differentiation between mitosis, they have a short life span, e.g. basal cells of the oral mucous membrane, early precursor stem cells such as erythroblastic or spermatogenic series.
- *Differentiating intermitotic cells* are less radiosensitive. They divide regularly but less often and undergo some differentiation between divisions, e.g. intermediate dividing and replicating cells of the inner enamel epithelium of developing teeth, cells of hematopoietic series that are in the intermediate stages of differentiation, spermatocytes and oocytes.
- *Multipotential connective tissue cells* have intermediate radiosensitivity. They divide regularly with limited differentiation, e.g. vascular endothelial cells, fibroblasts and mesenchymal cells.
- *Reverting postmitotic cells* are radioresistant. They divide infrequently, have a long life span and die without dividing. These divide only under special conditions and are specialized in function, e.g. acinar and ductal cells of salivary glands and pancreas, and parenchymal cells of the liver, kidney and thyroid.
- *Fixed postmitotic cells*: Are most radioresistant. These do not divide even in functional demand, e.g. neurons, striated muscle cells and squamous epithelial cells that have differentiated and are close to the surface of the oral mucous membrane.

The relative radiosensitivity of various organs may be listed as follows:

- *High sensitivity*: Lymphoid organs, bone marrow, testes, intestines, mucous membrane.
- *Intermediate sensitivity*: Fine vasculature, growing cartilage, growing bone, salivary glands, lungs, kidneys, liver.
- *Low sensitivity*: Optic lens, mature erythrocytes, muscle cells, neurons.

In dental radiography the critical organs receiving scattered radiation include:

- *Bone marrow*: A maximum dose of 200 R is required for any damage to the marrow or blood forming organs. Hence, the risk of bone marrow damage from dental X-rays is small. The primary somatic risk from dental radiography is leukemia induction, especially in young individuals. This is because at birth all bones contain only red bone marrow, (one of the blood forming organs of the body), but with age some marrow changes to yellow (fatty) bone marrow, thus younger individuals are at a greater risk of developing leukemia.
- *Thyroid*: A dose of 10 R will produce thyroid cancer. All dental radiography gives scattered radiation to the thyroid, except cephalometry and curved surface tomography, where the thyroid is in the direction of the primary beam.
- *Gonadal*: A single intraoral radiograph gives 100–900 mR to the face. From this:
  - Male gonads receive 0.3 mR.
  - Female gonads receive 0.03–0.001 mR, as these are placed internally.

  A person on an average receives 0.3 mR by way of exposure from the sun and other radioactive materials. Thus, gonadal exposure is minimal with dental radiography. The radiation to the gonads is principally via scattered radiation.
- *Eye*: A series of full mouth intraoral periapical radiographs, will give only a few mR. Cataract of the lens is produced after 500 R of exposure.

GENERAL EFFECTS OF RADIATION

- *Skin*: The reaction of the skin to radiation may be categorized as:
  - Early or acute signs:
    - Increased susceptibility to chapping.
    - Intolerance to surgical scrub.
    - Blunting and leveling of finger ridges.
    - Brittleness and ridging of finger nails.
  - Late or chronic signs:
    - Loosening of hair and epilation.
    - Dryness and atrophy of skin, due to destruction of the sweat glands.
    - Progressive pigmentation, telangiectasis and keratosis.
    - Indolent type of ulcerations.
    - Possibility of malignant changes in tissue.

    All these changes in the skin are due to radiation trauma to:
    - The blood vessels
    - Connective tissue
    - Epithelium.

    Early erythema may appear from a single dose of about 450 rads.

    With lower doses no erythema occurs.
- *Hematopoietic injury*: The usual picture of blood reaction to radiation is leukopenia, which in some cases may progress to leukemia, anemia, lymphopenia, and loss of specific immune response.
- *Eyes*:
  - Epilation of eyelashes.
  - Inflammation, fibrosis and decreased flexibility of the eyelid.
  - Damage to the lacrimal glands, leading to dryness.
  - Ulceration of the cornea.
  - Initiation of cataract formation from the periphery towards the center.

- *Ears*:
  - Columnar epithelium of the middle ear may be desquamated.
  - Edema of the mucosa and collection of sterile fluid in the middle ear, which leads to obstruction of the eustachian tube—*radiation otitis media*.
  - Deafness due to rupture of the eardrums.
- *Testicles*:
  - Suppression of germinal activity.
  - Alteration in fertility.
  - Functional changes in the offspring may be seen.
- *Ovary*:
  - The various cells respond differently to irradiation.
  - Increase in frequency of hemangioma in children receiving dose of radiation *in utero*.
- *Oral mucous membrane*:
  - Shows reddening and inflammation (mucositis).
  - The next step is the breakdown, with the formation of white to yellow pseudomembrane.
  - Sloughing of the mucosa.
  - Secondary infection is very common.
  - After termination of the therapy, the healing may be complete after about two months, but the mucous membrane tends to become atrophic, thin and relatively avascular, due to the obliteration of fine vasculature and fibrosis of the underlying connective tissue.
  - Patient is usually prone to oral ulcerations and is unable to tolerate dentures.
- *Taste buds*: These are sensitive to radiation and patient realizes a loss of taste in the second or third week of radiation therapy:
  - Posterior two-third of the tongue when irradiated effects the bitter and acid flavors.
  - Anterior third of the tongue when irradiated effects sweet and salty flavors.

  These changes in the taste perception may also be attributed to the salivary changes that occur due to radiation.
- *Salivary glands*: The parenchymal component of the gland is sensitive to radiation. The gland demonstrates progressive fibrosis, adiposis, loss of fine vasculature and simultaneous parenchymal degeneration.
  - There is marked decrease in the salivary flow.
  - The composition of saliva is affected.
  - There is increased concentration of sodium, chloride, calcium, magnesium ions and proteins.
  - The saliva loses its lubricating properties.
  - The mouth becomes dry and tender due to xerostomia.
  - The pH of saliva is decreased which may initiate decalcification of enamel.
  - A compensatory hypertrophy of the salivary gland may take place and the xerostomia may subside after six to twelve months after therapy. The xerostomia that persists beyond a year is less likely to show return to normal.

- *Teeth*: Adult teeth are resistant to the effects of radiation. When teeth are exposed to radiation in their developing stage, their development may be retarded.
  - Prior to calcification, the tooth buds get destroyed.
  - After initiation of calcification, there may be inhibition of cellular differentiation causing malformation or arrest of growth.
  - The pulp shows decreased vascularity, reduced cellularity and the tooth becomes more prone to pulpitis.

  Radiation caries: This is a rampant form of caries. These lesions occur secondary to changes in the salivary glands and saliva, due to the:
  - Decreased salivary flow
  - Decreased pH of saliva
  - Increased viscosity of saliva
  - Decreased lubricating properties of saliva.

  All of the following leads to the decalcification of the enamel and increased accumulation of the food debris. Clinically three types of radiation caries are seen:
  1. Primarily involving cementum and dentin in the cervical areas. This lesion progresses around the tooth circumference and ultimately results in the amputation of the crown.
  2. Generalized superficial lesions attacking the buccal, occlusal, incisal and palatal surfaces of the teeth.
  3. Dark pigmentation of the crown.
- *Bone*:
  - The primary damage to the mature bone is because of the damage to the fine vasculature which is already sparse in a dense bone such as the mandible.
  - Due to the loss of vasculature and hematopoietic elements, the marrow is replaced by fatty marrow and fibrous connective tissue.
  - The endosteum becomes atrophic, and shows lack of osteoblasts and osteoclastic activity.
  - The complication following irradiation is called osteoradionecrosis
    - In this, the bone becomes hypovascular, hypocellular and hypomineralized, with decreased blood supply.
    - It is more often seen in the mandible than the maxilla, this is commonly attributed to the fact that the mandible has a single blood supply.
    - On the radiograph, osteoradionecrosis does not show any periosteal reaction as that seen in the case of osteomyelitis.
    - Osteoradionecrosis of the bone usually occurs due to infection or necrosis of the bone following tooth extraction or a chronic denture sore.
- *Whole body irradiation*: When the whole body is exposed to low or moderate doses of radiation there are characteristic changes seen, called acute radiation syndrome (ARS) (**Table 5.1**); which may be followed by death within one month. Individuals surviving ARS may show late somatic effects which may be seen as:

Table 5.1 Acute effects following large whole body doses of radiation. (Acute radiation syndrome)

Dose	Whole body effect
0.25 Sv	No changes
0.25–1.0 Sv	• Prodromal symptoms. • Alteration in the blood components, e.g. decrease in WBC count. • Mild hematopoietic symptoms. • Vomiting (within three hours), fatigue, loss of appetite, blood changes. • Recovery in a few weeks.
2–6 Sv	• Severe hematopoietic symptoms. • Vomiting (within two hours), severe changes in the blood, loss of hair (within two weeks time). • Recovery in one month to one year for 70% of the patients.
6–10 Sv	• Gastrointestinal symptoms. • Vomiting (within one hour), intestinal damage, severe changes in the blood. • Death may occur in two weeks for 80–100% of the patients.
> 10 Sv	• Cardiovascular symptoms. • Complicated symptoms of the central nervous system, causing brain damage, coma, and eventual death.

- *Prodromal syndrome (1–2 Gy)*: Shortly after exposure the patient may develop nausea, vomiting, diarrhea and anorexia.
- *Latent period*: This is a period of apparent well being, the extent of which is dose related. Symptoms follow the latent period when the individuals are exposed in the lethal range (approximately 2–5 Gy) or the supralethal range (more than 5 Gy).
- *Bone marrow (hemopoietic) syndrome (2–7 Gy)*: Here severe damage may be caused to the circulatory system. The bone marrow being radiosensitive, results in fall in the number of granulocytes, platelets and erythrocytes. Clinically this is manifested as lymphopenia, granulocytopenia and or hemorrhage due to thrombocytopenia and anemia due to depletion of the erythrocytes.
- *Gastrointestinal syndrome (7–15 Gy)*: This causes extensive damage to the gastrointestinal tract, leading to anorexia, nausea, vomiting, severe diarrhoea and malaise. Injury to the basal cell epithelial cells of the intestines causes denuded mucosal surfaces, leading to loss of plasma and electrolytes, hemorrhage and ulcerations leading to diarrhoea, dehydration and loss of weight. Finally leading to septicaemia unusually leading to death.
- *Cardiovascular and central nervous system syndrome (more than 50 Gy)*: This produces death within one

or two days. Individuals show intermittent stupor, incoordination, disorientation and convulsions suggestive of extensive damage to the nervous system.

- *Shortening of the life span*: The life span is diminished following brief whole body radiation exposure, or a small amount of radiation given over a long period of time.
- *Radiation effect on embryos and foetuses*: Embryos and foetuses are significantly more radio-sensitive than adults because most embryonic cells are relatively undifferentiated and rapidly mitotic. The foetus of a patient exposed to radiation from dental radiography receives less than 0.25 mGy from a full mouth examination when a leaded apron is used.

The most sensitive period for inducing developmental abnormalities is during the period of organogenesis, between 18 and 45 days of gestation. These effects are deterministic in nature.

Irradiation during the foetal period (more than 50 days after conception) does not cause gross malformations. However, general retardation of growth may persist through life. There is also an bigger risk for childhood cancer, (leukemia and solid tumors), after irradiation *in utero*.

BIBLIOGRAPHY

1. Barr JH, Stephens RG. Radiological Health. In: Dental radiology. Pertinent Basic Concepts and their Applications in Clinical Practise. Philadelphia: WB Saunders; 1980.pp. 66-80.
2. Bushong SC. Radiologic Science for Technologist, Physics, Biology and Protection, 7th edition, St Louis, Mosby; 2001.
3. Dowd SB, Tilson ER. Practical Radiation Protection and Applied Radiology, 2nd edition, Philadelphia: WB Saunder; 1999.
4. Forrester SD. Principles of cancer management Part II, Surgery, Radiotherapy, Hyperthermia, Immunotherapy; 1997.
5. Frommer HH. Biological effects of radiation, In: Radiology for dental auxiliaries, 6th edition. St Louis: Mosby-Year book; 1996.pp.49-67.
6. Goaz PW, White SC. Health Physics. In: Oral Radiology, Principles and Interpretation, 3rd edition. St Louis: Mosby-Year Book; 1994.pp.48-68.
7. Johnson ON, McNally MA, Essay CE. Effects of Radiation Exposure. In: Essentials of Dental Radiography for Assistants and Hygienists, 6th edition. Norwalk, Appleton and Lange; 1999.pp.87-105.
8. Mason-Hing LR. In: Fundamentals of Dental Radiography, 3rd edition, Philadelphia: WB Saunders; 1993.pp.221-29.
9. Meredith WJ. Fundamental Physics of Radiology, 2nd edition, John Wright and Sons Ltd; 1972.
10. Reskin AB. Advances in Oral Radiology. PSG Publishing Co., 1980.
11. White SC. Assessment of radiation risks from dental radiology. Dentomaxillofac radiol. 1992;21:118.

Protection from Radiation | 6

Research studies measuring the risk of X-ray exposure for increased occurrence of cancer, birth defects, cataracts and life span shortening have been controversial and are not conclusive, while clinical cases of radiation damage from dental X-rays have not been reported. It cannot be proved that there is no possibility of a hazard to the patient. This situation has produced the concept of keeping radiation exposure 'as low as reasonably achievable'— The *ALARA Principle,* which recognizes the possibility that no matter how small the dose is, some stochastic effect may result.

The ALARA Principle should be followed:
- *Radiation workers*:
  - Occupationally exposed person—50 mSv in any one year
  - Women of reproductive age and pregnancy shall not exceed—10 mSv.
- *Members of the public*:
  - Annual effective dose for the public should not exceed—1 mSv
  - In any one year, members of public shall not receive an effective dose equivalent in excess of—5 mSv.
   The application of radiation protection principles is called *Health Physics.*

RADIATION PROTECTION

The principle of radiation protection is to do those things that will minimize exposure of patient and dental personnel and still provide benefits for the patient from use of diagnostic radiography.

PROTECTION IN GENERAL

For a given radiation source the amount of radiation at any point in the beam depends upon the distance from the point to the source of radiation (intensity is inversely proportional to the square of the distance) and the nature of thickness of the material through which the radiation is passed.

In addition, the average person is exposed to an additional 0.76-1.01 mSv per year from other sources, such as global fall out, occupational exposure, treatment and diagnostic radiation procedures and other miscellaneous causes.

Sources of Radiation Exposure

A wide variety of conditions and circumstances result in radiation exposure, they may be broadly classified into:

Natural or Background Exposure

Exposure to radiation from natural sources is known as background exposure. This radiation comes from a variety of sources.
- External:
  - *Cosmic (nonterrestrial)*: These include energetic subatomic particles, photons of extraterrestrial origin that reach the earth (primary cosmic radiation) and to a lesser extent the particles and photons (secondary cosmic radiation) generated by the interactions of primary cosmic radiations with atoms and molecules of the earth's atmosphere. Cosmic radiation also includes exposure resulting from airline travel.
  - *Terrestrial*: Exposure comes from radioactive nuclides in the soil, (potassium-40), and from radioactive decay products of uranium-238 and thorium-232.
       The total of much more than 13 mSv per year, represents the national average in India.
- *Internal*: These are radiations from radionuclides that are taken up from the external enviroment by inhalation and ingestion. This accounts for approximately 67% of the radiation exposure of the population.
  - Radon is a decay product in the uranium series.
  - Other internal sources is the second largest source (11%) of natural radiation which results from the ingestion of food and water that contain radio-nuclides.

Artificial Radiations

These are a result of the technological advances made by man. They are:
- *Medical*:
  - X-ray diagnosis
  - Nuclear medicine.
- *Consumer products*:
  - Occupational
  - Nuclear fuel cycle fall out
  - Miscellaneous.

Table 6.1 Approximate effective dose to the patient during various dental radiographic examinations*

Sr. No.	Type of examination	Approximate effective dose in μSv
1	Digital/F speed, with rectangular collimation FMX	34.9
2	Digital/F speed, with round collimation FMX	170.7
3	Conventional single IOPA	<8.3
4	Panoramic	2.7–24.3
5	Lateral cephalometric	2.3–5.6
6	CT maxillo-mandibular	180–2100
7	CT maxilla	1400
8	Intraoral radiographs (FMX), panoramic, and lateral cephalometric radiographs	43.2–200.6
9	CBCT large FOV	260–136
10	CBCT medium FOV	166–84
11	CBCT small FOV	122–92

*(Cone-beam computed tomography and radiographs in dentistry: Aspects related to radiation dose, Diego Coelho Lorenzoni, 1 AnaMaria Bolognese, 1 Daniela Gamba Garib, 2 Fabio Ribeiro Guedes, 3 and Eduardo Franzotti Sant'Anna 1 International Journal of Dentistry Volume 2012, Article ID 813768, 10 pages doi:10.1155/2012/813768)

Although the risk involved with dental radiography is small they are a common part of every day life. Despite the fact that the diagnostic radiation appears to be a weak carcinogen, the risk is increased because a large number of people are exposed. It is the responsibility of the practitioners to ensure that the patients avoid even the smallest unnecessary dose of radiation (**Table 6.1**).

The magnitude of biological effects produced depends upon how much radiation energy is absorbed by the irradiated material and hence the objective of X-ray dosimetry is the measurement of energy absorbed in any material with particular references on biological tissue.

DOSIMETRY

Dosimetry is the determination of the quantity of radiation exposure or dose (**Table 6.2**).

Radiation dosimetry: Deals with the measurement of the absorbed dose or dose rate resulting from the interaction of ionizing radiation with matter and particularly in different tissues of the body.

Dose: It is amount of radiation at a given point or the amount of energy absorbed per unit mass at the site of interest.

Erythema dose: It is that dose which produces in one sitting a reversible reddening of the skin (3–4 Gy).

Exposure: It is a measure of radiation quantity, the capacity of the radiation to ionize air (**Table 6.2**).

The SI unit of exposure in air is kerma (Kinetic Energy Released in Matter) and is expressed in units of dose gray (Gy), where 1 Gy equals 1 joule/kg. It has replaced the

Table 6.2 Summary of radiation quantities and units (New and old)

Amount	SI unit	Traditional unit	Conversion
Exposure	Air kerma	Roentgen (R)	1 Gy = 100 rad 1 rad = 0.01 Gy (1cGy)
Absorbed dose	Gray (Gy)	Rad	1 Gy = 100 rad 1 rad = 0.01 Gy (1cGy)
Equivalent dose	Sievert (Sv)	Rem	1 Sv = 100 rem 1 rem = 0.01 Sv (1cSv)
Effective dose	Sievert (Sv)	—	—
Radioactivity	Becquerel (Bq)	Curie (Ci)	1 Bq = 2.7 × 10⁻¹¹ Ci 1 Ci = 3.7 × 10¹⁰ Bq

Roentgen (R), the traditional unit of radiation exposure measured in air.

Absorbed dose (Tables 6.2 and 6.3): It is the measure of the energy absorbed by any type of ionizing radiation per unit mass of any type of matter. The SI unit is the Gray (Gy), was introduced which replaced the traditional unit Rad, where 1 Gy equals 1 joule/kg.

The unit of *equivalent dose/effective* dose is Sievert (Sv). The traditional unit of equivalent dose was 'rem' (**Table 6.2**).

For diagnostic radiology 1 Sv = 1 Gy.

Maximum permissible dose (MPD) 0.05 Sv/year.

- Operator accumulated dose (OAD)
- This is equal to 5(N – 18) where N = the age of the patient
- OAD is also called MAD or maximum accumulated dose.

Most of the *protection schemes* depend upon *distance and barriers*.

The greater the distances, atomic number and thickness of the barrier, the smaller the exposure rate.

Barriers may be against primary radiations (here a greater thickness of the barrier is used) or secondary radiation (in this case the thickness or the barrier is less).

The most commonly used material as a barrier is Lead, this is because lead has:

- Higher atomic number
- Higher density
- Higher linear coefficient of attenuation.

Lead can be used in form of:

- Viewing windows that are glass into which lead is incorporated
- As lead plywood that is lead sandwiched between layers of wood.

Before taking a radiographic exposure, it is necessary for both the operator as well the patient to become acquainted with the risks associated with ionizing radiation. It is also necessary for the operator to judge whether there is a justification for the radiograph being taken or the possibility of frequent treatment being done smoothly even without the radiograph.

SOURCES OF RADIATION IN A DENTAL RADIOLOGY DEPARTMENT (FIG. 6.1)

- Primary beam is defined as radiation originating from the focal spot
- Scattered or secondary radiation is the radiation originating from the irradiated tissues of the patient
- Leakage or stray radiation is the radiation from the X-ray tube head housing
- Scattered radiation is the radiation from filters and cones
- Scattered radiation is the radiation coming from the objects other than the patient such as the walls and furniture's that the primary beam may strike.

The means of protection can be divided into:

- Protection for the operator
- Protection for the patient
- Protection for the environment.

Protection for the Operator

The two most important sources of X-rays to which the operator is exposed to are the primary X-ray beam and scattered radiation originating from the irradiated tissues of the patient.

Other Sources of Lesser Importance Include

- Leakage radiation through the tube head housing
- Scattered X-ray from filters, cones
- Scattered radiation coming from objects other than the patient, such as walls and furniture that the primary beam may strike.

Protection against primary beam:

[*Primary beam*: It is defined as radiation emitted by the focal spot of the target]

- Effort must be made so that the operator can leave the room or take a suitable position behind a barrier or wall during exposure
- Dental operatory should be designed and constructed to meet the minimum shielding requirements
- Position distance rule—which states that the operator should stand at least six feet away from the source of radiation or the operator should be at an angle of 90°–135°, with respect to the direction of the central ray, (This rule takes advantage of the inverse square law to reduce the intensity and also considers that in this position the patient's head will absorb the most scattered radiation) (**Fig. 6.2**)

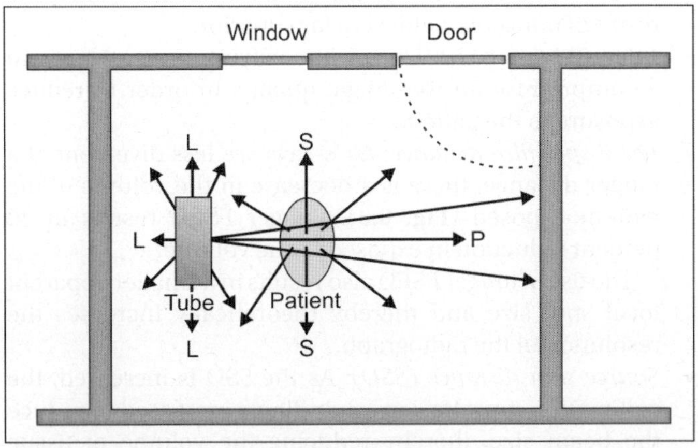

Figure 6.1 Primary: P. scattered; S. leakage; L. radiation during an X-ray exposure

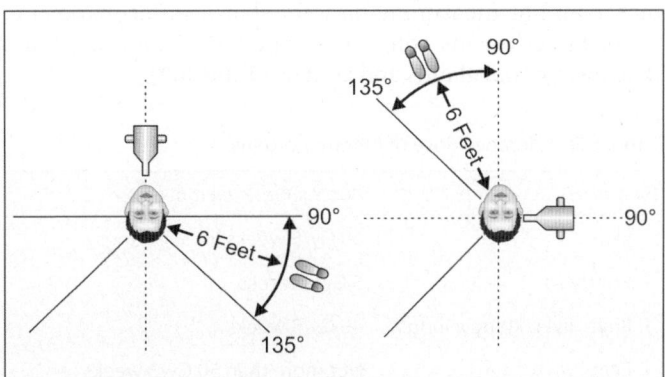

Figure 6.2 Position and distance rule. If no barrier is available, the operator should stand at least 6 feet from the patient, at an angle of 90°–135° to the central ray of the X-ray beam when the exposure is made

- Behind a barrier, made of suitable material, or
- If there is no shield or barrier the operator should use a lead apron
- The film should never be held by the operator. Ideally film holding devices should be used. If correct retention and placement is still not possible a parent or any other individual responsible for the patient must hold the film in position
- There should be no use of fluorescent mirrors in the oral cavity at the time of exposure
- Avoid holding the X-ray tube head of the machine. The suspension arms should be adequately maintained to prevent housing movement and drift.

Protection against leakage radiation:
[Leakage or stray radiation is defined as radiation emitted by any other part of the X-ray tube other than the focal spot].
- Neither the tube housing nor the cone should be hand held during exposure
- The machine should be periodically checked for leakage.

Protection from secondary and scattered radiation:
[Secondary radiation is defined as the radiation emitted by a substance through which X-rays are passing. Scattered radiation is defined as that radiation that has under gone change in direction during passage through a substance].
- Use of high speed films
- Replace the short plastic cone with an open ended lead lined cone
- Adequate filtration of the primary beam
- Use of collimator, to reduce the diameter of the beam
- Use of film badge/TLD badge/pocket dosimeter, for personnel radiation monitoring, to avoid accumulated over exposure.

Protection for the Patient

Patient dose from dental radiography is usually reported as the amount of radiation received by target organs. One of the most common measurements is the skin or surface exposure. Other target organs commonly reported include the bone marrow, thyroid glands and gonads (**Table 6.3**).

Table 6.3 Tolerance dose of different organs

Organ	Approximate tolerance dose
• Skin	60 Gy/5 weeks (in 30 sittings)
• Condyles	5 Gy/3 weeks
• Brain, liver, kidney, lungs	40 Gy/3 weeks
• Eyes	Not more than 50 Gy/3 weeks
• Gonads	Not more than 4 Gy in a single dose
– Male gonads	0.003 Gy
– Female gonads	0.005 Gy

- *Mean active bone marrow dose*: The dose derived as a specific dose relevant to a particular stochastic effect, e.g. leukemia. It is that dose of radiation that is averaged over the entire bone marrow.
- *Thyroid dose*: The proximity of thyroid gland to the X-ray beam is of crucial important in determining the magnitude of dose received. Particular concern has been expressed over the exposure of thyroid because it has one of the highest radiation induced cancer rates. Studies have reported that the dose to the gland from oral radiography is fairly low.
- *Gonad dose*: Radiographs that involve the abdomen result in the highest dose to the gonads. As a general category the dental X-ray examinations result in a generally insignificant dose to the gonads. The decision to use diagnostic radiography rest on professional judgment of its necessity for the benefit of the total health of the patient. Becoming aware of the potential risk associated with the use of ionizing radiation is the first step towards exposure and dose reduction in diagnostic radiography. Next is the use of the right techniques, materials and equipments that optimize the radiological process. It may be categorized as follows:

Patient selection: High yield or referral criteria, which is the clinical or historical findings that identify patients for whom a high probability exists that a radiographic examination will provide information affecting their treatment and prognosis.

Conduct of the examination: When the decision is made that a radiographic examination is justified, the way in which the examination is conducted greatly influences patient exposure to radiation. It is divided into:
- *Selection of the image receptor*: Use of high speed films, which will help reduce the exposure time. Although the image quality may be compromised, E speed films are routinely used without loss of diagnostic information.
- *Screen films*: The use of intensifying screens also helps reduce exposure time to the patient, but the diagnostic result of nonscreen films are far superior.
- *Intensifying screens*: Use of intensifying screens leads to a compromise on the image quality, in order to reduce exposure to the patient.
- *Focal spot film distance*: As X-rays are less divergent at a longer distance, there is a decrease in the volume of the patient exposed (**Fig. 6.3**). Longer FSFD results in 32 percent reduction in exposed tissue volume.

  The use of longer FSFD also results in a smaller apparent focal spot size and thereby theoretically increases the resolution of the radiograph.
- *Source skin distance (SSD)*: As the SSD is increased, the collimation must be correspondingly increased to reduce the beam size, thereby reducing the volume of tissue irradiated, thus reducing patient dose. The operating SSD depends on the kVp of the machine.

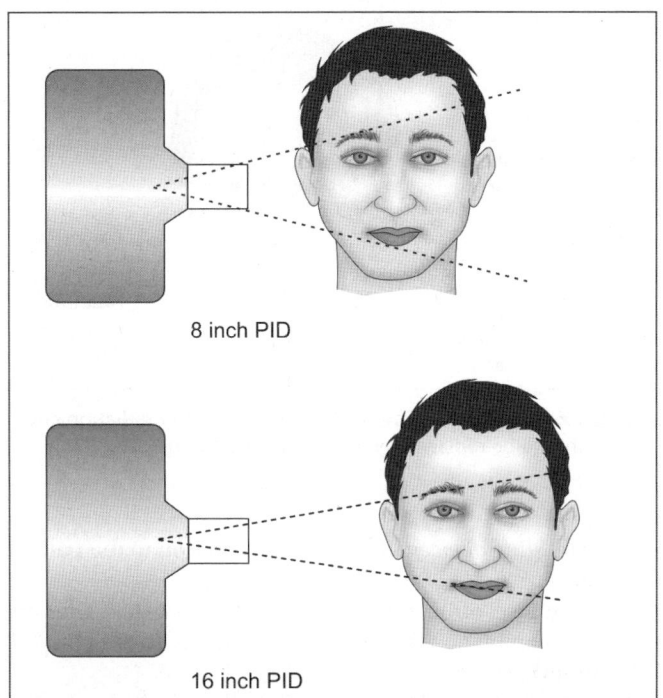

Figure 6.3 Compared to the short (8 inch) PID, the longer (16 inch) PID is preferred because it produces less divergence of the X-ray beam

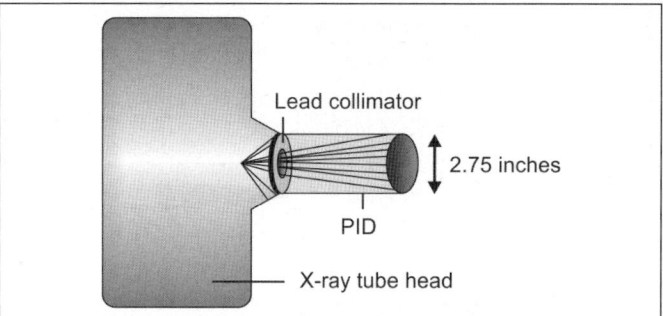

Figure 6.4 The federal regulations (in USA) require that the diameter of a collimated X-ray beam be restricted to 2.75 inches at the patient's face

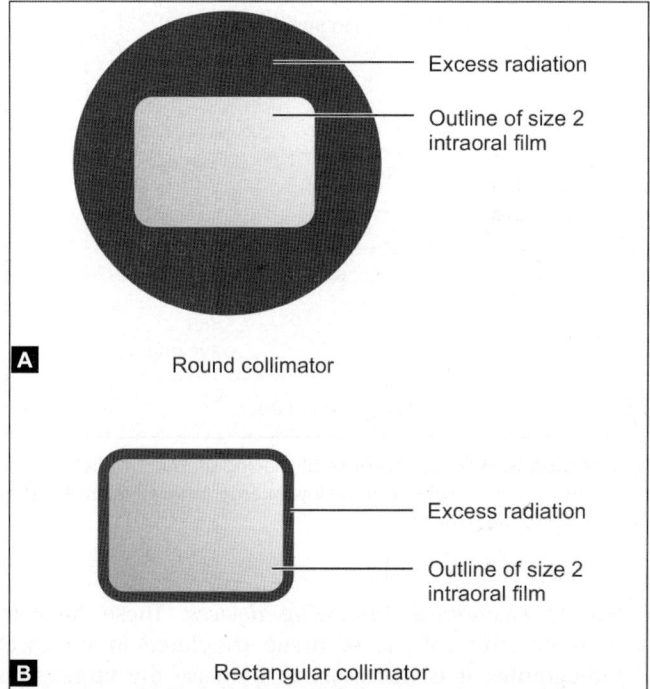

Figures 6.5A and B (A) The beam produced by a circular collimator is 2.75 inches in diameter, which is much larger than a size 2 intraoral film; (B) The beam produced by a rectangular collimator is just slightly larger than a size 2 intraoral film

Equipment operating below 50 kVp should have a minimum distance of 10 cm (4″) from the end of the PID to the focal spot.

Equipment operating above 50 kVp should have a minimum distance of 18 cm (7″) from the end of the PID to the focal spot.

- *Collimation of the beam*: Collimation helps to control the size and shape of the X-ray beam, allowing only the useful beam to emerge; (Useful beam is defined as that part of the primary radiation which is allowed to emerge through the collimating device). In intraoral machines there are fixed collimators and in extraoral machines there are adjustable collimators.

The beam should be limited to as small as an area possible for a particular radiographic examination. The recommended beam size is not more than 2 ¾″ in diameter at the patient's face, when the source film distance is 18 cm or more (**Fig. 6.4**). Collimation decreases the risk of radiation, minimises scattered radiation and decreases the fog, with a sharper image and better contrast (**Figs 6.5A and B**).

- *Filtration*: Filtration preferentially absorbs low energy photons which are undesirable as they add to the patient's skin dose but do not have enough energy to penetrate the tissue and bring about the image formation (**Figs 6.6A and B**).

The amount of filtration should be in accordance with the machine's operating range:

Below 50 kVp: 0.3–0.5 mm of (half value aluminum layer)
50–70 kVp: 1.2–1.5 mm of aluminum
Above 70 kVp: 2.1–4.1 mm of aluminum.

Rare earth materials like samariun, yttrium, niobium, etc. are also used in combination with aluminum filters, and help to reduce the patient exposure by 20 percent.

The disadvantage of using filters is that it leads to an increase in the exposure time and a decrease in the contrast.

- *Use of high kVp:* Higher kVp is used to keep the incident skin doses acceptable. The equipment should be capable of operating at a kilo voltage of 60 kVp or higher.

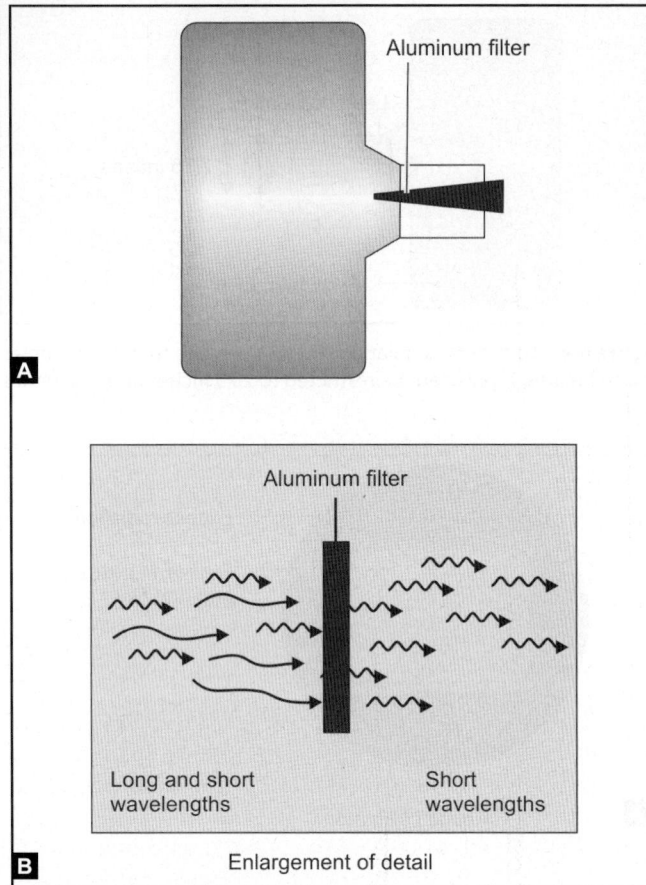

A

B Enlargement of detail

Figures 6.6A and B The purpose of placing aluminum discs in the path of the beam is to filter out the low energy, long wavelengths that are harmful to the patient

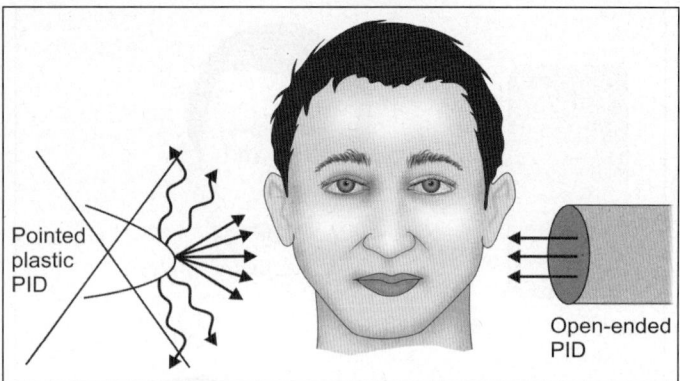

Figure 6.7 A plastic pointed PID produces scatter radiation and should be replaced by the open ended lead lined PID

- *Film holding devices*: These offer protection to the patient, because
  - Their use often reduces frequency of retakes, as the film can be positioned more accurately in the patient's mouth.
  - They also provide an external guide to indicate the film position.
  - The possibility of misaligning the X-ray tube and partially missing the film (cone cut), is also reduced.
  - Some of the holders also collimate the beam to the size of the film being used, which further reduces patient exposure.
  - The exposure to the patient's fingers is also reduced, as the patient does not have to hold the film.
- *Timers*: Most equipment are provided with 'dead man' timers. This timer requires a continuous pressure on the button (switch) during the exposure cycle in order to continue the operation of the X-ray machine. If the button is released the exposure is terminated.

  Dental X-ray machine timers generally automatically reset once the exposure has been terminated. Care should be taken that they are not capable of initiating another exposure until the switch is pressed again. Also, it should not make an exposure if the timer is set to zero or off position.

  The X-ray timer should be accurate (it should deliver the time exposure for which it is set) and reproducible (it should repeatedly deliver the same time interval at a given setting).

  The use of the electronic or synchronized timer permits exposure as low as 1/20 to 1/30 seconds, which was not possible with the traditional mechanical timer.
- *Use of protective barriers (Figs 6.8A to D)*
  - Leaded aprons should be used to protect the patient, especially in case of children, individuals of reproductive age and pregnant women. The lead apron provides more protective benefit to the males.

- *Use of positioning indicating devices*: These help to minimize the volume of tissue irradiated in intraoral radiography, it is necessary to increase the target film distance by using longer position indicating devices to direct the X-ray beam.

  One of the most widely used PID is the long open ended cylinder. This instrument reduces the more divergent rays that are inherent in the use of the short target film distance. As a result the diagnostic quality of the image is markedly improved and significantly smaller doses of radiation are delivered to the head and neck, this is due to the reduction of the beam divergence and concomitant reduction of the scattered radiation.

  If a change is made in the technique from short cone to long cone, it is important to simultaneously reduce the size of the collimator aperture.

  The use of open ended cylinders instead of a pointed plastic cone further reduces the scattered radiation that occurs when the X-ray beam passes through the plastic cone (**Fig. 6.7**).

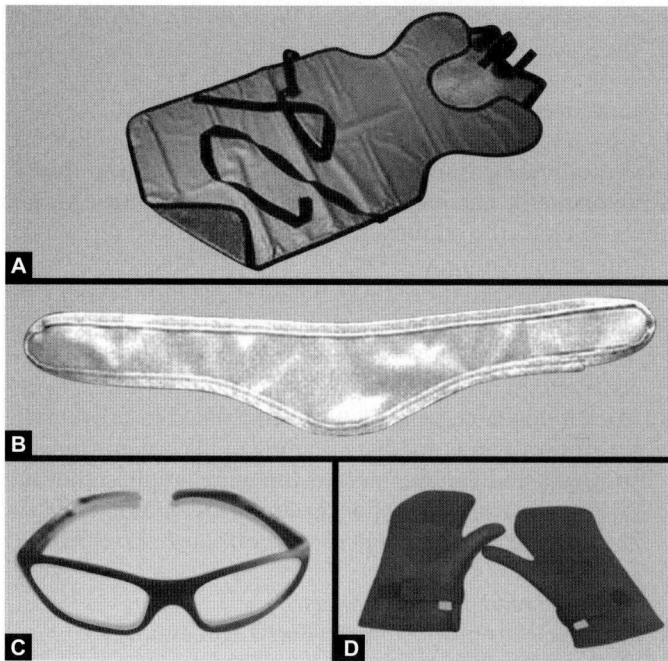

Figures 6.8A to D Protective barriers: (A) Lead apron; (B) Thyroid collar; (C) Protective glasses; (D) Shielding gloves

When used the lead apron should have a protective equivalent of 1/4th mm of lead.

It should be remembered that the lead aprons are a secondary measure to protect the patient and should not be substituted for use of fast films, lead collimation and aluminum filtration, which are the primary means of reducing exposure to the patient.

- Use of gonadal shields.
- Use of leaded thyroid shields, this is recommended especially when cephalometric examinations are carried out on children because of greater sensitivity of thyroid in young people. The thickness of the lead used should be 0.2 mm.
- Use of film holders with facial shields.
- *Use of proper technique*: The use of proper technique for the imaging of the particular anatomy of the patient.
- *Processing the image*: If films are not processed properly, retakes are required, increasing patient exposure and cost.
- *Interpretation of the image*: The radiograph should be viewed under proper conditions with an illuminated viewer. Proper interpretation precludes the necessity of retaking the images and subjecting the patient to additional exposure.

Protection for the Environment

The surrounding environment must be protected from radiation to avoid exposure to persons in the environment.

- Primary beam should never be directed at any one other than the patient.
- Patient should be positioned such that the X-ray beam is aimed at the wall of the room and not through a door or other opening where people may be located.
- Walls made of 3″ of concrete, 3″ × 16″ of steel or 1 mm of lead will suffice to protect adjacent rooms, even if the work load in the radiology department is high.
  - An alternative to lead is barium due to it's high atomic number, high density and high linear co-efficient of attenuation. Barium can be used in the form of barium plaster or barium concrete.
  - If it is not possible to incorporate lead or barium into the walls, they can be lined with lead plywood, 0.25 mm of lead sandwiched between layers of wood.
  - Primary barrier should be incorporated in any part of the floor or ceiling of the room at which the beam is fired.
  - Secondary barrier in the walls, provide protection against scattered or leakage radiation and as exposure rates are small they are ½ the thickness of the primary wall.
- *Windows*: It is necessary for the operator to see the patient as he is being irradiated, so a window is provided. This window should be situated such that the primary beam is not directed on it. Lead glass should be used.
- Doors of the radiology room should function as secondary barriers. They may have lead incorporated in them. Switches may be incorporated so that the beam is cut off as soon as the door is opened and not allow the beam to be switched on till the door is closed completely.
- Quality assurance may be defined as any planned activity to ensure that a dental office will consistently produce high quality images with the minimum exposure to patients and personnel.
- *Continuing education*: Practitioners should stay informed of new information on radiation safety issues as well as developments in equipment, materials and techniques and adopt appropriate items to improve radiographic practice.
- Regular radiation surveys, should be performed at regular intervals as the amount of exposure is dependent on many factors, such as:
  - The machine's kilo voltage
  - The work load of the X-ray machine
  - The X-ray absorbing ability of the walls (by using radiation measuring device)
  - The amount of time the adjacent areas are occupied by people.
- Radiation monitoring is measuring of the X-ray exposure of operators or associated personnel as a protective measure. There are various monitoring devices available.
  - Electrical
    - Ionization chamber
    - Thimble chamber

- Proportional counter
- Geiger counter
– Chemical
  - Film
  - Chemical dosimeter
– Light
  - Scintillation counter
  - Gerenkov counter.
– Thermoluminescence
  - Thermoluminescent dosimeter
– Heat
  - Calorimeter.

Personal monitoring devices:
• Pocket dosimeter
• Digital electronic dosimeter
• Film badge
• Thermoluminscent dosimeter.

Dosimeter Placement

Interpretation of the measured dose depends on the placement of the dosimeter. All personnel must wear their dosimeters correctly. The following list indicates where the dosimeters are to be worn:
• *Film badge with no TLD badge*: Wear the film badge above any protective clothing at collar level.

• *Film badge with a TLD badge*: Wear the film badge under the lead apron and the TLD above the apron at collar level.
• *Ring dosimeter*: Wear ring dosimeters so that the employee's name faces outwards.

Do not expose personnel monitoring devices to extreme heat or humidity. They are screened monthly. If any dosimeter has received a dose higher than the values shown below, the employee will be notified and the reason for the high reading will be investigated. Measures will be taken to keep radiation doses below these limits whenever possible:
Whole body: 125 mrem/calendar quarter
Extremities: 1875 mrem/calendar quarter
• Pocket dosimeter (**Figs 6.9A to F**) is used to provide the wearer with an immediate reading of his or her exposure to X-rays and gamma rays. As the name implies, they are commonly worn in the pocket. There are different types:
  – *Minometer or the condensor type or the indirect reading type*
  – *Direct read pocket dosimeter*
• Digital electronic dosimeter (**Figs 6.10A and B**)
  – *Arrow-tech dosimeters*
  – *Personal alarm dosimeter*
  – *Bubble detector dosimeter*
• *Film badges (**Figs 6.11A and B**)*
• *Thermoluminescence dosimeter (TLD)*

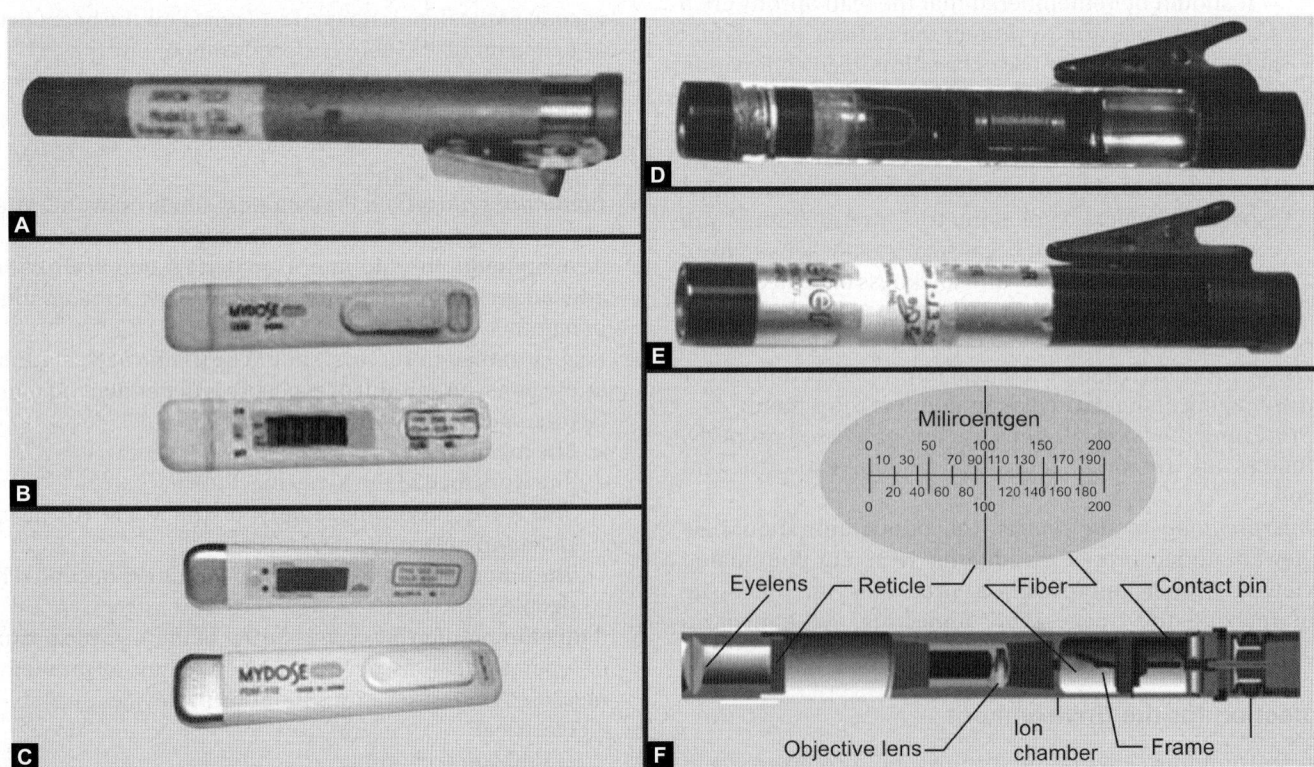

Figures 6.9A to F Pocket dosimeters

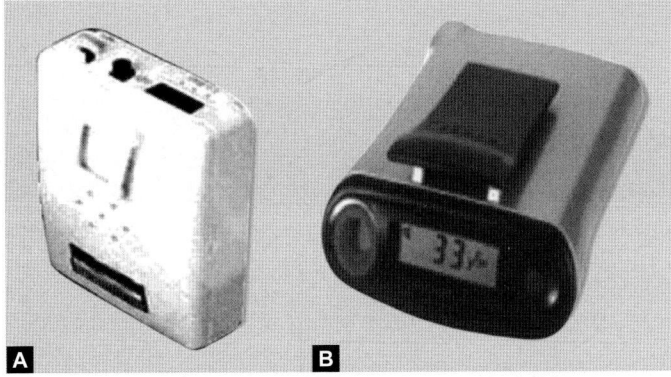

Figures 6.10A and B (A) Digital electronic dosimeter; (B) Personal alarm dosimeter

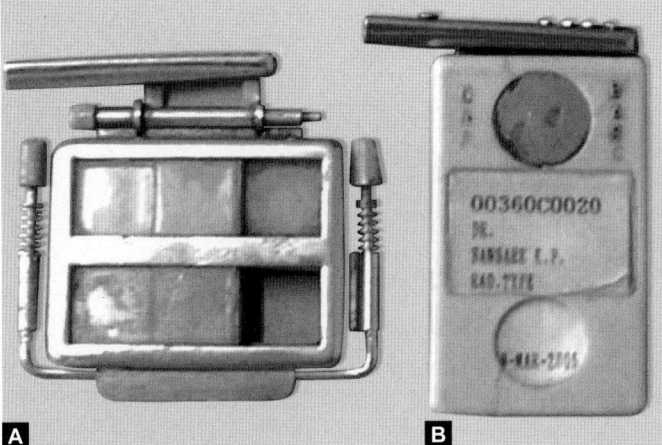

Figures 6.11A and B (A) Film badge; (B) TLD badge

BIBLIOGRAPHY

1. Barr JH, Stephens RG. Radiological Health. Dental radiology. Pertinent Basic Concepts and their Applications in Clinical Practise. Philadelphia: WB Saunders; 1980.pp. 66-80.
2. Brooks SL, Cho SY. Validation of a specific selection criterion for dental periapical radiography. Oral Surg Oral Med Oral Pathol. 1993;75(3):383-0.
3. Brooks SL. A study of selection criteria for intraoral dental radiography. Oral Surg Oral Med Oral Pathol. 1986;62(2):234-9.
4. Bushong SC. Radiologic Science for Technologist, Physics, Biology and Protection, 7th edition, St. Louis; 2001;7.
5. Dowd SB, Tilson ER. Practical Radiation Protection and Applied Radiology, 2nd edition, philadelphia; WB Saunder, Philadelphia; 1999.
6. Freeman JP, Brand JW. Radiation doses of commonly used dental radiographic surveys. Oral Surg Oral Med Oral Pathol. 1994;77(3):285-9.
7. Frommer HH. Radiation Protection. Radiology for Dental Auxiliaries, 6th edition St. Louis: Mosby-Year Book; 1996. pp.67-87.
8. Gibbs SJ, Pujol A Jr, Chen TS, et al. Patient risk from intra-oral dental radiography. Dentomaxillofac Radiol; 1988;17(1):15-23.
9. Gibbs SJ. Biological effects of radiation from dental radiography. Council on Dental Materials, Instruments, and Equipment. JADA; 1982;105(2):275-81.
10. Gibbs SJ. Effective dose equivalent and effective dose: comparison for common projections in oral and maxillofacial radiology. Oral Surg Oral Med Oral Pathol Oral Radiol Endod; 2000;90(4):538-45.
11. Goaz PW, White SC. Health Physics. In: Oral Radiology. Principles and interpretation, 3rd edition. St. Louis: Mosby Year Book; 1994.pp.47-68.
12. Hall EJ. Radiobiology for the Radiologist, 5th edition. Baltimore, Zero Lippincott, William and Wilker.
13. Health and Safety Executive. Occupational exposure to ionising radiation 1990-1996: Analysis of doses reported to the Health and Safety Executive's Central Index of Dose Information. Norwich, United Kingdom: Health and Safety Executive; 1998.
14. Johnson ON, McNally MA. Essay CE. Radiation Protection, inessentials of dental radiography for dental assistants and hygienists, 6th edition. Norwalk, Appleton and Lange; 1999.pp.105-30.
15. Mason-Hing LR. Fundamentals of Dental Radiography, 3rd edition. WB Saunders. Philadelphia; 1993.pp.221-9.
16. Meredith WJ. Fundamental Physics of Radiology, 2nd edition. John Wright and Sons Ltd, 1972.
17. Michel R, Zorn MJ. Implementation of an X-ray radiation protective equipment inspection program. Health Phys 2002;82(2 supplement):S51–S53.
18. National Council for Radiation Protection and Measurements. Radiation protection in dentistry. Bethesda, Md: National Council for Radiation Protection and Measurements; 2003.
19. Reskin AB. Advances in oral radiology, PSG Publishing Co.; 1980.
20. Sansare K, Vikram K, Karjodkar FR. Utility of thyroid collars in cephalometeric radiography, DMFR; 2011;40:471-5.
21. US Department of Health and Human Services, Food and Drug Administration. Performance standards for ionizing radiation emitting products.
22. US Department of Health and Human Services, Public Health Service, Food and Drug Administration; and American Dental Association, Council on Dental Benefit Programs, Council on Scientific Affairs. The selection of patients for dental radiographic examinations. Rev. ed. 2004. Available at: "www.ada.org/prof/resources/topics/radiography.asp". Accessed May 26, 2005.
23. van Aken J, van der Linden LW. The integral absorbed dose in conventional and panoramic complete-mouth examinations. Oral Surg Oral Med Oral Pathol; 1966;22(5):603.

Section **IV**

Imaging Principles

Ideal Radiographs | 7

An ideal radiograph is one that provides a great deal of information, the image exhibits proper density and contrast, has sharp outlines and is of the same shape and size as the object being radiographed.

Or in HM Worth's words: "An ideal radiograph is one which has desired density and overall blackness and which shows the part completely without distortion with maximum details and has the right amount of contrast to make the details fully apparent".

It is important to remember that an image on the radiograph is a two dimensional representation of a three dimensional object. Therefore, to obtain maximum value from the radiograph, the clinician must mentally reconstruct an accurate three dimensional image of the anatomical structures of interest from the radiograph.

Two terms are used to describe the black and white areas viewed on the dental radiograph: *radiolucent* and *radiopaque*, respectively.

Radiolucent refers to that portion of a processed radiograph that is dark or black. A structure that appears radiolucent on a radiograph lacks density and permits the passage of the X-ray beam with little or no resistance, e.g. air space, pulp tissue.

Radiopaque refers to that portion of the radiograph that appears light or white. Radiopaque structures are dense and absorb or resist the passage of the X-ray beam, e.g. enamel, dentin and bone.

The characteristics of an ideal radiograph are (**Table 7.1**):
- Visual characteristics:
  - Density
  - Contrast.
- Geometric characteristics:
  - Sharpness or detail, resolution or definition
  - Magnification
  - Distortion.
- Anatomical accuracy of radiographic images
- Adequate coverage of the anatomic region of interest.

VISUAL CHARACTERISTICS

Density

It is the overall blackness or darkness of a dental radiograph.

When a radiograph is viewed against a light source, the relative transparency of areas on the radiograph depends on the distribution of black silver particles in the emulsion. Darker areas represent heavier deposits of black silver particles. Density is this degree of silver blackening.

If the density is too dark, the film will appear too dark and the resulting images cannot be visually separated from each other. A radiograph with correct density enables the radiographer to view black areas (air spaces), white areas (enamel, dentin and bone) and gray areas (soft tissue).

Factors Affecting the Density of a Radiograph

First Degree Factors

- *Milliamperage (mA)*: An increase in milliamperage produces more X-rays that expose the film and as a result increase film density.
  - If mA increases then film density increases.
  - If mA decreases then film density decreases.
  Thus density varies directly and proportionately as the milliamperage or the tube current.
- *Exposure time*: An increase in the exposure time will increase the total number of X-rays that reach the film surface, thus the film density is increased.
  - If exposure time is increased, then film density is increased.
  - If exposure time is decreased, then film density is decreased.
  Exposure time and milliamperage are interchangeable and are thus considered as a single factor—mAs.
- *Operating kilo voltage peak (kVp)*: An increase in the kVp increases the energy of the X-rays, hence increases their power of penetration there by increasing the film density.
  - If kVp increases, then film density increases.
  - If kVp decreases, then film density decreases.
  - Thus density varies directly and in proportion to the square of the relative kVp.
- *Source film distance*: Since the intensity of an X-ray beam varies inversely as the square of the (S-F) distance, density also varies inversely as the square of the (S-F) distance.

Second Degree Factors

- *Subject thickness*: Fewer X-rays will reach the film in a patient with an increased amount of soft tissue or thick

Table 7.1 Factors affecting the radiographic quality of a diagnostic film

Image factors	Sharpness	Image size	Shape distortion	Film density	Radiographic contrast
• Factors related to the radiation beam					
– kVp				√	√
– mAs	√			√	√
– Collimation		√			
– Filtration				√	√
– Focal spot size	√	√		√	
– Equipment efficiency	√	√		√	√
• Factors related to the absorbing media or object					
– Object density	√			√	√
– Object shape	√			√	√
– Object thickness	√			√	√
• Factors related to the technique					
– Position of patient's head			√		
– Alignment					
i. Placement and position of the film			√		
ii. Angulation of the X-ray beam			√		
– Motion	√	√			
– Film speed	√			√	√
– Developing time				√	√
– Technique	√	√	√		
– Screen speed	√	√		√	√
• Factors related to recording of the roentgen image of the object					
– Reduction in secondary radiation	√			√	√
– Films and film storage				√	√
– Intensifying screens	√			√	√
– Film processing	√			√	√

dense bones. As a result the radiograph will appear light and have less density.
- If subject thickness increases, then density decreases.
- If subject thickness decreases, then density increases.

Adjustments in the operating mA, kVp or exposure time can be made to compensate for variations in size of the patient and subject thickness.

In case of a suspected pathology:
- If destruction is suspected then exposure time is decreased.
- If deposition is suspected then exposure time is increased.
  - In case of fair skinned individuals, they have increased circulation of blood per unit area of skin. Blood contains calcium ions and therefore exposure time should be increased when radiographing these individuals, and a lower kVp and/or mA setting should be used.

- Obese patients, have increased fat deposition and therefore exposure time should be increased when radiographing these patients, and a higher kVp and/or mA setting should be used.
- If patient is small and has a narrow facial bone structure, the next lower kVp and/or mA should be used.
- If the patient is edentulous, use the next lower kVp and/or mA setting.

• *Development conditions*: The radiograph may be light or dark depending on whether the films are under or over developed.
• *Type of film*:
  - *Film speed*: High speed films require less mAs in order to obtain a density change.
  - *Film latitude*: It is measured as a range of exposures that can be recorded as distinguishable densities on a film.

- *Radiographic noise*: It is the appearance of uneven density of a uniformly exposed radiographic film. It is seen on a small area of film as localized variations in density. The primary cause is radiographic mottle.
- *Screens*: Use of screens require less mAs in order to obtain a density change.
- *Grids*: The use of grids require more mAs in order to obtain a density change.
- *Amount of filtration used*: Reduction in the amount of added filtration used will increase the number of photons reaching the film and hence increase the density.
- *Fog*: Film fog may result in an undesirable form of darkening of the film.

Contrast

It is the difference in the degree of blackness (densities) between adjacent areas on a dental radiograph.

If a dental radiograph has very dark areas and very light areas, it is said to have a 'high contrast', as the dark and the light areas are strikingly different.

A radiograph that does not have very dark and very light areas, but instead has many shades of gray is said to have a 'low contrast'.

In dental radiography a film that is a compromise between low and high contrast is preferred.

The overall contrast of a dental radiograph is determined by film properties or film contrast and the object radiographed or the subject contrast:

- *Film contrast*: This refers to the characteristics of the film that influence the radiographic contrast. These characteristics include:
  - *Inherent qualities of a film*: These are under the control of the film manufacturer and cannot be changed by the dental radiographer.
    - Fast film requires less exposure but give decreased contrast and sharpness.
    - Double coated film with less exposure produce decreased contrast.
    - Films with thicker layer of emulsion, require more developing time and give increased contrast.
  - *Film processing*: This process is under the control of the dental radiographer.
    - Increase in the developing time will give increased contrast
    - Increase in the developer solution temperature will give increased contrast
    - Only Elon in the developing solution will give indistinct contrast
    - Only Hydroquinone in the developing solution will produce a harsh black and white image.

      Therefore a combination of Elon and Hydroquinone is used to produce better results and adequate contrast.

- Film fog, smothers the whole film with a dull gray shadow, giving a very poor contrast.
- *Subject contrast*: This refers to the characteristics of the subject, that influence radiographic contrast. Subject contrast is determined by:
  - Thickness of the subject.
  - Density of the subject.
  - Composition (atomic number) of the subject.
    - Subject contrast can be controlled by regulating the kilo voltage peak.
    - Increase in kVp (> 90 kVp) leads to decrease in subject contrast producing many shades of gray.
    - Decrease in kVp (65–70 kVp) leads to increase in the subject contrast producing areas of distinct black and white.
- *Operating kilo voltage peak (kVp)*: This is the only exposure factor which has a direct influence on the contrast of a dental radiograph.
  - Increase in kVp, leads to an increase in the energy of the X-rays produced.
    - This leads to increase in the penetrating power of the X-rays.
    - This leads to more variation in the tissue densities recorded.
    - This leads to production of various shades of gray.
    - This produces a decrease in the contrast obtained.
  - Decrease in kVp, produces many areas of black and white with increased contrast.
- *Exposure time*: An increase in the exposure time will produce increased contrast, but any *excessive increase or decrease* in the exposure time may decrease the amount of contrast obtained.

As mentioned earlier, the dental radiograph needs to have a compromise between the high and low contrast in order to produce a range of useful densities on a dental radiograph. This is called 'Scale of Contrast'.

  - Short scale contrast is produced by decreasing the kVp which produces black and white areas giving high contrast (**Fig. 7.1**).
  - Long scale contrast is produced by increasing the kVp which produces many shades of gray areas giving low contrast (**Fig. 7.1**).

    This scale of contrast can be illustrated by means of a Penetrometer, this is a radiographic testing device, made of aluminum and built up in steps.

For example:
    - Enamel has the highest density of all body tissues, but in the mandibular posterior teeth, the X-rays have to penetrate 8 mm of bone, and again on the same radiograph changes in the thin lamina dura around the teeth also has to be recorded.

      The lesions in enamel and lamina dura cause changes in the amount of X-rays absorbed by these tissues.

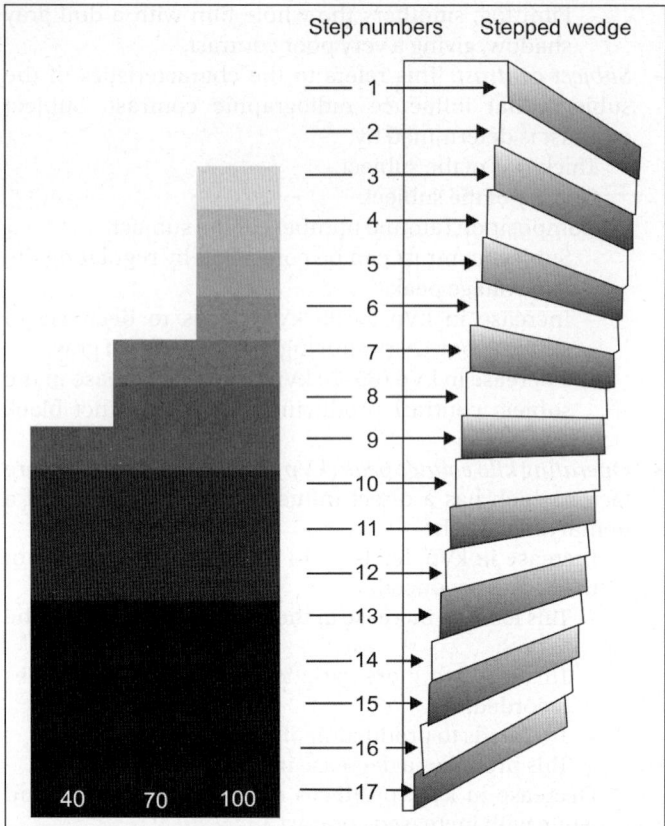

Figure 7.1 Radiographs taken at 40 kVp are predominantly black and white—that is they have high contrast or a short contrast scale. Those taken at 100 kVp show many shades of gray or a long contrast scale

As a result, the intraoral film density is a compromise between a less exposed film that will show the periodontal lesions optimally and a more exposed film which will show carious lesions clearly.
- X-rays are absorbed proportional to the total mass through which they may pass. Thus, a small amount of enamel may absorb the same amount of radiation as that absorbed by a large amount of soft tissue; for example the shadow of the nose and lips which appear on intraoral radiographs, where, the soft tissue mass has sufficient thickness to absorb enough X-rays to create an image.

Relationship between Contrast and Density

When contrast is altered, the density is also changed. However, when the radiographic density is altered by itself, there is no obvious change in contrast.

This is because:
- Change in kVp produces a change in contrast and density.
- Change in mA alone does not change the contrast.
Thus, if we change the contrast, density also changes, mAs is the prime factor in controlling density, but it is not a

controlling factor in contrast, therefore a change in mAs will produce a change in the radiographic density but with no noticeable change in contrast.

GEOMETRIC CHARACTERISTICS

Alterations in geometric characteristics are mainly due to:
- X-rays originate from a definite area rather than a point source.
- X-rays travel in diverging straight lines as they radiate from their source of origin which is an important source of magnification.
- Dental radiographs are a two dimensional representation of three dimensional structures. This results in unequal magnification of different parts of an object, because of the varying distances of these parts from the film.

Sharpness (Also Referred to as Detail, Resolution or Definition)

This refers to the capability of X-rays to reproduce distinct outlines of an object or to reproduce the smallest details of an object on a dental radiograph.

A certain degree of unsharpness is present in all dental radiographs. The fuzzy, unclear area that surrounds a radiographic image is termed 'Penumbra'. Penumbra is derived from two latin words: 'pene' meaning almost and 'umbra' meaning shadow.

Umbra is defined as that part of the shadow where all light is absorbed, or area of total darkness.

Penumbra is defined as that part of the shadow of an object which is larger than a point and yet represents a single point of the object. It is thus the unsharpness of the image seen at the edge of the image.

The various factors that control sharpness of an image on the X-ray film are:
- Geometric unsharpness
  - Size of the focal spot
  - Object film distance
  - Target film distance.
- Motion unsharpness
  - Patient
  - Tube
  - Film.
- Film unsharpness
  - Grain size
  - Single and double emulsion
  - Film thickness.
- 'Fog' unsharpness
  - Scattered radiation
  - Unsafe, safety light in the darkroom
  - Chemical fog.
- Intensifying screen unsharpness
  - Crystal size
  - Back screen scatter
  - Mottle.

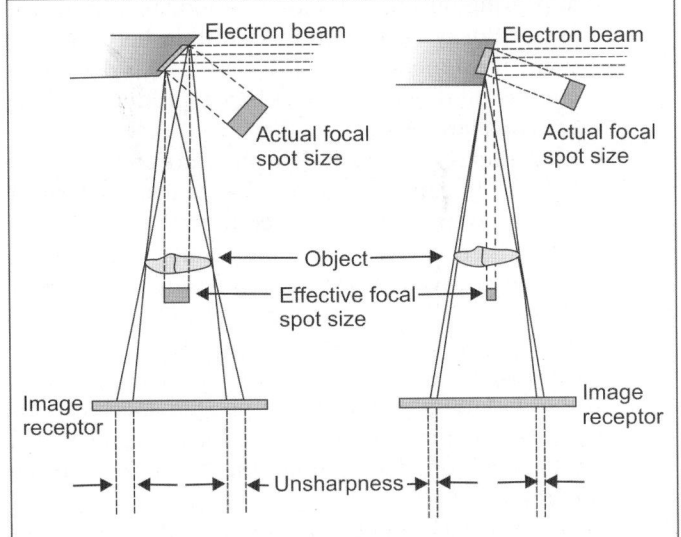

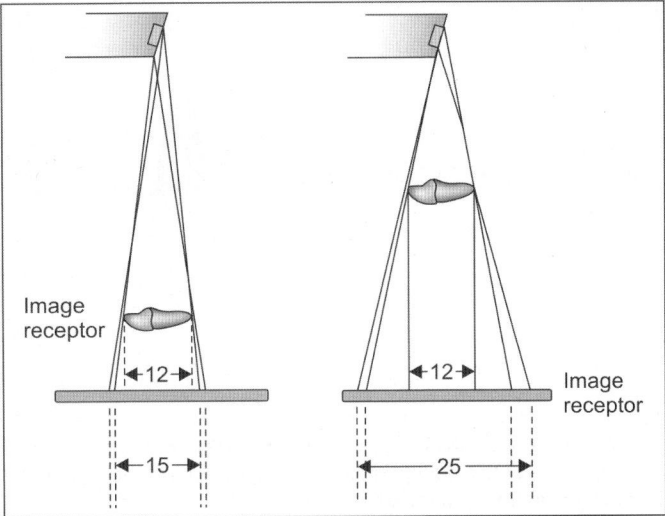

Figure 7.3 Decreasing the distance between the object and the film increases the sharpness and results in less magnification of the object

Figure 7.2 Decreasing the angle of the target perpendicular to the long axis of the electron beam decreases the actual focal spot size and decreases the heat dissipation and thereby tube life. It also decreases the effective focal spot size, thus increasing the sharpness of the image

- *Geometric unsharpness:* This type of unsharpness is due to criss-crossing of rays at the edges of the object, resulting in a fuzzy image border.
  - *Size of the focal spot (**Fig. 7.2**):* Smaller the focal spot, sharper the image produced. If a 'point source' is used, (normal focal spot size is 0.6–1 mm^2) no unsharpness is produced.
  - *Object film distance (**Fig. 7.3**):* This should be as small as possible, to get a sharper image.
  - *Target object distance (**Fig. 7.4**):* Should be as large as possible, to get a sharper image.

    In the dental radiographs, *the portion of the structures closest to the film will have greater sharpness,* therefore lingual cusps of teeth have a more sharper image than the buccal cusps, on the dental radiograph.
- *Motion unsharpness:* Any movement of either the patient, tube, or film, results in unsharpness of the image produced.

    A decrease in the exposure time will give less time for movement thus helping to obtain more sharpness on the radiograph.
- *Film unsharpness*
  - *Grain size:* The composition of the film emulsion influences the sharpness of the image produced, which is related to the grain size of the crystal.

    Faster the film speed, bigger the grain size of the crystal, produces decreased image sharpness.

    This is because larger crystals do not produce image outlines as well demarcated as smaller crystals.
  - *Single and double emulsion and film thickness (**Fig. 7.5**):* Use of double coated films leads to increased thickness, which produces unsharpness due to parallax.

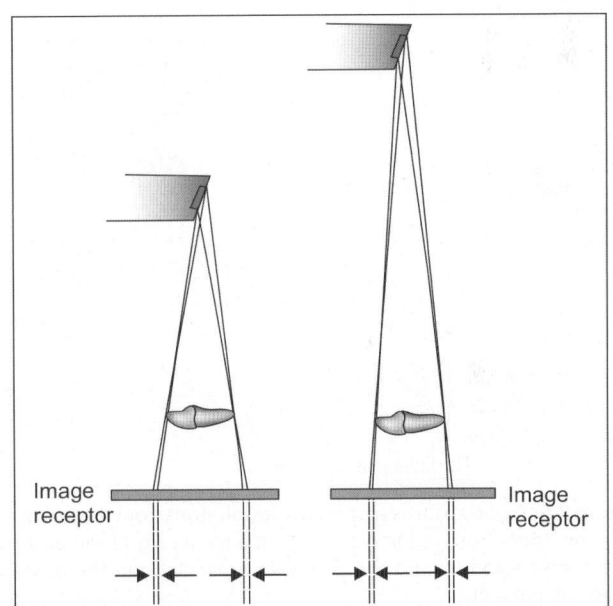

Figure 7.4 Increasing the distance between the focal spot and the object results in an image with increased sharpness and less magnification of the object

- *Fog unsharpness*
  - *Scattered radiation:* Scattered, stray, leakage or any other radiation not belonging to the primary beam is undesirable as it produces film fog.
    - For intra oral films, filtration, collimation and film packets with lead backed sheets should be used to reduce scattered and secondary radiation.
    - For extra oral films grids are used (**Fig. 7.6**).

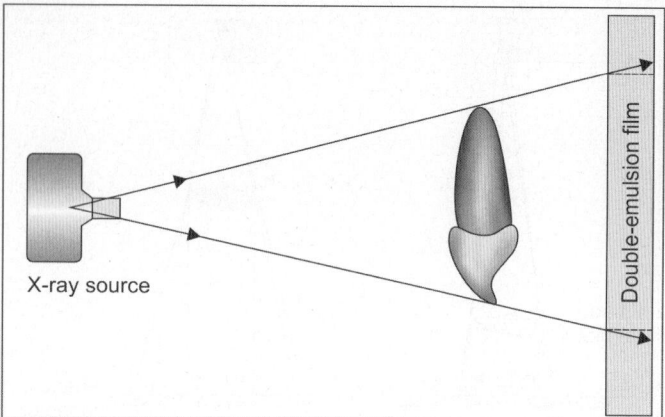

Figure 7.5 Parallax unsharpness results when double emulsion film is used because of the slightly greater magnification on the side of the film away from the X-ray source

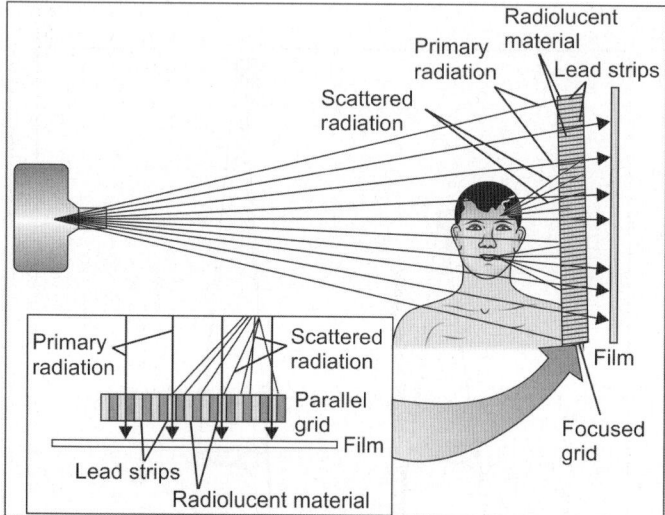

Figure 7.6 A grid absorbs scattered X-ray photons from the beam and prevents them from fogging the film. In a focused grid the absorber plates are angled toward the anode, in a parallel grid the absorber plates are parallel

A grid is a sheet of radiolucent material in which strips of lead are embedded. It is placed between the object and the film and allows only the X-rays which originate from the anode to pass through the object, without any change in direction to reach the film. The secondary radiations originating in the object and traveling in all directions is absorbed by the lead strips.

But, the disadvantage is that these lead strips produce white lines on the radiograph which decreases the contrast and produces distraction. Also the exposure time has to be increased when a grid is used. To prevent the grid lines from appearing on the radiograph, a moving grid called Potter Bucky Diaphram is used, but, here too due to the movement of the grid itself there is decreased contrast and density of the image produced, along with unsharpness.

- X-ray film is sensitive to light, pressure and any other type of ionizing radiation. The unexposed silver halide crystals slowly get converted to specks of silver. Therefore, it is important to safeguard the films from excessive temperature, humidity, exposure to chemicals and stray radiations. The films should be used preferably before their expiry date.

– *Unsafe, safety light in the darkroom*: The safe lights used in the darkroom should be as per the specifications given. Use of unsafe safe light produces fogging which can be verified by performing the 'Coin Test', in the dark room.

– *Chemical fog*: It is produced by prolonged development or development at high temperatures.

- Potassium bromide or the restrainers' prevents chemical fogging of the X-ray film by restraining the action of the developing agents on the unexposed silver halide crystals.

- If the radiograph is not adequately rinsed before putting it in the fixing solution, the alkaline developer will neutralize the acidic fixer and then the fixing and hardening action of the fixer solution is impaired, resulting in stains on the resultant radiograph.

- After fixing the radiograph should be thoroughly washed to remove all residual processing chemicals and silver salts from the film surface, as these may attack the silver image and/or certain products of fixation may decompose and produce a yellowish stain.

- If the temperature difference between the processing solutions and the rinsing water is more than 15°F, an orange peel appearance (reticulations) will appear on the film.

- The film must be adequately dried. If a wet film is touched or splashed with water during the drying process, it will produce spots that cannot be removed.

Potassium alum shrinks and hardens the gelatin so that the radiograph can withstand abuse of normal handling.

• *Intensifying screen unsharpness*: Intensifying screens are used in extraoral radiography in order to reduce the exposure to the patient. They may used singly or in pairs, placed in a metal cassette with the film sandwiched between them. They work on the principle of 'Fluorescence'.

Unsharpness may be caused due to:

– Improper film contact with the screens, thus when the X-rays strike the intensifying screen the fluorescent

crystals emit light in all directions, producing stray radiations and thus causing unsharpness
- Screen mottle
- Quantum mottle.

Use of the intensifying screens helps to reduce the exposure time, therefore there are less chances of any movement of patient, tube or film, hence reducing motion unsharpness.

Magnification

This refers to a radiographic image that appears larger than the actual size of the object it represents. This results because of the divergent path of the X-rays from the focal spot (**Fig. 7.7**).

Factors which influence magnification of the image are:
- *Target film distance*: This is determined in the intraoral machines by the length of the position indicating device (PID).
  - Longer the PID, more parallel X-rays from the middle of the beam strike the object, rather than the diverging rays from the periphery of the beam. Therefore, there is less magnification.
  - Shorter the PID, less parallel X-rays from the middle of the beam strike the object, and more of the diverging rays from the periphery of the beam strike the object. Therefore, there is more magnification.
- *Object film distance*:
  - Decrease the film to the object distance, lesser the magnification.

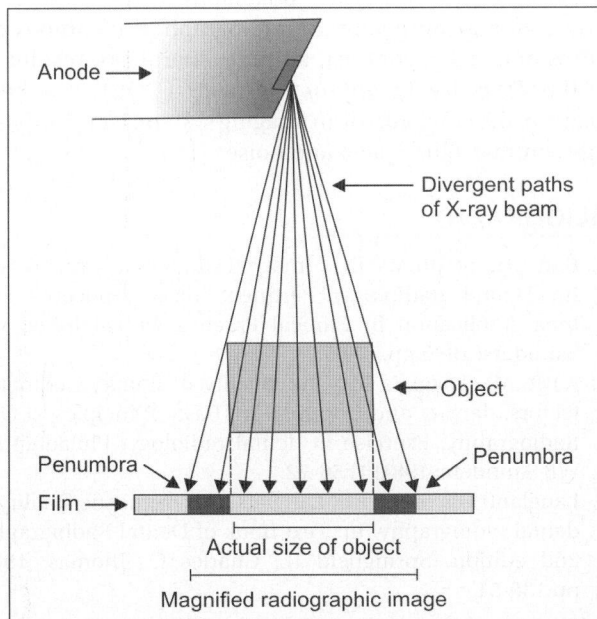

Figure 7.7 Diagram illustrating magnification as a result of the divergent paths of the X-ray beam

  - Increase the film to the object distance, more the magnification.
- *Use of intensifying screens*: The use of these screens increases the film to object distance, which produces a certain amount of magnification.
- *Magnification formulas*: The percentage of magnification of an object at any source film distance and object film distance can be determined by:

$$\frac{SFD}{SFD - OFD} - OFD \times 100\% = \text{Percentage of magnification}$$

- *Rule of magnification*: The actual size of the object is proportional to the size of the projected radiographic image of the object (tooth), as the S–O distance is to the S–F distance.

$$\frac{S_1 \text{ (size to object)}}{S_2 \text{ (size of image)}} = \frac{\text{S–O distance}}{\text{S–F distance}}$$

Distortion

Dimensional distortion of a radiographic image is a variation in the true size and shape of the object being recorded. A distorted image results from the unequal magnification of different parts of the same object.

This may occur due to:
- *Object-film alignment*: The object and the film should be placed parallel to each other, because if they are not parallel and if an angular relationship results, it will produce variation of the distances between the tooth and the film resulting in distortion. A distorted image may appear too long or too short.
- *X-ray beam angulation*: To minimize dimensional distortion the X-ray beam must be directed perpendicular to the tooth and the film, so as to record the tooth and adjacent structures in their true spatial relationship.
  - If the vertical angulation is increased there will be shortening of the image (**Fig. 7.8**).
  - If the vertical angulation is decreased there will be elongation of the image (**Fig. 7.9**).
  - If the horizontal angulation is increased mesially or distally there will be overlapping of structures.

    The teeth and the alveolar process are units of the facial bone, which are themselves fixed components of the skull. If the head is stabilized, the position of the teeth is automatically standardized.
    - The plane of occlusion should be parallel to the floor
    - The sagittal plane should be perpendicular to the floor.
    These two base lines if kept constant will help reduce errors in the angulation of the beam.

    If the height of the palatal arch is more the vertical angulation should be decreased.
- The film should never be bent in the direction of the long axis of the tooth, and the film holder should be used to prevent movement during exposure.

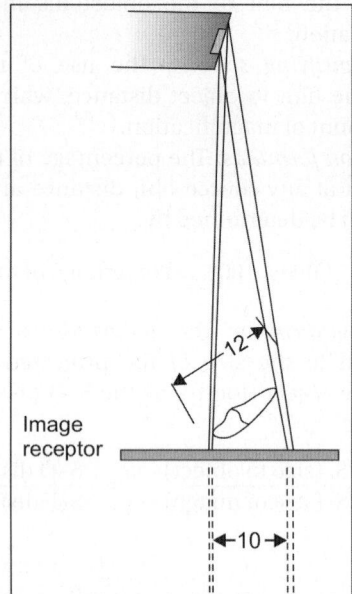

Figure 7.8 Foreshortening of a radiographic image result when the central ray is perpendicular to the film but the object is not parallel with the film

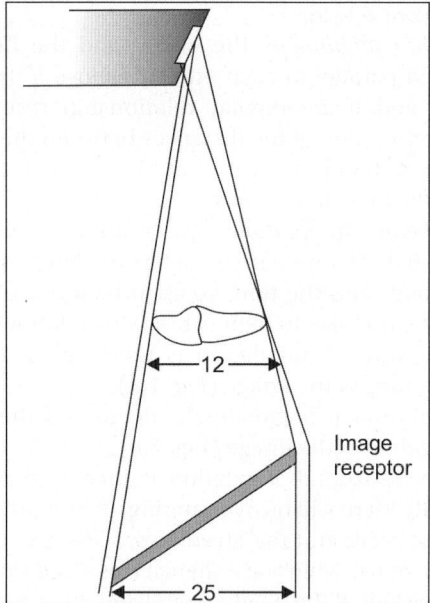

Figure 7.9 Elongation of a radiographic image results when the central ray is perpendicular to the object but not to the film

ANATOMICAL ACCURACY

This occurs when the anatomical structures are reproduced on the film in exact relationship as they normally appear.

A radiograph with anatomical accuracy will have a minimum of superimposition of images of adjacent tissues.

A radiograph is said to have anatomical accuracy when:

- Labial and lingual cemento enamel junctions of the anterior teeth are superimposed.
- Buccal and lingual cusps of the posterior teeth are superimposed.
- Contacts of the teeth are opened in at least one of the projections of a given area.
- Buccal portion of the alveolar crest is superimposed over the lingual portion of the alveolar crest.
- There is no superimposition of the zygoma over the roots of the maxillary molars.

    For intraoral periapical radiography, more accuracy is achieved by using the paralleling technique.

RADIOGRAPHIC COVERAGE

It is important that the area of interest is well covered in the radiograph. In case of the intraoral periapical radiograph, an adequate amount of bone surrounding the apices of the teeth should be revealed.

Adequate coverage of the area of interest depends upon several factors:

- Proper alignment of the film and the radiation beam to the area of interest
- Proper selection of the film types
- Proper selection of the film projection techniques.

Image Quality

This describes the subjective judgement by the clinician of the over all appearance of the radiograph. It combines the features of density, contrast, latitude, sharpness, resolution etc. The *Detective Quantum Efficiency* (DQE) is a basic measure of the efficiency of an imaging system. It encompases image contrast, blur, speed and noise.

BIBLIOGRAPHY

1. Barr JH, Stephens RG. Image Production with X-rays, In: Dental Radiology; Pertinent Basic Concepts and their Application in Clinical Practise. Philadelphia; WB Saunders; 1980.pp.53-65.
2. Kasle MJ, Lagglais RP. The Quality of Image, Geometric factors, density and Contrast. In: Basic Principles of Oral Radiography. Exercise in dental radiology, Philadelphia; WB Saunders; 1981(4):56-72.
3. Langland OE, Sippy FH, Langlais RP. Diagnostic Quality of dental radiography. In: Text Book of Dental Radiography, 2nd edition. Springfield IL, Charles C. Thomas; 1984. pp.130-51.

Faulty Radiographs | 8

Although film processing can produce radiographs of excellent quality, lack of attention to detail may lead to many problems and images that are diagnostically suboptimal. Poor radiographs contribute to a loss of diagnostic information, loss of professional and patient's time.

Causes of faulty radiographs can be broadly classified into:
- Projection errors
- Exposure and processing errors
- Automatic processing errors
- Miscellaneous technique errors.

With the advent of digital imaging the processing errors have become considerably less with reduced use of the dark room facilities. Radiographs can be manipulated with the help of tools available with the software provided which helps to improve the contrast etc. for better viewing and interpretation of the image.

PROJECTION ERRORS

- *Fault*: Apical ends of the teeth cut off (**Fig. 8.1**)
  - *Reason*: Film is placed too close to the teeth in the maxillary arch when using paralleling technique
    Rectification: Place the film away from the teeth

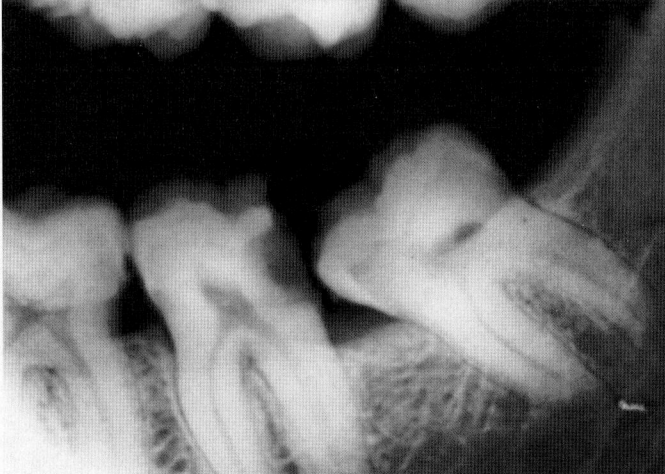

Figure 8.1 Apical ends of the teeth cut off

- *Reason*: Decreased vertical angulation which causes elongation
  Rectification: Increase the vertical angulation, especially in case of shallow vaults
- *Reason*: Film not positioned properly in the patient's mouth
  Rectification: Not more than 1/8th inch of the film edge should extend beyond the incisal-occlusal surfaces of the teeth.
- *Fault*: Overlapping of teeth (**Figs 8.2A and B**)
  - *Reason*: Plane of the film not parallel to the lingual surface of the teeth
    Rectification: Film should be placed parallel to the lingual surface of teeth
  - *Reason*: Incorrect horizontal angulation of the cone
    Rectification: Central ray of the X-ray beam should be directed perpendicular to the facial surfaces of the teeth
- *Fault*: The occlusal plane appears tipped or tilted (**Figs 8.3A and B**)
  - *Reason*: The edge of the film not placed parallel to the incisal-occlusal surfaces of the teeth
    Rectification: Ascertain that the edge of the film is parallel to the incisal-occlusal surface
  - *Reason*: Patient not instructed to hold the film firmly against the tooth, when the finger holding method is used
    Rectification: Instruct the patient to hold the film correctly.
- *Fault*: All of the specific region not showing (**Fig. 8.4**)
  - *Reason*: Faulty film placement
    Rectification: Center the film over the teeth to be radiographed
- *Fault*: Crowns of teeth not showing (**Fig. 8.5**)
  - *Reason*: Not enough film showing below or above the crowns of teeth
  - *Rectification*: Approximately 1/8th of the film should extend below or above the crown
  - *Reason*: Decreased vertical angulation causing elongation
    Rectification: Increase vertical angulation

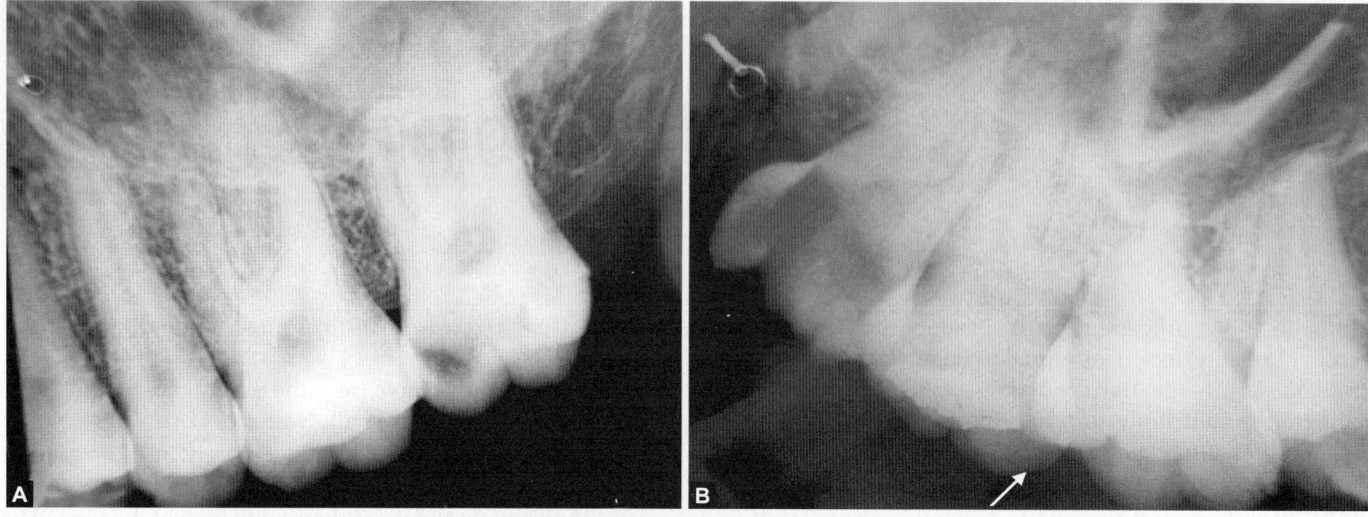

Figures 8.2A and B Overlapping of teeth

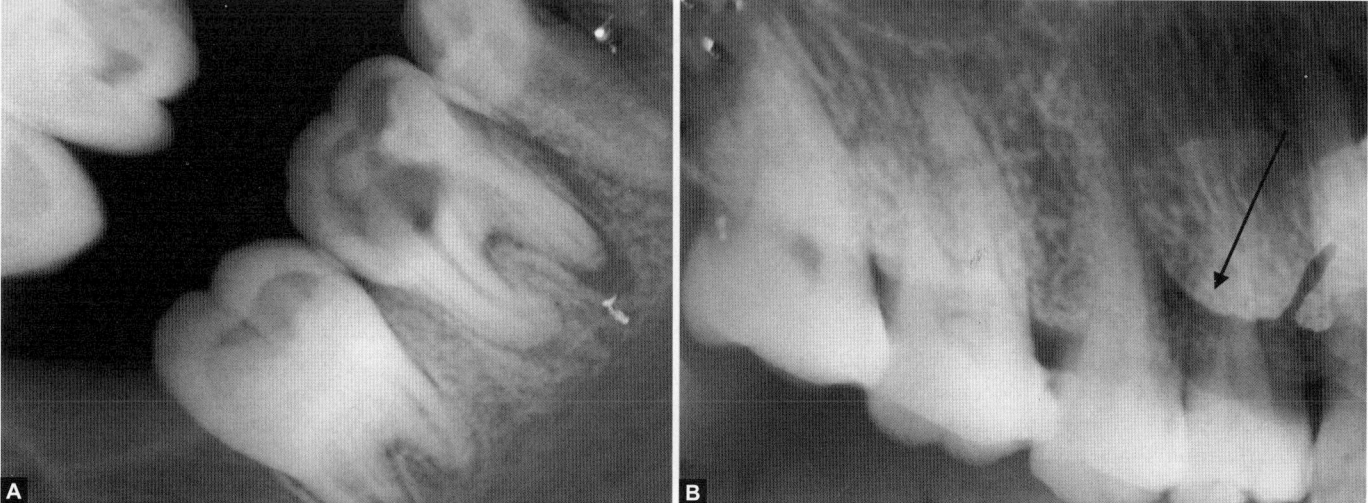

Figures 8.3A and B (A) The occlusal plane appears tipped or tilted; (B) Occlusal plain tilted with fixer stain (arrrow)

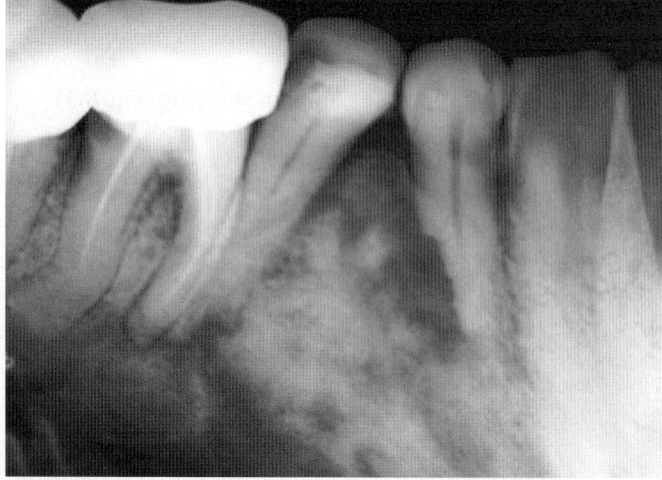

Figure 8.4 All of the specific region not showing that is the lower second molar for which the radiograph was prescribed

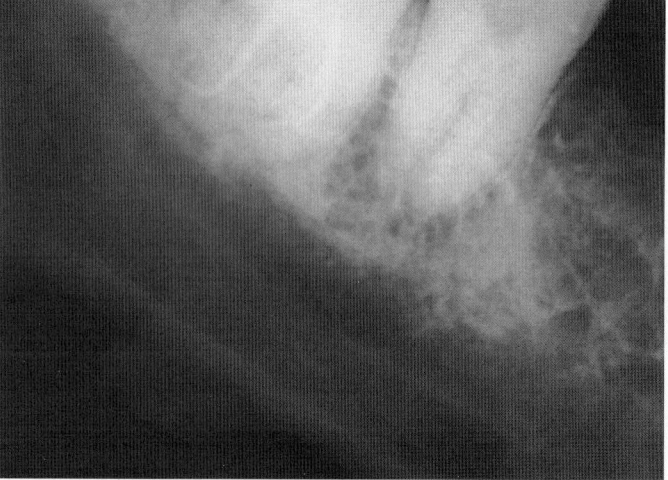

Figure 8.5 Crowns of teeth not showing, area beyond the periapex is covered

- *Fault*: Partial image
  - Cone cut (**Figs 8.6A and B**)
    - *Reason*: PID not covering area of interest, not using film holder
      Rectification: Make sure that the cone is properly centered over the area of interest and the film, both vertically and horizontally
    - *Reason*: Top of the film not immersed in the developing solution
      Rectification: Maintain the level of the solution in the processing tanks and ensure that the film is completely immersed during processing
  - Distal surface of canine not visible on bite wing film (**Figs 8.6C and D**)
    - *Reason*: The bite wing positioned too far posterior in the mouth; the front edge of the film not placed at the midline of the canine
      Rectification: Anterior edge of the bite wing film should be positioned at the midline of the mandibular canine
  - Third molar region not visible on the film (**Fig. 8.6E**)
    - *Reason*: Film was placed too far anterior in the mouth
      Rectification: Ascertain that the anterior edge of the film is positioned at the midline of the mandibular second premolar. Always center on the second molar, even when no erupted third molars are present
  - Only a portion of the film exposed, in panoramic films
    - *Reason*: Film cassette incorrectly positioned in the starting position
      Rectification: Place the cassette correctly

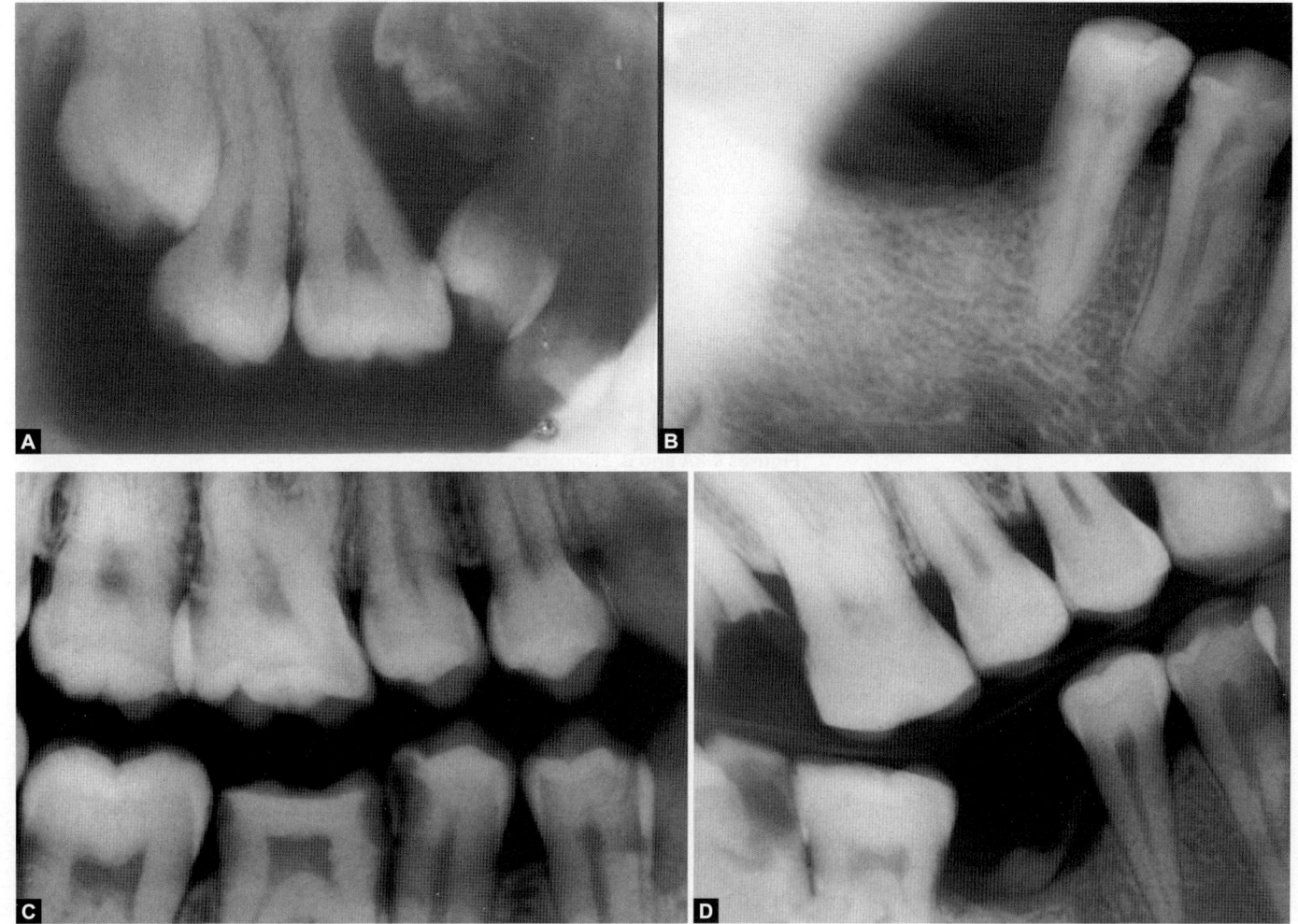

Figures 8.6A to D (A and B) Cone cut; (C and D) Distal surface of canine not visible on bite wing film

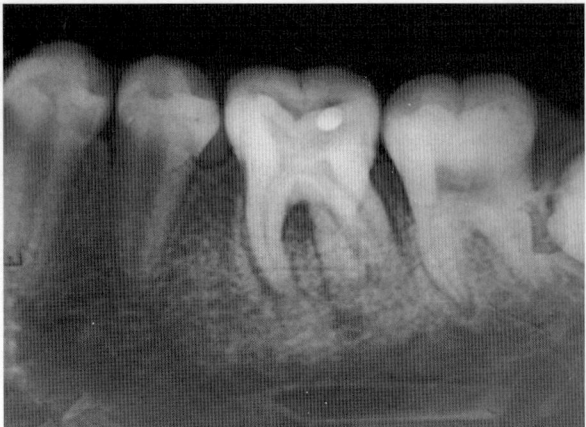

Figure 8.6E Third molar region not visible on the film

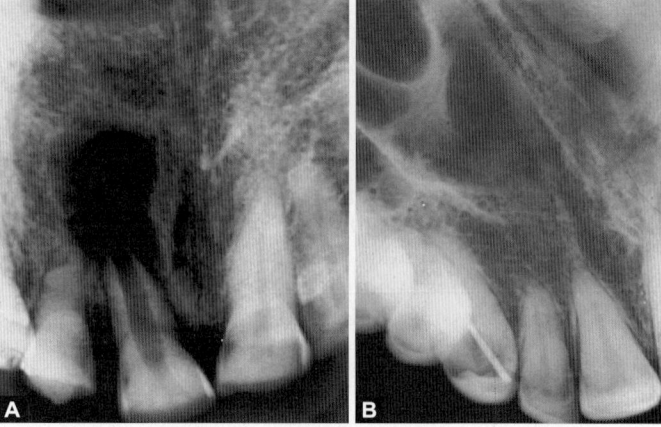

Figures 8.7A and B Foreshortening

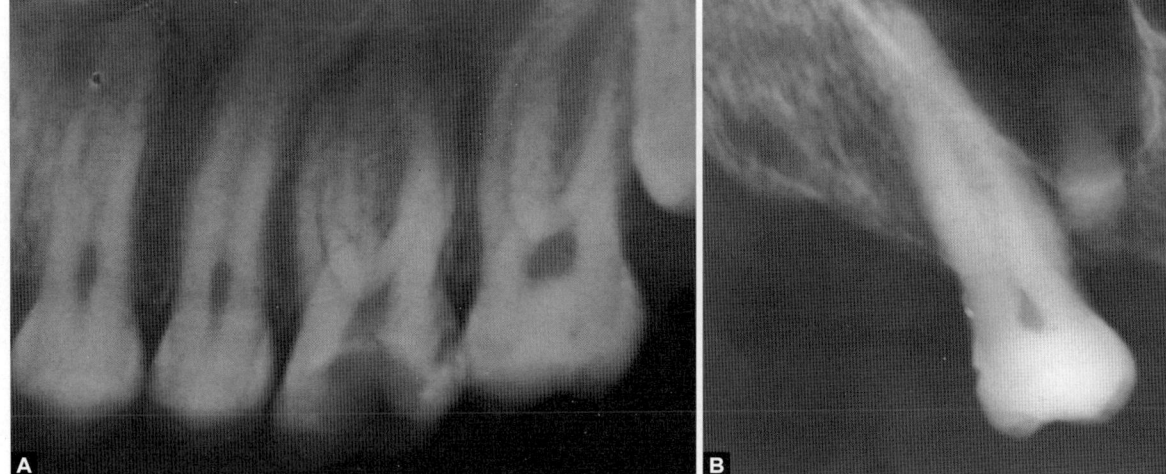

Figures 8.8A and B Elongation

- *Fault*: Shape distortion
  - Foreshortening (**Figs 8.7A and B**)
    - *Reason*: In the bisecting angle technique, there was increased vertical angulation of the cone
      Rectification: Reduce the vertical angulation
    - *Reason*: In the paralleling technique, the film not placed parallel to the long axis of the teeth or cone was not positioned properly
      Rectification: Place the film parallel to the long axis of the teeth. This is difficult in case of a shallow vault. Position the long cone so that the central ray strikes the film at right angles. Use position indicating devices
  - Elongation (**Figs 8.8A and B**)
    - *Reason*: In the bisecting angle technique, the vertical angulation of the cone was too flat
      Rectification: Increase the vertical angulation

  - *Reason*: In the paralleling technique, the film not placed parallel to the long axis of the teeth or cone not placed properly
    Rectification: Place the film parallel to the long axis of the teeth. This is difficult in case of a shallow vault. Position the long cone so that the central ray strikes the film at right angles. Use position indicating devices
  - Image distorted (**Figs 8.9A to D**)
    - *Reason*: Film is bent as the patient bites on the film holder, or as patient holds the film in the mouth.
      Rectification: Use a film backing
    - *Reason*: Negative vertical angulation used in bite wing technique
      Rectification: Always use +10° vertical angulation with bite wing technique

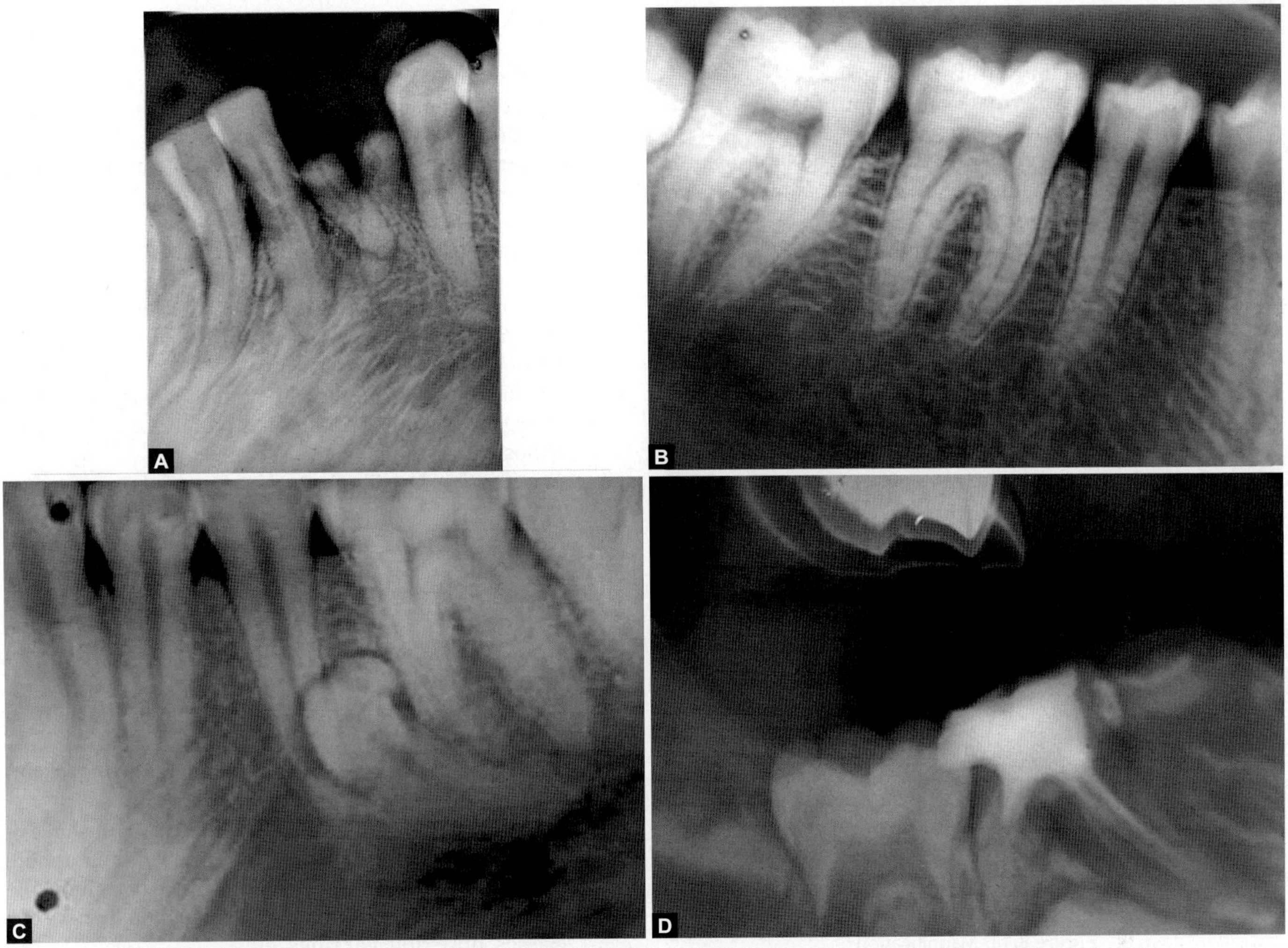

Figures 8.9A to D Image distorted: (A to C) Distortion due to bending of the film especially in the lower premolar region; (D) Radiograph of a small child

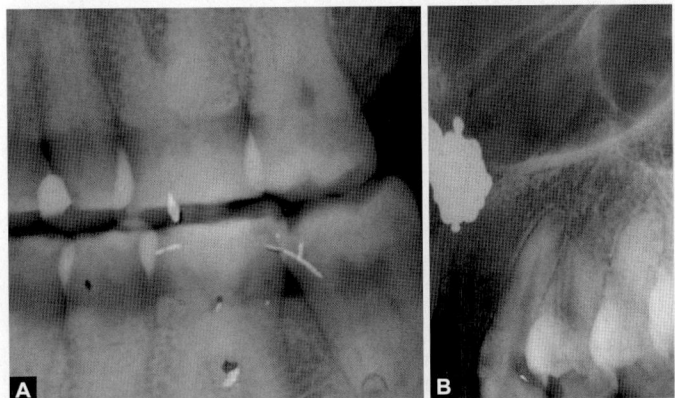

Figures 8.10A and B Overlapped contacts: (A) Due to improper horizontal angulation; (B) Due to improper placement of the film and angulation. There is a foreign body observed. Nose ring

- Overlapped contacts (**Figs 8.10A and B**)
  - *Reason*: Central ray was not directed through the inter proximal spaces
    Rectification: Direct the central ray through the inter proximal regions
- Magnification (**Fig. 8.11**)
  - *Reason*: Film to object distance is increased
    Rectification: Use the recommended film to object distance
  - *Reason*: A conical pointed cone is used which produces a divergent beam
    Rectification: Use open ended lead lined cones
- *Fault*: Herring bone effect or tyre track appearance (**Figs 8.12A and B**)
  - *Reason*: Back side of the film with the lead foil placed facing towards the cone

Rectification: Place the pebbled or the front side of the film towards the cone
- *Fault*: Black dot in the apical area (**Fig. 8.13**)
  - *Reason*: Identifying mark on the film placed towards the apical area of the teeth
  Rectification: Place the raised dot on the film towards the occlusal or the incisal surface of the teeth
- *Fault*: Artifacts on radiographs (**Fig. 8.14**)
  - Writing lines on the radiograph
    - *Reason*: Writing on the film packet with a ball point pen or a lead pencil
    - *Rectification*: Use a marker pen to mark the film packet

- Black lines on the radiograph
  - *Reason*: Bending of the film to reduce patient discomfort
  - *Rectification*: Avoid bending of the film
- Random artifacts on film
  - *Reason*: Contaminants (paper, dust, etc.) will prevent the X-rays from reaching the film
  - *Rectification*: Check and clean screens inside the cassettes for contaminants
- *Fault*: Double images on the radiograph (**Figs 8.15A and B**)
  - *Reason*: Film exposed twice to radiation
  Rectification: Place exposed film in separate labeled compartments
- *Fault*: Blurred image on the radiograph (**Figs 8.16A and B**)
  - *Reason*: Movement of the film, patient or tube during exposure
  Rectification: Use film holders.
        Ask the patient to keep steady
        There should be no play in the tube head
        Keep the tube ready before positioning the film in the patients mouth and pressing the exposure button so that no time is lost
  - *Reason*: Double exposure
  Rectification: Keep unexposed and exposed film in different receptacle and label the exposed film
- *Fault*: Radiopaque artifacts on the radiograph (**Figs 8.10B and 8.17**)
  - *Reason*: Dental appliances in the mouth, or presence of foreign bodies in and near the area being radiographed.
  Rectification: Instruct patient to remove all removable dental appliances and any other foreign bodies like eye glasses, nose ring, ear rings, etc.

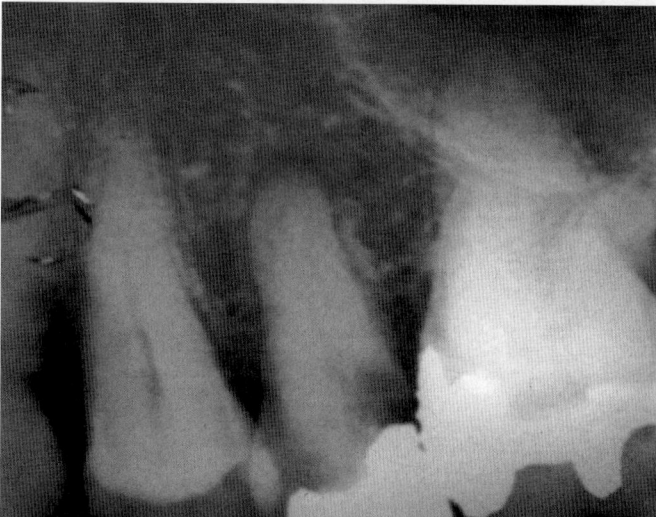

Figure 8.11 Magnification

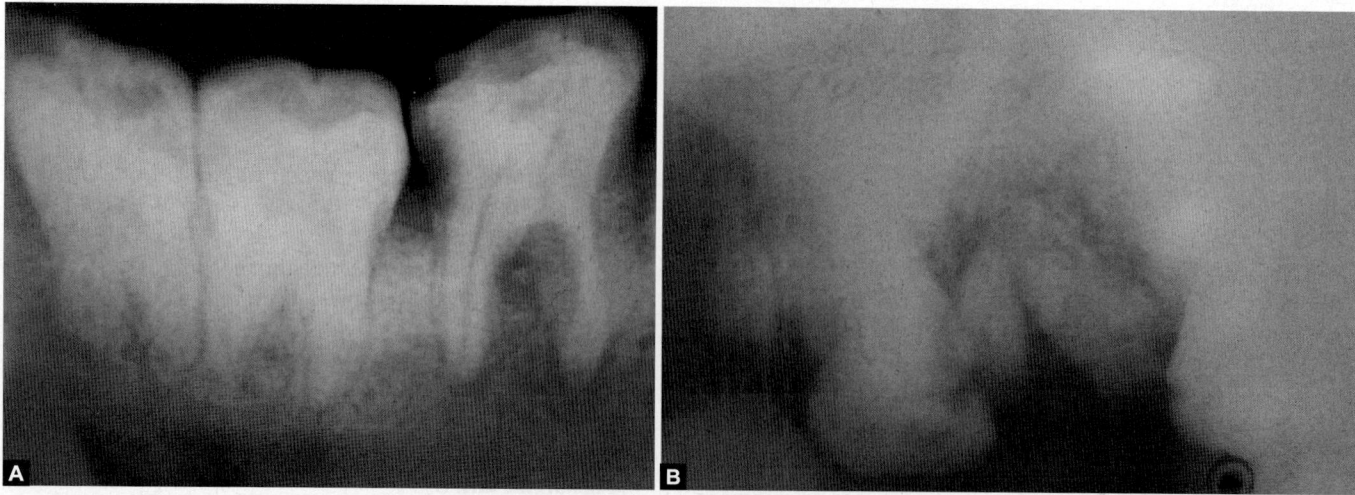

Figures 8.12A and B Herring bone effect or tyre track appearance

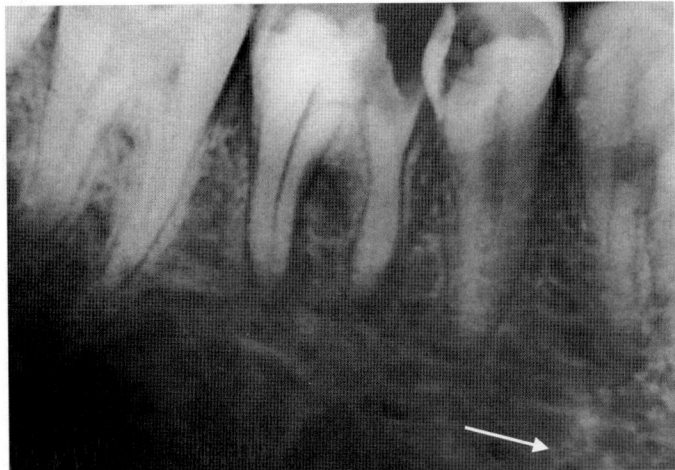

Figure 8.13 Black dot in the apical area and crowns of the teeth partially cut off

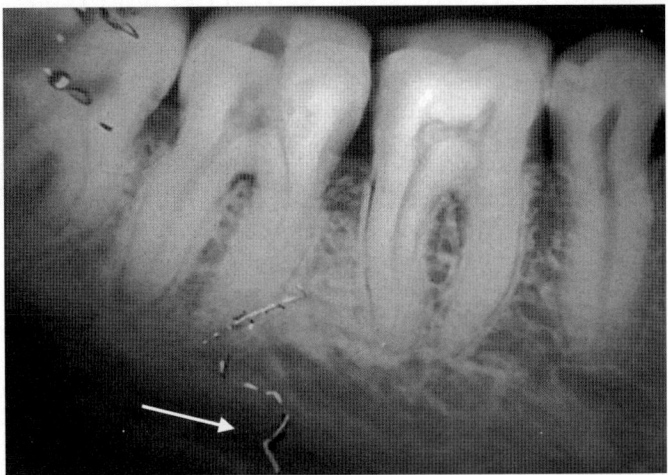

Figure 8.14 Artifacts on radiographs

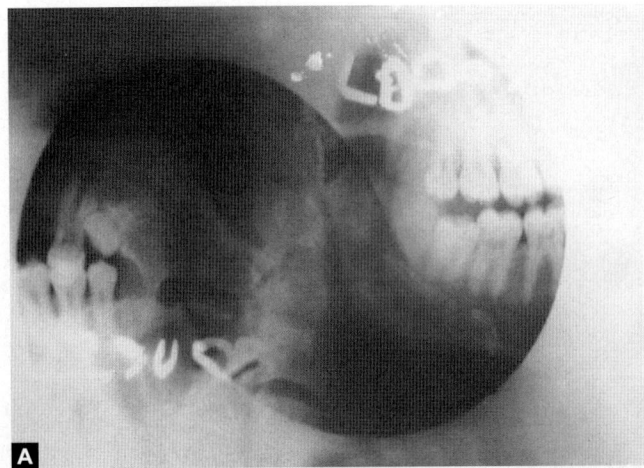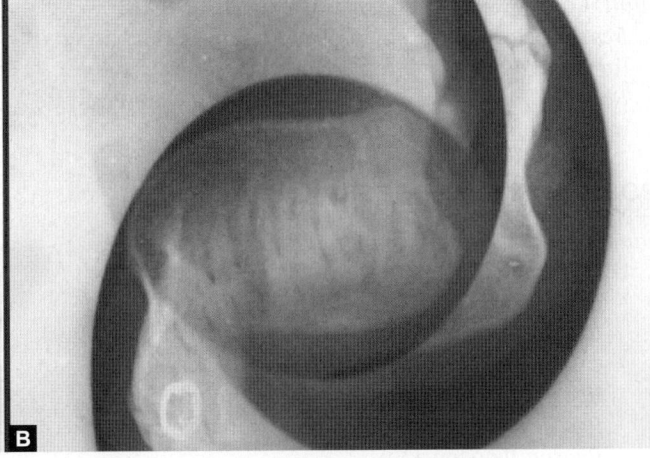

Figures 8.15A and B Double images on the radiograph: (A) Triple exposure; (B) Inverse exposure

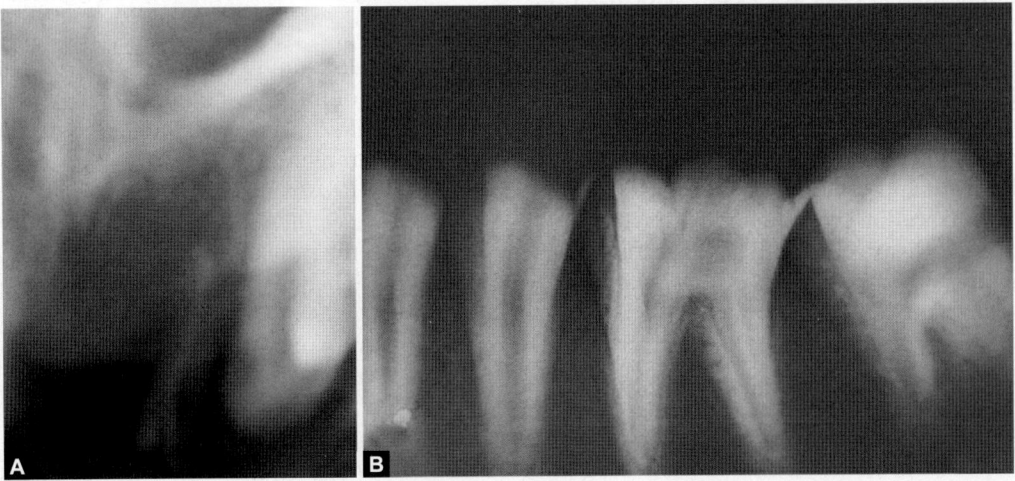

Figures 8.16A and B Blurred image on the radiograph

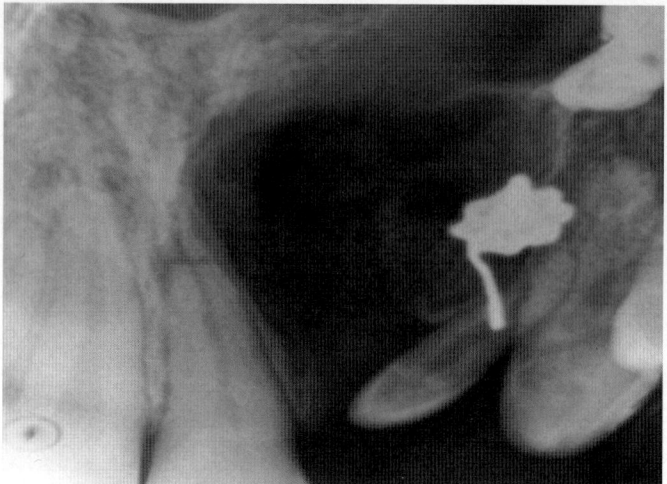

Figure 8.17 Radiopaque artifacts on the radiograph

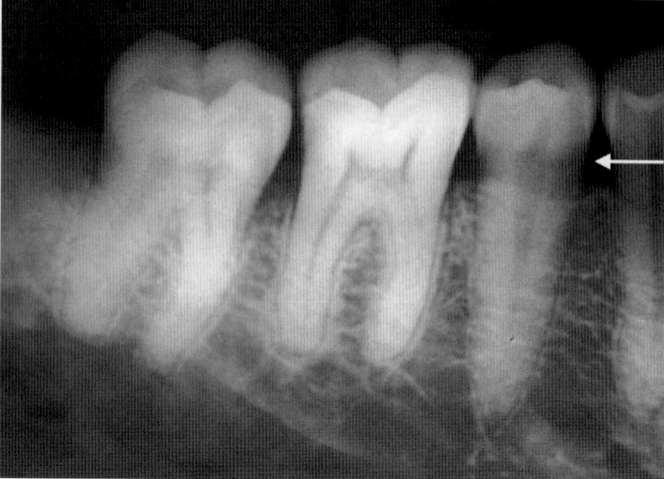

Figure 8.18 Adumbration (cervical burn out)

- *Fault*: Adumbration (cervical burn out) (**Fig. 8.18**)
  - *Reason*: Horizontal angle of the beam is not directed through the contact area of the teeth.
    Rectification: This is a relative radiolucency that may be mistaken for cervical caries or root caries.

EXPOSURE AND PROCESSING ERRORS

- *Fault*: Low density film (light radiograph) (**Fig. 8.19**)
  - Under exposure
    - *Reason*: Too short an exposure
      Rectification: Set exposure time correctly or check calibration of exposure time
    - *Reason*: Source film distance too great
      Rectification: Check the source film distance
    - *Reason*: Too low kVp
      Rectification: Increase kVp by approximately 5 kVp.
    - *Reason*: Too low mA
      Rectification: Increase the mA or the exposure time (mAs is one factor)
    - *Reason*: Film packet placed with the wrong side facing the tooth. Causing the image of the lead foil to be superimposed on the object image.
      Rectification: Place the pebbled side of the film facing the tooth and towards the cone.
    - *Reason*: Incorrect film screen combination used
      Rectification: Always use the right screen film combination
  - Under development
    - Improper development
      i. *Reason*: Time too short
         Rectification: Set darkroom timer correct (check accuracy)
      ii. *Reason*: Low developer temperature
          Rectification: Raise temperature to 70°F

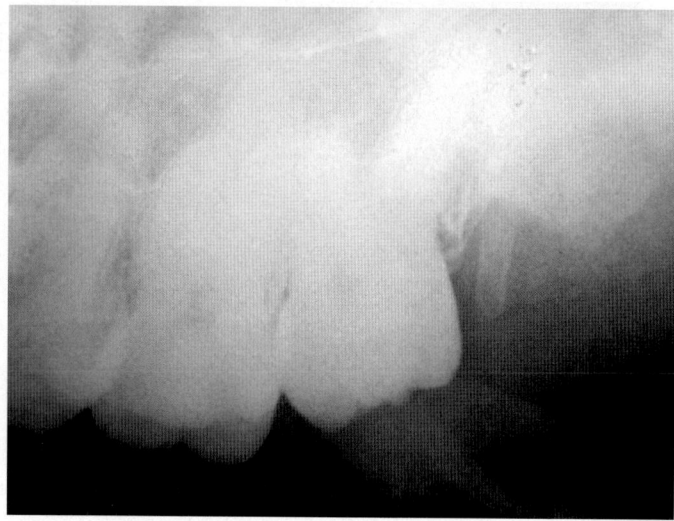

Figure 8.19 Low density film (light radiograph)

      iii. *Reason*: Exhausted and or contaminated and or diluted developer
           Rectification: Replace developer or add replenisher
      iv. *Reason*: Excessive fixation
          Rectification: Regulate the time for fixing as per the time table
- *Fault*: High density film (dark radiograph) (**Figs 8.20A and B**)
  - Exposure parameters
    - *Reason*: Exposure time too long
      Rectification: Set timer correctly and or reduce exposure time
    - *Reason*: kVp too high for the exposure time
      Rectification: Reduce kVp

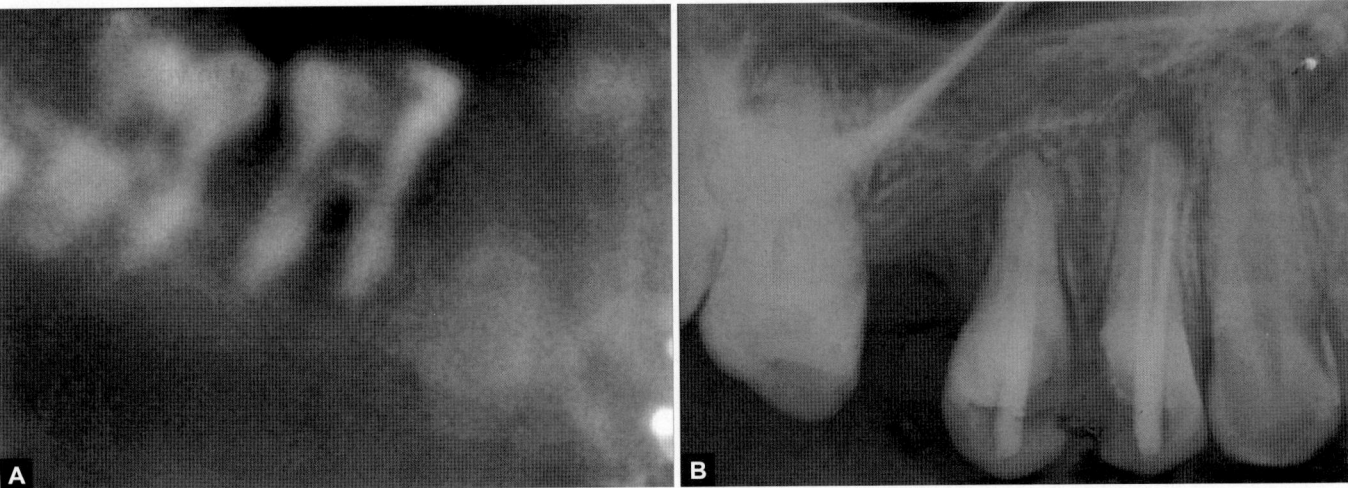

Figures 8.20A and B High density film (dark radiograph)

- *Reason*: Source film distance too short for the exposure time
  Rectification: Measure the source film distance and adjust the exposure time accordingly
- *Reason*: Timer inaccurate
  Rectification: Check the timer with spinning top and adjust the time accordingly
- *Reason*: mA too high for exposure
  Rectification: Reduce mA or exposure time
- Over development
  - *Reason*: Developing time too long
    Rectification: Use time temperature method with a darkroom timer
  - *Reason*: Developer temperature too high
    Rectification: Lower temperature to 70°F
  - *Reason*: Over strength developer
    Rectification: Check tank capacity and mixing instructions
  - *Reason*: Inadequate fixation
    Rectification: Fixation time should be standardized as per instruction
  - *Reason*: Accidental exposure to light or improper safe lighting
    Rectification: All darkroom procedures should be done in safelight only
- *Fault*: High contrast (**Fig. 8.21**)
  - *Reason*: Insufficient penetration
    Rectification: Increase kilo voltage
  - *Reason*: Over development
    Rectification: Use temperature method with a darkroom timer, lower temperature to 70°F
    Check tank capacity and mixing instructions. Fixation time should be standardized as per instruction. All darkroom procedures should be done is safelight only.

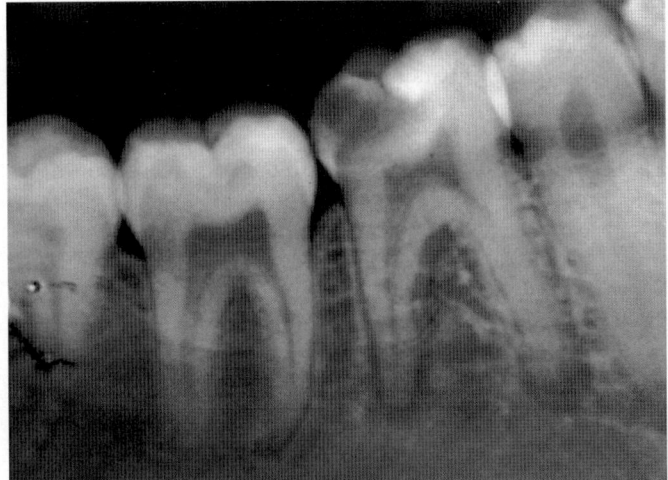

Figure 8.21 High contrast

- *Reason*: Use of film and/or intensifying screens of too high contrast
  Rectification: Use lower contrast film or slower speed screens
- *Reason*: Timer inaccurately set or timer out of calibration
  Rectification: Use proper timer
- *Fault*: Low contrast (**Fig. 8.22**)
  - *Reason*: Excessive penetration
    Rectification: Decrease kilo voltage
  - *Reason*: Under development
    Rectification: Set darkroom timer correct. Raise temperature to 70°F. Replace developer or add replenisher. Regulate the time for fixing as per the time table
  - *Reason*: Use of film having insufficient contrast and/or cassettes with too slow intensifying screens

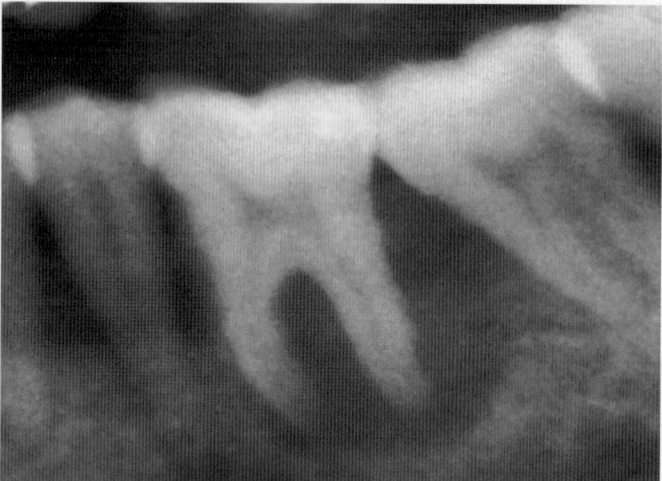

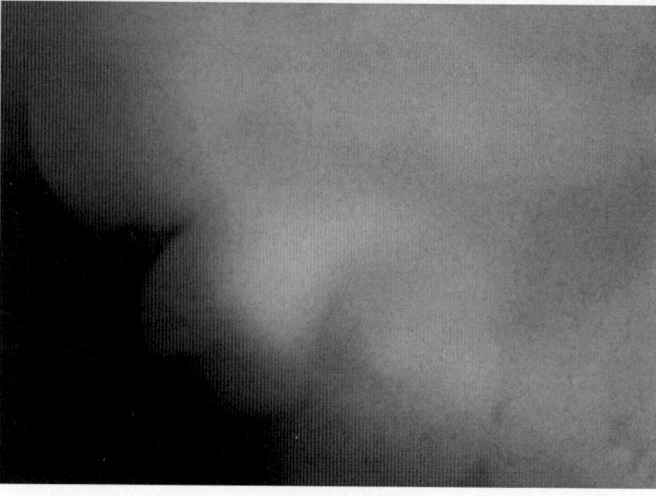

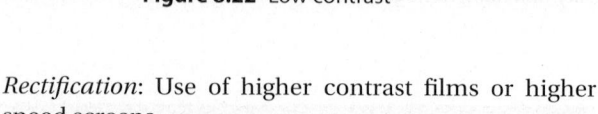

Figure 8.22 Low contrast   **Figure 8.23** Fog

Rectification: Use of higher contrast films or higher speed screens
- *Reason*: Scattered radiation
  Rectification: Check diaphragm size and use suitable cone
- *Reason*: Under exposure
  Rectification: Check exposure time and set the timer correctly
- *Reason*: Excessive film fog
  Rectification: Refer below Error: Fog
- *Fault*: Fog (**Fig. 8.23**)
  - *Reason*: Light leaks in the darkroom or improper safe lights or filter in safe light
    Rectification: Check vents, doors and walls for leaks, cracked safe light filter, use recommended safe light
  - *Reason*: Turning over head (white) light on too soon
    Rectification: Fix films for 1–2 minutes before turning on the light
  - *Reason*: Prolonged exposure of films to safe light
    Rectification: Reduce exposure time of films to the safe light
  - *Reason*: Smoking in the darkroom
    Rectification: Smoking should be banned
  - Chemical
    - *Reason*: Developer temperature too high, too concentrated, contaminated or prolonged development
      Rectification: Check concentration, temperature and clean the fixer tanks regularly. Use time temperature method
  - Deterioration of the film
    - *Reason*: Temperature of storage area too high
      Rectification: Store film in a cool place (70°F) or use the refrigerator for the storage of films
    - *Reason*: Humidity of storage area too high

Rectification: Store films in a dry place (50% relative humidity) Use the fridge
- *Reason*: Out dated film
  Rectification: Limit supply and use older films first
- Exposed to radiation
  - *Reason*: Insufficient protection
    Rectification: Store unexposed films in lead containers
  - *Reason*: Improper film screen combination
    Rectification: Especially when using high speed films the manufacturer's recommended combination should be followed
- *Fault*: Streaks on film
  - *Reason*: Failure to agitate during development
    Rectification: Agitate films on immersing them in the developer
  - *Reason*: Undue amount of inspection of film during development. When films are held in front of the safe light during development, the developer solution runs across the films producing uneven reduction of the emulsion.
    Rectification: Use time temperature method of development. This reduces the need to inspect the film during development.
  - *Reason*: Chemical deposits on hanger clips
    Rectification: Keep hanger clips clean
  - *Reason*: Excessive drying temperature
    Rectification: Reduce air flow over films
  - *Reason*: Insufficient fixing
    Rectification: Usually the fixing time should be twice the developing time
  - *Reason*: Dirty or contaminated wash water
    Rectification: Wash films in fresh running water
- *Fault*: Blisters on film
  - *Reason*: Unbalanced processing temperatures

Rectification: Control the temperature of water bath, which in turn controls temperature of processing solution

- *Reason*: Excessive acidity of fixer
  Rectification: Replace fixing solution
- *Reason*: Films not agitated when first immersed in fixer
  Rectification: Agitate
- *Fault*: Reticulation (orange peel appearance)
  - *Reason*: Sudden extreme temperature changes in processing
    Rectification: Maintain uniform processing temperatures
  - *Reason*: Weakened fixer solution
    Rectification: Replenish or replace fixer solution
- *Fault*: Frilling
  - *Reason*: Hot processing solution
    Rectification: Maintain correct processing temperature (70°F)
- *Fault*: Air bells
  - *Reason*: Air bubbles trapped on film surfaces preventing uniform reduction of the emulsion
    Rectification: Agitate film upon immersions into developer
- *Fault*: White spots and lines on films
  - *Reason*: Grit or dust present on the films or upon the screens
    Rectification: Keep darkroom clean to prevent dust and dirt particles from settling on films. Periodically clean screens with commercial screen cleaner.
  - *Reason*: Emulsion tears from rough handling of films in processing tanks
    Rectification: Do not rub films up against the sides of tanks or other film hangers
  - *Reason*: Film contamination with fixer before processing
    Rectification: Keep the dark room clean and dry
  - *Reason*: Excessive bending of film
  - *Reason*: Cracks in the intensifying screens
  - *Reason*: Finger contamination, where the contaminant is the fixer
  - *Reason*: Films handled roughly while being mounted on hangers
- *Fault*: Black spots on films
  - *Reason*: Grit or dust in contact with the undeveloped film
    Rectification: Prevent fine particles of developer coming in contact with film (dry chemicals)
  - *Reason*: Film splashed with developer before being placed in developer tank
    Rectification: Careful handling of solutions and clean work area
  - *Reason*: Films touching during developing
    Rectification: Films should not touch in the processing tank
  - *Reason*: Black wrapping paper sticking to film surface
    Rectification: Remove the black paper carefully, with dry hands

- *Reason*: Excessive bending of the film. Film is bent excessively owing to the curvature of the hard palate or heavy finger pressure on the film. As a result stretched and distorted images are seen on the radiograph
  Rectification: To avoid film bending always check the film placement before exposure. If the patient's finger pressure is excessive, instruct the patient to stabilize the film gently. If the film is bent because of the curvature of the hard palate, cotton rolls can be used with the paralleling technique, or the bisecting angle technique used. Film holding devices are helpful in preventing film bending
- *Reason*: Finger contamination where the contaminant is the developer
  Rectification: Wash hands properly
- *Reason*: Finger nail artifact
- *Fault*: Artifacts from processing
  - Black crescents
    - *Reason*: Rough handling of films
      Rectification: Handle films by edges only
  - Black smudge marks
    - *Reason*: Finger prints or finger abrasions
      Rectification: Have dry fingers when handling film (processing and mounting)
  - Black lines (**Fig. 8.24**)
    - *Reason*: Static electricity (naked tree, lightening marks). These are caused by electrical discharges that produce no visible light, but occur on the surface of the emulsion:
      - Rapid movement in removing film from the box
      - Film is removed rapidly from the interleaving
      - Paper
      - Film is touched by the fingers of the person
      - Processing the film

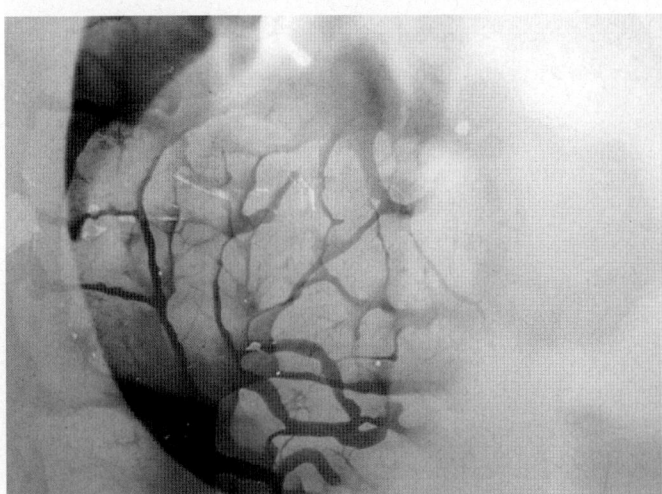

Figure 8.24 Static electricity (naked tree, lightening marks)

- Lack of moisture in the air (especially in winter).
- Static electricity. (Smudge markings), these may result from visible light produced by sparks caused by a relatively low potential electrical discharge in the air next to the film surface. The discharge follows a path induced by dust, lint, or a roughened intensifying screen

  Rectification:
  - Install an electric humidifier or cool vapor vaporizers in the dark room. The relative humidity in the dark room should be between, 50–75%
  - Do not remove the X-ray film too rapidly from the packet
  - Handle the film gently and let the paper fall away from the film, and place the film in the cassette gently.
  - Following exposure remove the film gently from the cassette
  - Coat the intensifying screens in the cassette with an antistatic solution
- *Reason:* Film creasing, and the film emulsion cracks. As a result a thin radiolucent line is seen on the radiograph.

  Rectification: Do not bend or crease the film excessively. Instead gently soften the corners of the film before placing it in the patient's mouth
- *Fault:* Stains on film (*see* **Fig. 8.3B**)
  - Yellow or brown (**Fig. 8.25**)
    - *Reason:* Exhausted or oxidized or contaminated developer or prolonged development

      Rectification: Use fresh developing solution and use recommended developing time
    - *Reason:* Insufficient rinsing

      Rectification: Rinse films for 15–20 seconds in fresh running water

- *Reason:* Exhausted or contaminated fixer solution

  Rectification: Use fresh fixer solution
- Dichroic (showing two colors) (**Fig. 8.26**)
  - *Reason:* Old exhausted or contaminated developer or fixer

    Rectification: Use fresh solutions
  - *Reason:* Film partially fixed in weak fixer, exposed to light and washed

    Rectification: Replace fixer solution and follow the recommended processing cycle
  - *Reason:* Prolonged intermediate rinse in contaminated rinse water

    Rectification: Use fresh, running water and recommended cycle
- *Fault:* Deposits on film
  - *Reason:* Exhausted, contaminated solutions, solutions not mixed in correct proportions, and contaminated rinsing water

    Rectification: Use fresh solutions, clean running water and follow manufacturers instruction when preparing the solutions
- *Fault:* Clear film (**Fig. 8.27**)
  - Film not exposed
    - *Reason:* Failure to switch on the X-ray machine, electrical failure, malfunction of machine

      Rectification: Ensure that the X-ray machine is working properly
    - *Reason:* Exposed film first put in the fixing solution

      Rectification: The position of the tanks containing the solutions should be fixed, as per the requirement of a darkroom
- *Fault:* Black film (**Fig. 8.28**)
  - *Reason:* Film exposed to light

    Rectification: Handling of the exposed and unexposed film should be done carefully

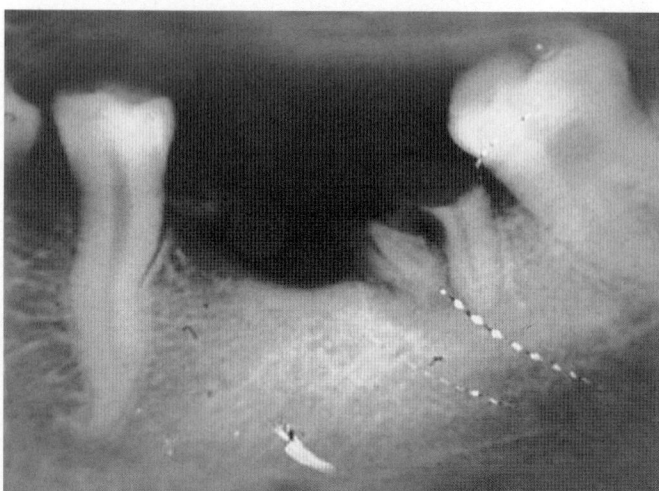

Figure 8.25 Yellow or brown stains
(*For color version see plate 1*)

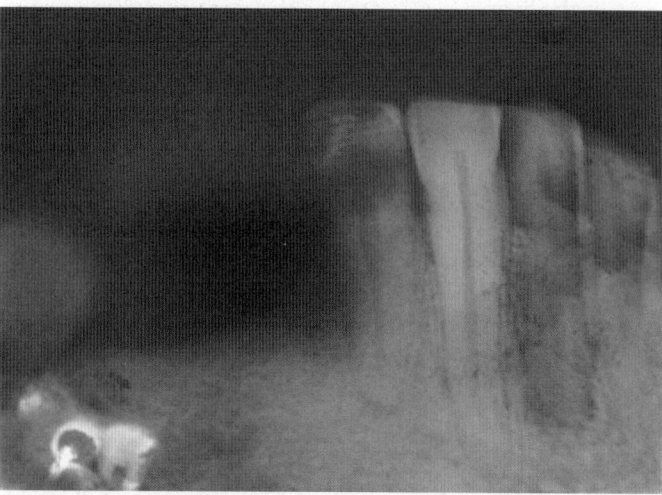

Figure 8.26 Dichroic (showing two colors)
(*For color version see plate 1*)

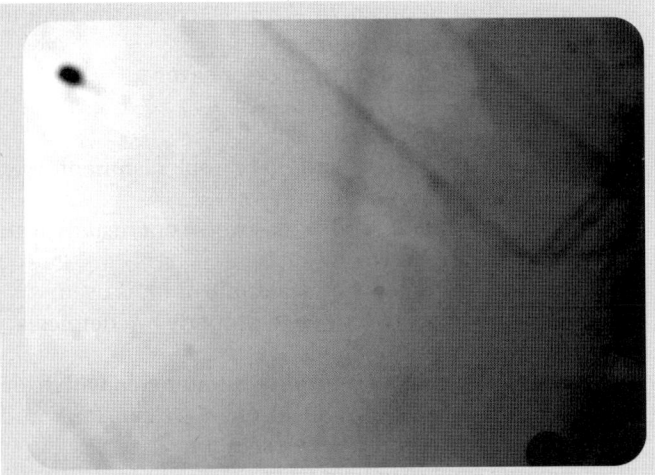

Figure 8.27 Clear film

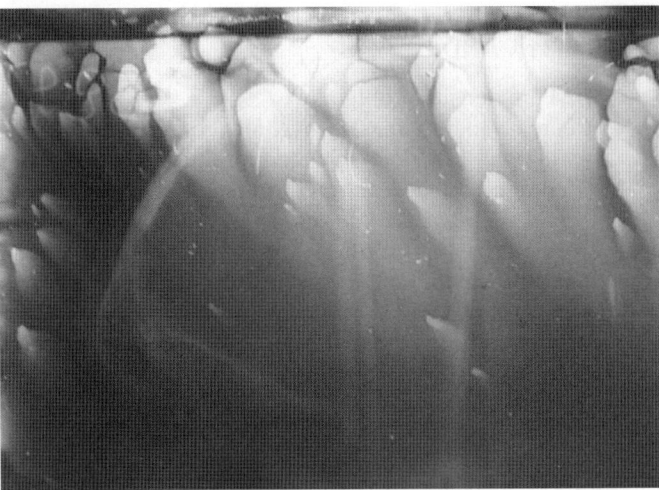

Figure 8.29 Dark flow marks

Figure 8.28 Black film

- *Fault*: Brittleness of finished radiographs
  - *Reason*: Excessive drying temperature
    Rectification: Reduce dryer temperature
  - *Reason*: Excessive drying time; incoming air too humid and cold air velocity too low
    Rectification: Use the dryer and reduce the drying time and adjust the incoming air. Use a wetting agent prior to placing films in dryer
  - *Reason*: Excessive fixer acidity
    Rectification: Replace fixer solution

- *Fault*: Faded image on finished radiograph (radiopaque appears radiolucent)
  - *Reason*: Exhausted fixer or inadequate fixing or insufficient final wash
- *Fault*: Dark flow marks (**Fig. 8.29**)
  - *Reason*: Vigorous agitation results in solution currents that may form dark flow marks. This is a common occurrence with a weak developer or high temperature development or insufficient agitation when the film is developed vertically, it may produce dark and light drainage streaks below low and high density areas respectively. Such streaks occur because alkali bromide, a by product of development, interferes with the developing process. An area of high density forms a local concentration of alkali bromide that drains downwards and restricts the development in the low density area. Conversely an area of low density contains less alkali bromide on development, hence relatively fresh developer drains down and increases development in the high density area
- *Fault*: Emulsion peel
  - *Reason*: Abrasion of image during processing or excessive time in wash water
- *Fault*: Grainy appearance (**Fig. 8.30**)
  - *Reason*: Developer solution too warm
- *Fault*: Vertical white line on panoramic radiograph
  - *Reason*: The push button on the exposure switch is accidently released and then pressed down for the remainder of the excursion, a blank space on the panoramic radiograph will result, as the radiation to the film is cut off.
    Rectification: Keep the exposure button properly pressed till the entire exposure cycle is through.

AUTOMATIC PROCESSING ERRORS (FIGS 8.31A AND B)

- *Fault*: Film density problems
  - Decrease in film density (over all light films)
    - *Reason*: Low developer temperature, exhausted or contaminated developer, no agitation in developer tank
      Rectification: Drain and thoroughly clean tank; install new developer. Be sure that the agitator paddle drive belt is in the proper position in the pulley
    - *Reason*: Processing too fast
  - Increase in film density (overall dark films)
    - *Reason*: Developer temperature too high
      Rectification: Check that the water is not turned off. Check temperature of the incoming water supply

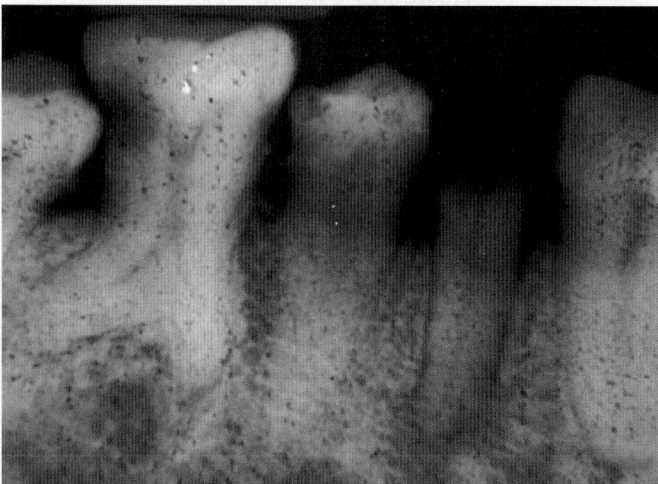

Figure 8.30 Grainy appearance

and adjust between 75°–78°F. Decrease the heat in the developing solution.
    - *Reason*: Light leaks in processor cover
    - *Reason*: Too much replenisher
  - Streaking (uneven density)
    - *Reason*: Developer and fixer replenishment low, unclean rinsing water
    - *Reason*: Rollers and crossovers encrusted with chemical deposits
    - *Reason*: Improper chemicals and/or films used
    - *Reason*: Films not hardened properly by chemicals
  - Fogged films
    - *Reason*: Developer solution contaminated with fixer
      Rectification: Drain and throughly clean tank and rack. Install new developer solution
    - *Reason*: Processor light leaks
      Rectification: Be sure processor cover is secure and firmly in place
    - *Reason*: Improper safe light and light leaks in dark room
    - *Reason*: Heat fog
      Rectification: Film storage area should not be excessively hot
    - *Reason*: Excessively high developer temperature
      Rectification: Readjust developer thermostat and water to proper temperature
- *Fault*: Film drying problems
  - Films are not dry
    - *Reason*: Depleted fixer or insufficient water flow (film not properly washed)
      Rectification: Install new fixer solution. Check incoming water line and valves
    - *Reason*: Dryer temperature setting too low, dryer thermostatic control or heater inoperative

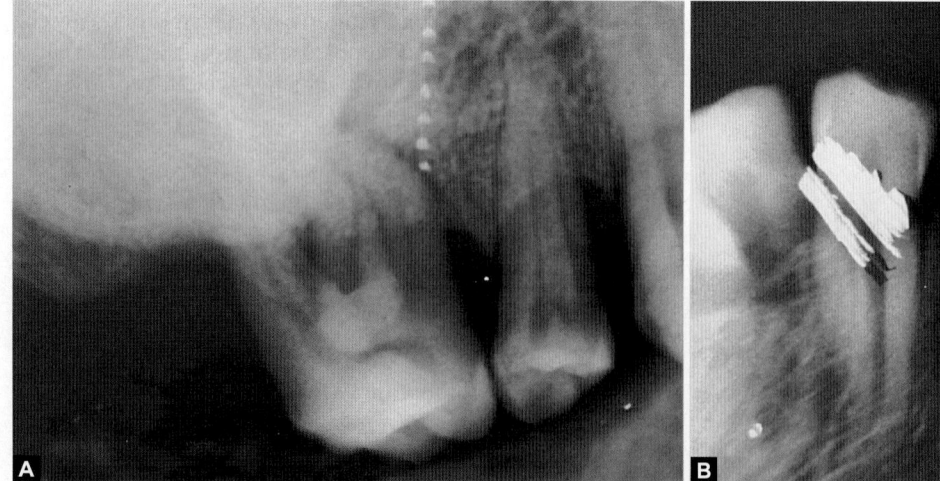

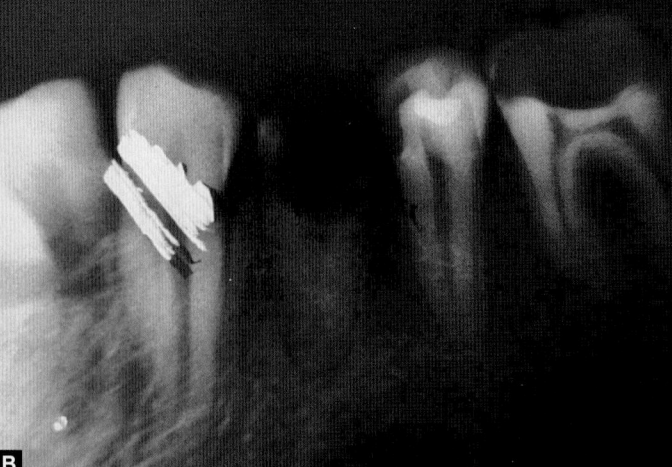

Figures 8.31A and B Artifacts due to automatic processor: (A) Roller marks; (B) Emulsion tear

- *Reason*: Chemical imbalance (either developer or fixer)
  Rectification: Replace with new solution
- *Reason*: Improper type of film for time cycle of processor
  Rectification: Check with dealer for information regarding proper type of film (it is not recommended for film with acetate film base or any other film not designed for automatic processing)
- *Reason*: Processing too fast
- *Fault*: Abnormal film surface marks
  - Peeling of the emulsion
    - *Reason*: Developer temperature too high
      Rectification: Reduce developer temperature to proper level
    - *Reason*: Improper fixer strength or depleted fixer
      Rectification: Replace fixer solution
    - *Reason*: Heavy developer deposits on developer rack rollers above solution level
      Rectification: Be sure to follow the recommended house keeping and cleaning procedures
    - *Reason*: Improper film
      Rectification: Check with the dealer for information regarding the proper type of film
    - *Reason*: Rough handling of films prior to processing
  - Pressure marks
    - *Reason*: Foreign material or rough spot on roller
      Rectification: Clean rollers and/or remove rough area on roller
    - *Reason*: Rough handling or excessive hand pressure on film before processing
      Rectification: Film emulsions are extremely sensitive, particularly after exposure and before the processing. Good habits in gentle handling of film must be practiced
  - Cloudy or smudge appearance on film surface (greenish or yellowish)
    - *Reason*: Depleted fixer
      Rectification: Replace fixer solution
    - *Reason*: Improper type of film for time cycle of processor
      Rectification: Check with dealer
  - White cloudy appearance over film surface
    - *Reason*: No water in water tank
      Rectification: Check incoming controls and lines
  - Scratches on film surface
    - *Reason*: Foreign material on roller(s)
      Rectification: Clean rollers
    - *Reason*: Improper handling of film before processing
      Rectification: Proper gentle handling of film must be practiced
    - *Reason*: Damaged or defective film
      Rectification: Hand develop film(s) of the same batch or box. This may pick up defects that could be characteristic of the particular box or batch of film

- *Reason*: Stalled or sticking roller
  Rectification: Inspect racks, gears and gear mesh. Correct as required
  - Drying pattern on film surface
    - *Reason*: Dryer too hot
      Rectification: Reduce dryer temperature
    - *Reason*: Characteristic of film
      Rectification: Process film of the same box through other processor and chemicals to determine consistency of pattern.
  - Dark spots or lines
    - *Reason*: Excessive roller pressure
      Rectification: Check with manufacturer or get the processor serviced
    - *Reason*: Dirty rollers in the processor
      Rectification: Clean rollers carefully
    - *Reason*: Contamination of the film by dirty work bench or water droplets
  - Broad horizontal white line
    - *Reason*: Irregularities on the surface of the rollers
  - Film discoloration
    - *Reason*: Fixer in developer (brown stains)
    - *Reason*: Processing too fast
  - Shiny films
    - *Reason*: Excessive hardening
      Rectification: Wash water not turned on
  - Films chalky or dirty
    - *Reason*: No wash water or dirty wash water
    - *Reason*: Precipitate in fixer
- *Fault*: Jam or failure of films to transport
  - *Reason*: Chemicals contaminated or diluted and or temperature too high
  - *Reason*: Films excessively soft and not adequately hardened, when enough gelatin lubricates the rollers, the films will jam up with one another
  - *Reason*: Dirty rollers and or dirty wash water
  - *Reason*: Incorrect dryer temperature
  - *Reason*: Racks not seated properly
  - *Reason*: Hesitation in drive assembly, causing film to pause in transit
  - *Reason*: Film not tracking through processor in straight course (improper feeding of films)

MISCELLANEOUS TECHNIQUE ERRORS

- *Fault*: Phalangioma (patient's finger on the film) (**Fig. 8.32**)
  - *Reason*: The patient's finger was incorrectly positioned in front of the film instead of behind the film. As a result the patient's finger appears on the radiograph. The term phalangioma was coined by Dr David F. Mitchell of the Indiana University of dentistry. It refers to the distal phalanx of the finger seen in radiographs. [A phalanx (phalanges) is any bone of a finger or toe]. This error occurs when the

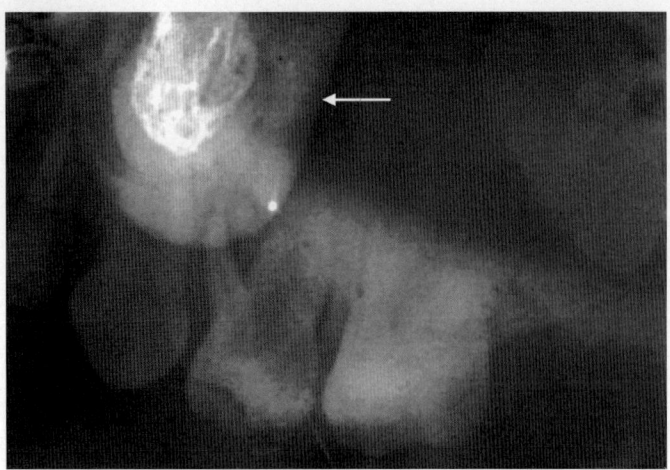

Figure 8.32 Phalangioma (patient's finger on the film)

finger holding method is used with the bisecting angle technique.

Rectification: To avoid phalangioma, make certain that the patient's finger used to stabilize the film is placed behind the film and not in front of it.

BIBLIOGRAPHY

1. A Look at X-ray Film Processing, Milwaukee, X-ray Department, General Electric Co.
2. Dark Room Technique for Better Radiographs. Wilmington, Delware, Photo Products Department, E.I. du Pont de Nemours and Co.
3. Mason and Hing LR. Radiographic Quality and Artifacts. In: Fundamentals of Dental Radiography, 3rd edition. Philadelphia, Lea and Fegiger; 1990. pp. 40-5.
4. Profexray's Automatic Dental Processor's Manual.

X-ray Films and Accessories | 9

The *X-ray film* is the image receptor system used in dental radiology. The image reception is modified by the composition of the film and also the use of intensifying screens and grids.

The X-ray films are *classified* according to:
- Their use:
  - Intraoral films
    - Periapical films
      1. No 0 for children.
      2. No 1 for anterior adult projections.
      3. No 2 for standard adult projections.
    - Occlusal films.
    - Bite wing films.
  - Extraoral films.
- The coating of emulsion
  - *Single coated*: These produce better and sharper images but the exposure to the patient is more, therefore mostly used in industrial radiography.
  - *Double coated*: These films have emulsion on both sides. Most dental films are double coated. These allow for less exposure to the patient.
- The speed of the film
  - *Slow films*: These have a very small grain of silver bromide and emulsion is on one side only. Therefore it gives better definition but the exposure required is more and are thus not routinely used. Their speeds are denoted by A, B, C.
  - *Fast films*: These have a larger grain size and the emulsion is on both sides. Their speeds are D-ultra speed, E-ekta speed and F-ultra ekta speed.
  - *Hyper speed G*: This is a 800-speed film that can half the patient exposure without blurring image quality.
- Packaging
  - *Single film packet*.
  - *Double film packet*: Two films are placed close to each other, when they are radiographed the second film serves as a duplicate.
- Use, nonuse of screens
  - Screen films
    - Sensitive to blue light, e.g. calcium tungstate screens.
    - Sensitive to green light, e.g. rare earth screens.
  - Nonscreen films.

- Barrier envelopes
  - *With barrier envelopes*: These ensure that there is no gross contamination in the dark room.
  - Without barrier envelopes.

COMPOSITION OF THE X-RAY FILM (FIG. 9.1)

The X-ray film is made up of:
- *Base*: It is a transparent supporting material upon which the emulsion is coated. The dental film base is composed of polyethylene terephthalate (a polyester) about 0.2 mm thick (0.007 inches). The film base should:
  - Have the proper amount of flexibility to allow ease of handling.
  - It should be translucent, casting no pattern on the resultant radiograph.
  - For optimal viewing of the diagnostic detail the film base should have a bluish tint
  - The base should be able to withstand exposure to processing solutions without distorting, heat, moisture and chemical exposure.

The film is known as a 'safe film' if the base is made up of acetate polyester, because this is not easily inflammable.

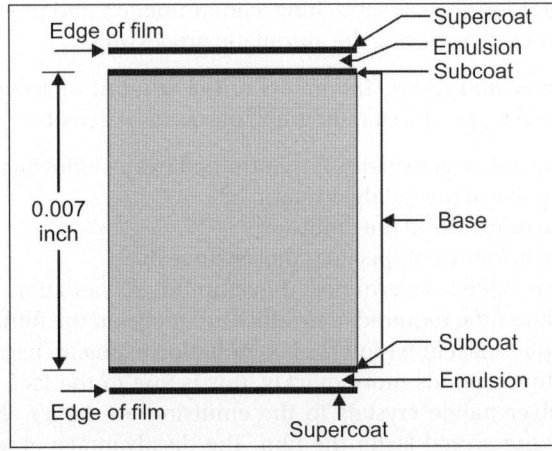

Figure 9.1 Schematic diagram of the components of a dental X-ray film. The film emulsion is coated on both the top and bottom surfaces of the polyethylene base

- *Substratum (subcoating)*: It is a thin adhesive material on both sides of the base, which ensures good adhesion between the sensitive emulsion and the film base.
- *Emulsion*: It is coated on both sides of the base, containing silver bromide crystals suspended in gelatin. This is photosensitive to visible light and X-rays. The films intended to be exposed to X-rays are called Direct Exposure Films. All intraoral dental films are 'Direct Exposure Films'. It helps to record the radiographic image. The emulsion layer consists of:
  - *Silver halide crystals*: These are photosensitive and composed primarily of silver bromide (80–99%) and to a lesser extent silver iodide crystals (1–10%). The mean diameter of the silver halide grain is about 0.70–0.75 mm. The presence of silver iodide crystals adds greatly to the sensitivity of the film emulsion, thereby reducing the radiation dose required to produce an adequate diagnostic image. The photosensitivity of the silver halide crystals is further increased by the incorporation of sulfur contamination during the manufacturing process. The silver halide crystals absorb radiation during X-ray exposure and store energy from the radiation.
  - *Gelatin matrix*: This supports the silver halide crystals, which are suspended in the gelatin framework applied to both sides of the supporting base. The gelatin is made from cattle bone and helps to keep the silver grains evenly dispersed. During processing the gelatin absorbs the processing solutions and helps to allow the chemicals to react with the halide grains.
- *Super coat*: It is a protective, transparent, nonabrasive layer over the emulsion. This is an additional layer of gelatin which is applied to the surface to serve as a protective barrier and protects the film from damage by mechanical handling such as scratching, contamination and pressure from rollers during the automatic processing.

Intraoral film speed: This refers to the amount of radiation required to produce a radiograph of standard density.

Film speed, or sensitivity, is determined by the following:
- The size of the halide crystal
- The thickness of the emulsion
- The presence of special radiosensitive dyes.

Film speed determines the amount of radiation and exposure time required to produce an image on the film. For example, a fast film requires less radiation exposure because the film responds more quickly, this is due to the fact, that the silver halide crystals in the emulsion are larger. Thus, larger the crystal faster the film. The disadvantage of using fast films is that though the amount of exposure to the patient is reduced, it is at the cost of the contrast quality which gets reduced.

An alphabetical classification is used to identify film speed. The films are given speed ratings from A speed (the slowest) to F speed (the fastest). Only D-speed and E-speed are used for intraoral radiography.

INTRAORAL FILMS

Intraoral films are available as (**Fig. 9.2**)

Periapical films: Usually used to record crowns, roots and periapical areas related to the tooth.
- No. 0 for children (22 × 35 mm).
- No. 1 for anterior adult projections (24 × 40 mm).
- No. 2 for posterior adult projections (31 × 41 mm).

Occlusal films: (also called 'bite film' or 'topographical film') Used to show larger areas of the maxilla or mandible. The size of the film is 57 × 76 mm.

Bite wing films: Used to record the crowns of maxillary and mandibular teeth in one film. These films have a paper tab projecting from the middle of the film on which the patient bites, to support the film.

They help in the detection of interproximal caries, visualize the alveolar crest and assessment of periodontal disease is more easier.

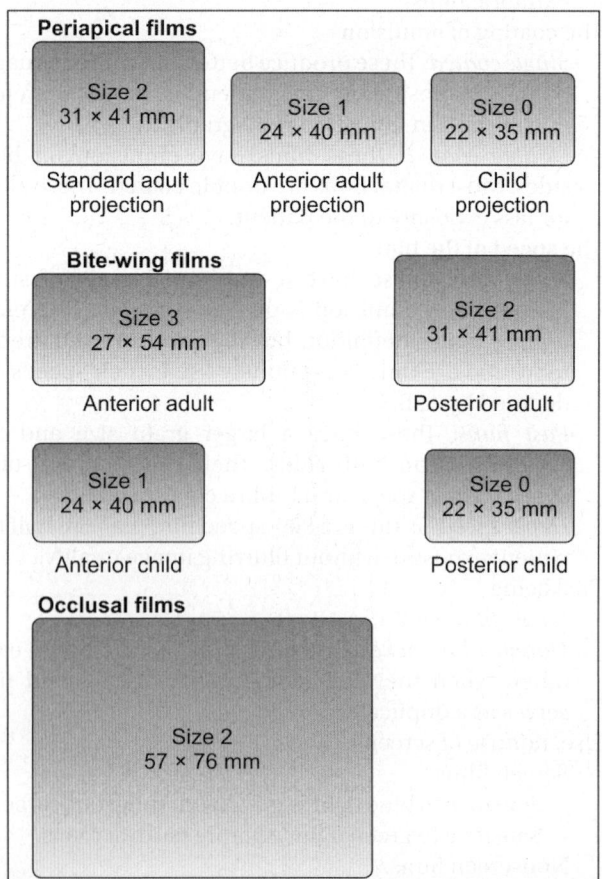

Figure 9.2 Schematic representation of the various intraoral film available and their sizes

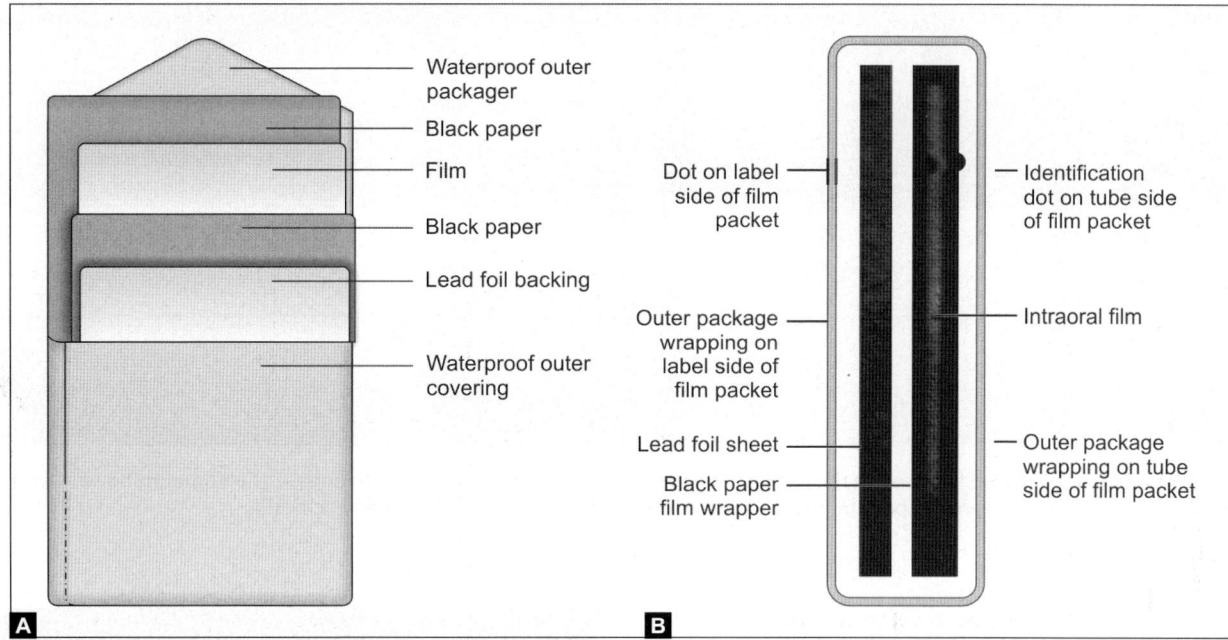

Figures 9.3A and B Schematic diagram of: (A) Contents of an intraoral X-ray packet; (B) Cross section of the contents of the film packet

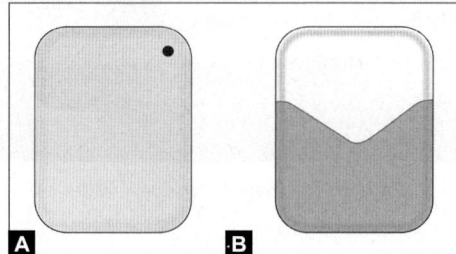

Figures 9.4A and B Film Packet: (A) Tube side (B) Label side

- Size 0 for child (posterior) (22 × 35 mm)
- Size 1 for child (anterior) (24 × 40 mm)
- Size 2 for adult (posterior) (31 × 41 mm)
- Size 3 for adult (anterior) (27 × 54 mm).

The intraoral films are available in plastic film packets. The film packet consists of (**Figs 9.3 and 9.4**):

- An outer plastic wrapping, made of white paper or soft vinyl which is hermetically sealed, semi-stiff, moisture proof, light proof and clearly indicates which side of the film should be directed towards the X-ray tube. This outer wrapper serves to protect the film from exposure to light and saliva.

The outer wrapper of the film packet has two sides, tube side and label side. The tube side of the plastic cover is solid white and bears a raised dot; this raised side should be placed towards the X-ray tube or the object to be radiographed. When inserted in the mouth, the edge carrying the dot should be placed at the incisive or occlusal margin of the tooth under consideration.

The dental X-ray film in the packet has a corresponding embossed dot on it which helps to identify the position of the film in relation to the patients mouth when mounting the radiograph.

The label side (**Fig. 9.4B**) of the film packet has a flap that is used to open the film packet to remove the film prior to processing. The label side is color coded to identify films outside of the plastic packaging container, color codes are used to distinguish between one film and two film packets, and between speeds of the film. When placed in the mouth the color coded side must face the tongue. The following information is usually printed on the label side of the film:

- A circle or dot that corresponds with the raised identification dot on the film
- The statement, "opposite side of the tube"
- The manufacturer's name
- The film speed
- The number of films enclosed.

The corners of the plastic packet and the enclosed film are rounded to avoid discomfort to the patient when the packet is introduced into the mouth.

A thin sheet of lead foil is placed in the plastic wrapper on the side of the film which is remote to the tooth under consideration and the X-ray tube. This foil absorbs most of the X-rays which pass through the film and prevent them from reaching the tongue and other oral tissues. It also absorbs the back scatter radiation and thus prevents fogging of the film which would otherwise cause loss of important diagnostic detail.

A secondary function of the lead foil is to give sufficient but not excessive rigidity to the whole film packet.

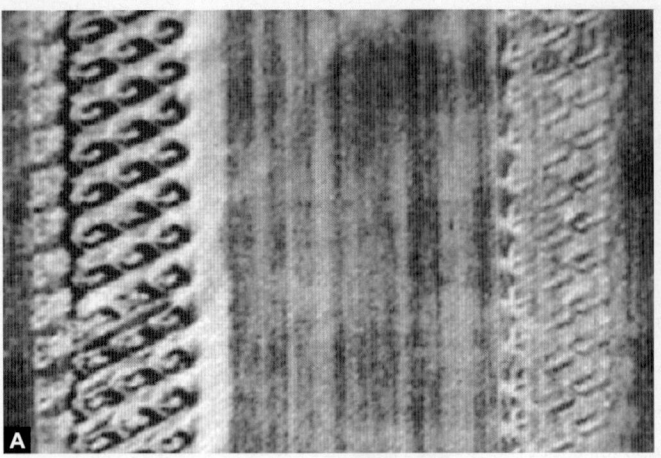
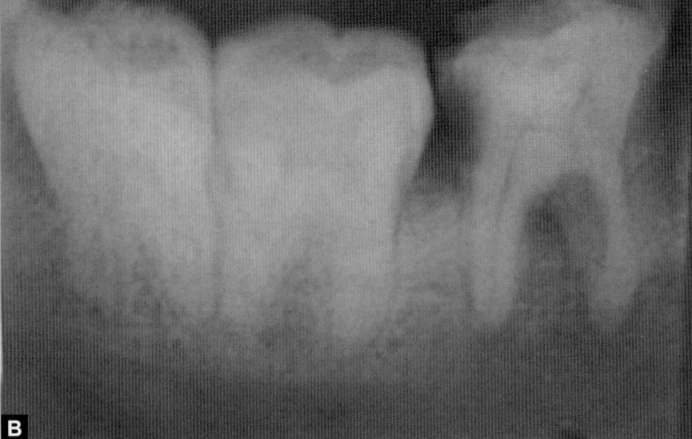

Figures 9.5A and B (A) The lead foil insert in the packet has a raised diamond packet across both ends; (B) Radiograph showing the raised diamond pattern from the lead backing when the film is positioned backwards

If the film packet is placed reverse in the mouth, the shadow of the foil is seen on the resultant radiograph as tyre track marks or herringbone appearance, which is the embossed pattern placed on the lead foil by the manufacturer (**Figs 9.5A and B**).

- A sheet of black paper wraps the film to protect it from any light leak.
- The X-ray film, which has rounded corners and an embossed raised dot for orientation.

The stabilization of these films may be done by various means:

- Finger holding technique
- Biting on the film or film tab
- Use of film holders.

FILM HOLDERS

Film holders are of various types:
- Blade type
  - Throat stick
  - Acrylic blade with slot
  - Snap-A-ray (**Fig. 9.6**).
- Bite block
  - Styrofoam block
  - Snap-A-ray
  - Artery forceps with bite block.
- Positioning indicating device:
  - Rinn XCP (extension cone paralleling) with normal or rectangular collimator
  - Precision X-ray holder.

Advantages of Film Holders

It allows the film to be placed parallel to the long axis of the teeth, maintaining a flat plane at all times, and retaining the film in position until it is properly exposed.

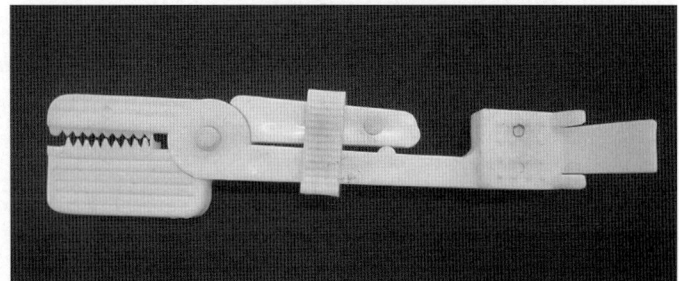

Figure 9.6 Snap-A-ray X-ray holder

Disadvantages of Film Holders

- Due to the presence of the bite block resting upon the teeth, the film may not extend far enough beyond the apical region to allow any latitude for examination of the apical tissues and structures.
- The mouth closing over the block prevents the operator from checking the position of the film in the mouth.
- It is difficult to angulate the tube to meet abnormal conditions. In many cases exposures with the use of film holders results in distortion of the teeth.

Sterilization and Disinfection of Film Holding Devices

The holders should be mechanically cleaned and well rinsed in running tap water to remove saliva before sterilizing.

The plastic XCP can only be steam autoclaved.

The Precision may be steam autoclaved or subjected to dry-heat sterilization. The bite blocks used with the precision instruments are disposable and should be discarded.

After sterilization, the instruments should be placed in 16″ × 10 ¾″ plastic bags (with new disposable bite blocks in the case of precision instruments) for storage and subsequent transport to the radiography area. The instruments must be placed in the bag with clean, gloved hands, working on a clean, disinfected surface.

The instruments to be taken to the radiography are in the given bags, and after using them they should be replaced in the same bag and brought back to the cleaning/sterilizing area.

EXTRAORAL FILMS

Extraoral films are those that are placed outside the mouth during X-ray exposure. These are used to examine large areas of the skull and jaws.

These films are of two types:
1. Nonscreen films
2. Screen films.

Both are available in various sizes:
- 4 ¾″ × 6 ½″
- 5″ × 7″
- 6 ½″ × 8″
- 8″ × 10″
- 6″ × 12″
- 10″ × 12″

Unlike intraoral films, extraoral films are designed to be used outside the mouth and therefore are not enclosed in moisture proof packets. Extraoral films commonly used in dentistry are of the sizes 5″ × 7″, 8″ × 10″, as well as panoramic, 5″ × 12″ and 6″ × 12″. Extra oral films are boxed in quantities of 50 or 100 films. Some manufacturers separate each piece of film with protective paper. Boxes of extraoral film are labeled with the type of film, film size, the total number of films enclosed and the expiry date.
- The films are usually placed in a film cassette, with or without intensifying screens.
- High contrast medium speed films are suitable for panoramic and skull radiography.

- Faster films which provide less image detail are used for panoramic radiography.
1. *Non-screen films*: These are used without the intensifying screens. The emulsion is sensitive to direct X-ray exposure rather than fluorescent light. These films are much slower and therefore require a longer exposure time but the detail of the image obtained on using these films are much sharper. These films are not recommended for dental use.
2. *Screen films*: These films are used in combination with intensifying screens, that emit visible light. These screens are placed in the film cassette, on either side of the film and are held under pressure in a rigid manner, so that the fluorescent layers of the screen and the emulsion of the film are pressed together closely. Poor contact produces a blurring of the image on the radiograph. When the cassette is exposed to X-rays, the screens convert the X-ray energy into light, which in turn exposes the screen film. Screen film is sensitive to fluorescent light rather than direct X-radiation.

Screen films are of two types, blue light sensitive (Kodak X-Omat and Ektamat films), and the other being green light sensitive (Kodak Ortho and T-Mat films). The Green light sensitive films are those used with the rare earth intensifying screens, and these are two or more times faster and provides sufficient clarity for most diagnostic tasks.

It is important to use the right screen film combination so that the emission and absorption characteristics of the screen and film are matched.

Extraoral film equipment: These films are used in combination with cassettes and intensifying screens (where applicable).

Cassette (Figs 9.7A and B)

This is a special device that is used to hold the extraoral film and the intensifying screens. Cassettes are available in a variety of sizes that correspond to the film and screen sizes.

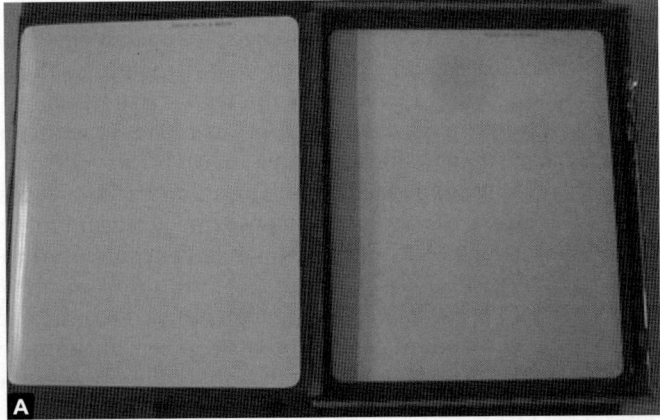

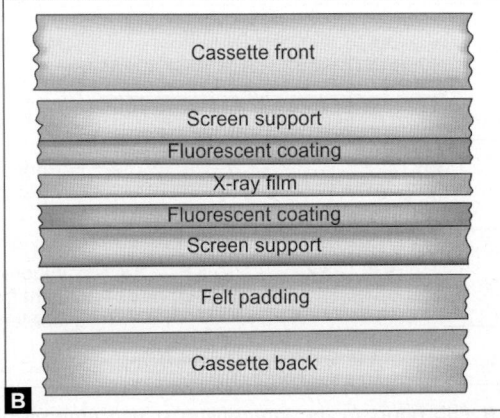

Figures 9.7A and B (A) Cassette for holding 8 × 10 inch film. When the cassette is closed, film is supported between two intensifying screens; (B) Diagram showing cross-section of components of a loaded cassette

A cassette may be flexible or rigid, most cassettes are rigid except for the panoramic cassette, which may be flexible.

A rigid cassette is more expensive, but it also lasts longer. A rigid cassette protects the screens from damage.

The film fits the rigid cassette exactly and cannot be loaded incorrectly, however, to load the flexible cassette properly, the film must be placed between the two screens and pushed to the end of the cassettes.

Both rigid and flexible cassettes must be light–tight, not only to protect the extraoral film from exposure but also to hold the intensifying screens in perfect contact with the extraoral film. This contact is critical, as lack of proper contact results in a loss of image sharpness.

A rigid cassette is like a book like container consisting of two aluminum or bakelite leaves which open and close on hinges. The front cover lid is placed so that it faces the tube head and is usually constructed of plastic or of low density metal and offers little resistance to the passage of the ray. The back plate is constructed of heavy metal and lined with lead to absorb X-rays which pass through the enclosed film and reduce scatter radiation. The intensifying screens are installed inside the front and back covers of the cassette. The film is positioned between the two intensifying screens. Each screen exposes one side of the film. The cassette is loaded and unloaded in the dark room.

The cassette must be marked to orient the finished radiograph, a metallic letter 'L' or 'R' is attached to the front cover of the cassette to indicate the patient's left or right side respectively.

Intensifying Screen

Intensifying screen (**Fig. 9.8**) is a device that transfers X-ray energy into visible light; the visible light, in turn exposes the screen film. These screens intensify the effect of X-rays on the film, thus less radiation is required to expose a screen film, and thus the patient is exposed to less radiation.

The action of radiation on photographic film is supplemented by means of special screens which intensify

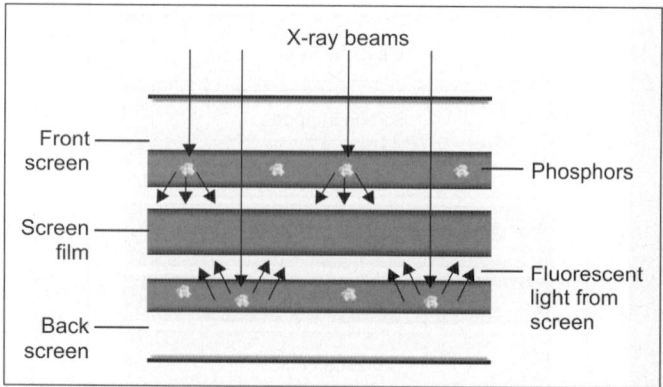

Figure 9.8 Phosphors in the intensifying screen emit visible light when hit by X-ray photons. Multiple visible light photons then strike and expose the film

the action of X-rays. Some materials are able to absorb X-rays and re-emit the energy in form of visible light photons. The amount of light emitted is strictly proportional to the amount of X-ray energy absorbed which in turn is proportional to the X-ray exposure to which the screen is subjected. It is then the sum effect of X-rays and visible light emitted by the screens that exposes the X-ray film. Such a combination of X-ray film with an intensifying screen results in an image receptor system ten to sixty times more sensitive to X-rays than the film alone. Thus, the duration of exposure is reduced, the contrast improved and radiation back scatter minimized.

In extraoral radiography, a screen film is sandwiched between the two intensifying screens of matching size and secured in a cassette.

An intensifying screen is a smooth plastic sheet coated with minute fluorescent crystals known as phosphors. When exposed to X-rays, the phosphors fluoresce and emit visible light in the blue or green spectrum, the emitted light then exposes the film.

Composition

- *Base*: Made of either a stiff sheet of cardboard or polyester plastic material (like the one used for the base of the radiographic film). It is about 0.25 mm thick. The base is the supporting component of the screen.
- *Reflecting layer*: This is a thin layer of white material (i.e. magnesium oxide or titanium dioxide) between the base and the luminiscent layer. It serves to redirect to the film a large fraction of the emitted visible light which is moving away from the film and which would therefore otherwise be lost. Thus, it increases the sensitivity but some degree of unsharpness is created because of divergence of light reflected back to the film.
- *Phosphor layer*: This layer consists of light sensitive phosphor crystals suspended in a plastic material.

When these crystals are struck by photons they fluoresce, that is, they emit visible light photons that expose the X-ray film. Even a single X-ray photon absorbed in an intensifying screen generates many light photons leading to increased film exposure. The speed of the screens increases as the crystal size increases but the overall image quality may be degraded. Types of phosphor used in dental screens are:

- Crystalline Calcium Tungstate, that fluoresces in the blue portion of the spectrum. Conventional screens (Kodak X-Omatic Regular screens) are used with blue sensitive films.
- Rare earth intensifying screens using terbium-activated gadolinium oxysulphide and thelium-activated lanthanum oxybromide, which fluoresce in the green portion of the spectrum.

The newer rare earth screens have phosphors that emit green light. The term 'rare earth' is used because it is difficult and expensive to separate these elements from earth and from each other and not because these elements are rare. Rare earth intensifying screens are four times more efficient than calcium screens and are considered faster, and thus less exposure is required when these rare earth screens are used. Rare earth screens (Kodak Lanex Regular and Medium screens) are designed for use with green sensitive films.

- *Coat*: This layer protects the phosphor layer from mechanical insult such as abrasion, scratching, etc. It is important to keep the intensifying screens clean, because any debris, spots which are opaque to visible light or scratches will result in light (under exposed) spots on the resultant radiograph.

Effect of the Screens

- *Unsharpness*: There are three types of screens available in the market:
  1. High definition.
  2. Normal.
  3. High speed.

  The manufacturer controls the screen thickness, crystal size and the amount of dye included in order to produce the optimum combination of intensification factor and screen unsharpness. The range of unsharpness produced by the screens varies from 0.15 mm for high definition to 0.45 mm for high speed screen.

  The use of the screen also produces an additional amount of image blurring over that which would occur if no screen is used. This extra blurring is greater for screens with a higher intensification factor.

  But, this fact is compensated for by the reduction in X-ray exposure so that the other type of unsharpness is reduced. Thus, the overall result is that the total unsharpness is less when screens are used than when they are not used.

- *Mottle*: This consists of faint irregular pattern of density variations which are not present in the X-ray beam.
  - *Screen mottle*: Nonuniformity in the fluorescent layer may show up on the radiograph since the intensification factor will vary over the surface of the screen. This effect is not as marked in the newer screens.
  - *Quantum mottle*: This is related to the actual number of X-ray photons which arrive at the cassette. With the advent of fast films, the actual numbers of X-ray photons which reach the cassette and form an image pattern on the radiograph are comparatively small. Emission of X-rays is a random process and so uneven is the primary beam, that the average number of X-ray photons directed at any part of the screens will not be the same. Hence, there is a variation in the X-ray intensity over the surface of the screen and it becomes apparent on the film. This is called quantum mottle.

  The use of fast films in combination with the screens reduces the exposure to the patient.

Care and Use of Screen

- There should be no gap between the screen and the film, so as to avoid excessive blurring of the image because of greater area of the film over which light can spread.
- The cassette after use may become buckled or bent, and then it is difficult even for the felt lining in the cassette to help maintain close contact between the screen and the film.
- Scratches, dust or grease will also prevent light photons passing from the screen to the film and thus, will show a pattern on the film. Thus, this should be prevented.

Lead intensifying screens: These are used only with high kV, radiography, i.e. with 250kV X-rays or cobalt 60 gamma rays.

Duplicating Film

A duplicate radiograph is one that is identical to the original. It is useful when the patient is referred to a specialist, for insurance claims and as teaching aids. A special duplicating film is required to make duplicate radiographs.

A duplicating film is a type of photographic film that is used to make an identical copy of an intraoral and extraoral radiograph, but unlike the radiographs, this duplicating film is used only in a dark room setting and is not exposed to X-rays.

The duplicating film has emulsion only on one side. The emulsion side of the film appears shiny, whereas the side without the emulsion appears dull. The emulsion side of the film must contact the radiograph during duplication process.

Radiographic duplicating films are available in periapical sizes as well as in 5″ × 12″ and 8″ × 10″ sheets.

A small photographic printer, can be used, by replacing the bulb with an ultra violet bulb, which may be used as the light source for duplicating.

Film Protection and Storage

- Film is adversely affected by heat, humidity and radiation.
- To prevent film fog, unexposed, unprocessed film must be kept in a cool, dry place.
- The optimum temperature for film storage ranges from, 50°–70°F.
- Optimum relative humidity level ranges from 30–50%.
- Film must be stored in areas that are adequately shielded from sources of radiation and should not be stored in areas where patients are exposed to X-radiation.
- To prevent film fog, lead-lined or radiation-resistant film dispensers and storage boxes are ideal.
- All dental X-ray film has a limited shelf life. Each box or container of film is clearly labeled with an expiration date.
- The 'first in, first out' rule of thumb should be applied to film use, the oldest film in stock always used before any new film.

GRIDS

These are devices which reduce the amount of scattered radiation reaching the film whilst still allowing the patterns containing the primary beams to reach the film.

The grid prevents the scattered radiation from reaching the film. Scattered radiation causes fog and reduces contrast of the film. This is because the scattered photon has lower energy than the primary photon and therefore is less penetrating and thus causes fogging of the film (**Figs 9.9 and 9.10**).

Types of Grids

- Focused grids and nonfocused grids.
- Stationary grids and moving grids.

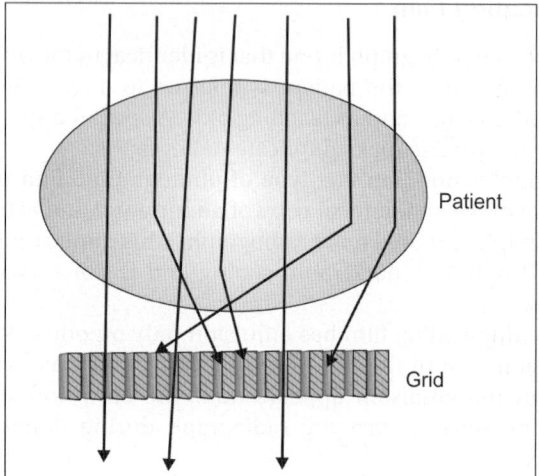

Figure 9.9 Obliquely moving scattered radiation is stopped by the grid, whilst the forward moving primary photons pass to the film

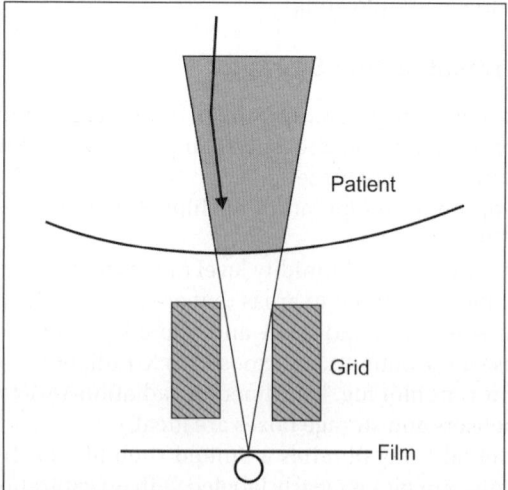

Figure 9.10 Scattered radiation produced within the shaded region of the patient and moving towards O is able to reach O unimpeded by the grid

Stationary Grids

As the name suggests, the grid is stationary and does not move. The presence of a grid between an object and the film causes the images of the radiopaque absorbing material to be projected onto the film.

- *The linear grid*: The strips of lead used are placed strictly parallel to each other. In this, the primary radiations traveling radially from the X-ray tube focal spot to the film will encounter the grid obliquely. Thus, the grid lines appear wider. At a sufficiently large distance from the center of the beam, a complete cut off of the primary radiation may occur. For all practical purposes the central beam should be in a plane parallel with the grid lines. This arrangement of the elements of the linear grid will eliminate the absorption of the more divergent primary photons at the margins of an X-ray beam, where their direction does not coincide with the alignment of the perpendicular lead strips in the grid.
- *The focused grid*: In this grid the strips of lead are angled progressively from the center to the edge so that interspaces point at the focal spot, thus their direction coincides with the direction of the path of diverging photons in the primary X-ray beam, thereby accommodating their passage through the grid. This helps to prevent the primary cut off.
- *The pseudo-focused grid*: In this grid the height of the strips is reduced progressively from the center resulting in a reduced grid ratio from the center to the edge (**Fig. 9.11**).
- *The crossed grid*: The linear grids are placed mutually at right angles so that even a small amount of scattered radiation gets blocked.

Moving Grid (Potter Bucky Grid)

In this the grid is moved sideways across the film during exposure. This leads to the blurring out of the shadows of grid strips, thus they are not visible on the film. Thus, the image of the radiopaque grid lines on the film can be deleted by mechanically moving the grid in a direction of 90° to the grid lines, (but not the object) during exposure. This results in evening (blurring) out the radiolucent lines and resulting in a more uniform exposure. It does not interfere with the absorption of scattered photons.

Composition

It is composed of a series of long parallel strips of an opaque material (usually lead) held apart and parallel to each other by an X-ray transparent interspace material (usually plastic (**Fig. 9.12**).

Working

The grid is placed between the patient's head and the film. During exposure, the grid permits the passage of the X-ray beam between the lead strips.

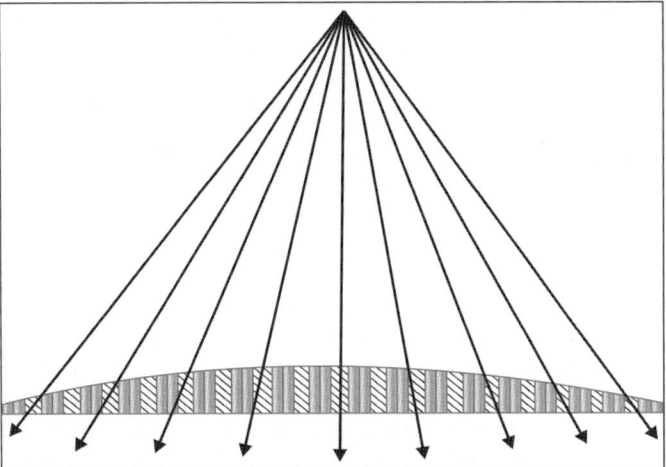

Figure 9.11 A pseudo focused grid

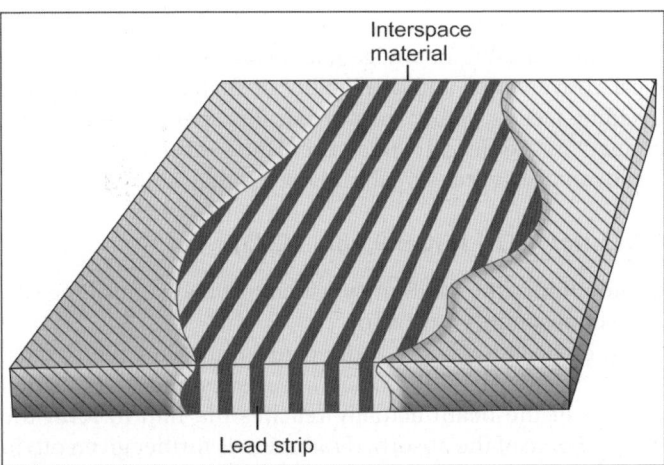

Figure 9.12 A grid showing the long, thin parallel lead strips separated by wider interspace material. The whole is enclosed in a metal outer covering

When some of the X-rays interact with the patient's tissues, scatter radiation is produced; this scatter radiation is then directed at the grid and film at an angle. As a result, scatter radiation is absorbed by the lead strips and does not reach the surface of the film to cause film fog.

The scattered radiation moves obliquely because of the change in direction which occurs in the scattering process. The majority of this radiation (scattered radiation) is stopped by the lead of the grid and hence it does not reach the film, on the other hand the majority of the primary radiation which is moving forward will pass through the interspace and reach the film upon which it will therefore impress the X-ray pattern.

The presence of the grid is usually able to remove as much as 80–90% of the scattered radiation. This largely helps to improve the contrast

Advantages of a Grid

- Scattered radiation exiting an irradiated object may be largely removed or reduced from the beam reaching the film by placing an X-ray grid between the object and the film. This helps to reduce film fog and increase radiographic (film) contrast.
- Some clinicians have found it useful to superimpose fine wire grids when exposing radiographs to aid in the measurement of relative bone height. Typically the grid form 1 mm squares, which appear as fine radiopaque lines on the resultant radiograph, that allow the quantitative measurement of the position of the alveolar bone with respect to the dentition. The procedure is particularly useful in evaluating osseous changes in radiographs made at different times with a reproducible positioning technique.

Disadvantages of a Grid

The exposure required to produce a radiograph when a grid is used approximately doubles compared to that used in the absence of a grid. This is to compensate for the presence of lead strips in the grid, an increased exposure time must be used to expose a film. Because of this increase in exposure time, a grid should be used only when improved image quality and high contrast are necessary.

FILTRATION

This involves removal of unwanted radiation whilst leaving the wanted radiation undiminished.

Radiation emitted by an X-ray tube is made up of photons of much different energy. The maximum photon energy depends only upon the kilovoltage used to generate the radiation. And the minimum energy depends upon the nature and thickness of the material of the wall of the X-ray tube. Because of their different energies, the photons have different penetrating powers. When the beam of radiation is incident upon the patient, the bulk of the low energy photons is absorbed in the superficial layers, which produce unwanted effects. Thus, these low energy radiations must be removed by a process called filtration.

Filtration of a beam is accomplished by:
- *Inherent filtration*: The primary beam of radiation passes through the glass wall of the tube, a layer of oil and the aperture window. As it passes through these components of the tube, a certain amount of filtration takes place, which is called inherent filtration.

  This filtration is usually not sufficient and additional filtration is required.
- *Additional filtration*: Additional materials are placed in the path of the primary beam to aid in further filtration.

  Total filtration is the sum of inherent filtration plus the added filtration.

Requirements of Filter Material

- It should be able to discriminate against the lower energy photons. It should attenuate principally by means of the photo-electric effect in the photon energy range being dealt with.
- The material should not have an absorption 'edge' at an energy close to the energies of the photons that are desired to be used.
- The thickness of the material must not be too small because in such cases, due to irregularities in thickness, the beam thus produced would be nonuniform. And 'pin holes' which occur easily would produce tiny completely unfiltered and unacceptable beams.

One quarter of a millimeter can be regarded as a minimum acceptable thickness.

Materials used for Filtration

The materials used may vary depending upon whether the beam is of high or low energy and therefore depending upon the generating voltage used. The generally accepted X-ray range for the materials used is:

- 30–120 kV   Aluminum (most commonly used)
- 100–250 kV   Copper (with appropriate backing)
- 200–600 kV   Tin (with appropriate backing)
- 600–2 mV   Lead (with appropriate backing)
- Above 2 mV   None

The aluminum filter is the one, most commonly used. The recommended total filtration must be equal to:

- 1.5 mm of aluminum for up to 70 kVp
- 2.5 mm of aluminum for all higher voltages.

Effects of Filtration

- It removes unwanted radiations and hardens the beam, thus increasing the penetrating power.
- If progressively thick layers of the filter material are introduced and the effects studied, it is found that initially there is a substantial increase in the quality accompanied by a substantial reduction in the beam intensity. Thus, there is a certain optimum thickness beyond which no further hardening occurs.
- It reduces unnecessary less penetrating radiation (skin dose) to the patient, which has no diagnostic value.

Patient exposure may be further reduced by removing low energy photons from the beam, leaving the mid range energy photons to expose the film. X-ray energies most effective in producing the image are between 35 keV and 55 keV.

The material used are rare earth elements like samarium, erbium, yttrium, niobium, gemdolium, terbium activated gadolinium oxysulfide and thulium activated lanthanum oxybromide.

The use of these in combination with aluminum will reduce the exposure by 20–80% more than when only aluminum is used. But there is 50% increase in the exposure time with decrease in contrast, sharpness and resolution of the resultant image.

Profile wedge filter: Reduction of the radiographic density of the soft tissue profile can also be accomplished by absorbing or removing some of the X-rays out of the part of the X-ray beam reaching the profile soft tissues. The absorbing device is a '*profile wedge filter*' consisting of a vertical bar that is wedge shaped anteroposteriorly. The thin edge of the filter is positioned posteriorly over the bone area of the patient to absorb less X-rays, while the thick edge is positioned in the soft tissue region. The wedge is usually made of aluminum and can be located in the cassette, in the X-ray beam between the patient and the X-ray source.

Wedge filter: These are used with mega-voltage radiations and in radiotherapy when it is desirable to treat from one side of the patient only, though it is necessary to use more than one beam. The material used for wedge filters is relatively unimportant, local convenience and availability of material are often the deciding factors, rather than physical properties. Aluminum, copper, brass or lead are often used, the denser materials have an advantage as they give thinner filters than aluminum.

COLLIMATION (FIGS 9.13A TO D)

Collimation is the method by which one can control the size and shape of the X-ray beam.

When an X-ray beam is directed towards a patient, most of it is absorbed by the overlying tissues and a very small portion of the beam actually reaches the film to form the image. Some of the absorbed radiation is further given out in all directions (compton effect). Thus, it may be observed that these radiations serve no useful purpose for the formation of the image on the film, but, instead add to the film fog. Therefore it is important to keep the size and shape of the beam just adequate to irradiate only the required area and no more. This method to control the size and shape of the primary beam is called collimation. This is achieved by placing a radiopaque barrier containing an aperture in the path of the beam. This reduces patient exposure and also ensures better film image quality.

Types of Collimators

They may be fixed type or adjustable type:

- *Diaphragm collimator*: It consists of a thick plate of radiopaque material (usually lead) with an aperture or an opening in it. The device is usually placed over the port in the X-ray head through which the X-ray beam emerges. The aperture may be of different size and shape as per the requirement.

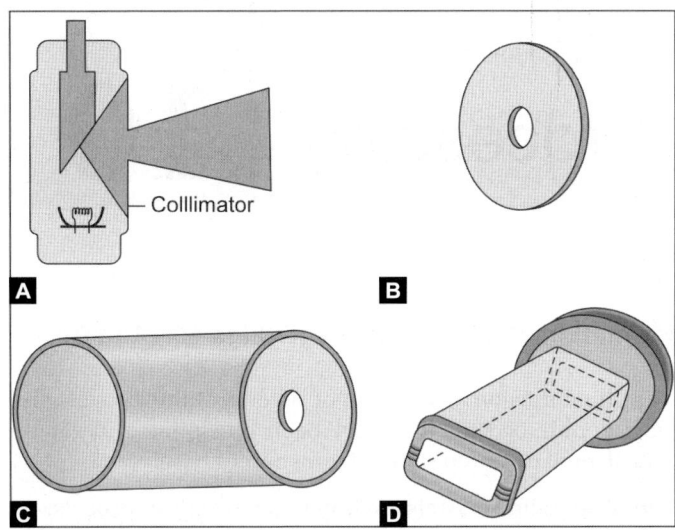

Figures 9.13A to D (A) Collimation of an X-ray beam (shown in color) is achieved by restricting its useful size; (B) Diaphragm collimator; (C) Tubular collimator; (D) Rectangular collimator

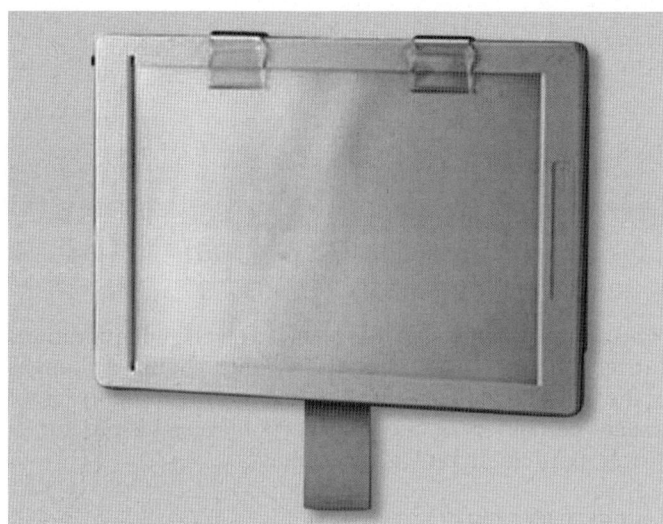

Figure 9.14 Film illuminator/viewer

- *Tubular collimator*: It is tube lined with or constructed of radiopaque material.

  A combination of tubular and diaphragm collimator can be used in which case, one end of the tube is in conjunction with the diaphragm collimator, which covers the X-ray port. This combination, also helps to reduce the penumbra at the periphery of the image. The longer the tube used, smaller is the penumbra.
- *Rectangular collimator*: These collimators limit the size, just larger than the size of the X-ray film. This rectangular collimation can also be incorporated in a film holding device.
- Slit collimator is used in OPG machines.

Film Illuminator (Fig. 9.14)

This is required for proper viewing and interpretation of the radiograph. The illuminator should have uniform brightness and luminance with a dimmer so that the light intensity can be monitored, with optimum reading capability even under conditions of various film densities and lighting of reading room. It should be flicker free to prevent eye strain.

BIBLIOGRAPHY

1. American National Standards Institute. Photography—intra-oral dental radiographic film—specification. New York: American National Standards Institute; 1997. ANSI/ISO 3665:1996, ANSI/NAPM IT2.49-1997.
2. Frommer HH. Image formation Image Receptors in Radiology for Dental Auxillaries, 6th edition. St. Louis; Mosby Year Book; 1996.pp.31-47.
3. Kaugars GE, Fatouros P. Clinical comparison of conventional and rare earth screen-film systems for cephalometric radiographs. Oral Surg Oral Med Oral Pathol. 1982;53(3):322-5.
4. Matteson SR, Whaley C, Secrist VC. Dental Radiology Practice and Equipment. In: Dental radiology, 4th edition. Chapel Hill, University of North Carolina Press; 1988. pp.14-16.
5. Meredith WJ, Massey JB. Fundamental Physics of Radiology, 2nd edition. Bristol: John Wright and Sons; 1972.
6. Miles DA, Van Dis ML, Jenson CS, et al. Radiographic Imaging for Dental Auxillaries. 2nd edition, Philadelphia; WB Saunders; 1993.pp.50-54,66,74,80,156.
7. Times of India, Mumbai, Friday, March. 2005;11-5.

Processing | 10

Processing is a collective title given to a series of operations carried out in the dark room, which effect chemical changes in the exposed radiographic film, making the invisible latent image, contained in the sensitized film emulsion into a visible, permanent radiographic image.

LATENT IMAGE

A radiographic film is a recording medium used in dental radiography. When this film is exposed to the information carrying beam of photons exiting an object, the photosensitive silver halide crystals in the film emulsion interact with these photons and are chemically changed. These chemically altered crystals are said to constitute the latent (invisible) image of the film.

These chemical changes in the crystals increase the liability of crystals to chemical action of the developing process that converts the latent image into manifest (visible) image.

Formation of the Latent Image (Figs 10.1A to D)

The film emulsion is made up of silver bromide crystals and silver iodide crystals that have been precipitated in gelatin and layered on a thin sheet of transparent base.

The silver halide crystals are imperfect in various aspects:
- *Interstitial silver ions*: These are free ions in the spaces between the crystalline lattice.
- Physical distortion are present in the regular rectangular array of silver and bromide ion crystals due to the presence of iodine atom occupying some of the bromide sites.
- The silver halide crystals are chemically sensitized by the presence of sulfur compounds which cause physical irregularities in the crystal produced by iodide ions, and these are called latent image sites.

The function of these latent image sites is to begin the process of image formation by trapping the electrons generated when the emulsion is irradiated.

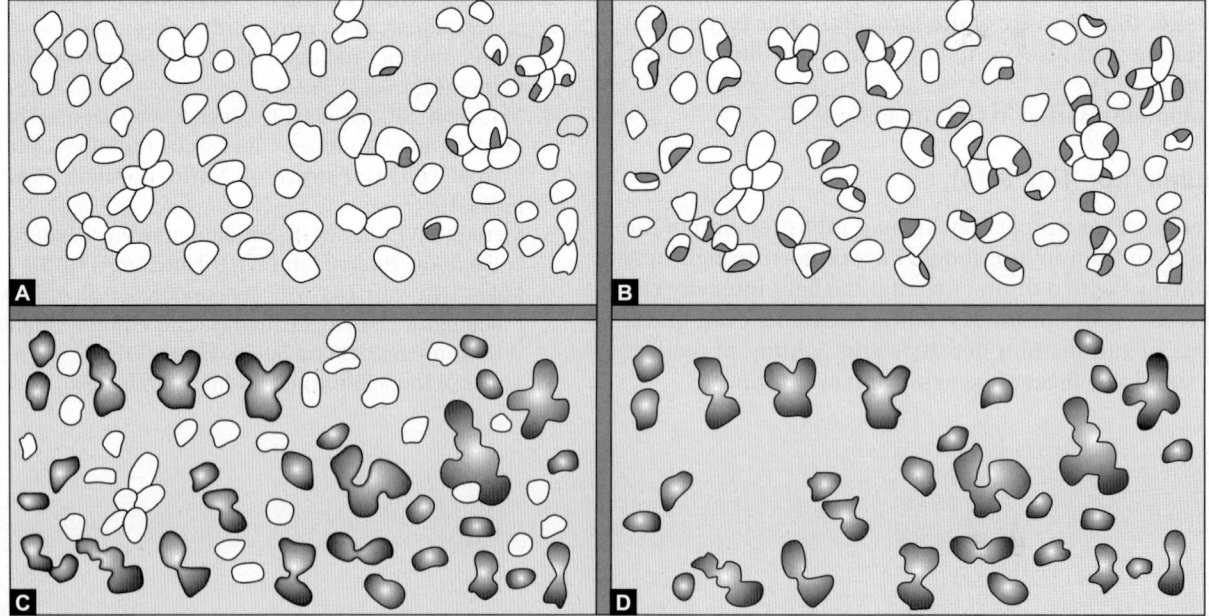

Figures 10.1A to D (A) Schematic of distribution of silver halide grains. The gray areas indicate a latent image produced by exposure; (B) Partial development begins to produce metallic silver (black) in exposed grains; (C) Development completed; (D) Unexposed silver grains have been removed by fixation

When the silver halide crystals are irradiated by X-ray photons it will result in the release of electrons usually by the bromide ions, (by compton and photoelectric interactions) which are converted to bromine atoms, by the removal of an electron (recoil electron). This recoil electron thus produced has sufficient kinetic energy with which it moves in the crystal and strikes the image site, imparting a negative charge to that region.

The free, positively charged interstitial silver ions are attracted to the negative latent image site and neutralize the image site with the result that an atom of metallic silver is deposited at the site.

After exposure of a film to radiation, the aggregate of silver atoms at the latent image sites, comprises the latent image. It is the metallic silver at each latent image site that catalyses the development of the halide crystal in which it formed and renders the crystal sensitive to development and image formation.

The primary action of the processing solutions is to convert the crystals with latent images into black metallic silver grains that can be visualized and to remove the unexposed silver bromide crystals.

FILM PROCESSING

This process makes the latent image produced in the film emulsion by exposure to radiation, visible.

Under special darkroom conditions, a chemical reaction takes place when a film with the latent image is immersed in a series of special chemical solutions. During processing a chemical reaction occurs, and the halide portion of the exposed, energized silver halide crystal is removed chemically, this is referred to as reduction. Reduction of the silver halide crystals results in precipitated metallic silver.

During film processing selective reduction of the exposed silver halide crystal occurs. Selective reduction refers to the reduction of the energized, exposed silver halide crystals into black metallic silver, while the unenergized, unexposed silver halide crystals are removed from the film.

Thus the latent image is made visible through the following processing procedure:

- The film is placed in a chemical known as the developer solution for a specific amount of time and at a specific temperature. The developer distinguishes between the exposed and unexposed silver halide crystals. The developer initiates a chemical reaction that reduces the exposed silver halide crystals into metallic silver and creates dark or black areas on a dental radiograph. At the same time the unexposed silver halide remains virtually unaffected by the developer.
- If the developer is allowed to remain in prolong contact with the silver bromide crystals that do not contain a latent image, it will slowly reduce them also and thereby over develop the film. Reduction of unexposed crystals results in the production of a chemical fog and not a dark radiograph.

- Following the developing process, the film is rinsed in water to remove any remaining developer solution. After development the film emulsion swells and becomes saturated with developer. At this point the films should be rinsed for 30 seconds with continuous, gentle agitation. Rinsing dilutes the developer, slowing down the developing process. It also removes the alkali activator, preventing neutralization of the acid fixer. The rinsing process is typical for the manual method but is not used in the automatic processing.
- Next the film is placed in a special chemical known as the fixer solution, for a specific amount of time. The fixer solution removes the unexposed silver halide crystals and creates white or clear areas on the dental radiograph. The undeveloped silver bromide gives the film a dense opalescent appearance and if exposed to light in this state the film will darken slowly. The black metallic silver is not removed and remains on the film. A second function of the fixer solution is to harden and shrink the film emulsion.
- Following the fixing process the film is washed in water to remove any remaining traces of the chemical solutions. Washing efficiency declines rapidly when the water temperature falls below 60°F. Warm water should not be used as the emulsion will soften and the film will be easily damaged. Any silver compound or thiosulfate that remains because of improper rinsing discolors and causes stains, which are most apparent on the radiopaque (light) areas. This discoloration results from the thiosulfate reacting with the silver to form brown silver sulphide, which can obscure diagnostic information (seen as yellow stains or white deposits). Washing time longer than 30 minutes should be avoided as this may also damage the film emulsion.
- *Drying*: After thoroughly rinsing the film is dried. The films may be placed in a drying cabinet or hung up in a well-ventilated dust free room. Care should be taken that the wet emulsion is not touched or damaged. Films should not be splashed with water during the drying cycle as this will produce spots which cannot be removed and reduce the diagnostic value of the film.

  After the films have been removed the hangers should be cleaned in running water to remove any traces of residual chemicals. Periodically hangers should be soaked overnight in acetic acid and scrubbed in warm soapy water. The hanger should be thoroughly clean and dry before a new film is loaded on it.
- *Mounting of the radiograph*: This helps to preserve and maintain the radiograph as these are important components of a patient's record. A mounted radiograph is more convenient for visualization. Each film mount should be correctly inscribed with the patient's name, and the relevant date for identification and indexing, for

record purpose. The convex side of the dot in the corner of the intra oral film should be placed towards the viewer.

The visible image that results on the radiograph is made up of black, white and gray areas.

Radiolucent structures are those that readily permit the passage of the X-ray beam and allow more X-rays to reach the film, more silver halide crystals in the film emulsion are exposed and energized, thus resulting in increased deposits of black metallic silver. A radiograph with large deposits of metallic silver appears black or radiolucent.

Radiopaque structures are those that resist the passage of the X-ray beam and restrict or limit the amount of X-rays that reach the film. If no X-rays reach the film, no silver halide crystals in the film emulsion are exposed, and no deposits of metallic silver are seen. A radiograph with areas of unexposed silver halide crystals that have been removed during processing and no metallic silver deposits appears white or radiopaque.

Film Processing Solutions

These may be obtained in the following forms:
- Powder
- Ready to use liquid
- Liquid concentrate.

The special chemical solutions are:
- Developer solution
- Fixing solution

Developer Solution

- *Reducing agents*
  - *Hydroquinone (para dihydroxy benzene)*: It is a benzene derivative and is concerned with the production of high contrast in the radiograph. Hydroquinone becomes relatively inactive in low temperatures.
  - *Metol or elon (mono methyl-para amine phenol sulfate)*: It is a by-product of analine dyes and helps develop the shadow areas or shades of gray on the film and brings out the details. It does not produce a high contrast. It is less sensitive to temperature changes.
  - When used together hydroquinone and metol produce an adequate contrast and detail, at 68°F or 20°C.
  - *Metolphenidone (1-phenyl-3-pyrazolidone)*: This serves as the first electron donor that converts silver ions to metallic silver at the latent image site. The electron transfer generates the oxidized form of phenidone. Hydroquinone provides an electron to reduce the oxidized phenidone back to its original active state so that it can continue to reduce silver halide grains to metallic silver.
  - This is an efficient activator for hydroquinone at a very low concentration and works at a lower alkalinity. It has longer keeping properties and is less likely to

cause dermatitis. A special restrainer should be used to prevent excessive fogging.This agent is used in automatic processing.
- *Preservative*
  - *Sodium sulphite*: This inhibits the tendency of the developing agent to combine with the oxygen dissolved in water or in the air. It therefore acts as a preservative and keeps the solution in an usable condition for several weeks. Oxidation of the developing agents forms colored substances which would stain the film and add to the film fog.
- *Activator*
  - *Potassium carbonate or sodium carbonate*: It is added to the developing solution to provide and maintain the degree of alkalinity in which the developing agent can function. This is also called the 'accelerator' because it speeds up the development. A low degree of alkalinity will slow down the process of development.

    Excessive alkalinity will cause rapid reduction even of unexposed silver bromide crystals and produce fog. It may also soften the gelatin which may swell and may even blister or frill.

    This component of the developing solution makes it 'soapy' to touch.

    Sodium hydroxide in conjunction with sodium carbonate may be used to give higher contrast.
- *Restrainer*
  - *Potassium bromide or benzotriazole*: It has a restraining action, in that it slows down the reduction action of the developing agents, and has it's greatest retarding effect on the development of unexposed crystals.

    It prevents excessive fogging of the film and increases the contrast.
- *Hardener*
  - *Glutaraldehyde*: This is added especially in automatic processing, to prevent the emulsion from softening and sticking to the rollers.
- *Fungicide*: To prevent bacterial growth.
- *Buffer*: To maintain the pH (+ 7)
- *Solvent*
  - *Water*: It is used as a solvent of the chemicals and as a medium in which they react with the silver bromide of the film emulsion. Normal water supply is usually satisfactory but water with a high calcium content may cause some precipitation. Water carries metallic impurities or hydrogen sulphide which may cause trouble, to avoid these inconveniences distilled water should be used.

    In automatic processing sulfate compounds are added to the developer to minimize the swelling of the emulsion so that the films can be transported by the rollers uniformly.

    The developer should always be made up in accordance with the instruction of the manufacturer.

The tank must be covered by a lid and the solution kept at 68°F or at the temperature recommended by the manufacturer.

If the developer is cold, its action will be slow and the time required for the full development is unduly long.

When the developer is too warm, the image develops quickly, the development time is short and it gives rise to uneven development and excessive fog. At very high temperatures the emulsion may be excessively softened.

– *Developer replenisher*: In the normal course of processing, phenidone and hydroquinone are consumed, and bromide ions and other by products are released into the solution. Developer also becomes inactivated by exposure to oxygen. These actions produce a 'seasoned' solution, and the film speed and contrast stabilize. The developing solution of both manual and automatic developers should be replenished with fresh solution each morning to prolong the life of the seasoned developer. The recommended amount to be added daily is 8 ounces of fresh developer (replenisher) per gallon of developing solution, if approximately thirty periapical films or five panoramic films are developed per day. Some of the used solution may need to be removed to make room for the replinisher.

Fixing Solution

- *Clearing agent*
  - *Ammonium thiosulfate or sodium thiosulfate (hypo)* is one of the few substances which will remove silver bromide without adverse effect on the film. The chemical reacts with the undeveloped silver bromide and converts it into a soluble substance which can be subsequently washed out of the film.
- *Preservative*
  - *Sodium sulphite*: It prevents the oxidation of the clearing agent, which is unstable in the acidic environment. It also binds with any colored oxidized developer carried over into the fixing solution, and thus prevents any oxidized developer from staining the film.
- *Acidifier*
  - *Acetic acid*: The acetic acid buffer system (pH 4–4.5) helps to keep the fixer pH constant. This acidic pH is required to promote good diffusion of the thiosulfate into the emulsion and of silver thiosulfate complex out of the emulsion.

    The acid solution also neutralizes any developing agent carried over, thereby blocking any further development of any unexposed crystals while the film is in the fixing tank.
- *Hardener*
  - *Aluminum chloride or aluminum sulfate or potassium alum*: These substances form complexes with the

gelatin during fixing and prevent further damage to the gelatin during subsequent handling. The hardeners also reduce the swelling of the emulsion during the final wash. This lessons mechanical damage to the emulsion and limits water absorption, thus shortening the drying time.

- *Solvent*
  - *Water*: The fixing solution should be made up in accordance with the manufacturer's instructions and used at a temperature of about 68°F (20°C). In order to clear completely films must remain in the fixer for at least twice the time they were kept in the developing tank. The clearing time will depend upon the type of film and the activity of the fixing solution. With usage the fixer becomes progressively slow in its action and when the clearing time for a given type of film has doubled, the fixer is considered exhausted. It should be replaced by a fresh solution.

It is not advisable to switch on the light until the film has been in the fixer for about 30 seconds, this will ensure that the development process has stopped.

No film should be exhibited for general viewing until it has been thoroughly fixed.

Reduction: An overexposed or grossly overdeveloped film will be too dark for convenient viewing, owing to the excessive deposit of silver which obscures the image detail.

A photographic reducer (Farmer's Reducer) contains an oxidizing agent, potassium ferricyanide which oxidizes the silver to silver ferrocyanide, which in turn is dissolved by the solution of sodium thiosulfate.

Chemical intensification of radiographs: A radiograph may be too light because of, underexposure, under development or both. Instead of repeating the radiograph, chemical intensification may be done. Most of the intensification methods act by converting the silver which forms the image into a compound which is more opaque, more colored or of a different physical form.

THE DARKROOM

The primary function of the darkroom is to provide a completely darkened environment where the X-ray film can be handled and processed to produce a diagnostic image in an efficient, precise and standardized procedure.

Since the processing operations are carried out in near total darkness, every piece of equipment must be in a specific place.

General Lay Out

The size of the darkroom for a dental office may be as small as 3' × 3' for an individual dentist, or may measure 16–20 square feet for a group practice or in an institution.

The size will vary depending upon:
- Volume of radiographs processed.
- Number of persons using the dark room.
- Type of processing equipment used (processing tanks or automatic processor).
- The space required for the duplication of films and storage.

The darkroom should have sufficient space to accommodate the processing tanks or automatic processors.

The darkroom work space must include an adequate counter area where films can be unwrapped prior to processing. This area should be absolutely clean, dry and free of processing chemicals, water, dust and debris. This should ideally be at least three feet away from the processing tank.

The darkroom storage space must include ample room for chemical processing solutions, film cassettes and other miscellaneous radiographic supplies.

The darkroom should be well ventilated, the use of an air conditioner is recommended, but during nonworking hours the windows and doors should be left open.

Fumes emitted from the chemical processing solutions may damage film emulsion of unexposed films, leading to film fog.

The temperature and humidity level of the darkroom must be controlled to prevent film damage. A room temperature of 70°F and humidity levels between 50–70% is recommended to be maintained.

The darkroom plumbing must include both hot and cold running water along with mixing valves to adjust the water temperature in the processing tanks.

A utility sink with running water is also useful in the darkroom.

As the term darkroom suggests the room must be completely dark and must exclude all visible light—light tight or light proof which may be accomplished:
- By exclusion of all external lights.
- By use of a light tight door or the door should have a lock to prevent accidental exposure of the film.
- Fluorescent lights should not be used in the dark room because there is often a short after glow that may fog.
- The first few films opened after the light is turned off.
- Use of both white light and safe light.
- White light illumination is required during cleaning tanks and preparing the solutions.

Safe Light Illumination

- Should be of low intensity, with a relatively long wave length (orange-red) that does not rapidly affect open film, but permits one to see enough of the work area.
- Films are sensitive to light until after fixation.
- Arrangement of safe light filter should be such that three zones of illumination are classified:
  - *Dimmest zone*: Area where the cassettes are loaded and intraoral films opened.
  - *Medium zone*: Area where the films are developed and fixed.
  - *Bright zone*: Area where the films are washed and placed in the drier.

This can be accomplished by placing one safe light above the working area and another on the wall behind the processing tanks.

Excessive exposure of film to safe light illumination will result in fog. The following three factors must be therefore considered:
- *Type of filter*: X-rays have the highest sensitivity in the blue green region of the spectrum and are less sensitive to light in the yellow and red region.

  Hence, safelights are safe when made of amber or red filters. The filters commonly used are:
  - Moralite filter (cannot be used for screen films)
  - Wratten Series 6 B filters
  - Red GBX-2 safe light filter.
- *Intensity of illumination*: To minimize fogging effect of prolonged exposure:
  - The wattage of the bulb should be 7½–15 watts.
  - The distance of the safe light above the work area should be four feet.

    The light illumination follows the inverse square law, which states that the intensity is inversely proportional to the square of the distance. Thus correct intensity can be obtained by adjusting either the distance of the bulb or wattage or both.
- *Time of exposure:* More the film is exposed to the safe light, more are the chances of film fogging. Film handling under a safelight should be limited to about 5 minutes before the film emulsion shows some sensitivity to light from a safe light with prolonged exposure.

Tests for Checking Unsafe Illumination

Film fogging can occur due to:
- Use of inappropriate safe light filters.
- Excessive exposure to safe light filters.
- Stray light.

i. Coin test/Penny test (**Figs 10.2A and B**) is a test to evaluate for fogging caused by inappropriate safe lighting conditions.
   - Shut all lights and put on the safe lights.
   - Open film packet and place the base film in the area where films are usually unwrapped.
   - Place a coin on the film and leave it in this position for approximately the time required to unwrap and mount a full mouth set of radiographs, usually 5 minutes.
   - Develop the test film as usual.
   - *Inference*: If the image of the coin can be seen on the resultant film, the room is not light safe for the particular film tested.

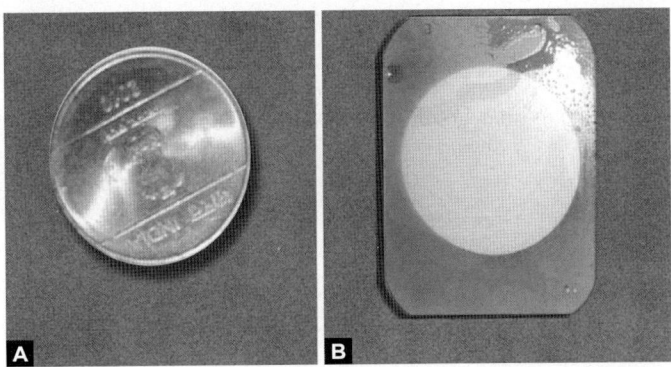

Figures 10.2A and B (A) Penny test or coin test for unsafe light illumination. Leave a coin on the exposed film on the working surface during the time that the film would be open (approximate 5 minutes); (B) If the processed radiograph shows the outline of the coin, the safe light conditions are inappropriate

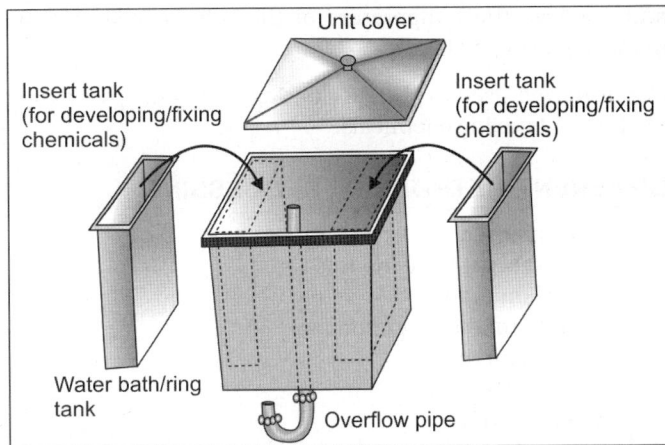

Figure 10.3 Processing tank, the developing and fixing tanks are inserted into the bath of running water with an over flow drain

ii. To check whether there is no light leak, shut the door and shut off all the lights in the dark room. A few minutes after you become accustomed to the darkness, carefully view all the areas, like periphery of doors and windows to check whether any light from outside is been seen inside the dark room.

Processing Equipment

Dental X-ray film is processed in the darkroom using manual processing techniques or an automatic film processor. Special equipment is required for both.

Manual processing (also known as Hand or Tank processing). This is the simplest and most efficient procedure for developing with accurate control.

The processing tank contains two parts (**Fig. 10.3**):
- *Master tank: Size 8″ × 10″*
  This serves as a heater jacket to hold the insert tanks and is large enough to provide space between the two insert tanks for rinsing and washing of the films when necessary. It also helps to maintain the temperature of the developer and the fixer in the insert tanks. An over flow pipe is used to control the water level in the master tank.
  Master tank should have a cover:
  – To reduce oxidation of the processing solution.
  – To protect the developing film from accidental exposure to light.
  – To minimize evaporation of processing solution.
  – To prevent contamination with dust.
  – There should be running cold and hot water facility. The ideal temperature is recommended to be 70°F.
- *Insert tanks*: These are removable containers for individual processing solutions. Developer is placed in the insert tank on the left side of the master tank and the fixer on the right side.

Insert tank should have a capacity of to hold one gallon of developer or fixer.

All three tanks may be made of:
- Stainless steel is preferred material as:
  – It does not react with the processing solution.
  – It accommodates more rapidly to change in temperature of the water in the master tank.
  – It is easy to clean.
- Enamel
- Earthenware
- Hard rubber.

Do not use tank or containers that have been soldered as reaction of the solution with the solder metals can cause chemical fogging.

Thermometer: A thermometer is required to check and maintain the temperature of the developing, fixing and washing solutions.

It may be clipped on to the side of the tank or left free floating in the tank.

Timer: is required to control the time of development and fixation.

Drying racks: Wet films are subjected to damage from scratching and abrasion if not handled properly.

Films should be dried in a dust free environment, by:
- Merely hanging a rack above a drip tray to catch the run of excess water.
- Electric fan can be used to speed the drying of films.
- Cabinet dryer using moderately dry air.

Stirring rod or stirring paddle: This is necessary for manual processing. A stirring rod is used to agitate the developer and fixer solution prior to developing, so as to mix the chemicals and equalize the temperature of the solutions. It may be made of plastic or glass.

Plastic apron: Used to protect clothing during the processing of films and mixing chemicals.

DIFFERENT METHODS OF PROCESSING

- Manual method
  - Time temperature method
  - Visual method
  - Rapid processing method.
- Automatic method
- Monobath method
- Day light method
- Digitized processing method
- Self-developing films.

Manual Method

Time Temperature Method

This method is best for mass processing of radiographs, keeping all other exposure parameters standard (kVp, mAs, exposure time, etc). The films do not have to be viewed during the developing process and a large number of films can be processed at one time.

This method ensures that the developing is standard thus any change in the image quality in regards to density or contrast reflects of disparity in the exposure parameters.

- *Replenish solutions*: The first step is to replenish the developer and fixer. Check the level of the solutions to ensure that the film on the top clips of the hanger will also be adequately immersed.
- Stir the solutions, with a separate paddle for the developer and fixer. Check the temperature of the developing solution, the optimum temperature is 68°–70°F. If the temperature of the solution is outside this range, the circulating water temperature must be adjusted accordingly, to reach the correct temperature (**Table 10.1**).
- Mount the film on hangers, label the hangers with the name of the patient and date. Close and lock the door of the dark room, turn off the over head white light and switch on the safe light.
  - For intraoral films, carefully unwrap each exposed film over a clean working surface using proper infection control procedures. Dispose of all film packet wrappings (**Figs 10.4 and 10.5**).
  - For extraoral film, remove the film from the cassette.
  - Handle all films by the edges only.
  - Clip each film to the labelled film hanger. Verify that each film is securely attached by running a finger along the film edge. Reattach any loose films.
  - Based on the temperature of the developing solution and the instructions of the manufacturer, set the timer. For intra oral film processing in conventional solutions,

Table 10.1 Processing temperature* and times* for time temperature method

Solution temperature	Time in developer (minutes)	Rinse time (minutes)	Time in fixer (minutes)	Wash time (minutes)
65°F (18.5°C)	6.0	0.5	10	20
68°F (20.0°C)	5.0	0.5	10	20
70°F (21.0°C)	4.5	0.5	10	20
72°F (22.0°C)	4.0	0.5	9	20
75°F (24.0°C)	3.0	0.5	7	20
80°F (26.5°C)	2.5	0.5	6	20

*It is important that the temperature and time be maintained and monitored with a calibrated thermometer and timer

the following development times are recommended (**Table 10.1**).

Processing at either higher or lower temperatures and for longer or shorter times than that recommended by the manufacturer reduces the contrast of the processed film. Processing for too long or at temperatures higher than those recommended can result in film fog, which will diminish film contrast and diagnostic information.

- Develop the films by first starting the timer mechanism and gently immerse the film hanger into the developing solution. Make sure that the films do not contact another film or the side of the processing tank. Gently agitate the hanger up and down to prevent air bubbles from clinging to the film. Hang the hanger on the film rack on the edge and leave it for the predetermined time without further agitation. Cover the processing tank.

  Before immersing the film in the developing solution it is advisable to wet the film uniformly in water, so that the action of the developing solution is uniform.

- When the timer goes off, uncover the processing tank, remove the film hanger, drain the excess developer in the wash bath. Place the hanger in the circulating water of the master tank. Agitate for 20–30 seconds. Remove and drain the excess water for several seconds. This will remove the excess developer, thus slowing the development and reducing the contamination of the fixer solution.

- *Fixation*: Based on the development time, the fixation time is determined and the timer is set. A time temperature chart is used to determine the time intervals. Fixation is usually approximately double the development time.

  Place the film hanger in the fixer solution for the given time. Agitate for 5 of every 30 seconds. This eliminates bubbles and brings fresh fixer into contact with the emulsion. Hang the hanger on the film rack on the edge of the insert tank, and cover the processing tank. When the timer goes off, uncover the processing tank, remove the hanger and allow the excess fixer to drain into the fixer tank. Place in circulating water.

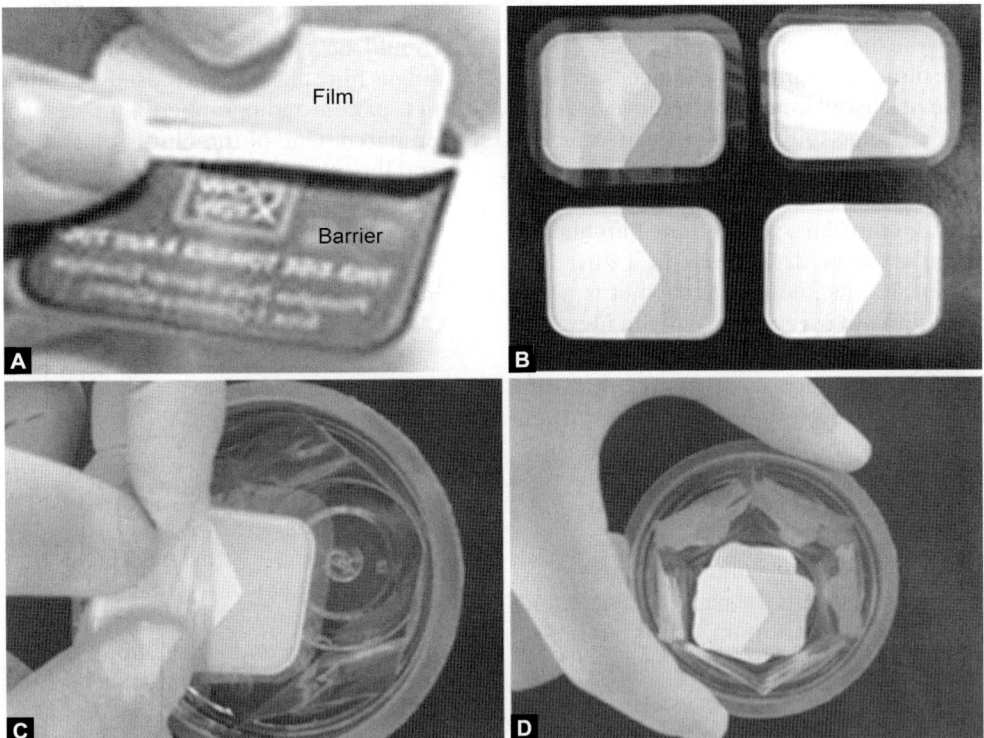

Figures 10.4A to D (A) Commercial barrier envelopes for infection control are available, in which the film is wrapped. Some companies prepackage the same and sell the product; (B) Film with protective plastic cover and films without the plastic cover; (C) Removal of the film after exposure from the plastic cover to prevent contamination; (D) Uncontaminated film, which can now be processed

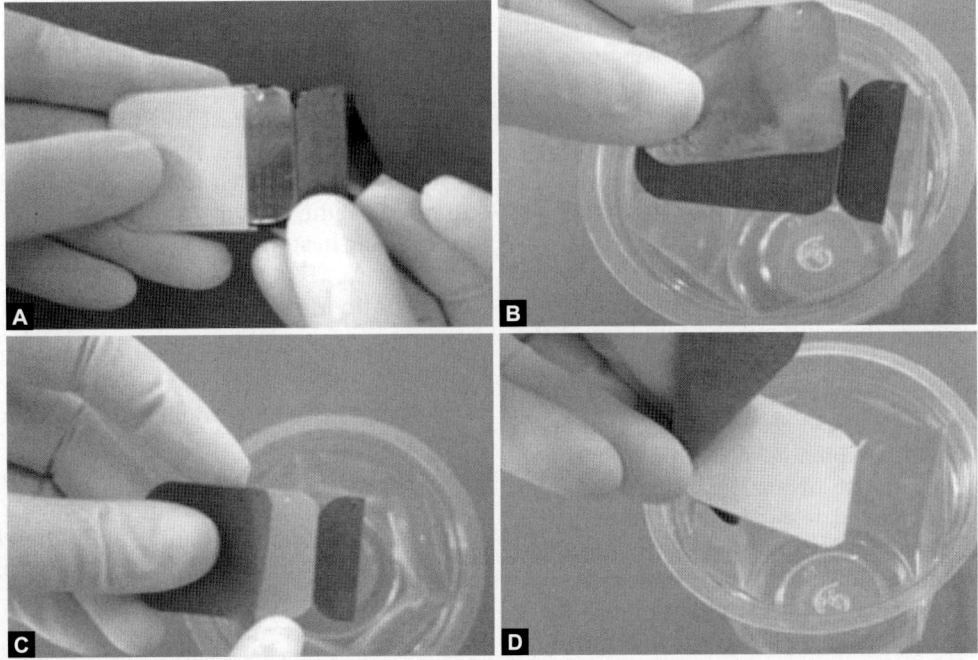

Figures 10.5A to D (A) Method of removing films from packet without touching with contaminated gloves. The tab is opened and the lead foil and black paper is slid out; (B) Rotate the foil away from the black paper and discard; (C) Open paper wrapping; (D) Allow film to be collected in a clean disposable cup

Excess fixation removes some of the metallic silver grains, diminishing the density of the film.

- After fixation of the films is complete, the hanger is placed in running water for at least 10 minutes to remove residual processing solutions. After the film has been washed, remove surface moisture by gently shaking excess water from the film and hanger. Cover the processing tank.
- Dry the film. To air dry the films, suspend the film hanger with the films from a rod or drying rack in a dust free area over a drip pan. If a heated drying cabinet is used, the temperature should not exceed 120°F. If the films dry rapidly with small drops of water clinging to their surface, the areas under the drops dry more slowly than the surrounding areas. This uneven drying causes distortion of the gelatin, leaving a drying artefact. The result is spots that frequently are visible and detract from the usefulness of the finished radiograph.

  After drying, the films are ready to mount.

- Remove the dry radiograph from the film hanger and place them in an envelope labeled with the patient's name and date of exposure. Out side the darkroom, use a view box to examine the radiograph and place them in a labeled film mount.
  - After the manual procedures have been completed, clean all processing equipment that was used and clean all work surfaces. A clean darkroom is essential for the production of diagnostic radiographs.
  - The interaction between the mineral salts in water and the carbonate in the processing solutions deposits on the inside of the insert tanks. Such deposits contaminate the processing solutions. The master and insert tanks must bc cleaned each time the solutions are changed. A commercial stainless steel tank cleaner or a solution of hydrochloric acid and water (1.5 ounces HCl to 128 ounces of water) can be used to remove the mineral salts and carbonate deposits. Abrasive type cleaners are not recommended as they may react adversely with the processing solutions.
- *Changing solutions*: All processing solutions deteriorate as a result of continuous processing and exposure to air. Replenishing prolongs their life but the build up of the reaction products eventually causes the solutions to cease functioning properly.

  Exhaustion of the developer results from oxidation of the developing agents, depletion of hydroquinone and builds up of bromide. Use of an exhausted developer results in films with reduced density and contrast.

  When the fixer becomes exhausted, silver thiosulfate complexes and halide ions build up. The increased concentration of the silver thiosulfate complexes slows the rate of diffusion of these complexes from the emulsion. The halide ions slow the rate of clearing of unexposed silver halide crystals. These changes result in films with incomplete clearing that turn brown with age.

A simple procedure can help determine when solutions should be changed. A double film packet instead of a single film packet is exposed on one projection for the first patient radiographed after new solutions have been prepared. One of the film is placed in the patients chart and the other is mounted on a corner of a view box in the darkroom. As successive films are processed, they are compared with this reference film. Loss of image contrast and density become evident as the solutions deteriorate, indicating when the time has come to change them. The fixer is changed when the developer is changed.

Visual Method

This manual method consists of placing the films in the developing solution and viewing them from time to time in the safe light, thus the degree of developing is at the operator's discretion.

The advantage of this method is that the film can be developed to the contrast and detail desired for the particular subject. And in case the film is over exposed it is possible to get good detail by under developing.

The disadvantage is that each film has to be processed individually and is very time consuming.

Rapid Processing Chemicals

In recent years manufacturers have produced rapid processing solutions that typically develop a film in 15 seconds at room temperature. They contain a higher concentration of hydroquinone and a more alkaline pH, which causes the emulsion to swell more, thus providing greater access to the developer. This has its applications in endodontics and emergency situations. The resultant images do not have the same degree of contrast and may discolor over a period of time if not fully washed. If these are kept in the conventional fixing solution (after viewing) for 4 minutes and washed for 10 minutes, the contrast is improved and the film becomes more stable in storage.

Automatic Method (Figs 10.6A and B)

This method uses equipment that automates all the processing steps. There are two types:

- Automatic dunking models that produces a washed film that still has to be dried.
- Miniature roller type that produces a dried film.

  The automatic processor may have a day light loading compartment for intraoral films thereby preluding the need to work in the darkroom (**Table 10.2**).

Advantages

- Rapidity of the operation, the entire process may take less than 4–7 minutes.
- Uniformity of results.

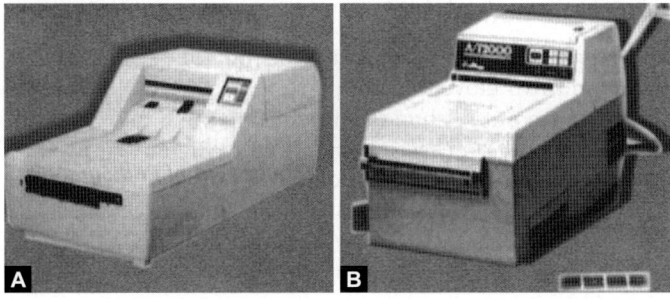

Figures 10.6A and B Automatic processor

Table 10.2 Guidelines for placement of films in the automatic processor

• Feed the film slowly and carefully, in a straight line, so as not to cause a jam-up in the processor
• If the film is bent, insert the unbent side of the film into the machine first
• Do not feed damp films into the machine as it will contaminate the rollers and cause streaking

- Less floor space required and have daylight loading capability.
- No wet films to be handled, no film hangers, and film dryer.
- No wet reading of films. A dry film is more useful diagnostically than a wet film.
- Density and contrast of the resultant radiograph are consistent.

Disadvantages

- Quality is not as high as that of a manually developed radiograph. More grain is evident in the final image.
- High cost of equipment and maintenance (**Table 10.3**).

Mechanism (Fig. 10.7)

The design is an in-line arrangement, consisting of a transport mechanism that picks up the unwrapped film and passes it through the developing, fixing, washing and drying sections. The transport system most often used is a series of rollers driven by a constant-speed motor that operates through gears, belts or chains. The rollers often consist of independent assemblies of multiple rollers in a rack, with one rack for each step. These assemblies are designed and positioned so that the film crosses over from one roller to the next, the operator may also be able to remove them independently for soaking, cleaning and repairing.

The function of the roller is to:
- Primarily move the film through the developing solutions.
- Their motion keeps the solutions agitated.

Table 10.3 Maintenance schedule for the automatic processor

- Daily.
  - Temperature of the developer should be from 80°–83°F depending on the time cycle.
    81°–83°F for a longer cycle.
    80°F for a 5 ½ minute cycle.
    83°F for a 4 minute cycle.
  - Drain water section daily. Run a cleaning film through each morning.
  - Transport sections should be checked for proper alignment.
  - Cover the processor at the end of the day leaving it slightly open to allow chemical fumes to escape.
- Weekly.
  - Soak and wash the roller sections with warm water thoroughly for 10–15 minutes, on a weekly basis. Run minimum two cleaning films through the processor before use.
  - Change/replenish solutions every 2–4 weeks depending on the work load. Use only automatic processing solutions, manual processing solution can damage the processor.
- Monthly.
  - Clean developer section with special developer cleaner (to prevent fogging of films).
  - Clean fixer section with warm water (to prevent formation of crystals on the rollers).
  - Clean wash section with household bleach/water solution (to prevent scum formation which form spots and artefacts on films).
  - Rinse all racks thoroughly with water after removing from cleaning solutions.
  - Visually check dryer and dust as required.
  - All moving parts like, gears, sprockets, idlers, bearings, drive mechanisms and ring points should be well lubricated to prevent excessive wear of moving parts. Take precaution that no oil spills on the rollers.

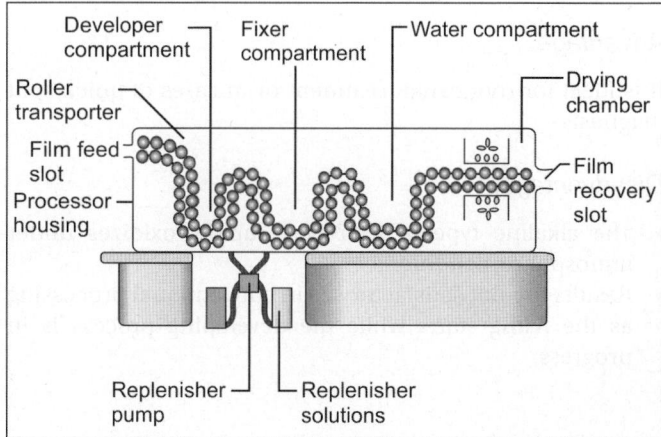

Figure 10.7 Component parts of the automatic processor

- In the developer, fixer and water tanks the rollers press on the film emulsion, forcing solution out of the emulsion. The emulsions rapidly fill again with solutions thus promoting solution exchange.
- The top roller at the cross over point between the developer and fixer tanks removes developing solution, minimizing carryover of the developer into the fixer tank. There by maintaining the uniformity of the processing chemicals.

The chemical composition of the developer and fixer is modified to operate at higher temperatures than used for manual processing and to meet the more rapid development, fixing, washing and drying requirement of automatic processing. The fixer has an additional hardener that helps the emulsion withstand the rigors of the transport system.

Replenishment

It is important to maintain the developer and fixer carefully to preserve the optimal sensitometric and physical properties of the film emulsion within the narrow limits of the speed and temperature of automatic processing. To compensate for the loss of activity some automatic processors include an automatic replenisher system. As in the manual processing, 8 ounces of fresh developer and fixer should be added per gallon of solution per day, assuming that 30 intraoral or 5 extraoral films are developed per day.

Insufficient replenishment of the developer results in a loss of contrast.

Exhaustion of the fixing solution causes poor clearing, insufficient hardening, and unreliable transport from the fixer assembly to the drying operation.

Monobath Method

In this method the developer and fixer are combined in one solution. The fixer is alkaline and does not neutralize the developer. This monobath is injected into a special water proof film packet and the film is developed by simply rubbing the film packet. There is no need of a darkroom.

Advantage

It is ideal for root canal treatment or in cases of quick spot diagnosis.

Disadvantages

- The alkaline type of fixer very rapidly oxidizes under atmospheric conditions.
- Results are not satisfactory as in conventional processing as the fixing starts while the developing process is in progress.

Day Light Method

This is carried out in a special device provided with safe light filters and two glove like compartments through which the operator can put his hands and develop the films. The films are opened and processed in subdued daylight.

- There is no need of the darkroom.
- This requires a special day light film by Kodak to be used.
- The emulsion consists of a yellow dye and the film appears yellow and black instead of the conventional blue white and black.

Digitized Processing Method

Digital images may be processed by two systems:
1. CR system or computed radiography system
2. DR system or digital radiography system.

CR system: In the CR system, instead of the cassette with an X-ray film, an IP cassette (**Fig. 10.8A**) is used. After exposing the cassette it is loaded into a Reader Unit (**Fig. 10.8B**). The image is read off the cassette and the cassette is cleared. The captured image is transferred to a workstation, where the operator can view the same on the monitor. The image may be enhanced, restored, analyzed, compressed, or synthesized as per the requirement and then stored in the computer or an output may be given on the printer (paper), Dry Laser Imager (**Figs 10.8C and D**), Compact disc. The image may also be transferred to the other departments/hospitals etc. via LAN/WAN connections and e-mail.

*DR system (**Fig. 10.9**):* Here the cassette is replaced by a sensor which is directly connected to the workstation, via cables or wireless devices. The image can be analyzed, interpreted, stored or sent to other departments in a manner similar to that used for the CR system.

Self-Developing Films (Figs 10.10A and B)

These are a recent advance in manual processing. The X-ray film is presented in a special sachet containing developer and fixer. Following exposure the developer tab is pulled, releasing developer solution which is milked down towards the film, and massaged around it. After about 30 seconds the fixer tab is pulled to release the fixer solution which is similarly milked down to the film. After fixing, the used chemicals are discarded and the film is rinsed thoroughly under running water for about 10 minutes.

Advantages

- No darkroom or processing facilities required.
- Time saving—the final radiograph is ready in about a minute.

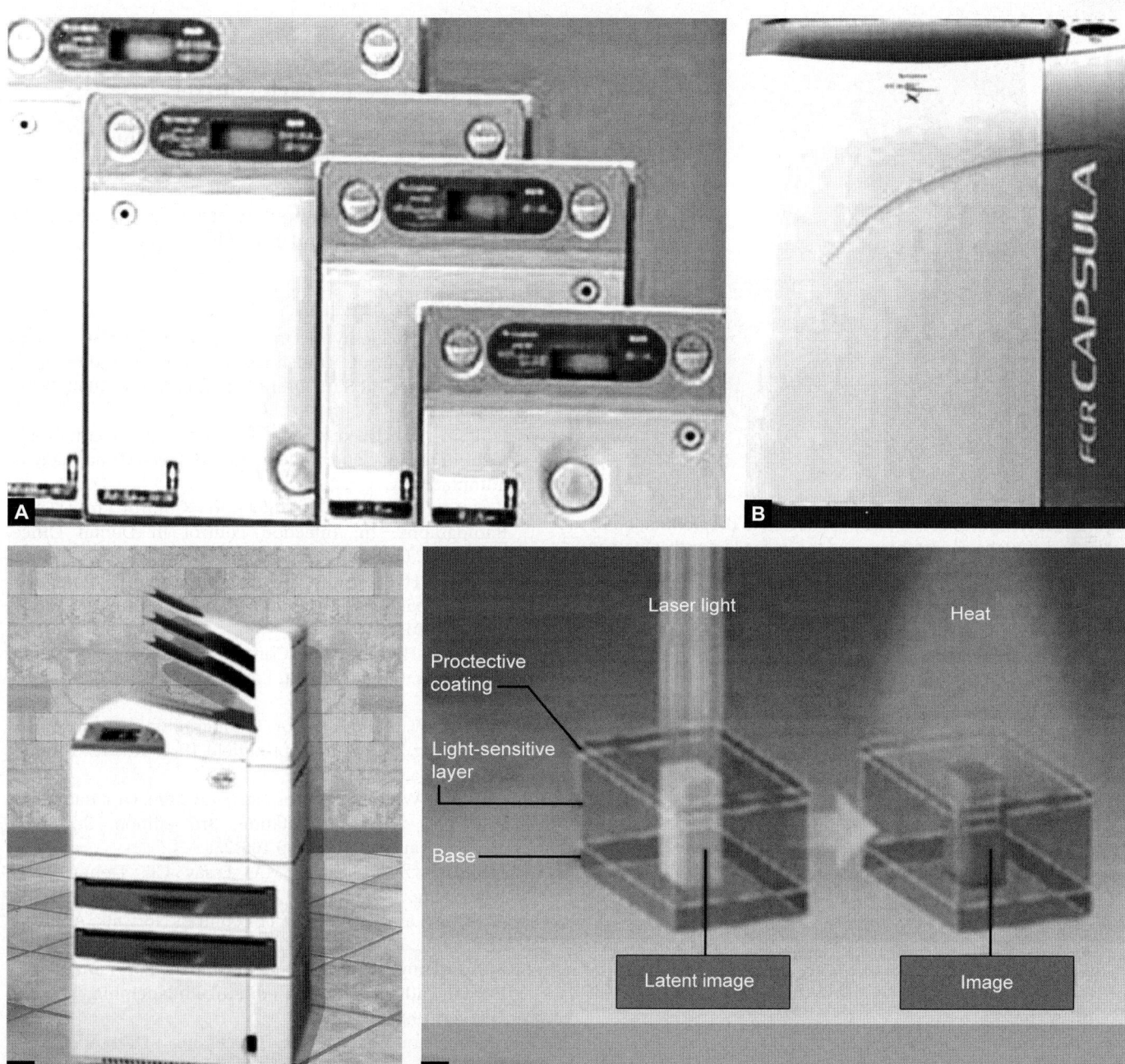

Figures 10.8A to D (A) IP cassettes laser imager; (B) Reader unit; (C) Printer-dry; (D) Dry laser imaging system; this process utilizes interpolation to magnify or reduce medical diagnostic images read from modalities, generating film image outputs in a variety of formats. Exposing the film surface to a modulating laser in accordance with the inputted data produces ultra-precise images while significantly reducing throughput time. There are no messy chemicals to handle or dispose off

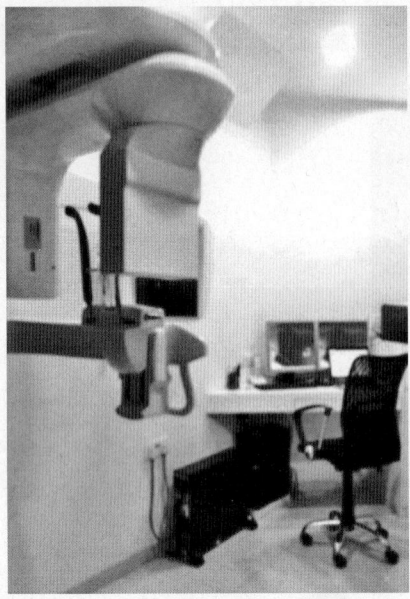

Figure 10.9 A CBCT unit is directly connected to the workstation by cables and after the patient is exposed the image is directly obtained on the monitor

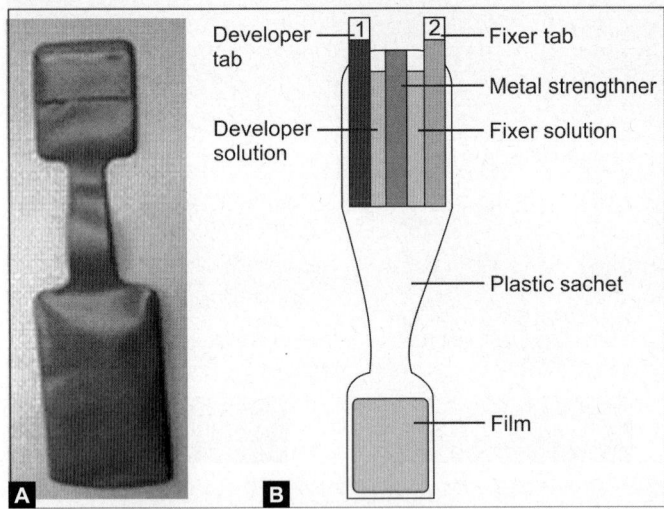

Figures 10.10A and B (A) Self-developing film; (B) Diagram showing the basic internal design

Disadvantages

- Poor overall image quality
- The image deteriorate rapidly with time
- There is no lead foil inside the film packet
- The film packet is very flexible and easily bent
- These films are difficult to use in positioning holders
- Relatively expensive (a rigid, plastic, backing support tray for the film is manufactured, which helps to reduce the problems of flexibility and lack of lead foil).

BIBLIOGRAPHY

1. American Academy of Oral and Maxillofacial Radiology infection control guidelines for dental radiographic procedures. Oral Surg Oral Med Oral Pathol. 1992; 73(2): 248-9.
2. DuPont EI, DeNemours and Co. Inc. Dark room techniques for better radiographs processed manually or automatically.
3. Eastman Kodak Co. Infection Control in Dental Radiography. In: Infection control in Dental Office, Rochester, Eastman Kodak Co. 1989;1-11.
4. Frommer HH. Film Processing - Darkroom. Radiology for Dental Auxillaries, 6th edition. St. Louis: Mosby-Year Book; 1996.pp.101-37.
5. Frommer HH. Infection Control in Radiology for Dental Auxillaries, 6th edition. St. Louis: Mosby Year Book; 1996. pp.89-99.
6. Fuchs AW. Principles of Radiographic Exposure and Processing, 2nd edition. Springfield, III, Charles C. Thomas, 1979.
7. Goaz PW, White SC. Processing X-ray Film. Oral Radiology, Principles and Interpretation, 3rd edition. St. Louis: Mosby-Year Book; 1994.pp.106-25.
8. Johnson ON, McNally MA, Essay CE. Dental X-ray Processing. Essentials of Dental Radiography for Dental Assistants and Hygienists, 6th edition. Norwalk, Appleton and Lange; 1999.pp.179-210.
9. Mason-Hing LR. Infection Control, In: Fundamentals of Dental Radiography, 3rd edition. Philadelphia: Lea and Febiger; 1990.pp.230-42.
10. Mason-Hing LR. Film Processing Darkroom and Duplicating. Fundamentals of Dental Radiography, 3rd edition. Philadelphia: WB Saunders; 1993.pp.20-35.

Developer tab
Fixer tab
Metal strengthner
Developer solution
Fixer solution
Plastic sachet
Film

Section V

Imaging Techniques

Intraoral Radiographic Techniques | 11

The basic principles of projection geometry (shadow casting) are:

- The focal spot (source of radiation) should be as small as possible (**Figs 11.1A to C**).
- The focal spot-object distance should be as long as possible (**Fig. 11.2**).
- The object-film distance should be as small as possible (**Fig. 11.3**).
- The long axis of the object and the film planes should be parallel (**Fig. 11.4**).
- The X-ray beam should strike the object and the film planes at right angles (**Fig. 11.5**).
- There should be no movement of the tube, film or patient during exposure. (Given by Mason and Lincoln) (**Fig. 11.6**).

There are three types of intraoral radiography:

- *Periapical*: Showing all of the tooth and the surrounding bone.
- *Bite wing*: Showing crowns of maxillary and mandibular teeth and adjacent alveolar crests.
- *Occlusal*: It shows images of the incisal edges and occlusal surfaces of teeth, and cross-section of the dental arches.

Intraoral localization techniques: Using the above techniques in combination we can help to localize objects in the oral cavity and jaws.

PERIAPICAL RADIOGRAPHY

Indications

- Detection of apical infection/inflammation
- Assessment of periodontal status
- After trauma to assess the teeth and alveolar bone
- Assessment of the presence and position of unerupted teeth
- Assessment of root morphology before extractions
- During endodontic therapy
- Preoperative assessment and postoperative appraisal of apical surgery
- Detailed evaluation of apical cysts and other lesions within the alveolar bone.
- Assessment of the position and prognosis of implants.

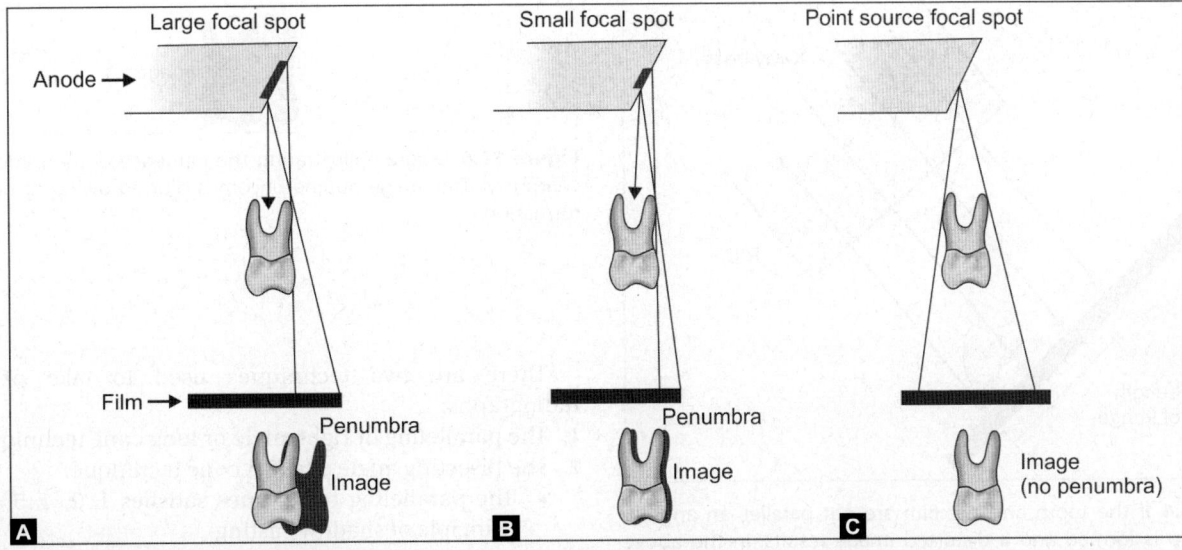

Figure 11.1 The smaller the focal spot area, the sharper the image. Larger the focal spot area, the greater the amount of penumbra and loss of image sharpness. Theoretical 'point source' of X-rays would produce a sharp image without penumbra

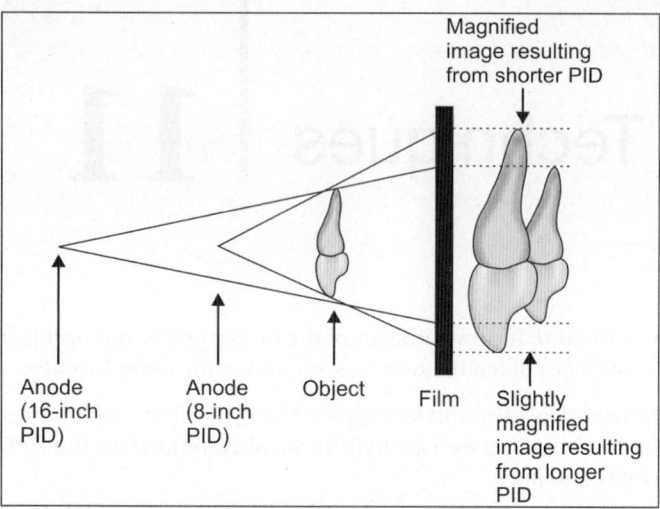

Figure 11.2 A longer PID and target film distance results in less magnification

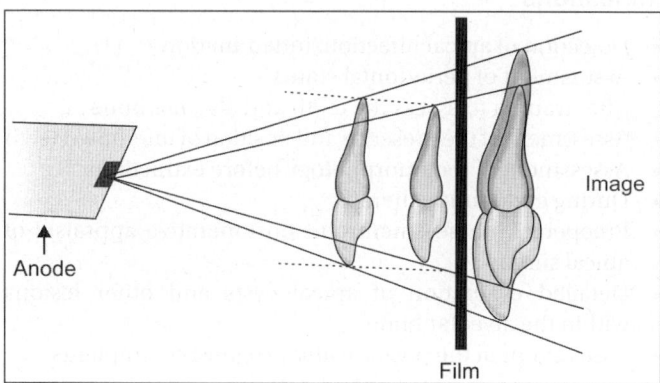

Figure 11.3 Diagram illustrating object film distance. The closer the proximity of the tooth to the film, lesser the image enlargement

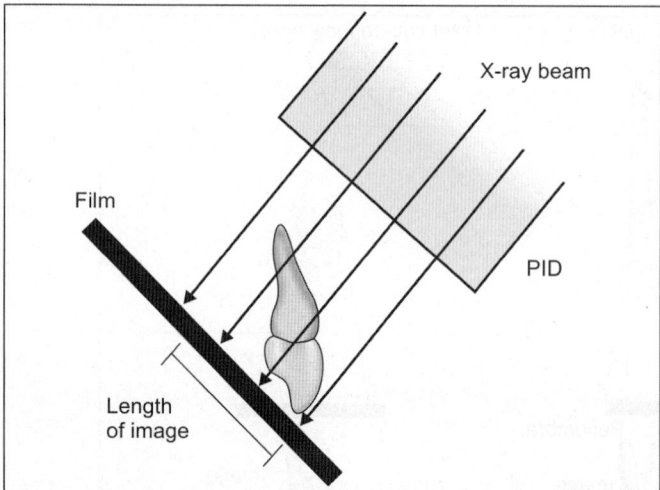

Figure 11.4 If the tooth and the film are not parallel, an angular relationship is formed and a distorted image results. In the above diagram the length of the image that appears on the film is shorter than the actual tooth

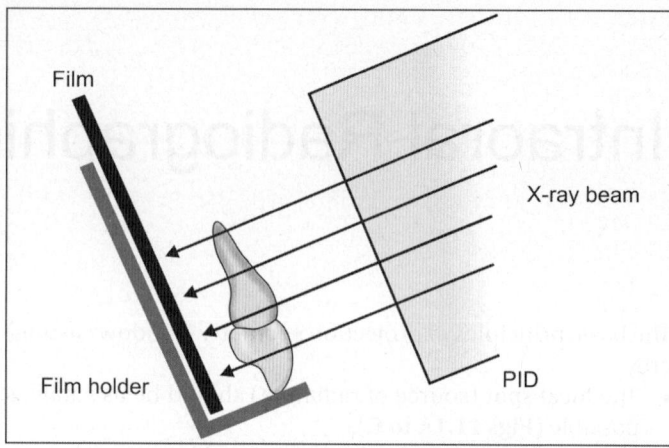

Figure 11.5 To limit distortion, the central ray of the X-ray beam must be perpendicular to the tooth and the film

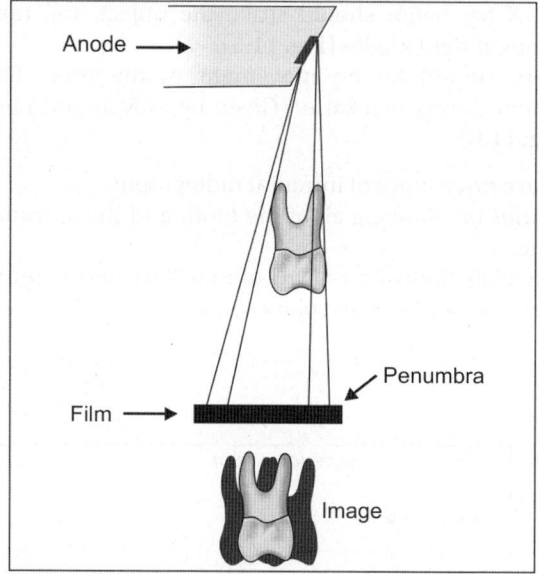

Figure 11.6 Diagram illustrating the influence of motion on image sharpness. The image outline becomes blurred owing to penumbra formation

There are two techniques used to take periapical radiographs:
1. The paralleling or right angle or long cone technique
2. The bisecting angle or short cone technique.
   - The paralleling techniques satisfies 1, 2, 4, 5 and 6th principle of shadow casting.
   - The bisecting angle technique satisfies 1, 3 and 6th principle of shadow casting.

PARALLELING TECHNIQUE (FIG. 11.7)

The essence of this technique is that the X-ray film is supported parallel to the long axis of the tooth and the central ray of the X-ray beam is directed at right angles to the tooth and film.

To achieve parallelism between the film and the tooth, the film must be placed away from the tooth and towards the middle of the oral cavity. Because of the anatomic configuration of the oral cavity (e.g. curvature of the palate), the object film distance must thus be increased to keep the film parallel with the long axis of the tooth. As the film is placed away from the tooth, image magnification and loss of definition results.

To compensate for image magnification, the target film distance must also be increased to ensure that only the most parallel rays will be directed at the tooth and the film. As a result a long (16 inch) target film distance must be used with the paralleling technique and hence this technique is also referred to as Long Cone Technique. The 'long' refers to the length of the cone or position indicating device (PID). The use of the long target film distance in the paralleling technique results in less image magnification and better definition.

Film holders: The paralleling technique requires the use of film holders. A film holder is defined as a device that is used to position an intraoral film in the mouth and retain the film in position during exposure. The film holder eliminates the need of the patient to stabilize the film.

The holder having the aiming rings help in the alignment of the PID with the film. Thus in long cone technique the horizontal and vertical angulations are determined and standardized by the aiming ring. The vertical angulation of the central ray is directed perpendicular to the film and the long axis of the tooth.

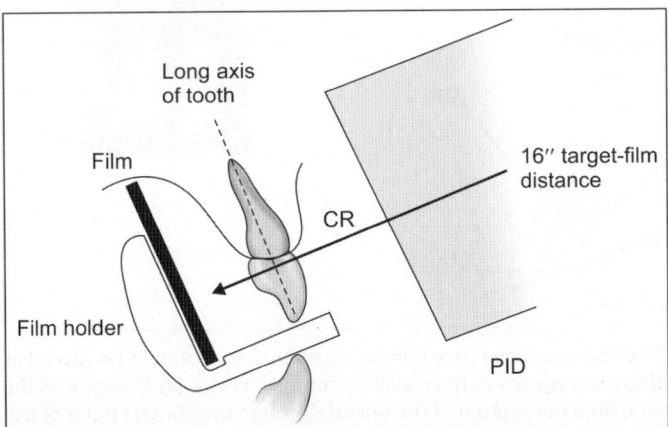

Figure 11.7 Positions of the film, tooth and the central ray of the X-ray beam in the paralleling technique. The film and long axis of the tooth are parallel. The central ray is perpendicular to the tooth and the film. An increased target film distance (16 inches) is required

Film: Ideally the size of the film used will depend upon the teeth being radiographed.
- *Size 1*: Film is used for anterior teeth, as this is a narrow film
- *Size 2*: Film is used for the posterior region.

Guidelines for Film Placement

- The white side of the film always faces the teeth.
- The film when used for anterior teeth is always placed vertically.
- The film when used for posterior teeth is always placed horizontally.
- The identification dot on the film is always placed in the slot of the film holder, or towards the occlusal end of the film.
- When positioning the film holder, always center the film over the area or tooth to be examined.

Patient Positioning for Paralleling Technique

- Briefly explain the procedure to the patient before you begin.
- Adjust the chair so that the patient is positioned upright in the chair. The level of the chair must be adjusted to a comfortable working height for the dental surgeon.
- Adjust the head rest to support and position the patient's head. The patient's head must be positioned so that the upper arch (occlusal plane) is parallel to the floor and the midsagittal (mid line) plane is perpendicular to the floor.
- Secure the lead apron and thyroid collar on the patient.
- Remove all objects from the mouth (e.g. dentures, retainers, chewing gum, etc.) that may interfere with the film exposure. Eye glasses must be removed also.

There are following basic rules to be followed in the paralleling technique:
- *Film placement*: The film must be positioned to cover the prescribed area of the teeth to be examined.
- *Film position*: The film must be positioned parallel to the long axis of the tooth. The film, in the film holder must be placed away from the teeth and towards the middle of the oral cavity.
  - *Maxillary incisors and canines*: The film packet is positioned sufficiently posteriorly, to enable its height to be accommodated in the vault of the palate.
  - *Maxillary premolars and molars*: The film packet is placed in the midline of the palate, again to accommodate its height in the vault of the palate.
  - *Mandibular incisors and canines*: The film packet is positioned in the floor of the mouth, roughly in line with the lower canines or first premolars.
  - *Mandibular premolars and molars*: The film packet is placed in the lingual sulcus next to the appropriate teeth.

- Alignment of the X-ray beam:
  - *Vertical angulation*: The central ray of the X-ray beam must be directed perpendicular to the film and the long axis of the tooth.
  - *Horizontal angulation*: The central ray of the X-rays beam must be directed through the contact areas between the teeth.
  - *Film exposure*: The X-ray beam must be centered on the film to ensure that all areas of the film are exposed. Failure to center the X-ray beam results in a partial image on the film or a 'cone-cut'.
- The exposure is made.

Specific positioning for different areas of the mouth, and the resultant radiographs are shown in **Figures 11.8 to 11.18** respectively.

Advantage of Long Cone Technique

- *Accuracy*: The paralleling technique produces an image that has dimensional accuracy (A profile view of the tooth with buccal and lingual roots projected in their normal respective lengths and buccal and lingual cusps correctly related on the same plane); the image is very representative of the actual tooth.

- The radiographic image is free of distortion and exhibits maximum detail and definition.
- There is no overlap of related structures (e.g. the zygomatic shadow), all shadows of anatomical structures are cast in their proper anatomic position.
- This accuracy is due to:
  - Increased source film distance.
  - Object and film are parallel to each other.
  - Central ray strikes perpendicular to the long axis of the tooth and film.
  - Though the object film distance is increased, it is compensated by increased source film distance and therefore there is decreased enlargement.
  - The increased kVp, to reduce exposure time, as the source film distance is increased, helps by reducing secondary and unwanted, short wave length radiations.
- *Simplicity*: This technique is simple and easy to learn and use. The film holder with a beam alignment device eliminates the need for all dental surgeons to determine horizontal and vertical angulations and also eliminates chances of dimensional distortion and coning off.
- *Duplication*: This technique is easy to standardize and can be accurately duplicated or repeated, when serial radiographs are indicated. As a result comparison of serial radiographs exposed using this technique have great validity.

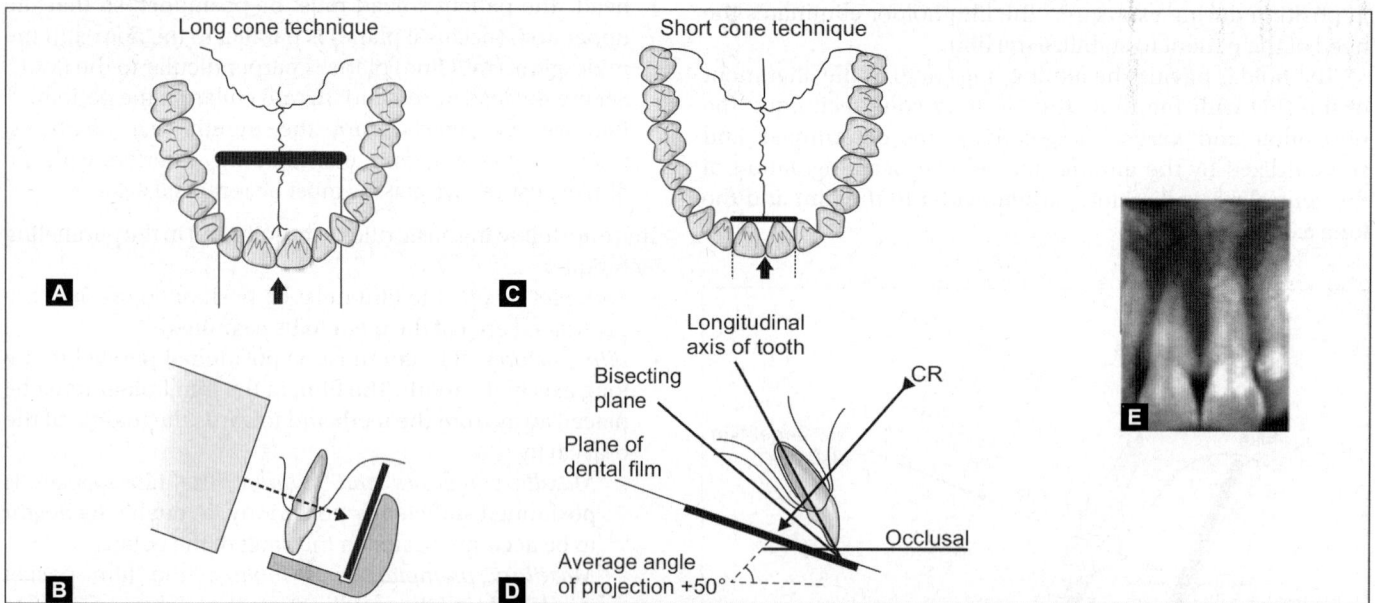

Figures 11.8A to E *Periapical technique for maxillary central incisor*: (A) *Film placement (Long cone paralleling technique)*: It should be placed at the level of the second premolars or first molars, with the long axis parallel to the long axis of the maxillary central incisors; (B) *Projection of the central ray (Long cone technique)*. Directed high on the lip, in the midline, just below the septum of the nostril. Through the contact point of the central incisors and perpendicular to the plane of the film and roots of the teeth. Because the axial inclination of the maxillary incisors is about 15° to 20°, the vertical angulation of the tube should be at the same positive angulation; (C) *Film placement (Short cone bisecting angle technique)*: The film is placed behind the maxillary central incisors in line with the midline of the arch. The film is placed with the superior border on the palate and the inferior border extending just beyond the incisal edges of the teeth; (D) *Projection of central ray (Short cone technique)*: The point of entry is through the midline, through the tip of the nose, through the contact point of the central incisors and perpendicular to the plane bisecting the angle between the long axis of the film and the roots of the teeth (+45° to +50°); (E) Radiograph of maxillary central incisor

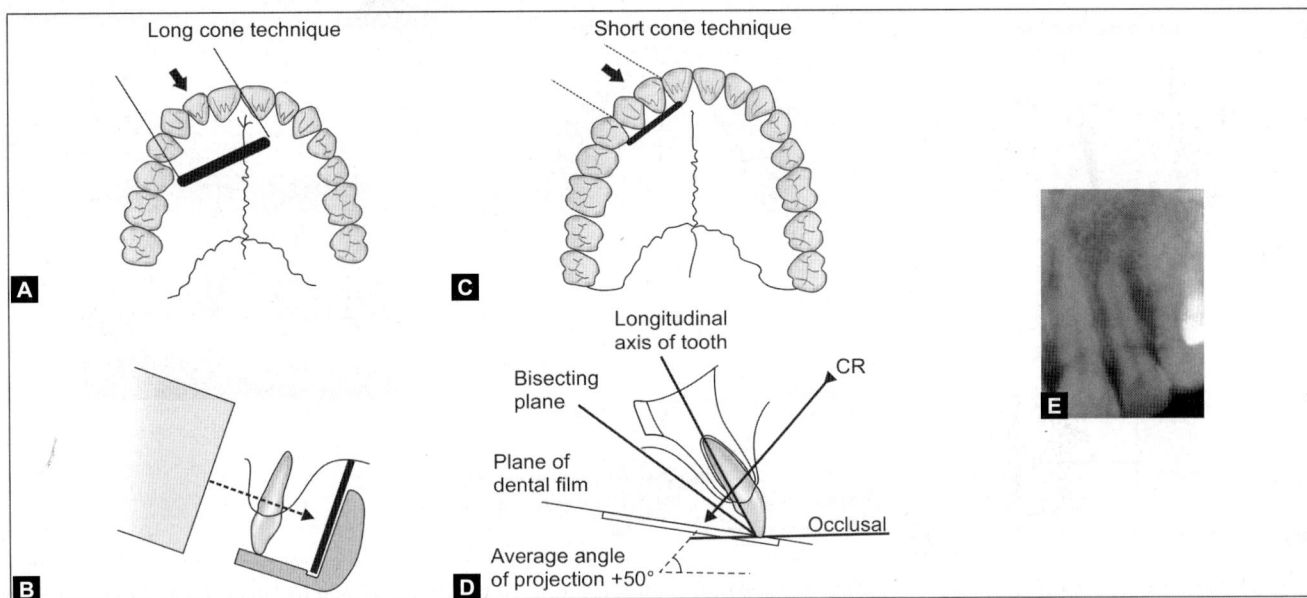

Figures 11.9A to E *Periapical technique for maxillary lateral incisor*: (A) *Film placement (Long cone paralleling technique)*: It should be placed parallel to the long axis and the mesiodistal plane of the maxillary lateral incisors; (B) *Projection of the central ray (Long cone technique)*: Directed high on the lip, about 1 cm from the midline. Through the middle of the lateral incisors, with no overlapping of the margins of the crowns at the interproximal space on its mesial aspect; (C) *Film placement (Short cone bisecting angle technique)*: The film is placed behind the maxillary lateral incisors. The film is placed with the superior border on the palate and the inferior border extending just beyond the incisal edges of the teeth; (D) *Projection of central ray (Short cone technique)*: The point of entry is through ala of the nose about 1 cm from the midline, through the middle of the lateral incisor and the open mesial contact area, and perpendicular to the plane bisecting the angle between the long axis of the film and the root of the tooth (+45° to +55°); (E) Radiograph of maxillary lateral incisor

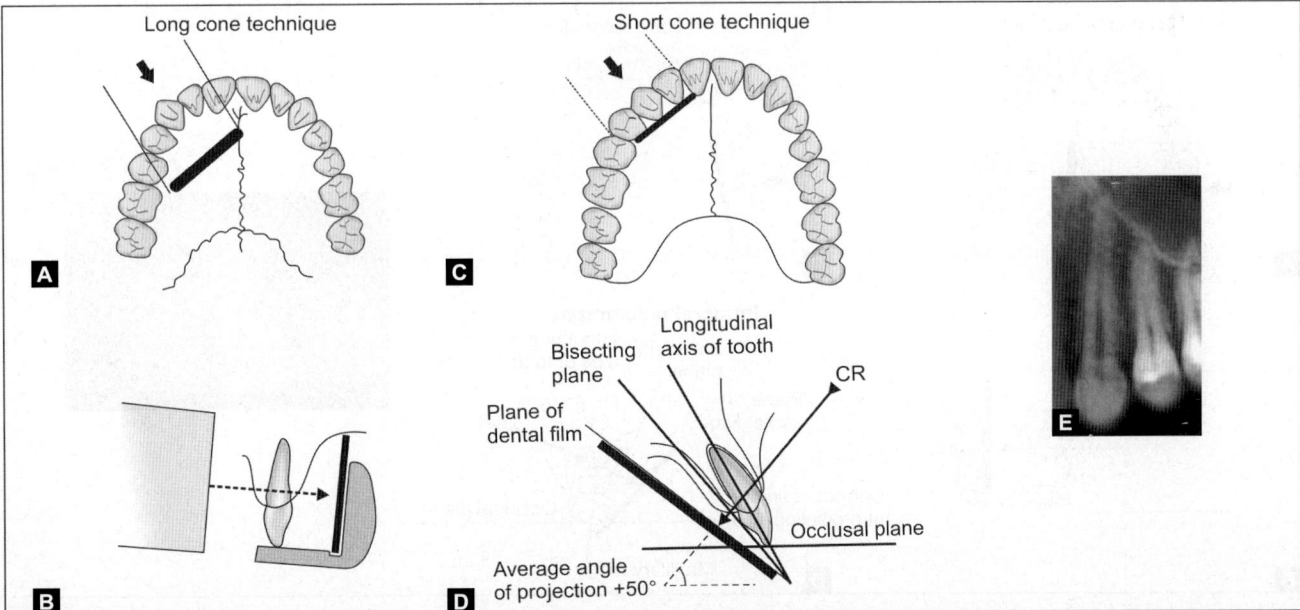

Figures 11.10A to E *Periapical technique for maxillary canine*: (A) *Film placement (Long cone paralleling technique)*: It should be placed against the palate, well away from the palatal surface of the teeth. Orient the film packet with its anterior edge at about the middle of the lateral incisor and its long axis parallel with the long axis of the canine; (B) *Projection of the central ray (Long cone technique)*: Directed through the canine eminence, at the intersection of the distal and inferior borders of the ala of the nose, through the mesial contact of the canine; (C) *Film placement (Short cone bisecting angle technique)*: The film is placed with the superior border against the palate and the inferior border extending just below the cusp of the canine, with the long axis of the tooth superimposed on the central long axis of the film; (D) *Projection of central ray (Short cone technique)*: The point of entry is through canine eminence, and perpendicular to the plane bisecting the angle between the long axis of the film and the root of the tooth (+40 to +45°). The horizontal angulation should be through the mesial contact of the canine; (E) Radiograph of maxillary canine

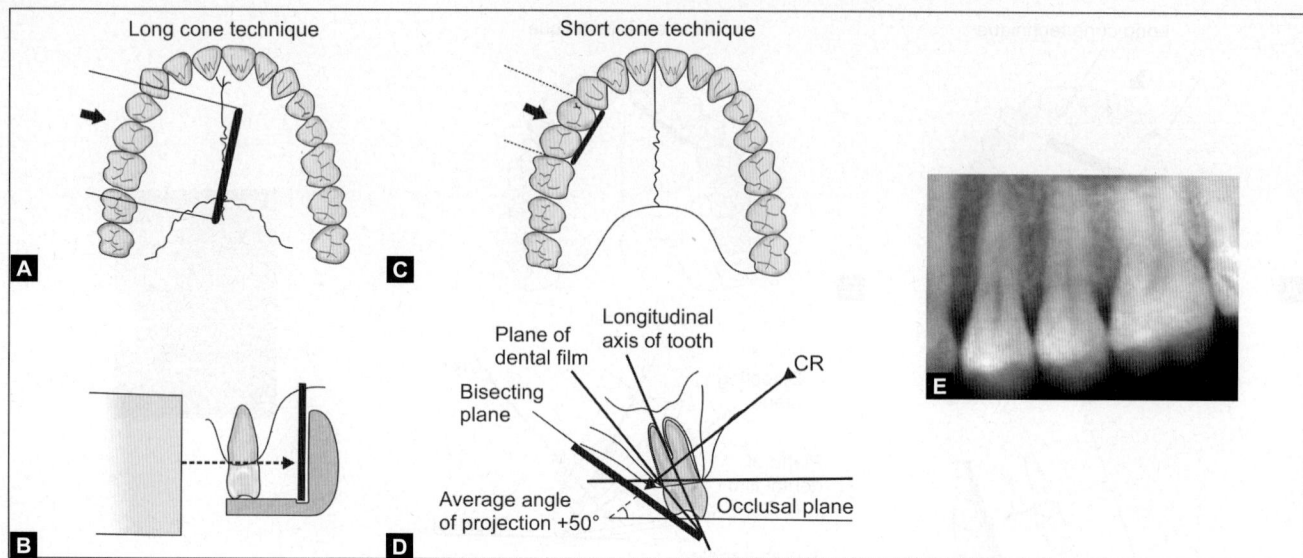

Figures 11.11A to E *Periapical technique for maxillary premolar*: (A) *Film placement (Long cone paralleling technique)*: Should be placed with the long dimension parallel with the occlusal plane and in the midline. It should cover the distal half of the canine, the premolars, and the first molar. The plane of the film should be nearly vertical to correspond with the long axis of the premolar teeth. (The long axis of the film should be approximately parallel to the mean buccal plane of the premolars); (B) *Projection of the central ray (Long cone technique)*: Directed through the center of the second premolar root, approximately below the pupil of the eye; (C) *Film placement (Short cone bisecting angle technique)*: The film is placed with the long dimension parallel with the occlusal plane and positioned with the superior border on the palate and the inferior border extending just below the buccal cusps of the premolars and first molar; (D) *Projection of central ray (Short cone technique)*: The point of entry is below the pupil of the eye, close to the level of the ala tragus line, and perpendicular to the plane bisecting the angle between the long axis of the film and the root of the tooth (+25° to +30°). The horizontal angulation should direct the beam between the first and second premolars; (E) Radiograph of maxillary premolars

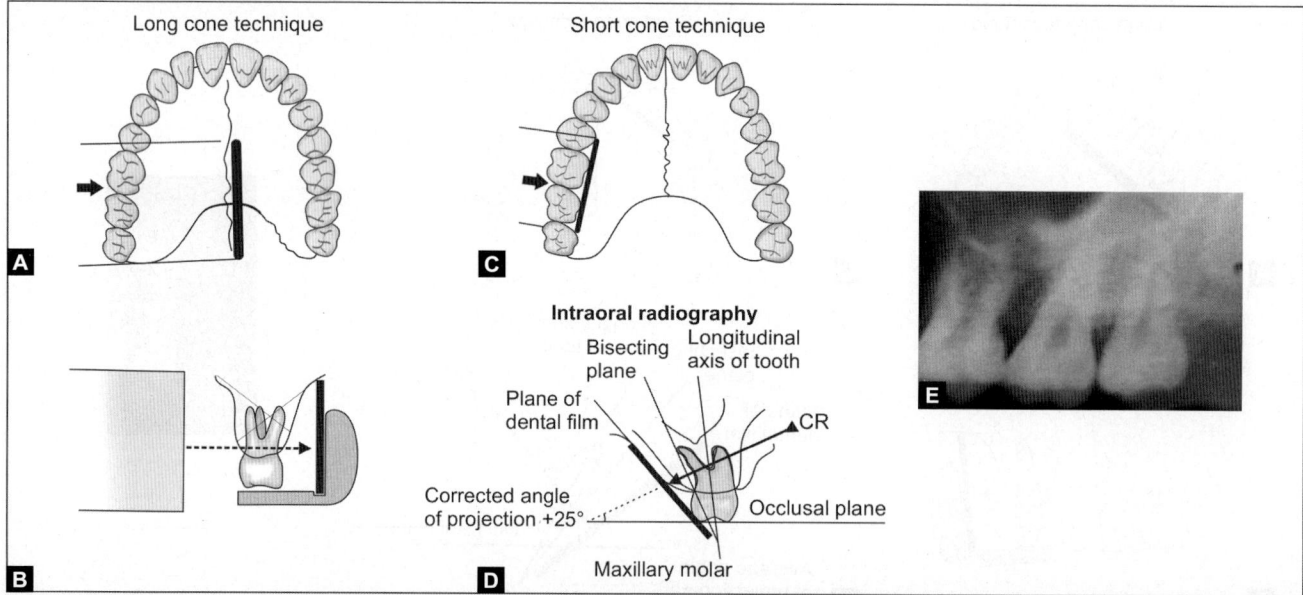

Figures 11.12A to E *Periapical technique for maxillary molar*: (A) *Film placement (Long cone paralleling technique)*: It should be placed parallel with the occlusal plane and in the midline, far enough posterior to cover the first, second and third molar areas and some of the tuberosity. The anterior border should just cover the distal aspect of the second premolar; (B) *Projection of the central ray (Long cone technique)*: Directed on the cheek below the outer canthus of the eye and the zygoma at the position of the maxillary second molar, perpendicular to the plane of the film; (C) *Film placement (Short cone bisecting angle technique)*: The film is placed with the long dimension parallel with the occlusal plane and far enough posteriorly positioned with the superior border on the palate and the inferior border extending just below the buccal cusps of the maxillary molars; (D) *Projection of central ray (Intraoral radiography) (Short cone technique)*: The point of entry is on the cheek in line with the outer canthus of the eye, below the zygoma and on an anteroposterior level with the second molar. The central ray should be perpendicular to the plane bisecting the angle between the long axis of the film and the root of the tooth (+30°). The horizontal angulation should direct the beam between the interproximal spaces between the molar teeth; (E) Radiograph of maxillary molars

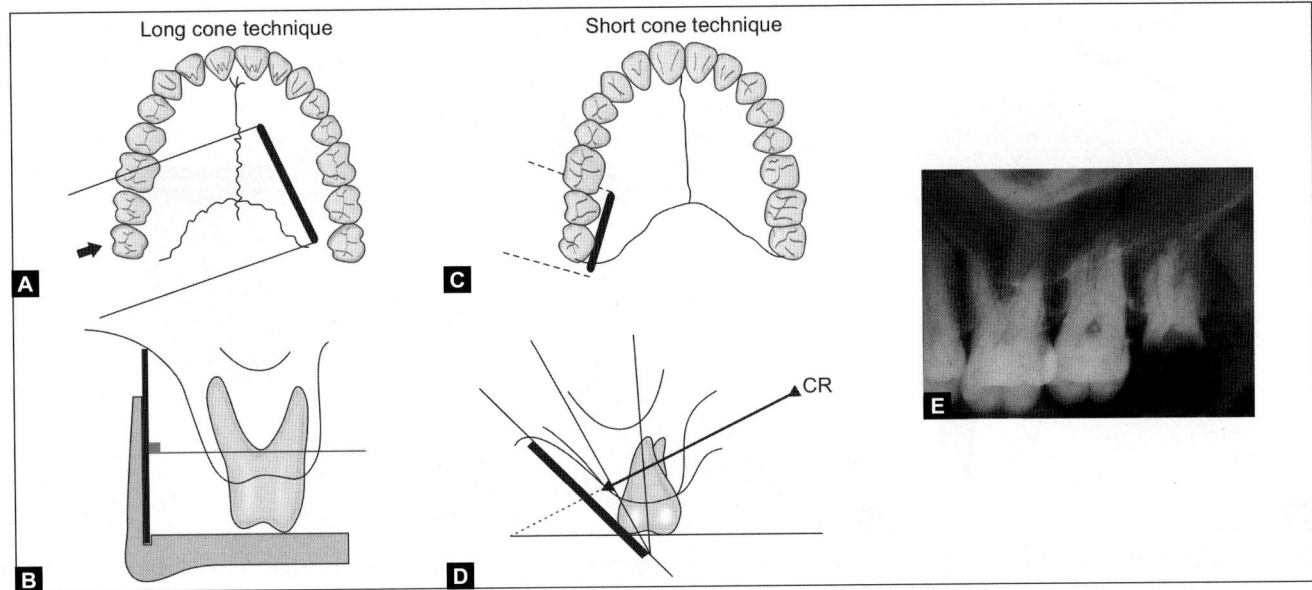

Figures 11.13A to E *Periapical technique for maxillary third molar*: (A) *Film placement (Long cone paralleling technique)*: It should be placed in the midline, far enough posterior to cover the tuberosity and area distal to it. The film should be angled across the midline so that the posterior border is away from the teeth of interest and the anterior border is near the molars on the side being radiographed; (B) *Projection of the central ray (Long cone technique)*: Directed through the maxillary third molar region just below the middle of the zygomatic arch, distal to the lateral canthus of the eye, perpendicular to the angled film; (C) *Film placement (Short cone bisecting angle technique)*: The film is placed with the long dimension parallel with the occlusal plane and far enough posteriorly positioned with the superior border on the palate and the inferior border extending just below the buccal cusps of the maxillary molars; (D) *Projection of central ray (Short cone technique)*: The point of entry is on the cheek in line with the outer canthus of the eye, below the zygoma and on an anteroposterior level between the second and third molar. The central ray should be perpendicular to the plane bisecting the angle between the long axis of the film and the root of the tooth (+25° to +30°). The horizontal angulation should direct the beam between the interproximal spaces between the molar teeth; (E) Radiograph of maxillary third molar

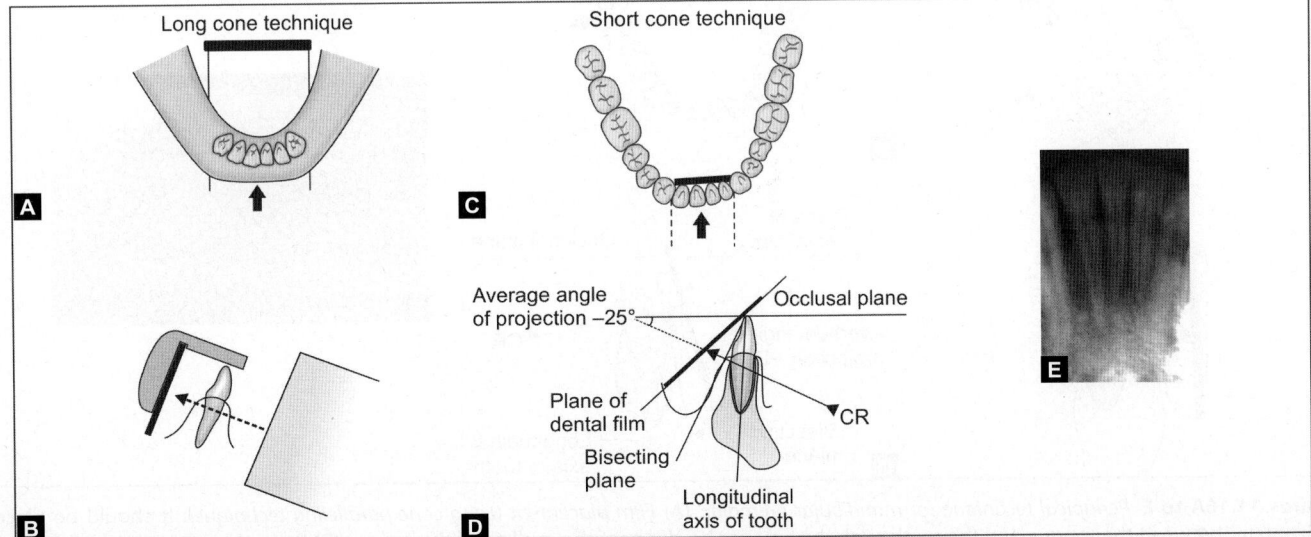

Figures 11.14A to E *Periapical technique for mandibular central and lateral incisors*: (A) *Film placement (Long cone paralleling technique)*: It should be placed vertically behind the central and lateral incisors with the contact area centered and the lower border below the tongue. The film should be placed as far back posteriorly, usually between the premolars; (B) *Projection of the central ray (Long cone technique)*: Directed below the lower lip, about 1 cm lateral to the midline, through the interproximal space between the central and lateral incisors; (C) *Film placement (Short cone bisecting technique)*: The film should be placed directly behind the central and lateral incisors with the superior border on the incisal edge of the teeth and the inferior border displaced distally, extending onto the lingual mucosa; (D) *Projection of central ray (Short cone technique)*: It should enter below the vermillion border of the lip. Approximately 1 cm from the midline. The central ray should be angled perpendicular to the bisector through the contact areas of the central and lateral incisors. The vertical angulation should be –15° to –25°; (E) Radiograph of mandibular central and lateral incisor

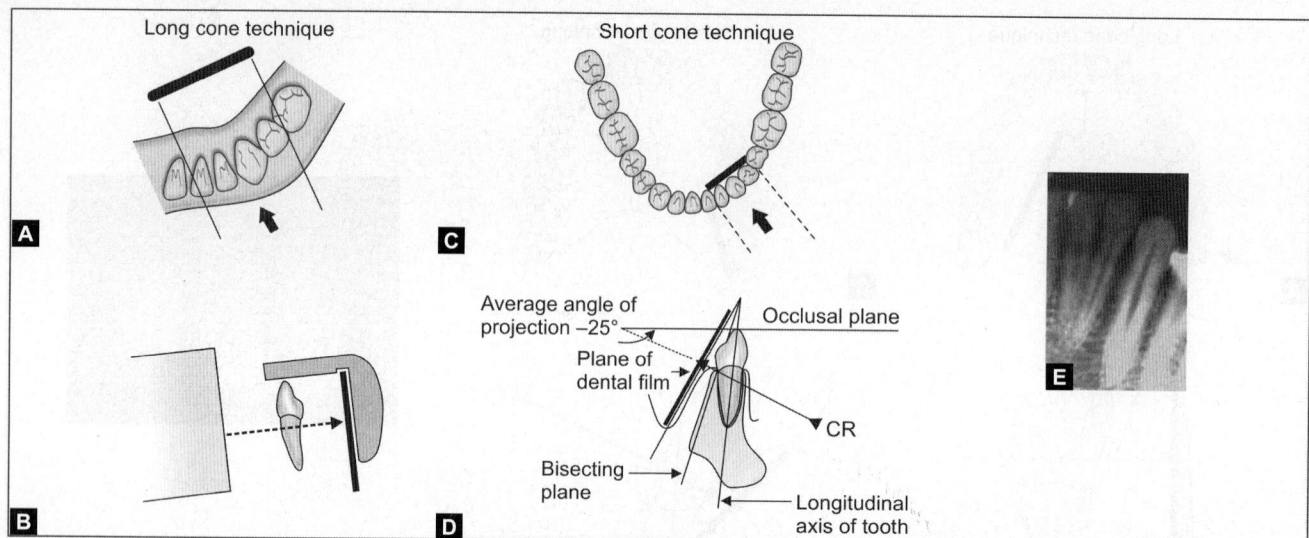

Figures 11.15A to E *Periapical technique for mandibular canine*: (A) *Film placement (Long cone paralleling technique)*: It should be placed vertically and the canine in the middle of the film. The film should be placed as far lingually as the tongue and contralateral alveolar process permit; (B) *Projection of the central ray (Long cone technique)*: Directed perpendicular to the ala of the nose, over the position of the canine, about 3 cm above the inferior border of the mandible, through the mesial contact of the canine; (C) *Film placement (Short cone bisecting angle technique)*: The film should be placed directly behind the canine with the superior border just above the cusp of the tooth and the inferior border extending onto the lingual mucosa of the mandible; (D) *Projection of central ray (Short cone technique)*: It should enter through the canine, approximately 3 cm from the midline. The central ray should be angled perpendicular to the bisector through the middle of the canine with a vertical angulation about –20° to –25°; (E) Radiograph of mandibular canine

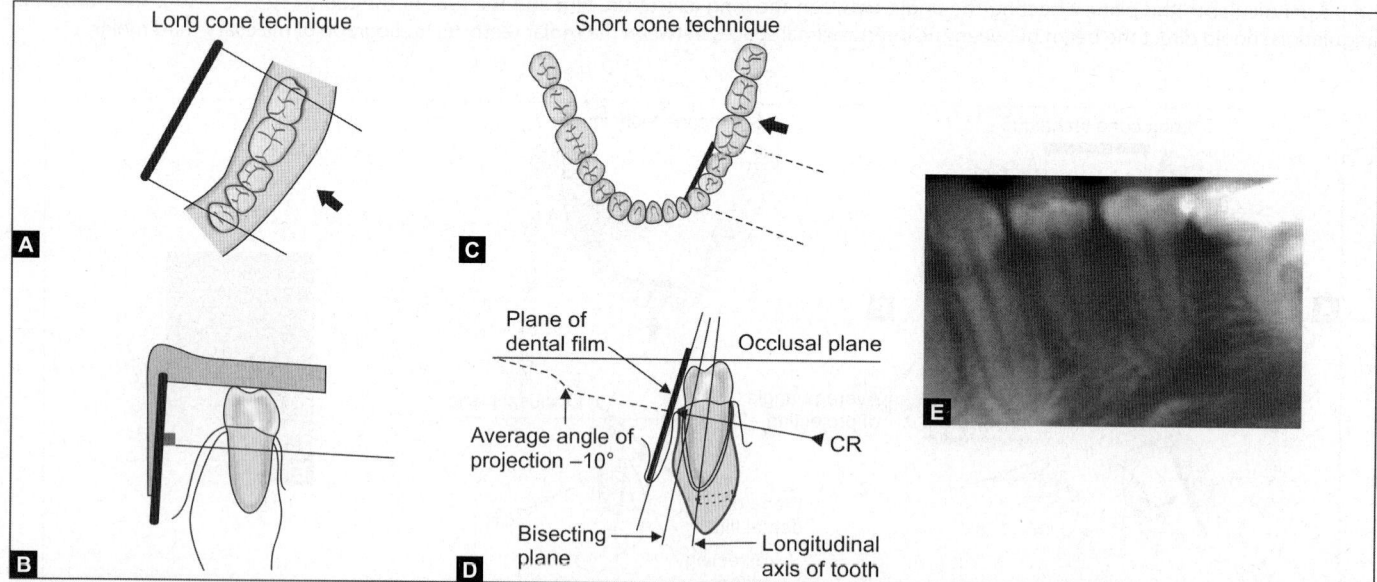

Figures 11.16A to E *Periapical technique for mandibular premolar*: (A) *Film placement (Long cone paralleling technique)*: It should be placed horizontally, between the tongue and the teeth, with the anterior border near the midline of the canine; (B) *Projection of the central (Long cone technique)*: Directed below the pupil of the eye and about 3 cm above the inferior border of the mandible, through the premolar contact area; (C) *Film placement (Short cone bisecting angle technique)*: The film should be placed with the inferior border positioned beneath the lateral border of the tongue and the superior border just above the cusp of the premolars. Care should be taken to extend the anterior border forward enough to cover the distal half of the canine; (D) *Projection of central ray (Short cone technique)*: It should pass through the interproximal space between the first and the second premolar. The point of entry is usually below the pupil of the eye, approximately 3 cm above the inferior border of the mandible. The central ray should be angled perpendicular to the bisector through the middle of the canine with a vertical angulation about –10° to –15°; (E) Radiograph of mandibular premolars

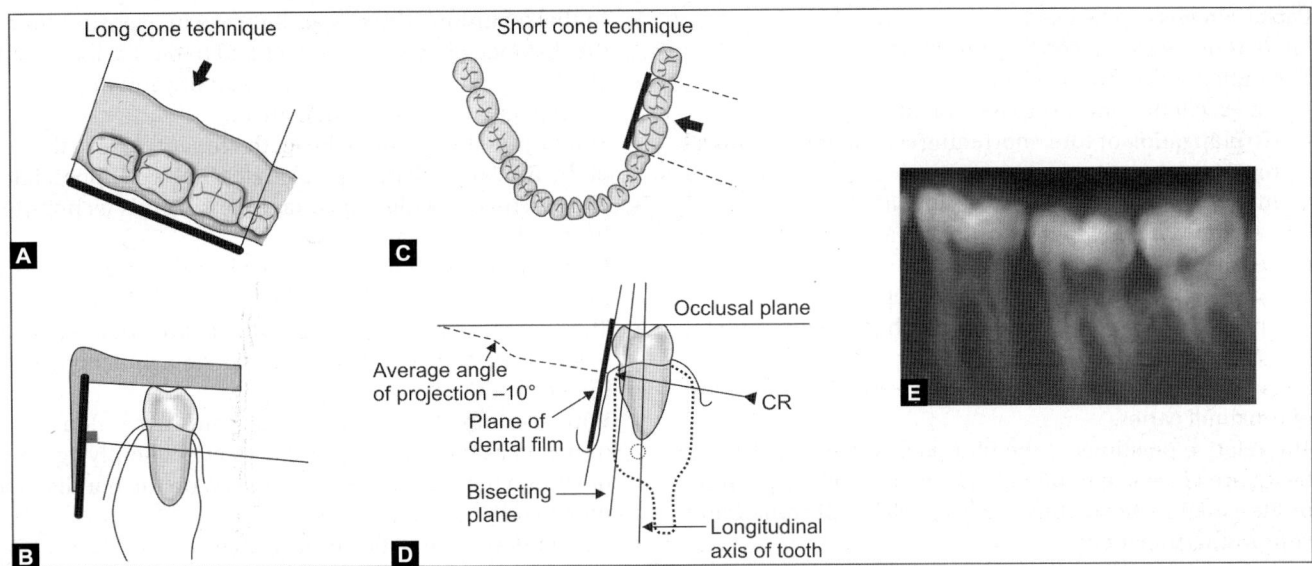

Figures 11.17A to E *Periapical technique for mandibular molar*: (A) *Film placement (Long cone paralleling technique)*: It should be placed horizontally, between the tongue and the teeth, with the anterior border near the middle of the second premolar; (B) *Projection of the central ray (Long cone technique)*: Directed below the outer canthus of the eye and about 3 cm above the inferior border of the mandible, through the molar contact area. Because of the slight lingual inclination of the molars, the central ray may have a slight positive angulation; (C) *Film placement (Short cone bisecting angle technique)*: The film should be placed with the inferior border positioned beneath the lateral border of the tongue and against the lingual surface of the mandible, and the superior border just above the cusps of the mandibular molars. The anterior border forward enough to cover the distal half of the second premolar; (D) *Projection of central ray (Short cone technique)*: It should pass through the interproximal space between the molar teeth. The point of entry is on the cheek below the lateral canthus of the eye, approximately 3 cm above the inferior border of the mandible. The central ray should be angled perpendicular to the bisector through the middle of the canine with a vertical angulation about –5° to –10°; (E) Radiograph of mandibular molars

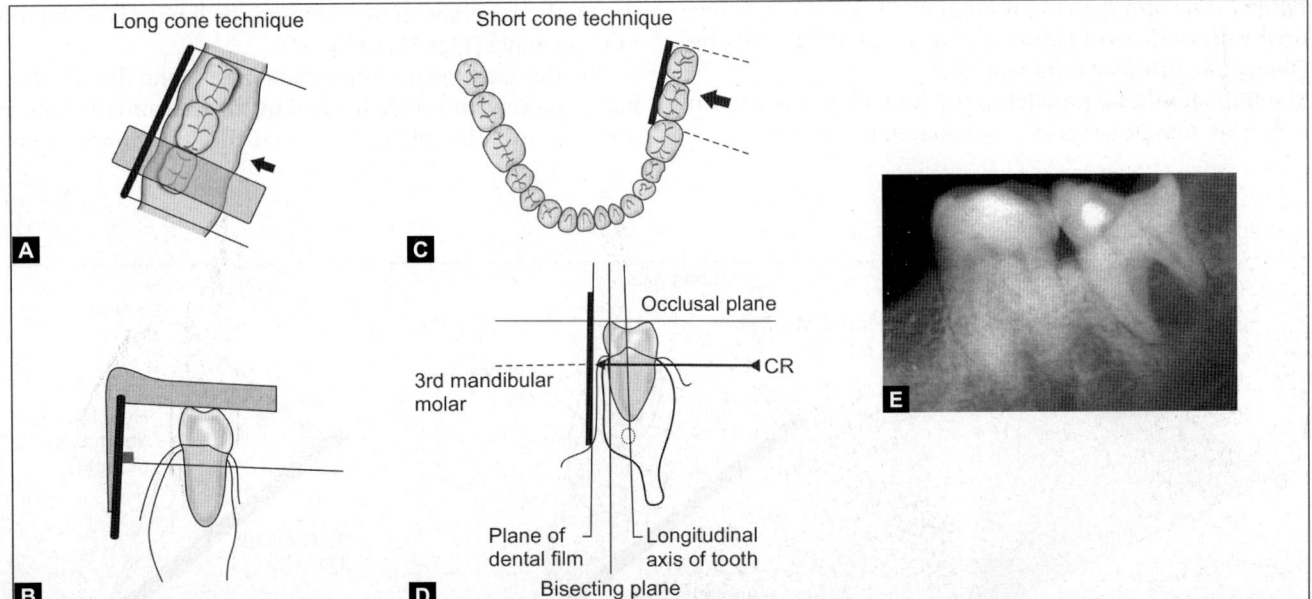

Figures 11.18A to E *Periapical technique for mandibular third molar*: (A) *Film placement (Long cone paralleling technique)*: It should be placed horizontally, between the tongue and the teeth, as far posteriorly, with the posterior border of the film angled towards the midline; (B) *Projection of the central ray (Long cone technique)*: Directed about 3 cm above the antegonial notch on the inferior border of the mandible, in line with the anterior border of the ramus. The beam is directed posteroanteriorly, through the third molar, so that the more distal objects are projected anteriorly onto the film; (C) *Film placement (Short cone bisecting angle technique)*: The film should be placed with the inferior border positioned beneath the lateral border of the tongue and against the lingual surface of the mandible, and the superior border just above the cusps of the mandibular molars. The anterior border should cover the mesial half of the first molar; (D) *Projection of central ray (Short cone technique)*: It should pass through the interproximal space between the molar teeth. The point of entry is on the cheek below, a little posterior to the lateral canthus of the eye, approximately 3 cm above the inferior border of the mandible. The central ray should be angled perpendicular to the bisector through the middle of the canine with a vertical angulation about –5° to –10°; (E) Radiograph of mandibular third molar

- Facial screens can be used.
- There is decreased secondary radiation.
- The radiographs produced give:
  - An excellent bone level assessment.
  - No elongation or fore-shortening seen in the periapical region.
  - Interproximal caries is clearly indicated.
- The shadow of the zygomatic bone appears above the apices of the molar teeth.
- The periodontal bone levels are well represented.
- The periapical tissues are accurately shown with minimal foreshortening or elongation.
- The crowns of the teeth are well shown enabling detection of proximal caries.
- The relative positions of the film packet, teeth and X-ray beam are always maintained, irrespective of the position of the patient's head. This is useful for handicapped and compromised patients.

Disadvantage of Long Cone Technique

The primary disadvantage is that of difficulty in film placement and patient discomfort.

- *Film placement*: The film holding device is difficult to place and adjust especially in child patients and adults with a small mouth or shallow palate.
- Positioning the holders within the mouth can be difficult for inexperienced operators.
- *Patient discomfort*: The film holding device may impinge on the oral soft tissues and cause discomfort and gagging.
- Object film distance is increased.
- The film should be parallel to the long axis of the tooth, only a 20° margin of error is considered permissible.

- In this technique there is an increase in exposure time as the distance between the target and patient is increased.
- The long cone is more space consuming and thus difficult to manage in a small dental office.
- Sometimes the apices of the teeth are very close to the edge of the film and the periapical area is not well appreciated.
- There is no particular advantage of using this technique in the lower molar region.
- Positioning the film in the third molar region can be difficult.
- The so-called long cones which are marketed are sometimes short which leads to gross magnification of the image produced.
- With certain X-ray machines, the heavy long cone unbalances the head which has to be frequently tightened or should have a counter balance put on the handle of the tube head.
- The holders need to be autoclavable.

ANGLE BISECTING TECHNIQUE

It is also called Short Cone Technique. It is based on the simple geometrical principle known as 'the rule of isometry' or "ciesenzky's rule of isometry", which states that two triangles are equal if they have two equal angles and share a common side.

In this technique the film is placed along the lingual surface of the tooth, and at the point where the film contacts the tooth, the plane of the film and the long axis of the tooth form an angle (**Figs 11.19A to C**).

The dental surgeon must visualize a plane that divides in half or bisects, the angle formed by the film and the long axis of the tooth. This plane is termed the 'imaginary bisector'

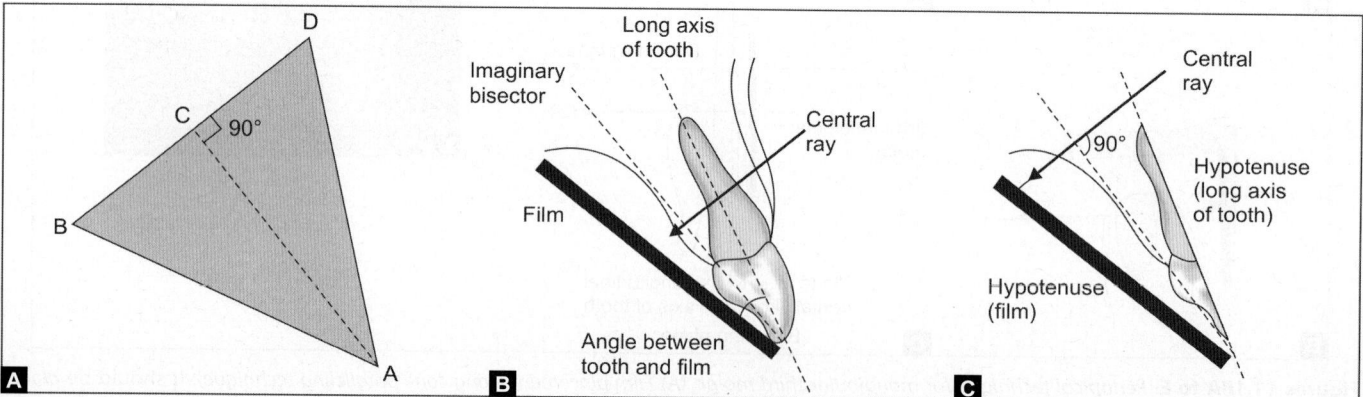

Figures 11.19A to C (A) The film (Line BA) is placed along the lingual surface of the tooth. At the point where the film contacts the tooth, the plane of the film and the long axis of the tooth (DA) form an angle (BAD). The imaginary bisector divides the angle into two equal angles (BAC and DAC). The central ray (BD) is directed perpendicular to the imaginary bisector and completes the third side, (BC and CD) of the two triangles; (B) Bisecting technique showing the central ray directed at right angle to the imaginary bisector; (C) The two imaginary triangles that result are right triangles and congruent. The hypotenuse of each triangle is represented by the long axis of the tooth and the plane of the film

and this bisector creates two equal angles and provides a common side for the two imaginary equal triangles.

The two imaginary triangles that result are right triangles and are congruent. The hypotenuse of one imaginary triangle is represented by the long axis of the tooth and the other hypotenuse is represented by the plane of the film.

When the rule of isometry is followed strictly, the radiographic image of the tooth is accurate.

Film stabilization: In bisecting angle technique the film holding instruments or the patient's finger may be used to position and stabilize the film.

Finger holding method or the digital method: Here the patient's finger or thumb is used to stabilize the film. The finger or the thumb is always placed behind the film and teeth.

The patient's thumb is used to position maxillary films and the index finger to stabilize mandibular films.

The patient's left hand is used for exposures on the right side of the mouth and right hand is used for exposures on the left side of the mouth.

Disadvantages

- Patient's hand is in the path of the primary beam, thus leading to unnecessary exposure.
- Patient may use excessive force to stabilize the film causing bending of the film which can cause image distortion.
- Patient may allow the film to slip from its position resulting in inadequate exposure of the prescribed area.
- Without the film holder and aiming ring, the dental surgeon may align the PID incorrectly, causing partial image or cone cut.

Films: The size 2 intraoral film is used.

Guidelines for Film Placement

- White side of the film always faces the teeth.
- Anterior films always placed vertically.
- Posterior films always placed horizontally.
- The incisal or occlusal edge of the film must extend approximately 1/8th inch beyond the incisal or occlusal surface of the tooth.
- When positioning the film, always center the film over the area to be examined or the tooth under consideration.
- When positioning the patient's finger to stabilize the film, instruct the patient to 'gently' push the finger against the lingual/palatal surface of the tooth.

Patient Positioning for Bisecting Angle Technique

- Briefly explain the radiographic procedure to the patient before the procedure begins.
- Position the patient upright in the chair. The chair level should be adjusted to a comfortable working height.

- Adjust the head rest to support the patient's head. The patient's head must be so positioned so that the arch being radiographed is parallel to the floor and the midsagittal plane is perpendicular to the floor.
- Place and secure the lead apron and thyroid collar over the patient.
- Remove all objects from the patient's mouth (e.g. dentures, retainers, chewing gum, etc.) that may interfere with film exposure. Eye glasses must also be removed.

PID Angulations

In bisecting angle technique the PID angulations are critical.

Angulation is a term used to describe the alignment of the central ray of the X-ray beam in the horizontal and vertical planes.

These angulations can be varied by moving the PID in either a horizontal or vertical direction.

The use of the bisecting angle instruments with aiming rings dictates the proper PID angulations. However, when finger holding method is employed the dental surgeon must determine the horizontal and vertical angulations.

Horizontal angulations: Refers to positioning of the tube head and direction of the central ray in a horizontal or side-to-side plane. This is the same for all techniques, be it long cone, bisecting angle or bite wing.

The correct horizontal angulation is achieved by directing the central ray perpendicular to the curvature of the arch and through the contact areas of the teeth.

As a result the contact area on the radiograph appears 'opened' (**Fig. 11.20**).

If the horizontal angulation is incorrect it results in overlapped (unopened) contact areas, in which inter proximal areas of the teeth cannot be evaluated (**Fig. 11.21**).

Vertical angulations (Table 11.1): Refers to the positioning of the PID in a vertical or up and down plane. Vertical angulation is measured in degrees and is registered on the outside of the tube head. The vertical angulation differs according to the technique used.

In short cone technique, the vertical angulation is determined by the imaginary bisector. The central ray is directed perpendicular to the imaginary bisector.

Correct vertical angulations result in a radiographic image that has the same length as the tooth. Some recommended vertical angulations for the bisecting angle technique are:

Incorrect vertical angulation results in a radiographic image that is not of the same length as the tooth. It may appear as:

- Foreshortened image, that is the image of the teeth appears shortened. This is due to excessive vertical angulation or when the central ray is directed perpendicular to the plane of the film rather than perpendicular to the imaginary bisector (**Fig. 11.22**).

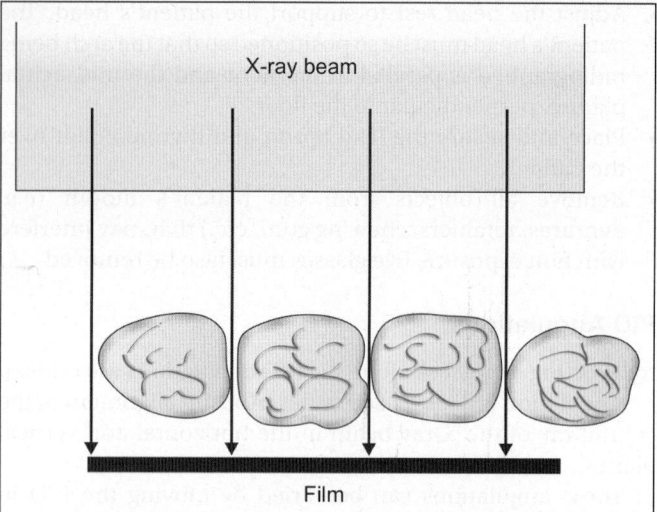

Figure 11.20 Correct horizontal angulation

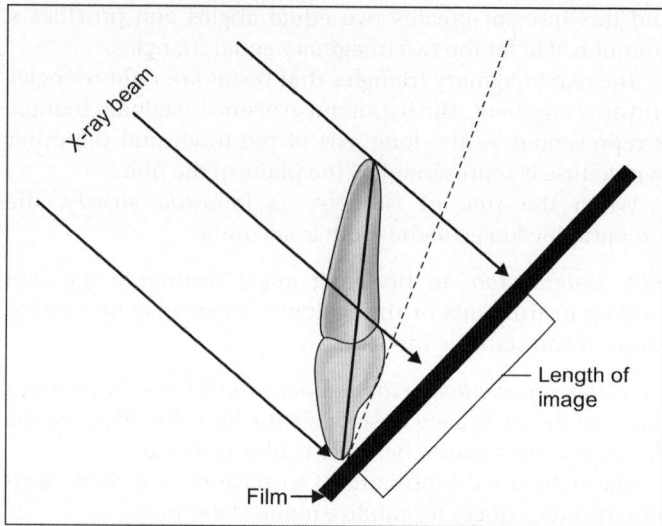

Figure 11.22 If the vertical angulation is too steep, the image on the film is shorter than the actual tooth

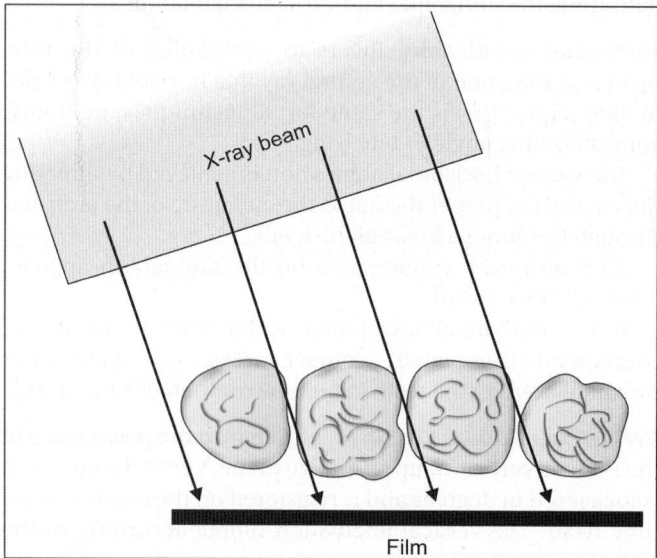

Figure 11.21 Incorrect horizontal angulation

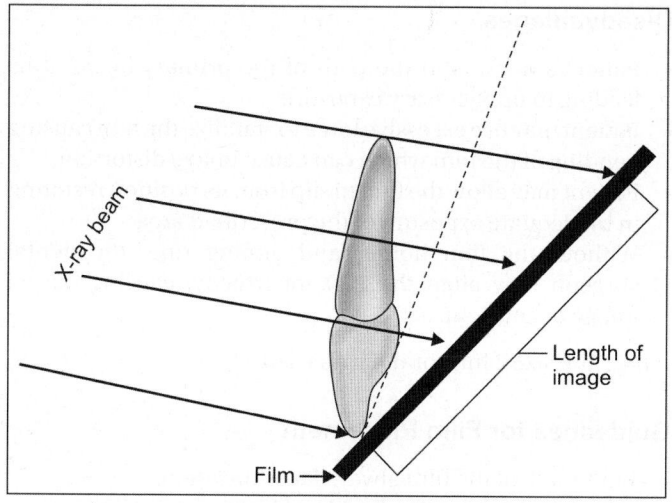

Figure 11.23 If the vertical angulation is too flat, the image on the film is longer than the actual tooth

Table 11.1 Vertical angulations recommended for bisecting angle technique

	Maxillary vertical angulation in degrees		Mandibular vertical angulation in degrees	
	Universal standard	Indian standard	Universal standard	Indian standard
Canines	+45 to +55	+45	−20 to −30	−25
Incisors	+40 to +50	+45	−15 to −25	−20
Premolars	+30 to +40	+30	−10 to −15	−15
Molars	+20 to +30	+30	−5 to 0	−10 to 0

- Elongated image, that is the image of the teeth appears too long. This is due to insufficient or flat vertical angulation or when the central ray is directed perpendicular to the long axis of the tooth rather than perpendicular to the imaginary bisector (**Fig. 11.23**).

Five basic rules that should be followed in bisecting angle technique:

1. *Film placement*: The film should be positioned to cover the prescribed area of teeth to be examined.
2. *Film position*: The film must be placed against the lingual surface of the tooth. The occlusal end of the film (indicated by the raised identification mark or dot) must extend

approximately 1/8th inch beyond the incisal or occlusal surfaces (**Fig. 11.24**). The apical end of the film must rest against the palatal or alveolar tissues if the finger holding method is used to stabilize the film. The patient must be instructed to press the film gently against the cervical portion (where the crown meets the roots) of the tooth (**Figs 11.25A to D**).

3. *Vertical angulation*: The central ray of the X-ray beam must be directed perpendicular to the image of the bisector that divides the angle formed by the film and the long axis of the tooth.
4. *Horizontal angulation*: The central ray of the X-ray beam must be directed through the contact areas between the teeth.
5. *Film exposure*: Center the X-ray beam on the film to ensure that all areas of the film are exposed. Failure to center the X-ray beam results in a partial image on the film or a cone cut.

*External guidelines for directing the central ray (**Figs 11.26 and 11.27**).*

A The line of concentration for maxillary teeth is indicated along a line approximately 1/4th inch above the ala tragus line.

B The line of concentration for mandibular teeth is indicated along a line approximately 1/4th inch above the lower border of the mandible.

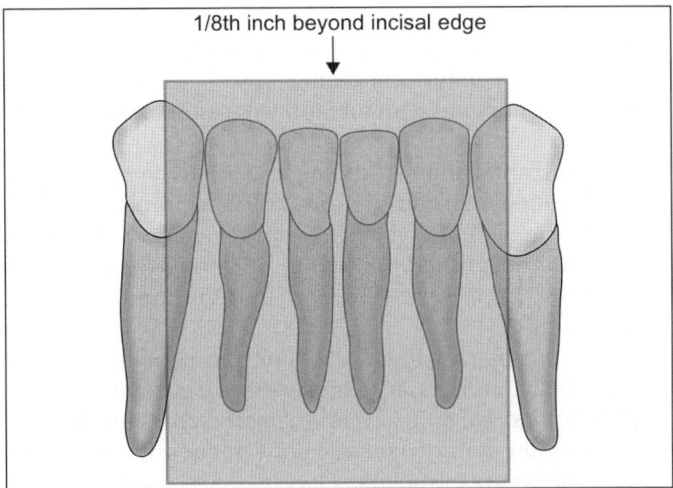

Figure 11.24 Approximately 1/8th inch of the film must appear beyond the incisal edges of the teeth

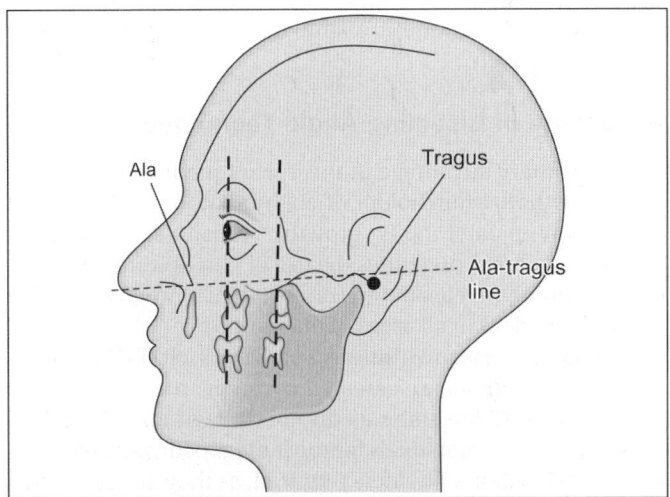

Figure 11.26 Location of apices of teeth as seen from side of the patient

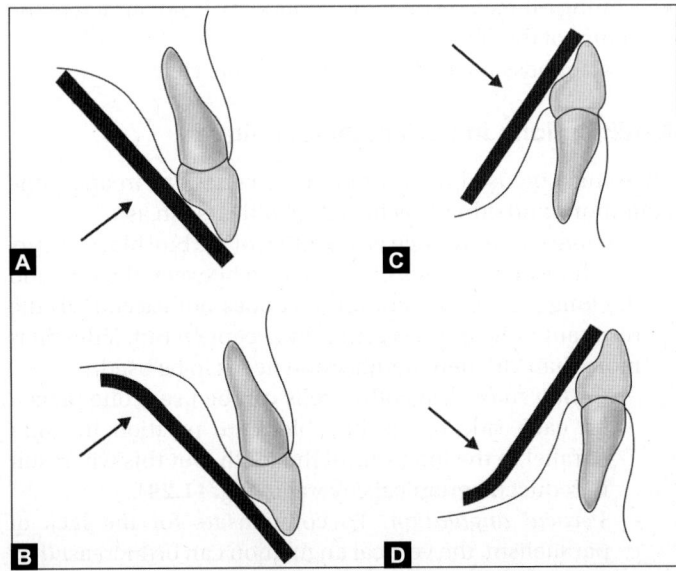

Figures 11.25A to D Correct and incorrect finger placement (arrows indicate finger pressure holding film in place): (A) Correct finger placement at crown gingival junction; (B) Incorrect finger placement on palatal tissues; (C) Correct finger placement at crown gingival junction; (D) Incorrect finger placement on alveolar tissues

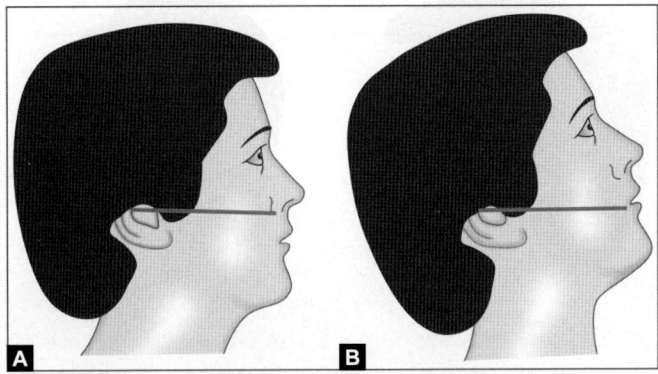

Figures 11.27A and B Correct position of the head for: (A) The maxillary teeth; (B) The mandibular teeth

Perpendicular Locating Lines (Fig. 11.28)

- *Maxillary and mandibular central incisors*: Point of intersection of a perpendicular line from the tip of the nose line CD to AB respectively.
- *Maxillary and mandibular lateral incisors*: Point of intersection of a perpendicular line from a point slightly distal to the tip of the nose. Point 6 to line AB respectively.
- *Maxillary and mandibular canines*: Point of intersection of a perpendicular line from the corner of the nose or inner canthus of the eye point 5 to line AB respectively.
- *Maxillary and mandibular premolars*: Point of intersection of a perpendicular line from the pupil of the eye (Patient asked to look straight ahead) point 4 to line AB repectively.
- *Maxillary and mandibular molars*: Point of intersection of a perpendicular line from the outer canthus of the eye to point 1 to line AB respectively.
- *Maxillary and mandibular third molars*: Point of intersection of a perpendicular line from distal to the outer canthus of the eye point 2/3 to line AB respectively.

The specific positioning for different areas of the mouth for bisecting technique are shown in the **Figures 11.9 to 11.18** respectively.

Advantage of Bisecting Angle Technique

- The primary advantage of this technique is that it can be used without a film holder when the anatomy of the patient (shallow palate, bony growths, sensitive mandibular premolar area) precludes the use of film holding device.
- Positioning is reasonably comfortable, simple and quick for the patient in all areas of the mouth.
- Decreased exposure time, as a short (8 inch) PID is used.
- If all angulations are assessed correctly, the image of the tooth will be the same as the tooth itself and should be adequate (but not ideal) for most diagnostic purposes.
- No sterilization of holders required, as they are not used.

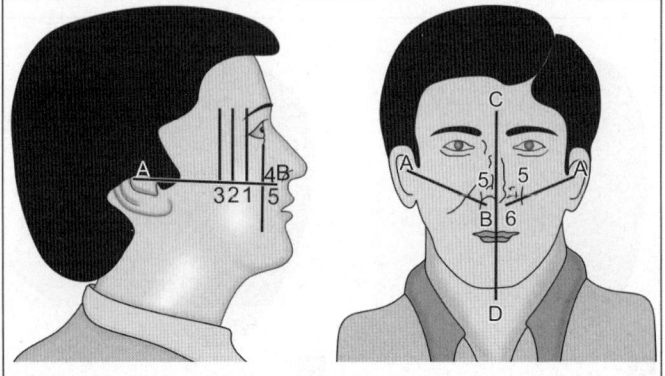

Figure 11.28 External landmarks which help in the location of the point of entry of the central ray for maxillary teeth

Disadvantage of Bisecting Angle Technique

- Image distortion, this occurs due to:
  - Use of short PID, as this results in the increase divergence of X-rays, leading to image magnification.
  - Due to the fact that the tooth (a 3 dimensional structure) is projected onto a film (a 2 dimensional structure), therefore structures further away from the film appear more elongated than those closer to the film.
- Angulation problems, without the use of film holders and aiming rings, it is difficult to visualize the imaginary bisector and determine the vertical angulation. Any error in the vertical angulation will result in distortion, leading to elongation or foreshortening.
- Incorrect horizontal angulation will result in overlapping of the crowns and roots.
- The horizontal and vertical angles have to be assessed for every patient and considerable skill is required.
- In the finger holding technique, the patient may shift the position of the film, before or during the exposure, leading to improper centering of the film, cone cut and/or blurring.
- When the patient holds the film, the patient's hand is exposed to unnecessary exposure to the primary beam.
- The periodontal bone levels are poorly represented.
- The shadow of the zygomatic bone frequently overlies the roots of the upper molars.
- The buccal roots of premolars and molars are foreshortened.
- The crowns of the teeth are often distorted, thus preventing the detection of proximal caries.
- Coning off may result if the central ray is not aimed at the center of the film.
- It is not possible to obtain reproducible views.

Modifications in periapical technique

These may be used to accommodate variations in anatomic conditions and other practical difficulties, such as:

- *Shallow palate*: In such cases tilting of the bite block occurs which results in a lack of parallelism between the film and the long axis of the tooth, if this does not exceed 20° the resultant radiograph is generally accepted. But, if the tilt is more than 20° then modification needs to be used.
  - *Cotton rolls*: Two cotton rolls can be used, one placed on each side of the bite block, to position the film parallel to the long axis of the tooth, but this will result in reduced periapical coverage (**Fig. 11.29**).
  - *Vertical angulation*: To compensate for the lack of parallelism, the vertical angulation can be increased by 5° to 15° more than the XCP instrument indicates, but due to this , image distortion may occur.
- *Bony growths*: Presence of mandibular or maxillary tori, interfere with the film placement, therefore modifications are necessary.

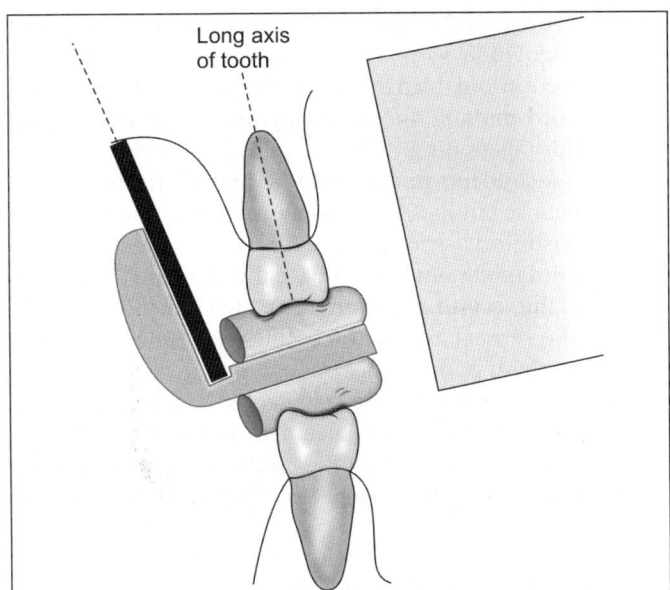

Figure 11.29 Two cotton rolls are used to position the film parallel to the long axis of the tooth

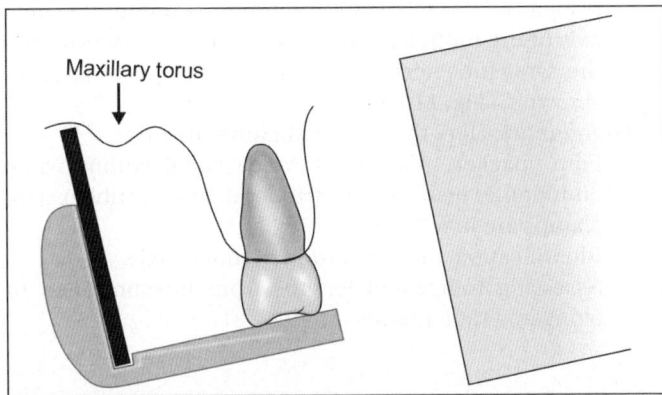

Figure 11.30 If a maxillary torus is present, the film must be placed on the far side of the torus and then exposed

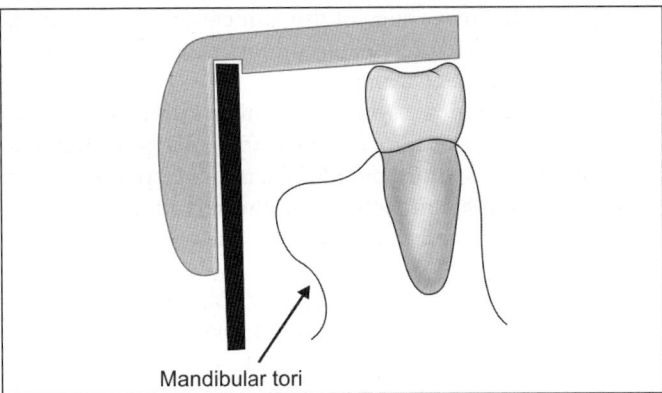

Figure 11.31 If mandibular tori are present, the film must be placed on the far side of the tori and then exposed

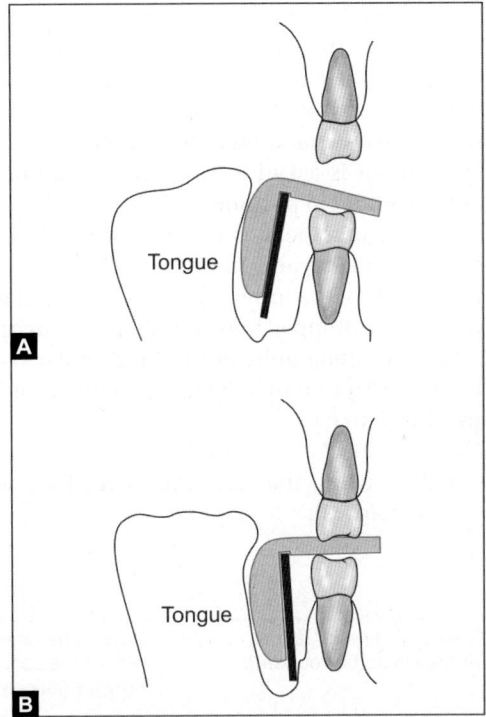

Figures 11.32A and B Positioning of the XCP instrument in the sensitive mandibular premolar area: (A) The film is tipped away from the tongue while the bite-block is placed firmly on the mandibular premolars; (B) When the patient closes on the bite block, the film is moved into the proper position

- *Maxillary torus*: The film must be placed on the far side of the torus (not on the torus) and then exposed (**Fig. 11.30**).
- *Mandibular torus*: The film must be placed between the torus and the tongue (not on the torus) and then exposed (**Fig. 11.31**).
- *Mandibular premolar region*: The floor of the mouth in this region is very sensitive and film placement causes great discomfort to the patient. Therefore certain modifications are necessary.
  - *Film placement*: The film must be placed under the tongue to avoid impinging on muscle attachments and the sensitive lingual gingiva. When inserting the film holder into the mouth, the film is tipped away from the tongue and toward the teeth being examined while the bite block is placed firmly on the mandibular premolars. When the patient closes on the bite block, the film is moved into proper position (**Figs 11.32A and B**).

- *Film*: The lower edge of the film can be gently curved or softened, to prevent discomfort. Bending or creasing the film must be avoided.
- *Mandibular third molar*: The main difficulty is the placement of the film packet sufficiently posteriorly to record the entire third mandibular molar (especially when it is horizontally impacted) and the surrounding tissues, including the inferior dental canal. The possible solutions include:
  - Using surgical needle holder to hold and position the film packet in the mouth, as follows:
    - Film holder is clipped securely on to the top edge of the film packet.
    - With the mouth open, the film packet is positioned gently in the lingual sulcus as far posteriorly as possible.
    - The patient is asked to close the mouth on the handles of the holders (so relaxing the tissue of the floor of the mouth) and at the same time the film packet is eased further back into the mouth, if required, until its front edge is opposite the mesial surface of the mandibular first molar.
    - The patient is asked to support the handles of the needle holder in position.
    - The X-ray tube head is positioned at right angles to the third molar and the film packet and centered 1 cm up from the lower border of the mandible, on a vertical line dropped from the outer canthus of the eye.
  - Taking two radiographs of the third molar using two different horizontal tube head angulations, as follows, (**Figs 11.33A to C**).
    - The film packet is positioned as posteriorly as possible (using the technique described with the needle holders).

- The X-ray tube head is aimed with the ideal horizontal angulation so the X-ray beam passes between the second and third molars. With horizontally impacted third molars, the apex may not be recorded using this positioning.
- A second film packet is placed in the same position as before, but the X-ray tube head is positioned further posteriorly aiming forward to project the apex of the third molar onto the film (in this position the crowns of the second and third molars become overlapped).
- The vertical angulation of the X-ray tube head is the same for both projections.

- *Problems of gagging*: The gag reflex is strong in some patients. This makes the placement of the film packet in the desired position particularly difficult, especially in the upper and lower molar regions. The probable solutions are:
  - Spraying the palate with local anesthetic before attempting to position the film packet.
  - Asking the patient to concentrate on breathing deeply while the film packet is in his mouth.
  - Placing the film packet flat in the mouth (in the occlusal plane) so it does not touch the palate, and applying the principles of the bisected angle technique; the long axis of the tooth and the film packet are assessed and the X-ray tube head's position modified accordingly as shown in (**Fig. 11.34**).
- *Endodontics*: Here the main difficulties involve:
  - Film packet placement and stabilization when endodontic instruments, rubber dam and rubber dam clamps are in position.
  - Identification and separation of root canals.
  - Assessing root canal lengths from foreshortened or elongated radiographs.

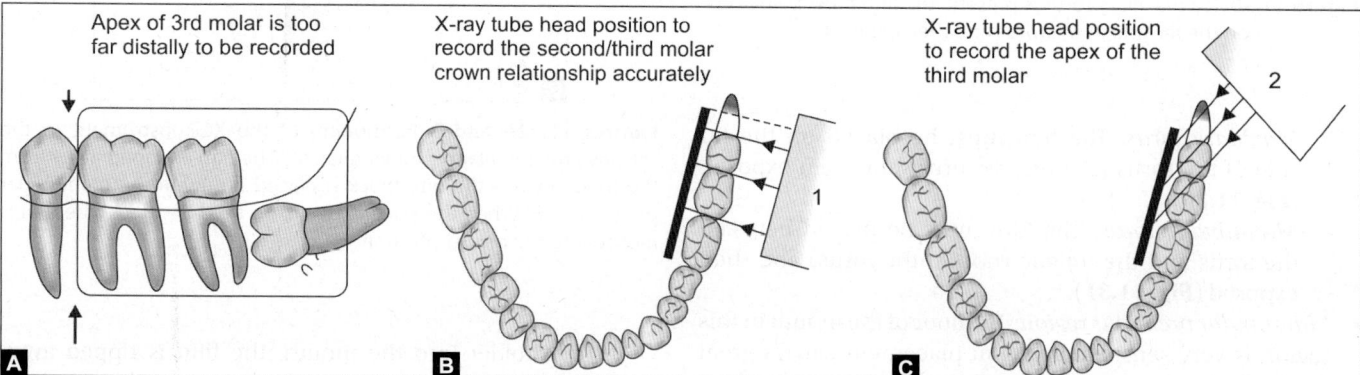

| Apex of 3rd molar is too far distally to be recorded | X-ray tube head position to record the second/third molar crown relationship accurately | X-ray tube head position to record the apex of the third molar |

A | **B** | **C**

Figures 11.33A to C The problem of the horizontal third molar: (A) Side view showing the often achievable film packet position; (B) Plane view showing X-ray tube head position-1; (C) Plane view showing X-ray tube head position-2

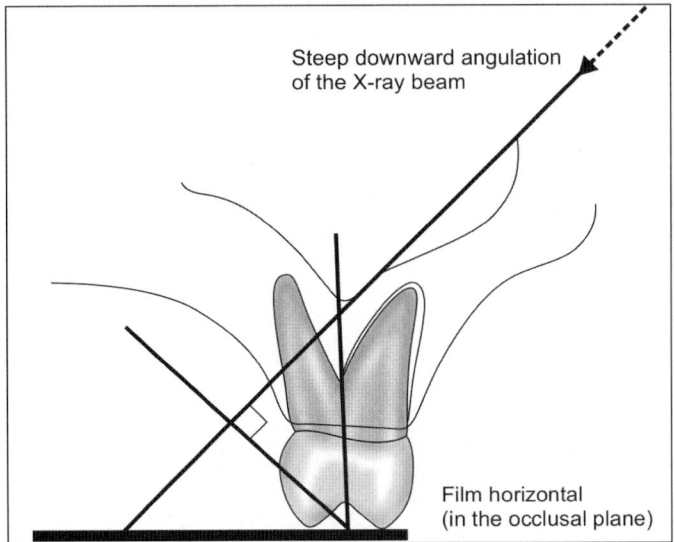

Figure 11.34 Diagram showing the relative position of the X-ray beam to the maxillary molar, when the film is placed in the occlusal plane

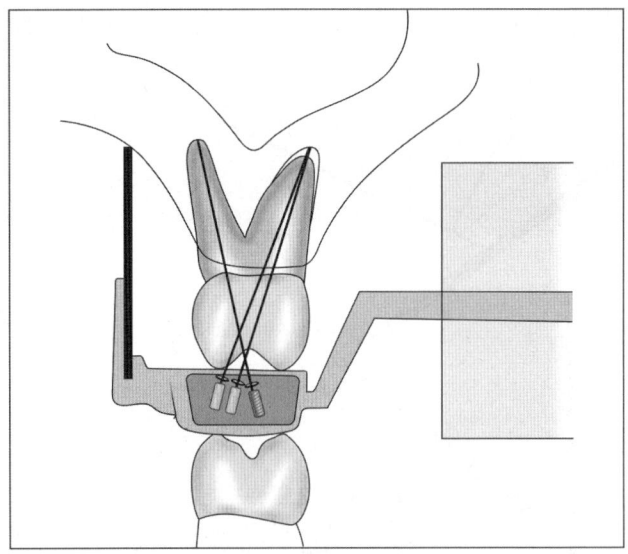

Figure 11.35 Diagram of especially designed film packet holder for use during endodontics, incorporating a basket to accommodate the handles of the endodontic instruments and a beam aiming device

The possible solutions are:
- – The problem of the film packet placement and stabilization can be resolved by:
  - Taping the intraoral film packet to one end of a wooden tongue spatula. This is positioned in the mouth and held in place by the patient.
  - Using the special endodontic film holders that have been developed. These incorporate a small basket in the bite platform area, to accommodate the handles of the endodontic instruments, while still allowing the film packet and the tooth to be parallel (**Fig. 11.35**).
- – The problem of identifying and separating the root canals can be solved by taking atleast two radiographs, using different horizontal X-ray tube head positions.
- – The problem of assessing root length can be solved by:
  - Taking an accurate paralleling technique periapical preoperatively and measuring the lengths of the root(s) directly from the radiograph before beginning the endodontic treatment. The amount of distortion on subsequent films can then be assessed.
- – Calculating mathematically the actual length of a root canal from a distorted bisecting angle technique periapical taken with the diagnostic instrument within the root canal at the clinically assessed apical stop.
- • *Edentulous ridge*: It is difficult to place the film packet. The solutions are:
  - – In the edentulous patient the lack of height in the palate, or loss of lingual sulcus depth, contraindicates the paralleling technique and all periapical radiographs should be taken using a modified bisected angle technique. The long axis of the film packet and

the alveolar ridge are assessed and the X-ray tube head position adjusted accordingly (**Figs 11.36A and B**).
- – In partially dentate patients, the paralleling technique can usually be used. If edentulous area causes the film packet holder to be displaced, the deficiency can be built up by using cotton rolls.
- • *Children*: The main problem is the size of the mouth and difficulty in placing the film packet intraorally.
  - – The paralleling technique is not possible in very small children, but can often be used (and is recommended) anteriorly, for investigating traumatized permanent incisors. The reproducibility afforded by this technique is invaluable for future comparative purposes.
  - – A modified bisected technique is possible in most children, with the film placed flat in the mouth (in the occlusal plane) and the position of the X-ray tube head adjusted accordingly.
- • *Handicapped patients*: The main problems encountered are in obtaining the patient's cooperation and in possible anatomical difficulties in relation to film packet placement, the possible options are:
  - – Only attempting radiographic investigations appropriate to the limitations imposed by the patient's handicap.
  - – Using the paralleling technique, if possible, for periapical radiography because, as mentioned earlier, with this technique the relative positions of the film packet, teeth and X-ray beam are maintained, irrespective of the position of the patient's head.
- • *Shadow of malar bone (Le Masters technique) (Fig. 11.37)*: When using the short cone technique sometimes due

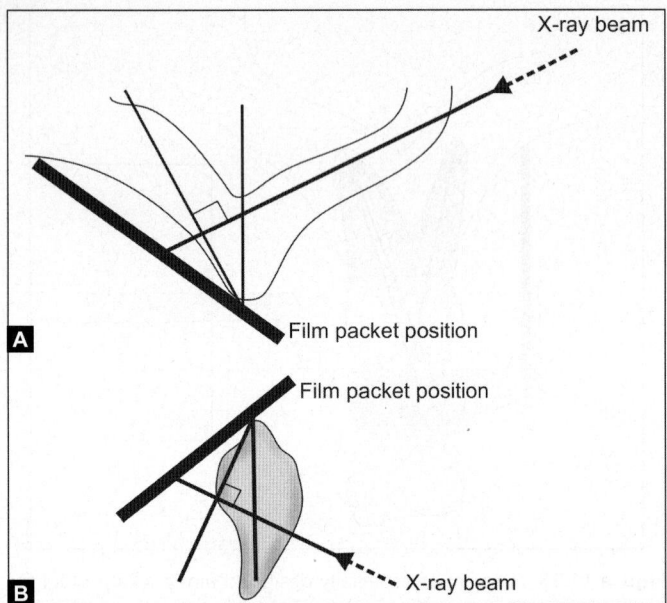

Figures 11.36A and B Diagram showing the relative position of the film packet and X-ray beam: (A) For the molar region of an edentulous maxillary ridge; (B) For the molar region of an edentulous mandibular ridge

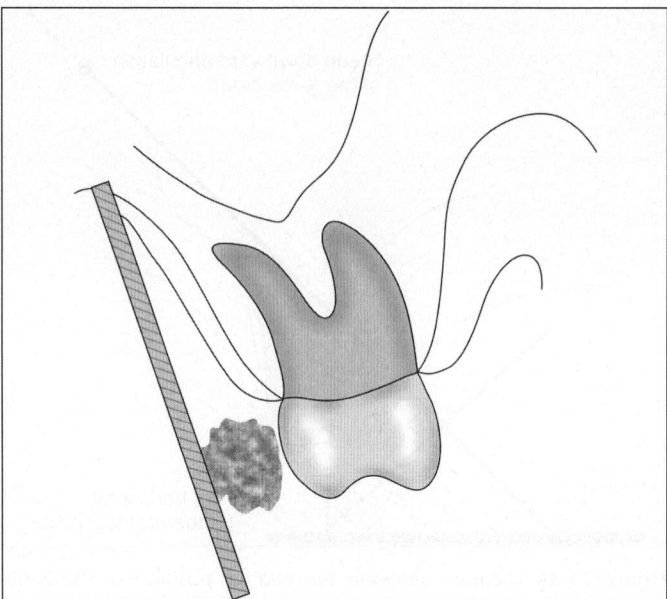

Figure 11.37 Le Masters technique; use of a cotton wool roll for the placing of the film in the upper molar region. The film and the tooth become more parallel

to prominence of the malar bone, X-rays projected in the molar area at the normal angle result in the superimposition of the malar bone over the roots of the maxillary molars.

- A cotton roll is fastened to the front side of the film. It rests against the palatal surface of the molars making the mean plane of the film more parallel to the plane of the tooth.
- The vertical angulation is decreased so as to avoid the malar bone.

The shadow of the malar bone on the apex of the maxillary molar can be avoided by reducing the vertical angulation of the Central ray, so that the ray passes below the malar bone onto to the tooth apex.

BITE WING RADIOGRAPHY

The bite wing technique or the interproximal technique is a method used to examine the interproximal surfaces of teeth.

Indications

- Detection of interproximal caries.
- Monitoring progression of dental caries.
- Detection of secondary caries below restorations.
- Evaluating periodontal conditions.
- Useful for evaluating alveolar bone crest and changes in bone height can be assessed by comparison with the adjacent teeth.

- For detecting calculus deposited in the interproximal areas (for better visualization, exposure should be reduced as calculus has relatively low density).

Principles

- The film is placed in the mouth parallel to the crowns of both the upper and lower teeth.
- The film is stabilized when the patient bites on the bite wing tab of bite wing film holder.
- The central ray of the X-ray beam is directed through the contacts of the teeth, using a +10° vertical angulation.

Film Holder and Bite Wing Tab

A film holder as already defined is used to stabilize the film. Those used for bite wing radiography are:
- Rinn XCP bite wing instruments
- Bite wing tab.

Films

Four sizes of bite wing films are available:
- *Size 0*: Used to study posterior teeth of children, always placed horizontally.
- *Size 1*: Used to examine posterior teeth in mixed dentitions or anterior teeth of adults. It is placed horizontally for the former and vertically for the latter.
- *Size 2*: Used to examine posterior teeth of adults and is always kept horizontally.

Position Indicating Device and Angulations

If the bite wing holder is used, the aiming ring dictates the proper PID angulations, but if the bite wing tab is used, then both the horizontal and vertical angulations must be precisely determined.

Horizontal angulations: The central ray is directed perpendicular to the curvature of the arch and through the contact areas of the teeth.

Vertical angulations: A +10° vertical angulation is recommended for the bite wing radiograph, to compensate for the slight bend of the upper portion of the film and the slight tilt of the maxillary teeth.

Patient Positioning

- Briefly explain the procedure.
- Patient is seated upright and the chair adjusted to a comfortable working position.

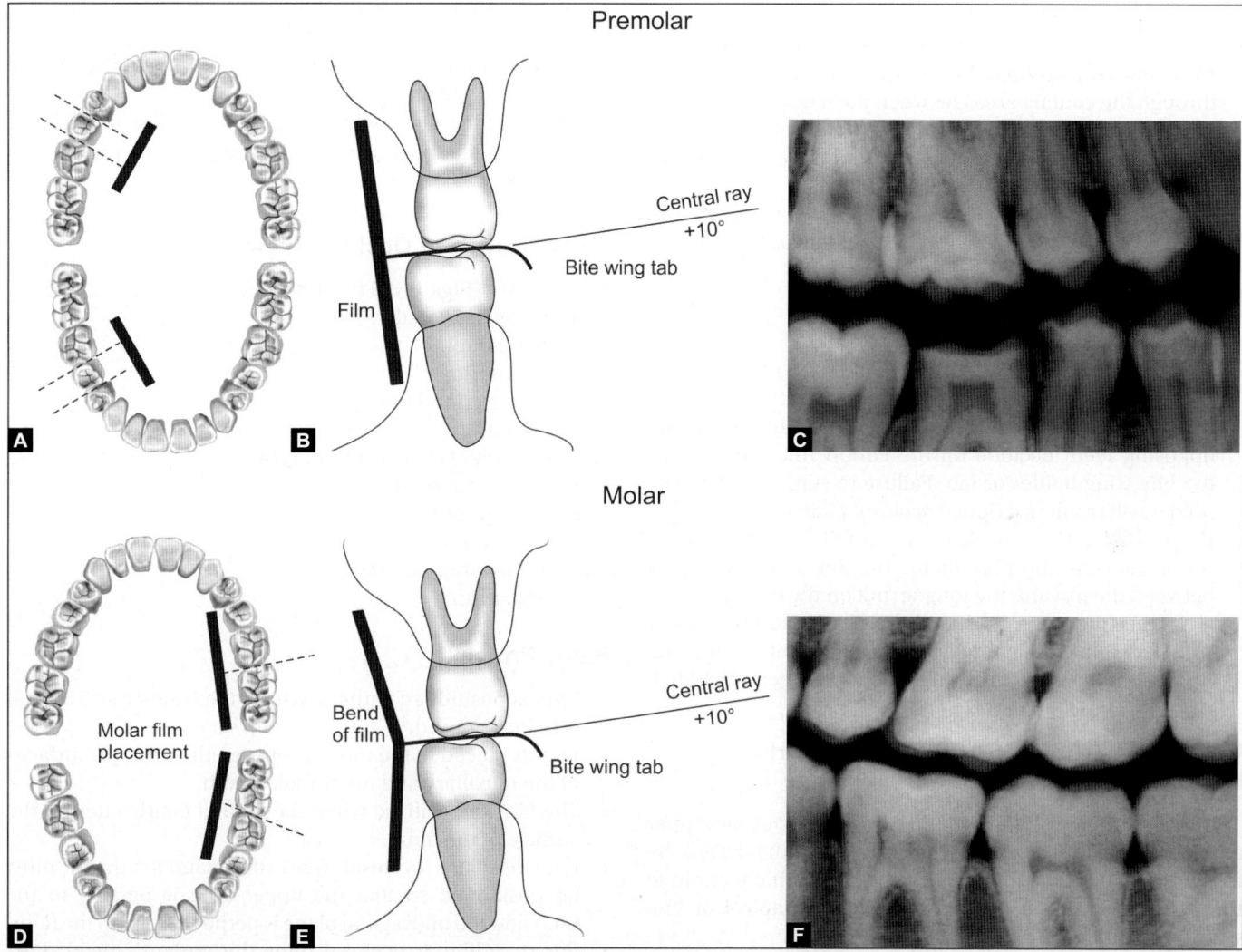

Figures 11.38A to F *Bite wing projection:* (A) *Film placement for premolars*—Place the film between the tongue and teeth, as far from the lingual surface of the teeth to prevent interference by the palate on closing and parallel to the long axis of the teeth as possible. The anterior border of the film should extend beyond the contact area between the mandibular canine and the lateral incisor; (B) Position of the film, bite wing tab and the central ray in the bite wing technique. The film is parallel to the crown of the upper and lower teeth. The central ray is directed diwnwards (+10° vertical angulation); (C) Bite wing radiograph of premolar region; (D) *Film placement for molars*—Place the film between the tongue and teeth, as far lingual as possible to avoid contacting the sensitive attached gingiva. The distal margin of the film should extend 1 to 2 mm beyond the most posterior erupted molar; (E) A + 10° vertical angulation is used to compensate for the slight bend of the upper portion of the film and the tilt of the maxillary teeth; (F) Bite wing radiograph of molar region

- Adjust the head rest to support and position the patient's head so that the upper arch is parallel to the floor and the mid sagittal (middle) plane is perpendicular to the floor.
- Secure the lead apron and thyroid collar.
- Remove all foreign objects from the face and mouth.

Five Basic Rules to follow in the Bite Wing Technique

- *Film placement*: The film must be placed to cover the prescribed area.
- *Film position*: The film must be positioned parallel to the crowns of both the upper and lower teeth and stabilized by biting on the film holder or tab.
- *Vertical angulation*: The central ray must be directed at +10°.
- *Horizontal angulation*: The central ray must be directed through the contact areas between the teeth.
- *Film exposure*: The X-ray beam must be centered on the film to ensure that all the areas of the film are exposed and thus partial image or cone cut is avoided.

The specific positioning for different areas of the mouth for bite wing technique are shown in the **Figures 11.38A to F**.

Modifications in Technique

May be used in cases where:
- *Edentulous spaces*: A cotton roll should be placed in the area of the missing tooth or teeth, to support the bite wing tab or film holder. When the patient closes the mouth, the opposing teeth occlude on the cotton roll and support the bite wing holder or tab. Failure to support the tab or holder will result in a tipped occlusal plane.
- *Bony out growths*: Especially a mandibilar tori, may cause problems with film placement. The film must be placed between the tori and the tongue, not on the tori.
  - In case the tori is large and the film is placed far from the teeth the patient may not be able to bite on the bite tab, in such cases bite wing holders are recommended.

OCCLUSAL RADIOGRAPHY (SANDWICH RADIOGRAPHY)

This technique is used to examine large areas of the upper and lower jaw. The palate and floor of the mouth may also be examined. This is a supplementary radiographic technique that is usually used in conjunction with periapical or bite wing radiographs.

Indications

- To locate retained roots of extracted teeth
- To locate supernumerary, unerupted or impacted teeth (especially impacted canine and third molars)
- To locate foreign bodies in the maxilla or mandible

- To locate salivary stones in the duct of the submandibular gland
- To locate and evaluate the extent of lesions (e.g. cysts, tumors, malignancies) in the maxilla or mandible. It is especially indicated to determine the mesial and lateral extent of the lesion and it is extent on the palate
- To evaluate boundaries of the maxillary sinus (anterior, mesial and lateral outline)
- To evaluate fractures of the maxilla and mandible. (location, extent and displacement)
- To aid in the examination of patient's who cannot open their mouths more than a few millimeters. Or in adults and children who are unable to tolerate periapical films
- To examine area of cleft palate
- To measure changes in the size and shape of the maxilla and mandible.
- As a midline view, when using the parallex method for determining the bucco/palatal position of unerupted canines.

Classification of Occlusal Views

1. Maxillary (**Figs 11.39 to 11.41**)
   - Cross-sectional
   - Topographic
     - Anterior
     - Posterior/lateral
   - Pediatric
2. Mandibular (**Figs 11.42 to 11.44**)
   - Cross-sectional
   - Topographic
     - Anterior
     - Posterior/lateral
   - Pediatric.

Basic Principle

- Film is positioned with the white side facing the arch that is being exposed.
- Film is placed in the mouth between the occlusal surfaces of the maxillary and mandibular teeth.
- The film is stabilized when the patient gently bites on the surface of the film.
- For maxillary occlusal films the patient's head must be positioned so that the upper arch is parallel to the floor and the midsagittal plane is perpendicular to the floor.
- For mandibular occlusal films the patient's head must be reclined and positioned so that the occlusal plane is perpendicular to the floor.

Film

Special occlusal films are marketed which are bigger than the intraoral films.

Occlusal Maxillary Views

- *Image field*: This projection shows the palate, the zygomatic process of the maxilla, the anterior-inferior aspects of each antrum, nasolacrimal canals, teeth from the right second molar to the left second molar and the nasal septum.
- *Film placement*: The film is placed cross wise into the mouth and gently pushed back until it contacts the anterior border of the rami.
- *Projection of the central ray*: The central ray is directed at a vertical angulation of +65° and a horizontal angulation of 0° towards the middle of the film. In general the central ray enters the patient's face through the bridge of the nose.

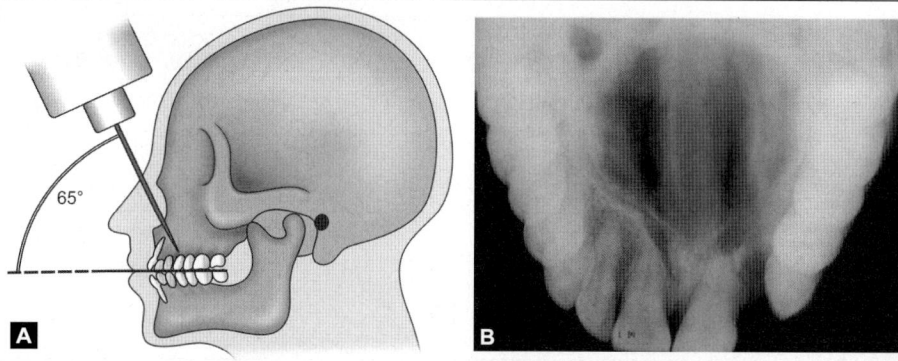

Figures 11.39A and B Maxillary cross-sectional view: (A) Projection of central ray with point of entry through the bridge of the nose; (B) Radiograph of maxillary cross-sectional view

- *Image field*: The primary field of this projection includes the anterior maxilla and it's dentition. It also includes the anterior floor of the nasal fossa and the teeth from canine to canine.
- *Film placement*: The film is placed with the exposure side towards the maxilla and the long dimension crosswise in the mouth.
- *Projection of the central ray*: The central ray is directed towards the middle of the film, the vertical angulation is +45° and horizontal angulation is 0°.
- In general the central ray enters the patient's face approximately through the tip of the nose.

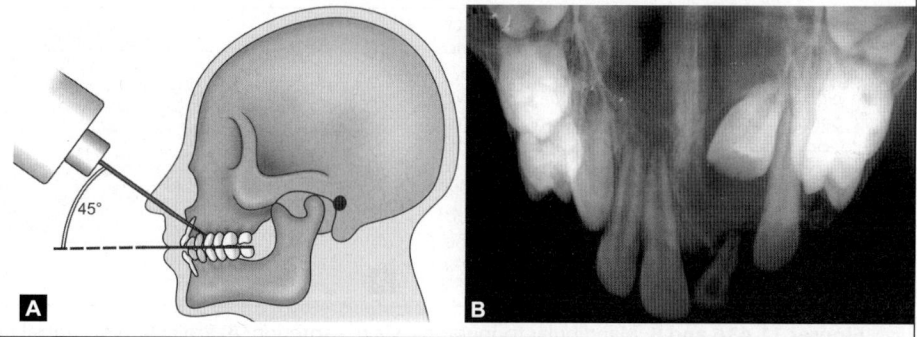

Figures 11.40A and B Maxillary topographic view—anterior: (A) Projection of central ray with point of entry through the tip of the nose; (B) Radiograph of maxillary topographic view–anterior

- *Image field*: This projection shows half of the alveolar ridge of the maxilla, infero-lateral aspect of the antrum, the tuberosity and the teeth from the lateral incisor to the third molar. It may also show the zygomatic process of the maxilla superimposed with the roots of the molar teeth.
- *Film placement*: The film is placed with it's long axis parallel to the sagittal plane and on the side of interest, with the pebbled side towards the maxilla in question. The lateral border should be positioned parallel to the buccal surfaces of the posterior teeth and extending laterally approximately 1/4th inch past the buccal cusps.
- *Projection of the central ray*: The central ray is projected to a point 2 cm below the lateral canthus of the eye and directed towards the center of the film, with a vertical angulation of +60°.

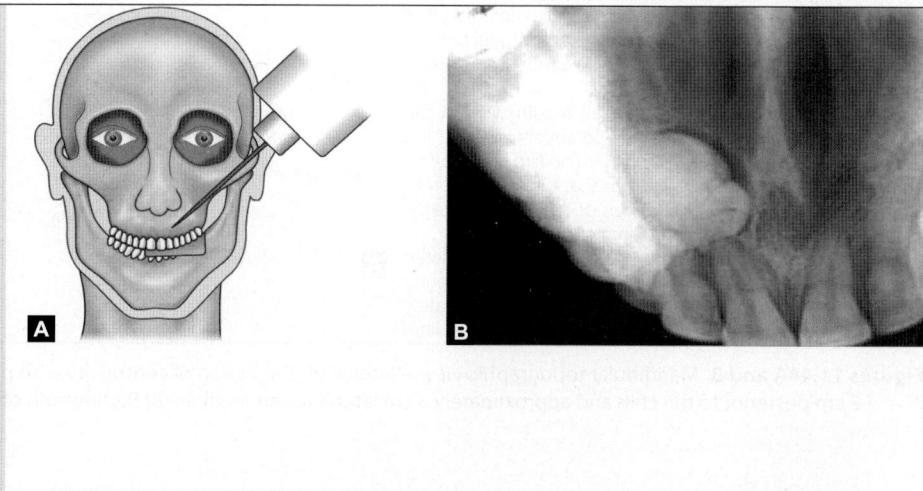

Figures 11.41A and B Maxillary topographic view—lateral: (A) Projection of central ray with point of entry at a point approximately 2 cm below the lateral canthus of the eye; (B) Radiograph of maxillary topographic view–lateral

Occlusal Mandibular Views

- *Image field*: This projection includes soft tissues of the floor of the mouth and delineates the lingual and buccal plates of the jaw bone and the teeth from second molar to second molar.
- *Film placement*: The film is placed in the mouth with its long axis perpendicular to the sagittal plane and the pebbled side towards the mandible. The anterior border of the film should be approximately ½ an inch anterior to the mandibular central incisors.
- *Projection of the central ray*: It is directed at right angles to the center of the film. The point of entry is in the middle through the floor of the mouth approximately 3 cm below the chin.

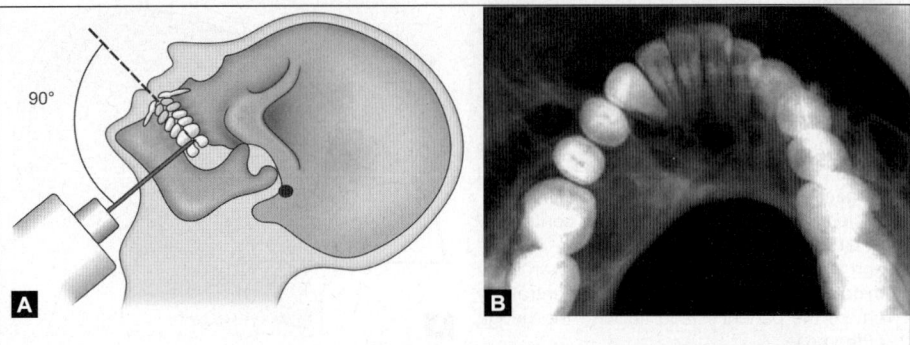

Figures 11.42A and B Mandibular cross-sectional view: (A) Projection of central ray with point of entry at a point approximately 3 cm below the chin; (B) Radiograph of mandibular cross-sectional view

- *Image field*: This projection depicts anterior portion of the mandible, the dentition from canine to canine and the inferior border of the mandible.
- *Film placement*: The film is placed with the long axis parallel with the sagittal plane and as far posteriorly as possible, with the pebbled side down.
- *Projection of the central ray*: The central ray is directed towards the middle of the film with −55° angulation in respect to the plane of the film. The point of entry of the central ray is in the midline and through the tip of the chin.

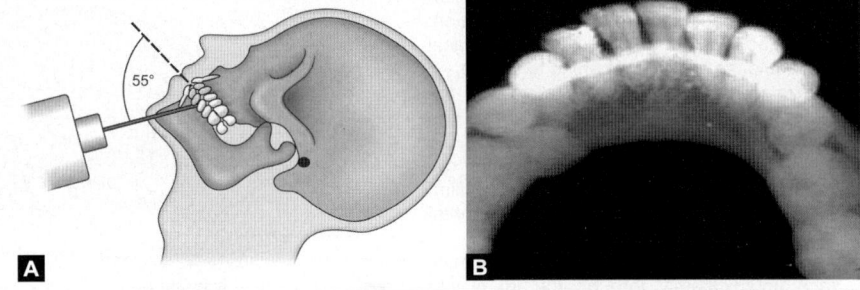

Figures 11.43A and B Mandibular topographic view—anterior: (A) Projection of central ray with point of entry at the tip of the chin; (B) Radiograph of mandibular topographic view—anterior

- *Image field*: This projection covers soft tissues of half of the floor of the mouth, and the buccal and lingual cortical plates of half of the mandible and teeth from lateral incisor to the third molar.
- *Film placement*: The film is placed length wise in the mouth with its long axis directed dorsoventrally and the pebbled side towards the mandible. The film is placed as far back posterior as possible, so that the lateral border is parallel to the buccal surfaces of the posterior teeth and extending laterally approximately 1 cm.
- *Projection of the central ray*: The central ray is directed perpendicular to the center of the film. The point of entry of the central ray is beneath the chin and approximately 3 cm posterior to the chin and 3 cm lateral to the mid line.

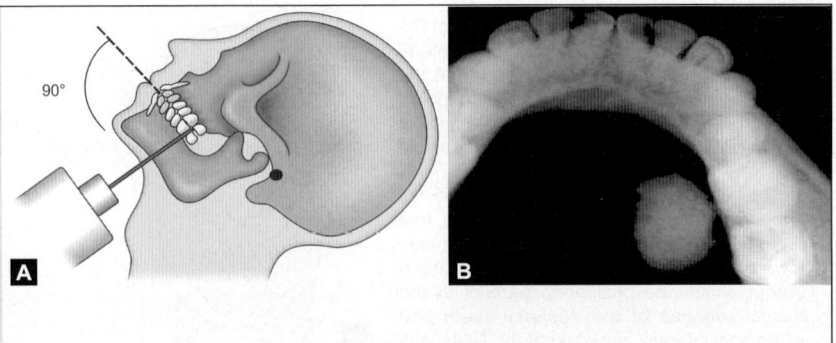

Figures 11.44A and B Mandibular topographic view—lateral: (A) Projection of central ray with point of entry beneath the chin, approximately 3 cm posterior to the chin and approximately 3 cm lateral to the midline; (B) Radiograph of mandibular topographic view—lateral

INTRAORAL LOCALIZATION TECHNIQUES

The dental radiograph is a two-dimensional picture of a three-dimensional object. It depicts the object in the superior-inferior and anterior-posterior relationship. It fails to depict the buccolingual relationship or depth of the object. Localization is used to overcome this lacuna.

Indications

- Foreign bodies
- Impacted teeth
- Unerupted teeth
- Retained roots
- Salivary stones
- Jaw fractures
- Broken needles and instruments
- Root positions
- Filling materials.

The methods used to locate the position of a tooth or object in the jaws are:
- Buccal object rule (Tube shift technique or Clark's rule) (**Figs 11.45 to 11.47**).
  - The basic principle is that the relative position of the radiographic images of two separate objects changes when the projection angle at which the projection was made is changed.
  - A different horizontal angle is used when trying to locate vertically aligned images, e.g. root canals.
  - A different vertical angulation is used when trying to locate a horizontally aligned image, e.g. mandibular canal.

Method

Two radiographs of the object are taken. First, using the proper technique and angulations as prescribed and the second, radiograph is taken keeping all other parameters constant and equivalent of those of the first radiograph, only changing the direction of the central ray either with a different horizontal or vertical angulation is used.

Interpretation

When the dental structure or object seen in the second radiograph appears to have moved in the same direction as the shift of the position indicating device (PID), the structure or the object in question is said to be positioned lingually.

But, if the object appears to have moved in a direction opposite to the shift of the PID, then the object in question is said to be positioned buccally. SLOB rule: Same side lingual. Opposite side buccal.

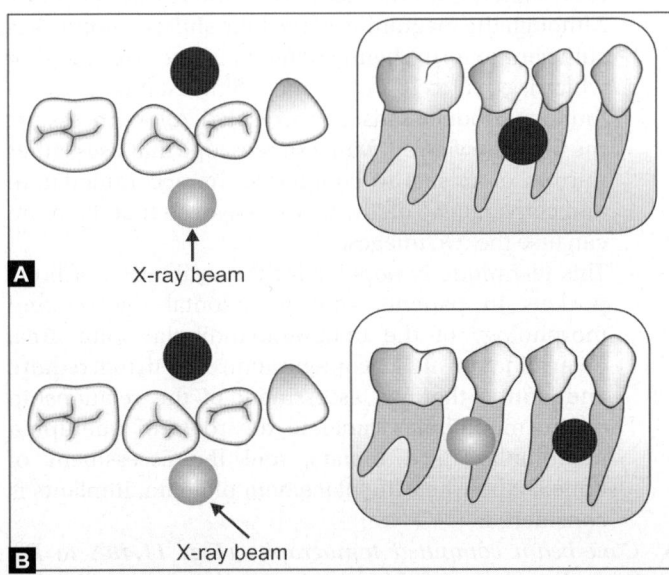

Figures 11.45A and B Buccal and lingual objects shift positions when the direction of the X-ray beam is changed: (A) Buccal (cross hatched circle) and lingual (black circle) are superimposed in the original radiograph; (B) If the tube head is shifted in the mesial direction, the buccal object moves distally and the lingual object moves mesially (Same direction = Lingual; Opposite direction = Buccal)

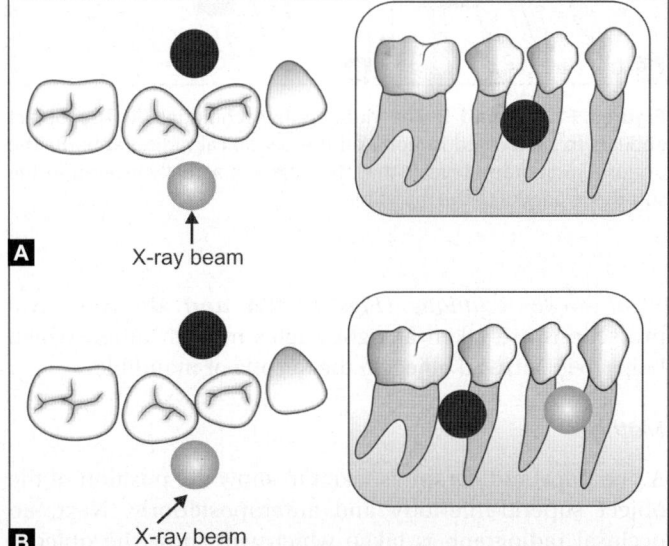

Figures 11.46A and B Buccal and lingual objects shift positions when the direction of the X-ray beam is changed: (A) Buccal (cross hatched circle) and lingual (black circle) are superimposed in the original radiograph; (B) If the tube head is shifted in the distal direction, the buccal object moves mesially and the lingual object moves distally (Same direction = Lingual; Opposite direction = Buccal)

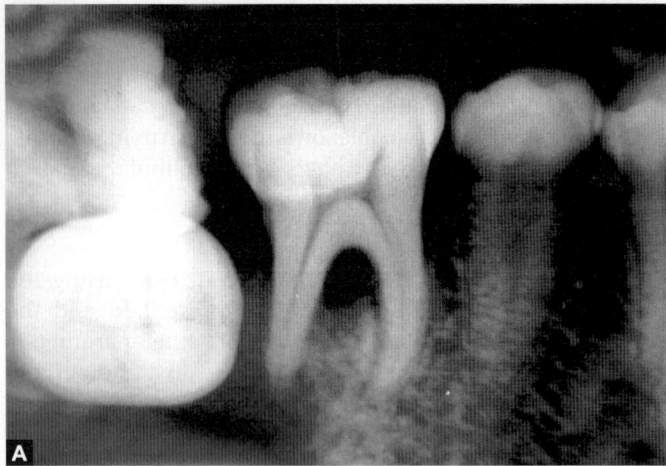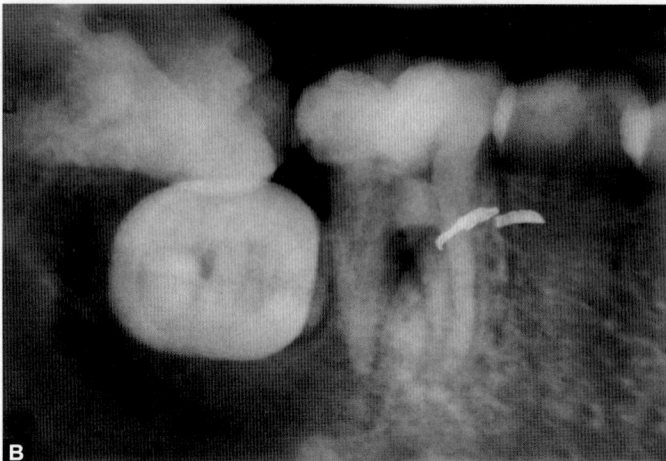

Figures 11.47A and B (A) Normal IOPA; (B) IOPA taken with mesial tube shift, the 2nd molar appears to have shifted mesially

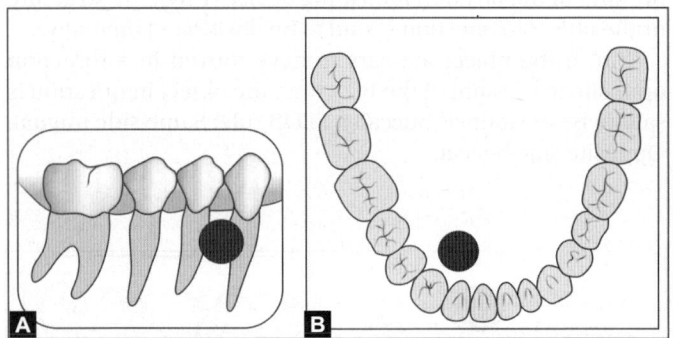

Figures 11.48A and B The right-angle technique: (A) The object appears to be located in bone on the periapical radiograph; (B) The occlusal radiograph reveals that the object is actually located in the soft tissue lingual to the mandible

*Right angle technique (**Figs 11.48A and B**):* Here two projections are taken at right angles to each other, which helps to localize an object in the maxilla or mandible.

Method

A periapical radiograph is taken to show the position of the object superio-inferiorly and anteroposteriorly. Next, an occlusal radiograph is taken which will show the object's buccolingual and anteroposterior relationship.

The two radiographs when studied together help to localize the object in all three dimensions.

- *Stereoscopy:* It has been used to determine the location of small intracranial calcifications and multiple foreign bodies in dense or thick section, and in cases in which the interpretation of images produced at right angles might be difficult and to evaluate the relationships of margins of bony fractures.
  - Stereoscopic imaging requires the exposure of two films, one for each eye, and thus delivers twice the amount of radiation to the patient. Between exposures the patient is maintained in position, the film is changed, and the tube shifted from the right eye to the left eye position. Although the magnitude of the tube shift is empiric, it is sufficient to form slightly different images (A tube shift which is equal to 10% of the focal-film distance has been found to produce satisfactory results). After processing, the films are viewed with a stereoscope that uses either mirrors or prisms to coordinate the accommodation and convergence of the viewer's eyes so that the brain can fuse the two images.
  - This technique is popular for the evaluation of bony pockets in patients with periodontal disease and morphology of the temporomandibular joint area, determination of root configuration of teeth that require endodontic therapy, assessment of the relationship of the mandibular canal to the roots of unerupted mandibular third molars, and the assessment of bone shape when the placement of dental implants is considered.
- *Cone-beam computed tomography (**Figs 11.49A to D**):* With the advent of this imaging technique, localization of any object or impacted tooth has become very simple. Once the scan of the patient is obtained the data can be manipulated with the help of the available software and the desired object/tooth can be studied in all aspects, superior, inferior, buccal, lingual.

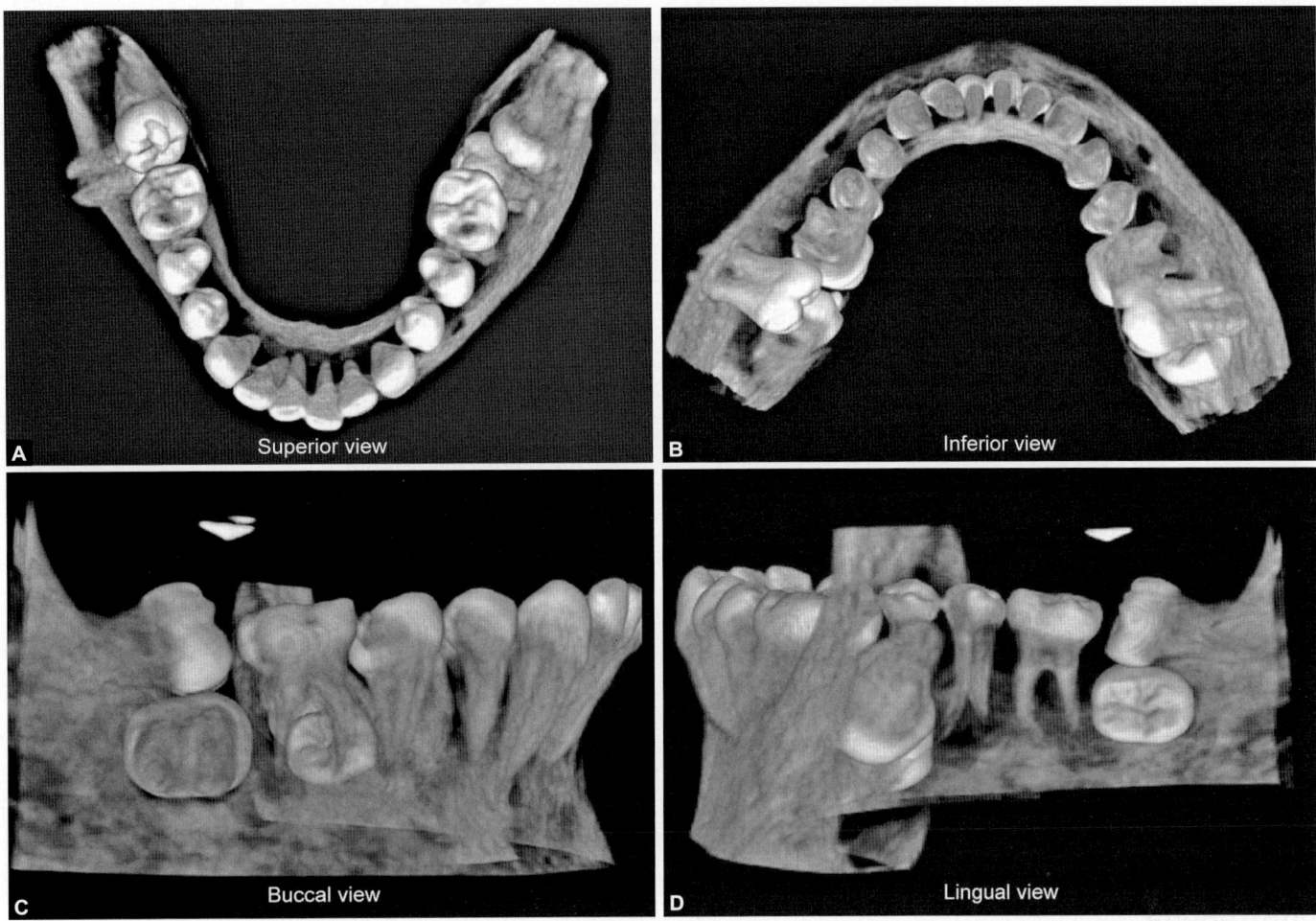

Figures 11.49A to D Cone-beam computed tomography showing superior, inferior, buccal and lingual view

BIBLIOGRAPHY

1. Frommer HH. Intraoral Radiographic Technique: The Paralleling Method in Radiology for Dental auxillaries, 6th edition. St Louis: Mosby-Year Book; 1996.pp.139-204.
2. Goaz PW, White SC. Intraoral Examination in Oral Radiology, Principles and Interpretation, 3rd edition St Louis: CV Mosby; 1994;102-05:151-212.
3. Johnson ON, McNally MA, Essay CE. The Periapical Examination Essentials of Dental Radiography for Dental Assistants and Hygienists, 6th edition. Norwalk: Appleton and Lange; 199;319-90.
4. Mason-Hing LR. In Fundamentals of Dental Radiography, 3rd edition. Philadelphia: WB Saunders; 1993.pp.1-139.
5. Matteson SR, Whaley C, Secrist VC. Intraoral Radiographic Techniques, In Dental Radiology, 4th edition. Chapel Hill: University of North Carolina Press; 1988.pp.77-105.

Extraoral Radiographs and Other Specialized Imaging Techniques

12

EXTRAORAL RADIOGRAPHIC TECHNIQUES

These techniques imply that the film is placed outside the oral cavity, against the side of the face to be radiographed and the X-ray beam is directed towards it.

INDICATIONS

- When it is not possible to place the film intraorally as during trismus
- To examine the extent of large lesions, especially when the area of pathology is greater than which can be covered by an intraoral periapical film
- When jaws or other facial bones have to be examined for evidence of disease lesions and other pathological conditions
- To evaluate skeletal growth and development
- To evaluate the status of impacted teeth
- To evaluate trauma
- To evaluate temporomandibular joint area.

DRAWBACKS

- Magnification occurs due to the greater object to film distance used

- Details are not well-defined due to the use of cassettes and intensifying screens. For optimum balance between loss of image detail and reduction of patient exposure medium or high speed screen film combinations should be used
- Contrast is reduced as the secondary radiation produced by the soft tissues is more.

An important aspect of the extraoral radiography techniques is the immobilization of the patient's head. This is achieved by the use of various devices like, compression bands, head clamps, craniostat.

Some Extraoral Landmarks Used for Patient Positioning (Figs 12.1A and B)

- The median plane of the head (Midsagittal plane)
- The infraorbital line
- The orbitomeatal line (Canthomeatal line)
- The frankfort horizontal line.

IMPORTANT PARAMETRES

The film focus distance is of paramount importance. An increase in the focus film distance will improve the image sharpness, but adequate collimation must be used to prevent scattered radiation.

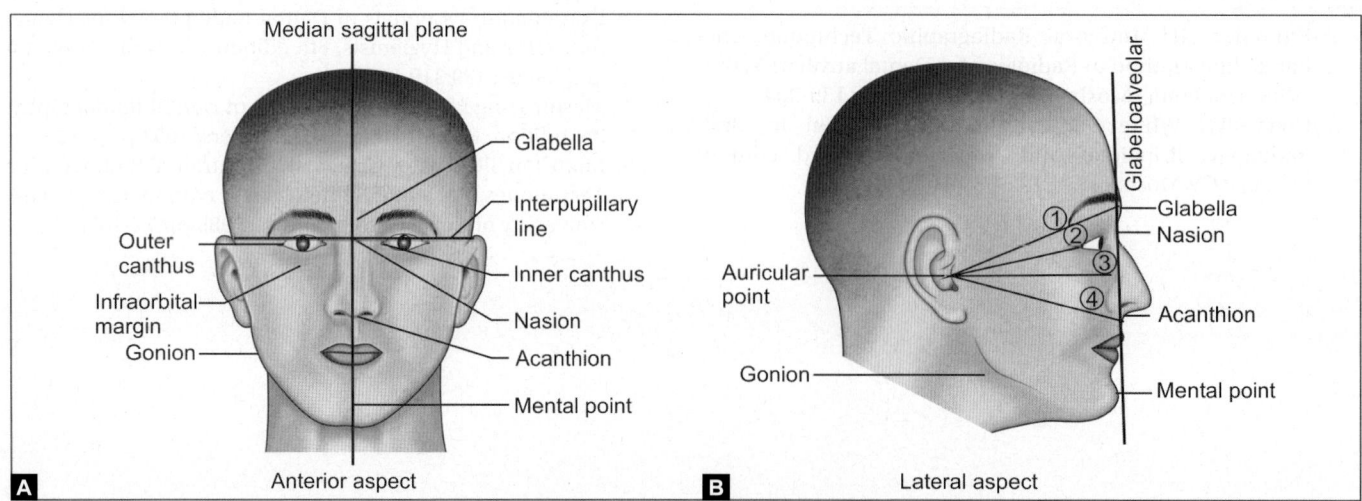

Figures 12.1A and B Diagram showing external guideline used for patient positioning: 1. Glabellomeatal line; 2. Orbitomeatal line; 3. Inframeatal line; 4. Acanthomeatal line

Most of the techniques for skull radiography use a film focus distance of approximately three feet (90 cm), in cephalometry a distance of five to six feet (150–180 cm) is used.

The centering point: The direction and angle of the central ray of the X-ray beam play an important and fundamental part in the clarity of the resultant shadow and the presence of distortion. The central beam should be so directed as to pass or project away from the dense structures which would over shadow the required details.

REQUIRED EQUIPMENT

- X-ray unit
  - Intraoral X-ray machine
  - Extraoral X-ray machine
  - Panoramic X-ray unit
  - Cephalometry X-ray unit
  - CBCT unit.
- Films
  - Extraoral nonscreen films
  - Extraoral screen films.
    - Sensitive to blue light
    - Sensitive to green light.
  - Panoramic films.
- Intensifying screens
  - Blue light
  - Green light.
- Film cassettes (Conventional/IP)
- Grids.

Procedure

- Equipment preparation
  - Load the extraoral cassette in the darkroom under safe light conditions. Place one extraoral film between two intensifying screens and securely close the cassette.
  - For digital processing
    - An IP cassette, make sure that the cassette has been read and cleared in the CR System
    - For DR system the sensor has to be readied
  - Set the exposure factors (kilo voltage, milliamperage, time) according to the manufacturer's recommendations.
  - Load the cassette into the cassette carrier.
  - Print in the date, patient's name, age, sex and the Case No.
- Patient preparation
  - Explain to the patient the radiographic procedure about to be performed.

- Place a lead apron without a lead collar over the patient and secure it. A double sided apron is recommended. The apron must be placed low around the back of the neck so that it does not block the X-ray beam. A thyroid collar is not recommended for extraoral radiography because it blocks part of the beam and obscures important diagnostic information.
- Remove all objects from the head and neck region that may interfere with film exposure. The patient must remove eyeglasses, ear rings, necklaces, napkin chains, hearing aids, hairpins and complete or partial removable dentures or any other removable appliance in the oral cavity.

MOST COMMONLY USED VIEWS FOR MAXILLOFACIAL IMAGING

- Radiography of paranasal sinuses
  - Posteroanterior projection (also known as occipito frontal projection of nasal sinuses)
    There are 2 methods for obtaining this projection.
    - Posterior anterior (Granger projection).
    - Modified method, inclined posterior anterior (Caldwell projection).
- Radiography of the maxillary sinuses
  - Standard occipitomental projection (0° OM)
  - Modified method (30° occipitomental projection)
  - Bregma menton
  - PA Water's
- Radiography of the mandible
  - PA mandible
  - Rotated PA mandible
  - Lateral oblique
    - Anterior body of mandible
    - Posterior body of mandible
    - Ramus of mandible
- Radiography of base of the skull
  - Submento vertex projection
- Radiography of the zygomatic arches
  - Jughandle view (A modification of submento vertex view)
- Radiography of the temporomandibular joint
  - Transcranial projection
  - Transpharyngeal projection
  - Transorbital projection
  - Reverse towne's projection
- Radiography of the skull
  - Lateral cephalogram
  - True lateral
  - PA cephalogram
  - PA skull
  - Towne's projection.

MODIFIED METHOD, INCLINED POSTEROANTERIOR (CALDWELL) PROJECTION (FIGS 12.2A AND B)

Structures Shown

This angulation will cause the petrous ridges to be superimposed on the maxillary sinuses, thus allowing more accurate examination of the orbits and ethmoidal air cells.

Film Placement

The cassette is placed perpendicular to the floor in a cassette holding device. The long-axis of the cassette is positioned vertically.

Position of Patient

The midsagittal plane is vertical and perpendicular to the cassette.

Only the forehead and nose touch the cassette, so that the canthomeatal line is perpendicular to the cassette. On the resultant radiograph the superior border of the petrous ridge is projected in the lower third of the orbit.

Central Ray

Is directed 23° to the canthomeatal line, entering the skull about 3 cm above the external occipital protuberance and exiting at the glabella.

Exposure Parameters

- Using extraoral machine
- kVp—70–80
- mA—60–50, seconds—1.6 (Bucky grid).

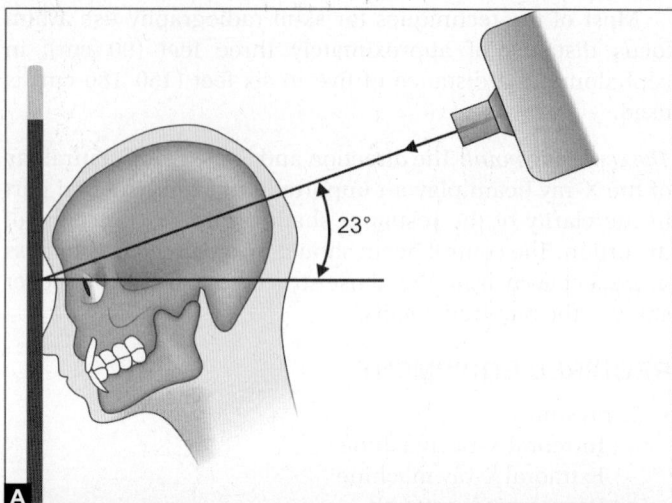

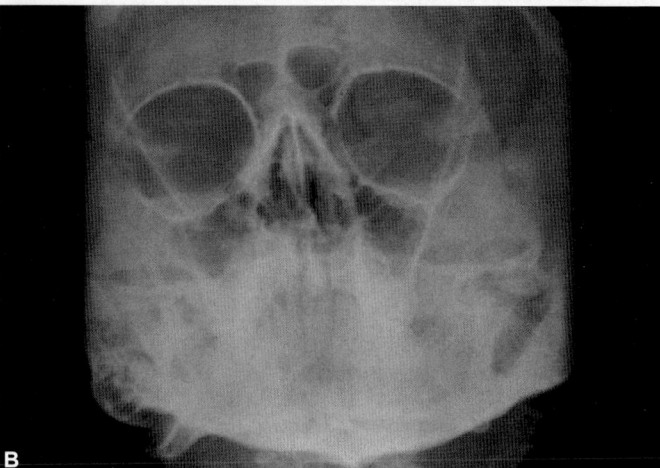

Figures 12.2A and B (A) Diagram of the positioning inclined posteroanterior (Caldwell) projection; (B) Caldwell projection

POSTEROANTERIOR WATER'S (FIGS 12.3A AND B)

Structures Shown

This projection is primarily used to demonstrate the maxillary sinus, frontal and ethmoidal sinuses.

The sphenoidal sinuses can be seen if the patient is asked to open his mouth, whereby the sphenoidal sinuses are projected on the palate.

The orbit, frontozygomatic suture, nasal cavity, coronoid process of the mandible and the zygomatic arch are also seen.

Film Placement

The cassette is placed perpendicular to the floor in a cassette holding device. The long-axis of the cassette is positioned vertically.

Position of Patient

The midsagittal plane should be vertical and perpendicular to the plane of the film.

The patient's head is extended so that only the chin touches the cassette.

The cassette is centered around the acanthion (anterior nasal spine).

The canthomeatal line should be at 37° to the plane of the film and the line from the external auditory meatus to the mental protuberance should be perpendicular to the film.

In this position the aim is to extend the patient's head just enough so as to place the dense shadows of the petrosae immediately below the antral floors.

When the head is extended too little, the petrosal shadows are projected onto the lower part of the antrum.

When the head is extended too much the antral shadows are foreshortened and results in failure to show the antral floor.

Water's (1915) specified that the tip of the nose should be 0.5 to 1.5 cm away from the cassette, Mahoney (1930) found that the petrosal shadows can be correctly placed by adjusting the orbitomeatal line at 37° to the horizontal.

An easy visual method is that a line extending from the external auditory meatus to the mental protuberance of the chin should be perpendicular to the cassette.

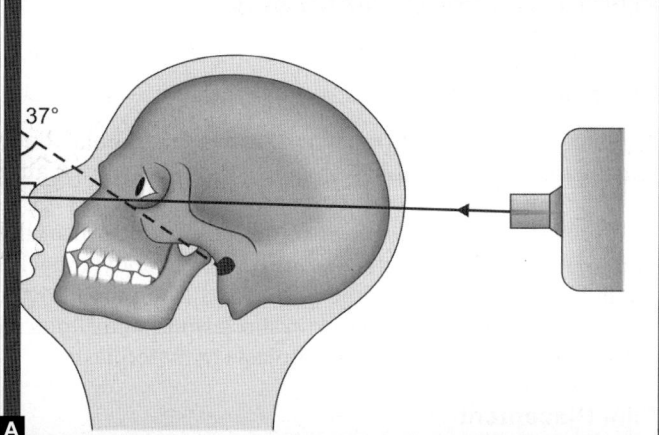

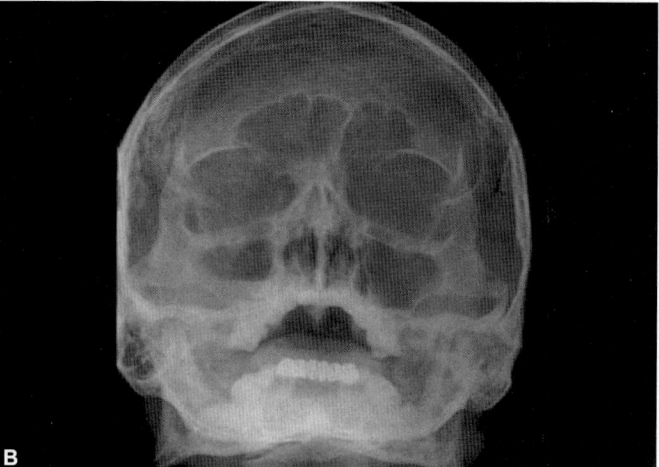

Figures 12.3A and B (A) Diagram for the positioning of posteroanterior Water's projection, the radiographic base line is at 37° to the film, and the X-ray is perpendicular to the film; (B) Posteroanterior Water's view

Central Ray

Central ray is directed perpendicular and to the mid point of the film. It enters from the vertex and exists from the acanthion.

Exposure Parameters

- Using extraoral machine
- kVp—70-80
- mA—60-50, seconds—1.6 (Bucky grid).

POSTEROANTERIOR MANDIBLE (FIGS 12.4A AND B)

Structures Shown

A posteroanterior (PA) projection of the mandibular body and the ramus. The symphysis region is not well seen because of the superimposition of the spine.

It is used to study fractures of the posterior third of the body of the mandible, angles, rami and lower condylar necks, mediolateral expansion of the posterior third of the body or the rami in case of tumors or cystic lesions, maxillofacial deformities and mandibular hypoplasia or hyperplasia.

Film Placement

The cassette is placed perpendicular to the floor in a cassette holding device. The long-axis of the cassette is positioned vertically.

Position of Patient

The sagittal plane should be vertical and perpendicular to the film.

The head is tipped downwards so that the forehead and nose touch the film. The radiographic base line is horizontal and perpendicular to the film.

The film is adjusted so that the lips are centered to the film.

Central Ray

Is directed at right angles to the film through the midsagittal plane through the cervical spine, at the level of the angles of the mandible.

Exposure Parameters

- Using extraoral machine
- kVp—65–80
- mA—60–80, seconds—1.6 (Bucky grid).

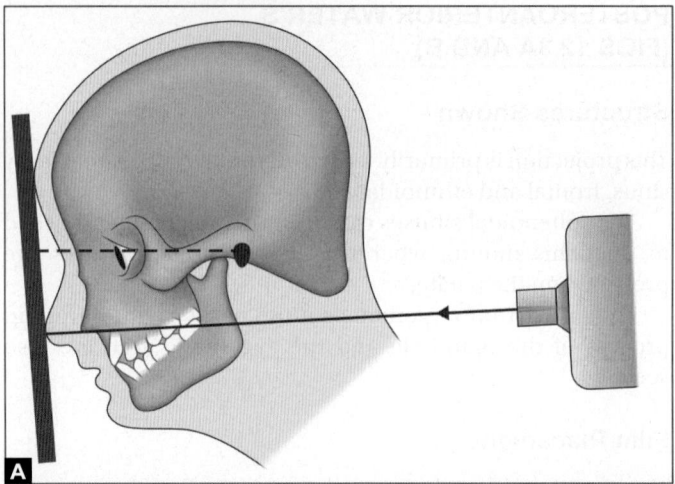

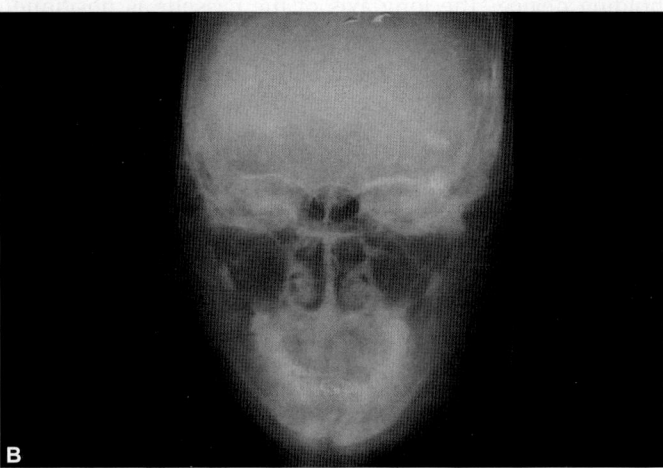

Figures 12.4A and B (A) Diagram for the positioning of posteroanterior mandible projection, the radiographic base line and the X-ray beam are perpendicular to the film; (B) Posteroanterior mandible view

ROTATED POSTEROANTERIOR MANDIBLE (FIGS 12.5A AND B)

Structures Shown

This projection is used to show the tissues of one side of the face and used to investigate the parotid gland and the ramus of the mandible. It is mainly used to demonstrate, stones or calculi in the parotid, to note the mediolateral expansion of lesions in the ramus and submasseteric infections.

Film Placement

The cassette is placed perpendicular to the floor in a cassette holding device. The long-axis of the cassette is positioned vertically.

Position of Patient

The patient is positioned facing the film, with the occlusal plane horizontal and the tip of the nose touching the film.

The head is rotated 10° to the side of interest. This rotates the bones of the back of the skull away from the side of the face under investigation.

Central Ray

It is directed at right angles to the film, aimed down the side of the face which is of interest.

Exposure Parameters

- Using extraoral machine
- kVp—65–80
- mA—60–80, seconds—1.6 (Bucky grid).

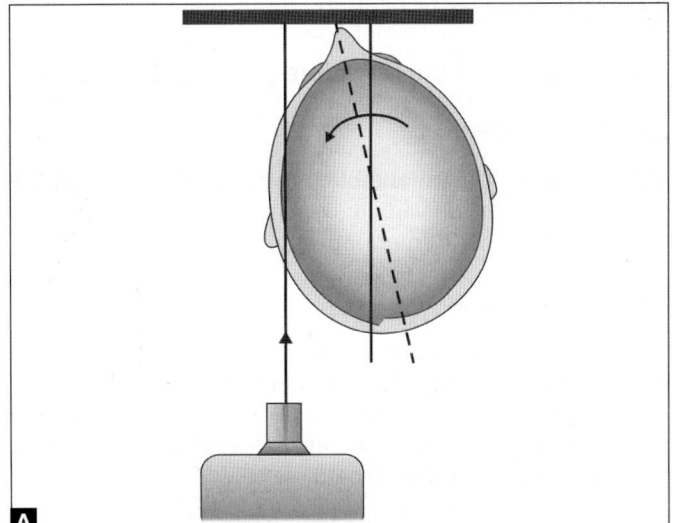

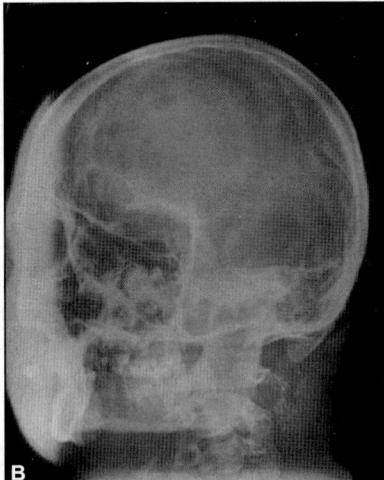

Figures 12.5A and B (A) Diagram for positioning rotated posteroanterior, from above, 10° rotation of the head to the side of interest and the X-ray beam aimed along the side of the face; (B) Rotated posteroanterior view showing parotid sialography, with the central ray passing through the glands

LATERAL OBLIQUE

Anterior Body of the Mandible (Figs 12.6A and B)

Structures Shown

Anterior body of the mandible, position of the teeth in the same area. Helps to evaluate impacted teeth, fractures and lesions located in the anterior portion of the mandible.

Film Placement

The cassette is placed flat against the patient's cheek and is centered over the body of the mandible, overlying the canine teeth. The patient must hold the cassette in position with the thumb placed under the edge of the cassette and the palm against the outer surface of the cassette.

Position of Patient

The patient's head is so adjusted, that the ala tragus line is parallel to the floor.

The mandible is protruded slightly to separate it from the vertebral column. The cassette is placed over the patient's cheek and centered over the area of interest.

The inferior border of the cassette should be parallel to the lower border of the mandible and below it.

The sagittal plane is tilted so that it is 5° to the vertical, and rotated 30° from the true lateral position.

For the bicuspid and incisor region, the patient's head should be turned slightly away from the tube so that the nose and chin approximate the cassette.

Central Ray

Is directed from 2 cm below the angle of the mandible opposite to the side of interest. The beam is directed upward (–10° to –15°) and centered on the anterior body of the mandible. The beam must be directed perpendicular to the horizontal plane of the film.

Exposure Parameters

- Using intraoral X-ray machine
- kVp—65–70, mA—7–10, seconds—0.8

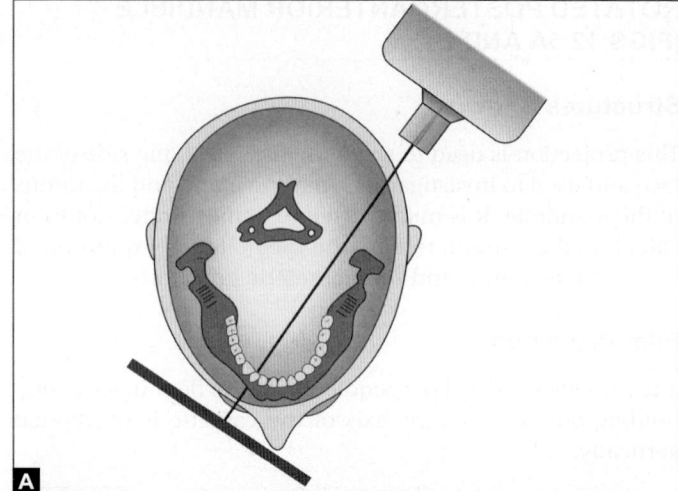

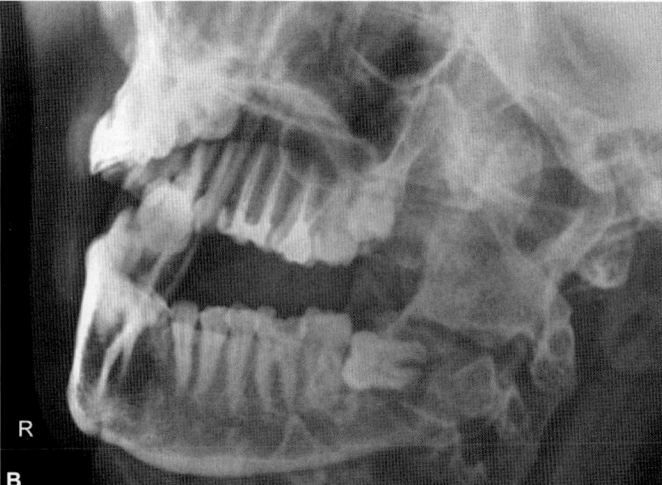

Figures 12.6A and B (A) Diagram for the positioning of lateral oblique projection for anterior body of the mandible, film is in contact with the cheek at the canine area, and the X-ray beam aims at the canine area, through the radiographic key hole; (B) Lateral oblique for the body of the anterior mandible

- Using extra oral X-ray machine
- kVp—40, mA—40, seconds—1.

LATERAL OBLIQUE

Posterior Body of Mandible (Figs 12.7A and B)

Structures Shown

Body of the mandible, position of the teeth in the same area, ramus of the mandible, angle of the mandible. Helps to evaluate impacted teeth, fractures and lesions located in the posterior border of the mandible.

Film Placement

The cassette is placed flat against the patient's cheek and is centered over the body of the mandible. The cassette also should be positioned parallel to the body of the mandible. The patient must hold the cassette in position with the thumb placed under the edge of the cassette and the palm against the outer surface of the cassette.

Position of Patient

The patient's head is so adjusted, that the ala tragus line is parallel to the floor.

The mandible is protruded slightly to separate it from the vertebral column. The cassette is placed over the patient's cheek and centered over the area of interest.

The inferior border of the cassette should be parallel to the lower border of the mandible and below it.

The sagittal plane is tilted so that it is 5° to the vertical and the head is rotated 10° to 15° from the true lateral position.

For the molar and ramus region, the head should not be turned away from the tube as this will place the ramus behind the vertebral column.

Central Ray

Is directed from 2 cm below the angle of the mandible opposite to the side of interest. The beam is directed upward (–10° to –15°) and centered on the body of the mandible. The beam must be directed perpendicular to the horizontal plane of the film.

Exposure Parameters

- Using intraoral X-ray machine
- kVp—65-70

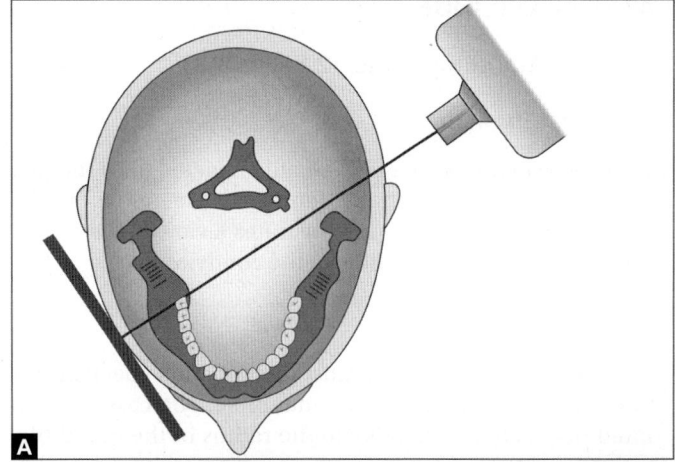

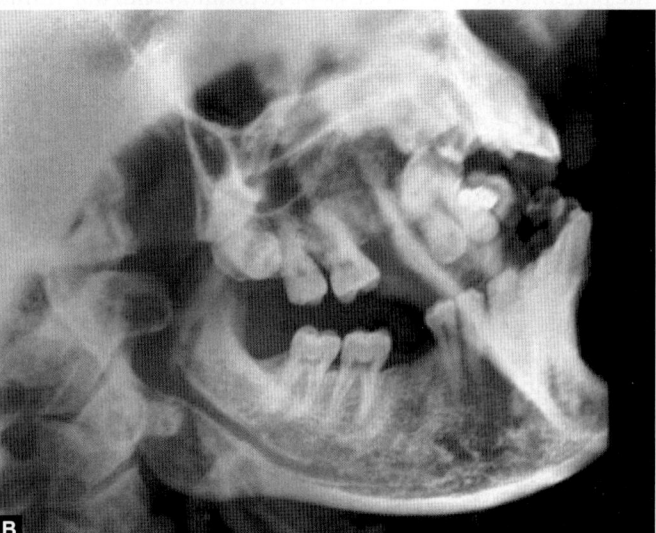

Figures 12.7A and B (A) Diagram for the positioning of lateral oblique projection for posterior body of the mandible, film is in contact with the cheek at the premolar area, and the X-ray beam aims at the premolar area, through the radiographic key hole; (B) Lateral oblique projection of the body of the mandible

- mA—7-10, seconds—0.8
- Using extraoral X-ray machine
- kVp—40
- mA—40, seconds—1.

LATERAL OBLIQUE

Ramus of Mandible (Figs 12.8A and B)

Structures Shown

The purpose of this view is to evaluate impacted third molars, large lesions, fractures that extend into the ramus of the mandible. This projection demonstrates a view of the ramus from the angle of the mandible to the condyles.

Film Placement

The cassette is placed flat against the patient's cheek and is centered over the ramus of the mandible. The cassette also should be positioned parallel to the ramus of the mandible. The patient must hold the cassette in position with the thumb placed under the edge of the cassette and the palm against the outer surface of the cassette.

Position of Patient

The patient's head is so adjusted, that the ala tragus line is parallel to the floor.

The mandible is protruded slightly to separate it from the vertebral column. The cassette is placed over the patient's cheek and centered over the area of interest.

The inferior border of the cassette should be parallel to the lower border of the mandible and below it.

The sagittal plane is tilted so that it is 10° to the vertical and the head is rotated 5° from the true lateral position.

Central Ray

Is directed from 2 cm below the angle of the mandible opposite to the side of interest, to a point posterior to the third molar region on the side opposite the cassette. The beam is directed upward (–10° to –15°) and centered on the ramus of the mandible. The beam must be directed perpendicular to the horizontal plane of the film.

Exposure Parameters

• Using intraoral X-ray machine
• kVp—65-70

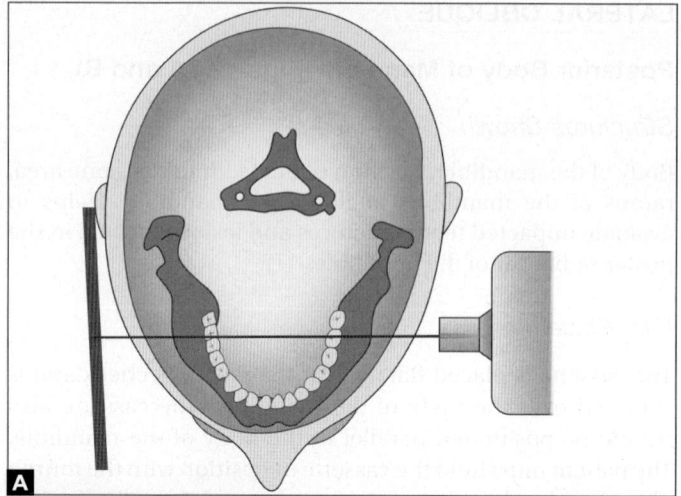

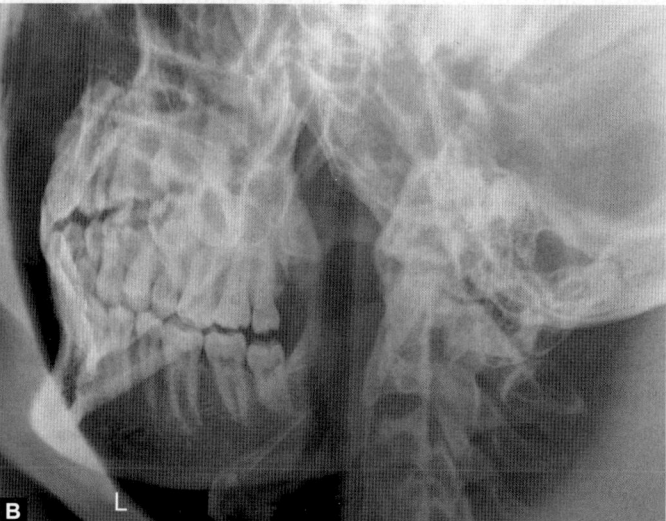

Figures 12.8A and B (A) Diagram for the positioning of lateral oblique projection for ramus of the mandible, film is in contact with the cheek at the ramus area, and the X-ray beam aims at the ramus area, between the cervical spine and mandibular ramus; (B) Lateral oblique projection of the mandibular ramus

• mA—7–10, seconds—0.8
• Using extra oral X-ray machine
• kVp—40, mA—40, seconds—1.

SUBMENTOVERTEX PROJECTION (FIGS 12.9A AND B)

Structures Shown

A full axial view of the base of the cranium showing a symmetrical projection of the petrosa, the mastoid process, foramen ovale, spinosum canals, carotid canals, sphenoidal sinuses, mandible, maxillary sinus, nasal septum, odontoid process of the atlas and the entire atlas, axial inclination of the mandibular condyles.

Helps to study destructive/expansile lesions affecting the palate, pterygoid region or base of the skull, sphenoidal sinus.

Film Placement

The cassette is placed perpendicular to the floor in a cassette holding device. The long-axis of the cassette is placed vertically.

Position of Patient

The head is centered on the cassette, with the patient's head and neck tipped back as far as possible, the vertex (top) of the skull touches the cassette. Both the midsagittal plane should be perpendicular to the plane of the film and the radiographic base line should be parallel to the film.

Central Ray

Is directed perpendicular to the film and through the midsagittal plane, between the angles of the mandible, perpendicular to an imaginary line joining the mandibular 1st molars (approximately 1 inch from the chin).

In order to view the petrous portion, the central ray is directed at right angles (or 5° to the horizontal) to the film midway between the external auditory meatus.

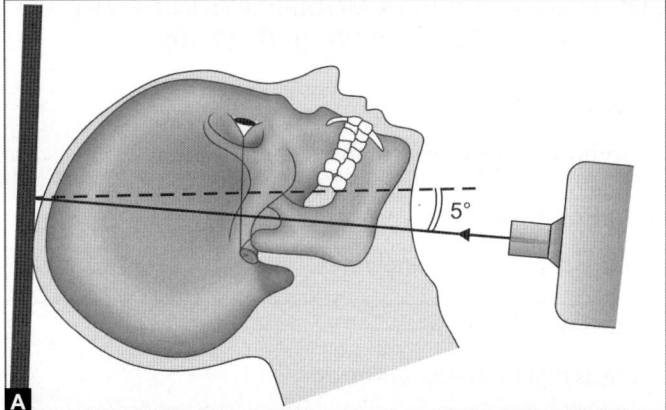

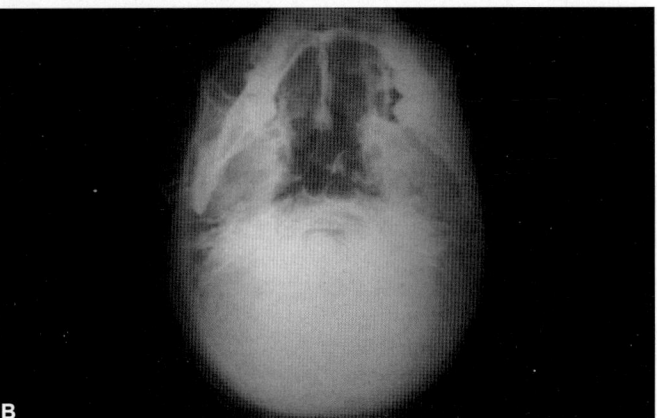

Figures 12.9A and B (A) Diagram for the positioning of submentovertex projection, the radiographic base line is parallel to the film, and the X-ray is perpendicular to the film; (B) Submentovertex view

Exposure Parameters

kVp—50
mA—20–30
seconds—0.4.

JUG HANDLE VIEW (A MODIFICATION OF THE SUBMENTOVERTEX VIEW) (FIG. 12.10)

Structures Shown

A symmetrical axial view of the zygomatic arches.

Film Position

Same as that in submentovertex.

Position of Patient

Same as that in submentovertex.

Central Ray

The cone is brought as close as possible to the patient (which leads to magnification of the structures at the base of the skull).

Exposure Parameters

- kVp—less than 50
- mA—20–30
- Seconds—0.4.

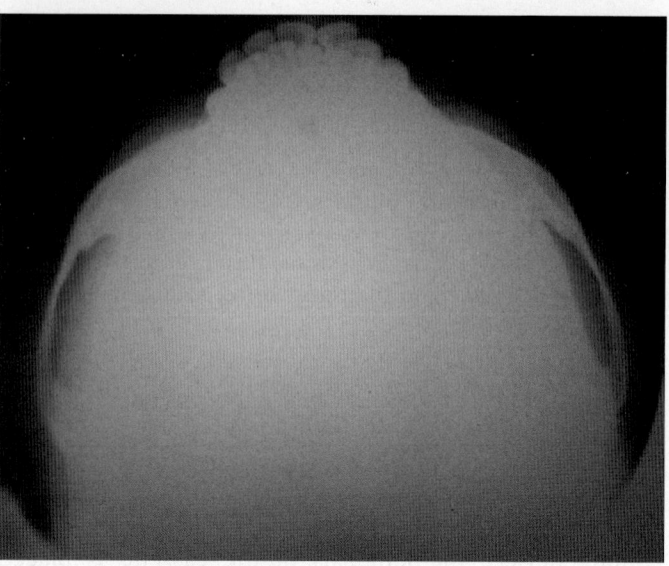

Figure 12.10 Jug handle view

The exposure time for the zygomatic arch is reduced to approximately one-third the normal exposure time for a submentovertex projection.

TRANSCRANIAL (FIGS 12.11A TO D)

Structures Shown

This technique is most useful in detecting arthritic changes on the articular surface. It helps to evaluate the joint's bony relationship. Changes on the central and medial surfaces are not seen.

Film Position

The cassette is placed flat against the patient's ear and centered over the TM joint of interest, against the facial skin parallel to the sagittal plane.

Position of Patient

The patient's head is adjusted so that the sagittal plane is vertical.

The ala tragus line is parallel to the floor.

This view is taken with the patient's mouth in three positions:
1. Open mouth.
2. Rest position.
3. Closed mouth.

Central Ray

The point of entry is different according to the technique used:
- Post auricular or Lindblom technique
  - Point of entry of the central ray is ½″ behind and 2″ above the auditory meatus.
  - According to Lindblom the central ray should be directed from posteriorly so that it passes along the long axis of the condyle. (The medial pole of the condyle is more posterior to the lateral pole).
- Grewcock approach
  - The central ray enters through a point 2″ above the external auditory meatus.
- Gill's approach
  - The central ray enters through a point ½″ anterior and 2″ above the external auditory meatus.
  - In all the three techniques the central ray is directed caudally at an angle of +20° to +25°.
  - The point of exit is through the TM joint of interest.

Exposure Parameters

- Intraoral X-ray machine
- kVp—70, mA—07, seconds—1.5.

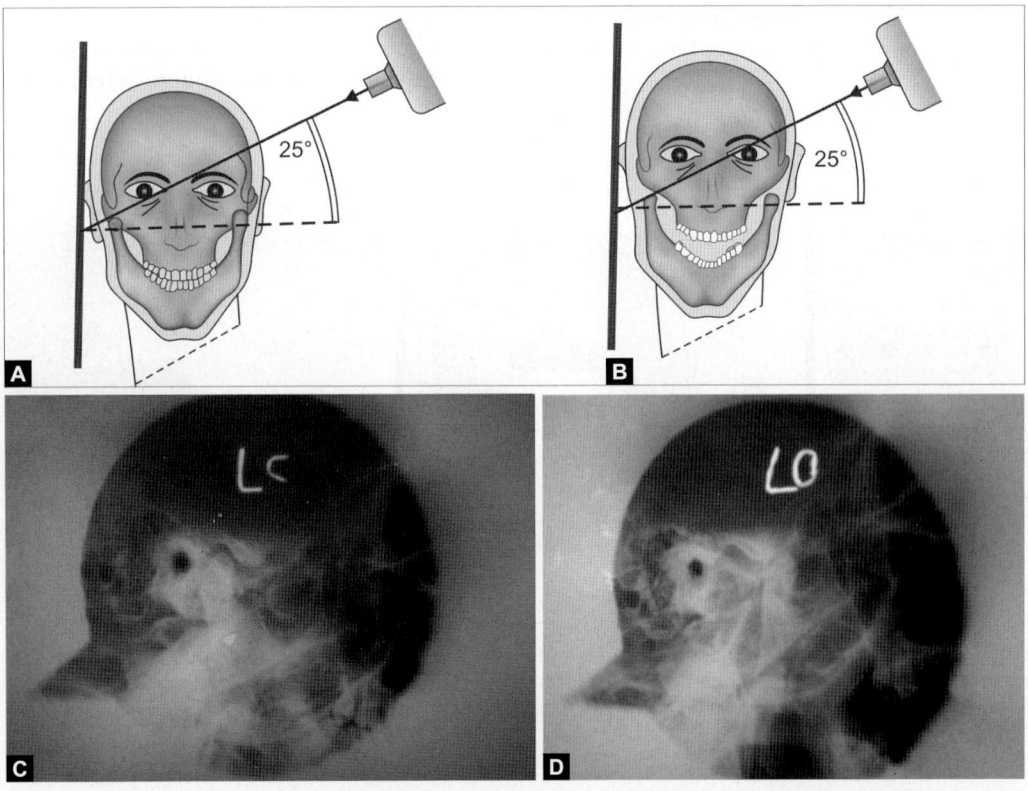

Figures 12.11A to D (A) Transcranial projection, the central ray is oriented at 25° positive angle from the opposite side and anteriorly 20°, centered over the TMJ of interest, mouth closed; (B) Transcranial projection, the central ray is oriented at 25° positive angle from the opposite side and anteriorly 20°, centered over the TMJ of interest, mouth open; (C) Transcranial view mouth closed position; (D) Transcranial view mouth open position

TRANSPHARYNGEAL (INFRACRANIAL OR McQUEEN DELL TECHNIQUE) (FIGS 12.12A to C)

Structures Shown

This view is a lateral projection showing medial surface of the condylar head and neck, usually taken in the mouth open position, so that the joint is projected into the shadow of air containing spaces of the nasopharynx, which helps to increase the contrast of the various parts of the joint.

Film Placement

The cassette is placed flat against the patient's ear and is centered to a point ½″ anterior to the external auditory meatus, over the TM joint of interest, against the facial skin parallel to the sagittal plane.

Position of Patient

The patient is positioned so that the sagittal plane is vertical and parallel to the film, with the TM joint of interest adjacent to the film.

The film is centered to a point ½″ anterior to the external auditory meatus.

The occlusal plane should be parallel to the transverse axis of the film so that the soft parts of the nasopharynx are in one line with the TM joint.

The patient is instructed to slowly inhale through the nose during exposure, so as to ensure filling of the nasopharynx with air during the exposure.

The patient should open his mouth so that the condyles move away from the base of the skull and the mandibular notch of the opposite side is enlarged.

Central Ray

It is directed from the opposite side cranially, at an angle of –5° to –10° posteriorly.

It is directed through the mandibular notch, that is a window between the coronoid, condyle and the zygomatic arch, of the opposite side below the base of the skull to the TM joint of interest.

Exposure Parameters

- Using intraoral X-ray machine
- kVp—65–70
- mA—7–10, seconds—0.8
- Using extra oral X-ray machine
- kVp—40, mA—40, seconds—1.

Parma Modification

The lead lined open ended cone is removed and the tube head is brought close to the skin surface, producing magnification of the tube side structures and there by reducing super imposition.

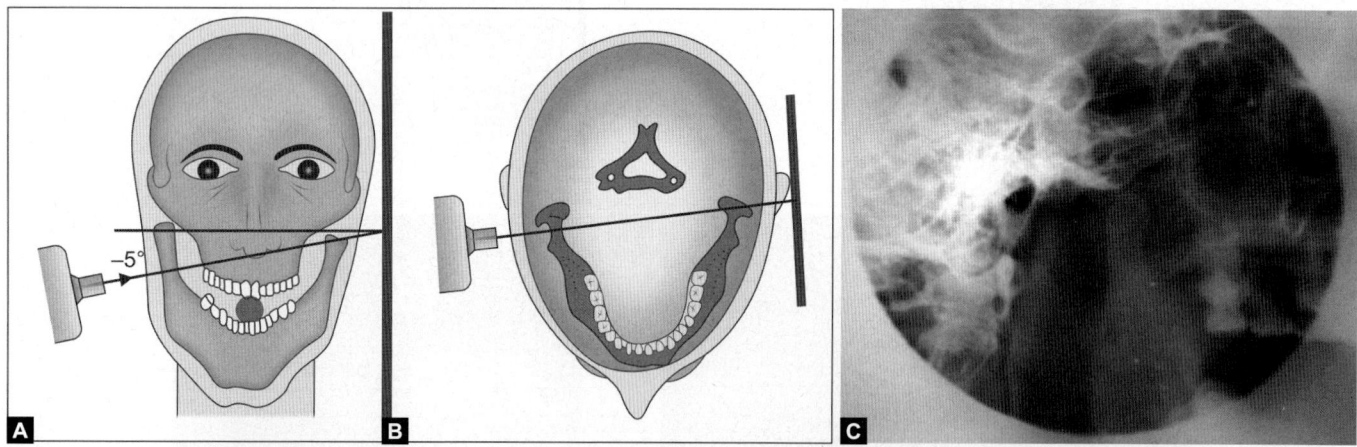

Figures 12.12A to C (A) Transpharyngeal projection. The central ray is oriented superiorly 5° to 10° and posteriorly approximately 10°, centered over the TMJ of interest. The mandible is positioned at maximal opening; (B) Transpharyngeal projection, showing positioning from above, showing the X-ray beam aimed slightly posteriorly across the pharynx; (C) Transpharyngeal view

TRANSORBITAL (ZIMMER PROJECTION) (FIGS 12.13A TO C)

This is the conventional frontal TM joint projection which is most successful in delineating the joint with minimal super impositions, leading to the production of a relatively true 'enface' projection.

Structures Shown

The anterior view of the temporomandibular joint and medial displacement of fractured condyle and fracture of neck of condyle are clearly seen in this view.

Film Position

The film is positioned behind the patient's head at an angle of 45° to the sagittal plane.

Position of Patient

The patient is positioned so that the sagittal plane is vertical.

The canthomeatal line should be 10° to the horizontal, with the head tipped downwards.

The mouth should be wide open.

Central Ray

The tube head is placed in front of the patient's face.

The central ray is directed to the joint of interest, at an angle of +20°, to strike the cassette at right angles.

The point of entry may be taken at:
- Pupil of the same eye, asking the patient to look straight ahead
- Medial canthus of the same eye
- Medial canthus of the opposite eye (**Fig. 12.13A**).

Exposure Parameters

- Using intraoral X-ray machine
- kVp—65–70
- mA—7–10, seconds—0.8
- Using extraoral X-ray machine
- kVp—40, mA—40, seconds—1.

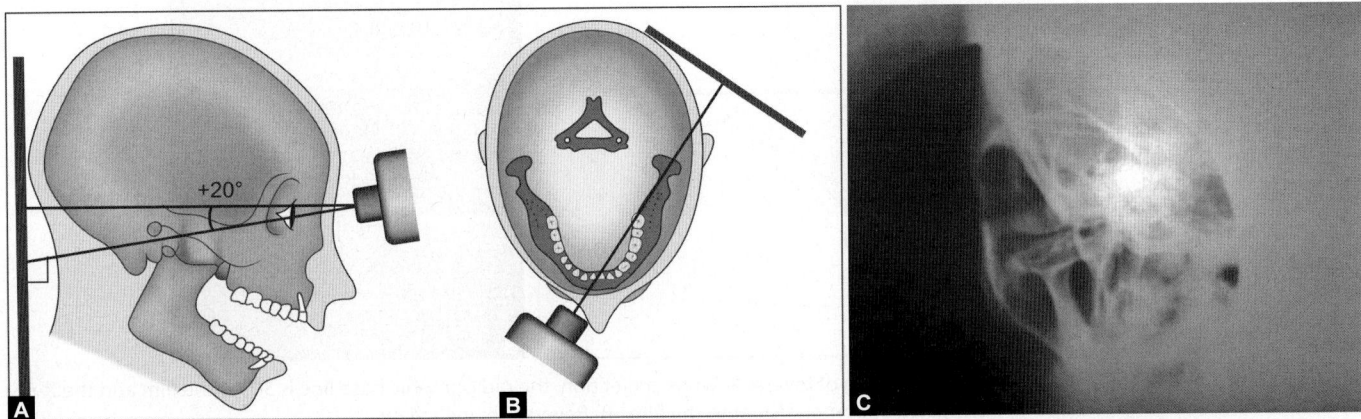

Figures 12.13A to C (A) Transorbital projection, the central ray is oriented downward approximately 20° and laterally approximately 30° through the contralateral orbit, centered over the TMJ of interest; (B) Transorbital projection, positioning from above, showing the cassette behind the condyle and X-ray beam aimed across the orbit; (C) Transorbital view

REVERSE TOWNE'S (FIGS 12.14A AND B)

Structures Shown

This view is primarily meant for viewing the condylar neck and head. High fractures of the condylar necks, intracapsular fractures of the TMJ, quality of articular surfaces, condylar hypoplasia or hypertrophy.

Film Position

The cassette is placed perpendicular to the floor in a cassette holding device. The long-axis of the cassette is placed vertically.

Position of Patient

The position of the patient is the same as that in PA mandible, that is:

- The sagittal plane should be vertical and perpendicular to the film
- The film is adjusted so that the lips are centered to the film
- Only the patient's forehead should touch the film.

The only difference being that the patient here is asked to keep his/her mouth wide open and the radiographic base line is at an angle of negative 30° to the film.

Central Ray

Central ray is directed through the midsagittal plane at the level of the mandible, and is perpendicular to the film.

Exposure Parameters

- Using extraoral machine
- kVp—70–80
- mA—60–50, seconds—1.6 (Bucky grid).

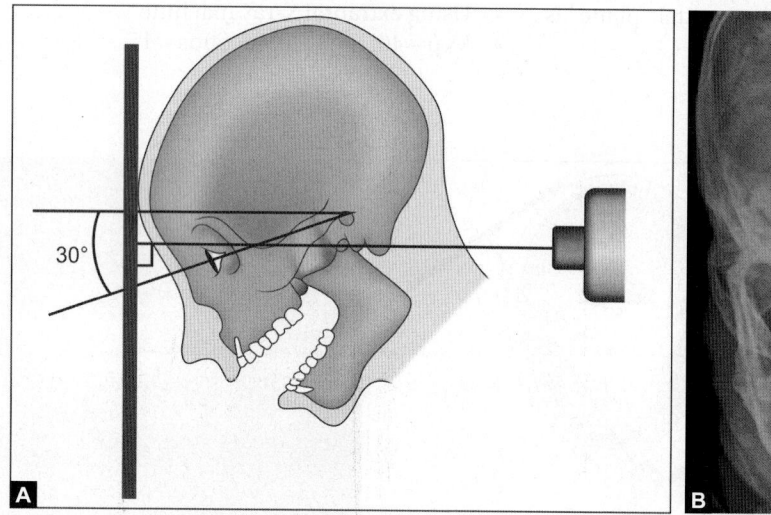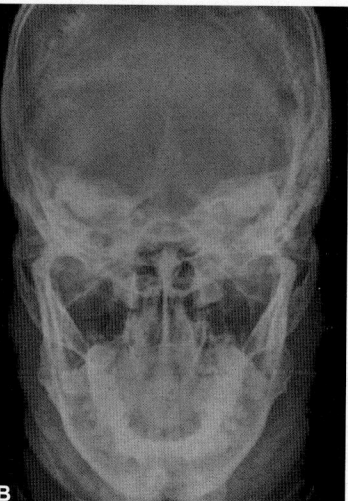

Figures 12.14A and B (A) Diagram for the positioning of reverse Towne's projection, the radiographic base line is 30° to the film and the X-ray is directed at perpendicular to the film; (B) Reverse Towne's view

LATERAL CEPHALOGRAM (FIGS 12.15A AND B)

Structures Shown

This view is used to evaluate facial growth and development, trauma, disease and developmental anomalies.

This projection demonstrates the bones of the face, skull as well as the soft tissue profile of the face.

The soft tissue outline of the face is more readily seen on the resulting radiograph when a filter is used. A filter is placed at the X-ray source, or between the patient and the film, and serves to remove some of the X-rays that pass through the soft tissue of the face, thus enhancing the image of the soft tissue profile.

In oral surgery and prosthetics it is used to establish pretreatment and post-treatment records.

Film Position

The cassette is placed perpendicular to the floor with the long axis of the cassette placed vertically. (FFD is the largest, 5 feet).

Position of Patient

The right side of the patient's head is positioned against the cassette.

The mid sagittal plane is perpendicular to the floor and parallel to the film/cassette.

The patient's head is stabilized with the help of the ear rods, nasion positioner and the orbital rod.

The patient is asked to keep the teeth in occlusion.

Central Ray

The central ray is directed perpendicular to the cassette through the porion.

The distance between the X-ray source and the midsagittal plane of the patient is 60 inches.

Exposure Parameters

- Using cephalometeric X-ray machine
- kVp—84
- mAs—13, seconds—1.6.

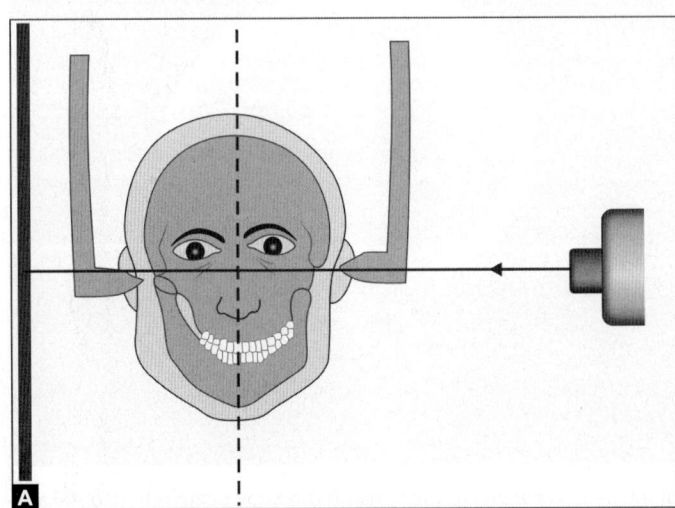 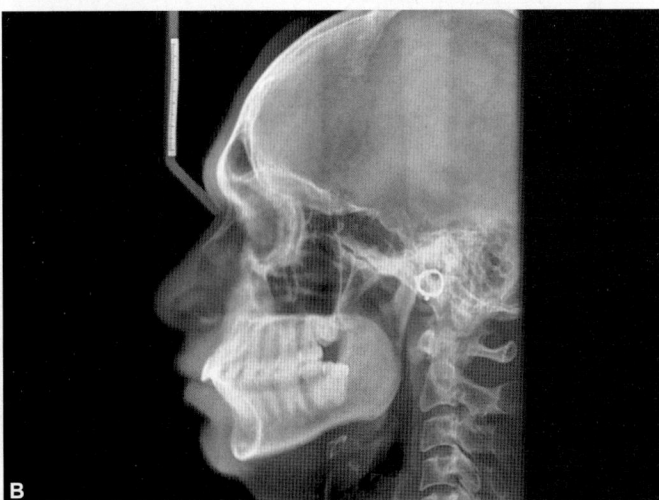

Figures 12.15A and B (A) Lateral cephalogram, the film is parallel to the midsagittal plane and the X-ray beam is directed perpendicular to the film; (B) Lateral skull radiograph (cephalometric technique). A cephalometric radiograph showing the relationship between the maxilla and the mandible in a patient, and demonstrating the soft tissue profile of the face. Note the broad radiopaque banding running vertically across the middle of the skull formed by part of the craniostat and also the circular ear-plugs

TRUE LATERAL (FIGS 12.16A AND B)

Structures Shown

It is used to survey the skull and facial bones for evidence of trauma, disease or developmental abnormality. This view reveals the nasopharyngeal soft tissues, paranasal sinuses and hard palate.

Conditions affecting the sella turcica, such as tumors of the pituitary gland in acromegaly.

Film Position

The film is held vertically against the patient's cheek and centered so that the entire skull along with the facial skeleton, is seen on the resultant radiograph.

Position of Patient

The sagittal plane should be vertical and parallel to the film.

The film is adjusted so that the upper circumference of the skull is ½ inch below the upper border of the cassette.

The patient here is asked to keep his/her teeth in occlusion, and the occlusal plane should be parallel to the floor.

Central Ray

The central ray is directed perpendicular to the cassette and the midsagittal plane and towards the external auditory meatus.

The distance between the X-ray source and the midcoronal plane of the patient is 36 to 40 inches.

Exposure Parameters

- Using extraoral machine
- kVp—70–80
- mA—60–50, seconds—1.6 (Bucky grid).

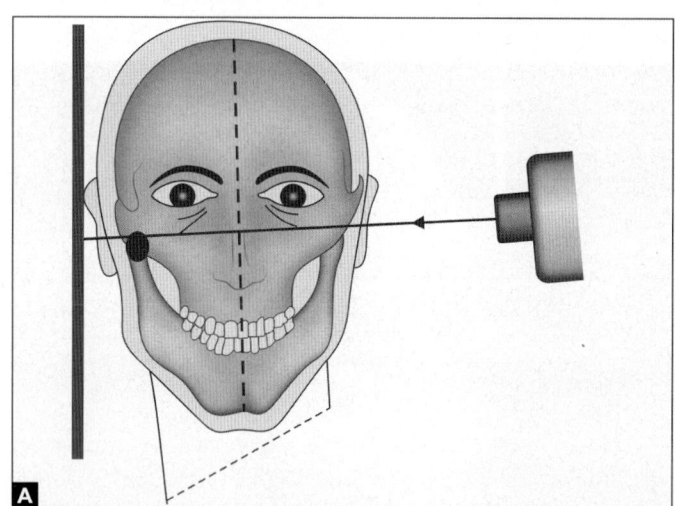 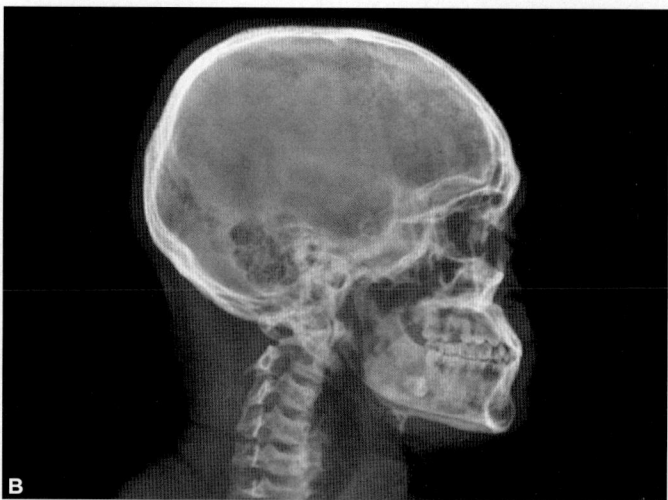

Figures 12.16A and B (A) True lateral skull projection, the sagittal plane of the head is parallel to the film and the X-ray beam is horizontal and perpendicular to the sagittal plane and the film; (B) True lateral view

POSTEROANTERIOR CEPHALOGRAM (FIGS 12.17A AND B)

Structures Shown

It is identical to posteroanterior (PA) view of the jaws except that it is standardized and reproducible. It is used for the assessment of facial asymmetries and for preoperative and postoperative comparisons in orthognathic surgeries involving the mandible.

Film Position

The cassette is placed perpendicular to the floor in a cassette holding device. The long-axis of the cassette is positioned vertically.

Position of Patient

The sagittal plane should be vertical and perpendicular to the film.

The head is tipped downwards so that only the nose touches the film. The radiographic base line is at 10° with the film.

The film is adjusted so that the lips are centered to the film.

Central Ray

Central ray is directed at right angles to the film through the midsagittal plane, centered at the level of the bridge of the nose.

Exposure Parameters

- Using Cephalometeric X-ray Machine
- kVp—84
- mA—13, seconds—1.5.

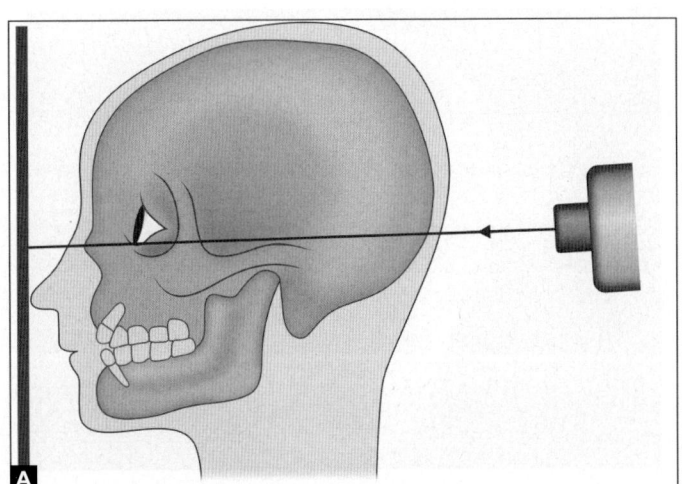 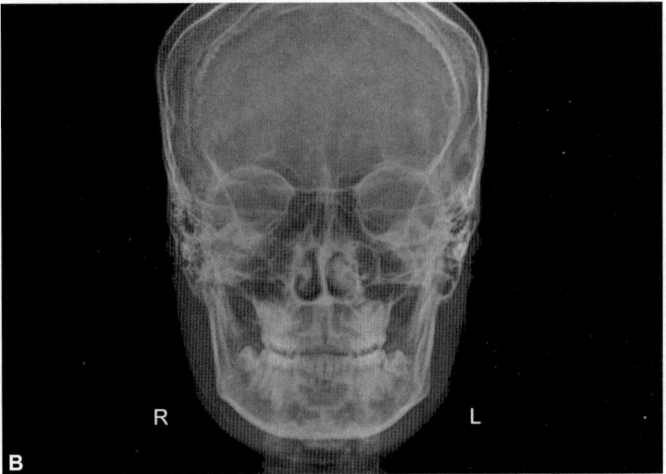

Figures 12.17A and B (A) Diagram for the positioning of posteroanterior cephalogram; (B) Posteroanterior cephalometric view

POSTEROANTERIOR SKULL (FIGS 12.18A AND B)

Structures Shown

Structure is used to survey the skull vault and primarily the facial bones for evidence of trauma, disease or developmental abnormality.

Fractures of the skull vault, investigation of frontal sinuses, conditions affecting the cranium (e.g. Paget's disease, multiple myeloma, hyperparathyroidism), intracranial calcifications.

Film Position

The cassette is placed perpendicular to the floor in a cassette holding device. The long-axis of the cassette is positioned vertically.

Position of Patient

The sagittal plane should be vertical and perpendicular to the film.

The head is tipped downwards so that the forehead and nose touch the film. The radiographic base line is horizontal and perpendicular to the film.

The film is adjusted so that the lips are centered to the film.

Central Ray

The central ray is directed at right angles to the film through the midsagittal plane through the occiput.

Exposure Parameters

- Using extraoral machine
- kVp—70–80
- mA—60–50, seconds–1.6 (Bucky grid).

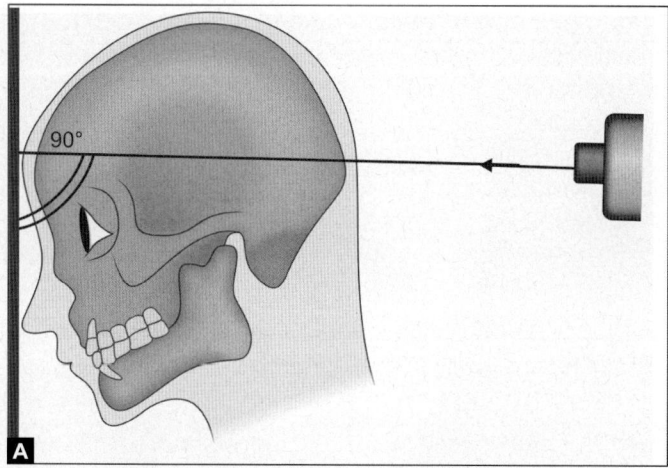
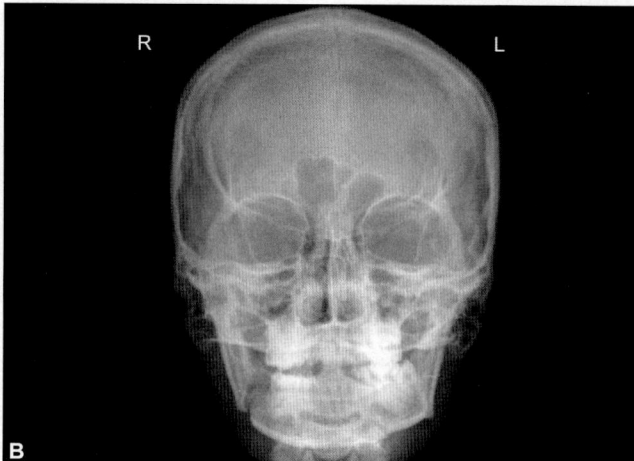

Figures 12.18A and B (A) Diagram for the positioning of posteroanterior skull projection, the radiographic base line is horizontal to the film and the X-ray beam is perpendicular to the film; (B) Posteroanterior skull view

TOWNE'S PROJECTION
(FIGS 12.19A AND B)

Structures Shown

It is primarily used to observe the occipital area of the skull. The necks of the condyloid process can also be viewed.

Film Position

The cassette is placed perpendicular to the floor in a cassette holding device. The long-axis of the cassette is positioned vertically.

Position of Patient

This is an anteroposterior view, with the back of the patient's head touching the film. The canthomeatal line is perpendicular to the film.

Central Ray

It is directed at 30° to the canthomeatal line and passes through it at a point between the external auditory canals.

Exposure Parameters

- Using extraoral machine
- kVp—70–80
- mA—60–50, seconds—1.6 (Bucky grid).

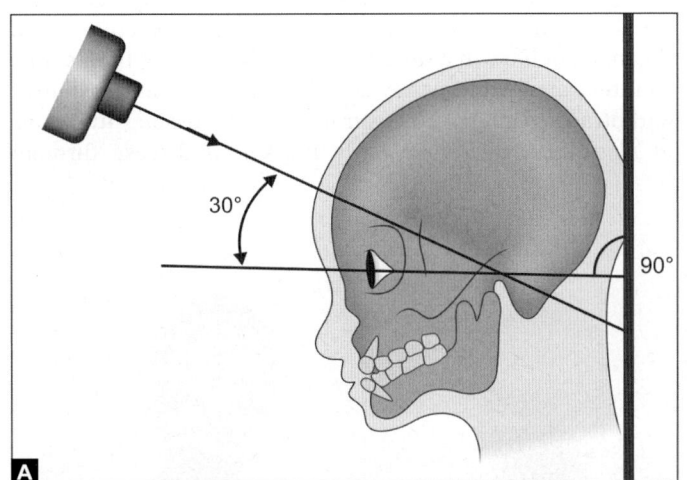 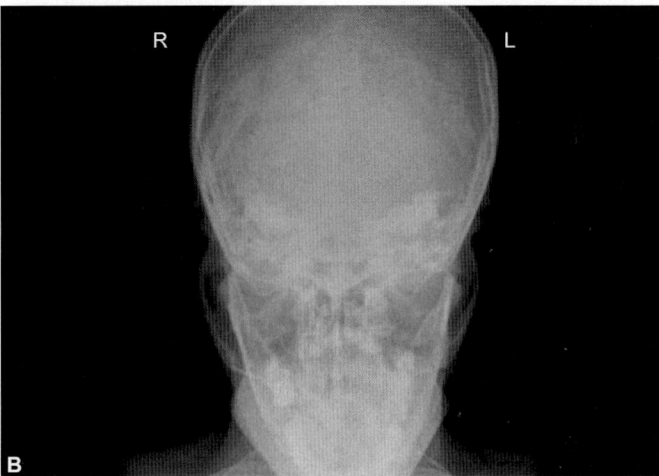

Figures 12.19A and B (A) Diagram for the positioning for Towne's projection, showing back of head of the patient touching the cassette and the central ray at an angle of 30° to the canthomeatal line; (B) Towne's view

OTHER SPECIALIZED IMAGING TECHNIQUES

Nuclear Medicine (Fig. 12.20)

Human disease can exist with no specific anatomic changes. Changes that are seen may simply be later effects of some biochemical process that remains undetected until physical symptoms develop. Radionuclide imaging (or functional imaging) provides the only means of assessing physiologic change that is a direct result of biochemical alteration.

Radioisotope imaging uses radioactive compounds that have an affinity for particular tissues so called target tissues. These radioactive compounds are injected into the patient, concentrated in the target tissue and their radiation emissions are then detected and imaged, usually using gamma camera. This investigation allows the function and/or the structure of the target tissue to be examined under both static and dynamic conditions.

Indications

- Investigations of salivary gland functions.
- Tumor staging—assessment of sites and extent of bone metastases.
- Evaluation of bone grafts.
- Assessment of continued growth in condylar hyperplasia.
- Investigation of the thyroid.
- Brain scans and assessment of the break down of the blood-brain barrier.

Nuclear medicine procedures are similar to those of conventional diagnostic radiology in that ionizing X-rays with energies of 20 to 510 kilo electron volt is used to generate an image, and a film looking some what like a radiograph is produced. However there are major differences:

- The patient, rather than the machine, is the source of radiation
- The detection instrument is different
- The sensitivities of nuclear medicine procedures are very great
- The specificities of the nuclear medicine procedures are very low.

Radionuclide imaging is based on the radiotracer method, which assumes that radioactive atoms or molecules in an organism behave in a manner identical to that of their stable counter parts because they are chemically indistinguishable. Radiotracers allow measurement of tissue functions *in vivo* and provide an early marker of disease through

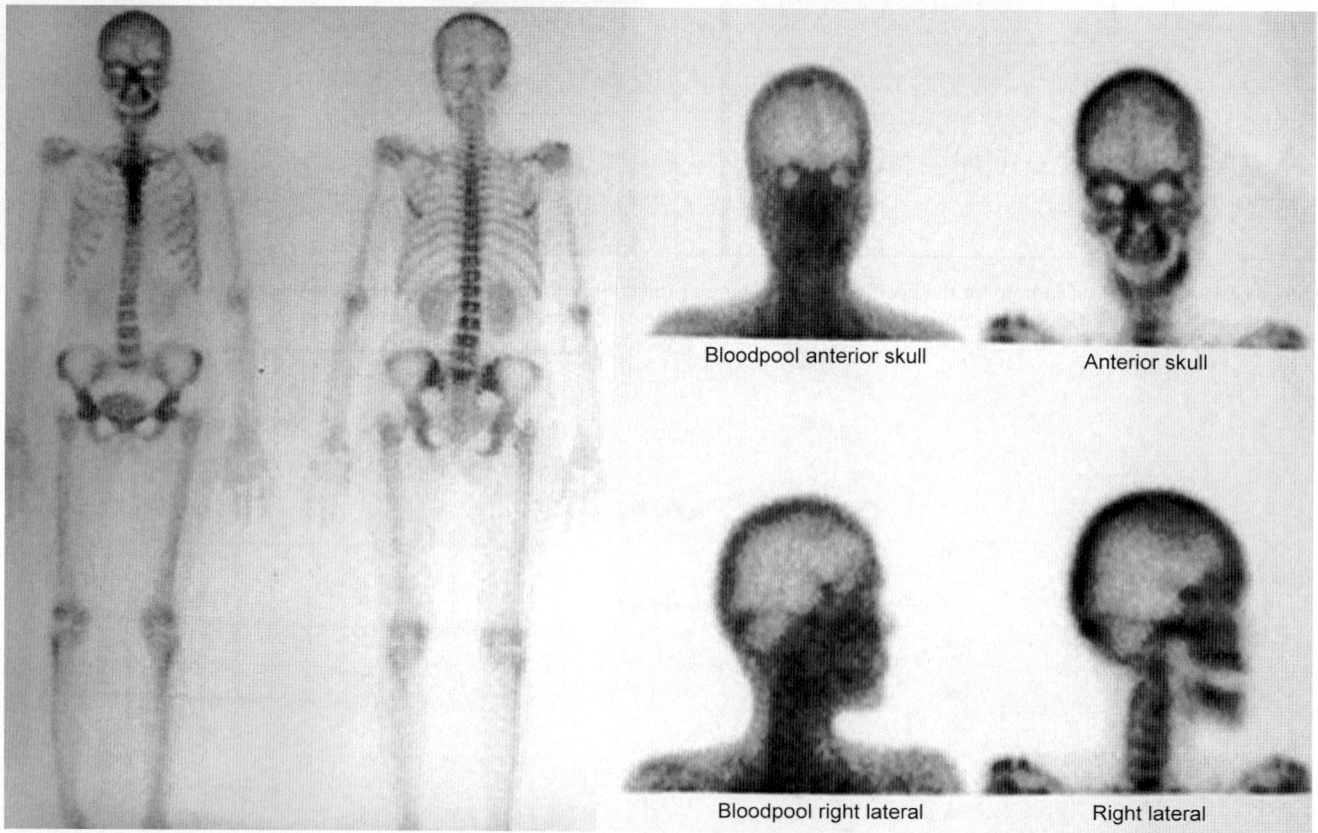

Figure 12.20 Bone scintigraphy showed increased radiotracer 99mTc-MDP uptake in left mandible. No similar lesion was found in other bones of the body, in a case of chronic osteomyelitis

measurements of biochemical change. Radionuclide-labeled tracers are used in quantities well below amounts that are lethal to cells.

The various radionuclide-label tracers which are used are:
- Technetium pertechnetate (99m Tc-pertechnetate)—salivary gland, thyroid, bone, blood, liver, lung and heart
- Iodine (131 I)—thyroid
- Gallium (67 Ga)—tumors and inflammation
- Selenium (74 Se)
- Krypton (81 Kr)—lung.

The use of tracers for diagnostic imaging became possible with the development of the rectilinear scanner and the gamma scintillation camera. Both these instruments record the gamma emissions from patients injected with appropriate tracers. The cameras use a scintillation crystal that has the ability to fluorescence on interaction with gamma rays. The fluorescence is detected by a photomultiplier tube that magnifies and amplifies the signal. The amplified signal is digitized and used to produce an image by computer algorithm. Use of a scintillation crystal for obtaining data for image formation has led to this technique being labelled as scintigraphy.

The newer procedures are those using:
- Single Photon Emission Computed Tomography (SPECT).
- Positron Emission Computed Tomography (PET).

Bone scan: In contrast to a radiograph, a bone scan gives no information on the morphology of a lesion, either internally or in areas of bone adjacent to the lesion. The scan does demonstrate, however, areas of altered bone metabolism within and around the lesion, thus allowing a reasonably accurate assessment of the growth of a lesion and extent of its borders. Bone scan also allows to view the entire skeleton with no additional radiation burden to the patient. Positive finding usually lead to conventional radiographs of the suspicious areas, allowing morphologic study of regions with altered metabolism.

Salivary scan: There is a substantial difference between salivary gland scanning and contrast sialography, the conventional radiographic technique most frequently used to examine the major salivary glands. A sialogram is primarily an anatomic study using conventional contrast radiography techniques while a salivary gland scan is primarily a functional study using a tissue specific radioactive scanner. The techniques complement each other significantly and, when used together, render more complete information on the salivary glands than either technique used alone. When used together the scan should be done first as sialography causes a mild diffuse inflammation of the gland, which may cause increased uptake of 99 m TcO4–, leading to spurious scan results.

Advantages

- Target tissue function is investigated
- All similar target tissue can be examined during one investigation, e.g. the whole skeleton can be imaged during one bone scan
- Computer analysis and enhancement of results is available.

Disadvantages

- Image resolution is poor—often only minimal information is obtained on target tissue anatomy
- The radiation dose to the whole body can be relatively high
- Images are not usually disease specific
- Some investigations take several hours
- Facilities are not widely available.

Diagnostic Ultrasound (Fig. 12.21)

Principle

As sound passes through any material, it encounters a certain level of impedance referred to as an 'acoustic impedance'. As sound passes from tissues of one sound acoustic impedance to another, some of it is reflected, some of it continues to penetrate and some energy is transferred to the particles of the medium as vibrational energy.

The greater the difference in acoustic impedance of the tissue, the greater is the sound reflected. This reflected sound (or echo) is picked up by the transducer and converted into electric impulses and finally displayed on the screen.

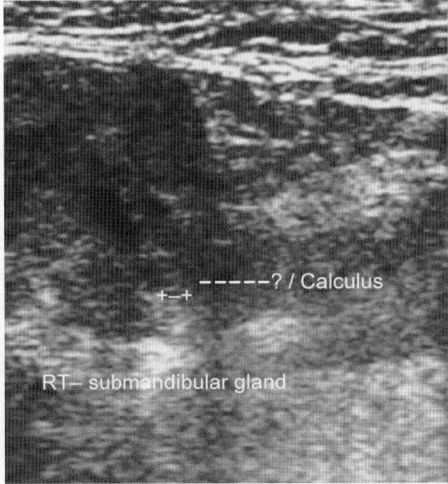

Figure 12.21 Ultrasound of right submandibular gland with hyper echoic area—calculus

By definition, ultrasound has a periodicity greater than 20 kHz. Diagnostic ultrasonography (sonography), the clinical application of ultrasound, uses vibratory frequencies in the range of 1–20 MHz.

Changes in echo pattern can delineate different tissues, but they can also be correlated with pathological changes in a tissue.

A-scan—is produced with the modulation of amplitude, the image appears as spikes extending towards the baseline. The height of each tracing is related to the intensity of each echo. A-scan shows the relationship between amplitude and depth, and are used for measuring the distances between boundaries of tissues with different acoustic properties. A-scan is used to distinguish between cystic and solid lesions and to measure the dimensions of structures such as the eye. It may be used to identify the location of the root apex.

B-scan—is displayed by brightness modulation, instead of a spike, a spot of variable brightness is produced on the cathode ray tube.

There are two types of B-scans:
1. Time position scan, which is more useful for the evaluation of dynamic structures, including components of the cardiovascular system.
2. The compound B-scan, this helps to produce a two dimensional image of the region under examination. It is useful for the evaluation of soft tissue swellings such as those which may be encountered in a salivary gland or thyroid.

Continuous ultrasound: Here the same change in frequency occurs with echoes that are coming from a moving interface within the body. Here two transducers are used, one to produce the sound and the other for the reception of the echo. This is useful for detecting heart sounds and for examining patterns of flow in blood vessels.

Clinical Applications

- Examination of the thyroid gland and the parathyroid glands and lymph nodes
- Examination of extracranial vessels of the neck, as a screening process to detect atheromatous plaques in the carotid artery, carotid artery aneurysms, venous thrombosis, stenosis and tumors of the carotid sheath
- Examination of the parotid glands. It helps to differentiate between cystic and solid lesions, localize lesions for biopsy, locate calculus in the ducts or parenchyma of the gland
- Examination of congenital inflammatory and neoplastic neck masses
- To detect fractures of the orbital wall and accompanying soft tissue
- Assessment of ventricular systems in babies by imaging through the open fontanelles.

Available data suggests that the benefits associated with ultrasound diagnosis outweigh any known risks.

It is now regarded as the investigation of choice for differentiating between solid and cystic lesions.

Advantages

- Sound waves are not ionizing radiations
- There are no known harmful effects to any tissues at the energies and doses currently used in diagnostic ultrasound
- Shows good differentiation between soft tissues
- Technique is widely available and inexpensive.

Disadvantages

- Ultrasound has limited use in head and neck region because sound waves are absorbed by bone
- Technique is very operator dependent
- Images can be difficult to interpret for inexperienced operators because image resolution is often poor.

Xeroradiography (Figs 12.22A to E)

This method is based on an electrostatic process similar to that used for xeroxing.

Conventional X-ray source is used in the production of xeroradiographs. The film is replaced by a selenium-coated photoreceptor (Xerox Plate), which has an uniformly distributed electrostatic charge. The charge is applied by a conditioner that also inserts the charged plate into a light-tight cassette. During an exposure, X-rays that penetrate a body part or object are absorbed by the surface of the selenium plate causing selective discharging. The distribution and the amount of discharge is related to the distribution and amount of radiation striking the xerox plate and, therefore, the information in the transmitted X-ray beam is left as a charged pattern on the plate. The pattern of electric charge, the latent image, is analogous to the latent image produced by the reduction of silver bromide molecules to free silver atoms in the sensitivity specks of a photographic emulsion.

The latent image is developed into a visible image. During development a cloud of charged powder particles of toner is exposed to the plate, and the powder particles are attracted to the charged pattern on the surface. The association between the toner and the plate is related to the distribution of charge. When the development is complete, the visible image is transferred to paper in a machine referred to as a developer.

Xeroradiograph can be viewed in reflected or transmitted light. When the latent image is transferred from plate to paper, the original image is reversed 180° and is seen as a mirror image.

Uses

- Mammography
- Cephalometry

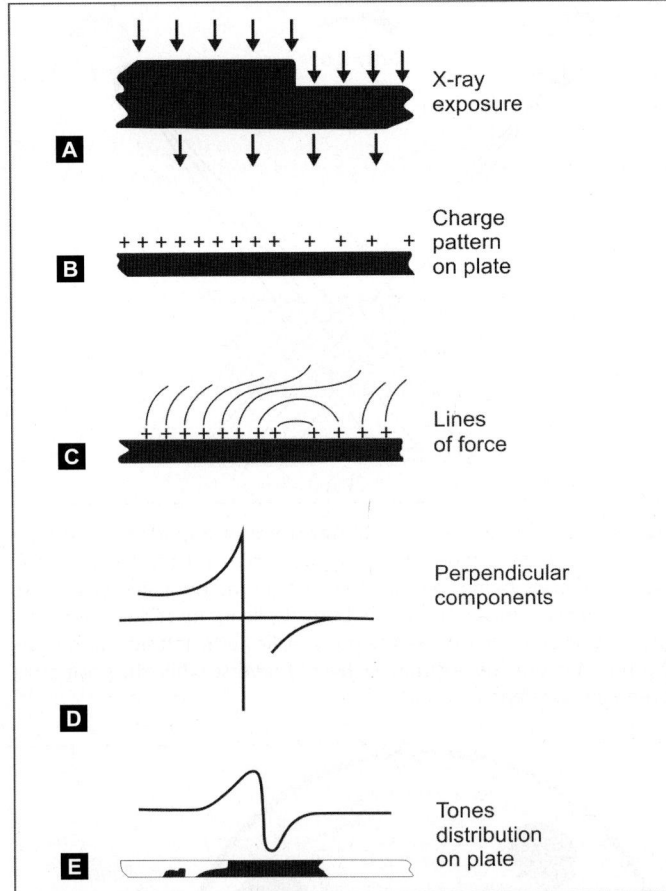

Figures 12.22A to E (A) An X-ray beam passing through an object is differentially attenuated according to the absorption characteristics of the object; (B) The disruption of transmitted X-ray photons alters the charge pattern on the Xerox plate; (C) Lines of the force produced as a result of the difference in charge densities on the plate surface; (D) These lines of forces have perpendicular components; (E) These components affect the distribution of the toner particles on the plate

- Evaluation of bone lesions in the mandible
- Sialography
- Study of variety of dental and nondental structures
- TM joint tomography.

The dental xeroradiograph system has a different physical design. The image receptor plates are the size no. 1 and 2 films and fit into the patient's mouth. The image receptors are charged and processed into a final permanent image in a single piece of equipment. To make an image, the photo receptor is charged at the output station. It is then put intraorally, exposed, and returned to the input station. The plate passes over a toner station, where charged toner particles suspended in a liquid vehicle are deposited on the plate to develop the image. Next the plate is dried to remove the liquid vehicle. The image is recovered from the plate by using a clear adhesive transfer station. The adhesive tape is brought into contact with the plate and pulls off all the toner particles. The image is protected by applying the adhesive with the image to a translucent backing strip.

Indications in Head and Neck Region

- Periodontal and periapical assessment to show good bony details
- Cephalometric radiography to show the required hard and soft tissue landmarks on one film
- Sialography to show fine duct structure
- Assessment of soft tissue shadows in the pharynx and larynx.

Advantages

- High contrast
- Greater ability to resolve fine structures
- They require 1/3rd the exposure of conventional radiographs
- Easy to use
- Produces permanent dry images for viewing in about 20 seconds after the exposed photoreceptor is returned to the machine
- Image is easily reversible
- For diagnostic purpose, as this method gives excellent definition of thin, fine structures due to edge enhancement,
  - Height of alveolar crest better visualized
  - Caries seen more readily
  - Useful in endodontics
  - Detection of cancer
  - Imaging biomaterials.

Disadvantages

- Edge enhancement artifacts
- Processors are expensive
- High radiation dose needed for extraoral techniques.

Tomography

Tomography is a generic term formed from the Greek words tomos meaning 'slice' or 'section' and graphia meaning 'picture' or 'describing'. Linear tomography (LT), a form of conventional tomography, is an alternative to the use of CT. This is a process by which an image layer of the body is produced, while the images of the structures above and below that layer are made invisible by blurring.

In normal radiography, the character of the pattern on the radiograph formed by the anatomical structures of interest is very often partially or sometimes even completely obscured by the shadows cast by the over lying or under lying structures. In many cases a distinction can be made by choosing appropriate orientation of the patient, but in others it is necessary to use a technique known as 'body section radiography' or 'Tomography'.

Conventional Tomography

Body section radiography is a special X-ray technique that enables visualization of a section of the patient's anatomy by blurring regions of the patient's anatomy above and below the section of interest. This is achieved by a synchronized movement of the film and the tube in opposite directions, about a fulcrum (i.e. the plane of interest in the patient's body) (**Fig. 12.23**).

Objects closest to the film are seen most sharply and objects farthest away are completely blurred.

Tomographic views are used to examine various facial structures:

- Tomography of sinuses
- Tomography of facial bones, to study facial fractures.
- Extent of orbital blow-out fractures
- Tomography of the mandible
- Tomography of the temporomandibular joint, especially when the patient is unable to open his mouth or in conjunction with arthrography
- For dental implant patients.

Computed Tomography

Computed Tomography (CT) imaging is also known as 'CAT scanning' (Computed Axial Tomography). CT scanners use X-rays to produce sectional images, but the radiographic film is replaced by very sensitive crystal or gas detectors. The patient's body to be scanned is interposed between the X-ray source and the detectors and a series of exposures are made over an arc of 180° to 360° with the X-ray beam collimated to determine the thickness of the slice (**Fig. 12.24**). The detectors measure the intensity of the X-ray beam emerging from the patient and convert this into digital data which is stored and manipulated by the computer. The numerical information is converted into gray scale representing different tissue densities, allowing a visual image to be generated. The image can then be reformatted into tomographic sections of the body, three-dimensional planes, it can be adjusted for optimal viewing to detect minute differences in tissue alterations and it gives highly accurate quantitative information about the tissues imaged (**Table 12.1**). The image scan is stored on magnetic tape or optical discs.

In the CT image, density values are represented as gray scale values. It comprise areas of high X-ray attenuation which are represented as the 'white areas' and areas of low attenuation which are represented as 'blackness'.

Indications

- Investigations of intracranial diseases including tumors, hemorrhage and infarcts
- Investigations of suspected intracranial and spinal cord damage following trauma to the head and neck

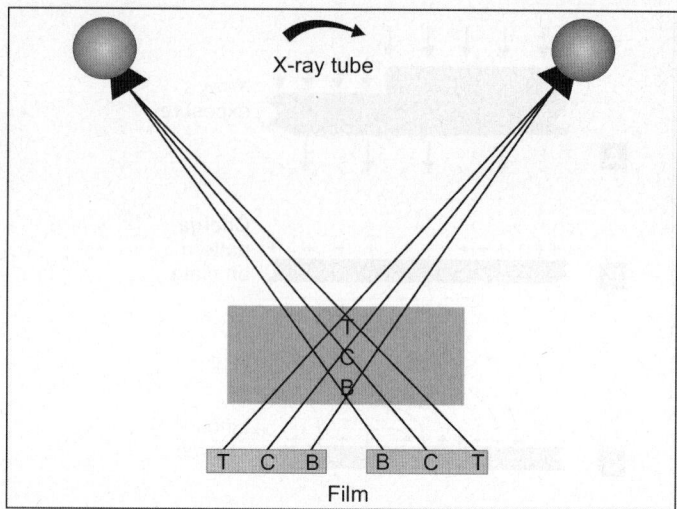

Figure 12.23 The tube and the film are rotated around the fulcrum(C) during an exposure. When the exposure is initiated, the objects at the top of the body being examined (T) are on the right side of the film while objects in the center of the body (C) lie in the center of the film and objects at the bottom of the body (B) lie at the left side of the film. During exposure, the positions of B and T reverse while the position of C remains constant

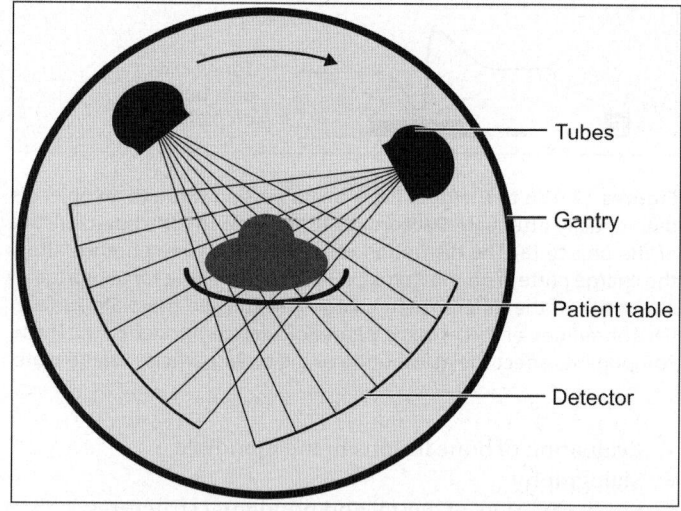

Figure 12.24 Mechanical geometry of CT scanners

- Assessment of fractures involving:
  - The orbits and nasoethmoidal complex
  - The cranial base
  - The odontoid peg
  - The cervical spine.
- Tumor staging–assessment of site, size and extent of benign and malignant tumors affecting:
  - The maxillary antra
  - The base of the skull
  - The pterygoid region

Table 12.1 Tissue characterization

Tissue	Hounsfield units
Air	– 1000
Water	0
Muscle	35–70
Fibrous tissue	60–90
Cartilage	80–130
Trabecular bone	300–500
Cortical bone	600–3000
Dentine	1600–2400
Enamel	2500–3000
Lung	– 300
Fat	– 90
White matter	30
Gray matter	40
Muscle	50

Table 12.2 Bone quality

Density	Hounsfield units
D1	1250
D2	850–1250
D3	350–850
D4	150–350
D5	<150

- – The pharynx
- – The larynx.
- Investigations of tumors and tumor like discrete swellings intrinsic and extrinsic to the salivary glands.
- Investigation of the TMJ.
- Preoperative assessment of maxillary alveolar bone height and thickness before inserting implants (**Table 12.2**).

Most CT scanners offer a choice of filters which may be selected by the operator to enhance either soft tissue features or bone detail in images. Sometimes these filters are referred to as algorithms. The algorithm can be defined as the mathematical formula used to process the scan data into the final image. The term kernel is also used.

The image reconstruction algorithms developed for X-ray CT can also be applied to gamma camera images (as in SPECT) to overcome limitations of planar nuclear imaging and to images generated using positron-emitting radioisotopes (as in PET).

Artifacts in Computed Tomography

CT artifacts can be defined as image degradation due to either physical, mechanical or computer malfunction or due to the physical state or condition of the patient. They are broadly classified into:

- System related artifacts
- Patient related artifacts.

System Related Artifacts

These can usually be related to the following:

- *X-ray tube*: If the quality or quantity of photons emerging from the tube varies, the image quality will also vary and a major cause of such a change is the aging of the tube. In addition, the physical damage to the rotor bearings, the glass insert, the anode surface or filament will all result in image degradation.
- *Detectors*: If the detector's elements are not geometrically aligned with the X-ray tube then only a part of the attenuated beam passing into the detector array will be collected. Artifacts will also occur, if the system of detectors has not been correctly calibrated or if there is a malfunction in the circuit.
- *Operator's fault*: Artifacts can also be related to an incorrect technique, e.g. on second generation scanners, the wrong size wedges may be fitted.

Patient Related Artifacts

- *Patient motion*: This can be due to:
  - – Patient movement
  - – Cardiac motion
  - – Peristalsis
  - – Breathing/Swallowing.
- *High density artefact's*: When scanning the head/brain, following can be seen on image and will cause artifacts on the image:
  - – Fillings in the teeth
  - – Surgical flaps/Clips
  - – Surgical shunts
  - – Hair pins/Hair grips
  - – Hearing aids.
- *Poor patient positioning*: The computer ideally requires a circular subject in order to reconstruct an image; this the radiographer can achieve by packing bolus material around the patient. It is also important to ensure that the patient is in the isocenter of the scan field, as artifacts will occur if the patient is too far to the left or right or is too high or too low.

Advantages

- Structural relationships of hard and soft tissues can be observed directly. Differences between tissues that differ in physical density by less than 1 percent can be distinguished
- The ability to rotate images and to add or subtract structural components permits relationships to be studied

- Contiguous structures can be separated and normal hidden surfaces examined in detail
- Accurate linear and volumetric measurements can be made
- Changes in linear or volumetric measures can be determined by sequential scans (e.g. remodeling of bone)
- Eliminates superimposition of images of structures outside the area of interest
- A single CT imaging procedure consisting of either multiple contiguous or one helical scan can be viewed as images in the axial, coronal or sagittal planes, depending on the diagnostic task (multiplanar reformatted imaging).

Limitations

- Since the measurements or pixels that form the image represent discrete subdivisions of space, the effect of blurring is much greater than in conventional radiographic systems
- The resolution of the image is also limited by the size represented by the pixel, which is generally greater than the size of the silver specks that form the conventional radiographs
- The detail of a computed tomographic image is not as fine as that obtainable on other radiographs

- Its application in longitudinal monitoring of implant prosthesis is limited and contraindicated because of the image artifact created by metals that would obscure the information
- Metallic objects such as fillings produce marked streak artifacts across the CT image
- The equipment is very expensive.

Generations

Since the introduction of the first clinical system by Hounsfield, several generations of scanners have been produced, with distinguishing tube-detector configuration and scanning motion.

Although numbered sequentially, the 3rd and 4th generation designs developed at approximately the same time. The concept of electron beam CT, which some authors have called 5th generation, followed later. Some authors have described up to 7 generations of CT design (**Table 12.3**).

Helical or Spiral CT

Helical, also called spiral, CT was introduced in the early 1990s. In helical CT the X-ray source are attached to a freely rotating gantry. During a scan, the table moves the patient smoothly through the scanner; the name derives

Table 12.3 Classification of CT scanners

Generation	Configuration	Detectors	Beam	Minimum scan time
First	Rotate translate	1–2	Pencil thin	2.5 min
Second	Rotate translate	3–52	Narrow fan	10 sec
Third	Rotate-rotate	256–1000	Wide fan	0.5 sec
Fourth	Rotate-fixed	600–4800	Wide fan	1 sec
Fifth	Electron beam	1284	Wide fan	33 ms
		Detectors	Electron beam	

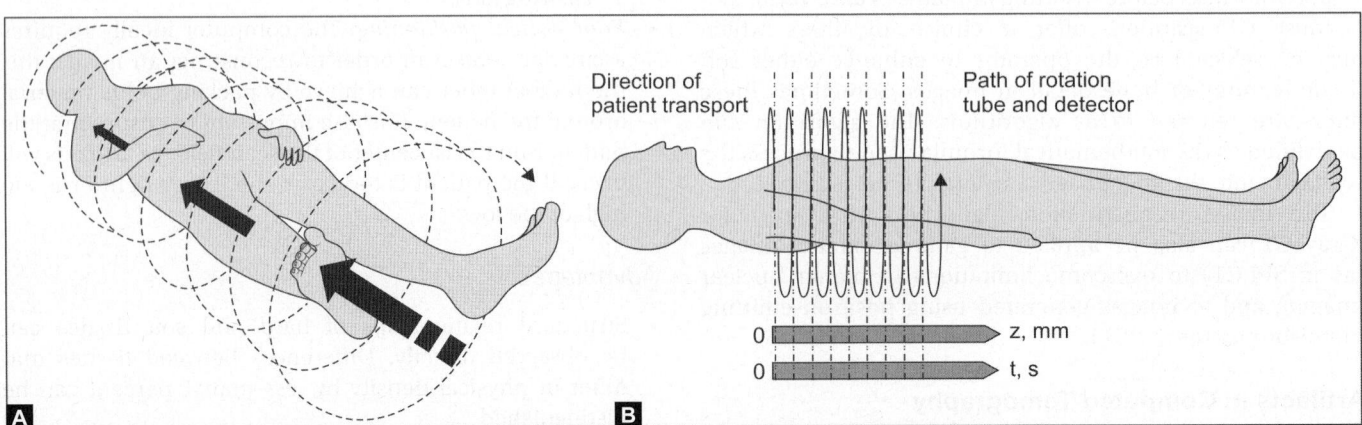

Figures 12.25A and B Principles of helical CT. As the patient is moved through the gantry, the continuously rotating X-ray tube and the detector describe a helical or spiral path about the patient, acquiring image data as they rotate

from the helical path traced out by the X-ray beam (**Figs 12.25A and B**).

Advantages

- Speed
- Often the patient can hold their breath for the entire study, reducing motion artifacts
- It allows for more optimal use of intravenous contrast enhancement
- The study is quicker than the equivalent conventional CT permitting the use of higher resolution acquisitions in the z-axis
- Decrease incidence of misregistration between consecutive axial slices
- Enhanced multiplanar (MPR) or three dimensional renderings.

These major advantages led to the rapid rise of helical CT as the most popular type of CT technology.

Multislice Spiral CT

Multislice CT scanners are similar in concept to the helical or spiral CT but there are more than one detector ring. The major benefit of multislice CT is the increased speed of volume coverage. This allows large volumes to be scanned at the optimal time following intravenous contrast administration; this has particularly benefitted CT angiography techniques.

256 Slice CT

The technology has demonstrated the potential to significantly reduce radiation exposure by eliminating the requirement for a helical examination in both cardiac CT angiography and whole brain perfusion studies for the evaluation of stroke.

Three-dimensional CT

These are computer programs that reformat the acquired data from axial CT scans into three-dimensional images (3D CT).

3D CT imaging techniques may be divided into the following groups:
- Multiplanar reformatting (MPR) and dental MPR
- Shaded surface display (SSD)
- Volume rendering
- Maximum intensity projection (MIP)
- Model production and virtual reality.

This is very useful for craniofacial reconstructive surgery and has been used both for treatment of congenital and acquired deformities and for evaluation of intracranial tumors, benign and malignant lesions of the maxillofacial complex, cervical spine injuries, pelvic fractures and deformities of the hands and feet. The availability of data in a three-dimensional format also has allowed the construction of life sized models that can be used for trial surgeries and the construction of surgical stents for guiding dental implants as well as creation of accurate implanted prostheses.

Advantages of Three-dimensional Displays

- Realistic display of volumes
- Presentation of the entire volume in one single image
- Improved recognition of diagnostically relevant details
- Helpful for more precise surgical planning
- CT image data as a basis for three-dimensional models
- Possible free rotation of 3D objects.

CT-Angiography (CTA)

CT-Angiography (CTA) enables the display of vascular structures aided by injections of contrast medium. The introduction of the multislice scanner has made it possible to display the entire vascular system with maximum contrast enhancement in extremely short scan times. Image post processing enables good display of the entire vascular system. Even small vascular exits and origins (branches) and embolisms or dissection membranes can be displayed. The physician can retrospectively select any projection and generate three-dimensional images, e.g. for surgical planning.

Dentascan Imaging

It was developed in 1987 by Schwarz, this is a Dental CT reformatting software programme which reformats axial CT images of jaw into panoramic and paraxial images and provides programmed reformation, organization and display of the imaging study. Dentascan is useful in oromaxillofacial imaging and is an excellent imaging modality.

A diagnostic template used for implant imaging is very useful.

Indications

- Preoperative evaluation for implants
- Post implantation complications like encroachment of canal, maxillary sinus, nasal cavity and peri-implantitis.
- Assess inflammatory diseases
  - Apical periodontitis
  - Sclerosingosteitis
  - Periosteal reaction
  - Reactive sinusitis.
- Tumors and cysts
  - Define the extent of lesion
  - Cortical involvement
  - Relationship with tooth
  - Relationship with mandibular canal, maxillary sinus
  - Differentiates benign lesions from the malignant.
- Oro-antral fistulas which are difficult to image on Conventional CT, the Dentascan provides the exact

size and location of the fistula and helps in planning for surgical repair.

- *Root fractures*: Vertical root fractures are best assessed by Dentascan.
- Plan surgical procedures like Sinus-lift procedure.
- Locate the foreign body in jaw, in caudo-cranial as well as bucco-lingual direction.

Advantages

- Minimum additional cost
- Low radiation dosage
- Multiplanar reformation
- Eliminate streak artifacts
- Exact information about the alveolar bone dimensions.
- Location of mandibular canal, maxillary sinus.
- Images in 1:1 ratio.
- In implant imaging Dentascan helps in measuring:
  - Height and bucco-lingual dimension of the ridge at the implant site (bone quantity)
  - Extent of bone resorption (bone volume)
  - Relative amount of bone and fat at the implant site (bone quality)
  - Precise location of the vital structures.

Limitations

- The image may not be of the true size and may require compensation for magnification
- It has a limited range of diagnostic gray scale
- Determination of bone quality requires other aids.

Tuned Aperture Computed Tomography

Only conventional CT can provide adequate cross sectional images for the identification of vital anatomic structures and available bone dimensions. An alternative method is based on optical aperture theory, known as TACT.

SPECT/CT and PET/CT

A more powerful approach is to use an X-ray CT scanner to generate the attenuation maps, numerous hybrid scanners have been produced as a result which combine nuclear medicine with CT imaging, as in SPECT/CT and PET/CT. An additional benefit of these developments is the simultaneous capability, with sufficient computing power, of blending the nuclear medicine and CT images so as to generate physiological images co-localized with images of patient anatomy and hence improve the diagnostic utility of nuclear medicine procedures.

Magnetic Resonance Imaging (MRI)

Magnetic Resonance Imaging (MRI) is based on totally different physical principles than Computerized Tomography

in that the radiant energy is in the form of radiofrequency waves, rather than X-rays (**Figs 12.26A to C**).

This technique relies on the phenomenon of nuclear magnetic resonance to produce a signal that can be used to construct an image. It uses the nonionizing radiation from the radiofrequency (RF) band of the electromagnetic spectrum. Because of its excellent soft tissue contrast resolution, MRI has proved useful in a variety of circumstances, diagnosing a suspected internal derangement of the TM joint and evaluating the treatment of the derangement after surgery, identifying and localizing orofacial soft tissue lesions and providing images of the salivary gland parenchyma.

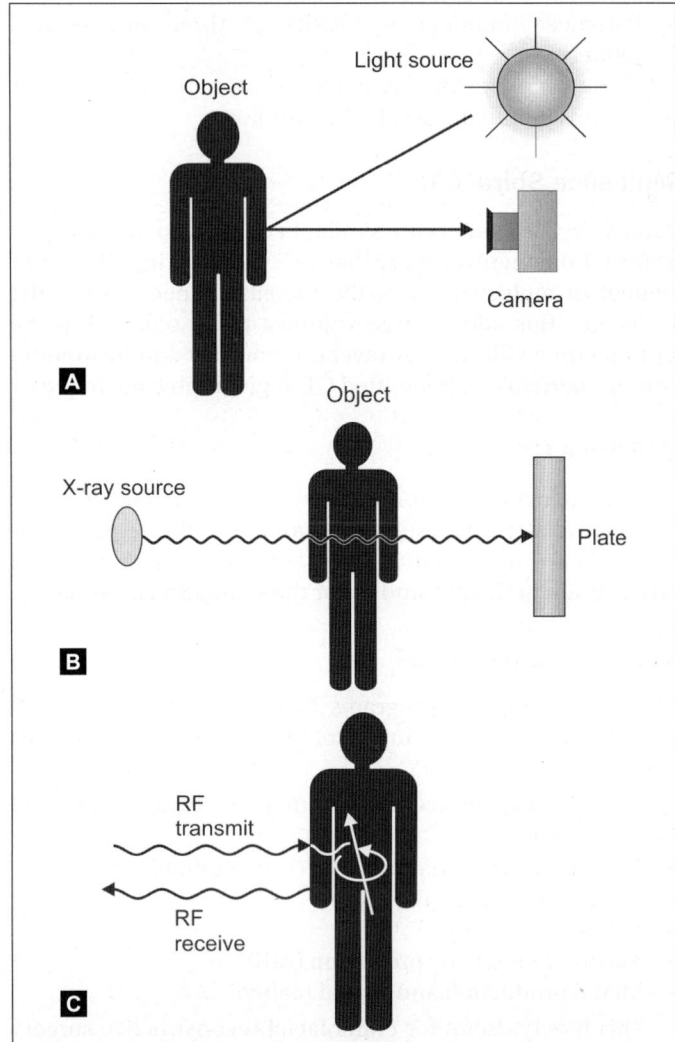

Figures 12.26A to C (A) In the photography, light is reflected off the object and is received by a photographic plate in a camera; (B) In X-rays, the radiation penetrates the object and reaches a photographic plate behind the object; (C) In MRI, a radiofrequency wave or a radiofrequency (RF) pulse is transmitted into the patient, and a signal is received from magnetized spins (protons) in the body

Indications

- Assessment of intracranial lesions and the pituitary
- The spinal cord
- Tumor staging—evaluation of the site, size and extent of soft tissue tumors and tumor like lesions, involving.
  - The salivary glands
  - The pharynx
  - The larynx.
- Investigations of the TMJ to show the marrow changes and soft tissue components of the joint including the disc.

Principles of Magnetic Resonance

The quantity and behavior of the protons in each tissue can be measured by resonance. Resonance is a transfer of vibration energy from one system to another. Every physical system can be made to vibrate, and each system has a frequency of vibration called resonance frequency. The resonance frequency is the frequency at which energy transfer is most efficient.

In MRI, the principle of resonance is used to transfer energy to the spinning hydrogen protons. The resonance frequency for the protons lies within the radiofrequency band of the electromagnetic spectrum.

The patient is placed inside a large magnet, which induces a relatively strong external magnetic field (usually 0.5–1.5 Tesla). Radio waves are pulsed into the patient by the body coil transmitter at 90° to the magnetic field. This causes the nuclei of many atoms of the body, including hydrogen, to behave like small magnets. When nuclei are subjected to the flux of an external magnetic field, two energy states result; spin-up, which is in the direction of the field, and spin-down which is in the opposite direction of the field. The combined effect of these two energy states is a weak net magnetic moment, or net magnetic vector (NMV), parallel with the applied magnetic field.

After application of an RF signal, energy is released from the body, detected by the receiver coil and used to construct the MR image by the computer.

Coil

A coil consists of one or more loops of conductive wire, looped around the core of the coil. A coil is used to create a magnetic field or to detect a changing magnetic field by voltage induced in the wire.

- Different types of MRI coils are used in MR systems
- Gradient coils
- Radio frequency coil.

Factors that Affect the Magnetic Resonance Signal

Several tissue-related factors influence the strength of the magnetic resonance (MR) signal. The most important factors are the relaxation times, but other factors of importance include proton density, magnetic susceptibility, chemical shift, flow and contrast agents.

- Relaxation times (T2 and T1)
- Flip angle
- FID (Free induction decay)
- Proton density
- Magnetic susceptibility
- Hemorrhage
- Flow
- Chemical shift.

Relaxation Times (T2 and T1) (Table 12.4)

As soon as the radio waves are turned off (the resonant RF pulse), two events occur simultaneously— the release of energy and the return of the nuclei to their original spin state at a lower energy. This process is called relaxation, and the energy loss is detected as a signal, which is called free induction decay (FID).

The time constant that describes the rate at which net magnetization returns to equilibrium by this transfer of energy is called the T1 relaxation time or spin-lattice time. T1 varies with different tissues and ability of the nuclei to transfer their excess energy to their environment. A tissue with a short T1 produces an intense MR signal, displayed as bright white in a T1-weighted image. A tissue with a long T1 produces a low intensity signal and appears dark in the MR image.

Magnetic resonance images are not produced from a single excitation of protons. The protons must be excited multiple times to produce enough data for the image. The time between excitations is called the repetition time (TR).

Table 12.4 Signal strength of various tissues within T1- and T2-weighted images

Tissue type	T1W image	T2W image
Fat	Bright	Bright
Aqueous liquids	Dark	Bright
Tumor	Dark	Bright
Inflammatory tissue	Dark	Bright
Muscle	Dark	Dark
Connective tissue	Dark	Dark
Hematoma, acute	Dark	Dark
Hematoma, subacute	No signal due to outflow effect	Bright
Blood, flowing		
Fibrous cartilage	Dark	Dark
Hyaline cartilage		Bright
Compact bone	Dark	Dark
Air	No signal	No signal

If the TR is long, than the protons can fully realign between excitations and produce a strong signal. However, if the TR is short, then there is only partial realignment.

Factors that influence the T1-value of a tissue are:

- The particular chemical substance and its physical state
- Field strength (T1 increases with field strength, therefore recovery is slower)
- Temperature (longer T1 with increased temperature in the biological samples)
- The liquid surrounding the protons
- The mobility of the protons.

For instance, fat has short T1 (200 to 300 msec) and appears bright. Tumors have longer time T1-relaxation times (e.g. 1000 msec) and appear darker.

T1-weighted images are called fat images, because fat has the shortest T1-relaxation time, and thus it appears bright in the image. T1 gives a good image contrast and T1-weighted images are helpful for depicting small anatomical regions like TM joint. In T1-weighted images, cerebrospinal fluid appears black. T1-weighed images with a strong longitudinal signal show normal tissue well.

The time constant that describes the rate of loss of transverse magnetization is called the T2-relaxation time or transverse (spin-spin) relaxation time. T2-relaxation relates to the incoherent exchange of energy among neighboring spins. Because of this, it is also called spin-spin relaxation. A T2-weighted image is acquired using a long repetition time between RF pulses and a long signal recovery time. A tissue with a long T2 produces a high intensity signal and a dark image.

T2-weighted images are called water images because water has the longest T2-relaxation time and appears bright in the image. These T2-weighted images are used when one is looking for inflammatory or pathologic changes.

In T2-weighted images cerebrospinal fluid appears white. T2 images with a strong transverse signal show disease well.

The T1 and T2 curves for different tissues will be:

- Fat has the shortest T1 and will have the steepest TI recovery curve
- Proteinaceous fluid also has a short T1
- H_2O has the longest T1 and will have the slowest T1 recovery curve
- Solid tissue has intermediate T1.

Signal strength of various tissues within T1- and T2-weighted images.

Basic Pulse Sequences

By varying the frequency and timing of the radio frequency input, the hydrogen protons can be excited to different degrees allowing different tissue characteristics to be highlighted on a variety of imaging sequences. In addition, tissue characteristics can be changed by using gadolinium as a contrast agent, which shortens the T1 relaxation time of tissues giving a high signal on a T1-weighted image.

- Spin-echo sequence (SE)
- Inversion-recovery sequence
- STIR Sequence (Short tau inversion recovery)
- Gradient-echo sequence
- Multi-echo sequences
- Fast Pulse sequences
- Fast or turbo Spin-echo sequences
- SSFSE and haste
- Fast or turbo inversion recovery sequences
- Fast gradient-echo sequences
- Echo-planar (EPI) sequences
- Hybrid sequences
- Grase (Gradient-echo and spin-echo)
- Spiral sequences
- Echo time and T2-contrast in fast sequences.

Magnetic Resonance Contrast Media

The signal intensity difference (SI-difference) of two tissues in the magnetic resonance (MR) image determines the image contrast. It depends on intrinsic (body related) factors, i.e. on the different tissue properties and on extrinsic (instrument related) factors, especially the particular pulse sequence applied.

Magnetic resonance (MR) contrast media are pharmaceuticals which, in order to improve diagnostic information, increase the SI-difference. They change the intrinsic tissue properties and in principle they can act in two ways:

1. Directly by changing the proton density of a tissue, or
2. Indirectly by changing the local magnetic field and consequently the T1- and/or T2-times.

Contrary to X-ray contrast media, we cannot see the contrast media (e.g. Gd compounds) themselves, but only their influence on the relaxation properties of the protons surrounding them.

There are four possibilities for such influence on the resulting image:

1. Influencing spin or proton density
2. Reducing the T1and the T2 relaxation times
3. Acceleration of dephasing by local field inhomogeneities (susceptibility effects)
4. Shifting of the resonance frequency (dysprosium)

The concentrations of most of the commercially available solutions are 0.5 mol/L. Thus the concentrations of gadolinium are standardized as well as the dose.

The least expensive oral contrast medium is water, which can also be used to demarcate the intestinal lumen. Water has a low signal for T1-weighted sequences while it displays a high signal for T2-weighted sequences.

Advantages

- No ionizing radiation
- No biological effects due to absence of radiation exposure
- Higher soft tissue contrast
- Excellent differentiation between soft tissues is possible between normal and abnormal tissues
- Blood vessels clearly seen
- The region of the body imaged in MRI is controlled electronically, direct multiplanar imaging is possible without reorienting the patient
- High resolution images can be constructed in all planes
- There is no need for enhancement of images using intravenous contrast media with their associated risks.

Limitations

- Expensive
- Potential hazard imposed by the presence of ferro-magnetic metals in the vicinity of the imaging magnet
- Patients with cardiac pace makers, insulin pumps and ferromagnetic implants cannot be investigated by MRI
- Metallic objects in the oral cavity such as appliances, crowns, etc. may cause artifacts
- Endotracheal tubes need to be replaced by plastic
- Claustrophobic procedure
- Relatively long imaging times
- Cortical bone is not imaged, the signal obtainable is only for the bone marrow
- The very powerful magnets pose problems with sitting of the equipment.
- Equipment is very expensive
- Facilities are not widely available.

BIBLIOGRAPHY

1. Bransetter BF, Weissman JL. Normal anatomy of the neck with CT and MR imaging correlation. Radiological clinics of North America. 2000:38(5);925-40.
2. Chen CN, Hoult D. Biomedical Magnetic Resonance Technology. New York, Adam Hilger; 1989.
3. Cohen MS, Weisskoff RM. Ultra-fast imaging. Magn Reson Imaging. 1991;9:1.
4. Delbaso AM. Maxillofacial Imaging. W.M. Saunders company, Philadelphia; 1990.
5. Edelstein WA, Hutchinson JMS, Johnson G, et al. Spin-warp NMR imaging and applications to human whole-body imaging. Phys Med Biol. 1980;25:751.
6. Evens RG, Evens JRG, AJR. 1991;157:603.
7. Goaz PW, White SC. Extraoral examination in oral radiology. Principles and Interpretation, 3rd edition. St Louis: CV Mosby; 1994.pp.299-313.
8. Hoult DI, Lauterbur PC. J Magnet Reson. 1979;34:425.
9. Johnson ON, McNally MA, Essay CE. The extra oral radiography in essentials of dental radiography for dental assistants and hygienists, 6th edition. Norwalk, Appleton and Lange; 1999.pp.443-9.
10. Langland OE, Langlais RP. Special Radiographic Techniques. In: Principles of Dental Imaging Baltimore, Williams and Williams; 1997.pp.265-87.
11. Laskin DM. Oral and Maxillofacial Surgery. CV Mosby Co. 1980;1:413.
12. Mason-Hing LR. Fundamentals of Dental Radiology. Lea and Febiger. 1979;113.
13. Mason-Hing LR. Occlusal and extra oral radiography. Fundamentals of Dental Radiography, 3rd ed. Philadelphia, WB Saunders; 1993.pp.144-54.
14. Misch EC, Rivcos LT. Contemporary Implant Dentistry, 2nd edition, Part I. Diagnostic Imaging and Techniques. 1999.pp.73-89.
15. Razmns JF, Williamson GF. An overview of oral and maxillofacial imaging. In current oral maxillofacial imaging, Philadelphia, WB Saunders; 1996.pp.1-22.
16. Reskin AB. Advances in Oral Radiology. PSG Computed Tomography 285 Publishing Co. 1980.
17. Richard CO' Brien. Dental Radiography: An Introduction for Dental Hygienists and Assistants. WB Saunders Co. 3rd edition. 1977.
18. Silver, Mawad, Hilal, Sane, Ganti. Computed tomography of the Nasopharynx and related spaces. Radiology. 1983; 147:725-31.
19. Smith NJD. Dental Radiography. Blackwell Scientific Publications; 1980.p.68.

Panoramic Radiography | 13

Panoramic radiography, is a radiographic procedure that produces a single tomographic image of facial structures including both maxillary and mandibular arches and their supporting structures.

There is greater ease and less time taken to produce a panoramic radiograph as compared to full mouth intraoral periapical radiographs, and the additional advantage is that there is visualization of areas of the body of the mandible, ramus, TM joint, and the maxillary sinus.

Panoramic radiographs are obtained using two methods:
1. *Intraoral source of radiation*: Status -X (**Fig. 13.1**)
2. *Extraoral source of radiation*: OPG (**Figs 13.2A and B**).

In panoramic radiography, the film and X-ray tube head move around the patient. The X-ray tube moves around the patient's head in one direction while the film rotates in the opposite direction. The patient may be seated or standing in a stationary position. The movement of the tube head and the film produces an image through the process known as tomography. (This is a curvilinear variant of conventional tomography, and is also based on the principle of the reciprocal movement of an X-ray source and an image receptor around a central point or plane, called the image layer). In panoramic radiography the image confirms to the shape of the dental arches.

PRINCIPLE

If the film moves at a speed that follows the moving projection of a certain point, this point will always be projected on the same spot on the film and will not appear unsharp.

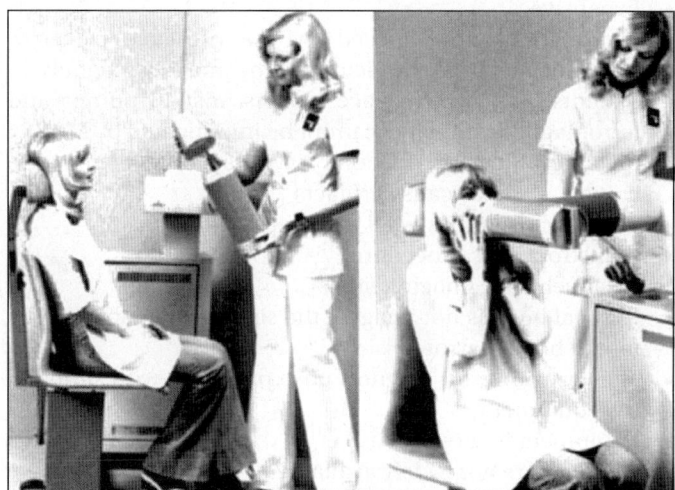

Figure 13.1 The status X-ray intraoral X-ray source machine (*Courtesy* of Siemens Corporation, Iselin, New Jersey)

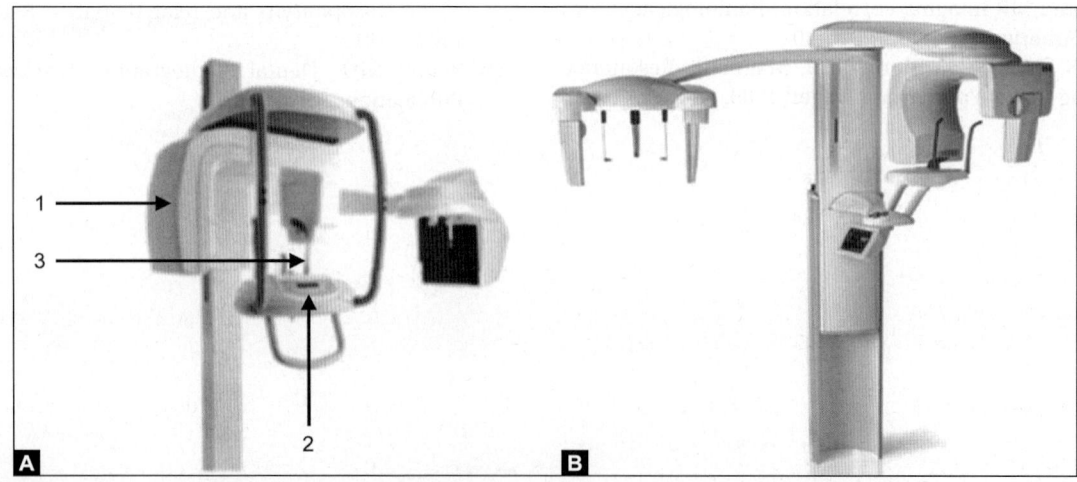

Figures 13.2A and B (A) Kodak OPG 8000C; (B) Planmeca Promax. The main components of the panoramic unit include: 1. The X-ray tube head; 2. The head positioner; 3. The exposure parameter panel

In panoramic radiography the film is attached to a rotating system and moves in the opposite direction to the beam. The film is given the correct speed by apposing this movement with a contrary movement relative to the beam.

FOCAL TROUGH OR IMAGE LAYER (FIG. 13.3)

It is defined as that zone which contains those object points which are depicted with optimum resolution in other words it is a three-dimensional curved zone in which structures lying within are clearly demonstrated on a panoramic radiograph.

In panoramic radiography the arches should be placed within the image layer.

The image layer thickness, depends upon the effective projection radius and the width of the beam. The size and shape of the focal trough varies according to the manufacturer. The closer the rotation center to the teeth, narrower the focal trough. In most machines the focal trough is narrow in the anterior region and wide in the posterior region.

Since the jaws are not circular, a variety of movement patterns for the beam have been developed.

ROTATION CENTER (FIGS 13.4A TO C)

In panoramic radiography, the film or cassette carrier and the tube head are connected and rotate simultaneously around a patient during exposure. The pivotal point or axis, around which the cassette carrier and X-ray tube head rotate is termed a rotational center.

- The earlier techniques used stationary rotation center of the beam, placed at one side of the jaws, projecting the other side of the jaws.
- *Single center of rotation*: e.g. The Rotagraph Machine.
- *Two centers of rotation*: This follows the principle that, the individual left and right sides of the arc formed by

the teeth and jaws closely form a part of a circle. It was suggested that the center of rotation be positioned some what anteriorly to the location of the third molar opposite the side being examined. This double rotational principle was used in the Panorex machine.

- *Three centers of rotation*: Three centers of rotation system divided the arc of the jaws into three areas:
  1. A condyle to first bicuspid posterior segment
  2. A cuspid-to-cuspid anterior segment
  3. A contralateral-posterior segment.
  e.g. Orthopantomograph, panoram, panora.
- *Moving rotational centers*: Systems described so far have rotation centers or X-ray beams which were positioned at one or more fixed locations during exposure. Pantomography is also achieved if the beam rotates around a fixed point or center, this system is also called 'Ellipso-pantomography'.

In all cases, the center of rotation changes as the film and tube head rotate around the patient. The rotational change allows the image layer to conform to the elliptical shape of the dental arches. The location and number of rotational centers influence the size and shape of the focal trough.

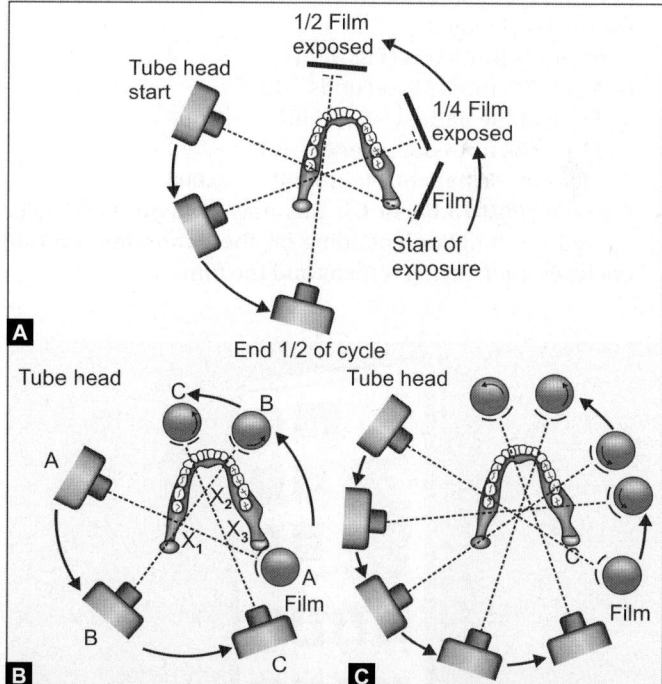

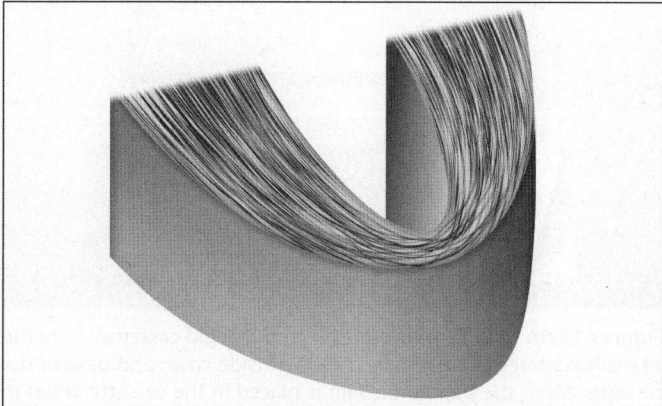

Figure 13.3 Focal trough. The closer to the center of the trough (dark zone) an anatomic structure is positioned, the more clearly it is imaged on the resulting radiograph

Figures 13.4A to C Types of panoramic X-ray machines: (A) Double center of rotation, machines have two rotational centers, one for the right and one for the left side of the jaws; (B) Triple center rotation machines have three centers of rotation and create an uninterrupted radiographic image of the jaws; (C) Moving center rotation machines rotate around a continuously moving center that is similar to the arches, creating an uninterrupted image of the jaws

EQUIPMENT

Panoramic X-ray unit: There are a number of units available, which differ in the number of rotational centers, the size and shape of the focal trough, and type of film transport mechanism. The main components of the panoramic unit include (*see* **Figs 13.2A and B**).

- *X-ray tube head*: This is similar to that of the intraoral machine except that:
  - The collimator used is a lead plate with a slit, and the X-ray beam thus emerges through the collimator as a narrow band. This beam passes through the patient and then exposes the film through another vertical slit in the cassette carrier (the metal holder that supports the cassette). This narrow beam gives minimal exposure to the patient.
  - The vertical angulation of the panoramic tube head is not varied. It is in a fixed position so that the beam is directed slightly upwards.
  - The panoramic tube head always rotates behind the patients head as the film rotates in front of the patient.
- *Head positioner*: Consists of a chin rest, notched bite-block, forehead rest and lateral head support guides.
- *Exposure controls*: The milliamperage and kilovoltage settings are adjustable and can be varied to accommodate patients of different sizes. The exposure time is fixed and cannot be changed.

  Exposure parameters (**Fig. 13.5**)
  - kVp—76, mA—15, seconds—15
  - Dose to the patient—0.103 mR +/– 0.008
  - kVp—80, mA—15, seconds—15
  - Dose to the patient—0.116 mR +/– 0.008.
- *Cassette (**Figs 13.6A to C**)*: This may be rigid or flexible, curved or straight, depending on the panoramic unit. It encloses intensifying screens and the film.

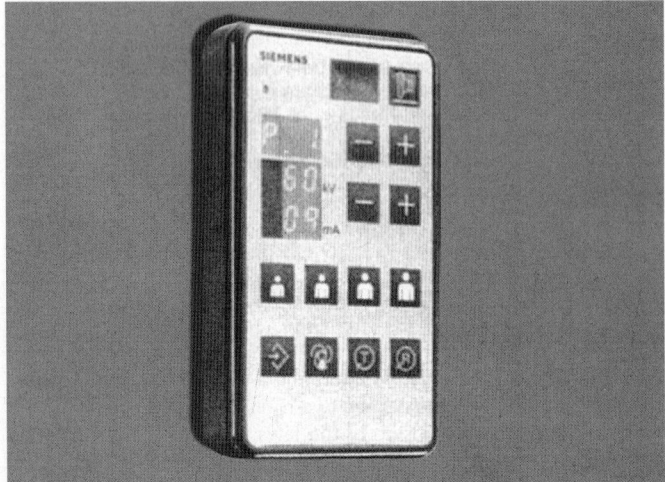

Figure 13.5 An example of exposure and control switch for a panoramic unit

PROCEDURE

- Explain the procedure to the patient.
- Make the patient wear a lead apron without a thyroid collar, and remove all objects from the head and neck region which will interfere with film exposure. Also have the patient remove jacket or bulky sweater, this allows more room between the bottom of the cassette holder and the patient's shoulder.
- Load the panoramic film in the dark room, and cover the bite block with a disposable plastic cover slip.
- Set the exposure factors and adjust the height of the machine to accommodate the patient.
- Center the lower border of the mandible on the chin rest and is equidistant from each side.
- Instruct the patient to sit or stand with the back straight and erect, and ask him to bite on the plastic bite block. The upper and the lower front teeth must be placed in an end-to-end position in the groove of the bite block.
- The midsagittal plane should be perpendicular to the floor and aligned with the vertical center of the chin rest, and the Frankfurt plane should be parallel to the floor, thus obtaining the correct position for the occlusal plane (The patient's head is tilted downwards so that the ala tragus

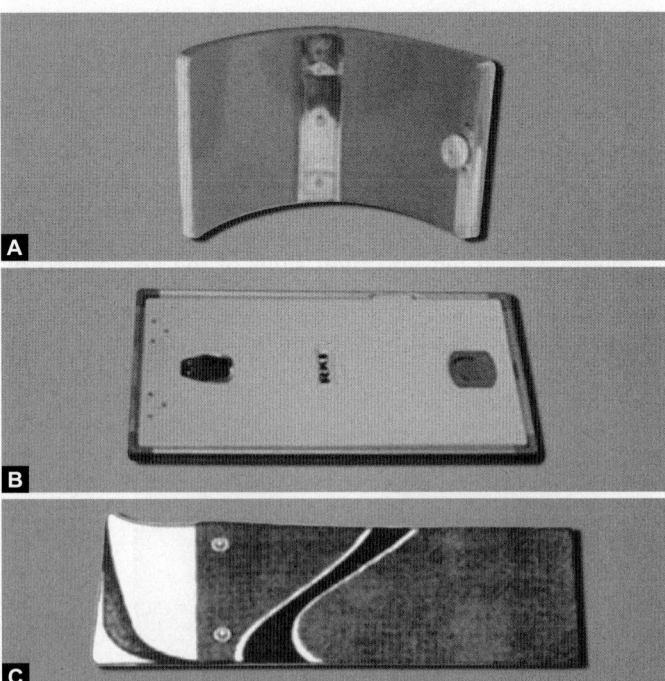

Figures 13.6A to C Film cassettes: (A and B) Rigid cassettes. Here the intensifying screens are attached to the inside cover and base of the cassette. When the panoramic film is placed in the cassette, it lies in between the screens; (C) Shows a flexible cassette that has an opening at one end creating a pouch. The panoramic film is placed between two removable, flexible intensifying screens which are then slid into the pouch

line is 5° down and forward). If the patient has a low palatal vault, increase the occlusal plane angulation slightly, if the patient has a high palatal vault decrease the occlusal plane slightly. The indicator lights in the machine help as a guide and the patients head should be immobilized by the head band.

- Instruct the patient to position the tongue on the palate and ask him to remain still while the machine is rotating during exposure. Also explain that the cassette holder will not strike him, although it may gently rub his ear and head at the limits of the excursion.
- After the exposure is complete the film is subjected to routine processing.

COMMON ERRORS

1. *Ghost images*: This is a radiopaque artifact seen on a panoramic film that is produced when a radiodense object is penetrated twice by the X-ray beam (**Figs 13.7A to G**).
   - The characteristics of a ghost image are:
     - A ghost image resembles it's real counterpart and has the same morphology.
     - It is found on the opposite side of the film from it's real counterpart.
     - It appears in distinct, the horizontal components are more blurred than the vertical components of a ghost image.
     - The ghost image is always larger than the real counterpart, the horizontal component is severely magnified, whereas the vertical component is not as severely magnified.
     - It is usually placed higher than its actual counterpart.
     - Ghost images are always reversed. Left and right being shifted.
   - Anatomical structures which are most often ghosted are:
     - Hyoid bone
     - Cervical spine
     - Inferior border of the mandible
     - Posterior border of the mandible
     - The Meatuses
     - The turbinates
   - Nonanatomical structures which are often ghosted are:
     - Chin rest
     - (R) or (L) Markers of the machine
     - Neck chains
     - Napkin chains
     - Earrings
     - Shoulder straps of protective aprons.
2. *Lead apron artifact (**Fig. 13.8**)*
3. *Patient positioning errors*:
   - *Positioning of the lips and teeth:* If the lips are not closed on the bite block, a dark radiolucent shadow obscures the anterior teeth.

- *Positioning of the frankfurt plane*:
   - *Upward (**Fig. 13.9**)*: If the patient's chin is positioned too high or tipped up (i.e. the chin is too far forward while the forehead is tilted towards the back):
     - The hard palate and the floor of the nasal cavity appear superimposed over the roots of the maxillary teeth
     - Loss of density in the middle of the radiograph, usually characterized by an hour glass shape
     - There is a loss of detail in the maxillary incisor region, magnification
     - The maxillary incisors appear blurred and magnified
     - Loss of one or both condyles at the side of the film
     - A 'reverse smile line' is seen on the radiograph (flattening of the occlusal plane).
   - *Downward (**Fig. 13.10**)*: Alatragus line greater than 5° downward, the patient's chin is positioned too low or is tipped down (i.e. chin positioned back and the forehead is positioned forward):
     - The mandibular incisors appear blurred.
     - There is a loss of detail in the anterior apical region of the mandible. The apices of the lower incisors are out of focus and blurred.
     - The condyles may not be visible, as they may be cut off at the top of the radiograph.
     - Shadow of the hyoid bone is superimposed on the anterior aspect of the mandible.
     - Premolars are severly overlapped.
     - An 'exaggerated smile line' is seen on the radiograph (severe curvature of the occlusal plane).
- *Positioning of the teeth*:
   - *Anterior to the focal trough (**Fig. 13.11**)*: Patient's head is positioned too far forward:
     - If the anterior teeth are not positioned in the groove of the bite block, the teeth appear blurred.
     - If the teeth are positioned too far forward on the bite block, the anterior teeth appear 'skinny' and out of focus (Blurred and narrow).
     - Spine is superimposed on the ramus areas.
     - Premolars are severely overlapped.
   - *Posterior to the focal trough (**Fig. 13.12**)*: Patient's head is positioned too far back:
     - If the anterior teeth are not positioned in the groove of the bite block, the teeth appear blurred.
     - If the teeth are positioned too far back on the bite block, the anterior teeth appear 'fat' and out of focus (blurred and wide).
     - Excessive ghosting of mandible and spine.
- *Positioning of the midsagittal plane (**Fig. 13.13**)*: If the patient's head is not centered, the ramus and the posterior teeth appear unequally magnified. The side farthest from the film appears magnified and the side closest to the film appears smaller.

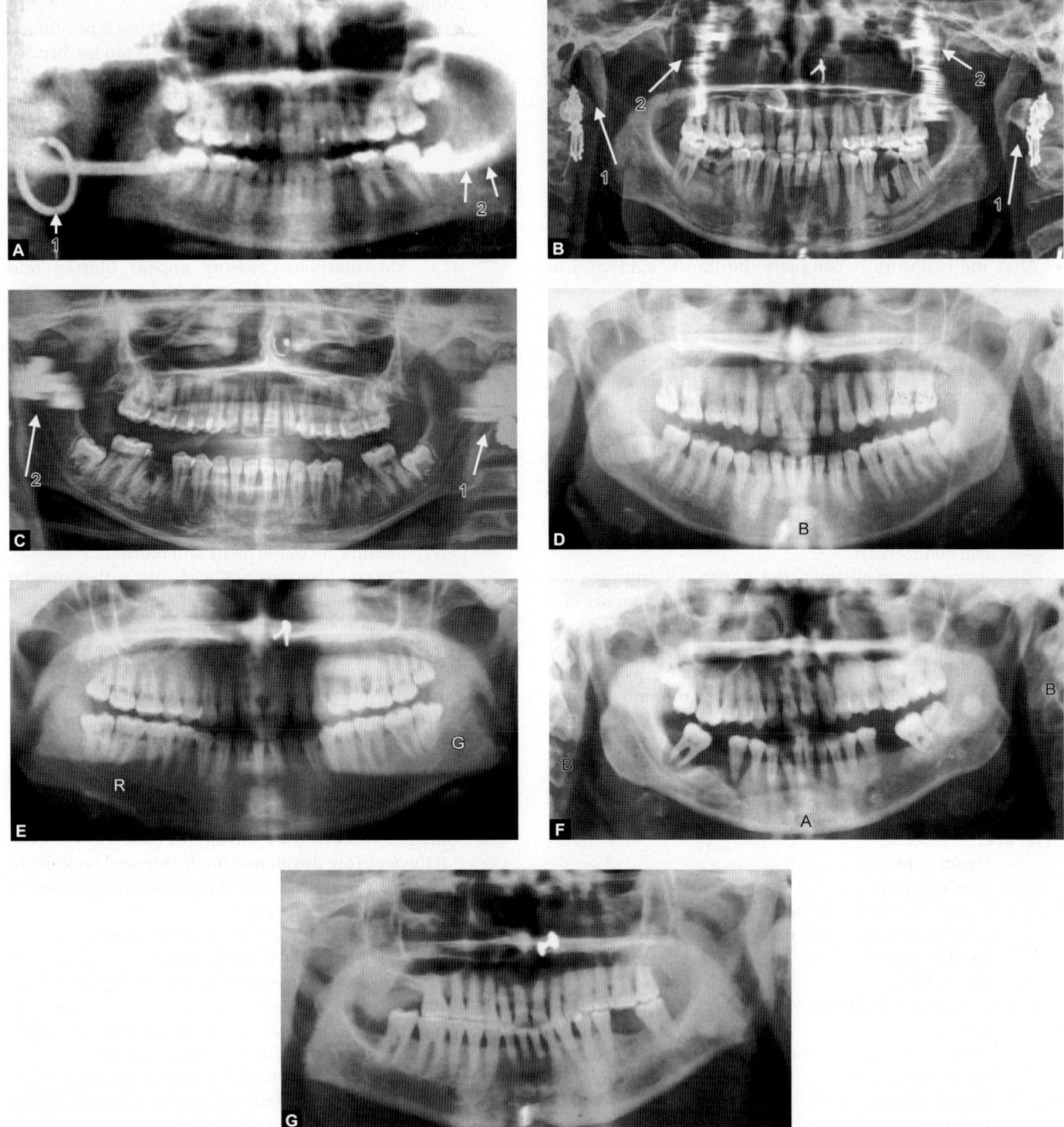

Figures 13.7A to G Ghost images: (A to C) Earrings: 1. True image of earring, 2. The ghost image of the earring appears on the opposite side of the film and is enlarged and laterally distorted, B; (D) 'B'; The ghost image of the neck chain appears near the apices of the lower central incisor region; (E) Ghost image of contra ramus R—Real images of ramus, G—Ghost images of contra ramus; (F) Ghost image of spine A—Ghost image of spine, B—Double real image of spine; (G) Nose ring lies in the 'diamond region' and is hence not ghosted

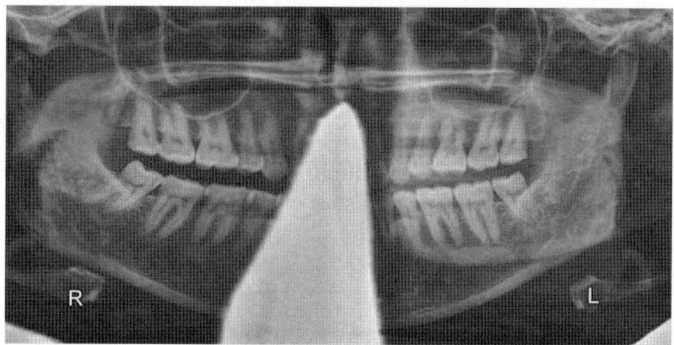

Figure 13.8 Lead apron artifact appears as a large cone shaped radiopacity obscuring the mandible

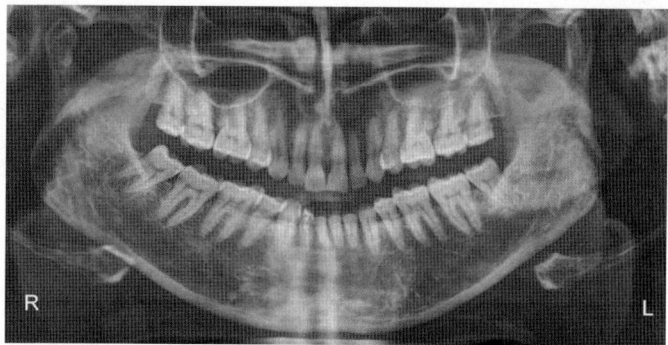

Figure 13.11 The anterior teeth appear narrow and blurred on a panoramic film when the patient is positioned too far forward on the bite block

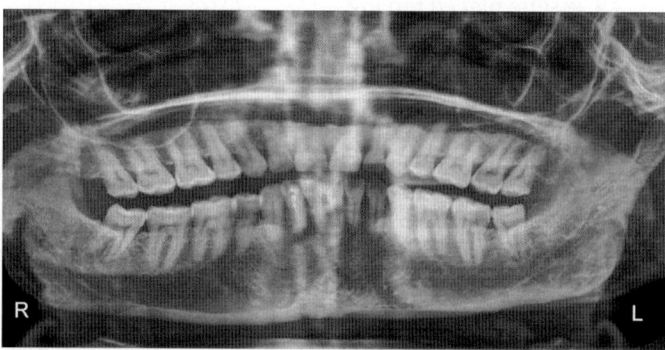

Figure 13.9 The chin and the occlusal plane are rotated upward, resulting in the overlapping of the images of the teeth and an opaque shadow (the hard palate) obscuring the roots of the maxillary teeth

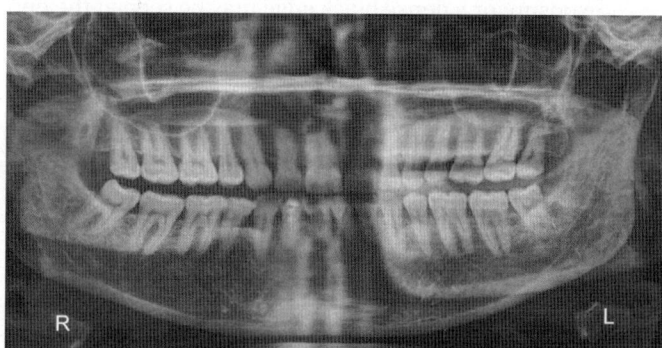

Figure 13.12 The anterior teeth appear widened and blurred on a panoramic film when the patient is positioned too far back on the bite block

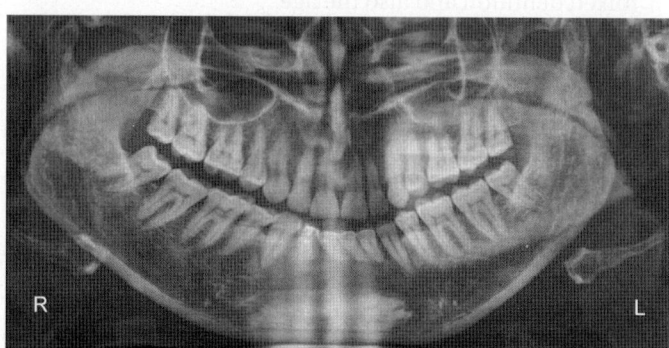

Figure 13.10 An exaggerated smile seen on a panoramic film when the patient's chin is tipped down

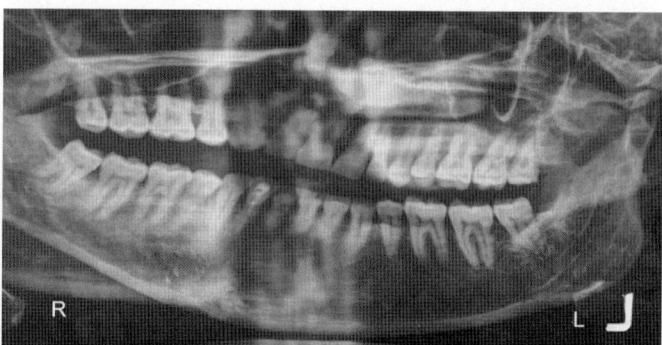

Figure 13.13 The patient's posterior teeth and ramus on one side appear to be magnified on the panoramic film when the head is not centered

- Patient's head is tilted to one side.
  - The side tilted towards the X-ray tube is enlarged
  - One condyle appears larger than the opposite one, the neck also appears longer on the larger side
  - Image appears to be tilted, one angle of the mandible is higher than the other.

- Patient's head is twisted to one side causing the mandible to fall outside the image layer, (one side is in front of the image layer while the other side is behind the image layer).
  - Teeth on one side of the midline appear wide and have severe overlapping of contacts, whereas the teeth on the other side appear very narrow.

- Ramus on one side is much wider than the other side.
  - Condyles differ in size.
- Whole head is off center position (patient biting the block off center with lateral incisors or cuspids).
  - The molar teeth and the mandibular ramus are magnified on the side farther from the film.
  - Anterior teeth are blurred with overlapping.
- *Positioning of the spine (Fig. 13.14)*: If the patient is not sitting or standing with a straight spine, the cervical spine appears as a pyramid shaped radiopacity in the center of the film and obscures diagnostic information.
- *Patient's shoulder touching the cassette during exposure*: This will slow the cassette rotation, resulting in prolonged exposure or completely stop the film movement.
  - Produces a dense black band, which is the area of overexposure or a dense black edge may be seen at the end of the radiographic image, due to eventual stoppage of rotation.
- *Position of patient's tongue during exposure (Fig. 13.14)*: If the tongue is not fully placed against the roof of the mouth.
  - A dark shadow appears in the maxilla below the palate, and the apices of the maxillary incisors are obscured.
- *Distortion due to patient movement*:
  - Movement in the same direction as the beam.
    - There is prolonged exposure of the same area, with increase in horizontal dimension of the image.
  - Movement in the opposite direction as the beam.
    - The horizontal dimension of the image in the region is decreased.
  - Sudden jerky movement in the same direction as the beam.
    - The area may be portrayed twice.
  - Sudden jerky movement in the direction opposite the beam movement.
    - A part of the object may be missing in the image.

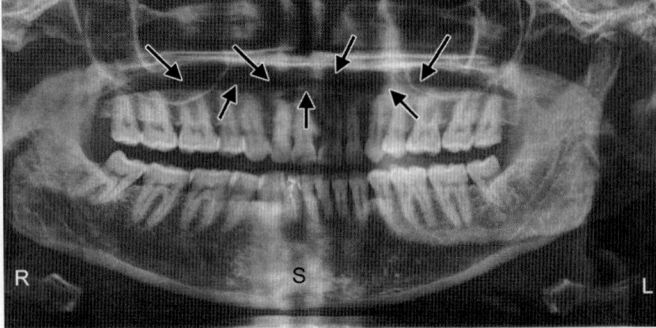

Figure 13.14 If the patient is not standing erect, superimposition of the cervical spine (S) may be seen on the center of the panoramic film and If the tongue is not placed on the roof of the mouth, a radiolucent shadow will be superimposed over the apices of the maxillary teeth (arrows)

- If the patient moves up or down during exposure.
  - Indentation in the lower border of the mandible (mimicing a fracture)
  - Blurring and unsharpness.
4. *Cassette positioning errors*:
   - Patient's shoulders touching the cassette during the movement in the exposure cycle.
   - This may happen if the patient has a short neck and well developed shoulders.
     - Alternating vertical dark and light bands appear on the radiograph due to improper movement of the cassette behind the slit in the cassette holder or the tube head cassette holder assembly around the patient's head.
   - Cassette placed too high.
     - Lower border of the mandible is cut off.
   - Cassette placed too low.
     - Diagnostic information in the maxilla will be cut off.
   - Two exposures on a single film.
   - Undiagnostic radiograph, with unnecessary exposure to the patient.
   - Cassette placed backwards.
     - This is common in panorex the X-rays must penetrate the metal latch, which will present as a radiopaque broad horizontal line through the middle of the radiograph.

CLINICAL INDICATIONS

- As a substitute for full mouth intraoral periapical radiographs.
- For evaluation of tooth development for children, the mixed dentition and also the age.
- To assist and assess the patient for and during orthodontic treatment.
- To establish the site and size of lesions such as cysts, tumors and developmental anomalies in the body and rami of the mandible.
- Prior to any surgical procedures such as extraction of impacted teeth, enucleation of a cyst, etc.
- For detection of fractures of the middle third face and the mandible after facial trauma.
- For follow-up of treatment, progress of pathology or postoperative bony healing.
- Investigation of TM joint dysfunction.
- To study the antrum, especially to study the floor, posterior and anterior walls of the antrum.
- Periodontal disease—as an overall view of the alveolar bone levels.
- Assessment for underlying bone disease before constructing complete or partial dentures.
- Evaluation of developmental anomalies.
- Evaluation of the vertical height of the alveolar bone before inserting osseointegrated implants.

Advantages

- Simple procedure requiring very little patient compliance.
- Convenient for the patient.
- Useful in patients with trismus and gagging problems.
- Time required is minimal compared to a full mouth intraoral periapical radiographs.
- That portion of the maxilla and the mandible lying within the focal trough can be visualized on a single film.
- The patient dose is relatively low.
- Panoramic radiographs taken for diagnostic purpose are valuable visual aid in patient education.
- A broad anatomic region is imaged. In addition to the teeth and the supporting structures, the entire maxillary region and the entire mandible extending distally up to the TM joint is visualized. Also seen in the same plate are the pharyngeal airspaces, hyoid bone and the styloid process.
- The anatomical structures are most identifiable and the teeth are oriented in their correct relationship to the adjacent structures and to each other.
- It allows for the assessment of the presence and position of unerupted teeth in orthodontic treatment.
- It demonstrates periodontal disease in a general way. Manifesting a generalized bone loss.
- All the parameters are standardized and repetitive images can be taken, on recall visits for comparative and research purposes.
- Useful for mass screening.
- This view helps in localization of objects/pathology in conjunction with a topographic occlusal view or an intraoral periapical radiograph.
- The radiation dose (effective dose equivalent) of app. 0.08 mSv is about one-third of the dose from a full mouth survey of intraoral films.

Disadvantages or Limitations

- Areas of diagnostic interest outside the focal trough may be poorly visualized, e.g. swelling on the palate, floor of the mouth.
- Comparatively this radiograph is of a poor diagnostic quality, in terms of magnification, geometric distortion, poor definition and loss of detail.
- There is an overlapping of the teeth in the bicuspid area of the maxilla and the mandible.
- In cases of pronounced inclination, the anterior teeth are poorly registered.
- The density of the spine, especially in short necked people can cause lack of clarity in the central portion of the film.
- Number of radiopaque and radiolucent areas may be present due to the superimposition of real/double or ghost images and because of soft tissue shadows and airspaces.
- Due to prescribed rotation, patient with facial asymmetry or patients who do not conform to the rotation curvature, cannot be X-rayed with any degree of satisfaction.

- If the patient positioning is improper, the amount of vertical and horizontal distortion will vary from one part of the film to another part of the film.
- The ease and convenience of obtaining an OPG may encourage careless evaluation of a patient's specific radiographic needs.
- Artifacts are easily misinterpreted and are more commonly seen, e.g. nose ring as a periapical radiopaque lesion, earring as a calcification in the maxillary sinus.
- OPG shows an oblique, rather than true lateral view of the condylar heads and hence, the joint space cannot be accurately assessed.
- The cost of the machine is very high.

INTERPRETING THE PANORAMIC IMAGE

Normal landmarks seen on the panoramic radiograph (**Fig. 13.15**).

The normal anatomical shadows that are evident on the panoramic radiographs vary from one machine to another, but generally they may be subdivided into:

- Real or actual shadows of structures in or close to the focal trough.
  - Hard tissue shadows
    - Teeth
    - Mandible
    - Maxilla, including the floor, anterior and posterior walls of the antra
    - Hard palate
    - Zygomatic arches
    - Styloid process
    - Hyoid bone
    - Nasal septum and conchae
    - Orbital rim
    - Base of skull.

    An additional real shadow is often cast by the vertical plastic head supports.
  - Soft tissue shadows
    - Ear lobes
    - Nasal cartilages
    - Soft palate
    - Dorsum of the tongue
    - Lips and cheeks
    - Nasolabial folds
  - Air shadows
    - Mouth/oral opening
    - Oropharynx.
- Ghost or artifactual shadows created by the tomographic movement, and cast by the structures on the opposite side or a long way from the focal trough. The 8° upward angulation of the X-ray beam means that these ghost shadows appear at a higher level than the structures that have caused them.
  - Cervical vertebrae
  - Body, angle and ramus of the contralateral side of the mandible
  - Palate.

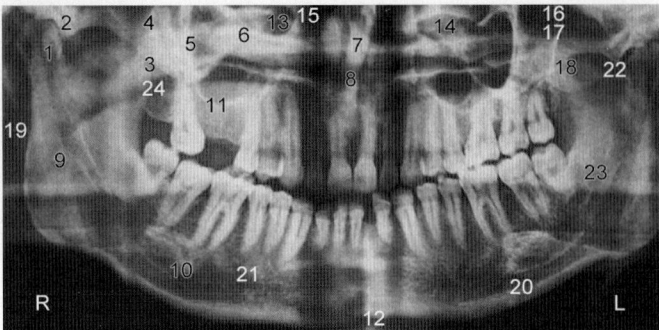

Figure 13.15 OPG radiographic view with anatomical landmarks outlined. It is a radiographic technique for producing a single image of the facial structures that includes both the maxillary and mandibular dental arches and their supporting structures. Various structures visible are: 1. Mandibular condyle; 2. Articular eminence; 3. Coronoid process of mandible superimposed on zygomatic process; 4. Posterior wall of maxillary sinus; 5. Posterior wall of zygomatic process of maxilla; 6. Hard palate; 7. Nasal septum; 8. Tip of nose; 9. Dorsum of tongue; 10. Hyoid superimposed over inferior border of mandible; 11. Inferior border of maxillary sinus; 12. Image of cervical spine; 13. Medial border of maxillary sinus; 14. Infraorbital canal; 15. Infraorbital rim; 16. Pterygomaxillary fissure; 17. Anterior border of the pterygoid plates; 18. Lateral pterygoid plates superimposed on soft palate and coronoid process of mandible; 19. Ear lobe; 20. Inferior border of mandibular canal; 21. Mental foramen; 22. Posterior wall of nasopharynx; 23. Inferior border of mandible superimposed from opposite side; 24. Shadow of soft palate

BONY LANDMARKS OF THE MAXILLA AND SURROUNDING STRUCTURES (FIGS 13.15 AND 13.16)

- *Mastoid process*: It is a marked prominence of bone located posterior and inferior to the temporomandibular joint, it is a part of the temporal bone.
    - On the radiograph it appears as a rounded radiopacity located posterior and inferior to the temporomandibular joint.
- *Styloid process*: It is a long pointed and sharp projection of bone that extends downwards from the inferior surface of the temporal bone. It is anterior to the mastoid process.
    - On the radiograph it appears as a long radiopaque spine extending from the temporal bone anterior to the mastoid process.
- *External auditory meatus (External acoustic meatus)*: It is an opening in the temporal bone located superior and anterior to the mastoid process.
    - On the radiograph it appears as a round to oval radiolucency anterior and superior to the mastoid process.
- *Glenoid fossa (Mandibular fossa)*: It is a concave, depressed area of the temporal bone, in which the mandibular condyle rests. It is located anterior to the mastoid process and the external auditory meatus.
    - On the radiograph it appears as a concave radiopacity superior to the mandibular condyle.

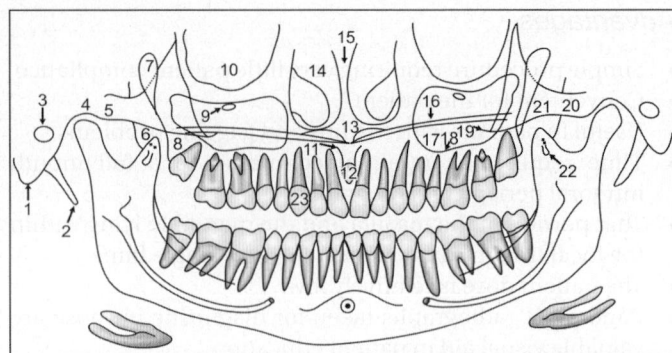

Figure 13.16 Normal anatomical landmarks of the maxilla and surrounding structures: 1. Mastoid process; 2. Styloid process; 3. External auditory meatus; 4. Glenoid fossa; 5. Articular eminence; 6. Lateral pterygoid plate; 7. Pterygomaxillary fissure; 8. Maxillary tuberosity; 9. Infraorbital foramen; 10. Orbit; 11. Incisive canal; 12. Incisive foramen; 13. Anterior nasal spine; 14. Nasal cavity and conchae; 15. Nasal septum; 16. Hard palate; 17. Maxillary sinus; 18. Floor of the maxillary sinus; 19. Zygomatic process of maxilla; 20. Zygomatic arch; 21. Zygoma; 22. Hamulus; 23. Dentition

- *Articular eminence (Articular tubercle)*: It is a rounded projection of the temporal bone located anterior to the glenoid fossa.
    - On the radiograph it appears as a rounded radiopaque projection of the bone located anterior to the glenoid fossa.
- *Lateral pterygoid plate*: It is a wing shaped bony projection of the sphenoid bone located distal to the maxillary tuberosity region.
    - On the radiograph it appears as a radiopaque projection of bone distal to the maxillary tuberosity region.
- *Pterygomaxillary fissure*: It is a narrow space or cleft that separates the lateral pterygoid plate and the maxilla.
    - On the radiograph it appears as a radiolucent area between the lateral pterygoid plate and the maxilla. The zygoma may superimpose and obscure the fissure.
- *Maxillary tuberosity*:
    - On the panoramic radiograph it appears as a radiopaque bulge distal to the third molar region.
- *Infraorbital foramen*: It is an opening in the bone found inferior to the border of the orbit.
    - On the panoramic radiograph it appears as a round or oval radiolucency inferior to the orbit.
    - It may be superimposed over the maxillary sinus.
- *Orbit*: It is the bony cavity that contains the eyeball.
    - On the panoramic radiograph it appears as
        - A round radiolucent compartment with radiopaque borders located superior to the maxillary sinus.
        - On most panoramic radiographs only the inferior border of the orbit is visible, where it appears as a radiopaque line.

- *Incisive canal (Nasopalatine canal)*: It is a passage through the bone that extends from the superior foramina of the incisive canal (located on the floor of the nasal cavity) to the incisive foramen (located on the anterior hard palate).
  - On the panoramic radiograph it appears as a tube like radiolucent area with radiopaque borders.
  - It is observed between the maxillary central incisors.
- *Incisive foramen (Nasopalatine foramen)*:
  - On the panoramic radiograph it appears as a small ovoid or round radiolucency located between the roots of the maxillary central incisors.
- *Anterior nasal spine*:
  - On the panoramic radiograph it appears as a 'V' shaped radiopaque area located at the inter-section of the floor of the nasal cavity and the nasal septum.
- *Nasal cavity*:
  - On the panoramic radiograph it appears as a large radiolucent area above the maxillary incisors.
- *Nasal septum*:
  - On the panoramic radiograph it appears as a vertical radiopaque partition that divides the nasal cavity.
- *Hard palate*: It is the bony wall that separates the nasal cavity from the oral cavity.
  - On the panoramic radiograph it appears as a horizontal radiopaque band superior to the apices of the maxillary teeth.
- *Maxillary sinus and floor of the maxillary sinus*:
  - On the panoramic radiograph it appears as a paired radiolucencies located above the apices of the maxillary premolars and molars.
  - The floor of the maxillary sinus is composed of dense cortical bone and appears as a radiopaque line.
- *Zygomatic process of the maxilla*:
  - On the panoramic radiograph it appears as a 'J' or 'U' shaped radiopacity located superior to the maxillary first molar.
- *Zygomatic arch*:
  - On the panoramic radiograph it appears as:
    - Posterior extension of zygoma.
    - Formed by temporal process of zygomatic bone (Anterior 1/3) and zygomatic process of temporal bone (Posterior 2/3).
- *Zygoma*:
  - On the panoramic radiograph it appears as a radiopaque band that extends posteriorly from the zygomatic process of the maxilla.
  - It is triangular in shape.
- *Hamulus*:
  - On the panoramic radiograph it appears as a radiopaque hook-like projection posterior to the maxillary tuberosity area.
- *Dentition*:
  - On the panoramic radiograph it appears as:
    - The complete dentition is demonstrated.

- Teeth should be evaluated for gross deformities, like caries, periapical and peridontal disease.
- Impacted molars can be observed for their orientation, number of roots, and the relationship of the roots to critical anatomical structures like floor and posterior wall of the maxillary sinus, maxillary tuberosity and adjacent teeth.
- The proximal surfaces of premolars often overlap which inteferes with the detection of caries.
- If the anterior teeth are excessively broad or narrow, it suggests the malpositioning of the patient.
- If the teeth are wider on one side than the other it suggests that the patient's sagittal plane was rotated.

BONY LANDMARKS OF THE MANDIBLE AND SURROUNDING STRUCTURES (FIGS 13.15 AND 13.17)

- *Mandibular condyle*: It is a rounded projection of bone extending from the posterosuperior border of the ramus of the mandible. It articulates with the glenoid fossa of the temporal bone.
  - On the panoramic radiograph it appears as a bony rounded, radiopaque projection extending from the posterior border of the ramus of the mandible.
- *Coronoid notch*: It is a scooped out concavity of bone located distal to the coronoid process of the mandible.
  - On the panoramic radiograph it appears as a radiolucent concavity located distal to the coronoid process on the superior border of the ramus.
- *Coronoid process*:
  - On the panoramic radiograph it appears as a triangular radiopacity posterior to the maxillary tuberosity region.
- *Mandibular foramen*: It is a round or ovoid opening on the lingual aspect of the ramus of the mandible.
  - On the panoramic radiograph it appears as a round or ovoid radiolucency centered within the ramus of the mandible.
- *Ramus*:
  - *On the panoramic radiograph*:
    - Shadows of other structures may be superimposed over the mandibular ramus area,
    - Pharyngeal air way shadow, especially when the patient is unable to expel air and place the tongue in the palate during exposure.
    - Posterior wall of the nasopharynx.
    - Cervical vertebrae, especially in patients with pronounced anterior lordosis (as seen in osteoporotic patients).
    - Ear lobe and ear decorations.
    - Soft palate and uvula.
    - Dorsum of the tongue.
    - Ghost shadows of the opposite side of the mandible.

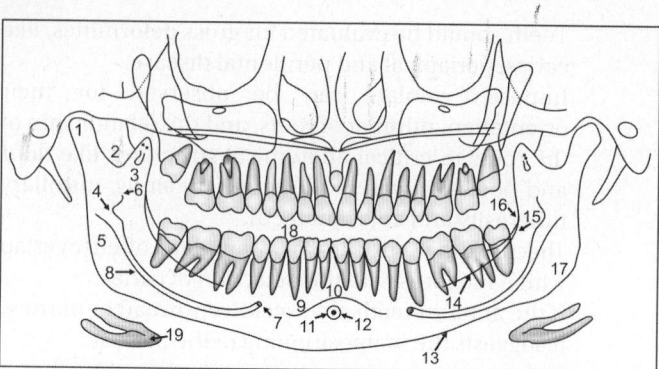

Figure 13.17 Normal anatomical landmarks of the mandible and surrounding structures: 1. Mandibular condyle; 2. Coronoid notch; 3. Coronoid process; 4. Mandibular foramen; 5. Ramus; 6. Lingula; mandibular canal; 7. Mental foramen; 8. Mandibular or inferior alveolar canal; 9. Mental ridge; 10. Mental fossa; 11. Lingual foramen; 12. Genial tubercles; 13. Inferior border of mandible; 14. Mylohyoid ridge; 15. Internal oblique ridge; 16. External oblique ridge; 17. Angle of mandible; 18. Dentition; 19. Hyoid bone

- *Lingula*: A small tongue shaped projection of bone seen adjacent to the mandibular foramen.
  - On the panoramic radiograph it appears as an indistinct radiopacity anterior to the mandibular foramen.
- *Mental foramen*:
  - On the panoramic radiograph it appears as a small ovoid or round radiolucency located in the apical region of the mandibular premolars.
- *Mandibular or inferior alveolar canal*:
  - On the panoramic radiograph it appears as a radiolucent band outlined by two thin radiopaque lines representing the cortical walls of the canal.
- *Mental ridge*:
  - On the panoramic radiograph it appears as a thick radiopaque band that extends from the mandibular premolar region to the incisor region.
- *Mental fossa*:
  - On the panoramic radiograph it appears as a radiolucent area above the mental ridge.
- *Lingual foramen*:
  - On the panoramic radiograph it appears as a small radiolucent dot located inferior to the apices of the mandibular incisors.
- *Genial tubercles*:
  - On the panoramic radiograph it appears as a ring shaped radiopacity surrounding the lingual foramen.
- *Inferior border of the mandible*: It is a linear prominence of cortical bone that defines the lower border of the mandible.
  - On the panoramic radiograph it appears as a dense radiopaque band that outlines the lower border of the mandible.

- *Mylohyoid ridge*:
  - On the panoramic radiograph it appears as a dense radiopaque band that extends downward and forward from the molar region.
- *Internal oblique ridge*:
  - On the panoramic radiograph it appears as a dense radiopaque band that extends downward and forward from the ramus.
- *External oblique ridge*:
  - On the panoramic radiograph it appears as a dense radiopaque band that extends downward and forward from the anterior border of the ramus of the mandible.
- *Angle of the mandible*: It is that area of the mandible where the body meets the ramus.
  - On the panoramic radiograph it appears as a radiopaque bony structure where the ramus joins the body of the mandible.
- *Dentition*: On the panoramic radiograph it appears as:
  - The complete dentition is demonstrated.
  - Teeth should be evaluated for gross deformities, like caries, periapical and peridontal disease.
  - Impacted molars can be observed for their orientation, number of roots, and the relationship of the roots to critical anatomical structures like the mandibular canal and adjacent teeth.
  - The proximal surfaces of premolars often overlap which interferes with the detection of caries.
  - If the anterior teeth are excessively broad or narrow, it suggests the malpositioning of the patient.
  - If the teeth are wider on one side than the other it suggests that the patient's sagittal plane was rotated.
- *Hyoid bone*:
  - On the panoramic radiograph it appears as bilateral, 'U' shaped radiopaque body, just below or at the level of the inferior border of the mandible in line with molars.

AIRSPACE IMAGES SEEN ON PANORAMIC RADIOGRAPHS (FIG. 13.18)

- *Palatoglossal airspace*: It is the space between the palate and the tongue.
  - On the panoramic radiograph it appears as a horizontal radiolucent band located above the apices of the maxillary teeth.
- *Nasopharyngeal airspace*: It is that portion of the pharynx located posterior to the nasal cavity.
  - On the panoramic radiograph it appears as a diagonal radiolucency located superior to the radiopaque shadow of the soft palate and uvula.
- *Glossopharyngeal airspace*:
  - It is that portion of the pharynx located posterior to the tongue and the oral cavity.
  - On the panoramic radiograph it appears as:

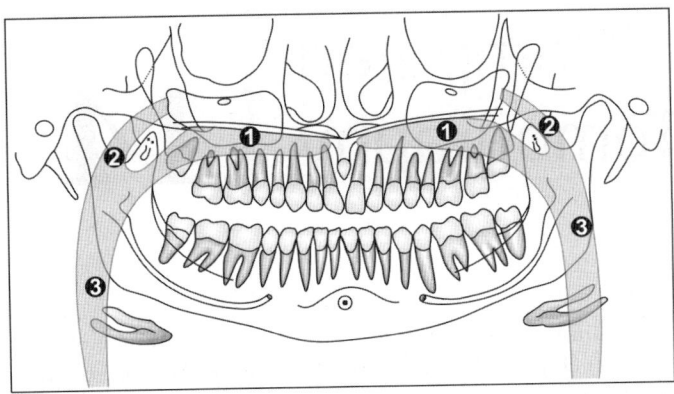

Figure 13.18 Airspace images seen on panoramic films: 1. Palatoglossal airspace; 2. Nasopharyngeal airspace; 3. Glossopharyngeal airspace

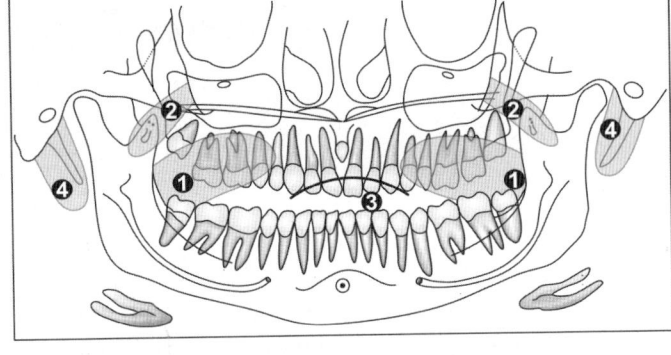

Figure 13.19 Soft tissue images seen on panoramic films: 1. Tongue; 2. Soft palate and uvula; 3. Lipline; 4. Ear

– A vertical radiolucent band superimposed over the ramus of the mandible.

– It is continuous with the nasopharyngeal airspace superiorly and the palatoglossal airspace inferiorly.

SOFT TISSUE IMAGES SEEN ON PANORAMIC RADIOGRAPHS (FIG. 13.19)

• *Tongue*: It is a movable muscular structure attached to the floor of the mouth.
  – On the panoramic radiograph it appears as a radiopaque area superimposed over the maxillary posterior teeth.

• *Soft palate and uvula*: These form a muscular curtain that separates the oral cavity from the nasal cavity.
  – On the panoramic radiograph it appears as a diagonal radiopacity projecting posteriorly and inferiorly from the maxillary tuberosity region.

• *Lip line*: It is formed by the position of the patient's lips.
  – On the panoramic radiograph it appears as:
    - The lip line is seen in the region of the anterior teeth.
    - The areas of the teeth not covered by the lips appear more radiolucent.
    - The areas of the teeth covered by the lips appear more radiopaque.

• *Ear*: On the panoramic radiograph it appears as:
  – A radiopaque shadow that projects anteriorly and inferiorly from the mastoid process
  – The ear is viewed superimposed over the styloid process.

BIBLIOGRAPHY

1. Goaz PW, White SC. Panoramic Radiography, Radiographic Examinations in Oral Radiology, Principles and Interpretation, 3rd edition. St Louis: Mosby-Year Book; 1994.pp.314-38.

2. Johnson ON, McNally MA, Essay CE. The Periapical Examination Essentials of Dental Radiography for Dental Assistants and Hygienists, 6th edition. Norwalk: Appleton and Lange; 1999.pp.319-90.

3. Karjodkar FR, Nahar P. Ghost Images which Haunt OPG, Dental Voice, IDA, 2002.

4. Karjodkar FR. Trouble Shooting Errors in Panoramic Techniques. Dental Voice, IDA, 1999.

5. Langland OE, Langlis RP, McDavid WD, et al. Panoramic Radiology, 2nd edition. Philadelphia, Lea and Febiger; 1989.pp.224-71.

6. Mason-Hing LR. In: Fundamentals of Dental Radiography, 3rd edition. Philadelphia: WB Saunders; 1993.pp.1-75.

7. Reskin AB. Advances in Oral Radiology, PSG Publishing Co. 1980.

Cone Beam Computed Tomography | 14

Cone beam computerized technology (CBCT) introduces a more complex and accurate imaging with 3-dimensional visualization as compared to the routinely used analog and digital radiographs. It is a precise technology for numerous clinical oral-maxillofacial indications, with the added advantage of lower radiation doses than computerized tomography.

3D cone beam technology shows up with different names according to countries and manufacturers:

- CBCT—Cone beam computed tomography
- DVT—Digital volumetric tomography
- VT—Volumetric tomography.

This technology is based on the principle of tomosynthesis, and the shape of the X-ray beam used for imaging is 'cone shaped' hence it is named Cone Beam Computed Tomography. The scanners used are ingenuously engineered to image and determine the anatomy of the maxillofacial region. In a single scan the X-ray source and a reciprocating X-ray sensor rotate around the head of the patient and acquire multiple images of the region of interest (ROI) (**Fig. 14.1**). The assimilated images are the raw data that subsequently undergo a primary reconstruction to mathematically replicate the patient's anatomy into a single,

three-dimensional volume that consists of volume elements (voxels) (**Fig. 14.2**). Each voxel is small in size (0.1–0.4 mm for each face) and hence the image has a reasonably high resolution. The field of view (FOV) can be customized to include a portion of or the entire maxillofacial region. The CBCT software permits reformatting and viewing the image data from multiple approaches; that is in straight or curved planes and in three-dimensions. With the help of these software tools the anatomy can be scrutinized layer by layer to localize and study the most desired anatomy.

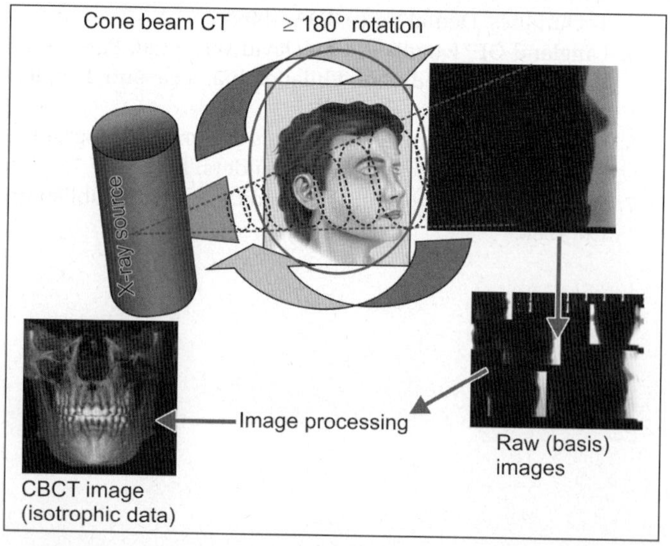

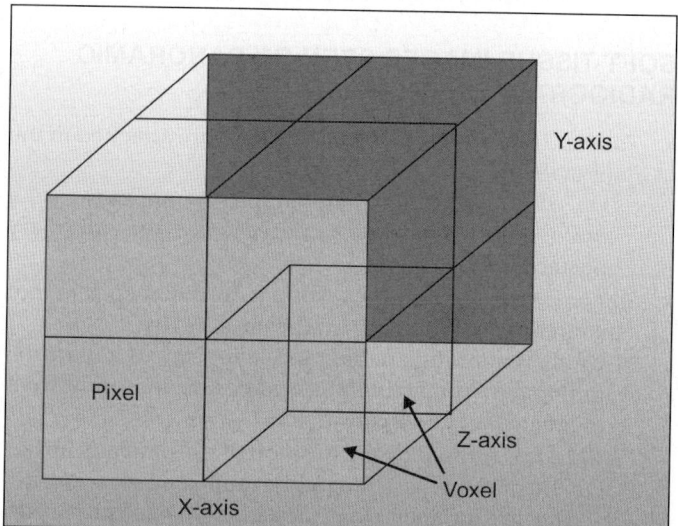

Figure 14.2 Voxel: The term pixel is a contraction derived from the words picture and element. Pixel represents the smallest single component of an image on a two-dimensional grid. The intensity, hue, and value of a pixel can vary, thus displaying multiple combinations of data elements that, when projected using an electronic display grid or printed on a photographic medium, will form an accurate rendering or image. The image can be viewed in color or as a black and white image using a gray scale. The attenuation of an X-ray signal by an object or tissue will determine the value and intensity of the individual pixels. A voxel is a volume pixel. The voxel adds the third dimension (3D) to the digital image by adding the Z-axis (depth) to the X-axis (width) and the Y-axis (height). Stacks of these volumetric boxes of data allow 360 degrees of virtual manipulation of imaged objects. The voxel becomes the smallest element in the 3D environment. When viewed as a digital image, the pixel size controls the resolution. The smaller pixel size yields a higher resolution image, and conversely, the larger the pixel size, the lower the resolution or quality of the image

Figure 14.1 Schematic sequence for cone beam computed tomography image acquisition

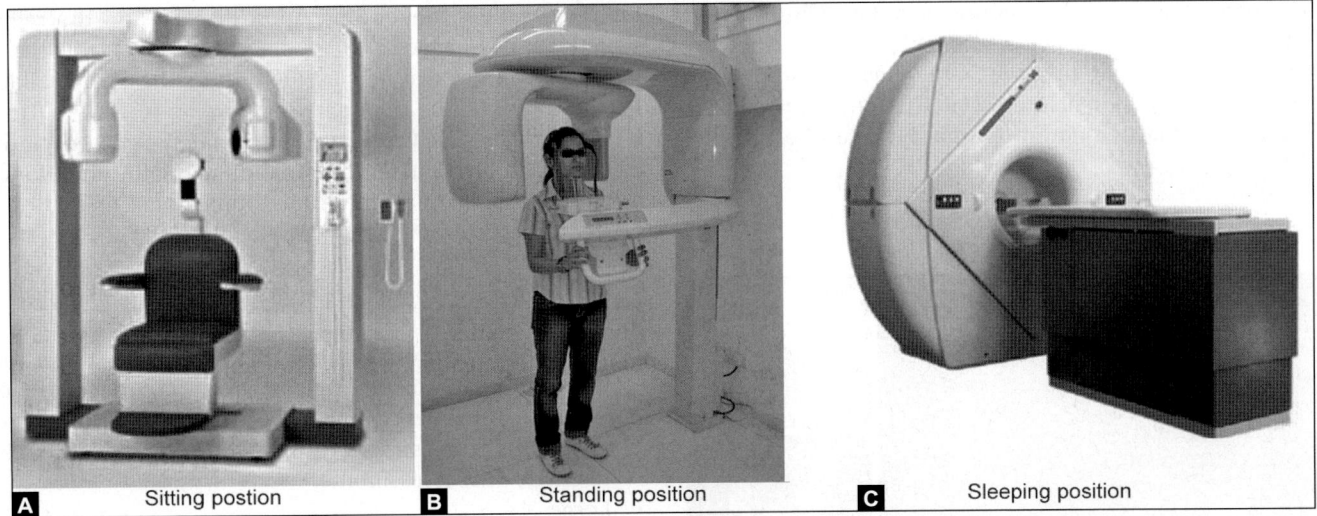

Figures 14.3A to C Cone beam machines

Cone-beam machines scan patients in three positions (**Fig. 14.3**):
1. Sitting.
2. Standing.
3. Supine.

The four basic constituents of CBCT image production are:
1. Acquisition configuration.
2. Image detection.
3. Image reconstruction.
4. Image display.

ACQUISITION CONFIGURATION

A single, partial or complete rotational scan from an X-ray source occurs when a corresponding reciprocating area detector moves synchronously around a fixed fulcrum within the patient's head.

X-ray Generation

During the scan rotation, each projection image is made by consecutive, single-image capture of attenuated X-ray beams by the detector. The X-ray beam is pulsed to coincide with the detector sampling, which means that actual exposure time is markedly less than scanning time. For example a 20-second scan usually exposes the patient to radiation for only 3.5 seconds. This technique reduces patient radiation dose considerably.

Field of View (Figs 14.3 to 14.9)

The dimensions of the FOV or scan volume generated depend principally on:
- The detector size and shape
- The beam projection geometry
- Collimation of the beam.

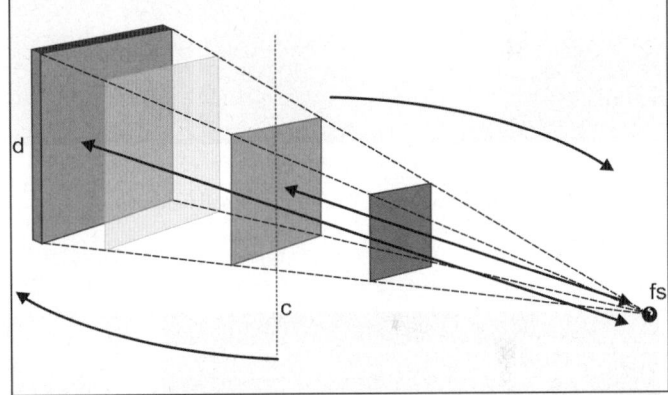

Figure 14.4 The field of view—FOV The FOV depends on: The detector size, the magnification ratio $D_{(fs/d)}/D'_{(fs/c)}$ The detector provides the n projections

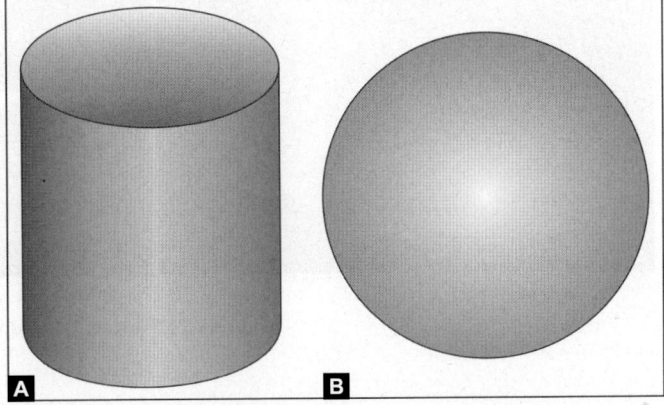

Figures 14.5A and B The shape of the scan volume (FOV) can be either cylindrical or spherical

The shape of the scan volume can be cylindrical or spherical.

Collimation of the primary X-ray beam restricts the irradiation to the region of interest (ROI). Hence the field size limitation safeguards that an optimal FOV can be selected for each patient, depending upon disease and the region selected to be imaged.

CBCT systems can be classified on the basis of available FOV as follows:

- *Small or localized region*: Approximately 5 × 5 cm or less (e.g. dentoalveolar, temporomandibular joint, endodontia, single implant placement, dis impactions, or any other treatment requiring a high level of detail (90 μm))
- *Medium*:
  - *Single arch*: Approximately 10 × 5 cm (e.g. mandible or maxilla)
  - *Interarch*: Approximately 10 × 10 or 8 × 8 cm (e.g. multiple implant placements, complicated dis impactions, pathologies involving both dental arches, mandible and superiorly to include the inferiorconcha, single TMJ assessments)
- *Large*:
  - *Maxillofacial*: Approximately 10 to 17 cm (17 × 11)
  - Mandible and extending to Nasion, Maxillofacila trauma)
  - *Craniofacial*: Approximately greater than 17 cm (17 × 13.5, 17 × 6) (e.g. complex treatment planning, pathologies extending from the lower border of the mandible upto the vertex of the head, sinus and airway analyses, orthodontia, orthognathic surgery, facial reconstruction, maxillofacial trauma, bilateral TMJ assessments)
- *Stitching*: Small or medium FOV and be stitched with software programes to enable visualization of larger areas.

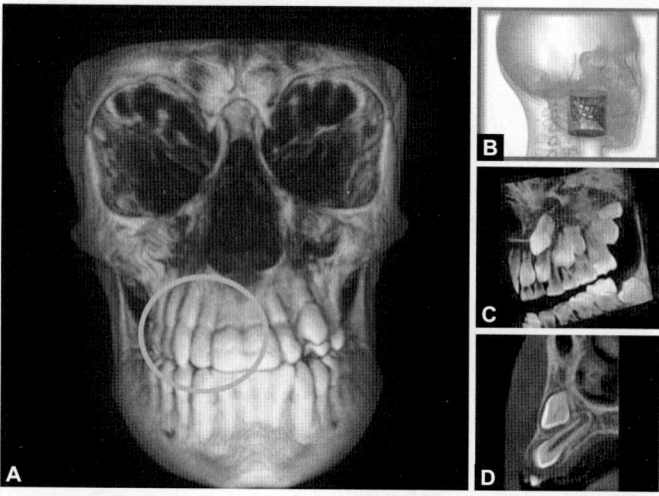

5 × 5 cm

Figures 14.6A to D CBCT system of small field of view

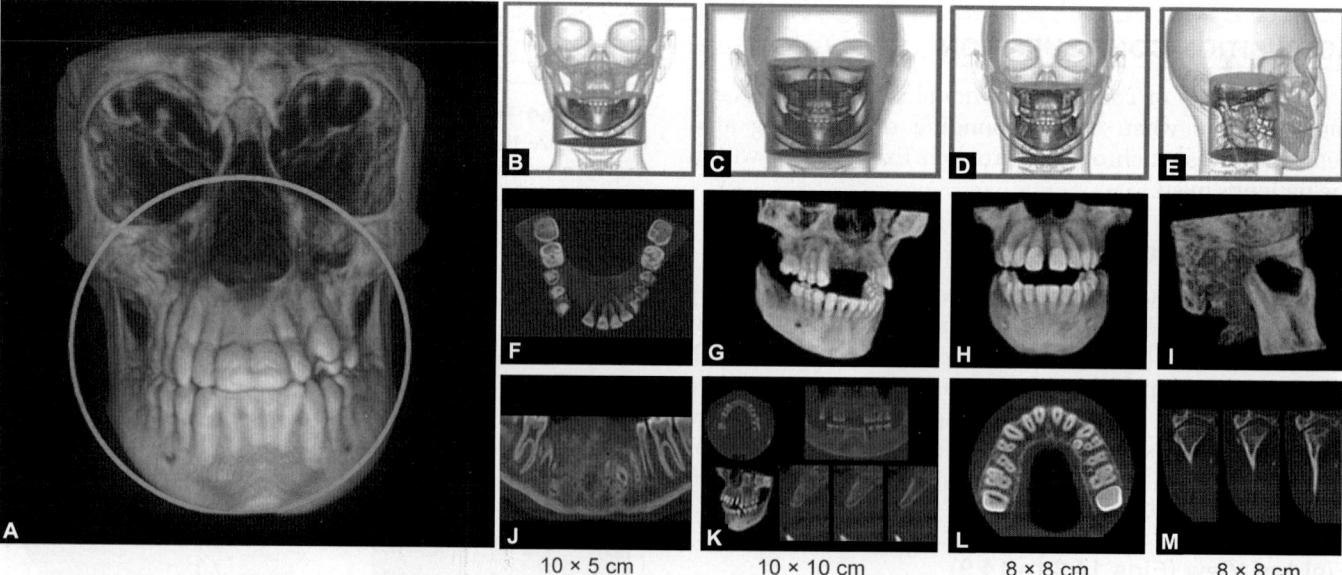

10 × 5 cm   10 × 10 cm   8 × 8 cm   8 × 8 cm

Figures 14.7A to M Medium FOV single arch and inter-arch

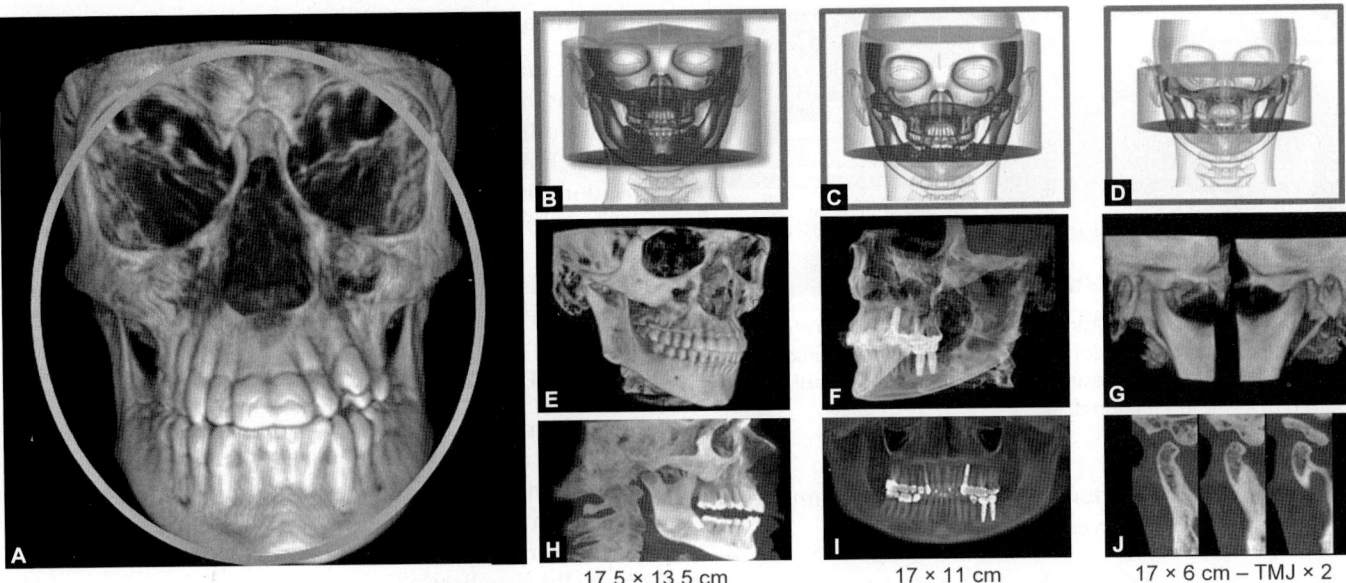

17 5 × 13.5 cm   17 × 11 cm   17 × 6 cm – TMJ × 2

Figures 14.8A to J CBCT system of large field of view

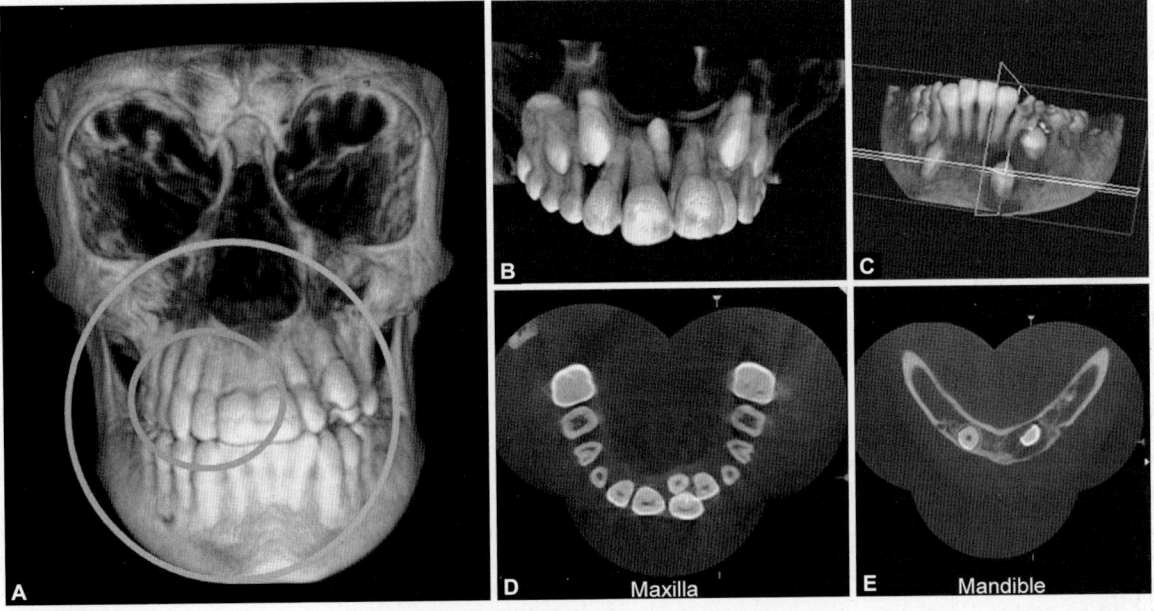

Figures 14.9A to E Stitched field of view

Scan Factors

As the scan progresses, single exposures are made at definite degree intervals, generating individual 2D projection images, known as '*basis*', '*frame*', or '*raw*' images which are comparable to lateral and posterior anterior '*cephalometric*' radiographic images, each slightly offset from one another.

The complete series of images is known as the '*projection data*'. (**Figs 14.10A and B**).

The number of images encompassing the projection data throughout the scan is determined by:
- The frame rate (number of images acquired per second)
- The completeness of the trajectory arc
- The speed of the rotation.

Frame Rate and Speed of Rotation

Higher frame rates provide images with fewer artifacts and better image quality. However, the greater number

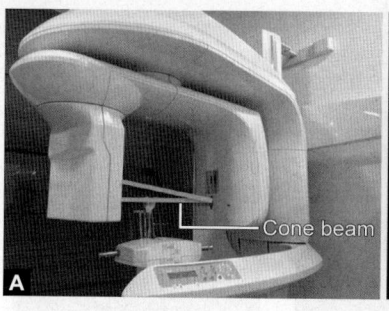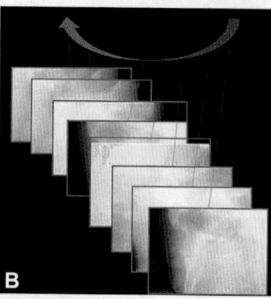

Figures 14.10A and B 'RAW' images. These images are similar to lateral and posterior-anterior 'cephalometric' radiographic images, each slightly offset from one another. The complete series of images is referred to as the 'projection data'

of projections proportionately increases the amount of radiation a patient receives.

Completeness of the Trajectory Arc

Most CBCT imaging systems use a complete circular trajectory or a scan arc of 360° to acquire projection data. This is usually necessary to produce projection data adequate for 3D reconstruction using the FDK algorithm.

IMAGE DETECTION

CBCT units are categorized into two groups, based on detector type:
1. An image intensifier tube/charge-coupled device (IIT/CCD) combination.
2. A flat-panel imager. (high-resolution, flat-panel detectors consisting of a large-area pixel array of hydrogenated amorphous silicon thin-film transistors).

Image Reconstruction

Once the basis projection frames have been acquired, data must be processed to create the volumetric data set. This process is called reconstruction.

The number of individual projection frames may vary from 100 to more than 600, each with more than one million pixels, with 12 to 16 bits of data designated to each pixel. The reconstruction of the data is therefore computationally complicated.

Reconstruction times vary, based on the acquisition parameters (voxel size, FOV, number of projections), hardware (processing speed, data throughout from acquisition to workstation computer), and software (reconstruction algorithms) used. Reconstruction is usually completed in less than 3 minutes for standard resolution scans.

Acquisition Stage

The raw images from CBCT detectors often show spatial variations of dark image offset and pixel gain due to the spatially differing physical properties of the photodiodes and the switching elements in the flat panel, and also because of variations in the X-ray sensitivity of the scintillator layer.

To compensate for this short coming, raw images require systematic offset and gain calibration and a correction of defect pixels. The sequence of the required calibration steps is known to as 'detector preprocessing'.

RECONSTRUCTION STAGE

After the images are corrected, they are related to each other and assembled using the FDK algorithm which is the most widely used filtered back projection algorithm for cone beam–acquired volumetric data. Once all the slices have been reconstructed, they are recombined into a single volume for visualization.

IMAGE DISPLAY

The CBCT technology comes in multiple image display formats. The volumetric data set is a compilation of all available voxels and, for most CBCT devices, it is displayed to the clinician on screen as secondary reconstructed images in three orthogonal planes (axial, sagittal, and coronal), (**Figs 14.11A and B**) usually at a thickness defaulted to the indigenous resolution. Optimum visualization of orthogonal reconstructed images is based upon the adjustment of window level and window width to favor bone and the application of specific filters.

Multiplanar Reformation (MPR) (Figs 14.12 to 14.19)

Multiplanar reformation (MRP) means the two-dimensional presentation of three-dimensional data in multiple projection planes. Spatial relationships between three simultaneous displayed planes are shown by projecting one plane onto the corresponding orthogonal planes as lines. Coronal, sagittal, and axial views are linked with synthesized views, such as oblique and/or curved slices planar reformation, and serial transplanar reformation. Slices or slab thickness also can be manipulated either directly or in real-time. Due to the large number of individual slices in any MPR image and the difficulty in relating adjacent structures, a number of methods have been developed to visualize adjacent voxels called Voxel Vision. There are essentially two techniques that can be applied to volumetric CBCT data to accomplish this:
1. *Ray sum or ray casting*: Any multiplanar image can be 'thickened' by increasing the number of adjacent voxels included in the display to obtain an image that is similar to a routine X-ray radiograph. This enables smoothing

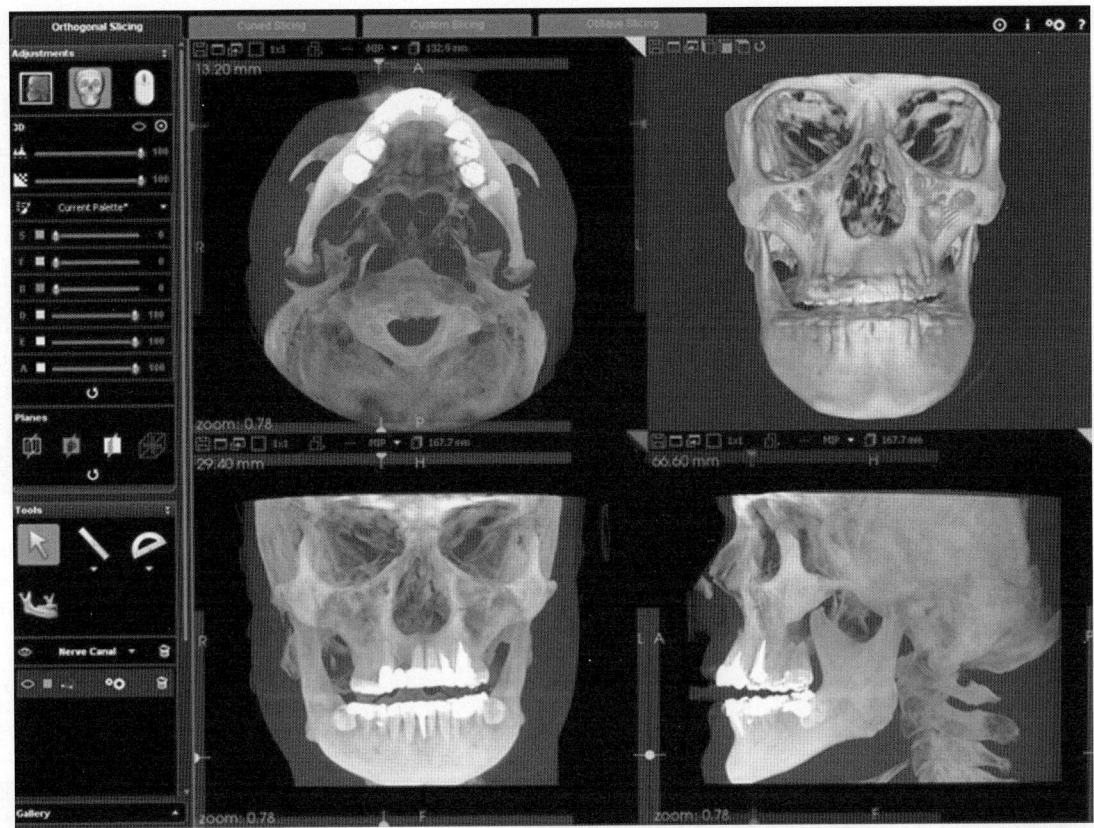

Figures 14.11 Monitor screen showing secondary reconstructed images in three orthogonal planes (axial, sagittal, coronal and 3D)

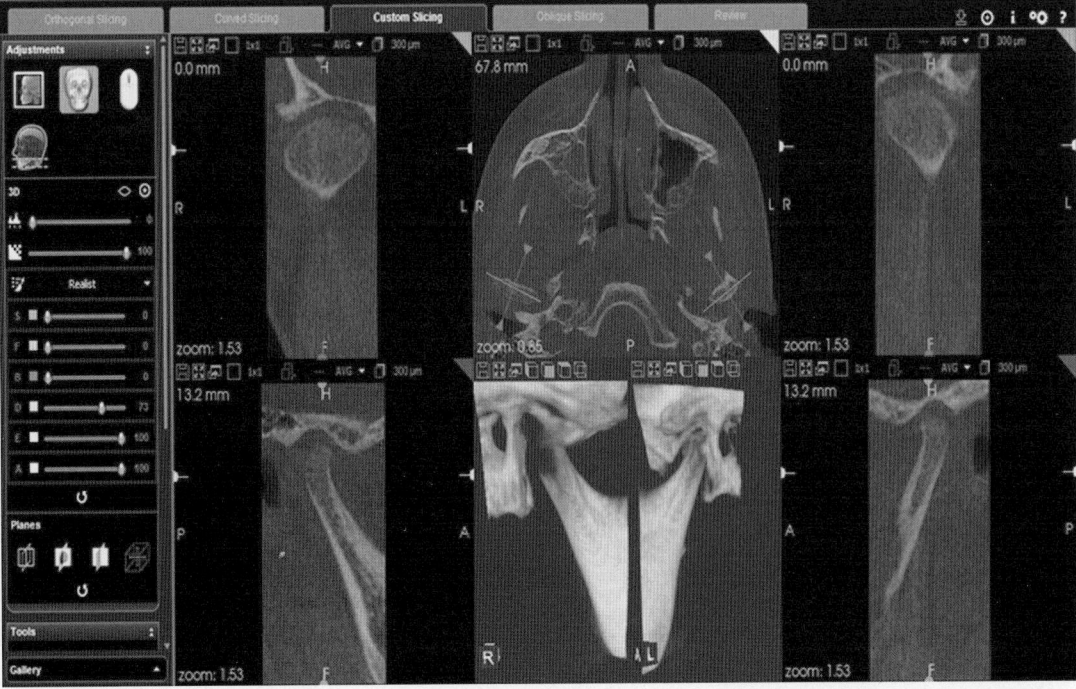

Figure 14.12 Oblique planar reformation. This mode is particularly useful for evaluating specific structures (e.g. TMJ, impacted third molars) as certain features may not be readily apparent on perpendicular MPR images

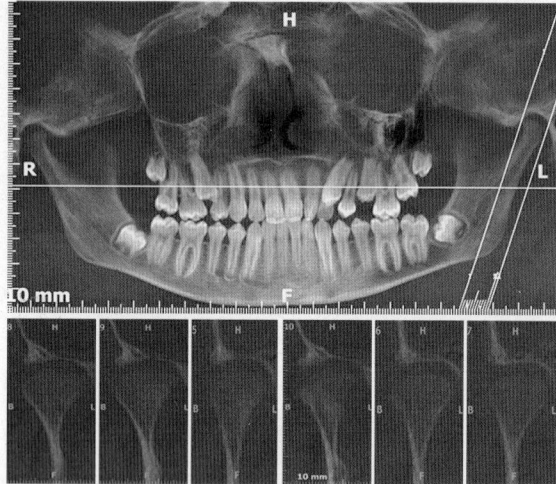

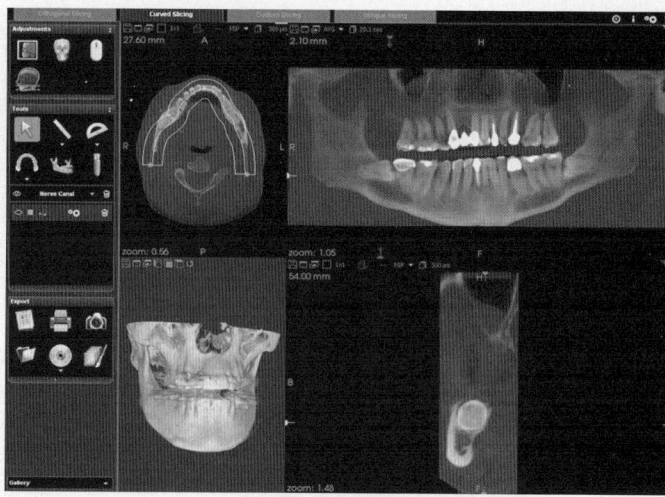

Figure 14.13 CBCT applications in TMJ assessment. Reformatted 'panoramic' image showing right and left condyles. Cropped paracoronal reformatted images clearly showing notching in surface of right condyle as compared to the left indicative of active degenerative joint disease

Figure 14.14 Curved planar reformation: This is a type of MPR accomplished by aligning the long axis of the imaging plane with a specific anatomic structure. This mode is useful in displaying the dental arch, providing familiar panorama—like thin slice images

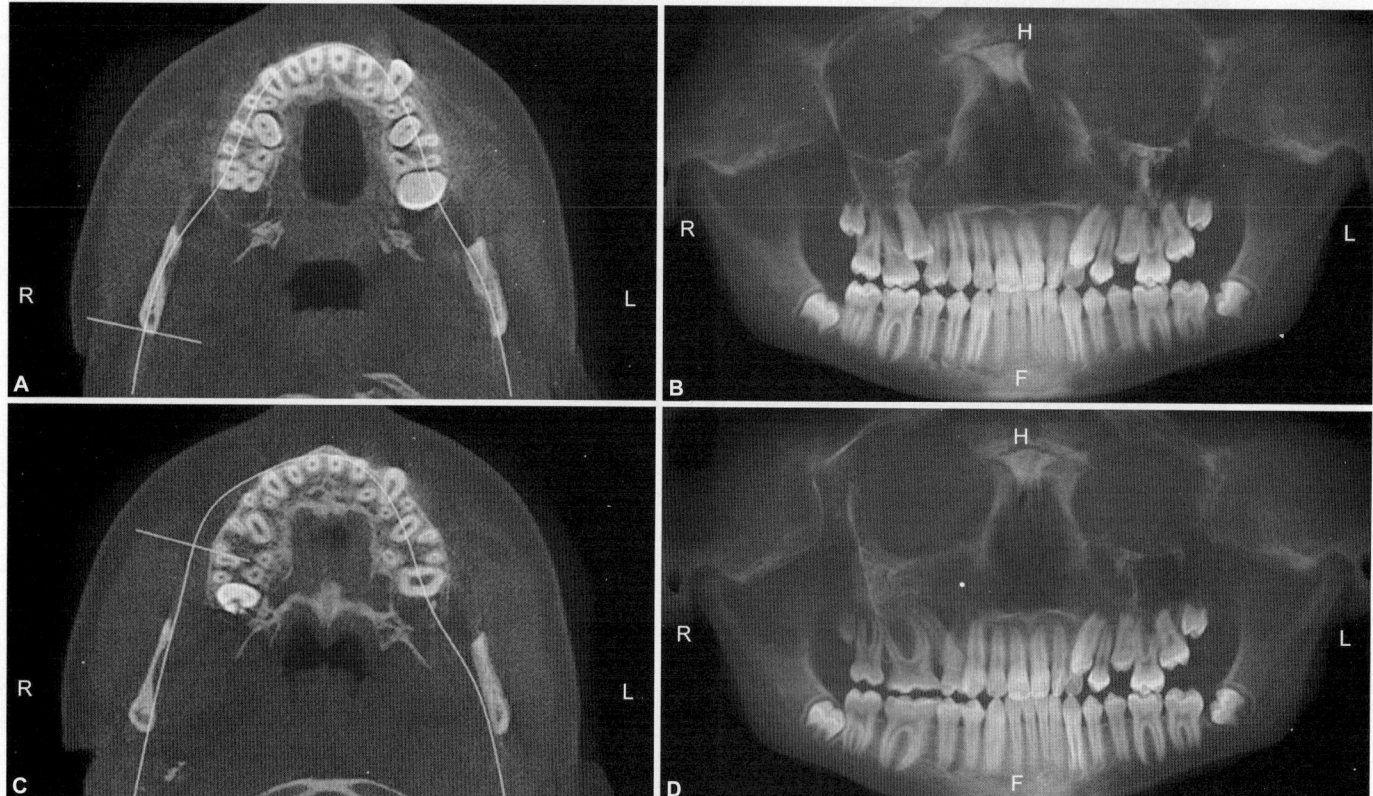

Figures 14.15A to D Curved planar reformation: (A and B) Images are undistorted so that measurements and angulations made from them have minimal error provided care is taken to trace the arch on the axial image; (C) Along the required area of pulp chambers of the teeth, when the arch is not traced correctly; (D) The image obtained may be distorted

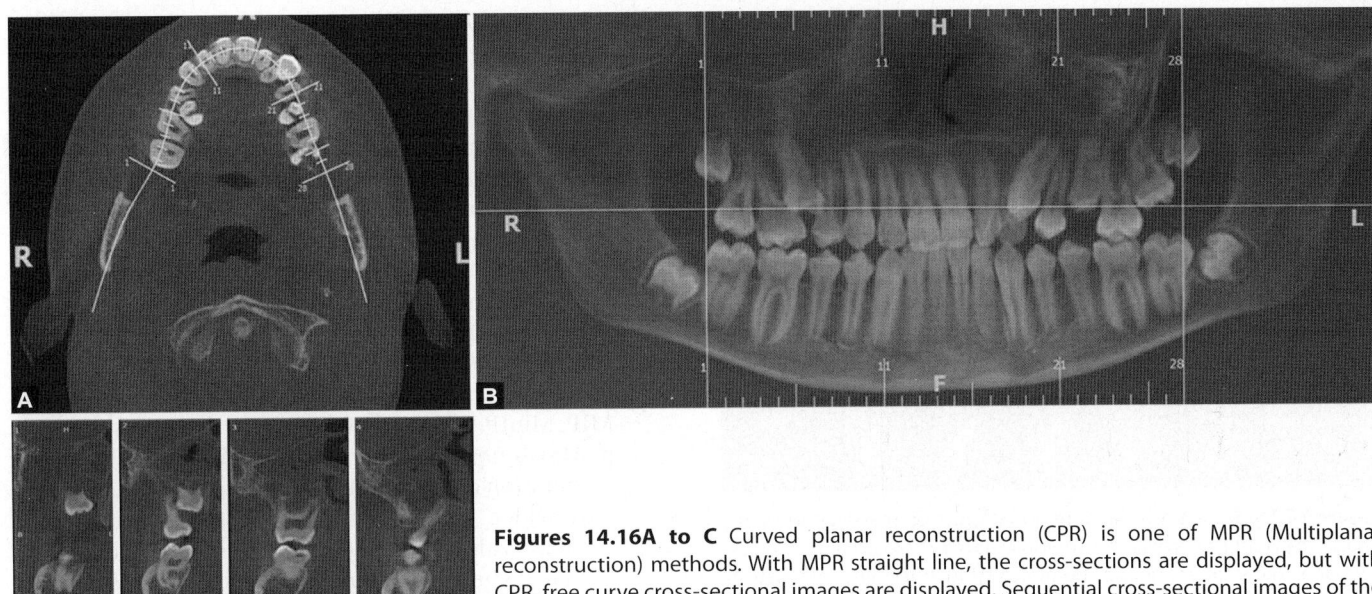

Figures 14.16A to C Curved planar reconstruction (CPR) is one of MPR (Multiplanar reconstruction) methods. With MPR straight line, the cross-sections are displayed, but with CPR, free curve cross-sectional images are displayed. Sequential cross-sectional images of the impacted tooth show the relation of the tooth with the adjacent teeth and vital structures

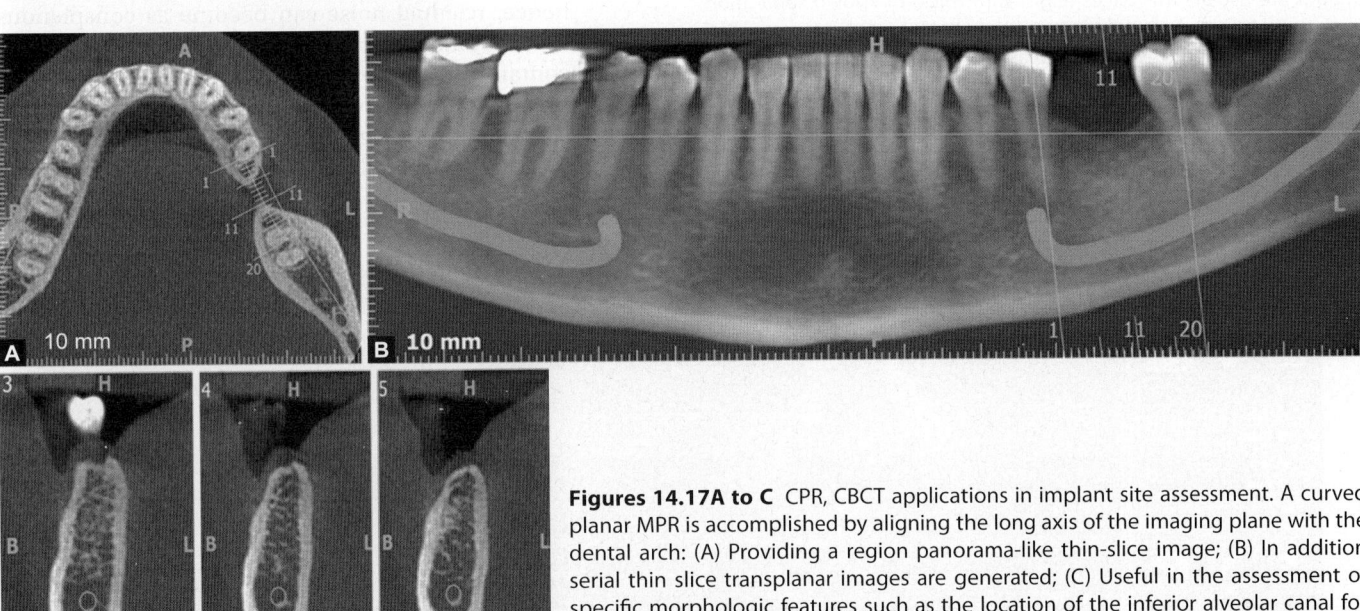

Figures 14.17A to C CPR, CBCT applications in implant site assessment. A curved planar MPR is accomplished by aligning the long axis of the imaging plane with the dental arch: (A) Providing a region panorama-like thin-slice image; (B) In addition serial thin slice transplanar images are generated; (C) Useful in the assessment of specific morphologic features such as the location of the inferior alveolar canal for implant site assessment as well as allowing measurement for the available alveolar bone height and width

coarse, grainy images with inter-patient variables of anatomy upon image quality (**Fig. 14.20**).

- The accumulation of intensity values of contiguous voxels throughout a particular slice by increasing the section thickness creates a 'slab' of the section known as a 'ray sum'. This mode can be utilized to create simulated projections such as lateral cephalometric images. These can be generated from full thickness (130–150v mm) perpendicular MPR images. These ray sum images have the advantage of being without magnification and are undistorted unlike conventional radiographs. However this technology utilizes the complete volumetric dataset and interpretation thus suffers from the problems of 'anatomic noise'—the superimposition of multiple structures.

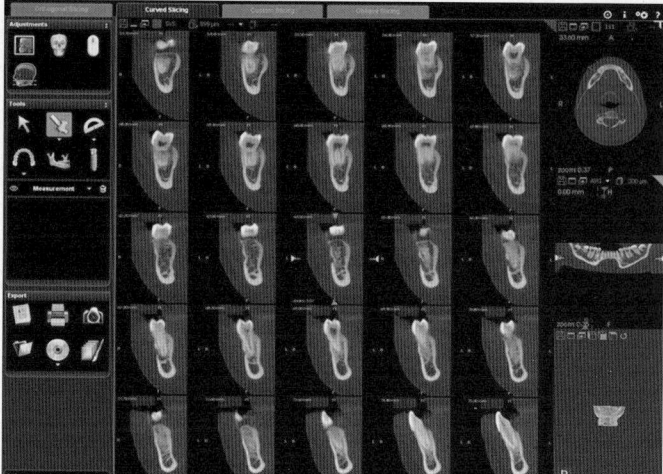

Figure 14.18 Serial transplanar reformation: Reformatted panoramic image providing reference for multiple narrow transaxial thin cross-sectional slices of mandible, demonstrating buccolingual relation. This technique produces a series of stacked sequential cross-sectional images orthogonal to the oblique or curved planar reformation. Images are usually thin slices (e.g. 1 mm thick) of known separation (e.g. 1 mm apart). Resultant images are useful in the assessment of specific morphologic features such as:

• Alveolar bone height and width for implant site assessment
• The inferior alveolar canal in relation to impacted mandibular molars
• Condylar surface and shape in the symptomatic TMJ or
• Evaluation of pathological conditions affecting the jaws

2. *Three-dimensional volume rendering*, signifies to technologies that allow the visualization of 3D data through integration of large volumes of adjacent voxels and selective display (**Figs 14.20 to 14.27**). Two specific techniques are available:

   i. *Indirect volume rendering (IVR):* It is a complicated process, requiring selecting the intensity or density of the grayscale level of the voxels to be presented within a complete data set (called segmentation). It delivers a volumetric surface reconstruction along with depth.

   ii. *Direct volume rendering (DVR):* It is however a simple process. The volume or section of image data can be visualized with different modes of display, including MIP, MinIP, SSR, and VR.

      a. *Maximum intensity projection (MIP):* It is the most common direct volume rendering technology which provides a presentation that stresses upon the areas with the highest CT values. This is displayed in a 3D image with gray scale. Voxel intensities that are below an arbitrary threshold are removed. All information is rendered at the same level of intensity hence, residual noise can become as conspicuous as anatomy. Though MIP images frequently contain 10% or less of the original data they are predominantly valuable in demonstrating the bony surface morphology of the maxillofacial region like locating the overall shape, implant area, etc.

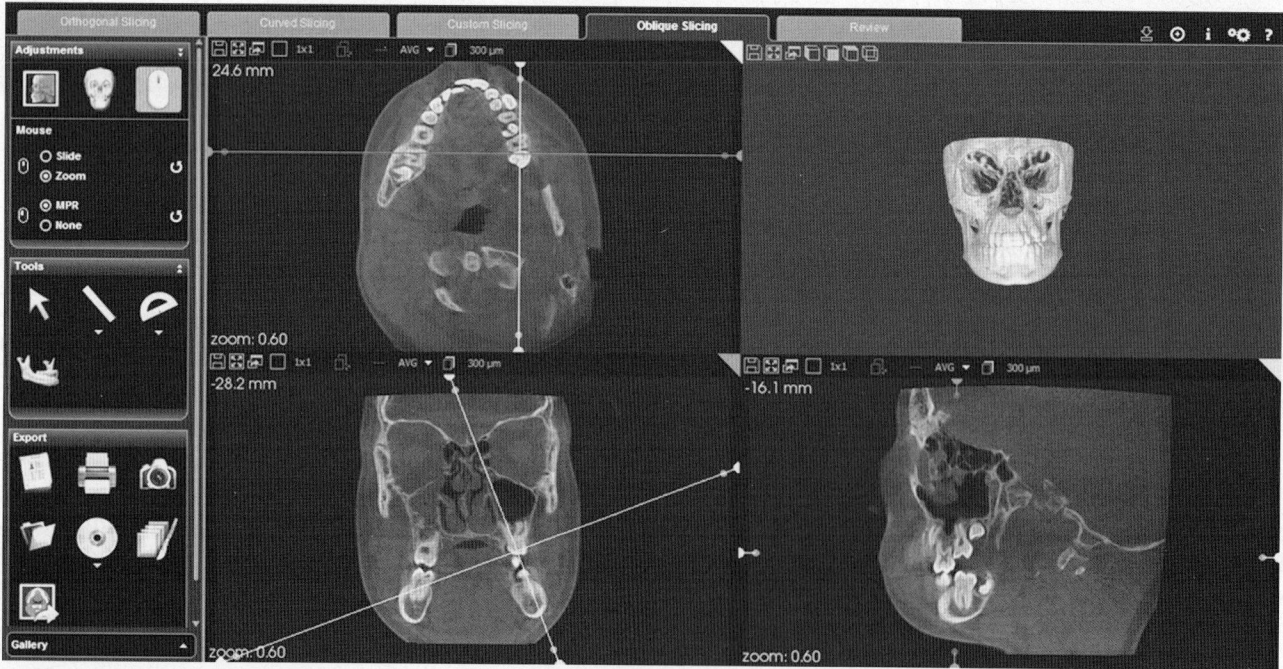

Figure 14.19 Double oblique: One of the MPR images which are sliced images cut out from any angle (direction) and may be obtained with double oblique function which is useful to make accurate diagnosis. The general single oblique fixes the cross line vertically, and hence cross-section images from the one fixed angle (direction) can be made with single oblique

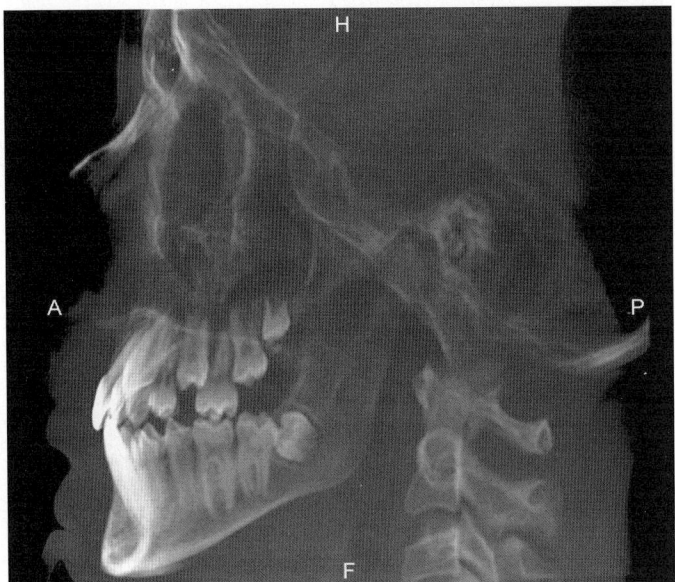

Figure 14.20 Multiplanar volume reformations: Plain projection images such as lateral cephalometric images can be created from full thickness (130–150 mm) perpendicular MPR images. These images can be exported and analyzed using third-party proprietary cephalometric software

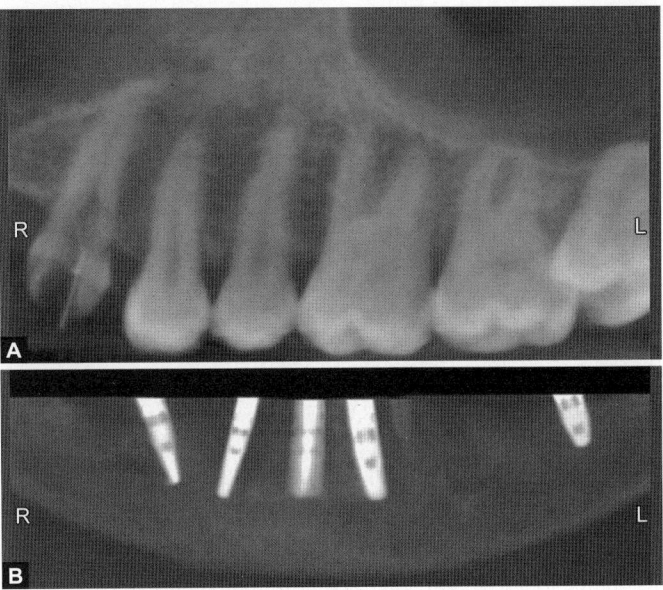

Figures 14.22A and B Maximum intensity projection (MIP): (A) 14.9 mm; (B) 20.2 mm

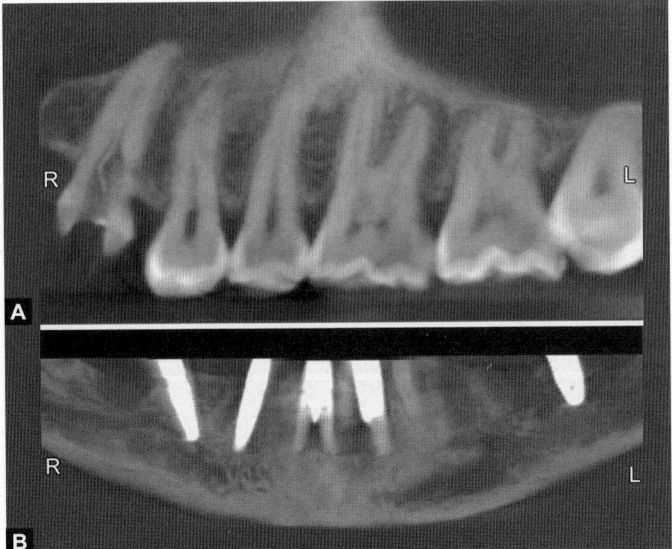

Figures 14.21A and B Ray sum or ray casting: (A) 3 mm thickness; (B) 2.2 mm

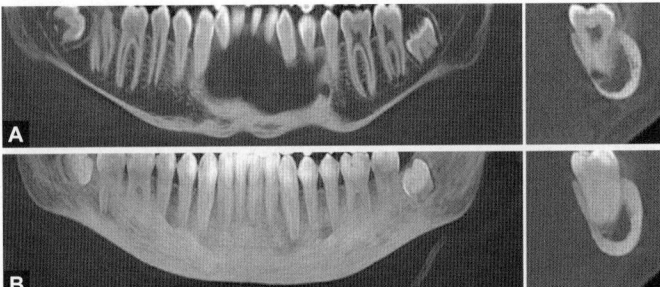

Figures 14.23A and B Panoramic and cross-sectional images in: (A) Minimum intensity projection; (B) Maximum intensity projection

    b. Techniques to overcome this intrinsic drawbacks are to decrease the thickness and/or volume which include:
-     - Limited Volume MIP
-     - Overlapping, limited volume (OLIVE) MIP.

    c. *Minimum intensity projection (Min IP)*: It delivers a display that stresses upon the areas with the lowest CT values like nerve canals and similar other lower density anatomical areas.

    d. *Shaded surface rendering (SSR)*: It is valuable for high-contrast imaging such as bone. SSR technology allows the operator to set a pixel or voxel intensity threshold that eliminates structures below the selected threshold, and renders all structures above the selected threshold. SSR generates a three-dimensional model that can be rotated as an object to be observed from any angle. When the tissue contrast is not high, then the selected threshold may not perfectly render the chosen anatomy.

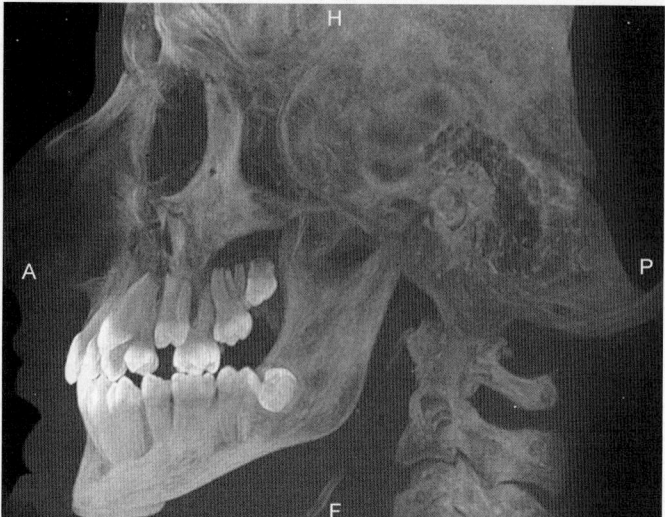

Figure 14.24 Multiplanar volume reformations: Another thickening technique is maximum intensity projection (MIP). These images are achieved by displaying only the highest voxel value within a particular thickness. This mode produces a 'pseudo' 3D structure and is particularly useful in representing the surface morphology of the maxillofacial region

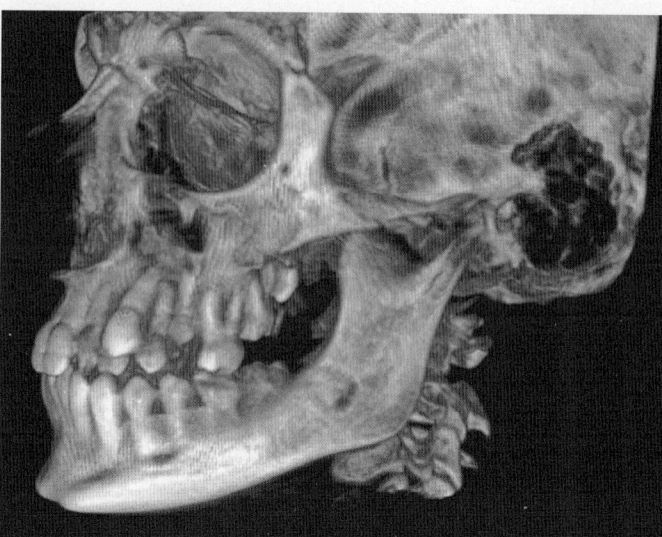

Figure 14.26 Multiplanar volume reformations: Shaded surface rendering of patient. More complicated shaded surface displays and volume rendering algorithms can be applied to the entire thickness of the volumetric data set to provide 3D reconstruction and presentation of data that can be interactively enhanced

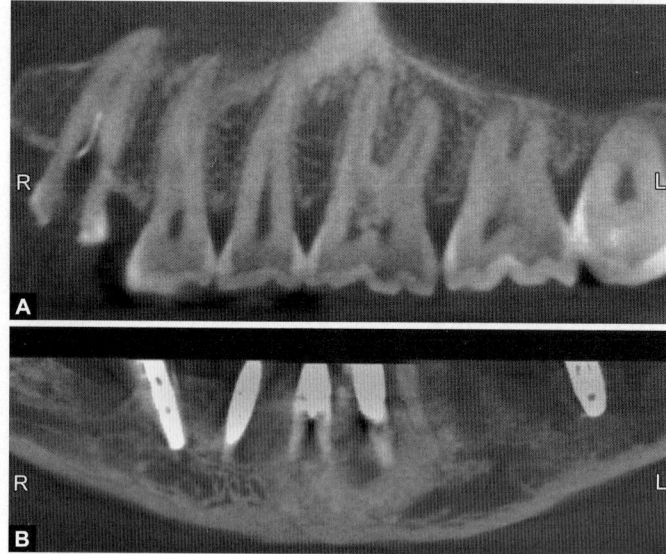

Figures 14.25A and B   Minimum intensity projection (Minimum IP): (A) 382 µm; (B) 200 µm

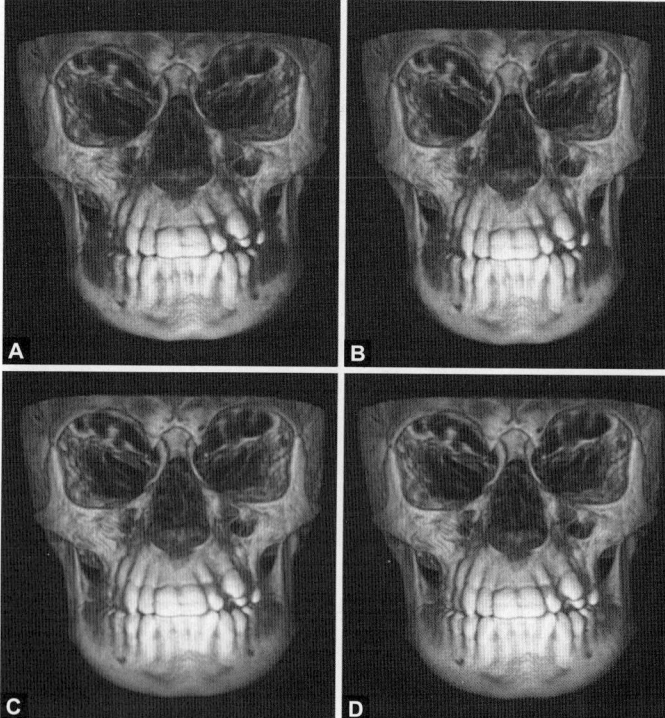

Figures 14.27A to D   VR stands for volume rendering. This is one of several types of visualization methods to render 3-dimensional pixels called voxels. VR is used to generate 3D images of the interior adding color and shadows based on the light penetration and reflection. Different degrees of VR seen in the figure

d. *Volume rendering (VR)*: It is used to create 3D images of the interior by adding color and shadows based on the light penetration and reflection. It also generates a three-dimensional model using pixel/voxel threshold for data exclusion. Basically, each voxel with a definite attenuation value (expressed in hounsfield units) will be allocated a distinct opacity value ranging from totally black (transparent) to totally white (opaque). So in place of sampling only the highest voxel value along the projection ray like in (maximum intensity projection) or only the lowest voxel value as in (minimum intensity projection) or taking the average as in (raysum projection), all of the acquired data may be used. The VR model can be rotated and the opacity levels altered, thus enabling viewing of the tissues layer by layer. VR is a good way to visually appreciate the anatomic relationships between structures, and can be used effectively for treatment planning and as a communication tool.

Advantages of CBCT

CBCT exhibits strong advantages over conventional radiographic methods, which includes controlled magnification, no superimposition, no geometric distortion, and appropriate multiplanar and 3-D displays. This technology offers improved structure visualization and diagnostic efficacy. Constant software and hardware developments allow ease and speed in data acquisition, reconstruction, and display. Commercially available cone beam scanners and third party software suppliers provide the dental practitioner a variety of options that can be tailored to their specific needs and applications (**Fig. 14.28**).

- CBCT offers a much superior alternative technology for numerous complex interpretative procedures currently used, for example, in parallax techniques [SLOB rule] for location of foreign bodies or unerupted/impacted teeth. CBCT, gives much more detail, with the added advantage of reduced exposure dose. The 3-D nature of the data

obtained permits simple and direct visualization of structures of the complex maxillofacial anatomy.

- CBCT imaging is synchronized for the craniofacial area, especially for assessing bone and dental hard tissue. In contrast to the medical CT, CBCT machines have been tailored for the head and face region, and the software has been explicitly streamlined to obtain the most suitable views using pre-determined factors. The data acquired is compatible with commercial maxillofacial imaging software's available in the market for implant planning, orthodontic analysis etc.
- X-ray beam limitation or collimation of the primary beam is used to reduce the size of the irradiated area thereby minimizing the radiation dose. Most CBCT units have the facility for the operator to select the FOV as per the region prescribed by the dental surgeon. Hence, a small FOV can be adjusted to scan small regions for specific diagnostic tasks and medium/large FOV for scanning the entire craniofacial complex.
- *Image accuracy*: CBCT units have isotropic voxel resolutions that is equal in all 3 dimensions (unlike Medical CT) representing a precise degree of X-ray absorption. The size of these voxels regulates the resolution of the image. This produces sub-millimeter resolutions (which is superior to the highest grade multislice CT) ranging from 0.4 mm to as low as 0.125 mm. Because of this characteristic, subsequent secondary (axial, coronal and sagittal) and MPR images realize a level of spatial resolution that is exact for measurement in maxillofacial applications where meticulous precision in all measurements is important for example facial growth in orthodontics analysis, implant site assessment etc.
- *Rapid scan time*: CBCT acquires all basis images in a single rotation, hence the scan time is less

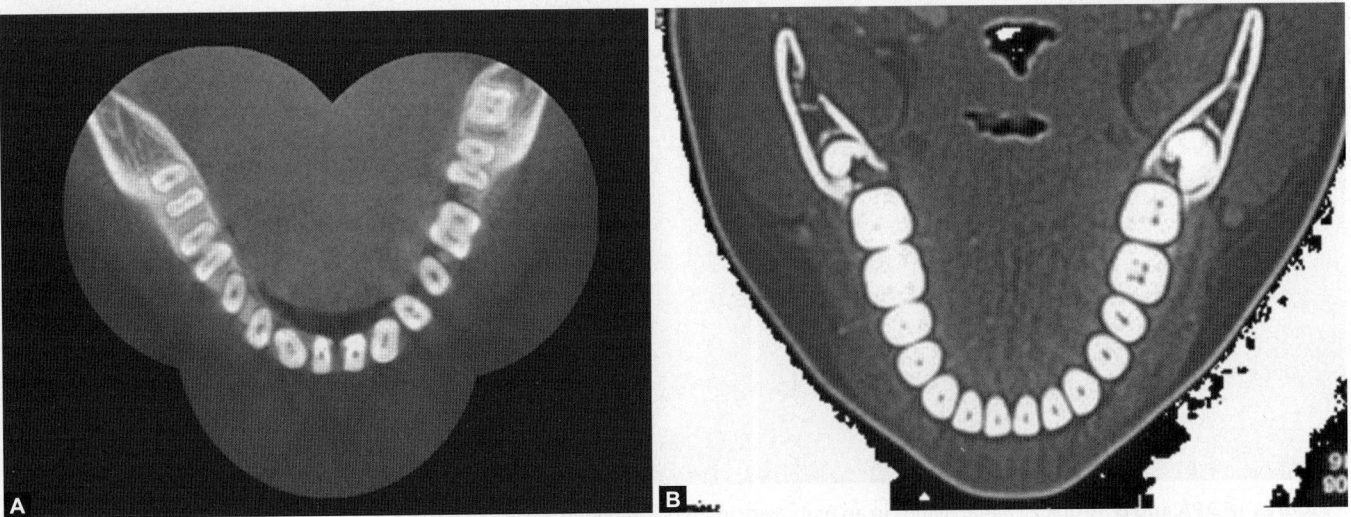

Figures 14.28A and B Details of dental structures are better appreciated on CBCT images (A) as compared to medical CT images (B)

(10–70 seconds) and subsequently motion artifacts due to subject movement are reduced. These scan times are analogous to conventional dental panoramic imaging and newer helical CT units.

Table 14.1 Comparative doses using different radiographic examinations

Sr. No.	Type of examination	Approximate effective dose in µSv
1	Digital/F speed, with rectangular collimation FMX	34.9
2	Digital/F speed, with round collimation FMX	170.7
3	Conventional single IOPA	<8.3
4	Panoramic	2.7–24.3
5	Lateral cephalometric	2.3–5.6
6	CT maxillo-mandibular	180–2100
7	CT maxilla	1400
8	Intraoral radiographs (FMX), panoramic, and lateral cephalometric radiographs	43.2–200.6
9	CBCT large FOV	260–136
10	CBCT medium FOV	166–84
11	CBCT small FOV	122–92

(Cone-Beam Computed Tomography and Radiographs in Dentistry: Aspects Related to Radiation Dose, Diego Coelho Lorenzoni,1 AnaMaria Bolognese,1 Daniela Gamba Garib,2 Fabio Ribeiro Guedes,3 and Eduardo Franzotti Sant'Anna1 International Journal of Dentistry Volume 2012, Article ID 813768, 10 pages doi:10.1155/2012/813768)

- *Dose reduction*: There is up to 98% reduction in the effective dose of radiation when compared with medical CT systems which consequently reduces the effective patient dose (**Table 14.1**).
- *Reduced image artifact*: CBCT images provide superior quality images of the oral anatomy as the secondary reconstructions are tailored for especially viewing the teeth and jaws, resulting in a low level of metal artifact as compare to the streak artifacts in CT images.
- *Interactive display modes applicable to maxillofacial imaging*: CBCT provides exclusive images representing features in 3D that conventional and digital intra oral and extra oral techniques cannot. CBCT units reconstruct the projection data to make available inter-relational images in three orthogonal planes (axial, sagittal, and coronal). Cursor-driven measurement algorithms deliver the clinician with an interactive capability for real-time dimensional assessment. Onscreen measurements offer distortion and magnification free dimensions.
- CBCT gives adequate information for dental procedures without the patient undergoing the claustrophobic CT procedure at a much reduced cost.

LIMITATIONS OF CBCT IMAGING (FIGS 14.29 TO 14.32)

The exact role of CBCT in head and neck imaging has yet to be critically evaluated. Factors limiting the usage include:

1. Cost for the equipment and imaging studies
2. Higher radiation dose as compared to conventional radiographs

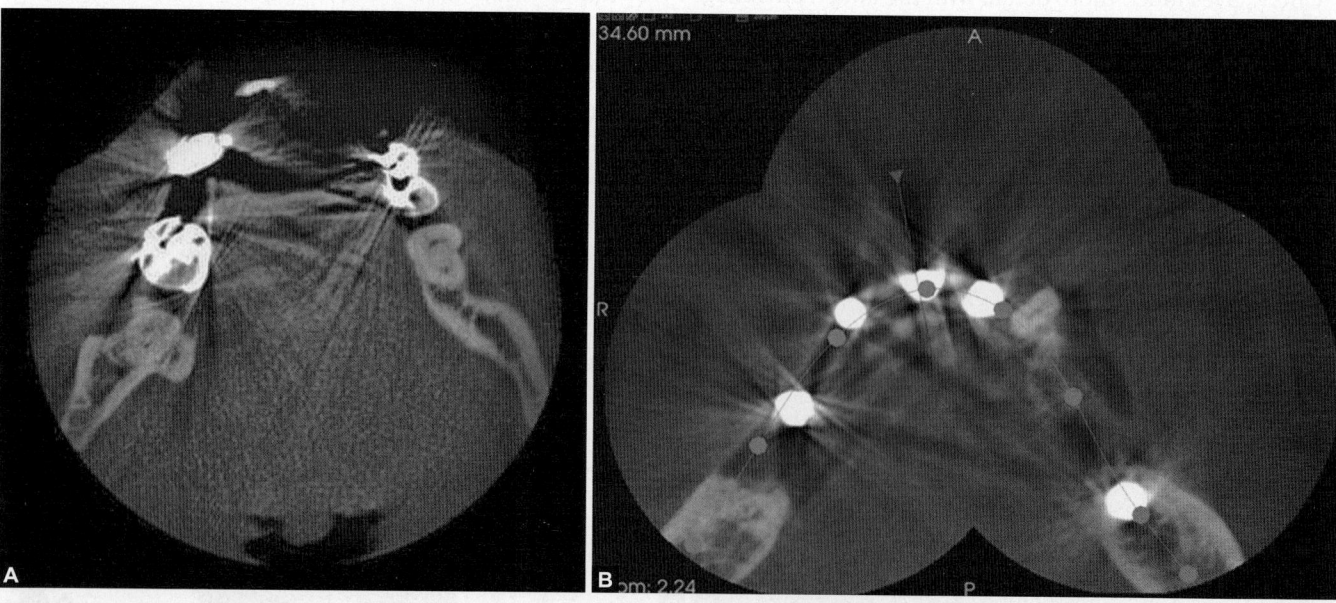

Figures 14.29A and B Artifacts: Metal fillings in an oral cavity influence X-rays in a ways that leads to streak artifacts. Streaking is less in a smaller FOV (A) as compared to a larger FOV (B)

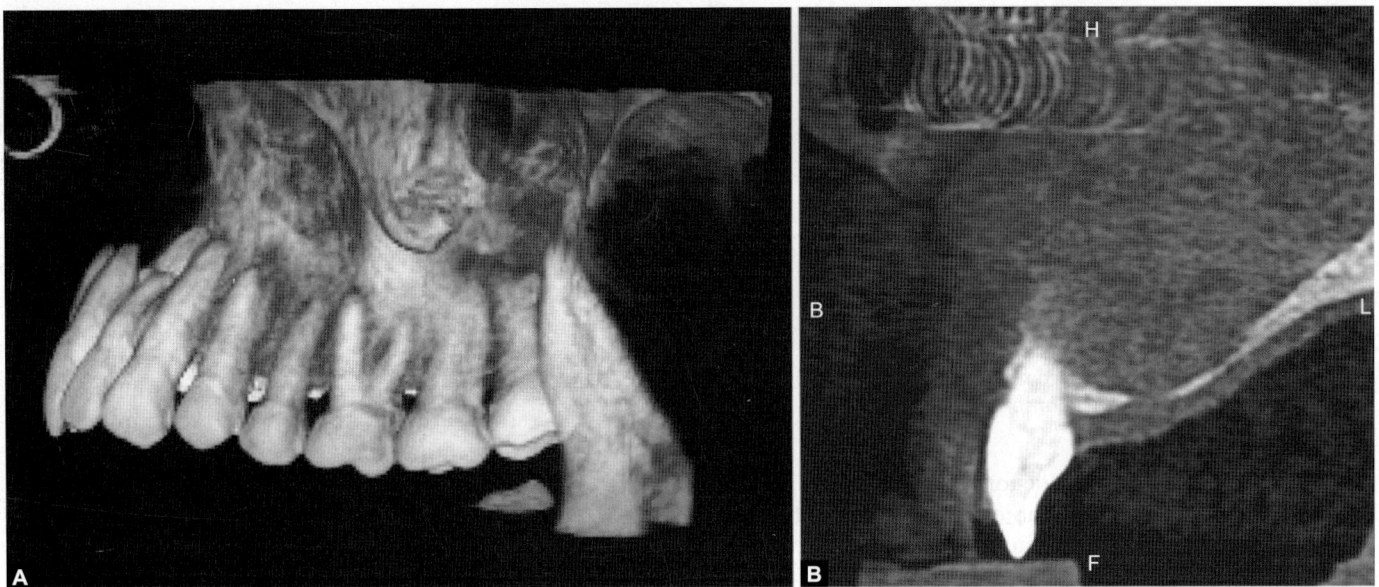

Figures 14.30A and B Nose ring causing circular ring like artifacts on the cross-sectional image

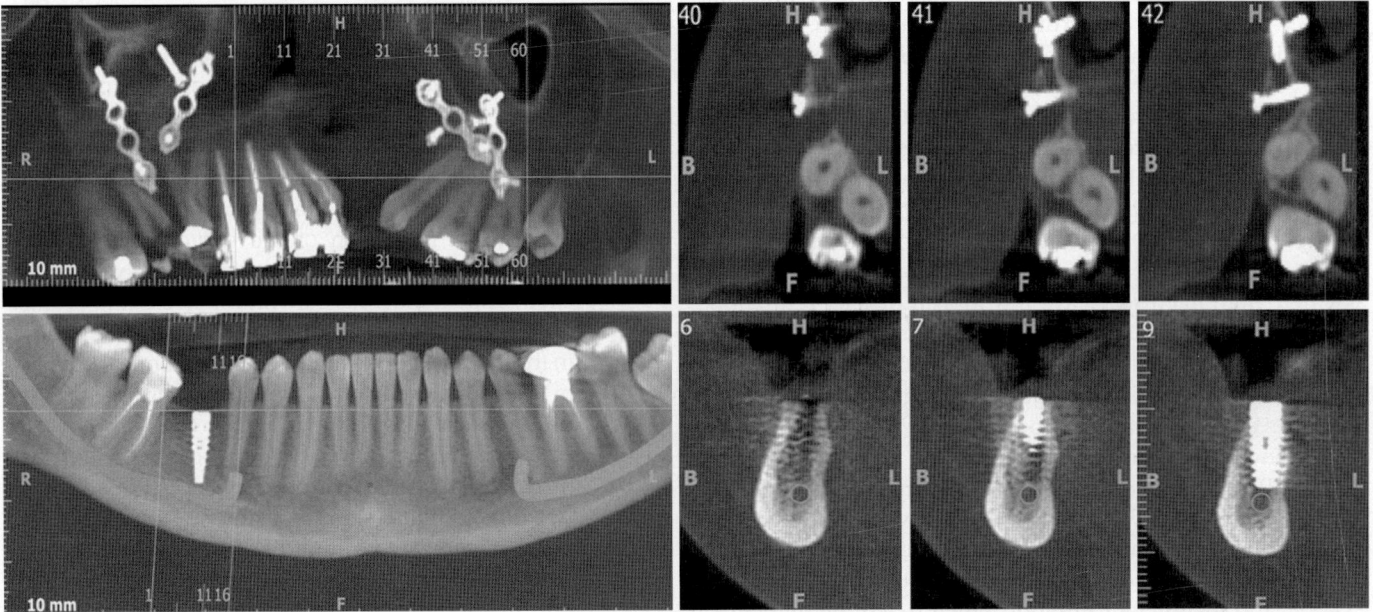

Figure 14.31 Artifacts: Distortion of metallic structures

3. Relative sophistication of operation, requires skilled and experienced personnel for interpretation of the resultant data. Especially when using a smaller FOV, as it is easy to become confused when scrolling through the images, inadequate orientation with the anatomical structures can make points of reference such as normal dental landmarks, or anomalous anatomy difficult.

4. Cone-beam technology centered on an image intensifier may create distortion of the periphery of the images.

5. Prolonged time required for image manipulation and interpretation.

6. Artifact is one of the foremost factors in corrupting the CBCT image quality and is thus a vital part in diagnostic precision.

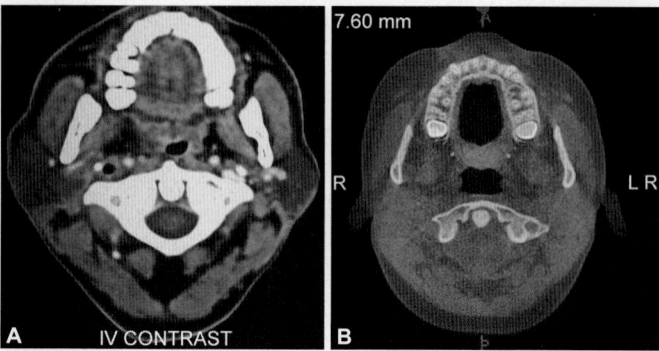

Figures 14.32A and B When compared to medical CT (A) CBCT (B) images give poor soft tissue contrast

Artifacts by definition; is any distortion or inaccuracy in the image that is disparate to the subject being studied. They are categorized according to their cause.

I. X-ray beam artifacts:
A. *Beam hardening*: CT image artifacts arise from the characteristic polychromatic nature of the projected X-ray beam which is a result of beam hardening
   i. Cupping artifact which is distortion of metallic structures due to differential absorption.
   ii. 'Streaks and dark bands' may appear between two dense objects.
   iii. It is desirable to reduce the FOV to circumvent scanning regions predisposed to beam hardening (e.g. metallic restorations, dental implants), which can be achieved by collimation, modification of patient positioning, or separation of the dental arches.

CBCT manufacturers have introduced artifact reduction technique algorithms within the reconstruction process which reduce image, noise, metal, and motion related artifacts and require fewer projection images.

However, these are computationally challenging and require increased reconstruction times.

B. *Photon starvation*: This is frequently seen in zones which highly attenuate the X-ray beam, resulting in serious streaking artifacts as the X-ray beam travels horizontally, the attenuation is maximum and insufficient photons which reach the detectors result in producing noisy projections at these tube angulations. This noise is in turn magnified by the reconstruction process causing horizontal streaking. Increasing the tube current could resolve the drawback of photon starvation but would require increased exposure to the patient.

II. *Patient based artifacts*:
A. *Motion artifacts*: Can cause unsharpness in the reconstructed image due to mis-registration of data. This unsharpness can be reduced by using a head stabilizer and a short scan time.

B. *Artifacts due to metallic objects*: The presence of metallic restorations in the FOV can cause major streaking artifacts due to extreme beam hardening or photon starvation resulting in horizontal streaks in the image and noisy projection reconstructions. This problem can be minimized by removing metallic objects and foreign bodies such as jewelry, removable artificial dentures etc. before scanning. It is important for the operator assessing and reporting regions especially for a potential implant site to be aware that the image quality adjacent to teeth having metallic and other dense materials is compromised. For example; Due to beam hardening and streak artifacts; the decalcification in teeth due to dental caries with adjacent metallic restorations and other dense prosthetic appliances are not well imaged by CBCT technology. Gutta percha may also appear as dense as amalgam and give rise to streak artifact as on a Medical CT.

III. *Scanner related artifacts*: Certain limitations and deficiencies in scanner detection or poor calibration may result in artifacts such as circular or ring-shaped defects.

IV. *Cone beam related artifacts*: The beam projection geometry of the CBCT and the image reconstruction method produce three types of cone-beam related artifacts:
   i. *Partial volume averaging*: It is a trait of conventional fan and CBCT imaging technology when the selected voxel resolution of the scan is greater than the spatial or contrast resolution of the object to be imaged. Boundaries in the ensuing image may present with a 'step' appearance. Partial volume averaging artifacts occur in regions where surfaces are rapidly changing in the Z direction (e.g. in the temporal bone). Selection of the smallest acquisition voxel may reduce the presence of these effects.
   ii. *Undersampling*: Can arise when too insufficient basis projections are delivered for the reconstruction. A reduced data sample leads to misregistration and sharp edges and noisier images where fine striations appear in the image. When resolution of minute detail is vital, undersampling artifacts need to be evaded by maintaining the number of basis projection images.
   iii. *Cone-beam effect*: It is a likely source of artifacts, particularly in the peripheral portions of the scan volume. Due to the divergence of the X-ray beam as it rotates around the patient in a horizontal plane, projection data are recorded by each detector pixel. The total amount of information for peripheral structures is condensed because the outer row detector pixels collect less attenuation, whereas more information is collected for objects projected

onto the more central detector pixels, which results in image distortion, streaking artifacts, and greater peripheral noise. This can be avoided by positioning the region of interest next to the horizontal plane of the X-ray beam and collimation of the beam to a suitable FOV.

V. *Image noise*: The cone-beam projection acquisition geometry results in a large volume being irradiated with every basis image projection. As a result, a large portion of the photons engage in interactions by way of attenuation. Most of this happens due to Compton scattering generating scattered radiation in all directions which is in turn recorded by pixels on the cone-beam area detector. This supplementary recorded X-ray attenuation, reflecting nonlinear attenuation, is known as noise. Because of the usage of an area detector, most of this nonlinear attenuation is recorded and adds to image degradation or noise.

7. Comprehensive selection criteria for utilization of CBCT technology for several dental applications have not yet been established.

8. *Viewing of lamina dura configuration or bony detail*: Both lamina dura and bony detail are best visualized on periapical radiographs compared to CBCT.

9. Cone-beam technology does not give much soft tissue detail and, although newer algorithms have been developed to improve this aspect, it cannot be compared to medical CT. This, definitely, confines the technique in the evaluation of head and neck malignancy where determining the soft tissue extent of the lesion is of paramount importance. Cancer staging will continue to be performed with conventional CT and/or MRI supplemented with newer imaging offered by CT/PET scan.

Poor soft tissue contrast: It is mainly due to three factors:
   i. Scattered radiation is a major feature in decreasing the contrast of the CBCT system.
   ii. Heel effect, produced by the divergence of the X-ray beam over the area detector. This effect creates a large variation in the incident X-ray beam on the patient and subsequent inhomogeneity in absorption, with greater signal-to-noise ratio (noise) on the cathode side of the image compared to the anode side.
   iii. Inherent flat-panel detector-based artifacts affect its linearity or response to X-radiation.

10. Dental CBCT systems do not use a standardized system for scaling the gray levels that signify the reconstructed density values which are arbitrary and do not allow for evaluation of bone quality. Hence it is demanding to infer the gray levels or relate the values resulting from different machines. CBCT systems do not appropriately display HU. [Hounsfield units (HU) are a quantitative measure of the radiolucency of different materials in a CAT scan enabling us to differentiate the relative densities of several biological structures. HU is the amount of material contrast relative to water]. The kV and mA (dosage) used in CBCT is less and hence the penetration power and the ability to resolve between different tissues is less. There is also only one sensor thus there is no internal reference in case of CBCT. These machines can only resolve bone, cartilage and tissues with similar densities and hence HU are not possible.

11. The ethical and legal ramifications regarding dentist and patient responsibilities and rights regarding pathologic findings outside the area of interest need to be discussed.

CLINICAL APPLICATIONS OF CBCT

- Implant planning and anatomical considerations (**Fig 14.33**):
  - Planning of precise implant position
  - Sinus lift procedures
  - Intra-alveolar distraction osteogenesis
  - Decreased vertical bone height
  - Decreased horizontal bone width
  - Vital anatomical structures and variations
  - Planning of templates.
- Maxillo facial surgery (**Fig. 14.34**)
  - Jaw pathology
  - The evaluation of impacted teeth, supernumerary, unerupted and their relation to vital structures
  - Alterations in the cortical and trabecular bone patterns
  - The assessment of bone grafts in analyzing and assessing paranasal sinuses
  - Obstructive sleep apnea.
- Periodontics (**Fig. 14.35**)
  - A detailed morphologic description of the bone
  - Assessing furcation involvements
  - To detect buccal and lingual defects
  - Measurements, intra-bony defects, dehiscence, fenestration defects and periodontal cysts
  - In assessing the result of regenerative periodontal therapy.
- Endodontics (**Fig. 14.36**)
  - Root morphology—shape, location, number of canals
  - Pathways of infection spread
  - Integrity of root canal filling
  - Exclude referred pain (sinus)
  - Proximal caries
  - Detecting vertical and horizontal root fracture,
  - Inflammatory root resorption,
  - External root resorption, external cervical and internal resorption,
  - Assessing root-canal fillings
  - Position of fractured instruments
  - Evaluation of teeth after trauma and in emergency situations.

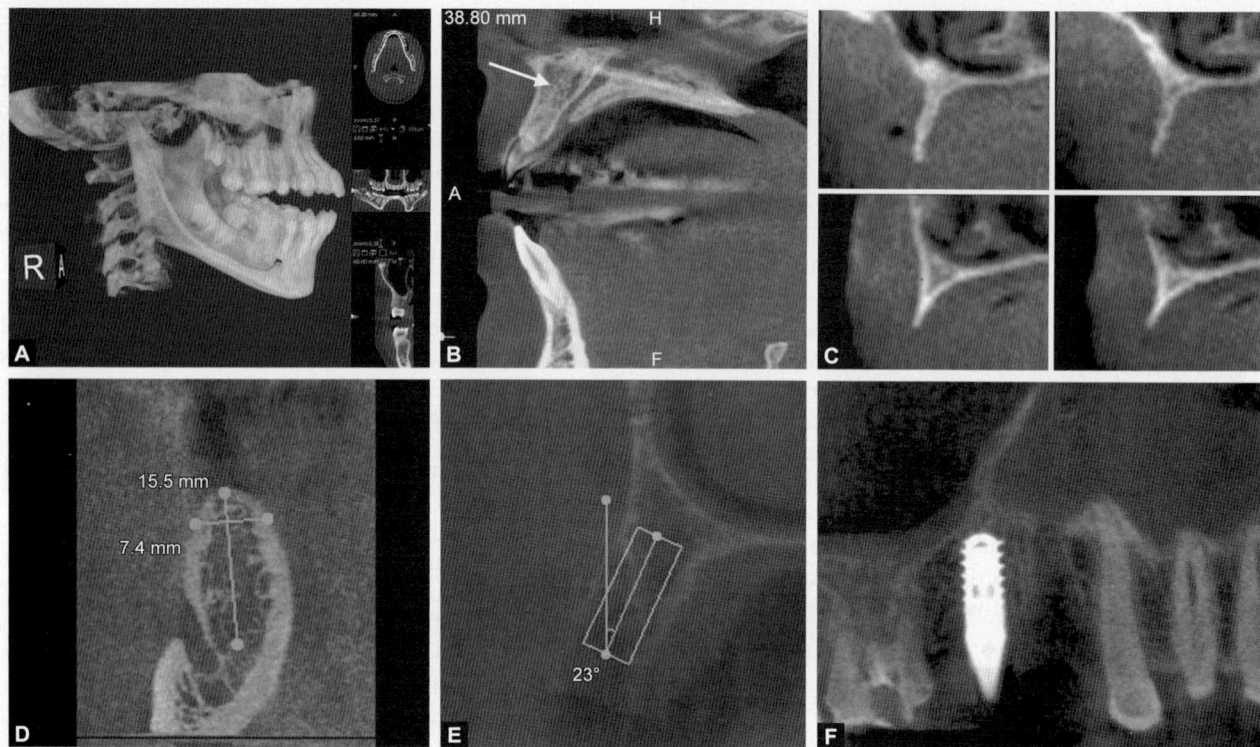

Figures 14.33A to F Implant planning and anatomical considerations: (A) Mandibular nerve tracing; (B) Nasopalatine canal; (C) Different widths of the alveolar process; (D) Precise measurements before implant placement; (E) Sagittal slice of the maxillary region which shows alignment of the planned implants in a trajectory that is consistent with the planned prosthetic buccolingual trajectories; (F) Visualization of implant placement via the simulation software

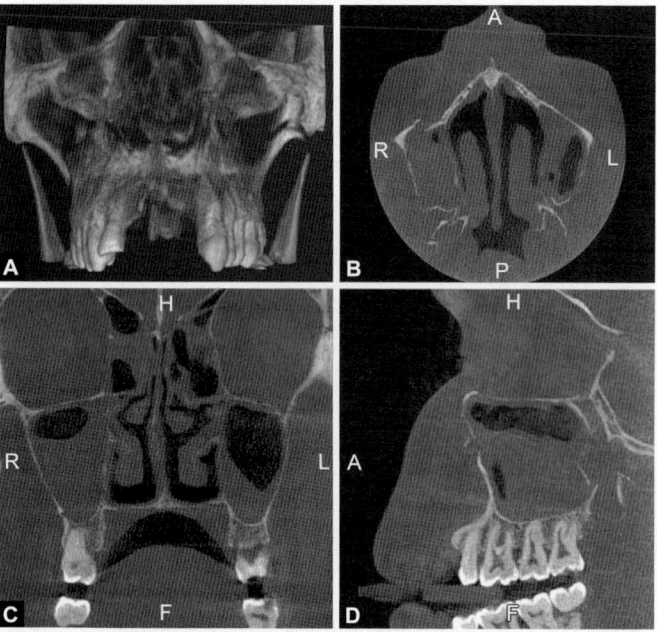

Figures 14.34A to D In maxillofacial surgery especially in cases of trauma e.g. Le Forte II fracture: (A) 3D; (B) Axial; (C) Coronal; (D) Sagittal view showing fractures of the lateral nasal wall, lateral and medial wall of the maxillary sinus and pterygoid plates

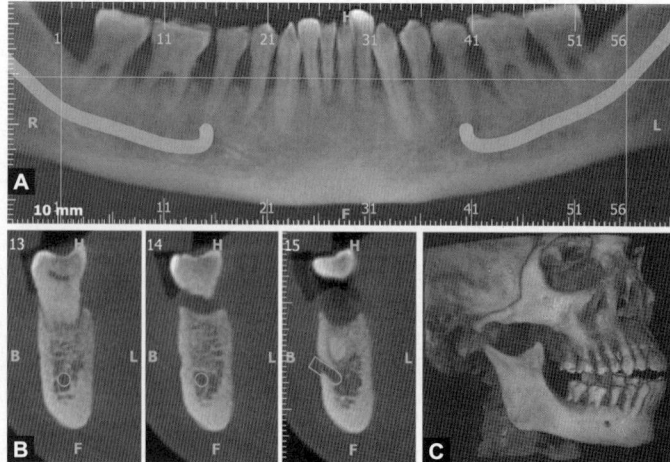

Figures 14.35A to C In periodontics, the buccolingual bone loss is better appreciated as compared to the diagnostic information available on any conventional radiograph: (A) Panoramic view; (B) Cross-sectional views; (C) 3D view

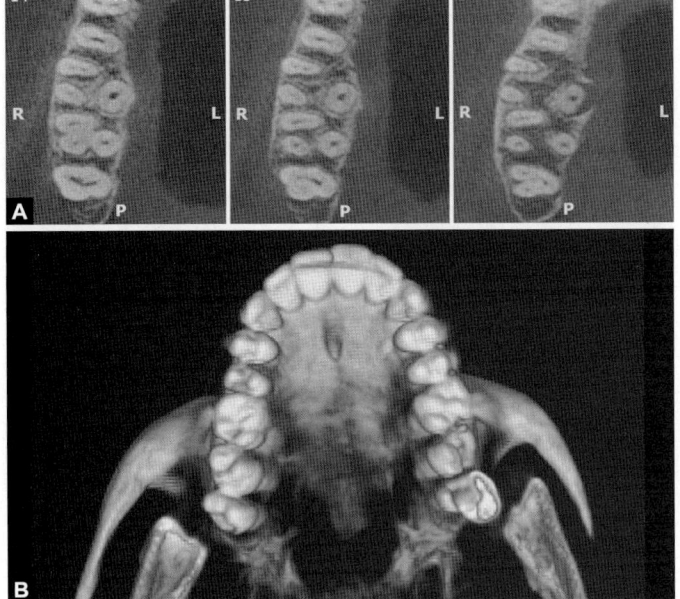

Figures 14.36A and B In endodontics is useful for locating the MB2 canals, which are inevitably superimposed and not detected on convention intraoral radiographs: (A) MB2 canal seen in the axial view at different levels of the root; (B) 3D axial view of the same patient

- Orthodontia (**Fig. 14.37**)
  - Orthodontic assessment and cephalometric analysis
  - Evaluation of maxillofacial growth, age, airway function and analysis
  - Disturbances in tooth eruption
  - Proximity to vital structures
  - Mini-screw implants
  - Developmental anomalies/asymmetries of the face and skull.
- TMJ (**Fig. 14.38**)
  - To delineate the true position of the condyle in the fossa
  - The degree of translation of the condyle in the fossa
  - Measurements of the roof of the glenoid fossa
  - In cases of maxillofacial trauma, pain, dysfunction, fibro-osseous ankylosis
  - In identifying presence of condylar cortical erosion and cysts
  - The image-guided puncture technique, can safely be performed
  - Visualize the TMJs and assess the maxillomandibular spatial relationships and occlusion.
- Oropharyngeal Volume (**Fig. 14.39**)
- Forensic Dentistry
- ENT.

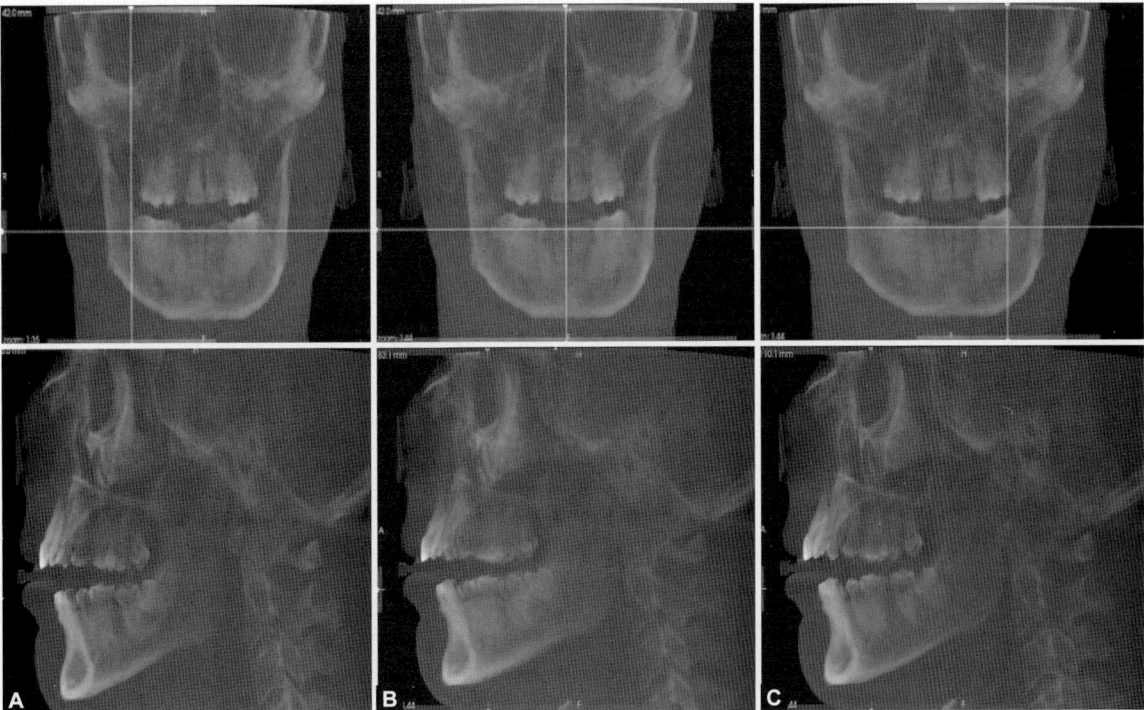

Figures 14.37A to C Orthodontia: Conventional lateral cephalogram has the limitation of overlapping of structures, using CBCT the captured image can be used to obtain lateral projections at different levels thereby reducing the inaccuracies in measurements and readings (A) Lateral cephalogram at the level of the right molar; (B) Lateral cephalogram at the midface (conventional radiograph); (C) Lateral cephalogram at the level of the left molar. The different positions of the right and left mandibular third molars may be appreciated in A and C as compared to the superimposition of the teeth in B

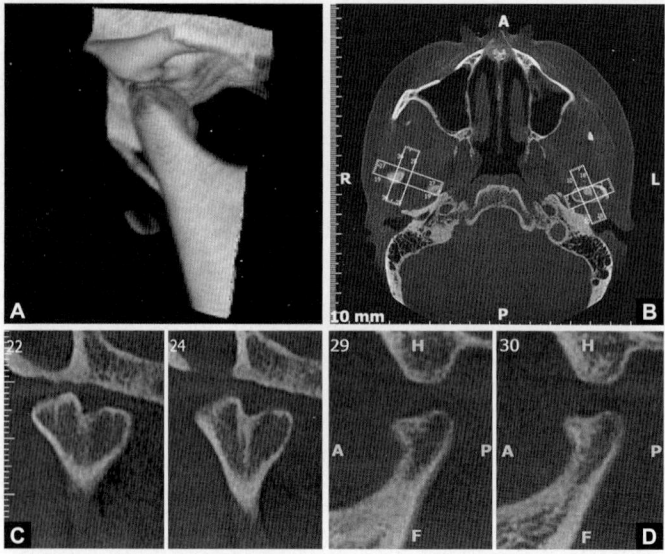

Figures 14.38A to D Study of hard tissue of the TMJ are very well appreciated on CBCT images (A) 3D view, (B) Axial view; (C) Coronal cros-sectional; (D) Sagittal cross-sectional views showing a bifid condyle

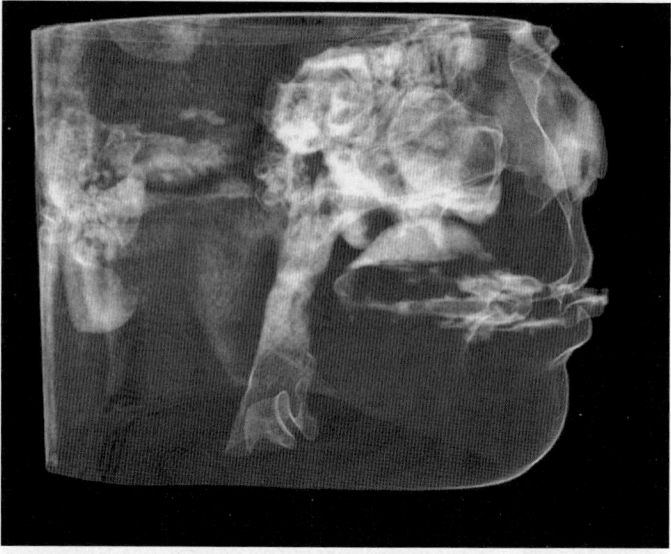

Figure 14.39 Measurement of the oropharyngeal volume using the data obtained from CBCT images with third party software is useful for diagnosis of and planning treatment for patients with sleep apnea

NORMAL LANDMARKS AS SEEN ON CBCT (FIGS 14.40 TO 14.63)

1. Anterior nasal spine
2. Coronoid process
3. Crista galli
4. Ethmoid sinus
5. Eustachian tube
6. External auditory canal
7. Foramen ovale
8. Foramen rotundum
9. Frontal bone
10. Frontal process of maxilla
11. Frontal sinus
12. Genial process of mandible
13. Glenoid fossa
14. Greater palatine canal
15. Greater palatine foramen
16. Greater wing of sphenoid bone
17. Hamulus of medial pterygoid plate
18. Hard palate
19. Hyoid bone
20. Incisive artery canal
21. Incisive canal
22. Incisive foramen
23. Inferior meatus
24. Inferior orbital fissure
25. Inferior turbinate
26. Infraorbital canal
27. Infratemporal fossa
28. Lacrimal bone
29. Lacrimal sac fossa
30. Lamina papyracea of ethmoid
31. Lateral pterygoid plate
32. Lateral recess of sphenoid sinus
33. Lesser palatine canal
34. Lingual septum
35. Mandible
36. Mandibular alveolar bone
37. Mandibular canal
38. Mandibular condyle
39. Mandibular foramen
40. Mandibular notch
41. Mandibular ramus
42. Mandibular tooth
43. Mandibular tooth 1, central incisor
44. Mandibular tooth 2, lateral incisor
45. Mandibular tooth 3, canine
46. Mandibular tooth 4, first premolar
47. Mandibular tooth 5, second premolar
48. Mandibular tooth 6, first molar
49. Mandibular tooth 7, second molar
50. Mandibular tooth 8, third molar
51. Mandibular tooth crown pulp
52. Mandibular tooth root
53. Mandibular tooth root canal
54. Mastoid process
55. Maxilla
56. Maxillary alveolar bone

57. Maxillary sinus
58. Maxillary tooth
59. Maxillary tooth I, central incisor
60. Maxillary tooth 2, lateral incisor
61. Maxillary tooth 3, canine
62. Maxillary tooth 4, first premolar
63. Maxillary tooth 5, second premolar
64. Maxillary tooth 6, first molar
65. Maxillary tooth 7, second molar
66. Maxillary tooth 8, third molar
67. Maxillary tooth crown pulp
68. Maxillary tooth root
69. Maxillary tooth root canal
70. Maxillary tuberosity
71. Medial pterygoid plate
72. Medial wall of maxillary sinus
73. Mental foramen
74. Middle meatus
75. Middle turbinate
76. Middle suture of hard palate
77. Mylohyoid line (ridge)
78. Nasal bone
79. Nasal cavity airway
80. Nasal septum
81. Nasal vestibule
82. Nasofrontal suture
83. Nasolacrimal canal
84. Nasopharynx
85. Olfactory recess
86. Orbit
87. Oropharynx
88. Palatal recess of maxillary sinus
89. Parapharyngeal space
90. Parotid gland
91. Parotid gland, accessory
92. Parotid gland, deep lobe
93. Parotid gland, superficial lobe
94. Perpendicular plate of ethmoid bone
95. Pterygoid fossa
96. Pterygoid process of sphenoid

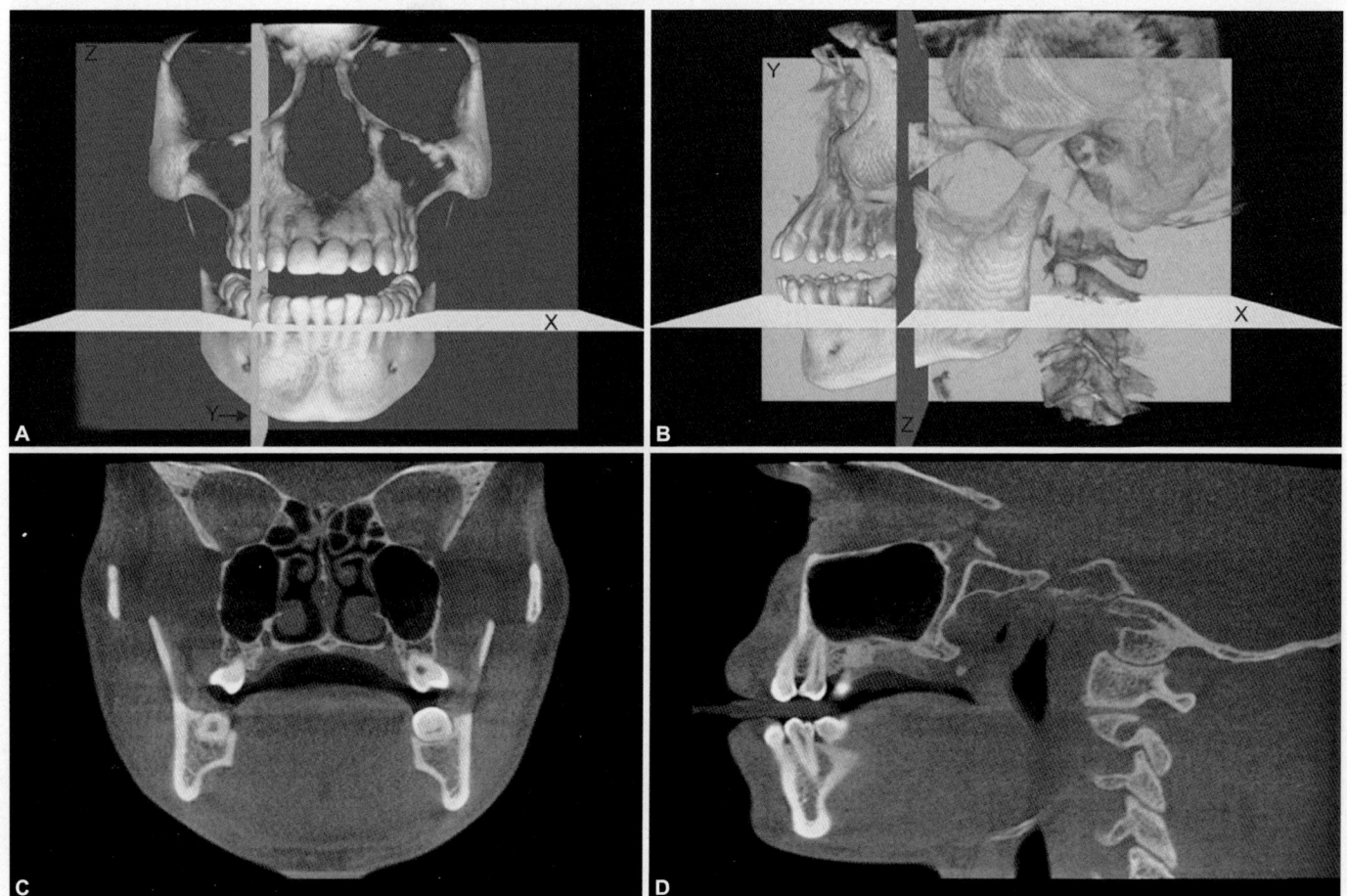

Figures 14.40A to D (A) 3D frontal view; (B) 3D lateral view showing X, Y and Z-axis (X-axis denotes axial view, Y-axis denotes sagittal view, Z-axis denotes coronal view); (C) Coronal section; (D) Sagittal section. All sections at 76 μm

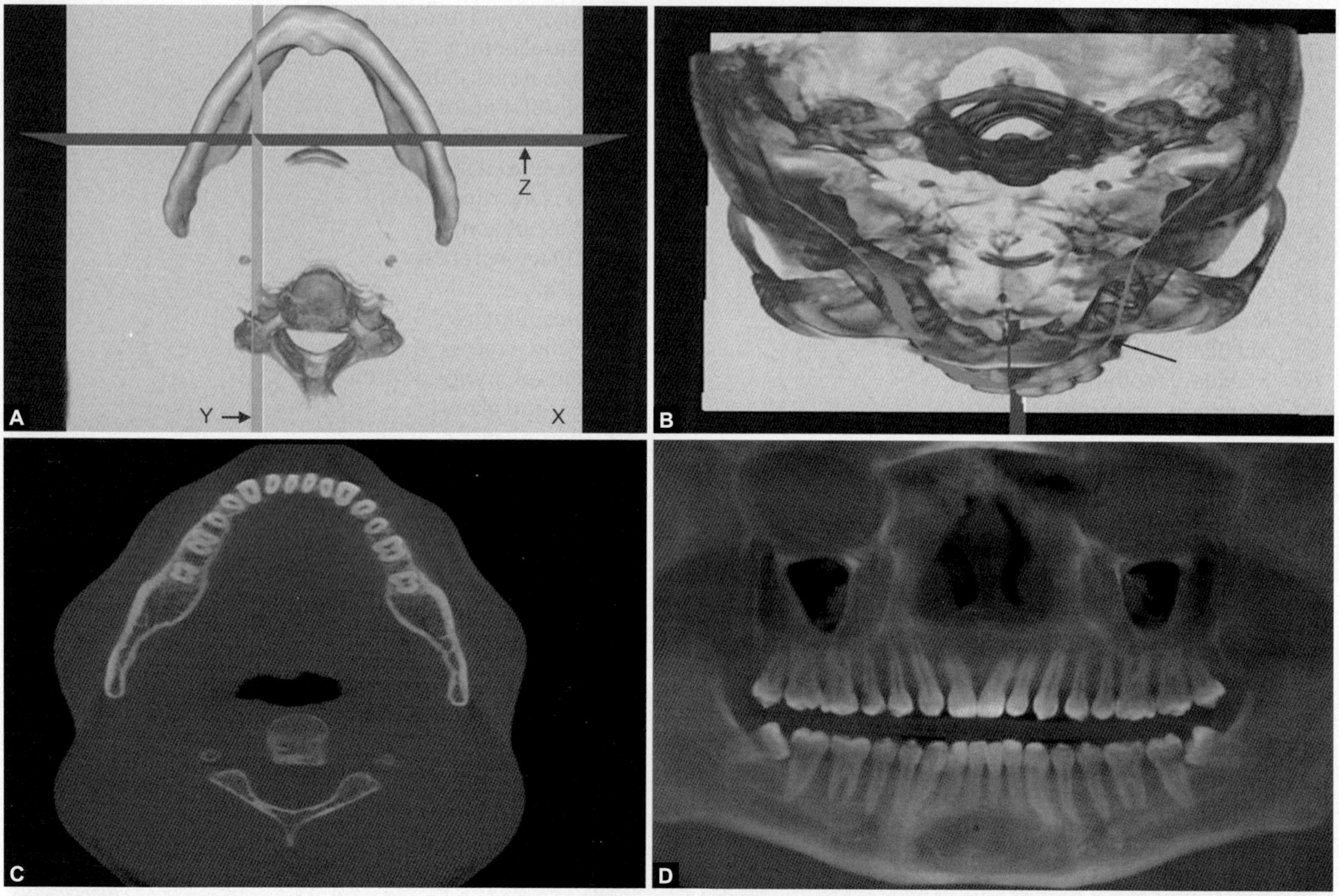

Figures 14.41A to D (A) 3D axial view showing X, Y, Z-axis. (X) axis denotes axial view, Y-axis denotes sagittal view, Z-axis denotes coronal view); (B) 3D panoramic view, arrow depicts manually created focal trough for the panoramic slice; (C) Axial section (76 μm); (D) Panoramic section (20 mm)

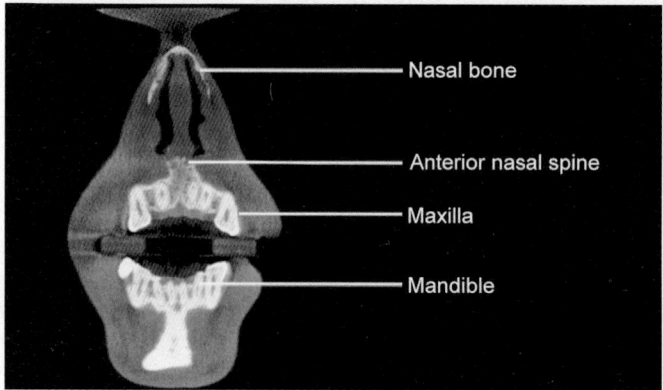

Figure 14.42 Coronal view, incisors and canine level

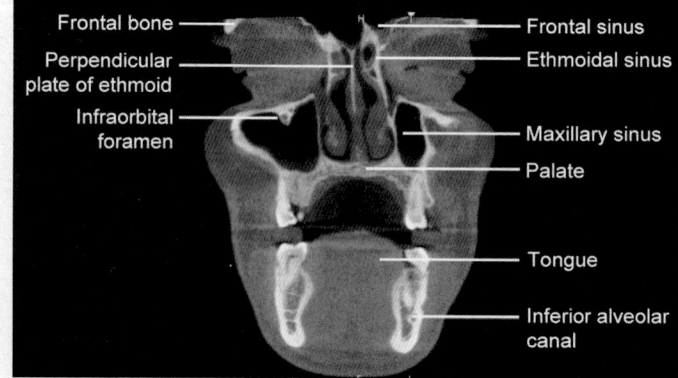

Figure 14.43 Coronal view, premolar level

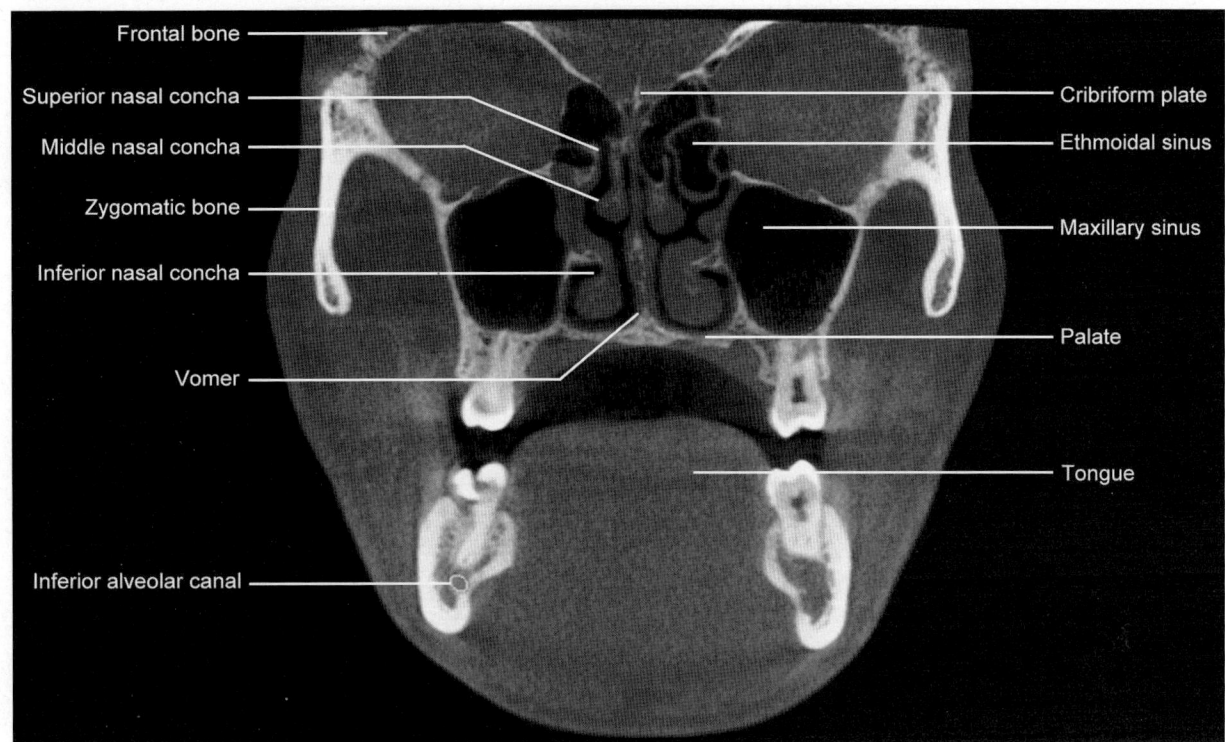

Frontal bone
Superior nasal concha
Middle nasal concha
Zygomatic bone
Inferior nasal concha
Vomer
Inferior alveolar canal

Cribriform plate
Ethmoidal sinus
Maxillary sinus
Palate
Tongue

Figure 14.44 Coronal view, molar level

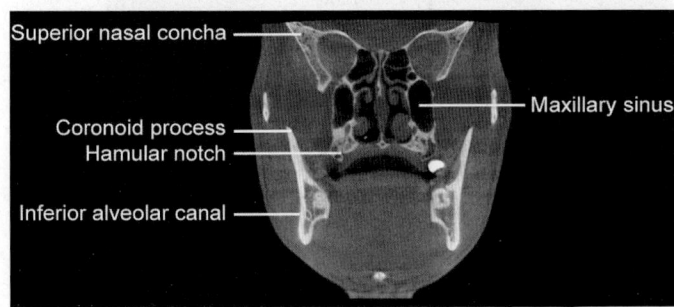

Superior nasal concha
Coronoid process
Hamular notch
Inferior alveolar canal
Maxillary sinus

Figure 14.45 Coronal view, coronoid process level

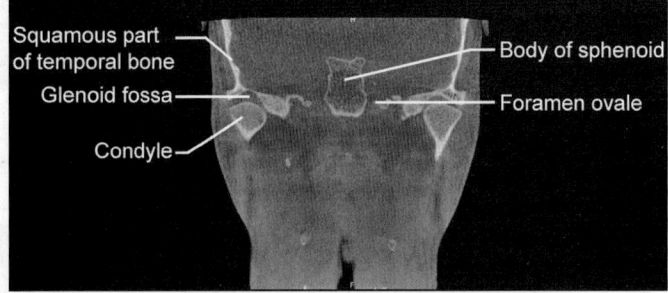

Squamous part of temporal bone
Glenoid fossa
Condyle
Body of sphenoid
Foramen ovale

Figure 14.47 Coronal view, condyle level

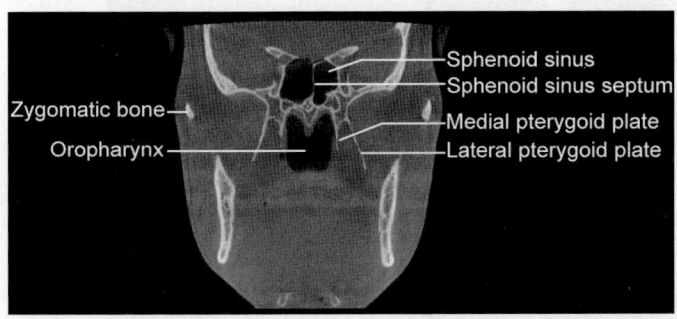

Zygomatic bone
Oropharynx
Sphenoid sinus
Sphenoid sinus septum
Medial pterygoid plate
Lateral pterygoid plate

Figure 14.46 Coronal view, mid ramus level

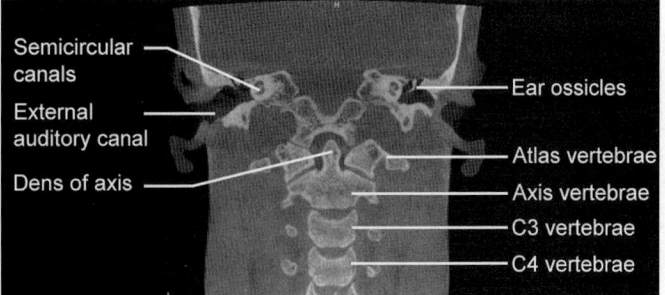

Semicircular canals
External auditory canal
Dens of axis
Ear ossicles
Atlas vertebrae
Axis vertebrae
C3 vertebrae
C4 vertebrae

Figure 14.48 Coronal view, vertebrae level

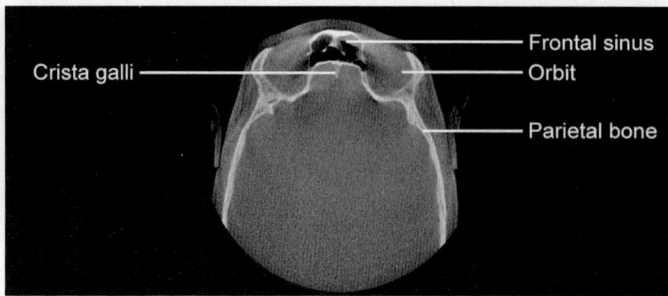

Figure 14.49 Axial view, frontal sinus level

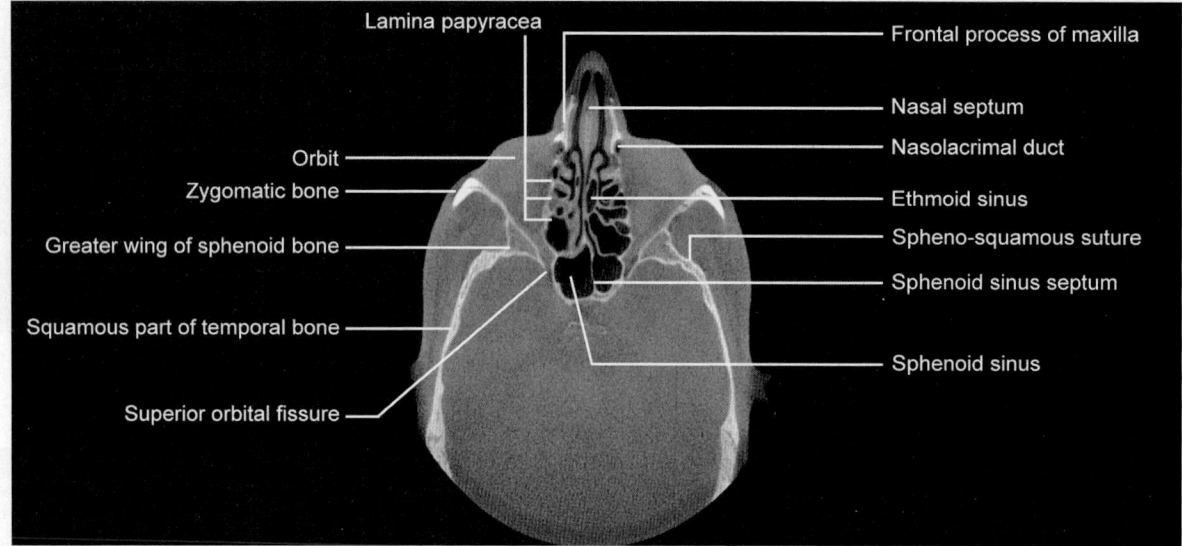

Figure 14.50 Axial view, mid orbital level

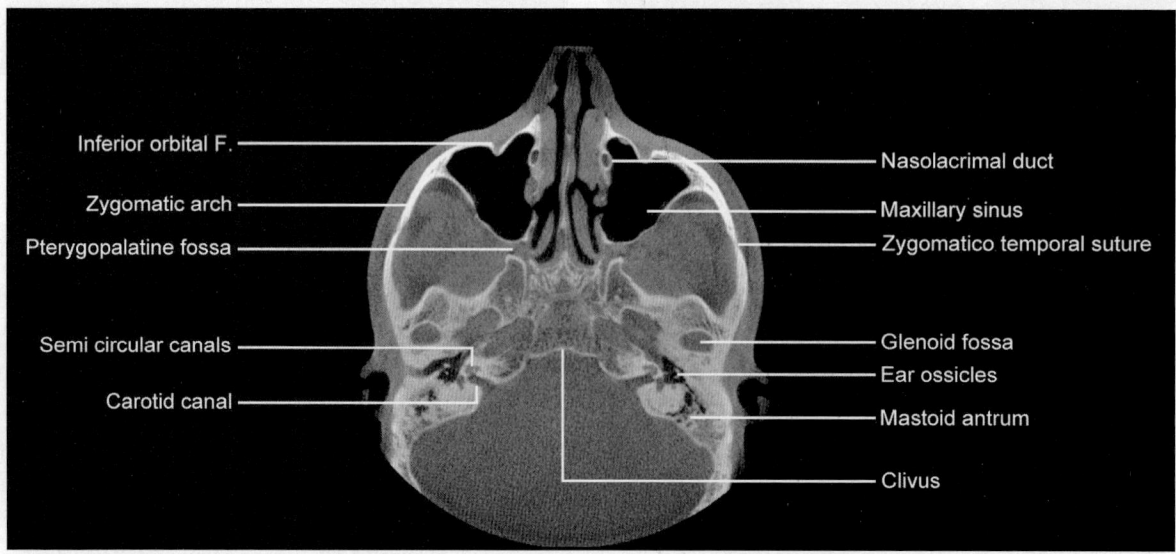

Figure 14.51 Axial view, inferior orbital foramen level

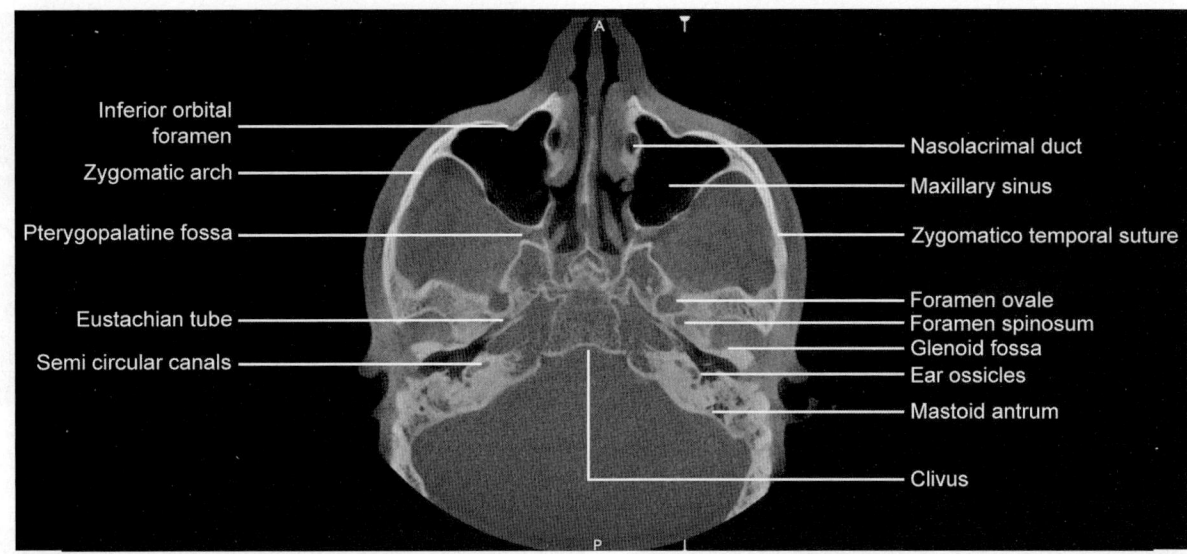

Figure 14.52 Axial view, below inferior orbital foramen level

Inferior orbital foramen
Zygomatic arch
Pterygopalatine fossa
Eustachian tube
Semi circular canals

Nasolacrimal duct
Maxillary sinus
Zygomatico temporal suture
Foramen ovale
Foramen spinosum
Glenoid fossa
Ear ossicles
Mastoid antrum
Clivus

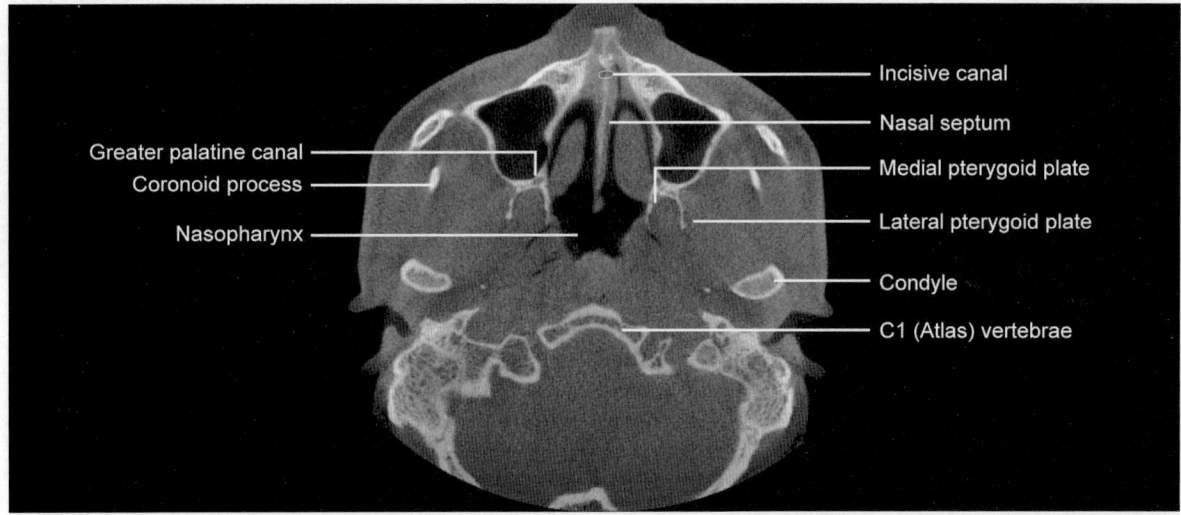

Figure 14.53 Axial view, maxillary sinus level

Greater palatine canal
Coronoid process
Nasopharynx

Incisive canal
Nasal septum
Medial pterygoid plate
Lateral pterygoid plate
Condyle
C1 (Atlas) vertebrae

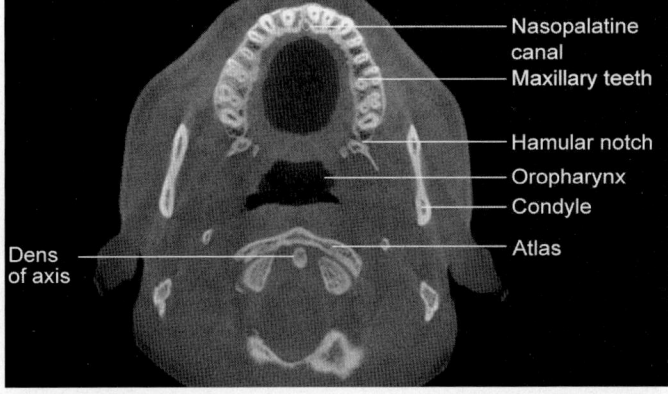

Nasopalatine canal
Maxillary teeth
Hamular notch
Oropharynx
Condyle
Atlas
Dens of axis

Figure 14.54 Axial view, maxillary dentition level

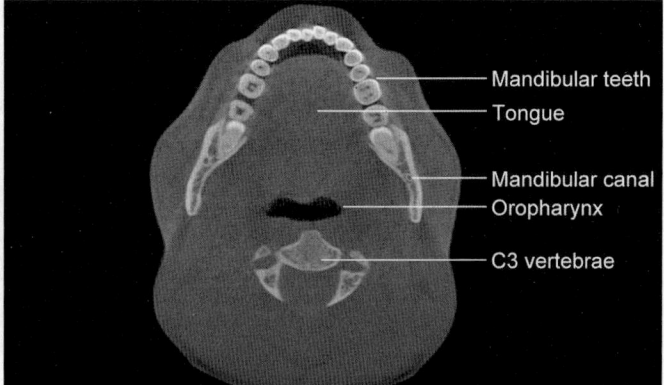

Mandibular teeth
Tongue
Mandibular canal
Oropharynx
C3 vertebrae

Figure 14.55 Axial view, mandibular dentition level

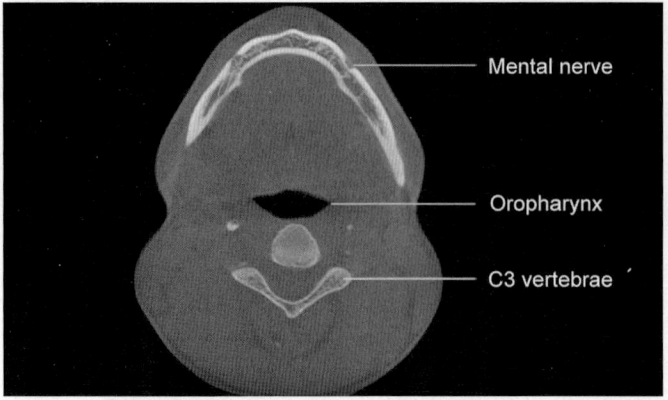

Figure 14.56 Axial view, mental foramen level

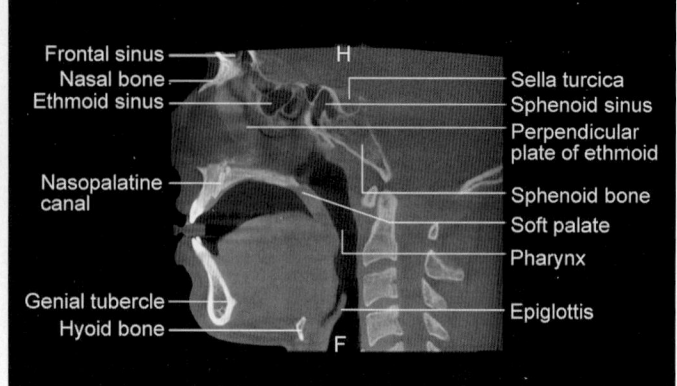

Figure 14.58 Sagittal view, mid sagittal plane level

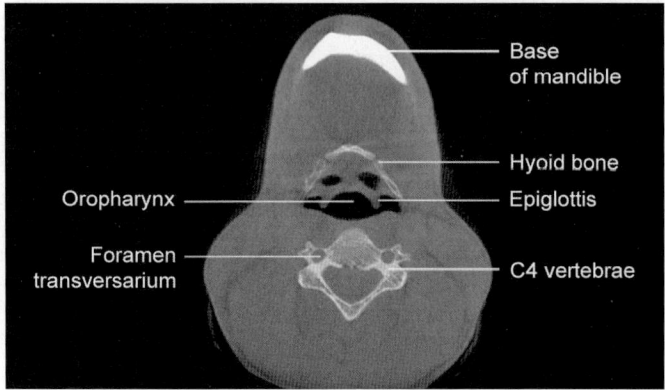

Figure 14.57 Axial view, floor of mandible level

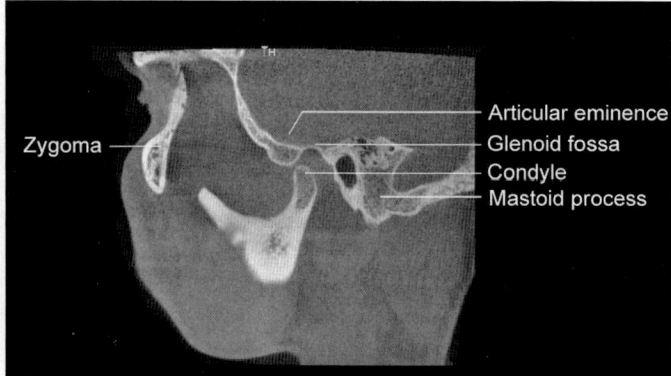

Figure 14.59 Sagittal view at the condyle level

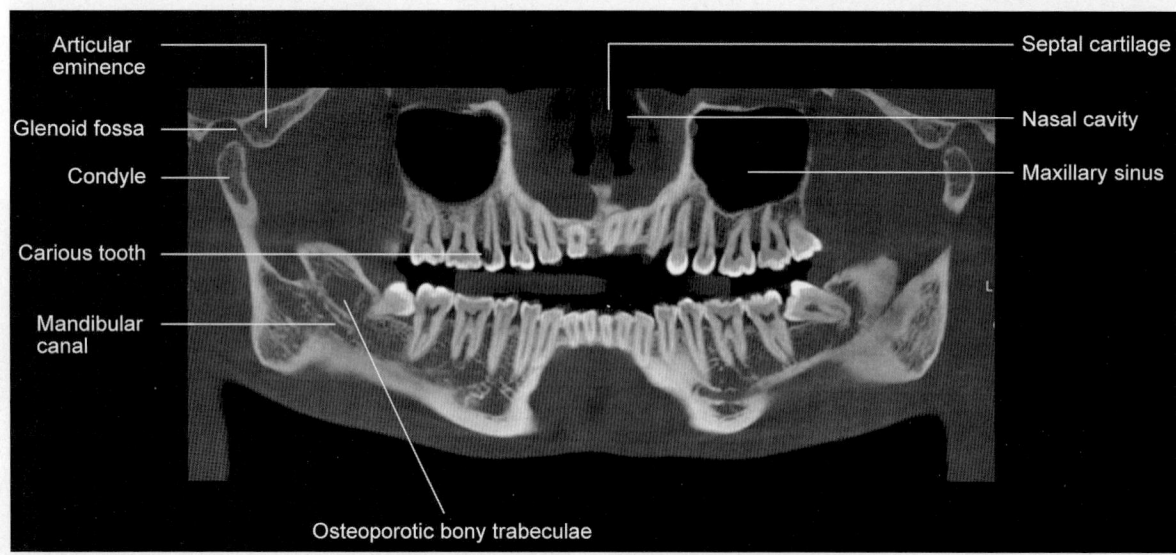

Figure 14.60 Panoramic view, thickness 0.3 mm

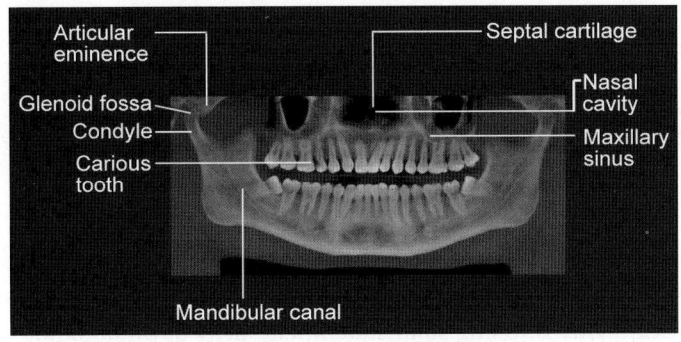

Figure 14.61 Panoramic view

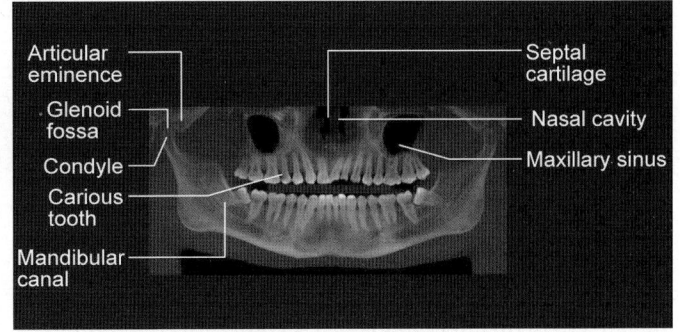

Figure 14.62 Panoramic view

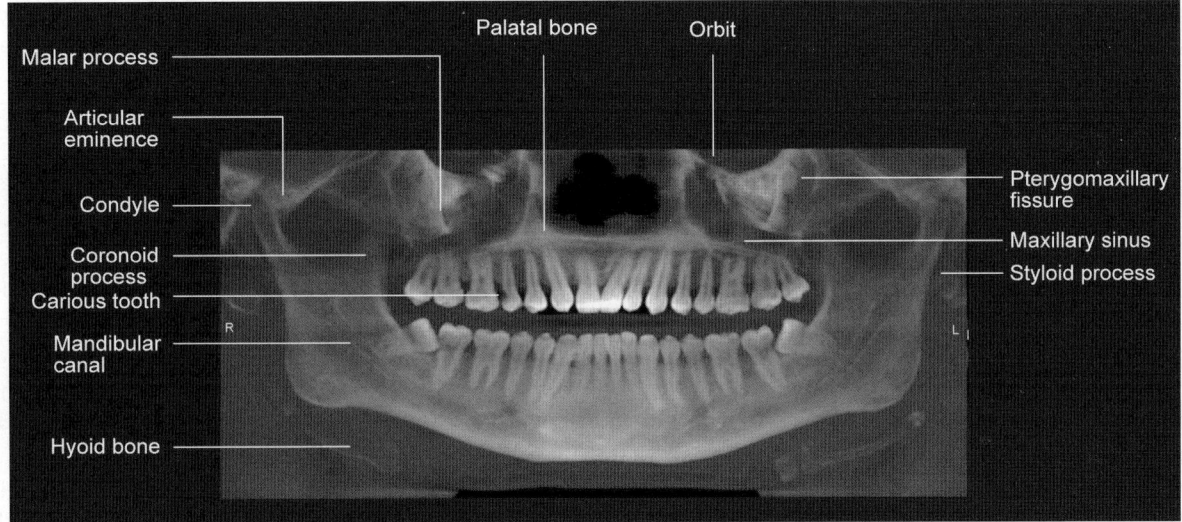

Figure 14.63 Panoramic view, thickness 50.0 mm

97. Pterygomandibular space
98. Pterygopalatine fossa
99. Retromolartrigone
100. Sphenoid bone
101. Sphenoid sinus
102. Sphenoid sinus septum
103. Sphenozygomatic suture

104. Styloid process
105. Sublingual space
106. Submandibular space
107. Submental space
108. Superior turbinate
109. Torus tubarius

Digital Radiography | 15

The advent of digital imaging has revolutionized radiology.

The term digital radiography refers to a method of capturing a radiographic image using a sensor, breaking it into electronic pieces and presenting and storing the image using a computer. This system is not limited to intraoral images; panoramic and cephalometric images may also be obtained.

RADIATION EXPOSURE

Digital imaging requires less X-radiation than conventional radiography, because the sensor is more sensitive to X-rays than a conventional film. Exposure time for digital radiography is 50–80 percent less than that required for conventional radiography using E-speed film, and thus the absorbed dose to the patient is much lower.

METHODS TO OBTAIN AN INTRAORAL DIGITAL IMAGE

- *Direct digital imaging*: Here a sensor is placed in the patient's mouth and exposed to radiation. The sensor captures the radiographic image and then transmits the image to a computer monitor, and within seconds the image appears on the computer screen.
- *Indirect digital imaging*: In this method an existing X-ray film is digitized using a CCD camera, which scans the image, digitizes or converts the image and then displays it on the computer monitor.
- *Storage phosphor imaging*: It is a wireless digital radiography system. A reusable imaging plate coated with phosphors is used. These plates are flexible and fit into the mouth. The storage phosphor imaging records diagnostic data on the plates following exposure to the X-ray source and uses a high-speed scanner to convert the information to electronic files which can be displayed on the computer screen.

METHODS TO OBTAIN AN EXTRAORAL DIGITAL IMAGE

PSP based radiography: It is applied to CR (Computed Radiography) system and has been used for extraoral projections and image analysis including dental panaromic radiography.

CCD systems: Using solid state linear array of photoiodides (DR system) (**Fig. 15.1**).

Extraoral digital imaging is available using both systems. However the larger CCD sensors are extremely expensive and usually requires the purchase of new X-ray generators, although a 'retro-fit' system has been developed. These constrictions effectively mean that the PSP method is the most commonly used.

EQUIPMENT

The essential components of a direct imaging system include:
- X-radiation source
- Sensor
- Digital image display.

X-RADIATION SOURCE

Most digital radiography systems use a conventional X-ray unit as the radiation source. The X-ray unit timer has to be adapted to allow exposures in a time frame of 1/100th of a second. A standard X-ray unit that is adapted for digital radiography can still be functional for conventional radiography.

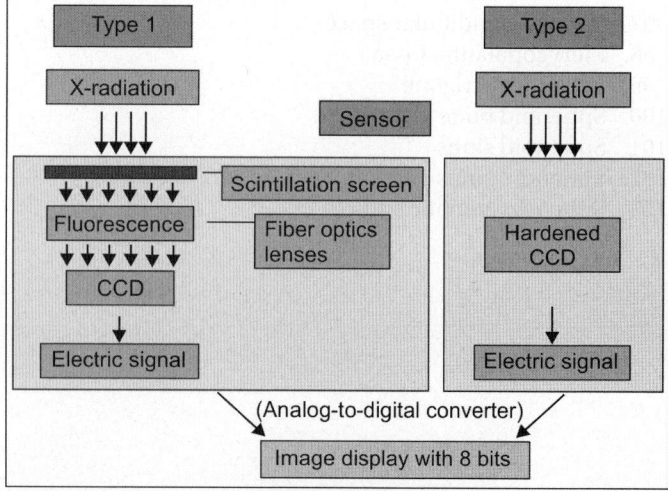

Figure 15.1 Scheme of direct digital image acquisition using two types of CCD-based systems

SENSOR

- *Extraoral*: PSP plates
- *Intraoral*: Intraoral sensor is used instead of the intraoral film. It is a small detector that is placed in the mouth of the patient and used to capture the radiographic image.

DIGITAL DETECTOR CHARACTERISTICS (TABLE 15.1)

- *Contrast resolution*: It is the ability to distinguish different densities in a radiographic image. This is the function of the interaction of the attenuation characteristics of the tissues that are being imaged, the capacity of the image receptors to distinguish differences in the numbers of X-ray photons coming from different areas of the subject, the ability of the computer to display or other output to portray differences in density, and the ability of the observer to recognize those differences.
- *Spatial resolution*: It is the capacity for distinguishing fine detail. The theoretical limit of resolution is a function of picture element (pixel) size for the digital imaging systems. Resolution is often measured and reported in units of line pairs per millimeter. A line and its associated space are called a line pair (lp). At least two pixels are required to resolve a line pair, one for the line and one for the space.
- *Detector latitude*: The ability of an imaging receptor to capture a range of X-ray exposures is termed latitude. The latitude of CCD and CMOS detectors is similar to film and can be extended with digital enhancement of contrast and brightness. Photostimulable phosphor receptors enjoy larger latitudes and have a linear response to five orders of magnitude of X-ray exposure.
- *Detector sensitivity*: It is the ability to respond to small amounts of radiation. Useful sensitivity of digital receptors is affected by a number of factors including detector efficiency, pixel size and system noise. High resolution CCD and CMOS systems achieve less dose reduction than lower resolution PSP systems.

The different type of sensors or digital detectors currently available are shown in **Figures 15.2A to D** (**Tables 15.2 and 15.3**).

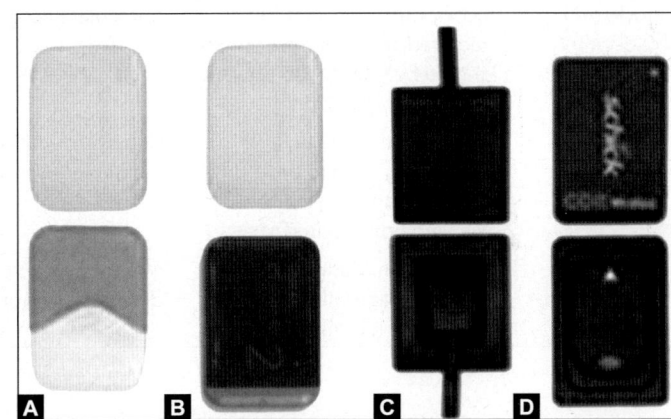

Figures 15.2A to D (A) Kodak film; (B) PSP Plate; (C) CCD Sensor; (D) Cordless sensor

Table 15.1 Terminology

Film-based imaging	Digital imaging
Density: The overall degree of darkening of an exposed film.	*Brightness*: Digital equivalent to density or overall degree of image darkening.
Latitude: Measure of the range of exposures that will produce usefully distinguishable densities on a film.	*Dynamic range*: The numerical range of each pixel; in visual terms it refers to the number of shades of gray that can be represented.
Film speed: Amount of radiation needed to produce a standard density; refers to the sensitivity of the film to radiation. The faster the film, the less radiation required.	*Linearity*: Linear or direct relationship between exposure and image density (*see* Fig. 17.1); contrast is not affected but density can be altered after image acquisition.
Contrast: The difference in densities between various areas on a radiograph; high contrast images have few shades of gray between black and white while low contrast will demonstrate more shades of gray.	*Contrast resolution*: The ability to differentiate small differences in density as displayed on an image.
Resolution: Ability to distinguish between small objects that are close together; measured in line pairs per millimeter.	*Spatial frequency*: Measure of resolution expressed in line pairs per millimeter. *Modulation transfer function*: Measure of image fidelity as a function of spatial frequency; how close the image is to the actual object.
Radiographic mottle (Noise): Appearance of uneven density of an exposed film or graininess.	*Background electronic noise*: Small electrical current that conveys no information but serves to obscure the electronic signal.
Sharpness: Ability of a radiograph to define an edge or display density boundaries.	*Signal to noise ratio*: Ratio between the fraction of the output signal (voltage or current or charge) that is directly related to the diagnostic information (signal) and the fraction of output that does not contain diagnostic information (noise).

Table 15.2 Comparison of intraoral imaging alternatives and their clinical applications

Procedure	Film	CCD/CMOS	PSP
Receptor preparation	None	Placement of plastic sleeve and connect to the computer along with patient data and registration number.	Erase previous image and put the plate in a disposable plastic cover.
Flexibility	Most flexible	Least flexible	More flexible than CCD
Receptor placement	Film may be held in place by the finger holding method or X-ray film holders. The film may be bent to accommodate anatomy.	Specialized film holders are used and the receptor is very hard and inflexible. The receptor cable needs to be carefully place so that the patient does not bite on it. Cordless receptors are more bulky and uncomfortable.	This is more flexible than CCD/CMOS, but bending may irreversibly damage the receptor, thus a receptor holder should be used.
Exposure	Simple	Computer activation required	Simple
Processing	Darkroom and chemicals required, all aseptic precautions should be followed to prevent saliva contamination.	Immediate image acquisition	Prior programming of processor, dim light and loading of plates required. All aseptic precautions should be followed to prevent saliva contamination.
Display	The films after drying and processing need to be mounted and labeled. Viewing box required.	Computer with adequate software helps to aid in viewing. The image obtained can be manipulated to achieve maximum diagnostic information.	
Image duplication	Duplication produces an inferior image with loss of diagnostic information.	Multiple copies can be made, either electronic which may be stored in the back up devices. A film or paper print out can also be obtained.	

- Charged couple device (CCD)
- Complementary metal oxide semiconductors (CMOS)
- Charge injection device (CID)
- Photostimulable phosphor plates (PSP)
- *Flat panel detectors*: These provide a relatively large matrix areas with pixel sizes less than 100 microns. This allows direct digital imaging of larger areas of the body, including the head. These are of two types: Indirect detectors that are sensitive to visible light, and an intensifying screen is used to convert X-ray photons to light. Direct detectors which used a photoconductor material (selenium) with properties similar to silicon and a higher atomic number that permits more efficient absorption of X-rays.

Advantages

- Superior gray scale resolution
- Easy reproducibility
- Reduced exposure to radiation
- Increased speed of image viewing
- Lower equipment and film cost
- Increased efficiency
- Enhancement of diagnostic image
- Excellent quality image with no loss of quality commonly associated with conventional chemical processing
- Image processing, enlargement and reconstruction for specific diagnostic purpose is possible
- With the aid of the computer, detection of defects and three dimensional visualization of dental structures based on radiographic data is possible
- Effective patient education tool.

Disadvantages

- Initial set-up is costly
- Image quality is still a source of debate
- Sensor size is thicker than intraoral films and therefore not patient compliant
- Infection control, the sensor has to be covered adequately in a disposable plastic wrapper
- Legal issues, because the original digital image can be manipulated, it is debatable whether digital radiographs can be used as evidence in lawsuits.

Digital Image Processing Tools for Dental Applications

- Image enhancement
  - Contrast enhancement
  - Filtering
  - Subtraction
  - Color.
- Image restoration
  - System defects
  - Geometric transformation.

Table 15.3 Comparison of physical properties of imaging receptors

Feature	Film	CCD/CMOS	PSP
Spatial resolution		.	
i. Intraoral Film > CCD = CMOS > PSP	Film has the best resolution	The limits of resolution for digital systems are readily appreciated when magnifying these images	
ii. Panoramic systems: Film = CCD = PSP	Resolution of panoramic systems is limited by mechanical motion to about 5 lp/mm	With magnification a 'blocky' or 'pixilated' appearance is evident.	
iii. Cephalometric systems Film > CCD = PSP	Film has the best resolution	With magnification a 'blocky' or 'pixilated' appearance is evident	
Exposure latitude PSP >> CCD = CMOS ≥ film			Because of the wide latitude of PSP and the automatic brightness and contrast 'optimization' by image acquisition software, use of more X-ray exposure than is necessary is possible.
Receptor dimensions For equivalent imaged area, Film = PSP < CCD = CMOS		The 'active area' of CCD and CMOS receptors is smaller than the surface area because of other electronic components within the plastic housing	
Time for image acquisition CCD = CMOS << PSP = film	Time consuming all the procedures have to be followed from placement of film, exposure, processing, drying, mounting and viewing on the illuminator.	Much faster. This rapid image acquisition is important for endodontic procedures or during implant placement	Easier than film but takes more time than CCD/CMOS, as the film has to be scanned before the image is obtained.
Image quality	Subjective quality is best with film when carefully exposed and well processed	Digital and film imaging are not significantly different when used for common diagnostic tasks	
Image adjustment/ processing		Improves appearance of digital images but may not improve diagnostic performance	
Cost	Recurring cost of films and processing chemicals besides maintenance of the machines.	Initial costs of digital systems are greater than film. Subsequent costs vary greatly depending on receptor wear and tear or abuse. Manufacturer's estimate of life expectancy of reusable receptors are perhaps overly optimistic	
Reliability	Mechanical problems may affect the film systems.	Mechanical problems affect digital PSP systems. Software reliability varies greatly among manufacturers. Changes in unrelated computer components and software can cause digital systems to malfunction. Digital systems fail when problems occur with receptors during image acquisition, or with computers during image processing, archiving, and display.	
Image storage and retrieval	Films can be misfiled and lost or be damaged by poor storage conditions.	Data backup is critical for digital systems. Digital data can be lost as a result of failures in power supplies and/or storage media, as well as operator error.	
Transmitting images	Physical transfer of film is difficult.	Rapidly done with digital images. Facilitates communication between colleagues or with insurance companies.	

- Image analysis
  - Measurement
  - Segmentation
  - Feature extraction
  - Object classification.
- Image compression
  - Lossless
  - Lossy.
- Image synthesis
  - Tomosynthesis
  - TACT
  - Localized CT.

Digital Subtraction Radiography (Figs 15.3A to C)

The diagnostic problem in a radiographic examination lies primarily in the identification of buried findings in a back ground of normal anatomical structures. During interpretation, the desired part has to be separated from the irrelevant distribution of other structures. The 'other structures' which do not contain diagnostic information of interest have been termed as 'noise'.

Technique

The reference radiograph is digitized and converted into its positive image by the computer. The subsequent radiograph is then displayed on the same server and aligned to the reference image and then digitized.

Subtraction of the gray levels between the two images is then performed. Any change that has occurred between the original radiograph and the subsequent radiograph shows up as light or dark areas. Loss of bone is seen as dark areas and gain of bone as light areas.

Applications

- Diagnosis of stuble changes in bone, e.g. it can be used to assess bone levels before and after periodontal therapy.
- Study of the periapical region.
- Study of the superior surface of the condyle.

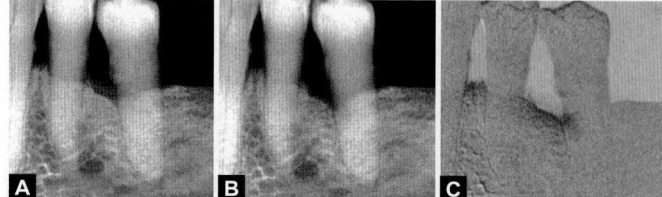

Figures 15.3A to C Use of digital subtraction radiography for detection of periodontal bone healing: (A) Image before surgery; (B) Image after 6 months; (C) Subtraction image showing the bone formation

BIBLIOGRAPHY

1. Brennan J. An Introduction to Digital Radiography in Dentistry—Journal of Orthodontics. United Kingdom; 2002 (29).
2. Christensen GJ. Why switch to Digital Radiography? JADA; USA. 2004;(135).
3. Cybula-Tahmazian, K. RDH: Dental Diagnosis with Digital Radiography http://www.umdnj.edu/idsweb/tech_reviews/Kathy—University of Medicine and Dentistry of New Jersey, USA.
4. Dunn SM, Kantor ML. Digital radiology: facts and fictions. JADA. 1993;124(12):38-47.
5. Farman AG. Guest Editorial, Dimensions in Computed Maxillofacial Imaging. J Ind Acad Oral Med Rad. 2004;16(2): 91-95.
6. Florman M. The Practice of Digital Dental Radiography; The Academy of Dental Therapeutics and Stomatology, Chesterland, Ohio, USA; 2005.
7. Haring JI, Howerton LJ. Dental Radiography, Principles and Techniques, 3rd edition, USA; 2006.
8. Kantor ML. Dental Digital Radiography. More than a fad, less than a revolution—JADA. USA; 2005(136).
9. Langland OE, Langlais RP. Special Radiographic Techniques. In: Principles of Dental Imaging. Baltimore, Williams and Wilkins; 1997. pp. 265-87.
10. Levato C. Are you ready for digital radiography? Dental Practise and Finance. 1999;7:17-24.
11. Lusk LT. Comparison of film based and digital radiography. J Prac Hyg. 1998;7:45-50.
12. Miles DA, Van Dis ML, Jenson CW, et al. Digital Imaging. In: Radiographic Imaging for Dental Auxillaries, 3rd edition. Philadelphia, WB Saunders; 1999. pp. 149-63.
13. Molander B, Grondahl HG, Ekestubbe A. Quality of film-based and digital panoramic radiography. Dentomaxillofac Radiol. 2004;33(1):32-6.
14. Parks ET, Williamson GF. Digital radiography: an overview. J Contemp Dent Pract. 2002;3(4):23-39.
15. Sansare K, Singh D, Farman A, et al. Dicom awareness of oral and maxillofacial radiologists in India. Dig Imag. JDI-12-02-0022.R1 OnLine July 2012.
16. Tsang A. DMD, et al. Potential for Fraudulent use of Digital Radiography. JADA. USA; 1999(130).
17. Van der Stelt. Filmless Imaging, The uses of Digital Radiography in Dental Practice, JADA. 2005(136).
18. Wenzel A, Grondahl HG. Direct digital radiography in the dental office. Int Dent J. 1995;45(1):27-34.
19. Wenzel A. Two Decades of Computerized Information Technologies in Dental Radiography. JDR. Denmark; 2002.

Section **VI**

Radiographic Diagnosis of Pathology Affecting the Jaws

Normal Anatomy on Intraoral and Extraoral Radiographs and Basics in Interpreting Radiographs

16

The radiographic recognition of disease requires knowledge of the radiographic appearance of normal structures. A good diagnosis mandates appreciation of a wide range of variation in the appearance of normal structures. Similarly most patients demonstrate many of the normal radiographic landmarks, but it is a rare patient who shows them all. Hence the absence of one or several landmarks in any individual should not be necessarily considered abnormal.

The radiographic appearance of various structures which can be visualized on the intraoral periapical radiograph can be classified as under:

- Teeth
- Supporting structures
- Maxilla
- Mandible
- Other restorative materials.

All these structures appear either radiopaque or radiolucent.

However, there are many structures which may not be visible on the intraoral periapical radiographs, these may be studied and observed on:

- Panoramic radiographs
- Cephalometric radiographs
- Skull projections.

Normal anatomical landmarks seen on the intraoral periapical radiographs may also be classified as:

- Radiopaque
- Radiolucent.

RADIOPAQUE

Maxilla	Mandible
• Enamel	• Enamel
• Dentin	• Dentin
• Cementum	• Cementum
• Lamina dura	• Lamina dura
• Alveolar crest	• Alveolar crest
• Cancellous bone	• Cancellous bone
• Nasal septum	• Genial tubercles
• Anterior nasal spine	• Mental ridge
• Floor of the nasal cavity	• Mylohyoid ridge
• Inferior nasal conchae	• External oblique ridge
• Nasolabial fold	• Inferior border of the
• Floor of the maxillary sinus	mandible

- Septa in maxillary
- Inverted Y in maxillary sinus
- Zygomatic process of the maxilla
- Zygoma (malar bone)
- Pterygoid plates
- Hamular process
- Maxillary tuberosity
- Coronoid process
- Internal oblique ridge

RADIOLUCENT

Maxilla	Mandible
• Pulp	• Pulp
• Periodontal ligament space	• Periodontal ligament space
• Nutrient canals	• Nutrient canals
• Intermaxillary suture	• Lingual foramen
• Nasal fossa (nasal cavity)	• Symphysis
• Incisive foramen	• Mental fossa
• Superior foramina of nasopalatine canal	• Mental foramen
• Incisive fossa (lateral or canine fossa)	• Mandibular canal
• Nasolacrimal canal	• Submandibular fossa
• Maxillary sinus	
• Nose	

Tooth

The tooth structure that can be viewed on the radiograph are (**Fig. 16.1**):

- *Enamel*: This is the densest structure found in the human body. It is seen as the outer most radiopaque layer of the crown of a tooth on the radiograph.
- *Dentin*: This is found beneath the enamel layer of a tooth and surrounds the pulp cavity. It appears radiopaque and comprises most of the tooth structure. Dentin is less radiopaque than enamel.
- *Cementum*: This is not usually apparent on the radiograph because the cemental layer is very thin and the contrast between the cementum and dentin is very low.

Diffuse radiolucent areas with ill-defined borders may be apparent radiographically on the mesial and distal aspects of the teeth in the cervical region between the edge of the enamel cap and the the crest of the alveolar ridge, (cementoenamel junction), this is called cervical burn out, which may be mistaken for cervical or root caries.

- *Pulp cavity*: This consists of the pulp chamber and the root canals. It contains the blood vessels, nerves and lymphatics and appears relatively radiolucent on the radiograph.

The size of the pulp chamber is generally large in children than in adults because it decreases with age owing to the formation of secondary dentin. Great variation exists between individuals in size of the pulp chambers and extent of the pulp horn.

The root canal may be apparent (**Figs 16.2A and B**).
- Extending to the apex of the root.
- In some teeth the canal may appear constricted in the region of the apex and thus not discernible in the last few millimeter or so of its length.
- In the above mentioned cases the canal may exit on the same side of the tooth, just short of the radiographic apex.

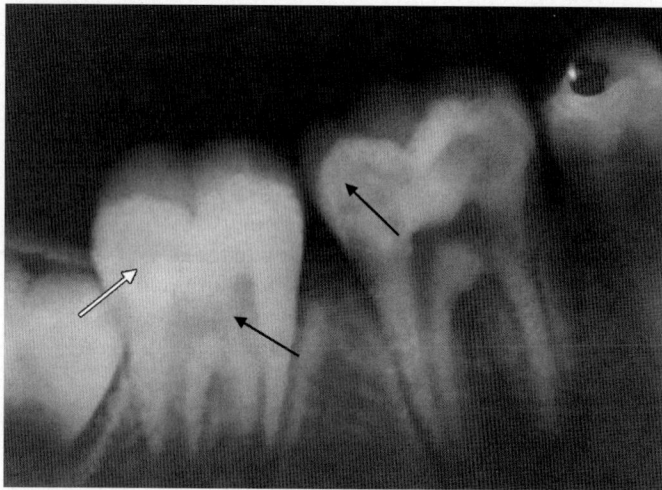

Figure 16.1 Teeth are made of various components, pulp (black arrow on second molar, enamel (arrow on first molar) dentine (white arrow on second molar) and cementum which is not regularly detected on the radiograph

- At the end of the developing tooth root, pulp canal diverges and the walls of the root rapidly taper to a knife edge. In the recess formed in the root walls and extending a short distance beyond is a small rounded, radiolucent area in the trabecular bone, surrounded by a thin layer of hyperostotic bone. This is the dental papilla surrounded by its bony crypt. The papilla forms the dentin and primordium of the pulp (**Figs 16.2C and D**).

In mature teeth the shape of the pulp chamber may change. With aging occurs a gradual deposition of dentin. This process begins apically, proceeds coronally, and may lead to pulp obliteration. Trauma may also stimulate dentin production leading to reduction of the size of the pulp chambers and canals.

Supporting Structures

Lamina Dura (Figs 16.3A to D)

This is the wall of the tooth socket that surrounds the tooth. It is made up of dense cortical bone.

On the radiograph lamina dura appears as:
- A thin dense radiopaque line that surrounds the root of the tooth. It is continuous with the shadow of the cortical bone at the alveolar crest.
- It is slightly thicker than the trabeculae of the cancellous bone in the area.
- When the X-ray beam is directed through the relatively long expanse of the structure, the lamina dura appears radiopaque and well-defined.
- When the beam is directed more obliquely, the lamina dura appears more diffuse and may not be discernible.
- The thickness and density of the lamina dura will vary with the amount of occlusal stresses. It is wider and more dense around roots of teeth in heavy occlusion, and thinner and less dense around teeth not subjected to occlusion function.
- Double lamina dura image appears if the mesial or distal surfaces of the root present two elevations in the path of the X-ray beam.

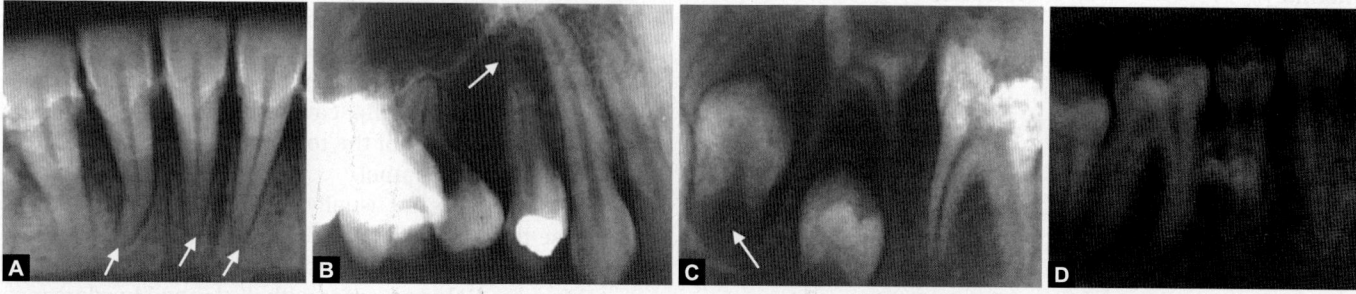

Figures 16.2A to D (A) Root canal lower incisors (arrow at the root apex); (B) Root canal not seen radiographically in the apical third (arrow) the canal may be actually present; (C) Developing root shown by arrow enclosed in a bony crypt; (D) Developing tooth crypt of supernumerary tooth near roots of premolar

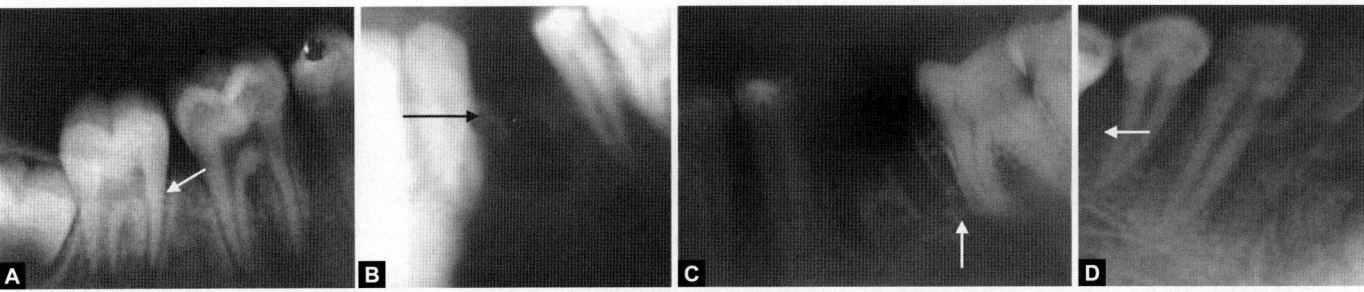

Figure 16.3A to D (A) Lamina dura is seen as a thin opaque layer; (B and C) Recent extraction socket showing lamina dura; (D) The arrow show poor visualization of lamina dura on the distal surface of the premolar

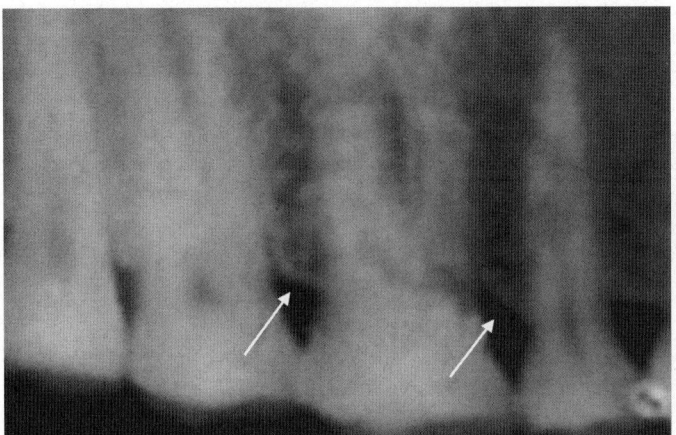

Figure 16.4 Arrows showing corticated crests of the alveolar bone (alveolar crests)

- Presence of an intact lamina dura around the tooth indicate a vital pulp, however in some cases its absence may be normal.

Alveolar Crest (Fig. 16.4)

This is the most coronal portion of the alveolar bone found between the teeth. It is made up of dense cortical bone and is continuous with the lamina dura.

On the radiograph the alveolar crest appears:
- Radiopaque and is typically located 1.5–2 mm below the junction of the crown and the root surfaces (cementoenamel junction).
- Anteriorly the crest is reduced to a point of bone and appears as a dense radiopaque line, whereas posteriorly, it is flat, parallel with or slightly below a line connecting the cementoenamel junction of adjacent teeth.
- The crest of the bone is continuous with the lamina dura and forms a sharp angle with it. Rounding of these sharp angles is indicative of periodontal disease.
- The alveolar crest may recede apically with age and show marked resorption with periodontal disease.

Periodontal Ligament Space (Figs 16.5A to C)

It is the space between the root of the tooth and the lamina dura. The PDL space contains connective tissue fibers, blood vessels and lymphatics.

On the radiograph the PDL appears as:
- A thin radiolucent line around the root of the tooth. It is usually of uniform thickness.
- It may be thinner in the middle of the root and slightly wider near the alveolar crest and the root apex, suggesting that the fulcrum of the physiologic movement is in the region where the PDL is thinnest.
- The thickness of the PDL is less around the roots of the embedded teeth and those that have lost their antagonists.
- The appearance of double PDL space is created by the shape of the tooth. When the X-ray beam is directed so that two convexities of a root surface appear on the film, double PDL space may be seen.

Cancellous Bone (Figs 16.6A to C)

This is soft spongy bone located between two layers of dense cortical bone. It is composed of numerous bony trabeculae that form a lattice like network of inter-communicating spaces filled with bone marrow.

On the radiograph the cancellous bone appears as:
- Predominantly radiolucent with the trabeculae appearing radiopaque in a criss cross pattern.
- In the maxilla:
  - Anteriorly the trabeculae are thin and numerous forming a fine, granular, dense pattern and the marrow spaces are small and relatively numerous.
  - Posteriorly the pattern is similar but the marrow spaces are larger.
- In the mandible:
  - Anteriorly the trabeculae are thicker, coarser and fewer than that in the maxilla with larger marrow spaces and are oriented more horizontally.
  - Posteriorly, the periradicular trabeculae and marrow spaces are larger than that in the anterior region.

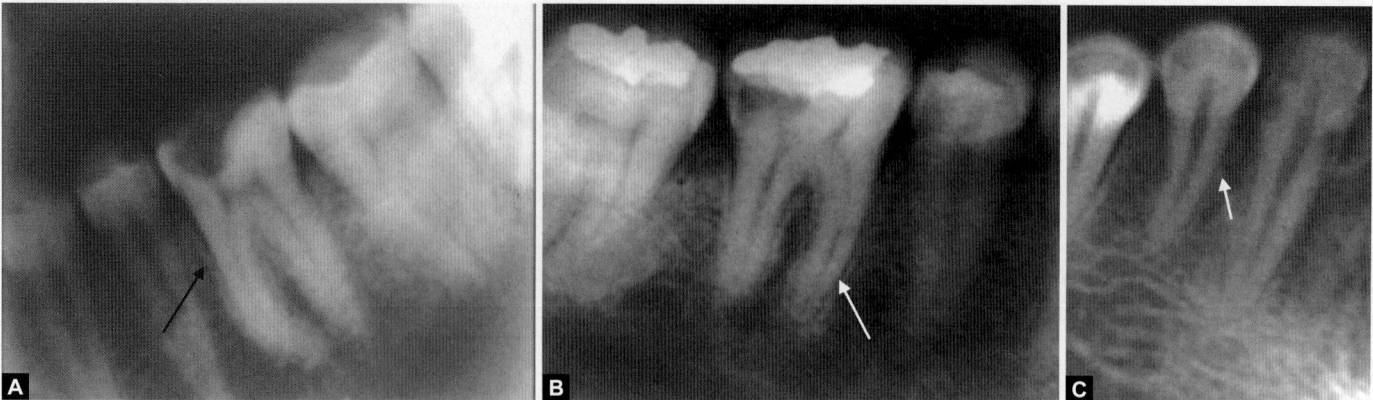

Figures 16.5A to C (A) Arrow showing double periodontal ligament space and lamina dura due to the convexity of the proximal surface of the root; (B) Arrow showing a narrow radiolucency between tooth root and lamina dura which is the periodontal ligament space; (C) Arrow show widened periodontal space on the mesial surface of the premolar, whereas it is thin on the distal surface

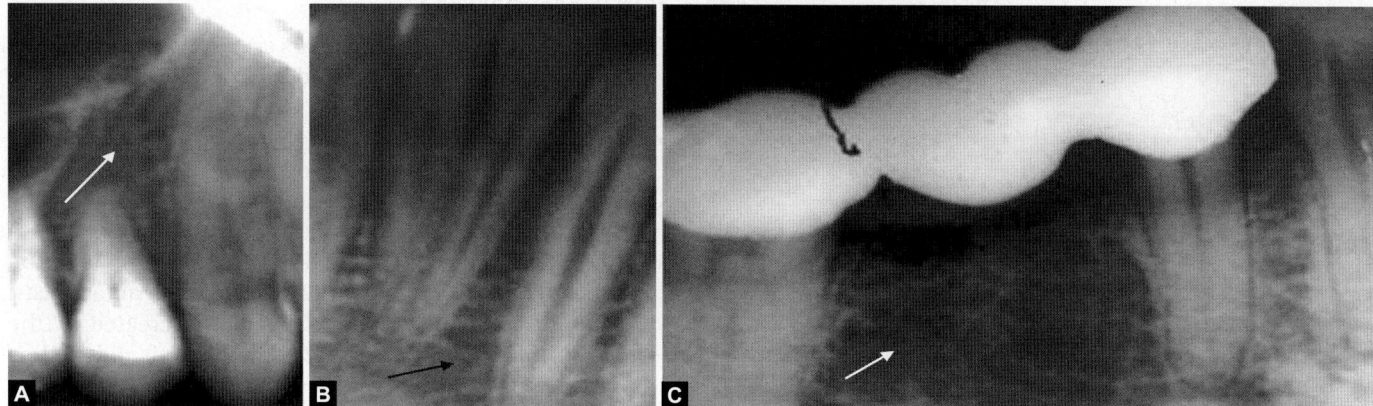

Figures 16.6A to C (A) Arrow showing characteristic fine trabecular plates and multiple small trabecular spaces in the maxilla; (B) Arrow showing coarse trabecular plates and larger marrow spaces in the anterior mandible; (C) Arrow showing variable, sparse trabecular pattern and large marrow spaces in the posterior mandible

- Occasionally the trabecular spaces in the region may be so irregular and large that they may mimic pathological lesions.
- Sparse trabecular pattern that is over exposed may get 'burnt out', suggesting the presence of disease.

Maxilla

The upper jaw is composed of two paired bones, the maxillae which meet at the center, to form the maxilla which is described as the architectural cornerstone of the face. The maxilla forms the floor of the orbit of the eyes, the sides and floor of the nasal cavities and the hard palate. The lower border of the maxilla supports the upper teeth.

Incisive Foramen (Nasopalatine or Anterior Palatine Foramen) (Fig. 16.7)

It is an opening located in the midline of the anterior portion of the hard palate, directly posterior to the central incisors.

The nasopalatine nerve exists the maxilla through this foramen.

On the radiograph it appears as a small ovoid or round radiolucent area located between the roots of the maxillary central incisors.

Superior Foramina of the Incisive Canal (Nasopalatine Canal) (Fig. 16.8)

These are two tiny openings or holes in bone that are located on the floor of the nasal cavity (foramina is the plural of foramen). The superior foramina are the openings of two small canals. These two small canals extend downward and medially from the floor of the nasal cavity, and join together to form the incisive canal and share a common exit, the incisive foramen. The nasopalatine nerve enters the maxilla through the superior foramina, travels down the incisive canal and exits through the incisive foramen.

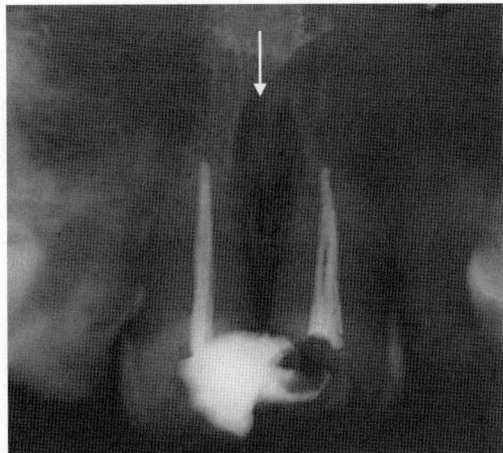

Figure 16.7 Ovoid shaped incisive foramen between the roots of the central incisors

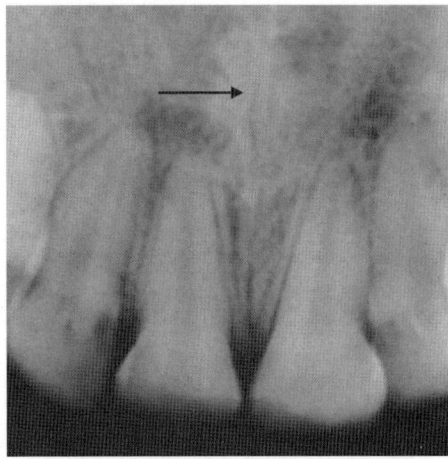

Figure 16.9 The median palatine suture appears as a thin radiolucent line

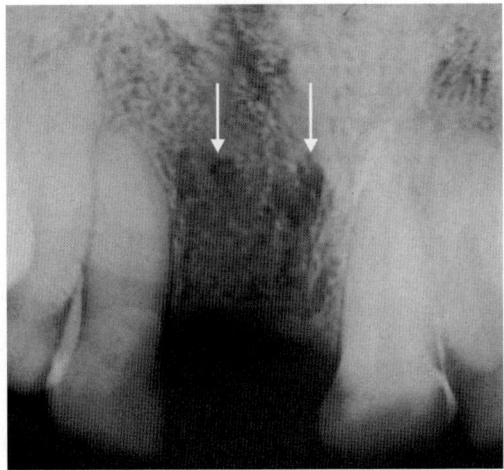

Figure 16.8 The superior foramen of the incisive canal appear as two small round radiolucencies

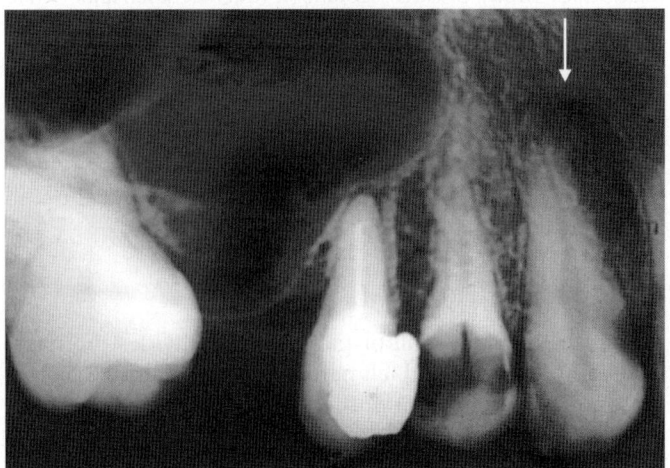

Figure 16.10 Arrow pointing to the lateral fossa, which may be misdiagnosed as a globulomaxillary cyst

On the radiograph the superior foramina appear as two small radiolucencies located superior to the apices of the maxillary central incisors, in the floor of the nasal cavity, near it's anterior border on both sides of the septum.

Median Palatine Suture (Intermaxillary Suture) (Fig. 16.9)

It is the immovable joint between the two palatine processes of the maxilla. It extends from the alveolar bone between the maxillary incisors to the posterior hard palate.

On the radiograph it appears as:
- A thin radiolucent line between the maxillary central incisors. This is bounded on both sides by dense cortical bone that appears radiopaque.
- The suture may terminate at the alveolar crest in a small rounded or V-shaped enlargement.

- As this suture fuses with age, it may appear less distinct radiographically.

Lateral Fossa (Incisive Fossa, Canine Fossa) (Fig. 16.10)

It is a smooth depressed area of the maxilla located just inferior and medial to the infraorbital foramen between the lateral incisors and canine.

On the radiograph it appears as a radiolucent area between the canine and the lateral incisors.

Nasal Cavity (Nasal Fossa) (Fig. 16.11)

It is a pearshaped, air filled compartment of bone located superior to the maxilla. The inferior portion, or floor of the nasal cavity is formed by the palatal process of the maxilla and the horizontal portions of the palatine bones. The lateral

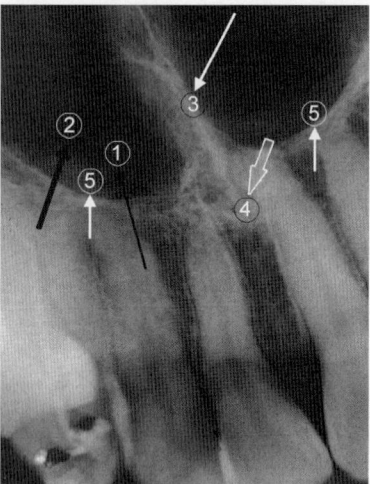

Figure 16.11 1. The nasal fossa (black arrow); 2. Inferior turbinates (black thick arrow); 3. Nasal septum; 4. Anterior nasal spine white hollow arrow); 5. Floor of the nasal cavity (white arrow)

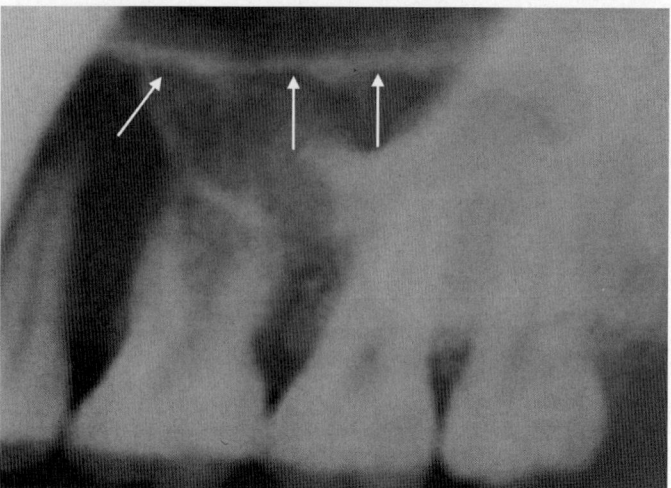

Figure 16.12 Arrows showing the floor of the nasal fossa which extends posteriorly and is superimposed with the maxillary sinus

walls of the nasal cavity are formed by the ethmoidal bone and the maxillae.

On the radiograph it appears as a large radiolucent area above the maxillary incisors.

Nasal Septum (Fig. 16.11)

It is a vertical bony wall or partition that divides the nasal cavity into the right and left nasal fossae. It is formed by two bones, the vomer and a portion of the ethmoid bone, and cartilage.

On the radiograph it appears as:
- A vertical radiopaque partition that divides the nasal cavity.
- The nasal septum may be superimposed over the median palatal suture.

Floor of the Nasal Cavity (Figs 16.11 to 16.13)

It is a bony wall formed by the palatal process of the maxilla and the horizontal portions of the palatine bones. The floor is made of dense cortical bone and defines the inferior border of the nasal cavity.

On the radiograph it appears as a dense radiopaque band above the maxillary incisors.

Anterior Nasal Spine (Figs 16.11 and 16.13)

It is a sharp projection of the maxilla located at the anterior and inferior portion of the nasal cavity.

On the radiograph it appears as a V-shaped radiopaque area located at the intersection of the floor of the nasal cavity and nasal septum.

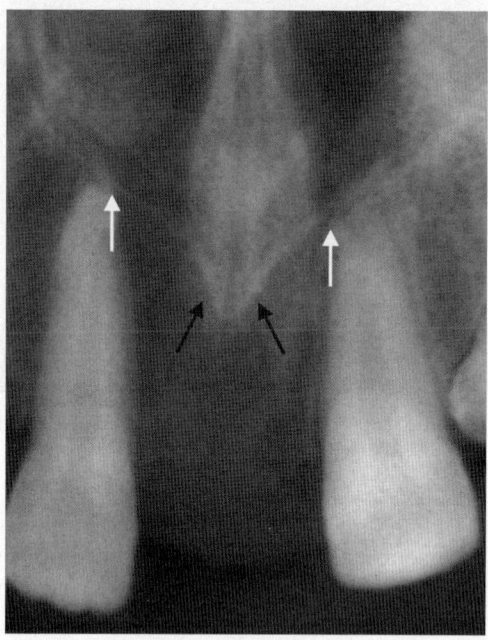

Figure 16.13 The anterior nasal spine appears as a 'V' shaped radiopacity at the midline of the floor of the nasal cavity (black arrows). Floor of the nasal cavity (white arrows)

Inferior Nasal Conchae (Figs 16.11 and 16.14)

These are wafer thin, curved plates of bone that extend from the lateral walls of the nasal cavity, in the lower lateral portions.

On the radiograph they appear as a diffuse radiopaque mass or projection within the nasal cavity.

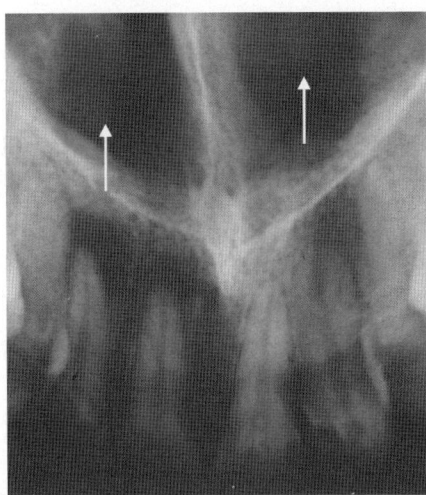

Figure 16.14 The inferior nasal conchae appear as diffuse radiopacities within the nasal cavity

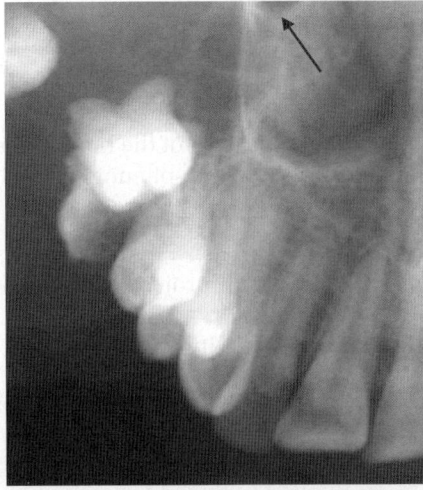

Figure 16.15 Arrow showing nasolacrimal canal (it may be seen at the apex of the canine if the vertical angulation is increased)

Nasolacrimal Canal (Fig. 16.15)

It is formed by the nasal and maxillary bones, running from the medial aspect of the anteroinferior border of the orbit inferiorly to drain under the inferior conchae of the nasal cavity.

On the radiograph it appears as:
- A well-defined slightly ovoid radiolucency, just above the apex of the maxillary canine, when a steep vertical angulation is used.
- It is seen more routinely on the maxillary occlusal projections.

Nose

The soft tissue of the nose is frequently seen in the projections of the maxillary central and lateral incisors, superimposed on the roots of these teeth. The image of the nose has a uniform, slightly opaque appearance with a sharp border. Sometimes, the radiolucent nares may be identified.

Nasolabial Fold

This is an oblique line demarcating a region that appears to be covered by a veil of slight radiopacity frequently seen in the premolar region. The line of contrast is sharp, and the area of increased radiopacity is posterior to the line. The line is the nasolabial fold, and the opaque veil is the thick cheek tissue superimposed on the teeth and the alveolar process. The image of the fold becomes more prominent with age.

Maxillary Sinus (Figs 16.16A to C)

These are paired three sided pyramidal cavities of bone within the maxilla. They are located above the maxillary premolar and molar teeth. Its three sides include; the superior wall forming the floor of the orbit, anterior wall extending above the premolars and posterior bulging above the molar teeth and maxillary tuberosity. Rarely does the

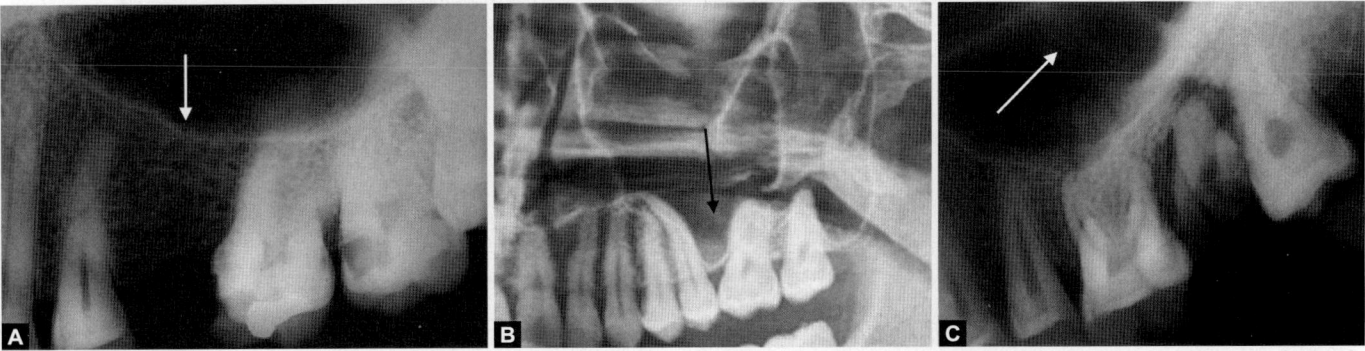

Figures 16.16A to C (A) The maxillary sinus floor appears as a radiolucent area above the maxillary posterior teeth; (B) Floor of the maxillary sinus dipping interdentally; (C) Septa within the maxillary sinus appear as radiopaque lines

sinus extend beyond the canine. The sinus at birth is the size of a small pea, but in adults it may extend to include interdental bone, molar furcation areas or the maxillary tuberosity region.

On the radiograph it appears as:
- A radiolucent area located above the apices of the maxillary molars.
- The borders of the maxillary sinus are composed of dense cortical bone and appears as a radiopaque line.
  - *Septa within the maxillary sinus (Fig. 16.16B)*: These are bony projections or partitions that appear to divide the sinus into compartments, their presence and number varies from person-to-person (**Fig. 16.16C**).

On the radiograph they appear as:
- Radiopaque lines within the sinus.
  - *Nutrient canals within the maxillary sinus*: These are tiny tube like passages through the bone that contain blood vessels and nerves that supply the maxillary teeth and interdental areas.

On the radiograph they appear as a narrow radiolucent band bounded by two thin radiopaque lines.

When the rounded sinus floor dips between the buccal and palatal molar roots and is medial to the premolar roots, the projection of the apices is superior to the floor, and this appearance conveys the impression that the roots project into the sinus cavity, which is an illusion.

Inverted 'Y' (Figs 16.17A and B)

This refers to the intersection of the maxillary sinus and the nasal cavity as seen on the radiograph.

On the radiograph it appears as:
- A radiopaque upside down 'Y' formed by the intersection of the floor of the nasal fossa and the anterior border of the maxillary sinus.
- The inverted Y is usually located above the maxillary canine.

Maxillary Tuberosity (Figs 16.18A and B)

This is a rounded prominence of bone which extends posterior to the third molar region. Blood vessels and nerves to the posterior teeth enter the maxilla from this region.

On the radiograph it appears as a radiopaque bulge posterior to the third molar region.

Pterygoid Plates (Figs 16.19A and B)

The medial and lateral pterygoid plate lies immediately posterior to the tuberosity of the maxilla.

On the radiograph they appear as:
- A single radiopaque homogeneous shadow without any evidence of trabeculation.
- It may not be seen on all radiographs.

Hamulus (Hamular Process) (Fig. 16.20)

It is a small hook-like projection of the bone extending from the medial pterygoid plate of the sphenoid bone. It is located posterior to the maxillary tuberosity process.

On the radiograph it appears as:
- A radiopaque hook-like projection posterior to the maxillary tuberosity area.
- The length, shape and density is variable.

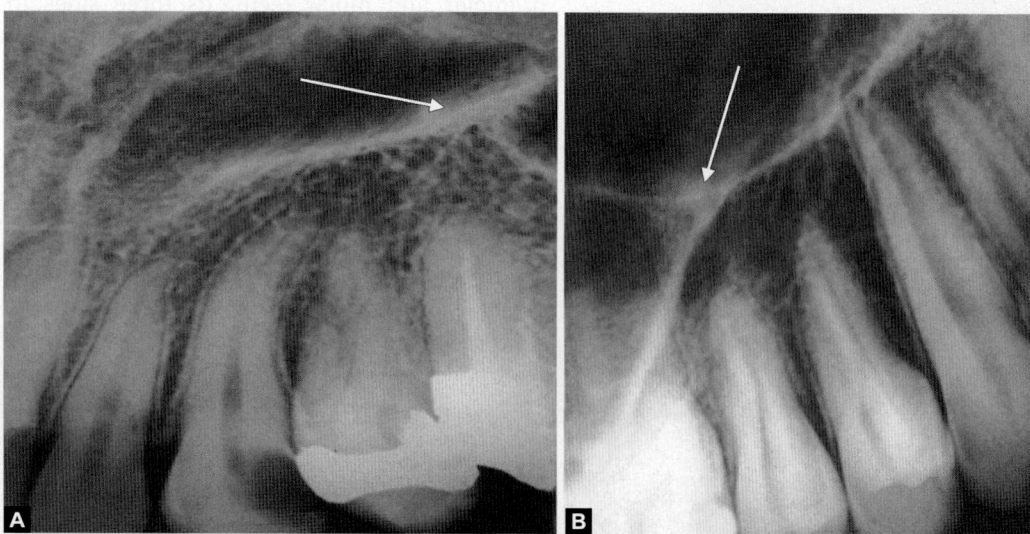

Figures 16.17A and B The floor of the nasal fossa and the maxillary sinus resemble the arms of the letter 'Y' and the bony walls separating the two structures resembles the leg of that letter

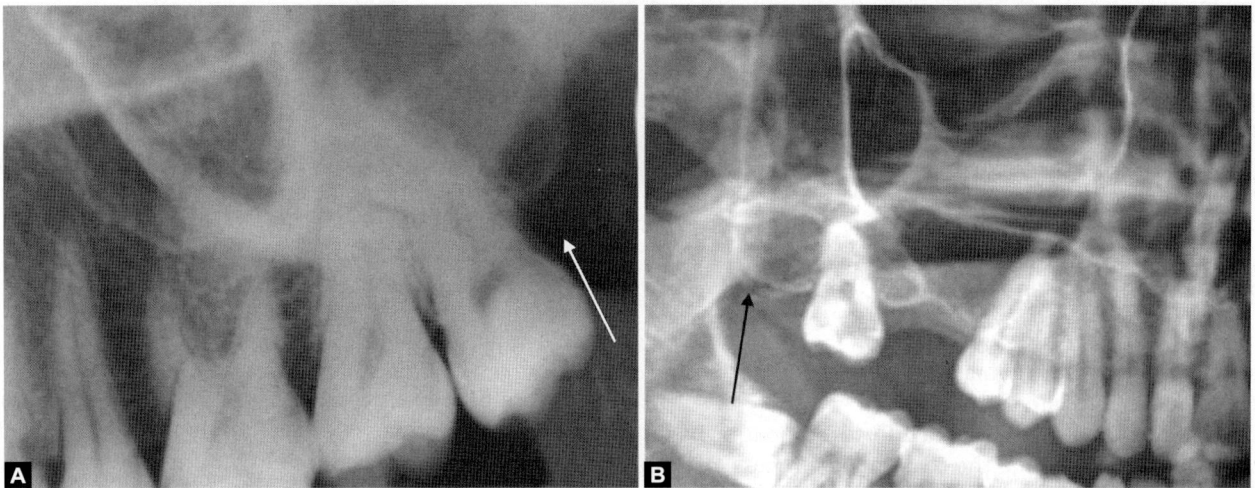

Figures 16.18A and B The maxillary tuberosity appears as a radiopaque bulge distal to the third molar region

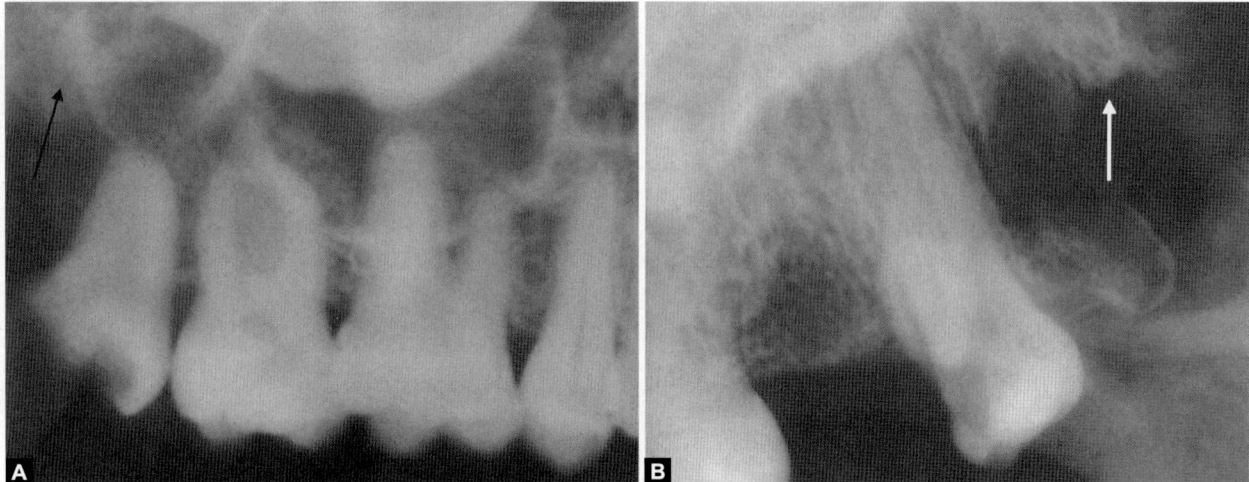

Figures 16.19A and B The medial plate of the pterygoid process: (A) (black arrow); (B) (solid arrow)

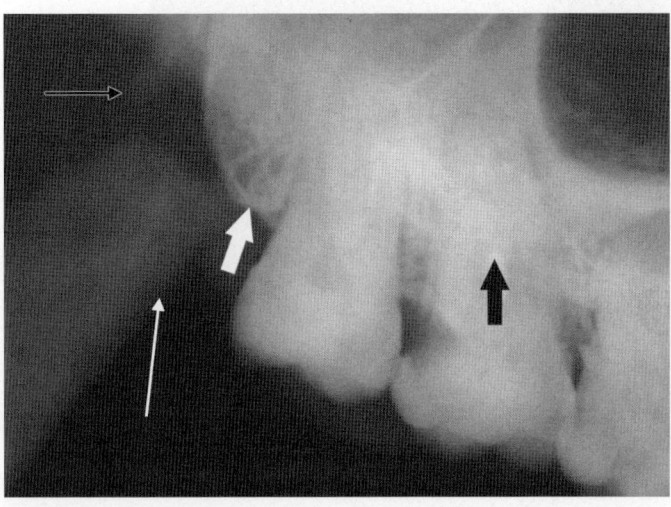

Figure 16.20 The hamulus appears as a hook-like radiopacity distal to the maxillary tuberosity area (black thin arrow), coronoid process (white thin arrow), zygoma (black solid arrow). White solid arrow shows the maxillary tuberosity

Zygomatic Process of the Maxilla (Figs 16.21A and B)

It is the bony process of the maxilla that articulates with the zygoma, and is composed of dense corticated bone.

On the radiograph it appears as a 'J' or 'U' shaped radiopacity located superior to the maxillary first molar region.

Zygoma (Zygomatic Bone, Malar or Cheek Bone) (Fig. 16.20)

This articulates with the zygomatic process of the maxilla and is made of dense corticated bone.

On the radiograph it appears as a diffuse radiopaque band extending posteriorly from the zygomatic process of the maxilla.

Mandible

The mandible or the lower jaw is the largest and strongest bone of the face. It can be divided into three parts:
1. The ramus which is the vertical portion of the mandible, found posterior to the third molar. The mandible has two rami, one on each side.
2. The body which is the horizontal 'U'-shaped portion of the mandible which extends from one ramus to the other.
3. Alveolar process which is that portion of the mandible that encases and supports the teeth.

Genial Tubercles (Mental Spine) (Fig. 16.22)

These are tiny bumps of bone on the lingual side of the mandible, approximately in the midline, that serve as attachment for the genioglossus and the geniohyoid muscles

On the radiograph they appear as ring shaped radiopacities below the apices of the mandibular incisors.

Lingual Foramen (Fig. 16.23)

It is a tiny opening in the bone located on the internal surface of the mandible, near the midline and surrounded by the genial tubercules.

On the radiograph it appears as a small radiolucent dot inferior to the apices of the mandibular incisors.

Nutrient Canals (Fig. 16.24)

These are tube like passages through the bone that contain nerves and blood vessels that supply the teeth. Interdental nutrient canals are seen more in the anterior mandible.

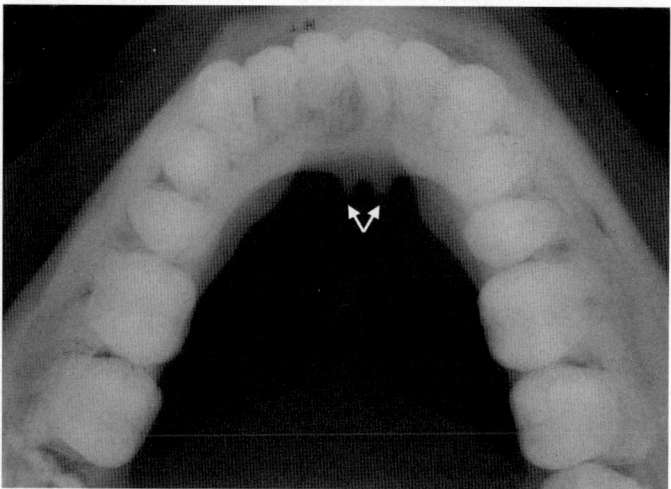

Figure 16.22 Arrow showing genial tubercules

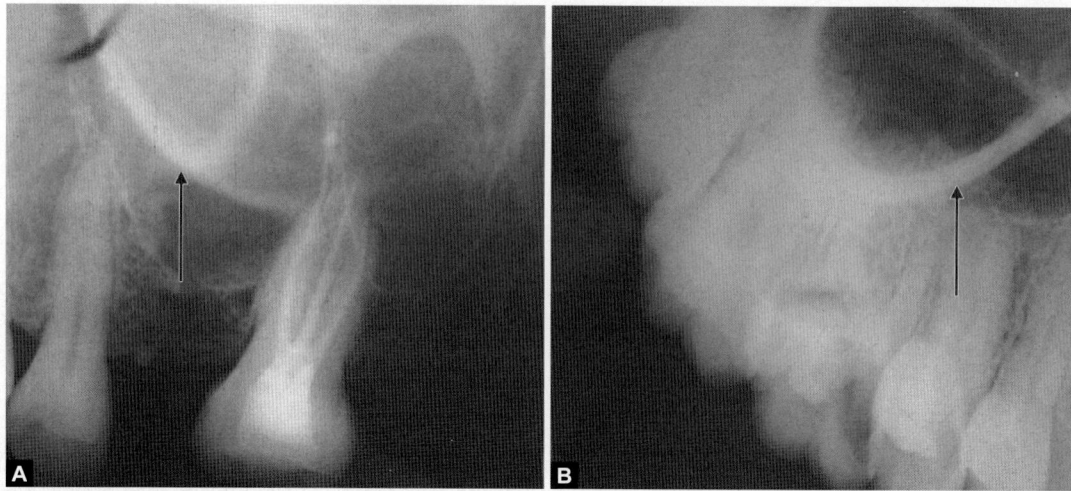

Figures 16.21A and B The zygomatic process of the maxilla appears as a 'J' or 'U' shaped radiopacity superior to the maxillary molars

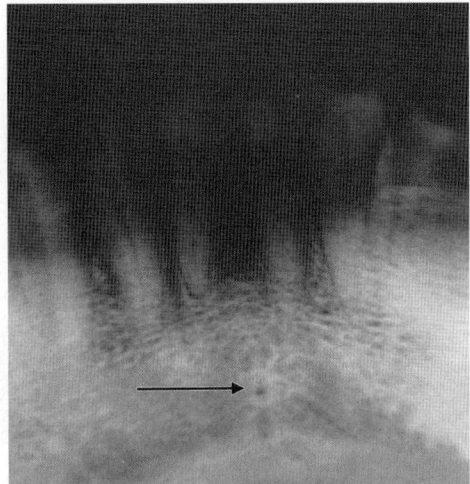

Figure 16.23 The lingual foramen

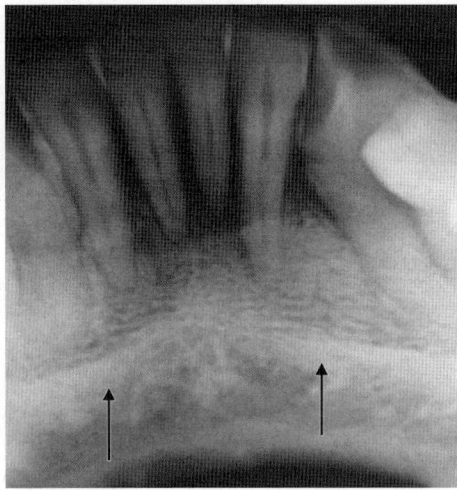

Figure 16.25 The mental ridge (solid arrows)

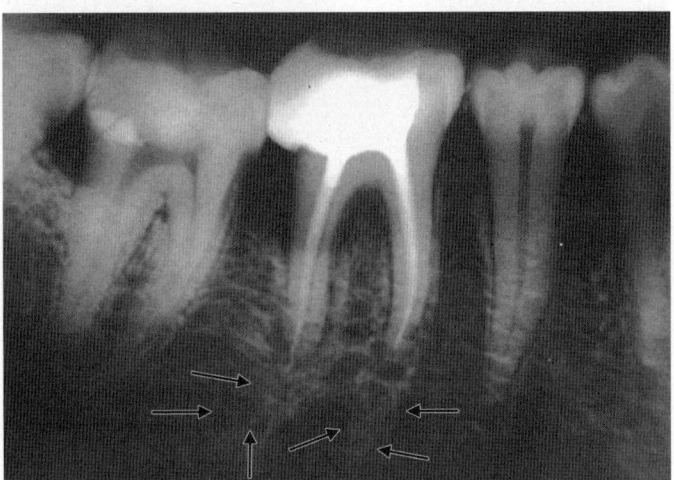

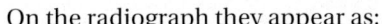

Figure 16.24 Nutrient canals (arrows)

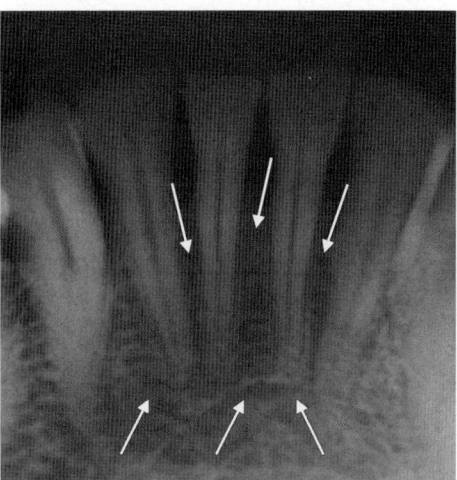

Figure 16.26 The mental fossa appears as a radiolucent area above the mental ridge

On the radiograph they appear as:
- Vertical radiolucent lines.
- These are more prominent in the anterior region and in the edentulous mandible.

Mental Ridge (Fig. 16.25)

This is a linear prominence of cortical bone, located on the external surface of the anterior portion of the mandible, from the premolar to the midline and slopes slightly upwards.

On the radiograph it appears as:
- A thick radiopaque band that extends from the premolar to the incisor region.
- It may appear superimposed on the mandibular anterior teeth.

Mental Fossa (Fig. 16.26)

This is a scooped out depressed area of the bone located on the external surface of the anterior mandible. It is located above the mental ridge in the mandibular incisor region.

On the radiograph it appears as:
- A radiolucent area above the mental ridge.
- The appearance varies and is determined by the thickness of the bone in the anterior region.

Mental Foramen (Fig. 16.27)

It is an opening in the bone located on the external surface of the mandible, in the region of the mandibular premolars. Blood vessels and nerves that supply the lower lip exit through the mental foramen.

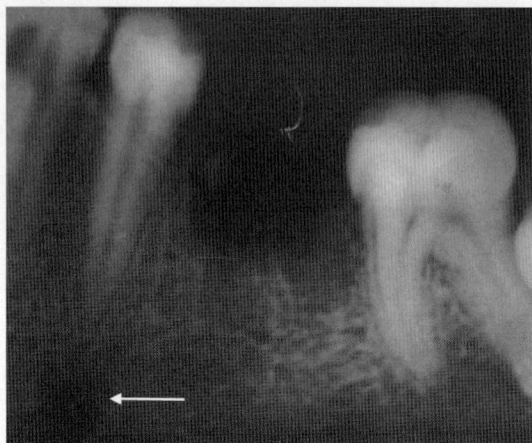

Figure 16.27 The mental foramen at the apex of the premolar

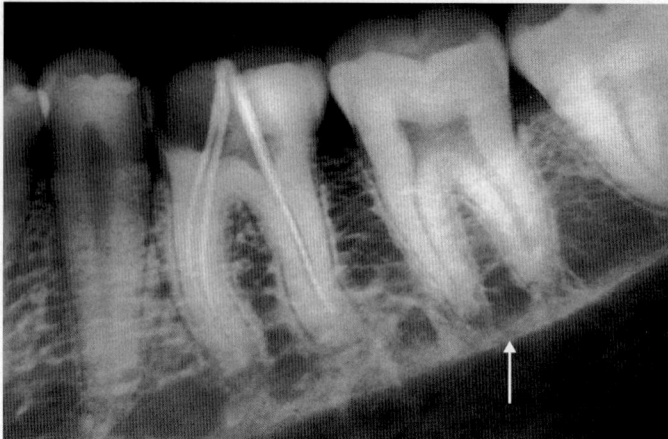

Figure 16.28 The mylohyoid ridge appears as a radiopaque band in the mandibular molar region

On the radiograph it appears as:
- A small ovoid or round radiolucent area located in the apical region of the premolars.
- It is frequently misdiagnosed as a periapical lesion because of its apical location.

Symphysis

The mandibular symphysis is the suture in the midline of the mandible. This suture fuses by the end of the first year of life, after which it is not radiographically apparent.

On the radiograph it appears as a radiolucent line through the midline of the jaw.

Mylohyoid Ridge (Fig. 16.28)

This is a linear prominence of the bone located on the internal surface of the mandible, extending from the molar region downwards and forward towards the lower border of the mandibular symphysis. It serves as an attachment for the mylohyoid muscle.

On the radiograph it appears as:
- A dense radiopaque band that extends downwards and forward from the molar region.
- It usually appears more prominent in the molar region and may be superimposed over the roots of the mandibular teeth.
- It may appear continuous with the internal oblique ridge.

Internal Oblique Ridge (Internal Oblique Line) (Fig. 16.29)

This is a linear prominence of bone located on the internal surface of the mandible extending downwards and forwards from the ramus. It may end in the region of the third molar or it may continue on as the mylohyoid ridge.

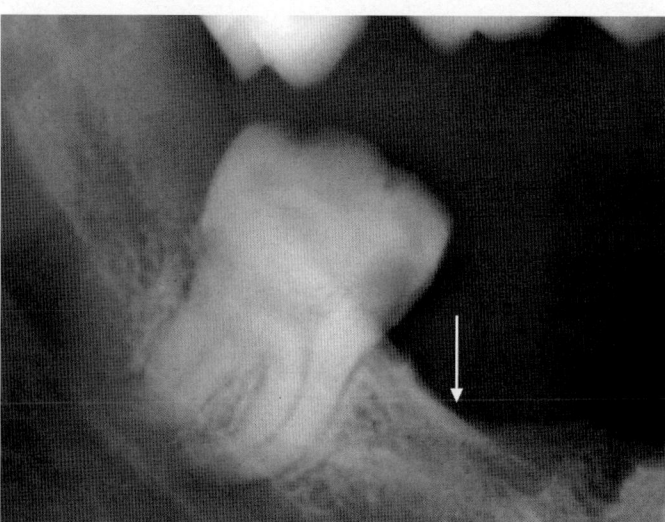

Figure 16.29 The internal oblique ridge appears as a radiopaque band

On the radiograph it appears as:
- A radiopaque band that extends downwards and forward from the ramus.
- Depending on the technique used the internal and external oblique ridge may appear superimposed on one another. When the ridges appear separate, then the superior radiopaque band is the external oblique ridge and the inferior radiopaque band is the internal oblique ridge.

External Oblique Ridge (External Oblique Line) (Fig. 16.30)

It is a linear prominence of bone located on the external surface of the body of the mandible. The anterior border of the ramus ends in the external oblique ridge.

On the radiograph it appears as:
- A radiopaque band extending downwards and forwards from the anterior border of the ramus of the mandible.
- It typically ends in the mandibular third molar region.

Mandibular Canal (Figs 16.31A and B)

It is a tube-like passage through the bone that travels the length of the mandible. It extends from the mandibular foramen to the mental foramen and houses the inferior alveolar nerve and the blood vessels.

On the radiograph it appears as:
- A radiolucent band, outlined by two thin radiopaque lines that represent the cortical walls of the canal.
- It may appear below or superimposed on the mandibular molar teeth.

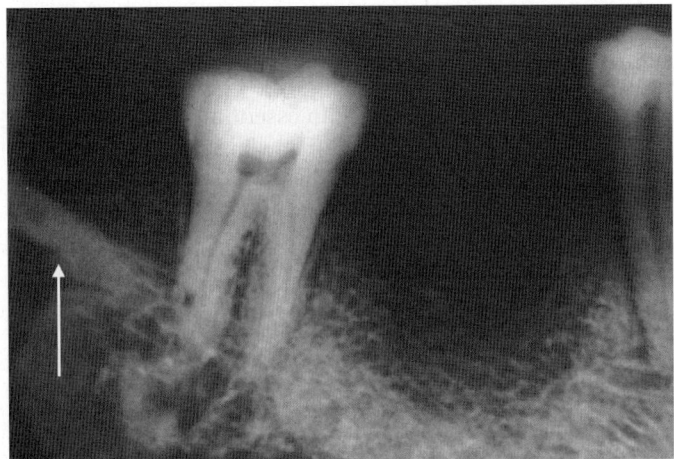

Figure 16.30 The external oblique ridge appears as a radiopaque band

Inferior Border of the Mandible (Fig. 16.32)

As the name suggests is the lower border of the mandible. It is rarely seen on the periapical projections.

On the radiograph it appears as a dense radiopaque band of bone.

Coronoid Process (Fig. 16.33)

It is a marked prominence of bone on the anterior ramus of the mandible. It is the site for attachment of the muscles of mastication.

On the radiograph it appears as:
- A triangular radiopacity superimposed over or inferior to the maxillary tuberosity region.
- It is seen on the maxillary molar periapical radiograph, and not a mandibular periapical radiograph.

Submandibular Fossa (Mandibular Fossa or Submaxillary Fossa) (Fig. 16.34)

It is a scooped out depressed area of the bone located on the internal surface of the mandible inferior to the mylohyoid line. It houses the submandibular salivary gland.

On the radiograph it appears as:
- A radiolucent area in the molar region below the mylohyoid ridge.
- Few bony trabeculae are seen in this region.

Other Restorative Materials

Restorative materials vary in their radiographic appearance, depending primarily on:
- Thickness
- Density
- Atomic number.

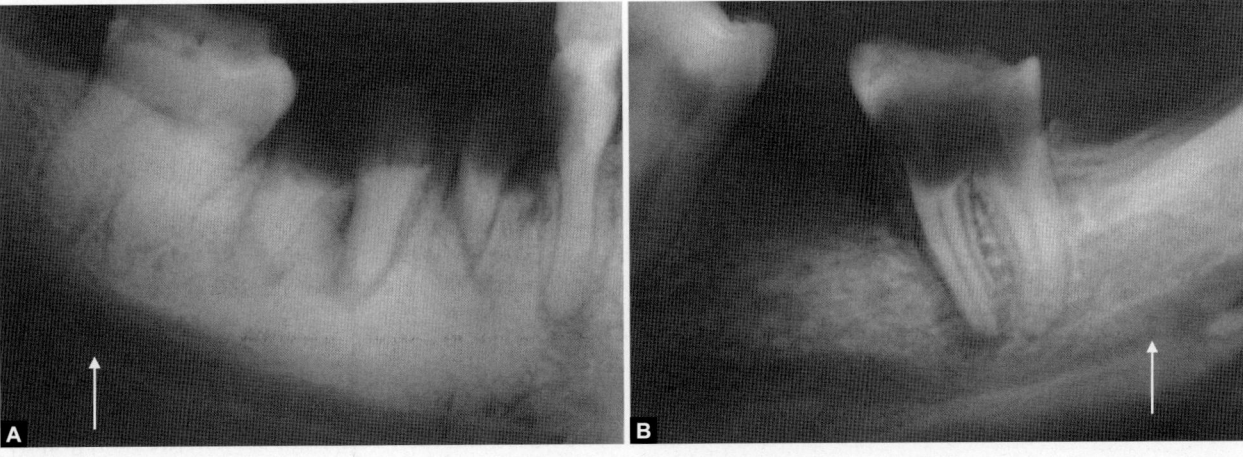

Figures 16.31A and B The mandibular canal

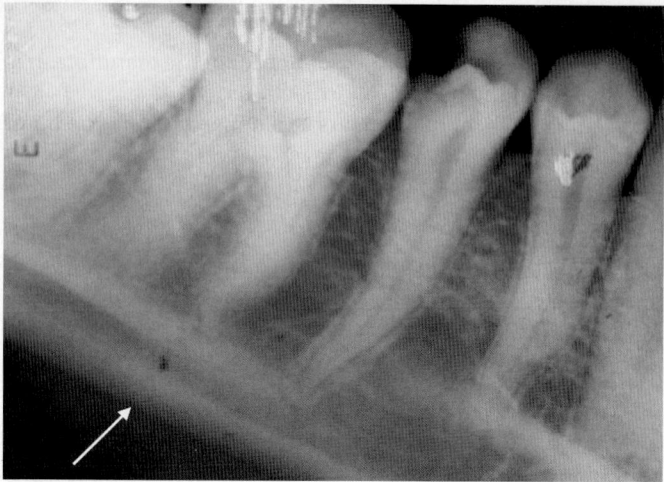

Figure 16.32 The inferior border of the mandible is seen as a dense, broad radiopaque band

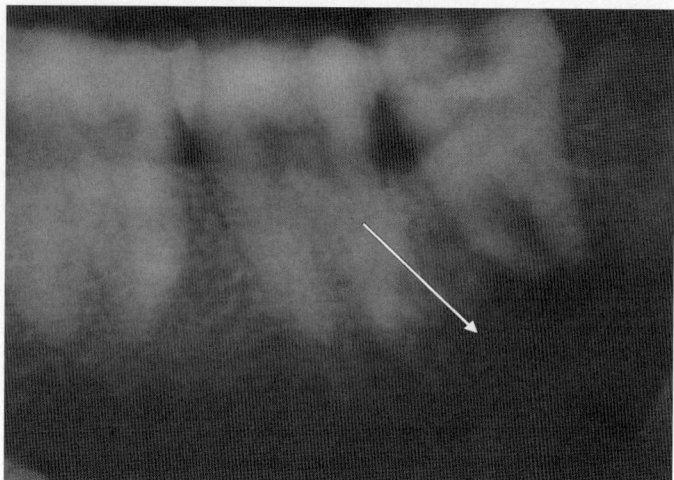

Figure 16.34 Submandibular fossa

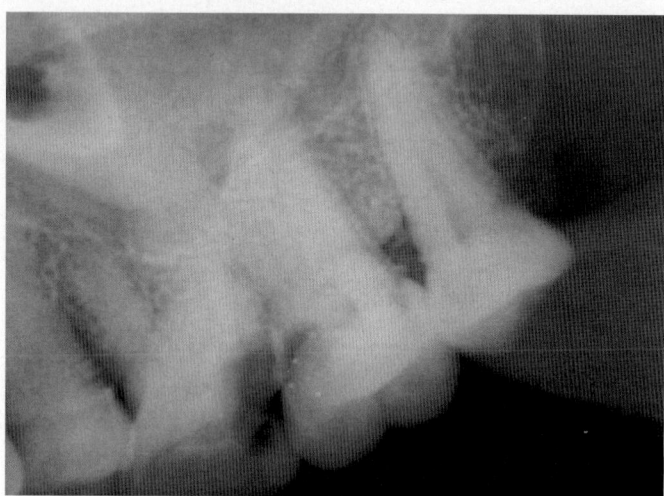

Figure 16.33 Coronoid process is seen as a triangular radiopacity superimposed over or inferior to the maxillary tuberosity region

Various restorative materials recognized on an intraoral radiographs are (**Figs 16.35A to G**):

- Silver amalgam : Completely radiopaque
- Gold : Completely radiopaque
- Stainless steel : Completely radiopaque
- Calcium : Generally radiopaque, but hydroxide base may be radiolucent
- Gutta percha : Radiopaque
- Silver points : Completely radiopaque
- Silicates : Completely radiolucent
- Composites : Appears radiolucent, may occasionally be radiopaque
- Porcelain : Appears radiolucent

BASICS IN INTERPRETING RADIOGRAPHS

Radiographic interpretation is an essential part of diagnostic process. The ability to recognize what is revealed by a radiograph enables a dental professional to play a vital role in the detection of diseases, lesions and conditions of the jaw that cannot be identified clinically.

One has to define the difference between:
- *Interpretation*: Refers to an explanation of what is viewed on the radiograph.
- *Diagnosis*: Refers to the identification of disease by examination or analysis.

In dentistry, a diagnosis is made by the dentist after a thorough review of medical history, dental history, clinical examination, radiographic examination, and clinical or laboratory tests.

For accurate diagnostic information to be interpreted there should be ideal viewing conditions:
- Reduced ambient light in the viewing room
- Intraoral radiographs should be mounted in a film holder
- Light from the view box should be of equal intensity across the viewing surface
- The size of the view box should accommodate the size of the film
- An intense light source is essential for evaluating dark regions of the film
- A magnifying glass allows detailed examination of small regions of the film.

In order to correctly and competently interpret a radiograph, the dental professional must be well versed in identification and recognition of the normal anatomical structures and their variations seen in the radiographs taken of the various regions.

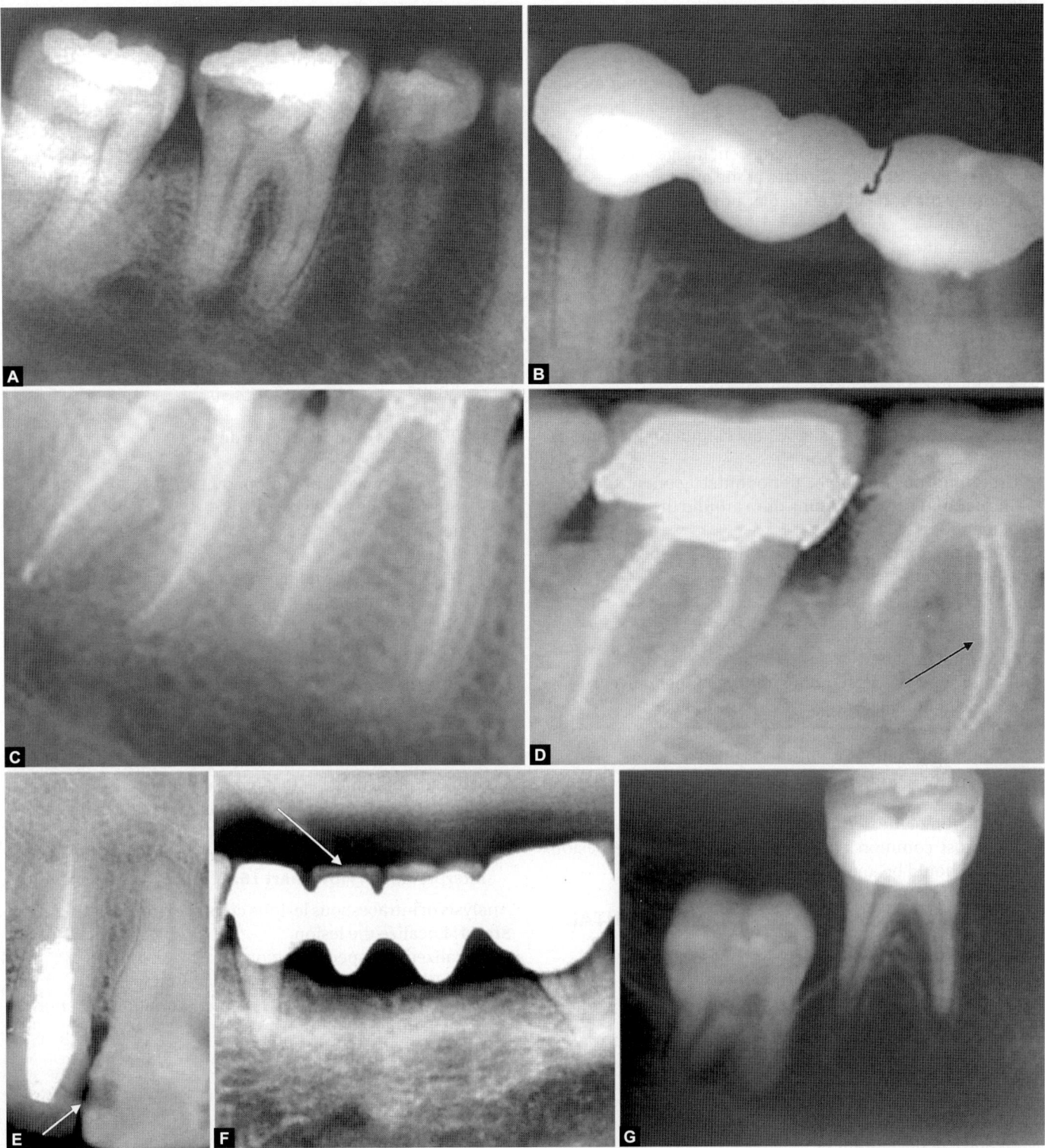

Figures 16.35A to G (A) Amalgam restorations seen as radio opacities; (B) Cast crowns appear completely radiopaque; (C) Radiopaque gutta percha material used for root canal filling; (D) Radiopaque silver points; (E) Silicate restorations appear radiolucent; (F) Porcelain appears radiolucent over metal capping; (G) Characteristic radiopaque appearance of orthodontic appliances

For intraoral images:
- Examination of the periapical image should be done before that of the bitewing image.
- Identify the normal anatomical landmarks of that region.
- Examine the character of the trabeculae of bone, the density, size, etc.
- Compare the same areas on adjacent images and with the corresponding area on images of the other side.
- Examine the bone of the alveolar process:
  - Height
  - Cortication
  - Erosion
  - Trabecular pattern of the alveolar bone.
- Examine each tooth in sequence:
  - The crown for normal development of enamel, caries, especially interproximal areas.
  - Check restorations for recurrent caries.
  - Examine the pulp chamber for size.
  - Examine roots for shape, developmental anomalies and external resorption.
- Uniformity of width of the periodontal ligament space.
- The continuity of the lamina dura around the entire length of the root.
- The most common abnormalities found in bone are either:
  - Radiolucent lesions
  - Radiopaque lesions.
    which need to be analyzed.

For extraoral images:
- A thorough understanding of the appearance of the normal anatomical structures on the image.
  - The absence of a normal anatomic structure may be the most important finding on the image.
- Examination and identification of normal soft tissues shadows.
- Evaluation of the dentition and supporting bone.
- The most common pathologies are intraosseous lesions which should be analyzed.

SYSTEMIC SEQUENCE FOR VIEWING A DENTAL PANORAMIC RADIOGRAPH

- General overview of the entire film.
  - Note the chronological and developmental age of the patient
  - Trace the outline of all normal anatomical shadows and compare their shape and radiodensity.
- The teeth.
  - Number of teeth present
  - Stage of development
  - Position
  - Condition of the crowns.
    - Caries
    - Restorations.

- Condition of the roots.
  - Length
  - Fillings
  - Resorption
  - Crown/root ratio.
- The apical tissues.
  - Integrity of lamina dura
  - Any radiolucency or radiopacity associated with the apices.
- The periodontal tissues.
  - The width of the periodontal ligament
  - The level and quality of crestal bone
  - Any vertical or horizontal bone loss
  - Any furcation involvements
  - Any calculus deposits.
- The body and the ramus of the mandible.
  - Shape
  - Outline
  - Thickness of the lower border
  - Trabeculae pattern
  - Any radiolucent or radiopaque areas
  - Shape of the condylar heads.
- Other structures.
  - The antra
    - Outline of the floor, and anterior and posterior walls
    - Radiodensity.
  - Nasal cavity
  - Styloid process.

Analysis of Intraosseous Lesions

There are two basic approaches:
1. *Aunt minnie method*: This involves trying to match the radiographic image with a mental picture.
2. *Five step, step-by-step analysis method*: This helps ensure recognition and collection of all the information contained in the image and in turns improves the accuracy of the interpretation (**Flow chart 16.1**).

Analysis of intraosseous lesions consist of the following steps:
Step 1: Localize the lesion.
- Localized to a specific region
  - *Unilateral*: More likely to be a pathology.
  - *Bilateral*: More likely to be variation of normal structures.
- Generalized
  - Metabolic disturbance
  - Endocrinal disturbance.
- Position in the jaws
  - Within the jaws
  - In the soft tissue.
- Position of the epicenter.
  - *Coronal to the tooth*: Composed of odontogenic epithelium

Flow chart 16.1 An algorithm representing the diagnostic process that follows evaluation of the radiographic features of an abnormality

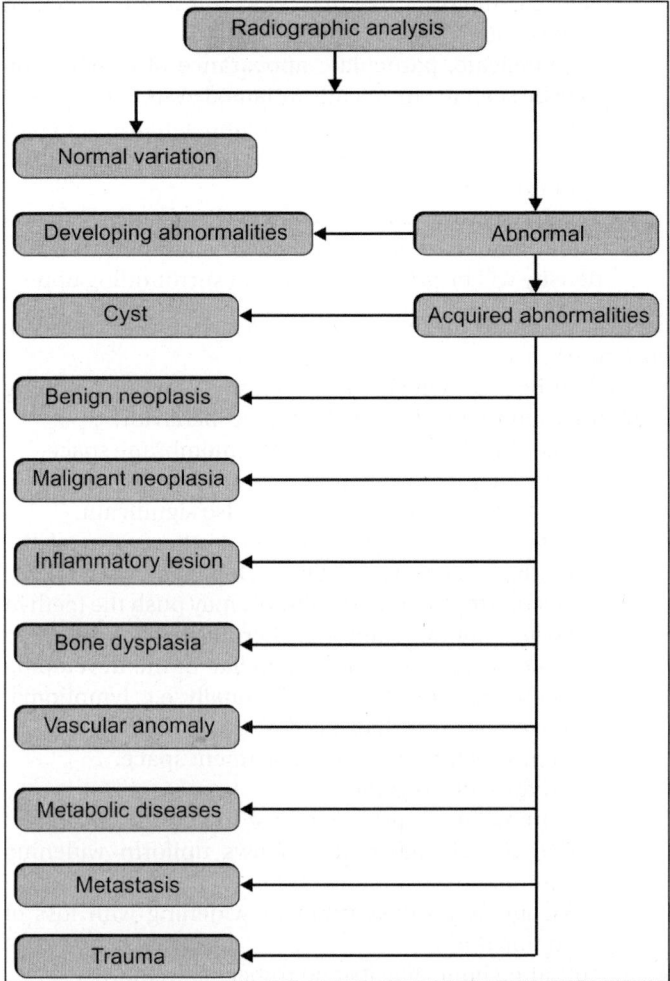

– *Above the inferior alveolar nerve*: Composed of odontogenic tissue.
– *Below the inferior alveolar nerve*: Unlikely to be composed of odontogenic tissue.
– *Within the inferior alveolar nerve*: Composed of neural or vascular tissue.
– *In the condylar region*: Cartilaginous lesions and osteochondromas.
– Within the maxillary antrum not of odontogenic tissue.
– *Grown into the antrum from the alveolar process*: Of odontogenic origin.

Some lesions have specific locations and epicenters:
– Central giant cell granuloma, the epicenter is located
  - Anterior to the first molars in the mandible
  - Anterior to the cuspid in the maxilla.
– Periapical cemental dysplasia occurs in the periapical region of the teeth.

– Osteomyelitis occurs in the mandible and rarely in the maxilla.
• Number
  – Single
  – Multifocal
    - E.g. periapical cemental dysplasia
    - Metastatic lesions
    - Multiple myeloma.
• *Size*: There are few size restrictions for a particular lesion, but it may aid in differential diagnosis, e.g. A dentigerous cyst is often larger than an erupting follicle.

Step 2: Evaluate the periphery and shape.
• Periphery
  – *Well-defined*: This is one in which most of the periphery is well-defined.
    - Punched out border, is a sharp border with no apparent bone reaction in the adjacent region, e.g. multiple myeloma.
    - Corticated margin, is a thin fairly uniform radiopaque line of reactive bone at the periphery, e.g. cysts.
    - Sclerotic margin, is a wide radiopaque border of reactive bone, not necessarily of uniform width, e.g. periapical cemental dysplasia.
    - Radiolucent line around radiopaque lesions, indicates a soft tissue capsule which may be in conjunction with a corticated periphery, e.g. odontomas, cementomas.
  – *Ill-defined*: This is one in which it is difficult to draw an exact delineation around most of an ill-defined periphery.
    - Blending border, it is ill-defined because of gradual transition between normal appearing bone trabeculae and abnormal appearing trabeculae of the lesion, e.g. fibrous dysplasia, sclerosing osteitis.
    - Invasive border or permeative border, is usually associated with rapid growth, e.g. malignancy.
• *Shape*: A lesion may have a particular shape or it may be irregular.
  – Circular or fluid filled, e.g. cyst.
  – Scalloped shape, this is a series of arcs or semi circles which may reflect the mechanism of growth, e.g. odontogenic keratocyst, benign tumors.

Step 3: Assess the internal structure (**Tables 16.1 to 16.3**).
• *Radiolucent*: e.g. air, fluid, soft tissue, bone marrow.
• *Mixed*: E.g. trabecular bone.
• *Radiopaque*: E.g. cortical bone, dentin, enamel, metal.

Common mixed density lesions:
• Orange peel or ground glass appearance as in fibrous dysplasia.
• Presence of septa (residual bone) may divide the internal structure into compartments (multilocular);

Table 16.1 Commonly occurring radiopaque lesions

Abnormalities of teeth
- Unerupted and misplaced teeth including supernumeraries.
- Odontomes
  - Compound
  - Complex
- Root remnants
- Hypercementosis

Conditions of variable radiopacity effecting the bone
- Developmental
  - Exostoses including tori-mandibular or palatal
- Inflammatory
  - Low grade infections
  - Sclerosing osteitis
  - Osteomyelitis—sequestra and involucrum formation
- Tumors
  - Odontogenic (late stages)
    - Calcifying epithelial odontogenic tumor (CEOT)
    - Adenomatoid odontogenic tumor
    - Calcifying odontogenic cyst
  - Nonodontogenic
    - Benign
      i. Osteoma
      ii. Chondroma
    - Malignant
      i. Osteosarcoma
      ii. Osteogenic secondary metastases
- Fibro-osseous lesions (late stages)
  - Fibrous dysplasia
  - Ossifying fibroma
  - Cementifying fibroma
  - True cementoma (cementoblastoma)
  - Periapical cemental dysplasia
  - Gigantiform cementoma
- Others
  - Paget's disease
  - Osteopetrosis

Superimposed soft tissue calcifications
- Salivary calculi
- Calcified lymph nodes
- Calcified tonsils
- Phleboliths
- Calcified acne scars

Foreign bodies
- Intrabony
- Within the soft tissues on or overlying the skin

- Curved coarse septa, giving an internal pattern of soap bubble appearance, e.g. ameloblastoma, odontogenic keratocysts.
- Wipsy or granular septa seen in giant cell granuloma.
- Small straight septa, tennis racket appearance, as seen in odontogenic myxoma.

- Dystrophic calcification, is one which occurs in damaged soft tissue.
  - Dense cauliflower like masses in soft tissue—calcified lymph nodes.
  - Very delicate, particulate appearance of calcification may be seen in chronically inflamed cysts.
- Cementum may have a homogeneous, dense, amorphorous structure and sometimes may be organized into round or oval shapes.
  - Tooth structure, can be recognized by the organization into enamel, dentin and pulp chamber. Internal density will be greater than that of surrounding bone.

Step 4: Evaluate the effects of the lesion on surrounding structures.

Evaluating the effects of the lesion on surrounding structures allows the observer to infer its behavior.
- Teeth, lamina dura and periodontal membrane space.
  - Displacement of teeth; indicates a slow growing lesion. The direction of displacement is also significant.
    - Lesion with an epicenter above the crown of the tooth, displace it apically, e.g. follicular cysts.
    - Lesions that start in the ramus, may push the teeth in an anterior direction, e.g. cherubism.
    - Lesions that grow in the papillae of the developing tooth, may push the tooth coronally, e.g. lymphoma, leukemia, langerhan's cell histiocytosis.
  - Widening of the periodontal ligament space.
    - Uniform or irregular
    - Lamina dura is present or lost
    - Orthodontic movement shows uniform widening without loss of lamina dura
    - Malignancy shows irregular widening with loss of lamina dura.
- Surrounding bone density and trabecular pattern.
  - The presence of reactive bone at the periphery, whether corticated or sclerotic signifies a slow benign growth.
- Inferior alveolar nerve and mental foramen.
  - Superior displacement of inferior alveolar canal—fibrous dysplasia.
  - Widening of the inferior alveolar canal with maintenance of cortical boundary—benign lesion of vascular or neural origin.
  - Irregular widening with cortical destruction—malignant neoplasm in the canal.
- Outer cortical bone and periosteal reactions.
  - Expanded bone with an outer cortical plate—slow growing lesion.
  - Expanded bone without the cortical plate—rapidly growing lesion.
  - Onion peel appearance, where the exudates from an inflammatory lesion lifts the periosteum off the surface of cortical bone and then stimulate periosteum to lay down new bone, and this process occurs more

Table 16.2 Commonly occurring radiolucent lesions

Unilocular	Multilocular or psuedolocular	Lesions which may develop internal radiopaque calcifications
Radicular cysts	Odontogenic keratocyst	Calcifying epithelial odontogenic tumor
Dentigerous cyst	Ameloblastoma	Adenomatoid odontogenic tumor
Nasopalatine duct cyst	Ameloblastic fibroma	Calcifying odontogenic cyst
Median mandibular cyst	Odontogenic fibroma	Chondroma
Solitary bone cyst	Odontogenic myxoma giant cell lesions	Fibro-osseous lesions
Secondary (metastatic) tumor	Granuloma brown tumor cherubism	Osteogenic sarcoma
Calcifying epithelial odontogenic cyst	Aneurysmal bone cyst	Cancellous osteoma
Adenomatoid odontogenic tumor		Fibrous dysplasia
Multiple myeloma		Ossifying fibroma
Eosinophillic granuloma		Cementifying fibroma
Fibro-osseous lesions		Gigantiform cementoma
Stafne's bone cavity		Periapical cemental dysplasia
		True cementoma (cementoblastoma)

Table 16.3 Typical radiographic description of various oral lesions as seen on the radiograph

Contd...

Ball in hand appearance	Benign salivary gland tumors
Balloon like appearance	• Follicular cysts • Aneurysmal bone cyst
Candlestick appearance	Pyknodysostosis
Cart wheel appearance	Central hemangioma
Chalk-like appearance	• Osteopetrosis • (Marble bone disease) • Hyperparathyroidism • Pyknodysostosis
Cherry blossom pattern	Sialograph of Sjögrens syndrome
Codman's triangle	Osteosarcoma
Cotton-wool appearance	• Fibrous dysplasia • Odontogenic fibroma • Pagets disease
Driven snow appearance	Pindborg's tumor (CEOT)
Egg shell appearance	• Ameloblastoma • Multilocular cyst
Filling defect	Salivary gland tumor
Floating teeth appearance	Squamous cell carcinoma • Malignant lymphoma • Eosinophillic granuloma • Osteomyelitis • Periodontitis • Papillon-Lefevre syndrome
Ghost teeth	Odontogenesis dysplasia
Ground glass appearance	• Fibrous dysplasia • Ossifying fibroma • Osteosarcoma • Hyperparathyroidism • Paget's disease • Rickets

Hair on end appearance	• Thalassemia • Sickle cell anemia
Heart shaped radiolucency	Incisive canal cyst
Honey comb appearance	• Ameloblastoma • Central hemangioma • Dentigerous cyst • Central giant cell granuloma
Moth eaten appearance*	• Squamous cell carcinoma • Malignant lymphoma • Chronic osteomyelitis
Mottled appearance	• Fibrous dysplasia • Ossifying fibroma
Onion-peel appearance	• Garre's osteomyelitis • Eosinophilic granuloma • Ewing's sarcoma • Infantile cortical hyperostosis • Osteogenic sarcoma • Ossifying subperiosteal hematoma
Orange peel appearance	• Fibrous dysplasia • Hyperparathyroidism • Paget's disease • Rickets
Permeated appearance	• Carcinoma of the gingiva carcinoma of the maxilla • Malignant lymphoma
Pear shaped appearance	• Globulomaxillary cyst • Radicular cyst
Pencil like appearance	Artheritic condyle
Pressure type appearance	Carcinoma of the gingiva
Punched out appearance	Multiple myeloma

Contd...   *Contd...*

Contd...

Sand like appearance	• Adenoameloblastoma • Gorlin's cyst • Pindborg tumor
Salt and pepper appearance	Hyperparathyroidism
Scalloping pattern (margins)	• Dentigerous cyst • Traumatic bone cyst • Aneurysmal bone cyst • Giant cell granuloma
Shell teeth	Dentinogenesis imperfecta
Soap bubble appearance**	• Ameloblastoma • Giant cell tumor • Central hemangioma • Aneurysmal cyst
Spiked root	• Malignant histiocytoma • Burkitttumor
Spokes wheel appearance	Central hemangioma
Sunray (burst) appearance	• Osteosarcoma • Ewing's sarcoma
Tennis racket appearance	Odontogenic myxoma
Worm eaten appearance*	• Carcinoma • Malignant lymphoma • Chronic osteomyelitis

*Moth eaten appearance and worm eaten appearance are used interchangeably. Moth eaten refers to a smaller circular cysts like radiolucencies of even sizes.
**Soap bubble appearance refers to circular cyst like radiolucencies of various sizes, bigger than those in 'moth-eaten'

than once, inflammatory lesion and in rare malignant lesions (leukemia) and Langerhans cell histiocytosis.
– Some periosteal reactions are specific:
  - Spiculated new bone formed at right angles to the outer cortical plate
  - Hair on end appearance, thalassemia, sickle cell anemia
  - Radiating pattern—osteogenic sarcoma.
– Root resorption (**Table 16.4**).

Step 5: Radiographic interpretation.
• *Normal versus abnormal*: Normal or variation from the normal requires no treatment.
• *Developmental versus acquired*: If the abnormality is developmental, no further assessment required.

Table 16.4 Causes of external resorption of tooth

Physiological	*Pathological*
Deciduous dentition	• Reimplanted teeth • Nonvital teeth • Unerupted teeth • Retained roots • Impacted teeth • Orthodontic treatment • Traumatic occlusion • Foreign body • Tooth fracture • Cyst • Giant cell lesion • Hyperparathyroidism • Idiopathic

• *Classification*: If the abnormality is acquired, then the next step is to classify it, into cyst, benign or malignant tumor, inflammatory lesion, bone dysplasia, vascular abnormalities, metabolic diseases or physical changes.
• *Advanced investigations*
  – Any other radiographs
  – Biopsy
  – Put the patient under observation.

BIBLIOGRAPHY

1. Atchison KA, White SC, Flack VF, et al. Assessing the FDA guidelines for ordering dental radiographs. JADA. 1995;126(10):1372-83.
2. Brand RW, Isselhard DE. Osteology of the skull. In: Anatomy of Orofacial Structures, 4th edition. St Louis: CV Mosby; 1990.pp.117-3.
3. Goaz PW, White SC. In: Oral Radiology, Principles and Interpretation, 3rd edition. St Louis: CV Mosby; 1994.
4. Haring JI, Lind LJ. Normal anatomy. In: Radiographic Interpretation for Dental Hygienist. Philadelphia: WB Saunders; 1993.pp.25-81.
5. Miles DA, Van Dis ML, Jensen CW, et al. Interpretation: Normal versus abnormal and common radiographic presentation of lesions. In: Radiographic Imaging for Dental Auxiliaries, 3rd edition. Philadelphia: WB Saunders; 1999.pp.231-80.
6. Recommendations in radiographic practices: an update, 1988.
7. Worth HM. Principles and Practice of Oral Radiologic Interpretation. Chicago: Mosby; 1972.

Dental Caries | 17

Dental caries is an infectious microbial disease of the calcified tissues of the teeth characterized by demineralization of the inorganic portion and destruction of the organic substance of the tooth. 'Caries' is a Latin word which means to 'rot'. It affects nearly 95% of the population.

Since caries causes demineralization of the tooth, it can be diagnosed on the radiograph (after approximately 40% demineralization is achieved), as the lesion allows greater passage of X-rays as compared to the surrounding structures and hence appears more radiolucent.

Intraoral radiography can reveal caries lesions that otherwise might go undetected, especially in case of proximal lesions. However, it must be kept in mind that both clinical and radiographic examinations play a vital role in the detection of dental caries.

Various radiographs for caries detection:
- *Bitewing*: Aids in detecting caries in interproximal areas and distal ends of premolars and molars, and caries at CE junction.
- *Periapical*: Aids in detecting gross carious lesions, root caries and changes in the apical and inter-radicular bone due to caries.
- *OPG*: Useful to examine a case with multiple carious teeth or rampant caries.

Dental panoramic tomographs and CBCT are not recommended for the diagnosis of caries.

The limitation of a radiograph is that it is a two-dimensional representation of a three-dimensional object, thus, the exact site of caries cannot be located.

Digital image receptors are now available but the disadvantage of using the sensor is that the sensor is smaller than the size 2 film, thus, fewer interproximal tooth surfaces per bitewing image are seen, the stiffness and thickness of these sensors may result in projection errors and retakes.

Radiographic appearance of caries may be studied as (**Figs 17.1A to J**):
- According to the severity and extent of the lesion:
  - Incipient
  - Moderate
  - Advanced
  - Severe.
- According to the location on the tooth:

- Pit and fissure caries
  - Occlusal
  - Buccal/Lingual pit.
- Smooth surface caries
  - Proximal
  - Buccal or lingual surfaces
  - Root surface caries.
- Recurrent caries
  - According to etiology
    - Recurrent caries
    - Rampant caries
    - Radiation caries.

*Proximal caries (**Fig 17.1 A to J**)*: Caries found on the smooth surfaces between two teeth. On a dental radiograph, interproximal caries is typically seen at or just below (apical to) the contact point. This area is difficult, if not impossible, to examine clinically with an explorer. Lesions confined to the enamel may not be evident radiographically until approximately 30–40% demineralization has occurred. It is found in the area between the contact point and the free gingival margin. The fact that the lesion does not start below the gingival margin helps distinguish a carious lesion from cervical burn out.

*Incipient interproximal caries (**Fig. 17.2**)*: This appears as a classical triangle with its broad base at the tooth surface spreading along the enamel rods; it may also appear as a 'notch', a dot, a band or a thin line. The early lesions do not extend more than half the thickness of enamel. A magnifying glass may be used for precise results.

*Moderate interproximal caries (**Fig. 17.3**)*: These lesions are those that involve more than the outer half of the enamel but are not seen extending into the DE junction.

These lesions may present three different appearances:
1. Triangular in shape with its base at the surface of the tooth (67%)
2. Diffuse radiolucent image (16%)
3. Combination of the above two (17%).
- *Advanced interproximal caries (**Fig. 17.2**)*: These lesions are those that have invaded the DE junction. It appears triangular and diffuse and in addition there is spreading of demineralization process at the DE junction, undermining

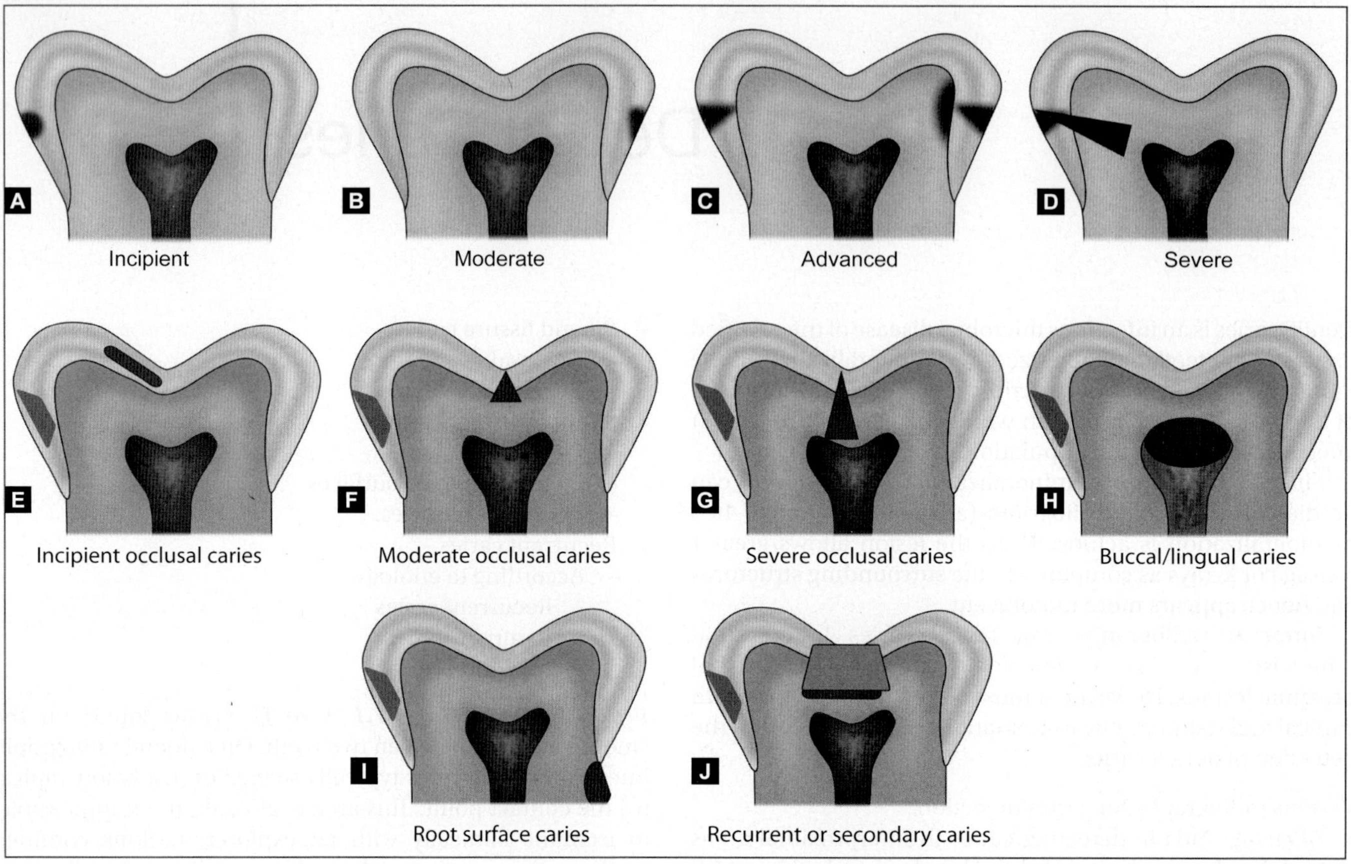

Incipient

Moderate

Advanced

Severe

Incipient occlusal caries

Moderate occlusal caries

Severe occlusal caries

Buccal/lingual caries

Root surface caries

Recurrent or secondary caries

Figures 17.1A to J Diagrammatic representation of caries: (A to D) Proximal; (E to G) Occlusal; (H) Buccal; (I) Root surface; (J) Secondary caries

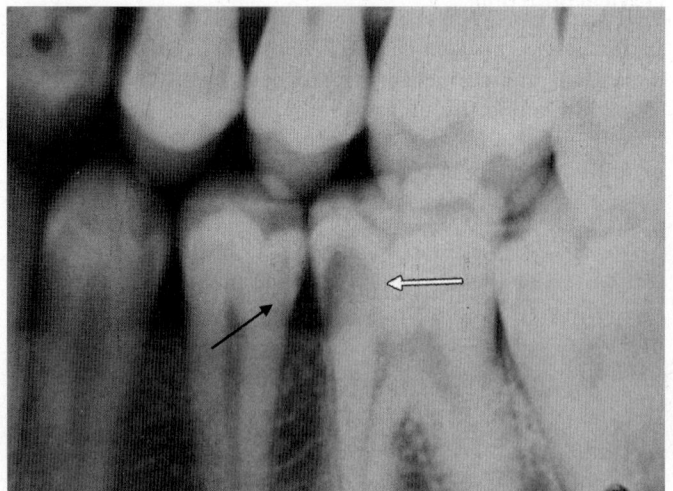

Figure 17.2 Radiographs showing incipient proximal lesion on mandibular premolar (black arrow) and advanced proximal caries molar (white arrow)

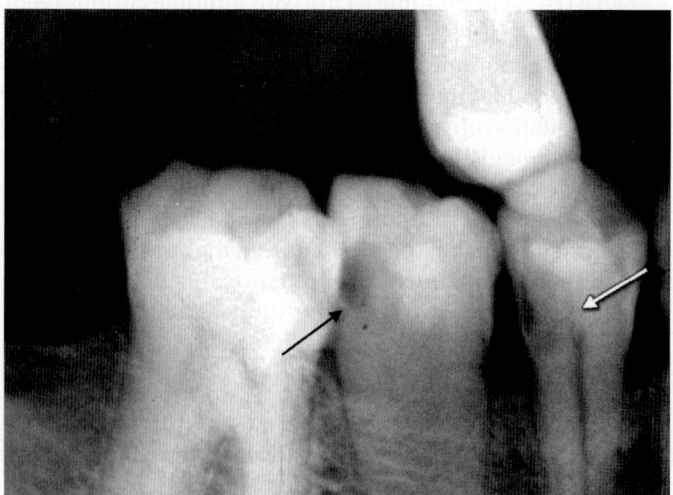

Figure 17.3 Radiographs showing severe proximal lesion on mandibular molar (black arrow) and moderate proximal caries premolar (white arrow)

the enamel and extending into the dentine and this forms a second triangular radiolucent image in the dentine with the base at the DE junction and the apex of the triangle is directed towards the pulp chamber. Usually the lesion does not spread beyond more than half the thickness of the dentine.

- *Severe proximal lesions (**Fig. 17.3**)*: The carious lesion are seen radiographically to have penetrated through more than half of dentine and is approaching the pulp chamber. The image usually reveals a narrow path of destruction through enamel; an expanded radiolucency at the DE junction. The lesion may or may not involve the pulp.

Occlusal caries or pit and fissure caries: Occlusal or pit and fissure caries usually involve the posterior teeth; the demineralization process originates in the enamel pits and fissures and is initially seen as a chalky white, yellow, brown or black discoloration of the occlusal fissures.

Three common errors in interpretation of occlusal caries:

1. Failure to recognize caries of enamel, because of superimposition of heavy cuspal enamel over the fissured (carious) areas.
2. Failure to carefully observe a thin radiolucency that first appears at the DE junction as the sign of occlusal caries.
3. Failure to distinguish between occlusal and buccal caries, because many a times the buccal grooves of the molars are superimposed over the occlusal areas and simulate occlusal lesions.

- *Incipient occlusal lesions (**Fig. 17.4**)*: Usually not detected on the radiograph unless the lesion has reached the dentine. The only change which may sometimes be detected is a fine grey shadow just below the DE junction. However, a similar but usually less broad shadow is frequently apparent on the image of the unaffected teeth

below or above the occlusal enamel, this line of increased density at the junction is an optical illusion called 'MACH BAND' effect. This phenomenon occurs along boundaries of relatively sharp contrast and is more pronounced when the contrast between adjacent areas is greater. This may also occur between a metallic restoration and sound enamel, such that it may be perceived as recurrent caries.

- *Moderate occlusal lesions (**Fig. 17.5**)*: These lesions have a classical radiographic change as a broad based thin radiolucent zone in the dentine with little or no change apparent in the enamel. Another manifestation of occlusal caries in the dentine is a band of increased opacity between the carious lesion and the pulp chamber. The band represents calcification within the primary dentine.
- *Severe occlusal lesions (**Fig. 17.6**)*: These lesions are readily observed clinically as a large cavity in the crown. It is important to note that pulp exposure cannot be determined by radiographs, and clinical examination should substantiate the X-ray impression.

*Buccal/facial/lingual/cervical caries (**Figs 17.7A and B**)*: It is difficult to differentiate between buccal and lingual caries on a radiograph, a clinical observation of the same is usually more direct and definitive. These occur in enamel pits and fissures. They appear as small round radiolucencies and become elliptical or semi lunar as the lesion enlarges. They have sharp well defined borders, with a uniform noncarious region of enamel surrounding the apparent radiolucency. It may be necessary to take more than one radiograph to rule out superimposition of the lesion on the DE junction which may suggest occlusal lesions. Occlusal lesions are usually more extensive and not as well defined. If the lesion extends up to the distal line angle it may project onto the proximal surface and appear as a proximal lesion.

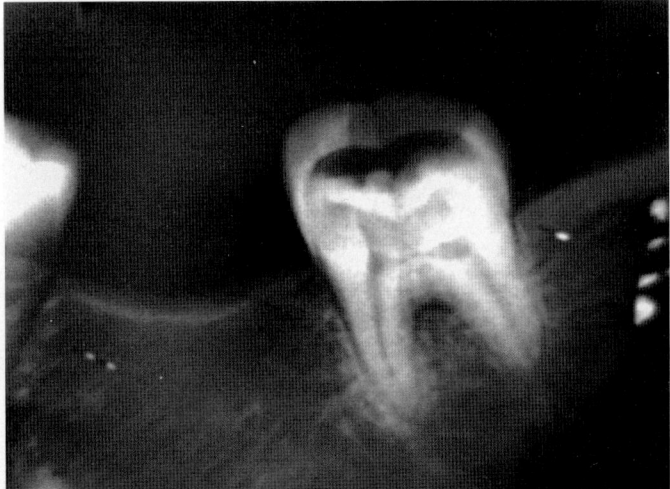

Figure 17.4 Radiographs showing incipient occlusal lesion in the mandibular molar

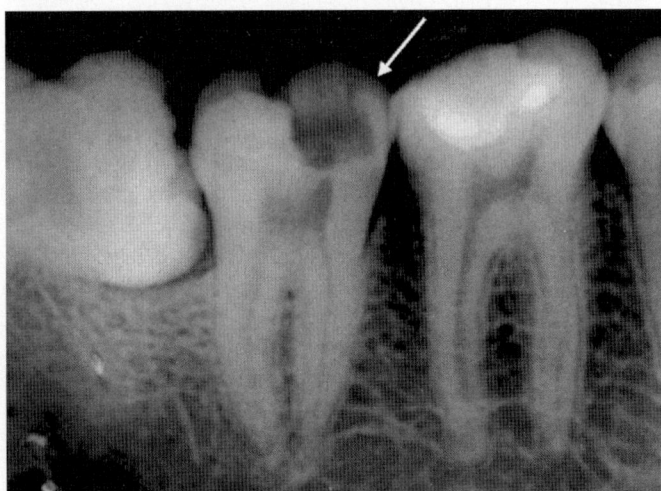

Figure 17.5 Radiographs showing moderate occlusal lesion in the mandibular molar (white arrow)

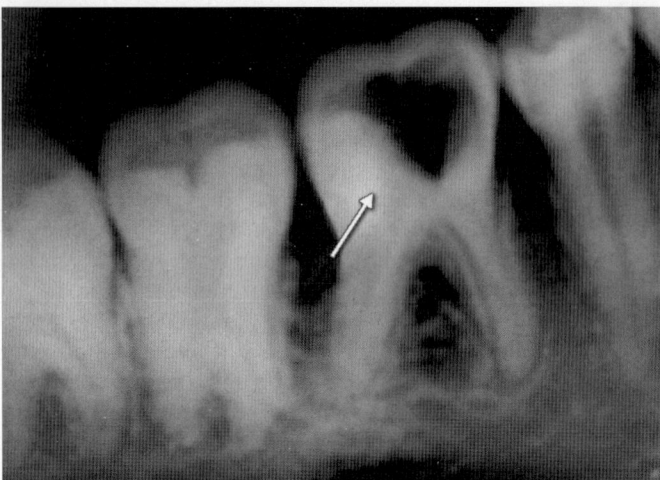

Figure 17.6 Radiographs showing advanced occlusal lesion in the mandibular molar (white arrow)

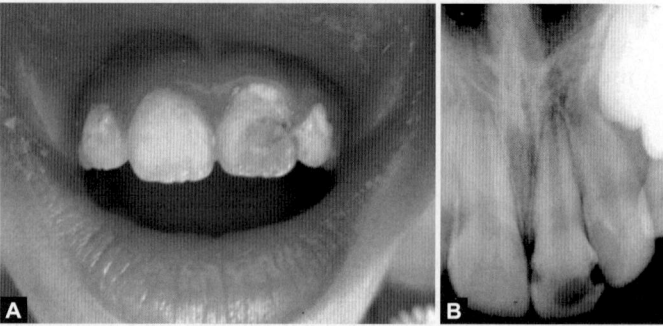

Figures 17.7A and B Facial caries on the labial aspect of the central incisor seen as a circular radiolucency overlapping the pulp chamber in the radiograph. The central also shows proximal caries on mesial and distal surface involving the enamel and dentine (*For color version see plate 1*)

*Root surface caries or cemental caries (**Fig. 17.8**)*: It involves both cementum and dentine. It is more common in mandibular molar and premolar region, most frequently affected tooth surfaces are buccal, lingual followed by the proximal surface. It develops due to the degradation of the exposed cementum by attrition, abrasion and erosion. The caries process is best described as a 'scooping out', which results in a radiographic appearance of an 'ill-defined saucer like crater' or when the peripheral surface area is small it appears 'notched'. Root caries does not generally involve the enamel except by extension into the dentine immediately under the enamel along the DE junction.

- Cervical burnout may simulate root caries, and should be distinguished from the true carious lesion by the absence of an image of the root edge and by the appearance of a diffuse rounded inner border where the tooth substance has been lost.

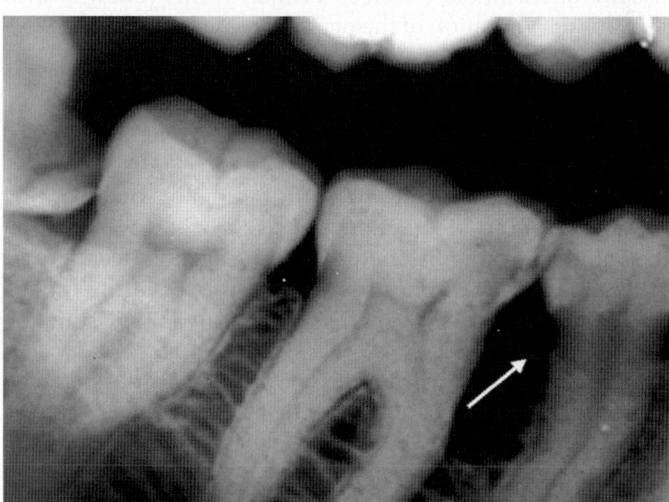

Figure 17.8 Radiographs showing root caries in mandibular premolar (white arrow)

*Recurrent caries or secondary caries (**Figs 17.9 and 17.10**)*: This usually develops at the margins of an existing restoration, which may be a direct result of poor marginal adaptation of the restoration or faulty shaping and inadequate extension.

- A lesion next to the restoration may be obscured by the radiopaque image of the restoration.
- Recurrent lesions of the mesiogingival and distogingival margins are most frequently detected radiographically.
- Restorative materials vary in their radiographic appearance depending on thickness, density, atomic number and the X-ray energy used to take the radiograph. Some materials may be confused with caries.

Rampant caries: This is commonly seen in children with poor dietary habits and poor oral hygiene, however, with water fluoridation and wide spread enlightening of good nutrition and oral hygiene the incidents of this type of caries is on

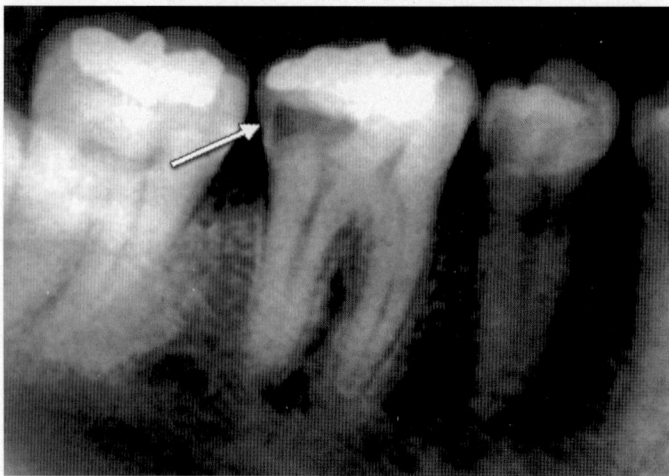

Figure 17.9 Radiographs showing secondary caries in mandibular first molar (white arrow)

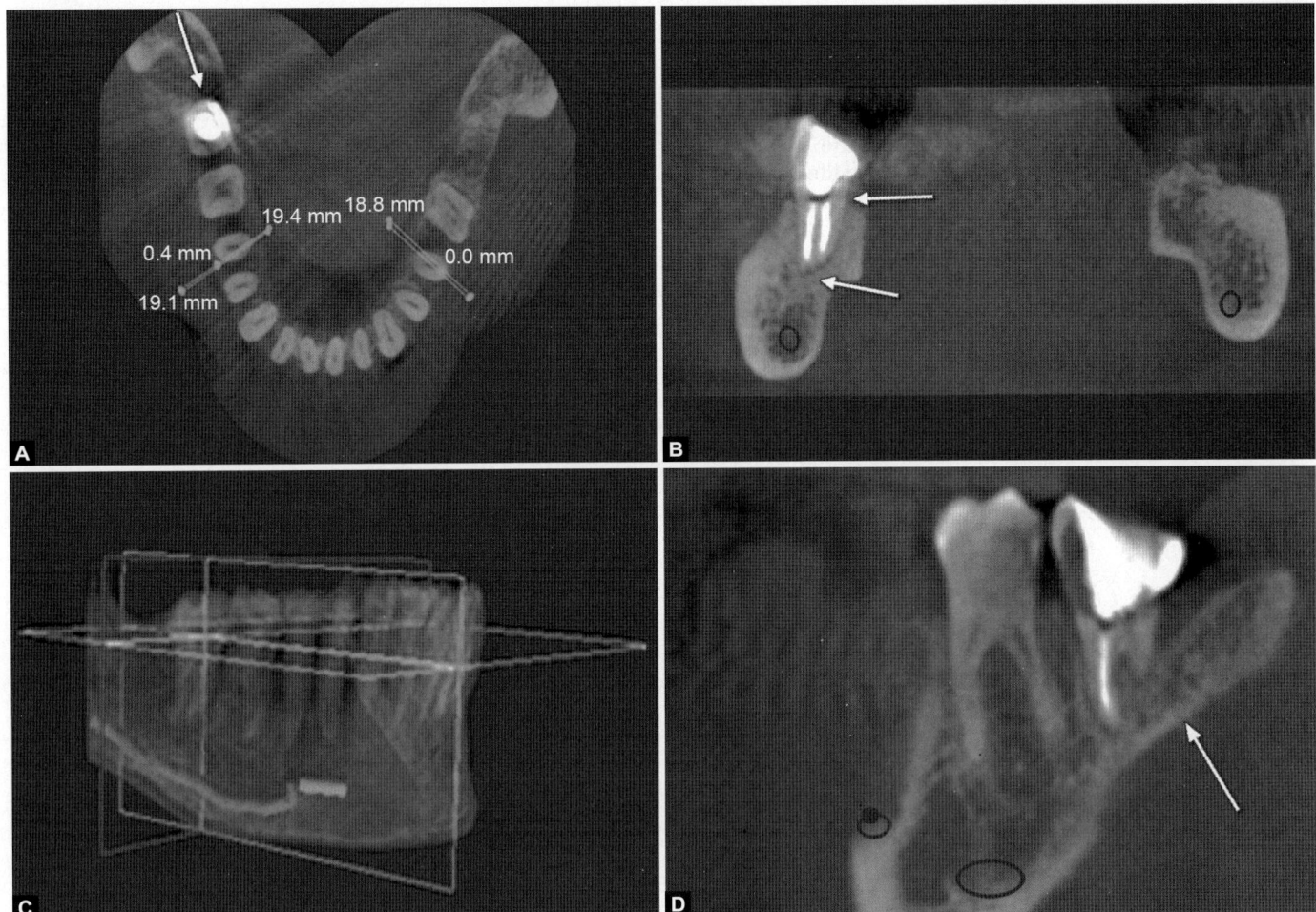

Figures 17.10A to D CBCT showing axial/coronal/3D/sagittal view. The mandibular second molar shows a large filing with root canal treatment, with recurrent caries below the radiopaque filling and a persistent radiolucency at the periapex

the decline. Radiographically it is seen as an extensive inter proximal caries involving almost the whole of the primary dentine.

Nursing bottle caries: This is caused due to prolonged bottle feeding, leading to early carious involvement especially of the maxillary anterior teeth, the maxillary and mandibular first permanent molars and the mandibular canines. Sometimes only the root stumps remain.

Pre-eruptive caries: This defect on the crowns of developing dental teeth are evident radiographically, even though no infection of the primary tooth or surrounding area is evident.

RADIOGRAPHIC DIFFERENTIAL DIAGNOSIS OF DENTAL CARIES

- *Erosion cavity*: These are saucer shaped and have sloping margins on the radiograph.
- *Nonopaque filling*: It should be distinguished by the sharpness and uniformity of the margins.

- *Cervical burn out*: It is usually located at the neck of the teeth, demarcated above by the enamel cap or restoration and below by the alveolar bone level, triangular in shape, gradually becoming less apparent towards the center of the tooth, the axial border fades or follows anatomical contour and the peripheral border appears intact. Usually all the teeth on the radiograph will appear to be affected.
- *Internal resorption*: The margins are well-defined and the normal margins of the pulp chamber are effaced.
- *External resorption*: Here the line of demarcation between the adjacent tooth substance and the defective area is sharp.
- *Hypoplasia of enamel*: Here the radiolucent areas are not single; several small dark spots are seen across the tooth.
  Unfortunately, radiographic interpretation of dental caries is not always straightforward. It is often complicated by two additional radiographic shadows:
- Radiolucent cervical burnout or translucency
- The radiopaque zone beneath amalgam restorations.

Radiolucent Cervical Burnout

This radiolucent shadow is often evident at the neck of the teeth, as illustrated in **Figures 17.11A and B**.

It is an artifactual phenomenon created by the anatomy of the teeth and the variable penetration of the X-ray beam. Cervical burnout can be explained by considering all the different parts of the tooth and supporting bone tissues that the same X-ray beam has to penetrate (**Figs 17.12A and B**):

- In the crown—the dense enamel cap and dentine
- In the neck—only dentine
- In the root—dentine and the buccal and lingual plates of alveolar bone.

Thus, at the edges of the teeth in the cervical region, there is less tissue for the X-ray beam to pass through. Less attenuation therefore takes place and virtually no opaque shadow is cast of this area on the radiograph. It therefore appears radiolucent, as if some cervical tooth tissue does not exist or that it has been apparently burnout. Cervical burnout is of diagnostic importance because of its similarity to the radiolucent shadows of cervical and recurrent caries.

However, burnout can usually be distinguished by the following characteristic features:

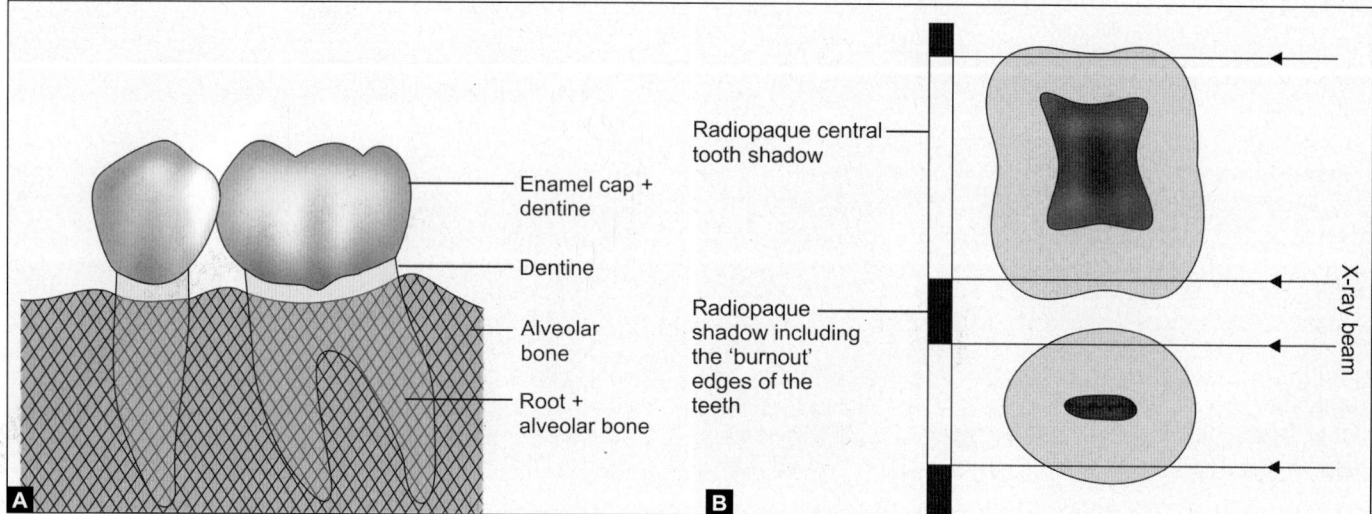

Figures 17.11A and B (A) Diagrammatic representation of lower premolar and molar showing the three-dimensional structures involved in the formation of the radiographic image. Note that there is less tissue present in the cervical region; (B) Axial view at the level of the necks of the teeth. Through the center of the teeth there is a large mass of dentine which absorbs the X-ray beam, while at the edges of the necks of the teeth there is only a small amount hence not dense enough to stop the X-ray beam, so their normally opaque shadows do not appear on the final radiograph

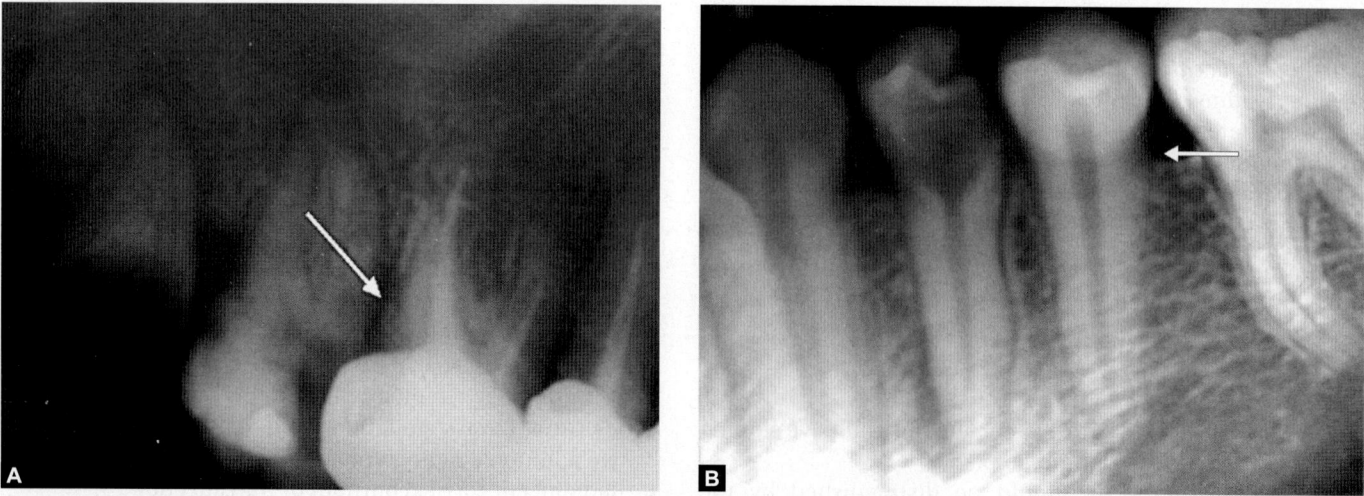

Figures 17.12A and B Cervical burn out: (A) Below the margin of the crown; (B) At the CE junction

- It is located at the neck of the teeth, demarcated above by the enamel cap or restoration and below by the alveolar bone level.
- It is triangular in shape, gradually becoming less apparent towards the center of the tooth.
- Usually all the teeth on the radiograph are affected, especially the smaller premolars.

In contrast, root and recurrent carious lesions, although they also often affect the cervical region, have no apparent upper and lower demarcating borders. These lesions are saucer-shaped and tend to be localized. If in doubt, the diagnosis should be confirmed clinically.

Important Points to Note

- Burnout is more obvious when the exposure factors are increased, as required ideally for detecting proximal caries.
- It is also more apparent by the perceptual problem of contrast if the tooth contains a metallic restoration, which may make the zone above the cervical shadow completely radiopaque. As this area is also the main site for recurrent caries, diagnosis is further complicated.

LIMITATIONS OF RADIOGRAPHIC DIAGNOSIS OF CARIES

In addition to the problems of diagnosis caused by the radiolucent and radiopaque shadows mentioned earlier, further limitations are imposed by the radiographic image. The main problems include:

- Carious lesions are usually larger clinically than they appear radiographically and very early lesions are not evident at all.
- Technique variations in film and X-ray beam positions can affect considerably the image of the carious lesion.

- Varying the horizontal tube head angulations can make a lesion confined to enamel appear to have progressed into dentine (**Figs 17.13A and B**)—hence the need for accurate, reproducible techniques
- Technique variations in vertical tube head position may cause recurrent carious lesions to be obscured (**Figs 17.14A to C**).
- Exposure factors can have a marked effect on the overall radiographic contrast and thus affect the appearance or size of carious lesions on the radiograph.
- Superimposition and a two-dimensional image mean that the following features cannot always be determined:
  - The exact site of a carious lesion, e.g. buccal or lingual
  - The buccolingual extent of a lesion
  - The distance between the carious lesion and the pulp horns. These two shadows can appear to be close together or even in contact but they may not be in the same plane.
  - The presence of an enamel lesion
  - The density of the overlying enamel may obscure the zone of decalcification
  - The presence of recurrent caries
  - Existing restorations may completely overlie the carious lesion (**Figs 17.15A to D**)
  - Only part of a restoration can be assessed radiographically
  - A dense radiopaque restoration may totally obscure a carious lesion in another part of the tooth
  - Recurrent caries at the base of an interproximal box may not be detected (**Figs 17.16A and B**).
- Cervical burnout shadows tend to be more obvious when their upper borders are demarcated by dense white restorations because of the increased contrast differences.

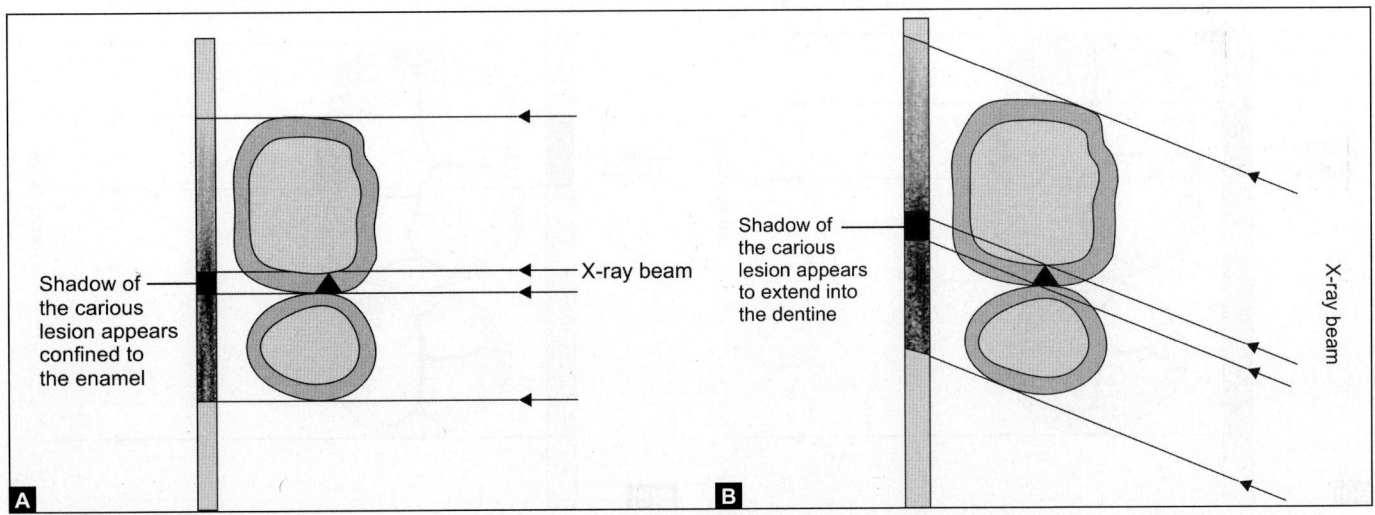

Figures 17.13A and B Diagrams showing how the appearance and extent of a carious lesion confined to enamel alter with change in horizontal X-ray beam angulations: (A) Ideal horizontal X-ray beam angulation; (B) Incorrect horizontal X-ray beam angulation

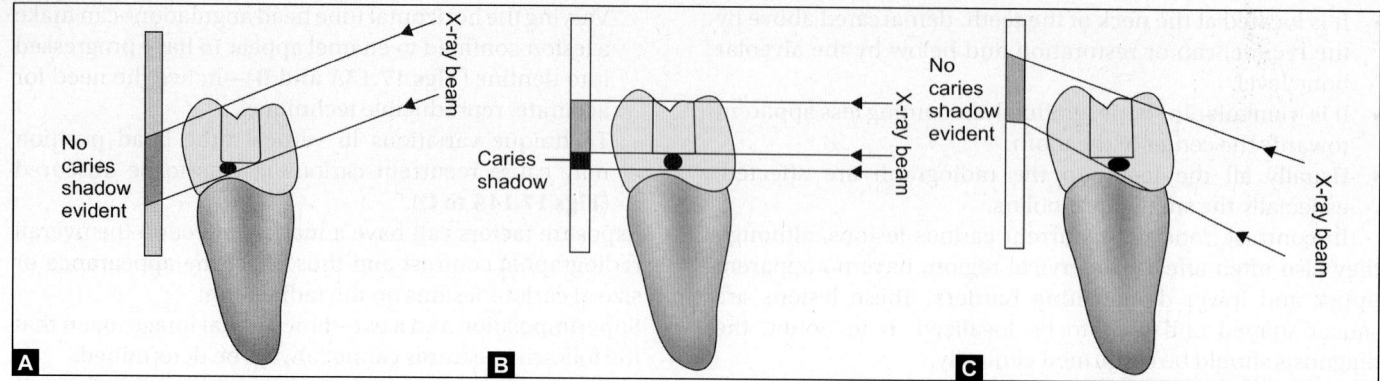

Figures 17.14A to C Diagrams showing the effect of incorrect vertical X-ray beam angulations in diagnosing recurrent lesions at the base of a restoration

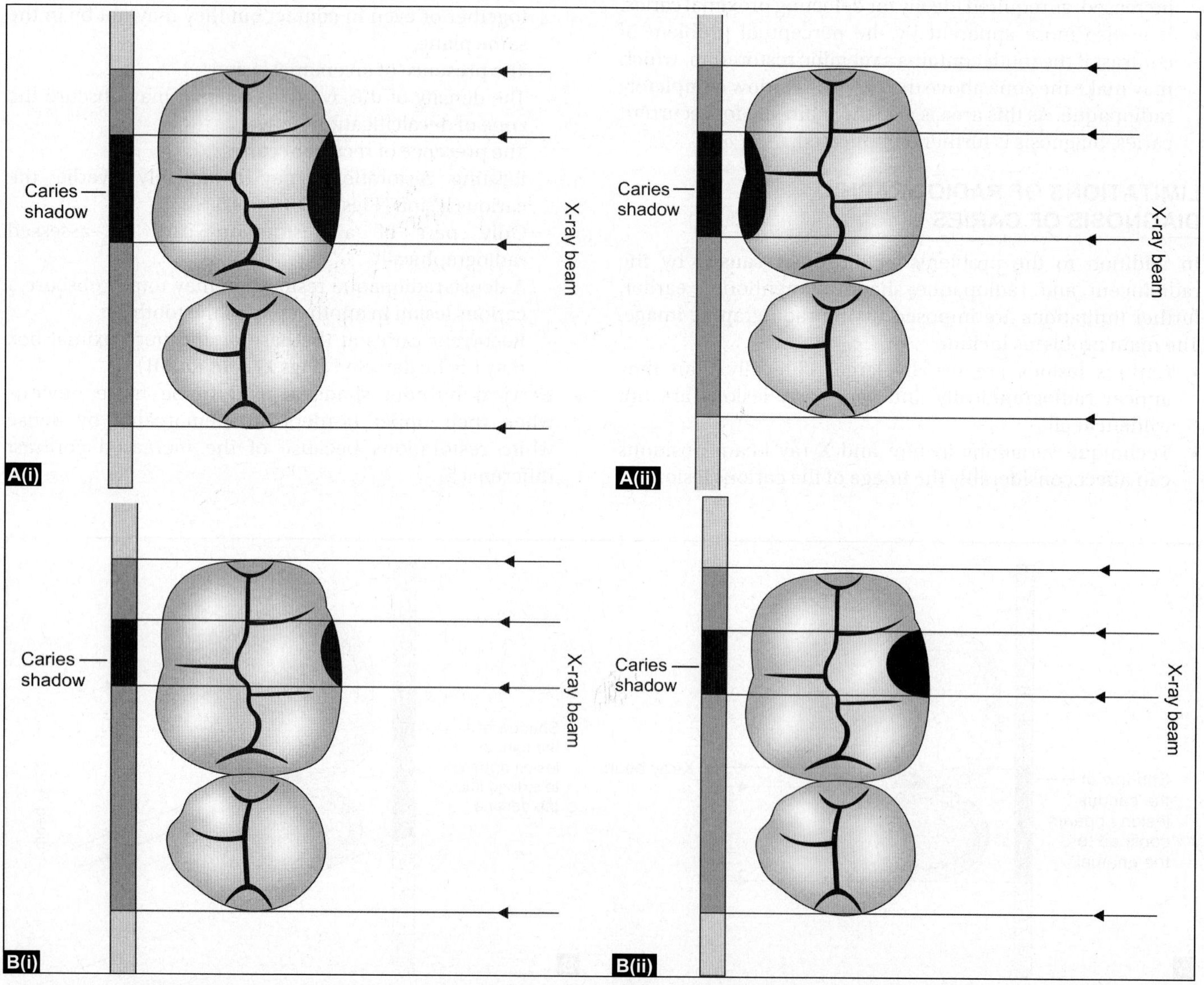

Figures 17.15A and B (A) Diagrams showing differently positioned lesions i. Buccal, ii. lingual, producing similar radiographic shadows; (B) Diagrams showing different sized buccal lesions; i. Shallow, ii. Deep, producing similar radiographic shadows

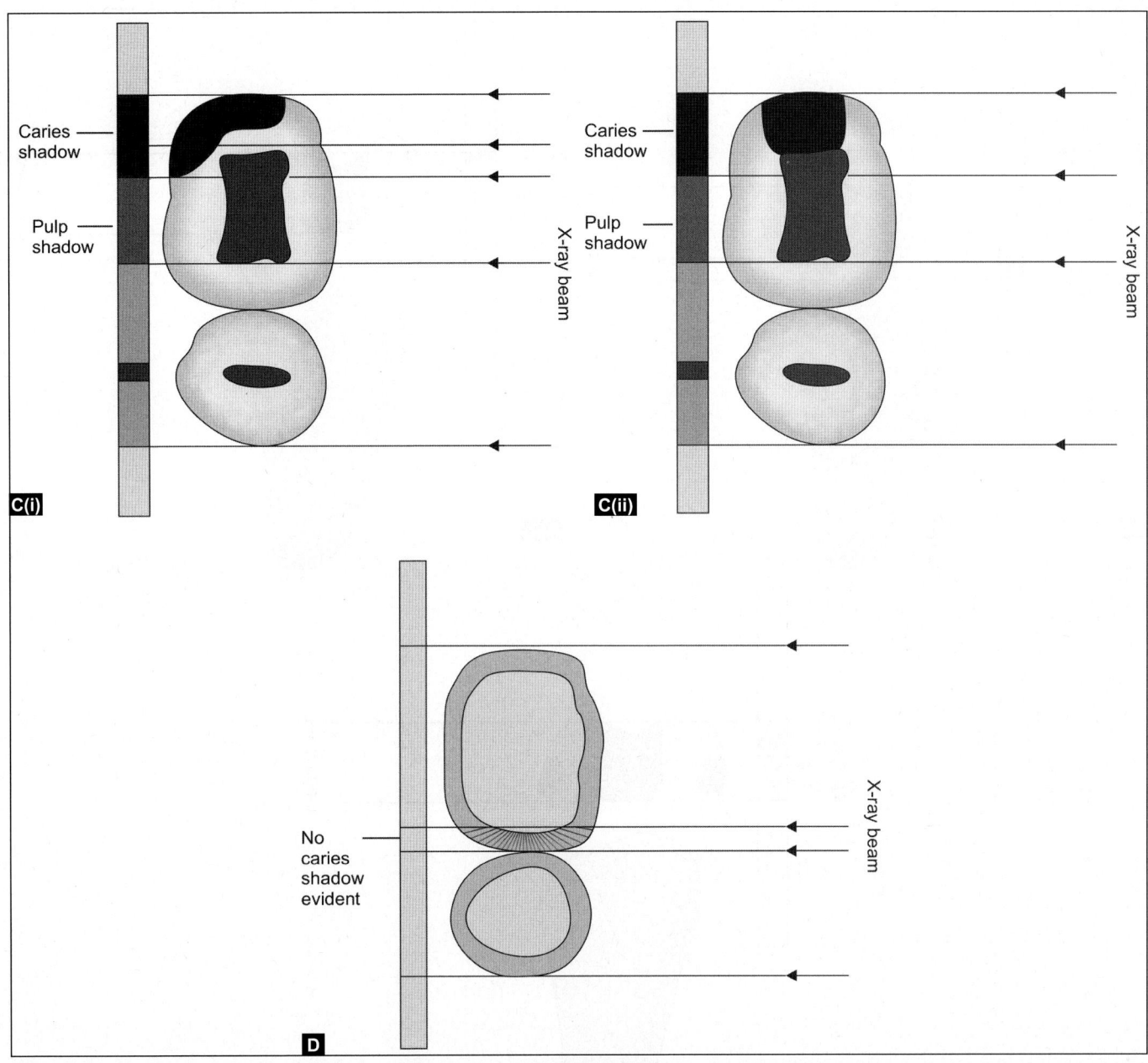

Figures 17.15C to D (C) Diagrams showing: i. A large proximal lesion superimposed over, but not involving the pulp; ii. A large proximal lesion involving the pulp, both producing similar radiographic shadows; (D) Diagram showing how a small lesion may not be evident radiographically if dense radiopaque enamel shadows are superimposed

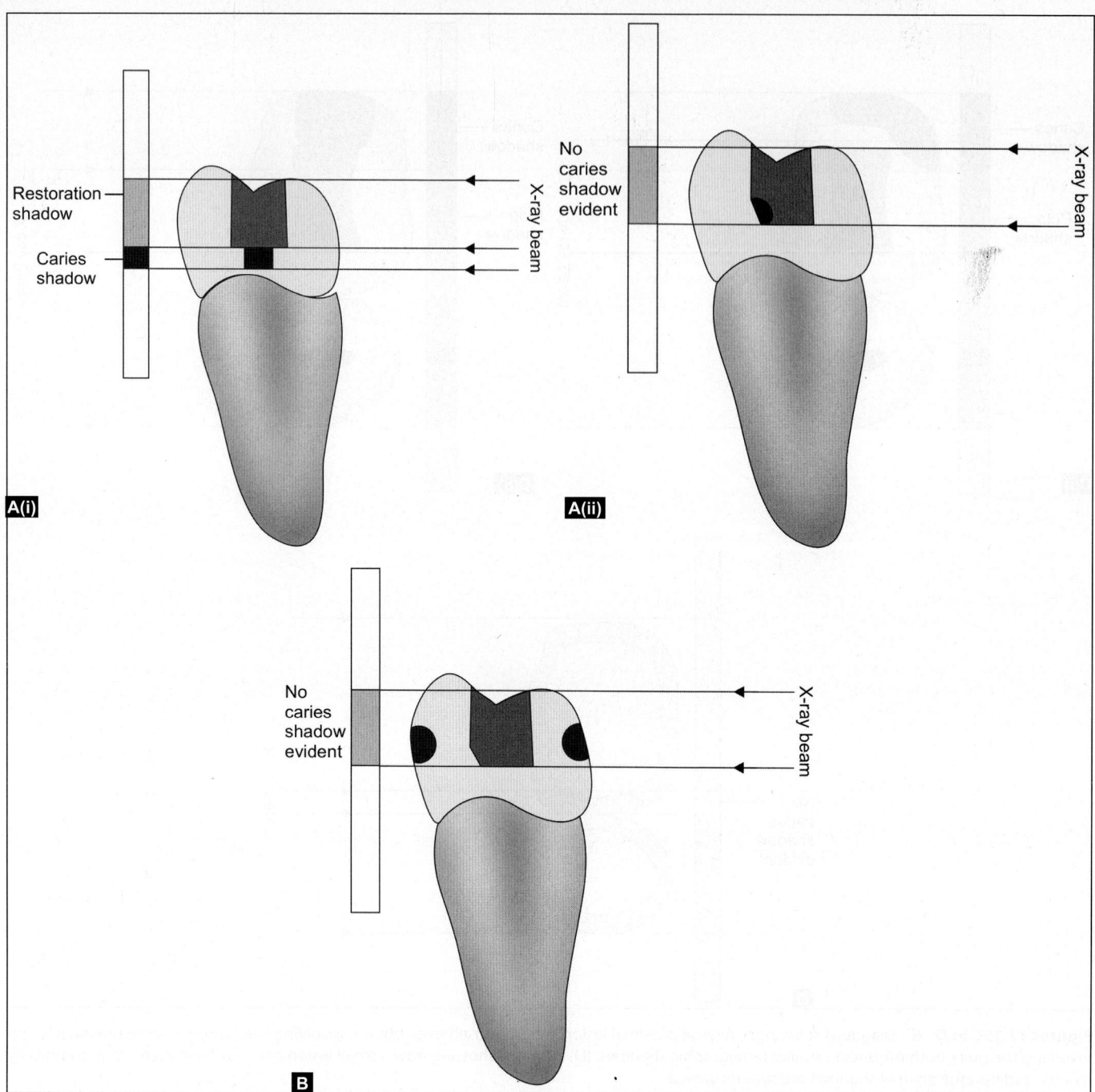

Figures 17.16A and B (A) Diagrams illustrating the difficulty of assessing caries beneath a restoration; (B) Diagram showing the difficulty of assessing buccal and lingual lesions in restored teeth

BIBLIOGRAPHY

1. De Araujo F, et al. Diagnosis of approximal caries: radiographic versus clinical examination using tooth separation. Am J Dent. 1992;5:245.

2. Kidd EAM, Pitts NB. A reappraisal of the value of the bitewing radiograph in the diagnosis of posterior proximal caries. Br Dent J. 1990;1689:195.

3. Miles DA, Van Dis MJ, Jensen CW, et al. Interpretation normal versus abnormal and common radiographic presentations of lesions. In: Radiographic and Imaging for Dental Auxillaries, 3rd edition. Philadelphia: WB Saunders; 1999.pp.231-80.

4. Shafer WG, et al. A Text Book of Oral Pathology. Philadelphia: WB Saunders; 1983.p.86.

5. Syriopoulos K, Sanderink GC, Velders XL et al. Radiographic detection of approximal caries: a comparison of dental films and digital imaging systems. Dentomaxillofac Radiol. 2000;29(5):312-8.

6. Wenzel A, Pitts N, Verdonschot EM, et al. Developments in radiographic caries diagnosis. J Dent. 1993;21:131.

7. Wenzel A. Current trends in radiographic caries imaging. Oral Surg Oral Med Oral Pathol Oral Raddiol. Endod. 1995;80:527.

8. Wood NK, Goaz PW. Differential diagnosis of oral lesions, 4th edition. CV Mosby: St Louis; 1991.pp.552-48.

9. Wood RE. Handbook of signs in dental and maxillofacial radiology. 2nd edition. Warthog Publications, Toronto; 1988.

10. Worth HM. Principles and Practice of Oral Radiographic Interpretation. Year Book Medical Publishers, Chicago; 1963.pp.215-300.

Periodontal Diseases | 18

Several distinct yet related disorders of the periodontium are collectively known as periodontal disease. The most common being gingivitis, which is a sequela of infection limited to the marginal gingiva and periodontitis which is also the result of various specific infections with involvement and loss of the alveolar bone. It may be localized or generalized, juvenile or adult periodontitis.

Radiographs play an integral role in the diagnosis and assessment of periodontal disease. They help to assess:

- The amount of bone present
- Condition of the alveolar crests
- Bone loss in furcation areas
- Width of the periodontal ligament space
- Local irritating factors that cause or intensify periodontal disease:
  - Calculus
  - Poorly contoured or over extended restorations.
- Root length and morphology and the crown to root ratio
- Anatomical considerations:
  - Position of the maxillary sinus in relation to a periodontal deformity
  - Missing, supernumerary or impacted teeth.
- Pathological considerations:
  - Caries
  - Periapical lesions
  - Root resorption.

Radiographs also provide a permanent record of the condition of the bone throughout the course of the disease. It is important to note that clinical and radiographic examinations are complimentary, as radiographs are an adjunct to the diagnostic process. Although a radiograph may demonstrate advanced periodontitis well, other equally important changes in the periodontium may not be seen radiographically.

LIMITATIONS OF RADIOGRAPHS

- Bony defects overlapped by existing bony walls are difficult to perceive on the radiographs, as the radiograph provides a restricted (two-dimensional) representation of the (three-dimensional) situation.
  - It is difficult to differentiate between the buccal and lingual crestal bone levels.
  - Only part of a complex bony defect is shown.

- One wall of a bone defect may obscure the rest of the defect.
- Dense tooth or restoration shadows may obscure buccal or lingual bone defects, and buccal or lingual calculus deposits.
- Bone resorption in the furcation area may be obscured by an overlying root or bone shadow.
- Early (incipient) destructive lesion in the bone (where there is not sufficient alteration in bone density), are not detected on the radiograph.
- Density of the root superimposed on the image, tends to obscure the bone height.
- Radiographs show less severe destruction than actually present.
- Bone loss is detectable only when sufficient calcified tissue has been resorbed to alter the attenuation of the X-ray beam. As a result, the histological front of the disease process cannot be determined by the radiographic appearance.
- Radiographs do not demonstrate the soft tissue to hard tissue relationships.
- Information is provided only on the hard tissues of the periodontium, since the soft tissue gingival defects are not normally detectable.
- Radiographs will not identify successfully managed case as opposed to an untreated one.
- Technique variation and X-ray beam position can affect the appearance of the periodontal tissues. Hence the need for accurate, reproducible techniques.
- Overexposure can cause burn out.
- Complete reliance cannot be placed on images of dental panoramic tomographs although they do provide a reasonable overview of the periodontal status (**Fig. 18.1**).

RADIOGRAPHS FOR DETECTION OF PERIODONTAL DISEASES

- The bitewing and periapical radiographs are useful for evaluating the periodontium. For radiography of the alveolar bone, 80 kVp or more is recommended, as the increased penetration provides better visualization of the extent of bony defect and tooth roots. Films that are slightly light are useful for examining cortical margins of bone.

- Intraoral grids may be used to evaluate the bone height.
- Computers and image-processing techniques have been used to enhance radiographs to achieve improved detection of alveolar bone loss associated with periodontal disease.
- Digital subtraction radiography including subtraction radiography and densitometric image analysis which assist in showing and measuring subtle changes in fine alveolar and crestal bone pattern. It allows for better detection of small amounts of bone loss between radiographs made at different times.
- In CBCT, the axial, coronal and sagiital sections obtained help to evaluate the extent of bone loss without the superimposition of the buccal/labial and palatal/lingual cortical plates, helping to better evaluate the bone defects (**Figs 18.2A to D**).

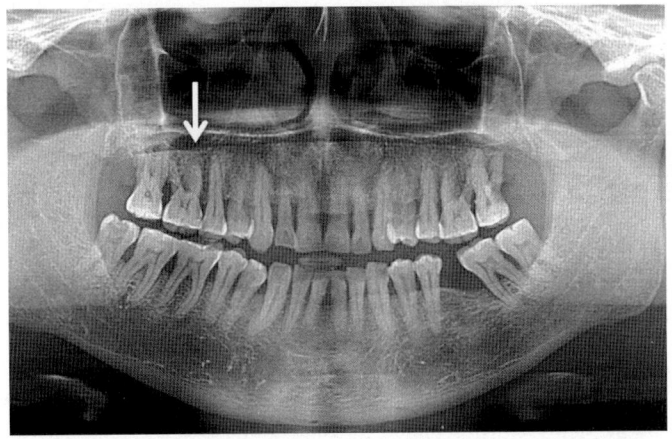

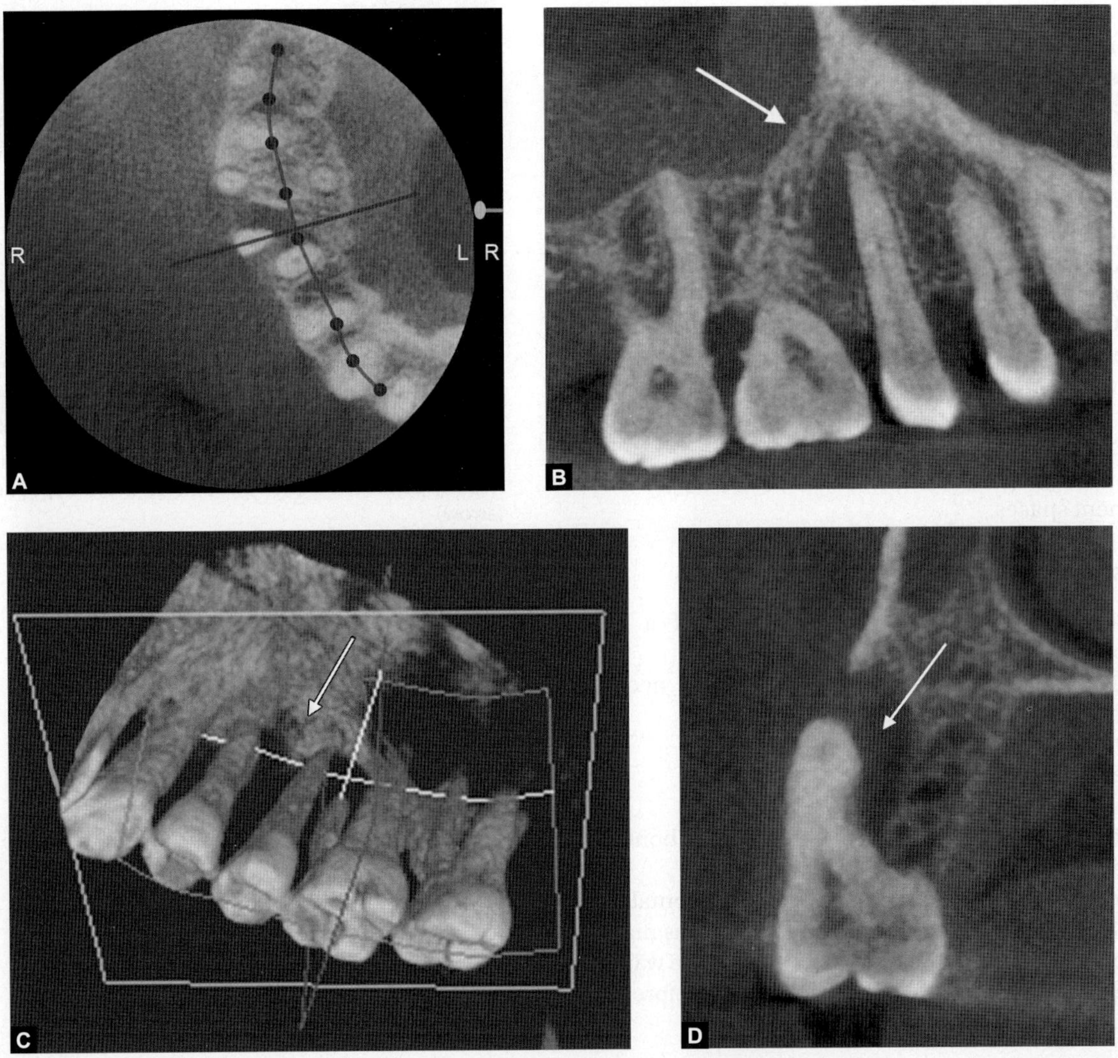

Figures 18.1 Panoramic radiograph showing bone loss (white arrow)

Figures 18.2A to D CBCT: (A) Axial; (B) Panoramic; (C) (3D); (D) (Sagittal) sections showing detailed extent of bone loss and defects

Normal Anatomy

A healthy periodontium can be regarded as periodontal tissue exhibiting no evidence of disease. Unfortunately, health cannot be ascertained from radiographs alone, clinical information is also required. However, to be able to interpret radiographs successfully clinicians need to know the usual radiographic features of healthy tissues where there has been no bone loss.

A thin layer of opaque cortical bone often covers the alveolar crest, the height of which is 1–1.5 mm below the level of the CE junction of the adjacent teeth. Between the posterior teeth the alveolar crest is usually pointed and has a dense cortex and is within 1–1.5 mm of a line connecting the CE junctions. A well mineralized cortical outline of the alveolar crest indicates the absence of periodontitis. The alveolar crest is continuous with the lamina dura of adjacent teeth.

The only reliable radiographic feature is the relationship between the crestal bone margin and the cementoenamel junction (CEJ). If this distance is within normal limits (2–3 mm) and there are no clinical signs of loss of attachment, then it can be said that there has been no periodontitis.

The usual radiographic features of healthy alveolar bone are shown in **Figures 18.3 and 18.4** and include:

- Thin, smooth, evenly corticated margins of the interdental crestal bone in the posterior regions.
- Thin, even, pointed margins of the interdental crestal bone in the anterior regions. Cortication at the top of the crest is not always evident, owing mainly to the small amount of bone between the teeth anteriorly.
- The interdental crestal bone is continuous with the lamina dura of the adjacent teeth. The junction of the two forms a sharp angle.
- Thin even width of the mesial and distal periodontal ligament spaces.

Important Points to Note

- Although these are the usual features of a healthy periodontium, they are not always evident.
- Their absence from radiographs does not necessarily mean that periodontal disease is present.
- Failure to see these features may be due to:
  - Technique error
  - Over exposure
  - Normal anatomical variation in alveolar bone shape and density.
- Following successful treatment, the periodontal tissues may appear healthy clinically, but radiographs may show evidence of earlier bone loss when the disease was active. Bone loss observed on radiographs is therefore not an indicator of the presence of inflammation.

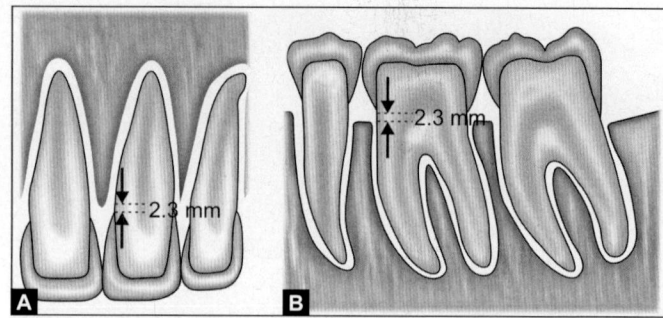

Figures 18.3A and B Diagrams illustrating the radiographic appearances of a healthy periodontium. (A) The upper incisor region; (B) The lower molar region. The normal distance of 2–3 mm from the crestal margin to the cementoenamel junction is indicated

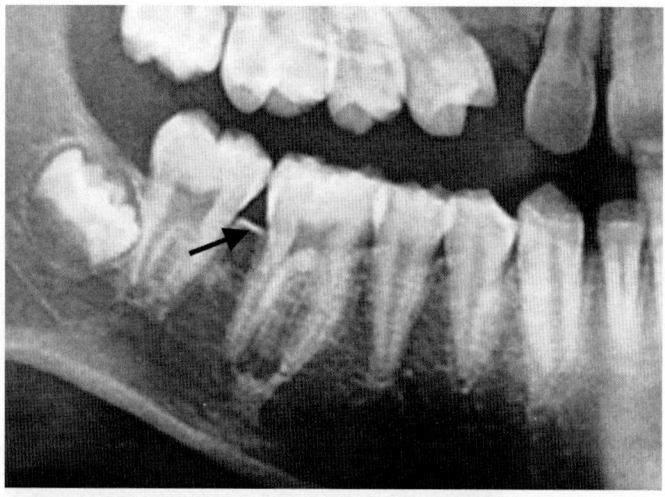

Figure 18.4 Radiograph showing the radiographic features of a healthy periodontium (arrowed) note the radiopaque coated margin (arrow)

Inflammatory Periodontal Diseases are Classified as: (Figs 18.5A to E)

Gingivitis

- Acute
  - Caused by trauma
  - Acute ulcerative gingivitis
  - Acute herpetic gingivostomatitis
  - Acute nonspecific
- Chronic
  - Hyperplastic
  - Desquamative.

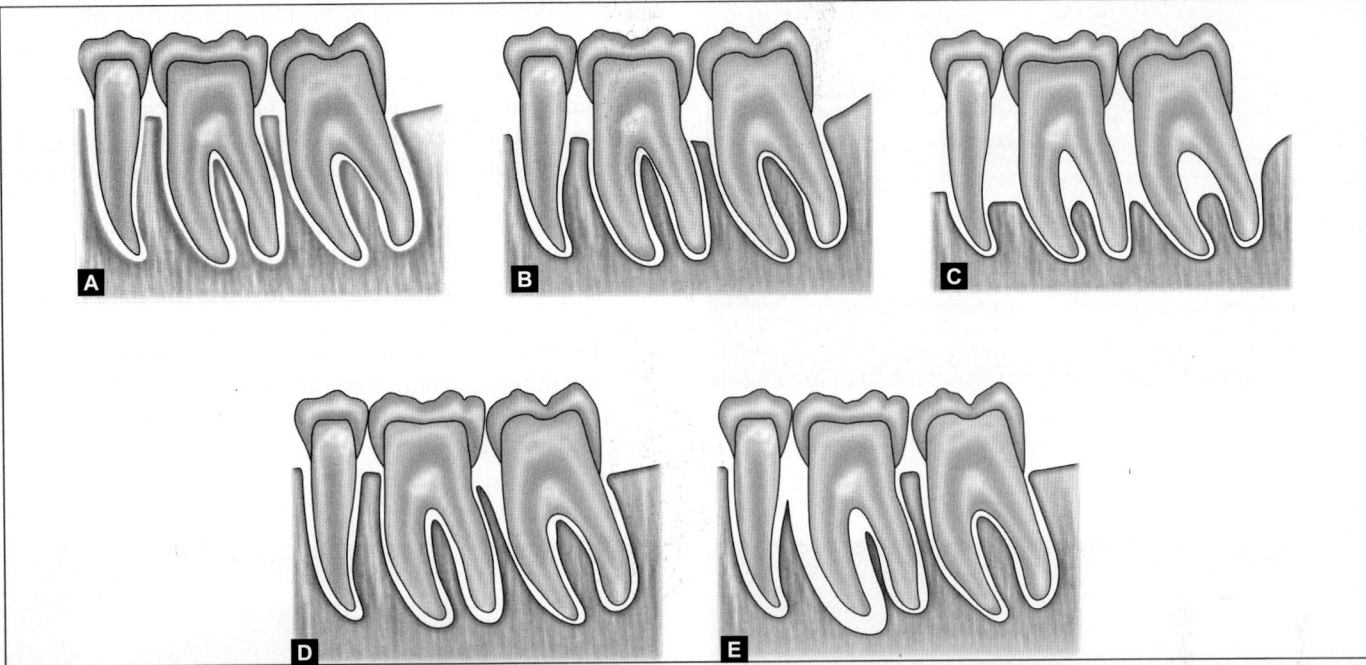

Figures 18.5A to E Diagrams illustrating the various radiographic appearances of periodontitis. (A) Early loss of the corticated crestal bone, widening of the periodontal ligament and loss of the normally sharp angle between the crestal bone and the lamina dura; (B) Moderate horizontal bone loss; (C) Extensive generalized horizontal bone loss with furcation involvement; (D) Localized vertical bone loss affecting lower second molar; (E) Extensive localized bone loss involving the apex of mandibular first molar—the so called perio-endo lesion

Periodontitis

- Acute
  - Acute periodontal abscess
- Chronic periodontitis
  - Early
  - Moderate
  - Severe
- Early onset periodontitis
  - Prepubertal
  - Juvenile
  - Rapidly progressive

Systemic or Generalized Conditions that can Affect the Periodontium

Including amongst Others

- Pregnancy
- Uncontrolled diabetes
- Drugs, e.g. epanutin, nifedipine
- HIV
- Leukemia
- Down's syndrome
- Langerhans' cell disease (histiocytosis X)
- Papillon-Lefevre syndrome
- Secondary metastases.

ACUTE AND CHRONIC GINGIVITIS

Radiographs provide no direct evidence of the soft tissue involvement in gingivitis.

However, in severe cases of acute ulcerative gingivitis (ANUG) where there has been extensive cratering of the interdental papilla, inflammatory destruction of the underlying crestal bone may be observed.

PERIODONTITIS

Early or mild periodontitis is represented as an area of localized erosion of the alveolar bone crest. In the anterior region it is seen as the blunting of the alveolar crests. In the posterior region there may be a loss in the sharp angle between the lamina dura and the alveolar crest, with loss of the cortical margin and appears rounded off with an irregular diffuse border.

It is important to note that significant loss of attachment must be present for 6–8 months before there is radiographic evidence of bone loss, therefore even when only slight radiographic changes are detected; it means that the disease is not of recent onset.

Moderate periodontitis (**Figs 18.6 and 18.7**) is said to occur when the destruction of the alveolar bone extends beyond the early changes on the alveolar crest and may induce a

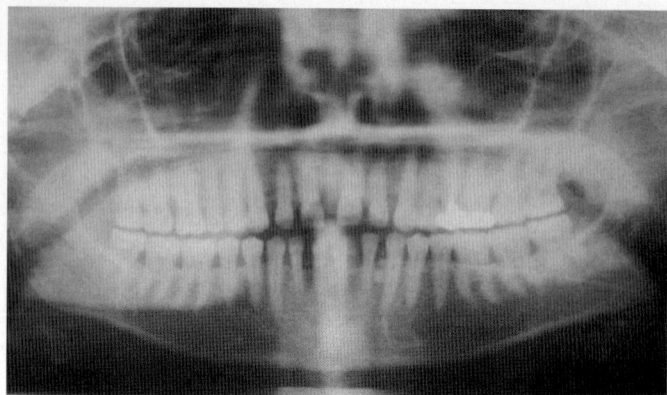

Figure 18.6 Radiograph showing the typical radiographic features of moderate bone loss and horizontal bone loss

variety of defects. The buccal and lingual cortical plate may resorb or there may be bone defects of bone between the buccal and lingual plates. It may be seen on the radiograph as generalized horizontal erosion or as a localized vertical (angular) defect. There may be clinical mobility of the tooth. Many a times the complete extent of bone loss is not evident on the radiograph.

Horizontal bone loss is the loss of height of the alveolar bone with the crest still horizontal or parallel to the occlusal plane. This may be local involving limited teeth or generalized, involving a quadrant or more. It may be further classified into mild, moderate or severe depending upon the extent. In horizontal bone loss the buccal and lingual cortical plates and the intervening interdental bone is resorbed (**Figs 18.8 and 18.9**).

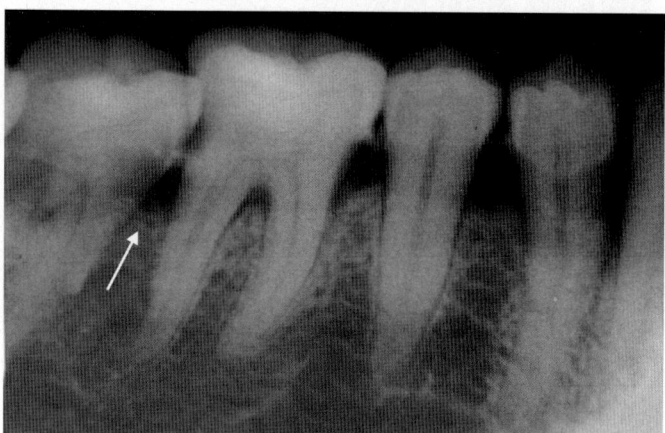

Figure 18.7 Radiographs showing the typical radiographic features of moderate horizontal bone loss (arrowed) in chronic periodontitis affecting posterior teeth. Also seen calculus 'spurs' at the cervical margin of the molars

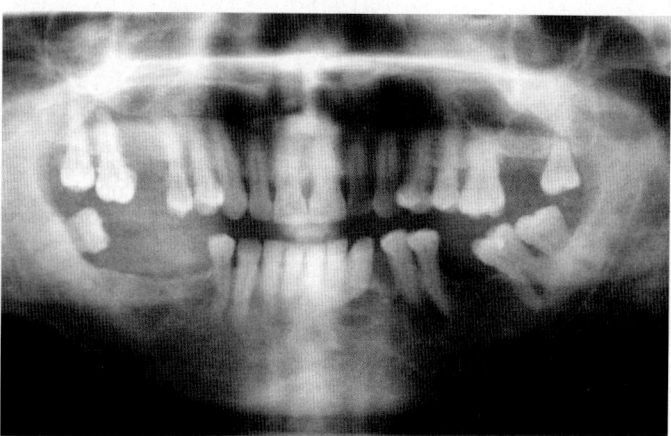

Figure 18.8 Periapical radiographs showing the typical radiographic features of severe bone loss and horizontal bone loss in periodontitis affecting maxillary teeth

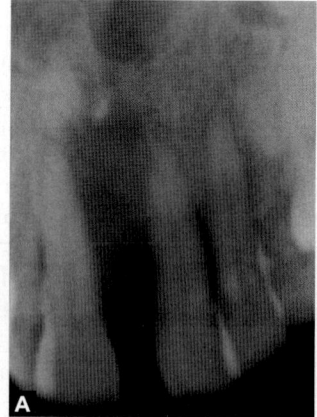
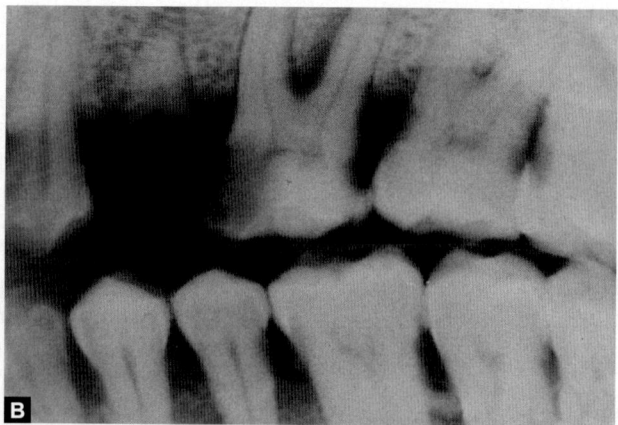

Figures 18.9A and B Horizontal bone loss: (A) Radiograph of upper anterior region showed horizontal alveolar bone loss up to apex of roots with periodontal ligament space widening and loss of Lamina dura; (B) Horizontal bone loss affecting the maxillary and mandibular posterior teeth

Vertical osseous defects (**Figs 18.10 to 18.13**): These are vertical (angular) bony lesions that are localized to one or two teeth. These appear as an oblique angulation of the alveolar bone in the area of the involved teeth. These defects are often difficult to diagnose on a radiograph because one or both of the cortical bony plates remains superimposed with the defect. There are four common types of osseous defects:

1. *Interproximal crater*: It is a trough like depression that occurs on the crests of the interproximal septal bone between adjacent teeth. It has two walls, buccal and lingual cortical plates and two additional walls created by the roots of the adjacent teeth.

   The coronal limits of the buccal and lingual walls are seen radiographically. The image of the wall which is more coronal will show reduced density compared to the apical image of the superimposed walls. If the crestal edges of the two walls are exactly superimposed, it may appear as an irregular linear area of reduced density between

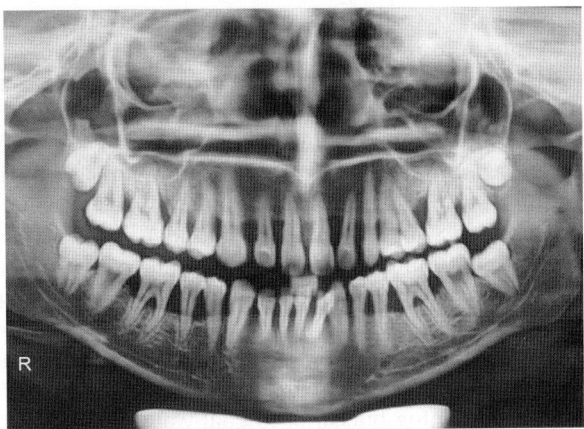

Figure 18.10 Radiographs showing the typical radiographic severe generalized angular bone loss extending to more than half the root length. Arc shaped bone loss extending to the apical portion with 16, 26 radiolucency seen in the furcation region of 36, 46

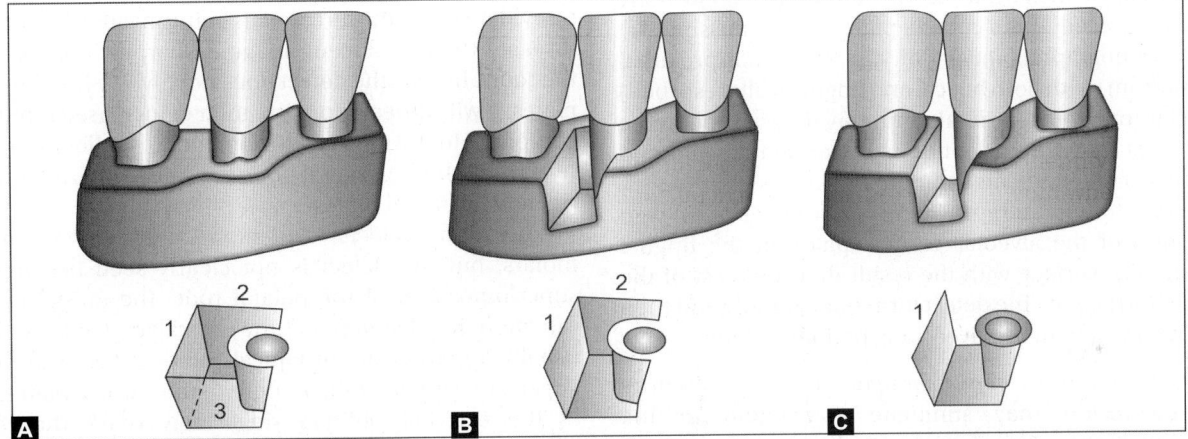

Figures 18.11A to C (A) Three-walled defect: 1. Distal, 2. Lingual, 3. Facial; (B) Two-walled defect: 1. Distal, 2. Lingual; (C) One-walled defect: 1. Distal

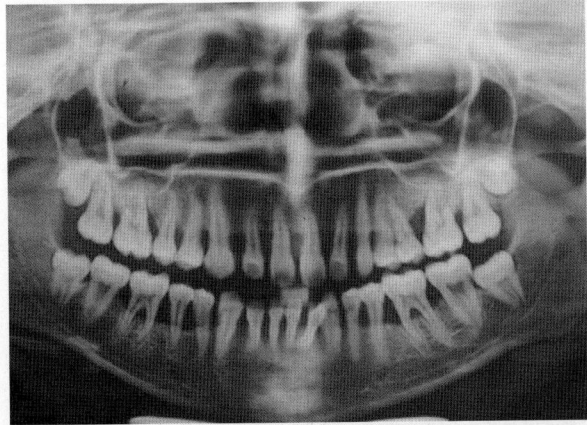

Figure 18.12 Panoramic radiograph showing generalized severe angular bone loss with furcation involvement with respect to 16, 26, 36, 46 and generalized spacing between 11, 12, 13, 21, 22, 23, 31, 32, 33, 41, 42, 43.

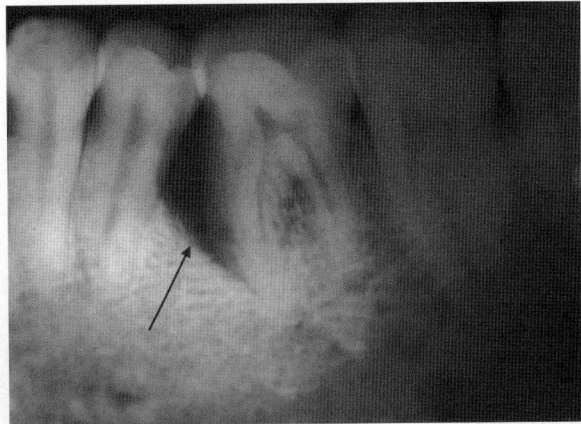

Figure 18.13 Periapical radiograph showing an extensive area of bone loss (arrowed) associated with lower first molar, this is called a endo-perio lesion. Clinically the patient may be having a periodontal abscess

adjacent teeth. Craters which are radiograhically detected are 1 mm or more deep. The apical margin of the defect is ill-defined and blends with the normal bone apical to it. In the mandible the external oblique ridge may obscure interproximal craters involving third molars.

2. *Proximal intrabony defect*: This is a three walled vertical deformity within the bone. It extends apically along the root from the alveolar crest. Surrounded by three walls, a hemisepta and lingual and buccal cortical plates. Radiographically the infrabony defect is generally 'V' shaped and sharply outlined, lying immediately next to the root surface of the affected tooth. A crestal lamina often appears coronal to the defect and represents the coronal limits of the highest remaining buccal or lingual wall. Visualization of the depth may be aided by inserting a gutta-percha point.

3. *Two walled defects* (two walls remaining) next to the hemisepta are usually indistinguishable from a proximal intrabony defect.

4. *Interproximal hemisepta*: These are one wall defect when only mesial or distal portion of the interproximal bony septum is present. Both cortical plates will be missing.

   The radiographic image of one wall interproximal hemiseptum (with both buccal and lingual walls resorbed) is similar to that of proximal intrabony defect, though the defect next to the hemiseptum is better demarcated and may have a well corticated margin.

5. *Inconsistent bony margins*: These are a result of uneven resorption of the alveolar cortical plate on the lingual or vestibular surface with the result that the crest of the margin is irregular. The defect form quite rapidly and then remain constant for relatively long periods of time.

Surrounding internal bone changes the inflammatory periodontal lesion may stimulate a reaction in the surrounding bone. The peripheral bone may appear radiolucent which reflects loss of density and number of trabeculae, usually seen in acute lesions, many a times when the lesion resolves with successful treatment the trabeculae remineralize. The sclerotic (radiopaque) lesion is a result of deposition of bone on existing trabeculae at the expense of the marrow, which may eventually appear as a dense amorphous radiopaque mass. Usually the surrounding bone reaction is a mixture of the two.

Advance or severe periodontitis is where there is extensive bone loss with excessive mobility and drifting of the remaining teeth. This may be accompanied with extensive horizontal bone loss or extensive osseous defects.

OTHER PERIODONTAL PATHOLOGIES

Osseous deformities in the furcations of multirooted teeth (Figs 18.14A to C) is a result of bone resorption which extends down the side of the multirooted tooth, eliminating the marginal vertical bone over the root, it may reach the level of the furcation and beyond. The thickening of the periodontal ligament space at the apex of the inter-radicular bony crest, is an evidence that the furcation is being invaded by periodontal disease. The radiolucent image is sharply outlined between the roots. In case the defect does not involve both the cortical plates, it will appear more irregular of increased radiolucency compared to the normal adjacent bone. Radiographs will not reveal whether the septal bone has been lost from the buccal or lingual cortical plates.

Furcation defects are more common in maxillary molars, but the defect is not clearly seen because of the superimposition of the palatal root. The mesial and distal furcation involvement of the maxillary teeth is also not usually apparent on periapical radiographs because of the superimposition of one or more of the cortical plates.

The external oblique ridge may mask the furcation involvement of the third molar. Convergent roots may also obscure furcation defects in maxillary and mandibular second and third molars.

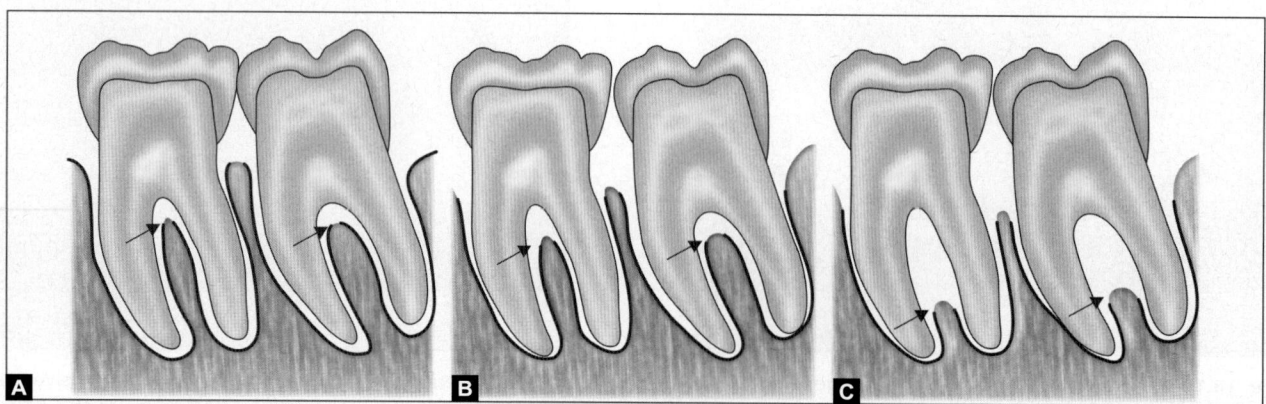

Figures 18.14A to C Diagrams illustrating the radiographic appearances of varying degrees of furcation involvement in lower molars (arrowed). (A) Very early involvement showing widening of the furcation periodontal ligament shadow; (B) Moderate involvement; (C) Severe involvement

Periodontal dehiscense results when the marginal bone dips apically and exposes the length of the root surface, and is not usually seen well on radiographs.

Periodontal abscess originates in a deep soft tissue pocket, when the coronal portion of the pocket becomes occluded or when foreign particles get lodged in it. If the lesion persists a generalized radiolucency may form. After treatment some reformation of bone may occur.

Aggressive periodontitis or early on-set perio dontitis (**Figs 18.15A and B**) includes three types: Localized juvenile periodontitis (LJP), Generalized juvenile periodontitis (GJP), and rapidly progressing periodontitis (RPP). This disease has a rapid onset and occurs in patients under the age of 30 years.

Localized aggressive peridontitis is associated with attachment loss involving the incisors and first molars, it commences around puberty, and usually there is no associated soft tissue inflammation or plaque accumulation. Radiographically there is vertical bone loss, with maxillary teeth (first molars and/or incisors more often involved) with strong left-right symmetry. There are arch or saucer-shaped defects, sometimes the bone loss is more generalized with migration of the incisors with diastema formation due to rapid rate of bone loss.

Generalized aggressive periodontitis may involve variable number of teeth, from a minimum of three to all the teeth in the dentition, it affects individuals under thirty. The gingiva may be normal or may present with an inflammatory response. Radiographically several teeth are seen to be involved with a rapid loss of bone which may be of the vertical or angular or horizontal pattern.

If there is an associated history of premature loss of deciduous teeth and the permanent teeth are rapidly lost soon after eruption, a possible diagnosis of Papillon-Lefèvre syndrome may be considered. This is usually associated with hyperkeratosis of the palmer and planter surfaces.

Dental conditions associated with periodontal diseases are a result of various changes in the dentition and the supporting structures due to various factors such as overhanging and faulty restorations, occlusal trauma, tooth mobility, open contacts and local irritation.

- *Occlusal trauma*: In addition to clinical symptoms such as increased mobility, wear facets, unusal response to percussion and a history of contributory habits, the radiographic evidences are:
  - Widening of the periodontal ligament space.
  - Decreased definition of the lamina dura.
  - Bone loss and altered trabeculation (increase in number and size).
  - Hypercementosis and root fractures.
- *Tooth mobility*: Widening of the periodontal ligament space suggests tooth mobility, due to occlusal trauma. In the case of a single root it may develop an hour-glass shape, and in multirooted teeth widening of the periodontal space is seen at the apices and in the region of the furcation.
- *Open contacts*: They are more associated with periodontal disease. Similar potential situations in which periodontal disease may develop include discrepancies in the height of two adjacent marginal ridges or tipped teeth. Abnormal tooth alignment does not cause periodontal disease, but provides an environment in which disease may develop. These areas show early and excessive bone loss.
- *Local irritating factors*: Radiographs help to reveal many local irritating factors which lead to periodontitis such as—calculus, defective restorations with over hanging or poorly contoured margins, crowns with insufficient contour below the gingival, etc. (**Fig. 18.16**).

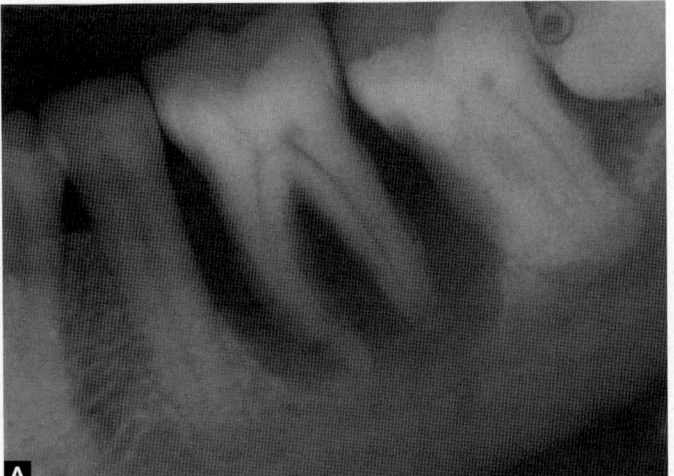 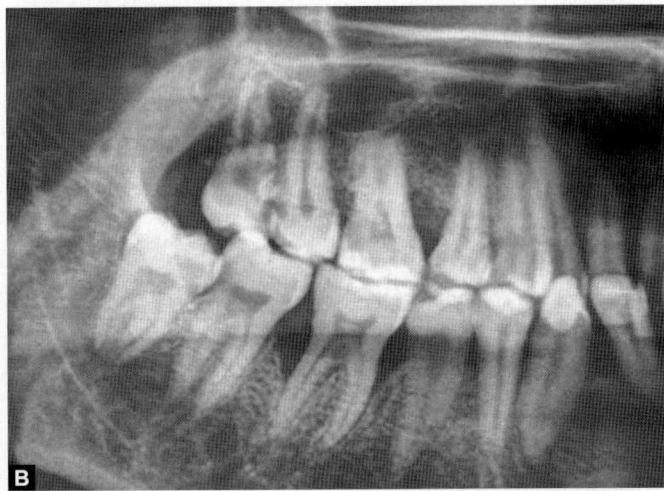

Figures 18.15A and B Juvenile periodontitis as seen on a part of a dental panoramic radiographs showing the typical bone defects affecting the first molars

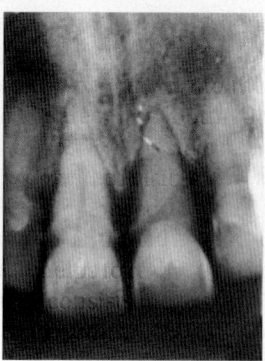

Figure 18.16 Supragingival calculus 'spurs' at the cervical margin seen on periapical film, of upper central incisors

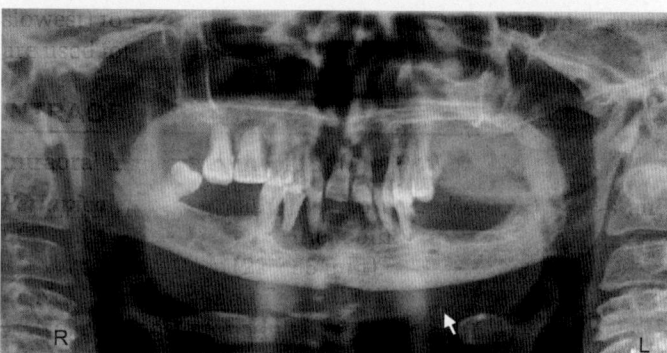

Figure 18.17 Severe bone loss w.r.t. 41, 42, 43 giving floating tooth appearance surrounded by the well-defined corticated borders and should be differentiated from carcinoma

- *Evaluation of periodontal therapy*: Radiographs may show signs of successful treatment of periodontal disease. The relative radiolucent margins of bone which were undergoing active resorption before treatment may become more sclerotic (radiopaque) after successful therapy. The enlarged marrow spaces are reduced and bone becomes denser, creating an illusion of vertical bone growth. The borders of the healthy bone have a well-defined corticated margin.

Radiographs do not reveal therapeutic elimination of (radiolucent) soft tissue periodontal pockets.

Sequential radiographs made with different beam angulations may give a false impression that bone has grown into periodontal pockets. The amount of exposure and processing time of the dental radiograph is also important too high an exposure and too long a developing time may create the impression of destroyed bone as a result of alveolar crest burnout. If the post-treatment radiograph is subjected to a low exposure and a short developing time the denser appearing image may suggest vertical bone growth.

The clinical crown to tooth ratio is a useful criteria for determining the nature of the restorative treatment to be performed and the prognosis of an individual tooth. An unfavorable crown to root ratio is when the length of the tooth out of the bone exceeds the length of the root supported by the bone.

Differential diagnosis: Periodontal disease should be differentiated from:
- *Squamous cell carcinoma*, which usually shows extensive localized destruction of bone, having a very invasive tendency, and should be correlated clinically (**Fig. 18.17**).
- *Langerhans' cell histiocytosis (Eosinophilic Granuloma)* is manifested as a single or multiple regions of bone destruction around the roots of teeth, usually no particular tooth is targeted and the midroot region is the epicenter of bone destruction which gives the lesion an 'ice cream scoop' appearance. The alveolar crest remains intact.

- *Effect of systemic diseases on periodontal disease*: Although systemic diseases do not cause periodontal disease, they do influence its cause by limiting the capacity of the individual to affect repair. The few diseases which appear to influence the periodontium and periodontal treatment are: diabetes mellitus, hematologic disorders (monocytic conditions, myelogenous leukemia, neutropenia, hemophilia, abnormal bleeding, nonhemophilic polycythemia vera), genetic and hereditary disturbances (Papillon-Lefèvre syndrome, Down's syndrome, hypophosphatemia, Chédiak-Higashi syndrome), hormonal changes (puberty, pregnancy, menopause) and stress.
- *AIDS* patients show an increase in the frequency and severity of periodontal disease. There is rapid progression that leads to bone sequestration and loss of multiple teeth. The patients do not respond to standard periodontal therapy.
- *Diabetes mellitus* is the most common systemic disease which influences the onset and course of periodontal disease. The altered glucose metabolism leads to protein break down, degenerative vascular changes, lowered resistance to infection and increased severity to infections. Patients with uncontrolled diabetes show severe and rapid alveolar bone resorption and are prone to develop periodontal abscesses.
- *Hyperkeratosis (Palmoplantaris)* also called Papillon-Lefèvre syndrome is a rare heritable condition (autosomal dominant) manifested by hyperkeratosis of the palms and soles. There is also extensive, prepubertal destruction of the periodontal bone which is manifested as extensive generalized horizontal bone loss. The condition may result in loss of the entire primary dentition by the age of 5 years and loss of secondary dentition before the age of 20 years. An interesting observation, on the radiographs of the affected patients is that bone loss appears to be arrested once the tooth is lost. Thus one school of thought suggests that since this condition cannot be treated, early removal of the tooth will arrest bone loss, thus providing sufficient healthy bone to seat a denture or an implant.

BIBLIOGRAPHY

1. Efficacy of the FDA selection criteria for radiographic assessment of the periodontium. J Dent Res. 1995;74(7): 1424-32.
2. Goaz PW, White SC. Principles and Interpretation, In: Oral radiology, 3rd edition. St. Louis: Mosby Year Book; 1994.
3. Gröndahl K, et al. Influence of variations in projection geometry on the detectability of periodontal bone lesions: A comparison between subtraction radiology and conventional radiographic techniques. J Clin Periodontol. 1984;11:411.
4. Gutteridge DL. The use of radiographic techniques in the diagnosis and management of periodontal diseases, Dentomaxillofac Radiol. 1995;24:107.
5. Miles DA, Van Dis MJ, Jensen CW. et al. Interpretation normal versus abnormal and common radiographic presentations of lesions. In: Radiographic and Imaging for Dental Auxillaries, 3rd edition. Philadelphia: WB Saunders; 1999.pp.231-80.
6. Pepelassi EA, Diamanti-Kipioti A. Selection of the most accurate method of conventional radiography for the assessment of periodontal osseous destruction. J Clin Periodontol. 1997;24:557.
7. Rushton VE, Honer K. The use of panoramic radiology in dental practice. J Dent. 1996;24:185.
8. Shafer WG, et al. A Textbook of Oral Pathology. Philadelphia: WB Saunders; 1983.
9. Wood NK, Goaz PW. Differential diagnosis of oral lesions. 4th edition. CV Mosby: St Louis; 1991.
10. Wood RE. Handbook of signs in dental and maxillofacial radiology. Warthog Publications, Toronto; 1988.
11. Worth HM. Principles and practice of oral radiographic interpretation. Year Book Medical Publishers, Chicago; 1963.

Dental Anomalies and Developmental Disturbances of the Jaws

19

Dental anomalies as the term indicates is a variation from the normal. This may occur due to developmental aberrations or due to acquired circumstances (**Table 19.1**).

Developmental anomalies indicate that it may have occurred due to any disturbance during the formation of the tooth/teeth, this may be attributed to various causes.

Acquired anomalies are changes in the dentition that are initiated after development of the tooth as a result of change due to normal function and faulty habits.

Developmental disturbances of the face and jaws affect the normal growth and differentiation of craniofacial structures. These conditions result in a variety of abnormalities, which affect the structure, shape, organization and function of the hard and soft tissues. The causes of most of the disturbances are of unknown etiology but some may be attributed to congenital (present at or before birth but not necessarily inherited), hereditary (these are apparent at birth, but some may become evident after many years) or genetic mutations caused due to altered environmental factors.

A multitude of such conditions exist that affect the morphogenesis of the face and jaws, many of which are rare syndromes (**Table 19.2**). This chapter briefly enumerates the various disturbances and discusses a few which may be encountered in dental practice.

Table 19.1 Classification of dental anomalies

- Developmental anomalies
  - Abnormalities in the number of the teeth
  - Abnormalities in the size of the teeth
  - Abnormalities in the shape (morphology) of the teeth
  - Abnormalities in the eruption of the teeth
  - Abnormalities in the structure of the teeth
- Acquired anomalies
  - Attrition
  - Abrasion
  - Erosion
  - Resorption
    - Internal
    - External
  - Secondary dentine
  - Pulp stones
  - Pulpal sclerosis
  - Hypercementosis

Table 19.2 Developmental abnormalities of the jaw bones

- Agnathia
- Agenesis
- Micrognathia
- Macrognathia
- Congenital unilateral hyperplasia of the face
- Congenital unilateral hypoplasia of the face (Craniofacial microsomia, goldenhar syndrome, oculo-auricular vertebral dysplasia)
- Progressive facial hemiatrophy (Parry-Romberg's syndrome)
- Facial hemihypertrophy (Friedreich's disease)
- Segmental odontomaxillary dysplasia (Hemimaxillofacial dysplasia)
- Accessory maxilla (Distomus)
- Abnormalities due to disturbance of growth:
  - Torticollis (Wry Neck)
  - Klippel feil syndrome (Affects the cervical spine)
  - Congenital elevation of scapula
  - Pterygium Colli (Web neck)
  - Turner's syndrome
  - Bonneric-Vilnick syndrome
  - Burns
- Facial clefts (Oral fissures)
  - Cleft lips
  - Double lip
  - Cleft palate
  - Mandibular clefts
- OsteogenesisImperfecta (Fragilitas ossium)
- Osteopetrosis (Marble bone disease, albers-schonberg's disease, osteosclerosis fragilis generalisata)
- Idiopathic hypercalcemia
- Pyknodysostosis
- Melorheostosis unilateral
- Progressive diaphyseal dysplasia (Engelmann's disease)
- Familial metaphyseal dyspalsia (Pyle's disease)
- Chondroectodermal dysplasia (Ellis-van Creveld disease)
- Achondroplasia (Chondrodystrophica foetalis)
- Lipochondrodystrophy (Gargoylism, dysostosis multiplex, Hurler's disease)
- Morquio's disease (Osteochondrodystrophy)
- Chondrodystrophia calcificans congenita (Dysplasia epiphysallis punctata)
- Cleidocranial dysostosis (Marie and Sainton disease, cleidocranial dysplasia)
- Congenital Craniosynostosis (Oxycephaly, acrocephaly)
- Anhidrocephaly
- Ocular hypertelorism

Contd...

Contd...

- Ocular hypotelorism
- Craniofacial dysostosis (Crouzon's disease)
- Apert's syndrome
- Mandibulofacial dysostosis (Treacher collins syndrome)
- Marfan's syndrome (Arachnodactyly)
- Laurence moon-biedl syndrome
- Microcephaly
- Macrocephaly
- Pierre robin syndrome
- Leri's pleonostenosis
- Dysmorphodystrophica mesodermalis congenita (Inverted Marfan's syndrome)
- Mental defectives
- Hyperplasia of maxillary tuberosity
- Hyperplasia of coronoid process
- Focal osteoporotic bone marrow defects
- Arhinencephaly
- Developmental lingual mandibular gland depression
- Abnormalities of the dental arches.

DEVELOPMENTAL ANOMALIES OF THE TEETH (FIGS 19.1A TO E)

Abnormalities in Number

Supernumerary Teeth (Hyperdontia, Distodens, Mesiodens, Para Teeth, Peridens and Supplemental Teeth) (Figs 19.2 to 19.5)

- These are teeth that develop in addition to the normal complement.

- When the extratooth has normal morphology it is called supplemental.
- The supernumerary teeth that occur between the maxillary central incisors are called mesiodens
- The supernumerary teeth that occur in the molar area are called paramolars
- The supernumerary teeth that erupt distal to the third molar are called distodens or distomolars.
- The supernumerary teeth that erupt ectopically either bucally or lingually to the normal arch are called peridens.

Clinical Features

- Occur in 1–4% of the population
- More common in permanent dentition
- Single supernumerary more common in the anterior maxilla and maxillary molar region
- Multiple supernumeraries more common in the premolar regions, in the mandible
- More often found in males, especially Asians and native Americans
- May be detected on a routine radiograph when not erupted
- May obstruct the path of eruption of the permanent tooth
- Usually positioned outside the normal arch.

Radiographic Features

- The tooth may vary from normal appearing to a conical form and in extreme cases, a gross deformed structure may be seen
- Size is usually smaller than the normal dentition
- It may be seen interfering with the path of normal eruption.

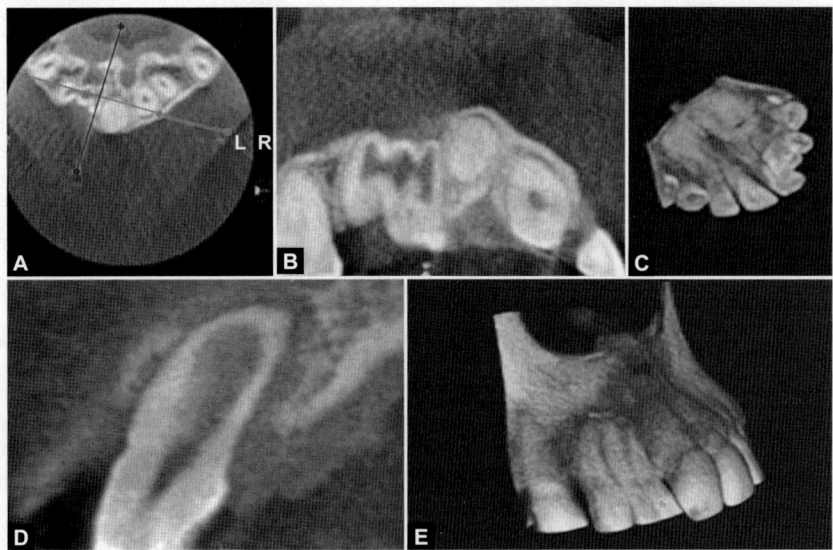

Figures 19.1A to E CBCT showing 6 dental anomalies in the same patient. Fusion, dilaceration, dilated odontome, spernumerary and talons cusp: (A) Axial view; (B) Coronal view showing continuous pulp chambers; (C and E) 3D views showing the lingual and labial aspect of the teeth involved; (D) Sagittal section showing the dilated odontome

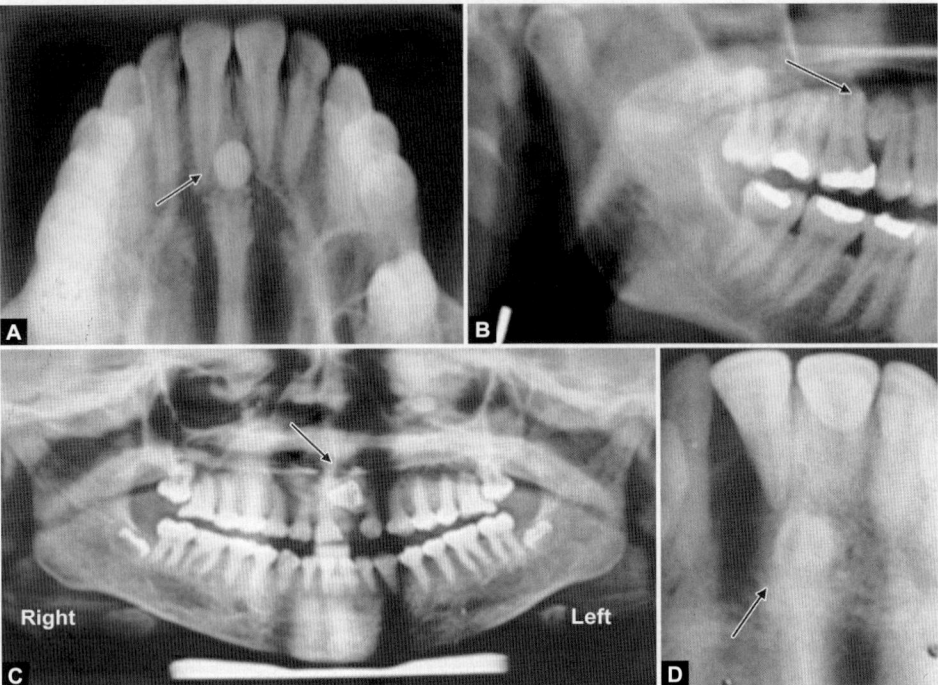

Figures 19.2A to D (A) Occlusal showing mesiodens between roots of central incisors; (B) Lateral oblique showing paramolar between upper first molar and second premolar; (C) OPG; (D) Intraoral periapical view showing mesiodens

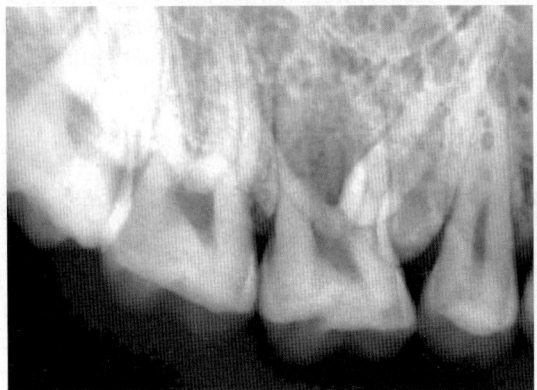

Figure 19.3 Periodontal abscess in the 26 region due to impacted supernumerary tooth

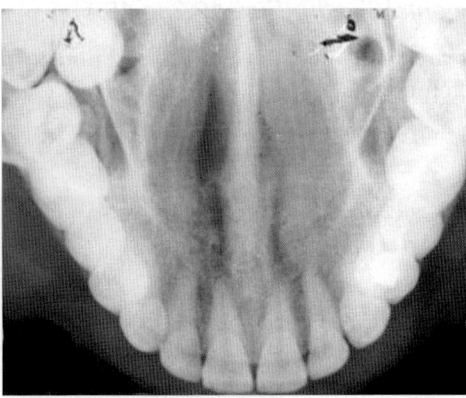

Figure 19.4 Para molars

Differential Diagnosis

- Cleidocranial dysostosis (**Fig. 19.6**)
- Gardner's syndrome.

Management

Treatment depends on many factors, including their potential effect on the developing normal dentition, their position and number, and the complications that may result from surgical intervention.

Missing Teeth (Hypodontia, Oligodontia and Anodontia)

- This may result due to various pathological mechanisms that may affect the orderly formation of the dental lamina (orofaciodigital syndrome), failure of tooth germ to develop, lack of space, etc.
- The absence of one or few teeth is called hypodontia (**Fig. 19.7**).
- The absence of numerous teeth is called oligodontia (**Fig. 19.8**).

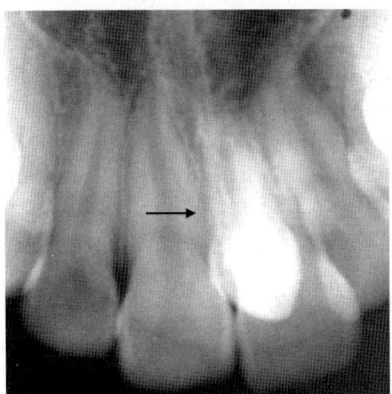

Figure 19.5 Mesiodens

- The failure of all teeth to develop is called anodontia.
- A tooth may be considered to be developmentally missing when it cannot be discerned clinically or radiographically and no history exists of its extraction.

Clinical Features

- In the permanent dentition, excluding the third molars, it is found in 3–10% of the population.
- More in Asians and native Americans.
- In the deciduous dentition missing teeth is rare, when seen the maxillary incisor is affected.
- In the permanent dentition the most common is the third molar, followed by the second premolars, maxillary laterals and mandibular central incisors.
- The absence may be unilateral or bilateral.

Radiographic Features

- Eruption of some teeth may be developmentally delayed by a number of years after the established time (especially the mandibular second bicuspid) and others may show evidence of development as late as a year after the contralateral tooth.
- Missing teeth are recognized by identifying and counting the existing teeth.

Differential Diagnosis

Anodontia or oligodontia occurs in patients with ectodermal dysplasia. This disorder results in the absence of at least two ectodermally derived structures such as sweat glands, hair, skin, nails and teeth. The severity of the condition is variable and may result in multiple missing teeth and malformed teeth, often having a conical shape and a notable decrease in size.

Management

Missing teeth, abnormal occlusion or altered facial appearance may cause some patients psychological distress.

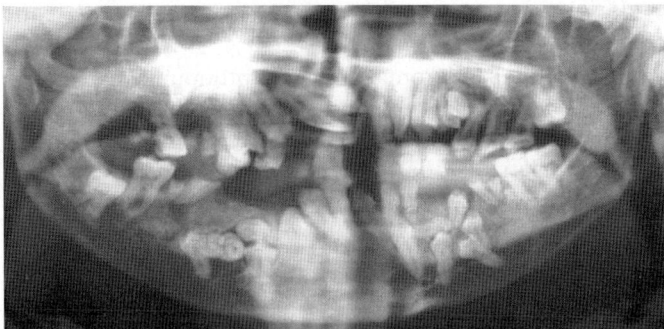

Figure 19.6 Cleidocranial dysostosis

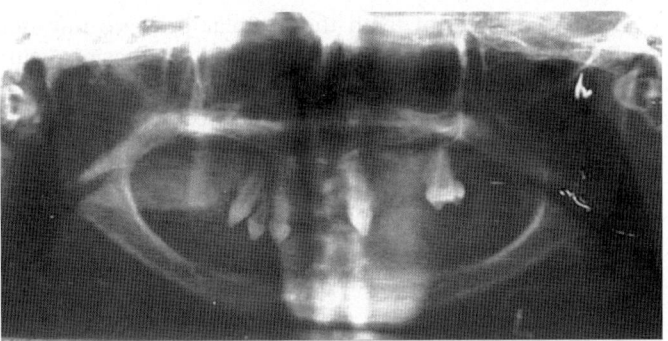

Figure 19.7 Hypodontia

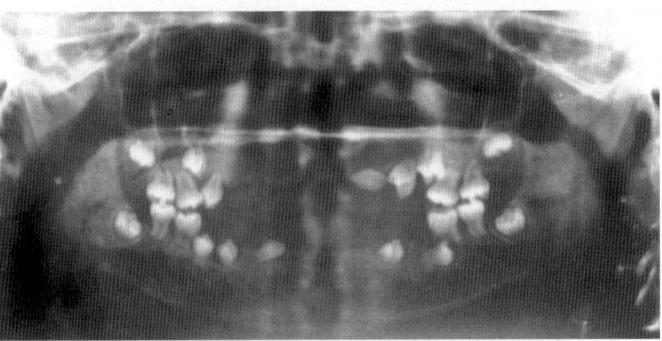

Figure 19.8 Oligodontia

If the extent of hypodontia is mild, then the associated changes may likewise be slight and manageable by orthodontics.

In more severe cases restorative, implant and prosthetic procedures may be undertaken.

Ectodermal Dysplasia [Hereditary Hypohidrotic (Anhidrotic) Ectodermal Dysplasia] (Figs 19.7 to 19.9)

It is an X-linked, recessive inherited disorder, associated with partial or complete absence of teeth.

Clinical Features

- Males are more affected.
- It is characterized by hypotrichosis, hypohidrosis and anhidrosis with saddle nose appearance.

- The hair of the scalp and eyebrows tend to be fine, scanty and blond.
- Supraorbital and frontal bossing is pronounced.
- The skin is usually dry and scaly with absence of sweat glands.
- These patients do not perspire and suffer from hyperpyrexia and intolerance to warm temperatures.
- The facial appearance of these individuals is so similar that they may be mistaken to be siblings.
- They usually have oligodontia or partial absence of teeth, with frequent malformation of the present deciduous or permanent teeth. The shape may be truncated or cone shaped.
- Due to absence of teeth the alveolar process may not develop, causing a reduced vertical dimension with protuberant lips.
- They usually have high arched palates. Clefts are also common among these patients.
- The salivary glands are sometimes hypoplastic leading to xerostomia and dry cracked lips and angular cheilitis.

Radiographic Features

Help to identify and confirm missing and present teeth.

Management

Prosthetic rehabilitation with supplementary mouth wetting agents.

Abnormalities in Size

A positive correlation exists between tooth size (mesiodistal diameter by buccolingual diameter) and body height.

Macrodontia (Megadontia)

- The involved teeth are larger than normal.
- It rarely involves the entire dentition, is usually limited to a single or group of teeth.

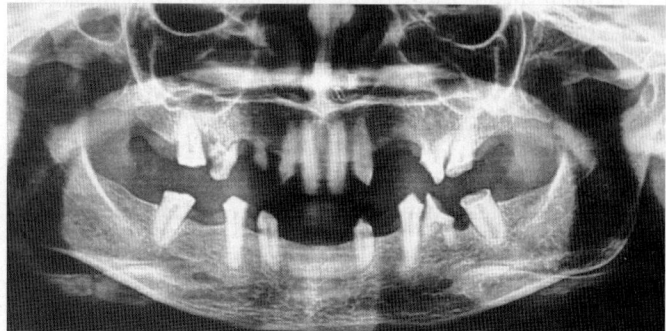

Figure 19.9 Ectodermal dysplasia: Radiograph shows conical cusped teeth. Multiple missing teeth. Generalized resorption of bone

- It may be classified as:
  - True generalized macrodontia (pituitary gigantism)
  - Localized true macrodontia (hemihypertrophy of the face)
  - Relative generalized macrodontia (when the teeth are of normal size but occur in a smaller than normal jaw)
  - Macrodontia of a single tooth (presence of an hemangioma).

Clinical Features

- Large size of teeth is apparent on clinical examination
- Crowding
- Malocclusion
- Impaction may be seen.

Radiographic Features

- Increased size of both erupted and unerupted tooth
- Crowding with impaction of other teeth
- Shape of the tooth is usually normal but may show mildly distorted morphology.

Differential Diagnosis

- *Fusion*: In this case there will be a missing tooth.
- *Gemination*: All the teeth may be present, but there may be evidence of a division or cleft of the coronal or root segment of the tooth.

Management

No treatment required, except in cases of malocclusion where it may be treated orthodontically.

Microdontia (Fig. 19.10)

It may be classified as:
- True generalized microdontia (pituitary dwarfism)
- Relative generalized microdontia (when the teeth are of normal size but occur in a larger than normal jaw)
- Microdontia of a single tooth (supernumerary teeth, laterals and third molars).

Clinical Features

- Involved teeth are smaller with an altered morphology.
- It rarely involves the entire dentition, is usually limited to a single or group of teeth.
- Microdent molars may have an altered shape—from 5 to 4 cusps in the mandibular molars and 4 to 3 cusps in the maxillary molars.
- Microdont lateral is smaller and usually peg shaped.

Radiographic Features

The shape may be normal but more frequently they are malformed.

Differential Diagnosis

The number and distribution of microdonts may suggest consideration of syndromes:
- Congenital heart disease
- Progeria.

Management

Restorative or prosthetic treatment may be considered to create a more normal appearance of the tooth.

Abnormalities in Shape (Morphology)

Fusion (Synodontia) (Figs 19.11A to C)

This results from the combining of adjacent tooth germs, before calcification. Pressure generated during development may cause contact of adjacent tooth buds, leading to their fusion.

Clinical Features

- Reduced number of teeth in the arch, except in cases where fusion is between a supernumerary and a normal tooth.

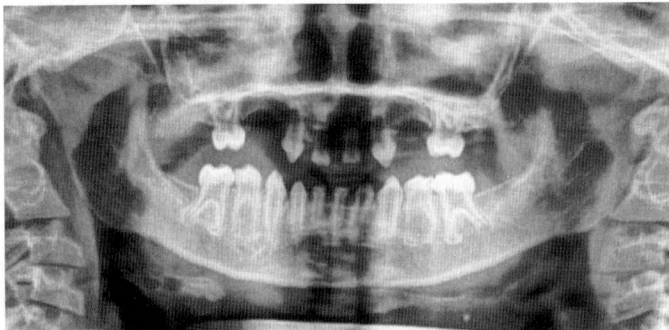

Figure 19.10 Generalized microdontia and oligodontia, know case of ectodermal dysplasia

- More common in deciduous dentition than the permanent dentition.
- When deciduous canine and lateral fuse together, the corresponding permanent lateral incisor is missing.
- More common in anterior teeth.
- It may be total or partial depending on the stage of odontogenesis and the proximity of the developing teeth.
- The crowns of the fused teeth usually appear to be large and single, or an incisocervical groove of varying depth or a bifid crown occurs.

Radiographic Features

- True nature and extent of the union is more apparent on the radiograph.
- The fused tooth may show unusual configuration of the pulp chamber, root canal or crown.

Differential Diagnosis

- Gemination
- Macrodontia.

Management

Deciduous teeth may be retained, and if extraction is planned then confirmation of the succedaneous tooth is a must. Fused crowns may be reshaped with a restoration that mimics two independent crowns.

Concrescence

It occurs when the roots of two or more teeth are united by cementum. Although its cause is unknown, it is suspected that space restriction during development, local trauma, excessive occlusal forces or local infection after development plays an important role.

If concrescence occurs during development it is called true concrescence.

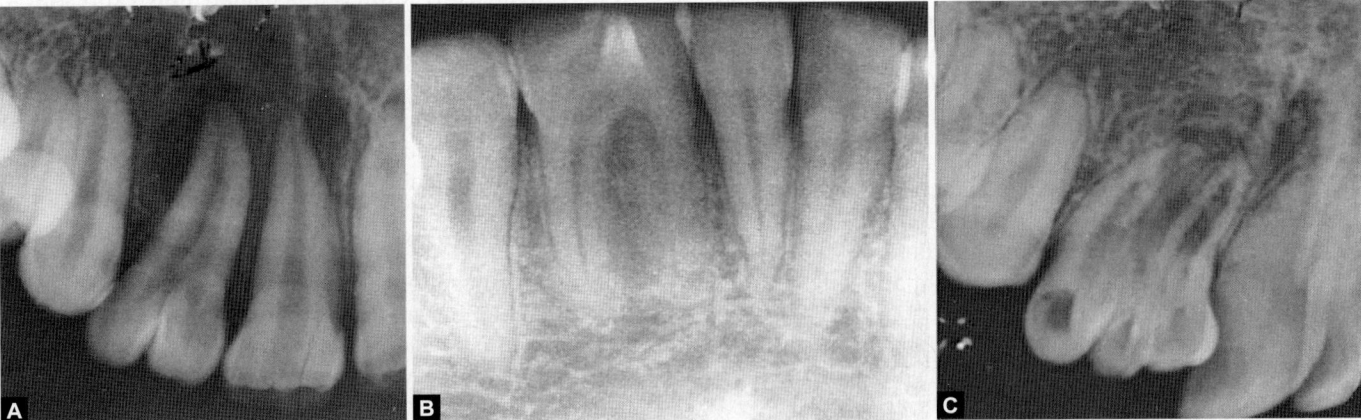

Figures 19.11A to C Fusion: (A) Fusion of upper lateral insicor with supernumerary; (B) Lower central and lateral incisor; (C) Fusion of upper central, supernumerary and lateral incisor

If concrescence occurs after development it is called acquired concrescence.

Clinical Features

- It may involve primary or secondary dentition
- Both sexes are equally affected
- Maxillary molars are most frequently involved, especially a third molar and a supernumerary
- The involved teeth may fail to erupt.

Radiographic Features

- Reveals the extent of fusion of roots.
- Sometimes the radiographic examination may not distinguish concrescence and teeth that are in close in contact or simply superimposed. In such a case additional projections at different angles must be obtained.

Differential Diagnosis

If the roots are joined radiographically it is difficult to tell whether the union is by cementum or by dentine (Fusion).

Management

The condition is of clinical importance only when extraction is contemplated.

Gemination (Twinning) (Fig. 19.12)

It is a rare anomaly where the tooth bud of a single tooth attempts to divide. This may result in an invagination of the crown, with partial division or in rare cases complete division throughout the crown and root.

Clinical Features

- More common in primary teeth
- Usually seen in the incisor region
- Occurrence in male and female is about equal
- Can be detected clinically after the anomalous tooth erupts
- The enamel and dentine of the geminated tooth may be hypoplastic or hypocalcified.

Radiographic Features

- Altered shape of the hard tissue and pulp chamber can be seen
- Radiopaque enamel outlines the clefts in the crowns and invaginations and thus accentuates them
- The pulp chamber is usually enlarged and single or may be partially divided
- In a rare case of premolar gemination, the tooth image may be suggestive of a molar with an enlarged crown and two roots.

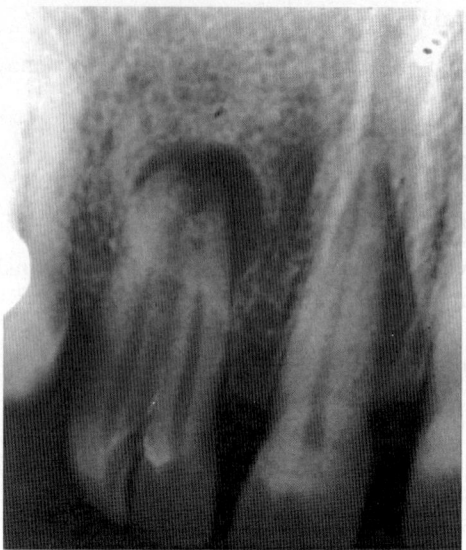

Figure 19.12 Gemination

Differential Diagnosis

- Fusion
- If the malformed tooth is counted as one, individuals with gemination have a normal tooth count, whereas those with fusion will have one less tooth.

Management

If affected tooth is deciduous it may be extracted. The crown may be restored or reshaped or the tooth may be kept under observation to preclude any development of complication.

Taurodontism (Figs 19.13A to C)

Clinical Features

- It may occur in primary or secondary dentition.
- It may involve any tooth but is usually fully expressed in the molars and less in premolars.
- It may involve single or multiple teeth, unilaterally or bilaterally and in any combination of teeth or quadrants.
- Because the body and the roots lie below the alveolar margins the distinguishing features of these teeth are not recognizable clinically.

Radiographic Features

- The distinct morphology is only seen on the radiograph.
- The pulp chamber has a rectangular appearance, with an extension into the elongated body.
- The size of the crown is normal but the root and root canals appear shortened.

Differential Diagnosis

- The developing molar should be distinguished by the presence of a wide apical foramina and incompletely formed roots.
- Taurodontism frequently occurs in Trisomy 21 or Down's syndrome.

Management

This does not require any treatment. But care should be taken when planning an extraction.

Dilaceration (Figs 19.14A to E)

It is a disturbance in tooth formation that produces a sharp bend or curve in the tooth. It is believed to be the result of mechanical trauma to the calcified portion of a partially formed tooth. The angular distortion may occur any where in the crown or root.

Clinical Features

- In most cases of radicular dilacerations it is not seen clinically, but may be manifested by the noneruption of the affected tooth.
- The crown dilacerations may be readily seen as a defect of the crown in the oral cavity.

- Most often affects the permanent maxillary molars.

Radiographic Features

- If the roots are bent mesially or distally it is clearly apparent on the radiograph.
- If the roots are bent bucally (labially) or lingually, the central ray passes more or less parallel to the dilacerated portion and it thus appears at the apical end of the unaltered root as a round opaque area with a dark shadow in its central region cast by the apical foramen and root canal—a "bull's eye appearance".
- The periodontal ligament space around the dilacerated portion may be seen as a radiolucent halo, and the radiopacity of this segment of the root is greater than the rest of the root.
- In the maxilla the geometry of the projection may prelude the recognition of a dilaceration.

Differential Diagnosis

It should be differentiated from:
- Fused roots
- Condensing osteitis
- A dense bone island.

This is achieved by taking radiographs from different angles.

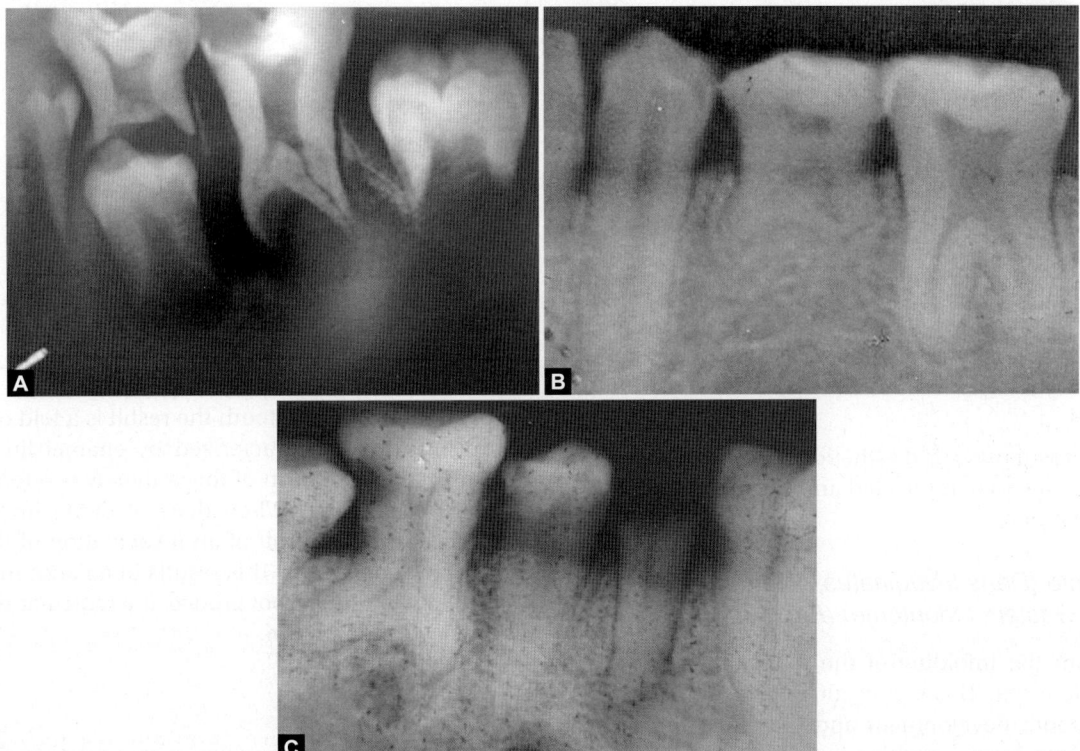

Figures 19.13A to C Taurodontism: These teeth have a longitudinally enlarged pulp chamber. The crown is of normal shape and size, but the body is enlarged and the roots are short. The pulp chamber extends from a normal position in the crown throughout the length of the extended body, leading to an increased distance between the cementoenamel junction and the furcation

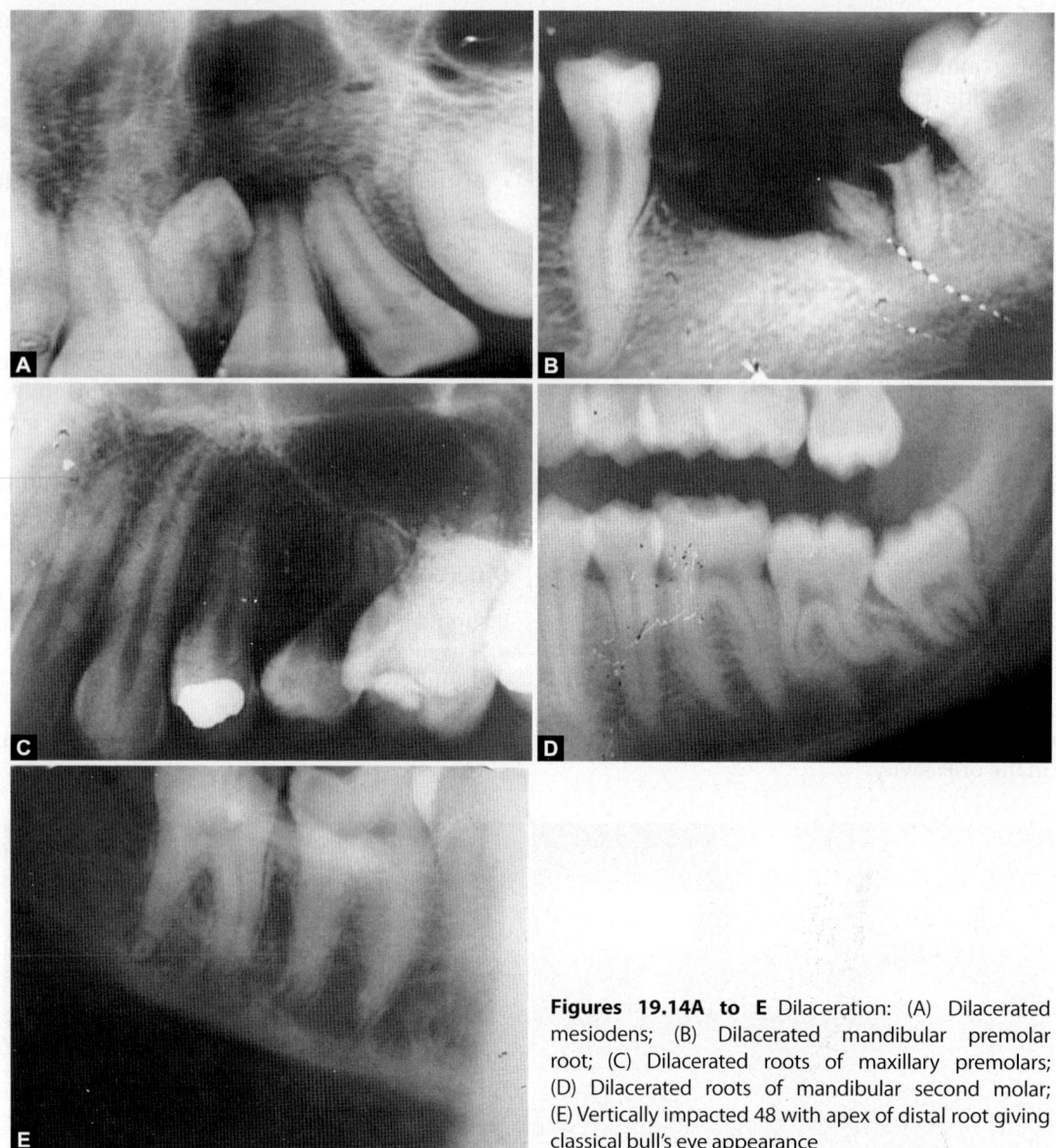

Figures 19.14A to E Dilaceration: (A) Dilacerated mesiodens; (B) Dilacerated mandibular premolar root; (C) Dilacerated roots of maxillary premolars; (D) Dilacerated roots of mandibular second molar; (E) Vertically impacted 48 with apex of distal root giving classical bull's eye appearance

Management

Dilacerated crown may need esthetic treatment. Dilacerated roots usually cause a complicated and difficult extraction or root canal treatment.

Dens in Dente (Dens Invaginatus, Dilated Odontome, Gestant Odontome) (Fig. 19.15)

It results from the infolding of the outer surface into the interior of the tooth. This can occur in either crown or the root during tooth development and may involve the pulp chamber or root canal, resulting in deformity either in the crown or the root.

Coronal invaginations usually originates from an anomalous infolding of the enamel organ into the dental papilla. In the mature tooth the result is a fold of hard tissue within the tooth characterized by enamel lining the fold. The most extreme form of this anomaly is referred to as the 'dilated odontome'. When dens in dente involves a root, it appears to be a result of an invagination of the Hertwig's epithelial root sheath. This results in an accentuation of the normal longitudinal root groove, the radicular type of defect is lined with cementum.

Clinical Features

- The anomaly is most often seen in the crown, involving most commonly the permanent maxillary lateral incisor, followed by the maxillary central incisors, premolars and canine and less often seen in the posterior teeth.

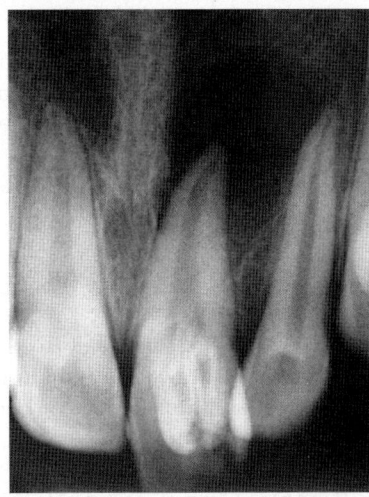

Figure 19.15 Central incisor showing dens in dente

- The coronal dens in dente are usually not large and the morphology of the crown may appear normal and is clinically seen as a pit at the incisal edge or cingulum.
- The pit in the cingulum may be broad and deep, which is often difficult to keep clean, which leads to caries, which rapidly involves the pulp.
- In addition there may be fine canals which extend between the invagination and the pulp chamber, resulting in pulpal disease even in the absence of caries.

Radiographic Features

- Dens in dente are usually detected on the radiograph, even before the tooth erupts.
- The infolding of the enamel lining is more radiopaque than the surrounding tooth structure and can easily be identified.
- Radicular invaginations appear as a poorly defined, slightly radiolucent structures running longitudinally within the root.
- If the coronal invagination is extensive, the crown is almost invariably malformed, with the apical foramen usually wide.
- In the most severe form (dilated odontome) the tooth is severely deformed having a circular or oval shape with a radiolucent interior.

Differential Diagnosis

The appearance especially in the incisors is so characteristic that once recognized, there is little place for confusion with any other condition.

Management

Early identification of the anomaly and prophylactic treatment can ensure a normal life span for the tooth.

Dens Evaginatus (Leong's Premolar, Evaginated Odontome, Occlusal Enamel Pearl)

This is the result of an outfolding of the enamel organ, which results in an enamel covered tubercle, usually in or near the middle of the occlusal surface of a premolar or occasionally a molar. The canine is rarely affected.

Clinical Features

- It appears clinically as a tubercle, usually in or near the middle of the occlusal surface of the affected tooth, appearing like a polyp in the central groove or lingual ridge of a buccal cusp, more often seen bilaterally in the mandible.
- The tubercle has a dentine core and a very slender pulp horn which extends into the evagination.
- After the tubercle is worn out by the apposing tooth, it appears as a small circular facet with a small black pit in the center.
- In rare cases a microscopic communication may occur between the pulp and the oral cavity through the tubercle. This may lead to the pulp becoming infected.

Radiographic Features

- It shows a dentine core usually covered with enamel, with an extension of a dentine tubercle on the occlusal surface.
- If the tubercle has been worn to a point of pulpal exposure or has fractured causing pulpal necrosis, it is shown by the presence of an open apical foramen and periapical radiolucency.

Differential Diagnosis

The appearance is characteristic, unless the tubercle has been worn down to the occlusal surface.

Management

If it is causing occlusal interferences, it should be removed under aseptic conditions and the pulp capped if necessary.

Talons Cusp (Figs 19.16A to C)

It is an anomalous hyperplasia of the cingulum of a maxillary or mandibular incisor.

Clinical Features

- It is a rare anomaly, found in either sex in both primary and secondary dentition.
- It varies in size from a prominent cingulum to that of a cusp like structure extending to the level of the incisal edge.
- When viewed from the incisal edge, the cusp appears 'T'-shaped with the top of the T represented by the incisal edge.

- The cusp blends smoothly with the tooth except if there is a deep developmental groove which may become caries prone.
- The cusp may or may not have an extension (horn) of the pulp.

Radiographic Features

- The cusp is apparent on the radiograph before eruption and may simulate the presence of a supernumerary tooth.
- Its outline is smooth and a layer of normal appearing enamel is seen.
- The radiograph may not reveal a pulp horn.

Differential Diagnosis

- It has a distinct appearance.
- To distinguish from a supernumerary, the parallex or buccal object technique may be used.

Management

If the cusp is large it may cause malocclusion or esthetic problems and needs to be treated accordingly. If the groove starts to decay, endodontic treatment may be required.

Supernumerary Roots (Figs 19.17A and B)

This developmental condition wherein there is presence of an extra root or roots is not a rarity.

Clinical Features

It may involve any tooth; single rooted teeth especially the mandibular cuspids often have two roots. Both the maxillary and mandibular molars, especially the third molars exhibit one or more supernumerary roots.

Radiographic Features

- May or may not be easily detected on the radiograph.
- The parallax or buccal object technique should be used to verify the presence if an extraroot is suspected.

Differential Diagnosis

It has a distinct appearance.

Management

It is important to diagnose the same before an extraction or endodontic treatment as if allowed to remain unrecognized after an extraction or not included in the root canal treatment may lead to persistent infection.

Enamel Pearl (Enamel Drop, Enamel Nodule, Enameloma) (Figs 19.18A and B)

Is a small globule of enamel 1.3 mm in diameter which occurs on the roots of molars. It is believed to be formed by Hertwig's epithelial root sheath, before the epithelium loses its enamel forming potential.

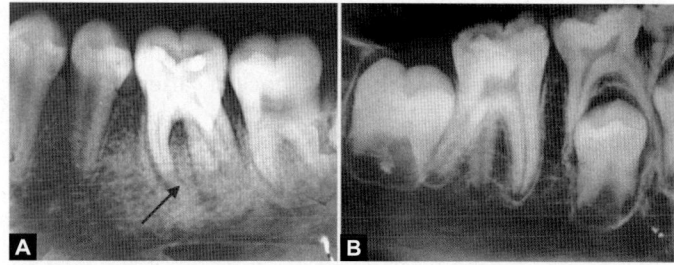

Figures 19.17A and B Mandibular first molars exhibiting supernumerary root

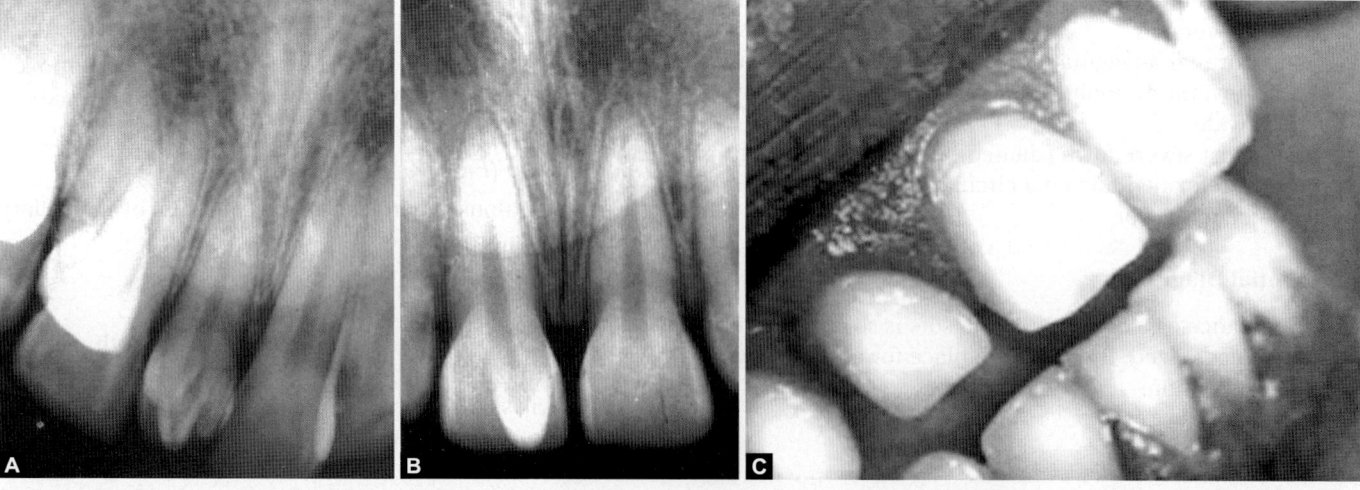

Figures 19.16A to C Talons cusp: Affecting the upper lateral incisor, and facial Talons cusp on the surface of the central incisor radiographic and clinical picture

Clinical Features

- It is found in approximately 3% of the population.
- It is made up of a core of dentine and rarely a pulp horn extending from the chamber of the host tooth.
- It is mostly found below the crest of the gingival, just apical of the cemento enamel junction, and may not be detected clinically.
- It may develop at the trifurcation of the maxillary molars (mesial or distal aspect) or the bifurcation of the mandibular molars (buccal or lingual aspects) (usually third molars in both the cases).
- Clinically symptom less, but may cause periodontal pocket formation.

Radiographic Features

- It appears smooth, round and comparable in radiopacity to the enamel covering the crown.
- The dentine casts a small radiolucent shadow in the center of the radiopaque sphere of enamel.

Differential Diagnosis

- Isolated piece of calculus, can be clinically verified.
- Pulp stone; an increase in the vertical angulations will move the image of the enamel pearl away from the pulp chamber.
- Radiopaque density due to superimposition of portions of the roots (of maxillary and mandibular molars) in the region of the furcation; take another image at a slightly different horizontal angle so as to eliminate the radiopaque region.

Management

The pearl needs to be removed, only if it is causing periodontal problems. Care should be taken to treat the pulp horn if present.

The presence of the pearl should be considered before an extraction of the tooth.

Abnormalities in Eruption

Premature Eruption

Neonatal teeth (teeth that erupt in the first 30 days) or natal teeth (deciduous teeth) which are present in the mouth of infants at birth.

Clinical Features

- Inconvenience during suckling
- Riga-Fede disease (trauma to the surrounding soft tissues).

Management

Treatment consists of extraction and/or rounding of the sharp edge of the tooth.

Transposition (Fig. 19.19)

It is a condition where two teeth have exchanged position or do not erupt in their normal position.

Clinical Features

- The most frequently transposed teeth are the permanent canines and first premolars.
- The second premolar, which frequently lies between the first and second molars.
- The transposition of the central and lateral is rare.

Radiographic Features

Radiographs reveal transposition when the teeth are not in their usual sequence.

Management

Transposed teeth are frequently altered prosthetically to improve function and esthetics. Orthodontically they may be brought to their correct position.

Embedded, Impacted and Submerged Teeth (Figs 19.20A to C)

Embedded teeth are individual teeth which are unerupted because of lack of eruption forces.

Impacted teeth are those prevented from erupting by some physical barrier in the path of eruption.

Submerged teeth are those which, lie below the plane of occlusion.

Clinical Features

The most common impacted teeth are the third molars (mandibular more often than the maxillary) and the maxillary cuspids.

Radiographic Features

Radiographs reveal the extent and type of impaction, imaginary Winter lines may be drawn to facilitate and plan the surgical extraction.

Management

Treatment includes extraction of the impacted teeth when they become symptomatic.

Abnormalities in the Structure

Amelogenesis Imperfecta (Figs 19.21A to D)

It is a developmental disturbance that interferes with normal enamel formation. It usually involves all the teeth, in both the dentitions. Most forms are autosomal dominant or

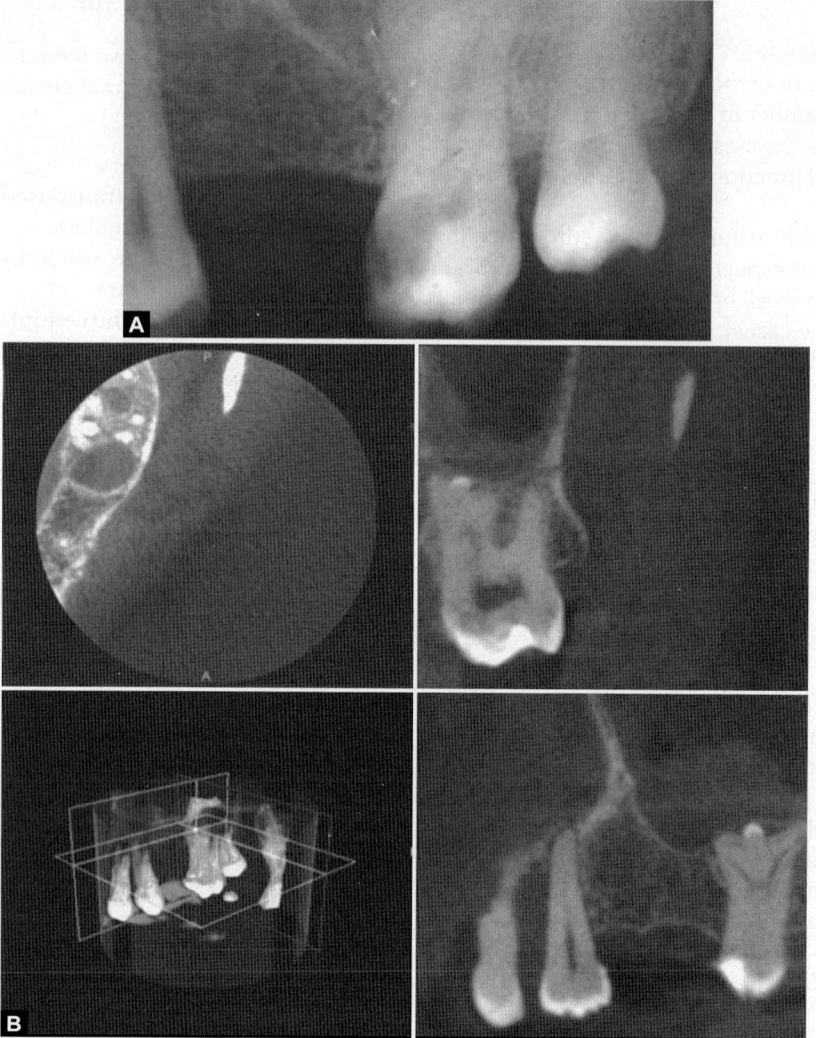

Figures 19.18A and B Enamel pearl: (A) Intra oral periapical radiograph showing a well-defined rounded radiopacity within the roots of the upper molar; (B) CBCT axial/coronal/3D/sagittal view of the same tooth showing the molar exhibiting taurodontism with an enamel pearl attached to its roots

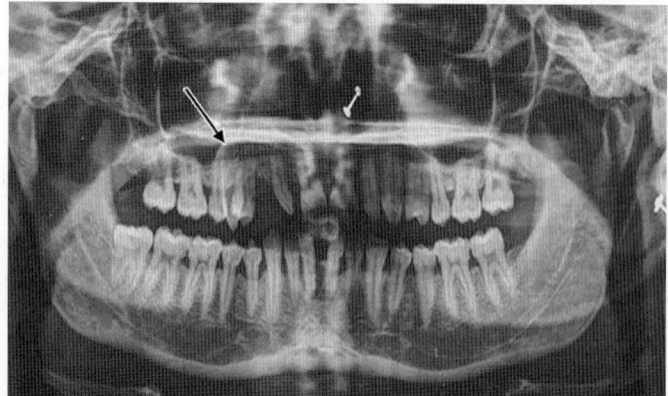

Figure 19.19 Panoramic radiograph showing trans position of right upper canine and premolar (black arrow) and peg shaped laterals

recessive, but two types are X-linked. The enamel lacks the normal prismatic structures, being laminated making it resistant to decay. The teeth may exhibit delayed eruption and a tendency to remain impacted. There are at least 14 variants of the said condition, the 4 most commonly seen are described; hypoplastic type, hypomaturation, hypocalcified type and hypomaturation-hypocalcified type associated with taurodontism.

Clinical Features

Hypoplastic Type

- The enamel fails to develop to its normal thickness, and is so thin that the dentine shows through giving a yellowish brown color to the tooth.

- The enamel may be pitted, rough or smooth and glossy.
- The crown contour is squarish, it is under sized with loss of contacts between adjacent teeth.
- The occlusal surfaces of the posterior teeth are relatively flat with low cusps which are easily attrited.
- An anterior open bite may be present.

Hypomaturation Type

- The enamel is of normal thickness but has a mottled appearance.

- The density of the enamel is comparable to that of dentine, thus it is softer than normal enamel and may chip away from the crown.
- The color varies from clear cloudy white, yellow to brown.
- In a particular form of hypomaturation the enamel appears white opaque giving a 'snow capped' appearance.

Hypocalcified Type

- This is a more common variety.
- The enamel is of normal thickness, thus the tooth that erupts has a crown of normal size and shape, but since

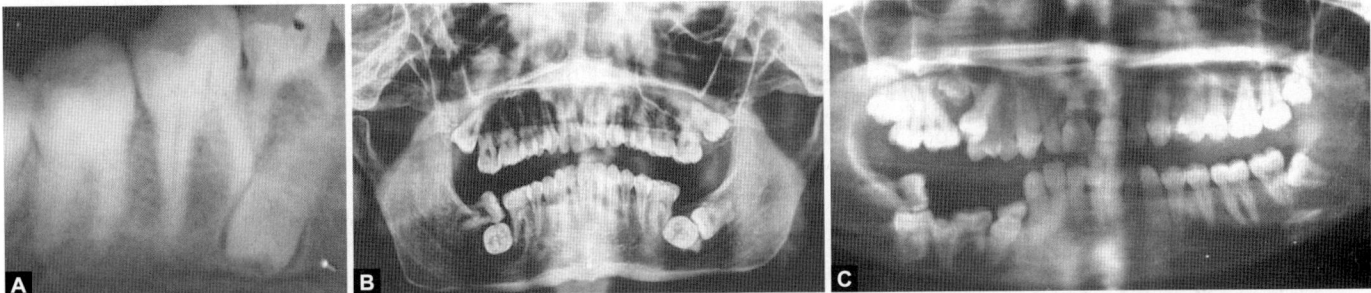

Figures 19.20A to C (A) Premolar erupting downwards; (B) Panoramic radiograph showing bilateral buccally impacted mandibular second molar; (C) Panoramic radiograph showing multiple unerupted teeth

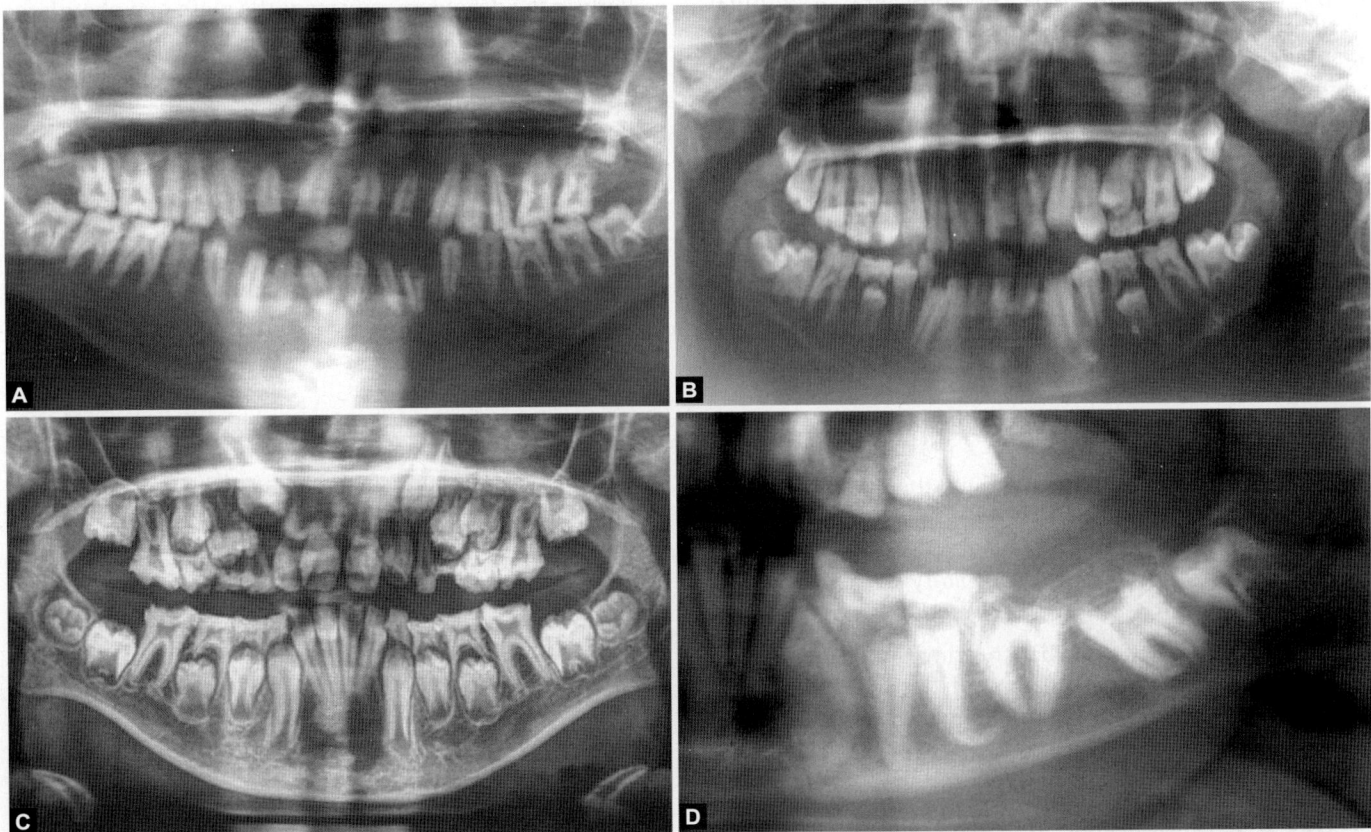

Figures 19.21A to D Amelogenesis imperfecta: (A to D) Panoramic radiographs showing generalized loss of the enamel on the occlusal surface, pitting of the occlusal surface of all the erupting erupted and developing permanent teeth

the enamel is poorly mineralized, and less dense than even the dentine, it starts to fracture away when the tooth comes into function.

- The soft enamel and dentine quickly wears away, resulting in the tooth being worn down to the level of the gingiva.
- The hypocalcified enamel has increased permeability and becomes stained and darkened, and appear dark brown due to food stains.

Hypomaturation-hypocalcified Type

- As the name suggests it is a combination of the above mentioned types.
- Hypomaturation-hypocalcified type has mottled and discolored (yellow and brown) enamel, which has the same radiopacity as the dentin.
- Hypocalcified-hypomaturation type has a similar appearance but the enamel layer is thinner.

Radiographic Features

- A square crown with relatively thin opaque layer of enamel with low or absent cusps.
- Pitted enamel appears as sharply localized areas of mottled density.
- The hypomaturation type demonstrates a normal thickness of the enamel, but the density is that of dentine.
- The hypocalcified type has normal enamel thickness but the density is even less than that of dentine.
- With advanced abrasion, obliteration of the pulp chamber may be seen.

Differential Diagnosis

Dentinogenesis imperfecta: Especially when there is increased abrasion leading to secondary dentine formation and obliteration of the pulp chamber. In dentinogenesis imperfecta the crown is more bulbous, narrow roots, obliteration of the pulp chamber and relative normal density of the enamel.

Management

Treatment includes restoration of the esthetics and function of the affected tooth.

Dentinogenesis Imperfecta (Hereditary Opalescent Dentine) (Figs 19.22A to D)

It is a developmental disturbance primarily of the dentin, with the enamel also being thinner. It is an autosomal dominant disturbance of high penetrance and occurs with equal frequency in males and females.

Two types of dentinogenesis imperfecta exist: Type I and Type II.
1. *Type I*: It is associated with osteogenesis imperfecta. Here the tooth roots and pulp chambers are small and

underdeveloped, and it affects the primary dentition more than the secondary dentition.
2. *Type II*: It is similar to type I but the lesion affects only the dentine with no skeletal defects. Type II may show enlarged pulp chambers in primary teeth.

Clinical Features

- It shows amber like translucency and a range of colors from yellow to blue-gray (depending on whether the affected teeth are observed by transmitted light or reflected light).
- The enamel easily fractures, and the crown wears down easily to the level of the gingiva.
- The exposed dentin becomes stained, and may be seen as dark brown to black.
- Some patients show an anterior open bite.

Radiographic Features

- The image of the crown size is normal, with a constriction of the cervical portion, giving a bulbous appearance.
- Marked attrition of the occlusal surface.
- The roots are short and slender.
- Type I and Type II show partial or complete obliteration of the pulp chamber.
- Early in the developmental stage the teeth may show large pulp chambers, but these are quickly obliterated by the formation of dentin. Ultimately the root canals may be absent or thread like.
- Periapical radiolucencies may be occasionally seen in association with sound teeth without evidence of pulpal involvement, which may occur via microscopic communication between the residual pulp and the oral cavity.
- The architecture of the bone in the maxilla and mandible is normal.

Differential Diagnosis

- Dentinal dysplasia where the crown size and shape is in proportion.
- Amelogenesis imperfecta.

Management

In children (5–15 years) extraction is not advised, prosthetic crowns (only if good root support is present) or over dentures may be placed to prevent alveolar resorption. In adults extraction with replacement is advised.

Osteogenesis Imperfecta (Brittle Bone Disease, Lobstein Disease)

It is a hereditary disorder characterized by osseous fractures. The pathogenesis is supposed to be an inborn error in the

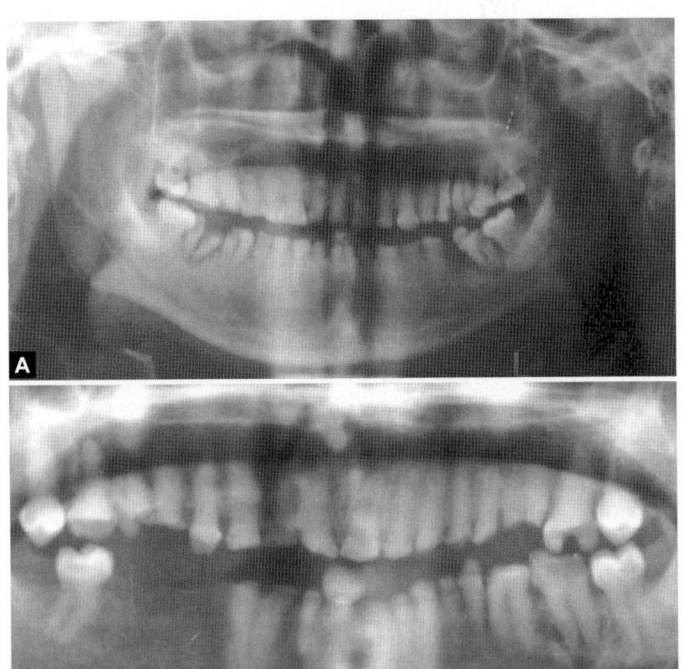

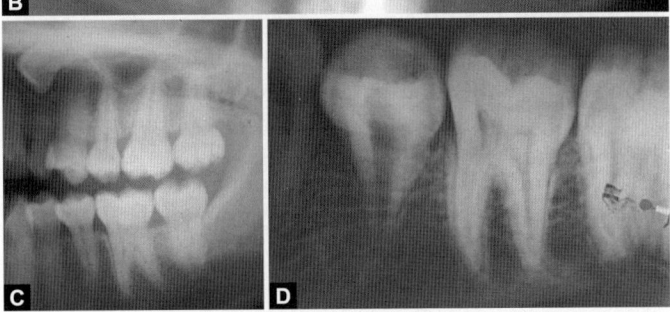

Figures 19.22A to D (A and B) Panoramic radiographs showing loss of enamel caps on all the teeth except on third molars. Complete obliteration of pulp chambers and canals of incisors, canines and premolars. Obliteration of pulp chambers of molars but thin radiolucent pulp canals could be seen. Diffuse ill-defined periapical radiolucencies in relation to multiple teeth; (C) Cropped OPG image showing dentinogenesis imperfecta (globular shape of the crowns). Taurodontism with mandibular molar; (D) Periapical radiograph showing fusiform shape of lower premolar

synthesis of type I collagen, which results in brittle bone. It is transmitted as an autosomal dominant trait. There are two types:

1. *Congenital or Vrolik's type*: This is present at birth
2. *Tarda or Lobstein's type*: This is recognized later in life, and is also known as osteopsathyrosis.

It may also be classified into clinical types:

- *Neonatal lethal type*: This is characterized by multiple fractures in infants and the child seldom survives.

- *Severe nonlethal type*: This is not evident till late childhood and the patient shows fracture of the bone with minimum trauma. The fracture may heal rapidly, but there is considerable skeletal deformity and dwarfed structure.
- *Moderate and deforming type*: This is associated with dentinogenesis imperfecta and blue sclera.
- *Mild and nondeformity type*: The patients are clinically normal, but they have an increased tendency for bone fracture, due to trauma.

Clinical Features

- Blue sclera, deafness, abnormal electric reaction of muscle and an increased tendency for capillary bleeding
- Wormian bones (skull sutures)
- Progressive osteopenia
- Dentinogenesis imperfecta is found in approximately 25% of the cases
- Enamel hypoplasia is sometimes seen
- Deciduous teeth are poorly calcified and semi-translucent or waxy. The teeth appear a faint dirty pink in color, half the normal size with globular crowns and relatively short roots in proportion to the other dimensions
- Class III malocclusions
- Increased incidence of impacted first and second molars
- The chin is sharply pointed, as a result of softening of bone, leading to flattening of the sides of the mandible.

Radiographic Features

- Patients may show wormian bones (skull sutures), skeletal deformities and progressive osteopenia.
- The bone is osteoporotic, with less density and fewer trabeculae.

Management

No known treatment.

Dentin Dysplasia (Fig. 19.23)

It is a rare autosomal dominant trait that resembles dentinogenesis imperfecta. There are two types: Type I (radicular) and Type II (coronal).

Clinical Features

- In type I (radicular) the teeth have normal color and shape in both the dentitions. A bluish brown translucency may be observed. The teeth are malaligned in the arch, with drifting and exfoliation on minimum or no trauma.
- In type II (coronal) the crowns of the primary teeth appear to be of the same size, shape and color as that in dentinogenesis imperfecta and these rapidly abrade. The permanent teeth are normal.

Radiographic Features

- Type I (Radicular), the roots of primary and permanent teeth are either short or abnormally shaped. The roots of the primary teeth may appear as thin spicules. The pulp chambers and root canals completely fill in before eruption. The 20% of these teeth which are usually noncarious have periapical radiolucencies which may be either cysts or granulomas.
- In type II (Coronal) obliteration of the pulp chamber and reduction in the calibration of the root canal occurs after eruption (at least 5-6 years). As the pulp chambers of the molars are filled with hypertrophic dentin, the pulp chambers become flame shaped and may have multiple pulp stones. The anterior teeth and premolars develop a pulp chamber that is 'thistle-tube' in shape because of its extension into the root. The roots of the coronal variety are normal in shape and proportion.

Differential Diagnosis

- Dentinogenesis imperfecta and dentin dyplasia, these two conditions seem to form a continuum, their differentiation may be difficult at first, as both produce altered color and occluded pulp chambers.
  - In type II dentinal dysplasia, the pulp chambers do not fill in before eruption, and the thistle-tube shaped pulp chamber in single rooted teeth is characteristic.
  - In dentinogenesis imperfecta the crowns have atypical bulbous appearance with a cervical constriction, whereas crowns appear normal in dentin dyspalsia.
  - The roots in dentinogenesis imperfects are short and narrow, whereas roots appear normal or practically no roots are suggestive of dentin dyspalsia.
  - Periapical rarefying osteitis in association with noncarious teeth is more common in dentin dysplasia.

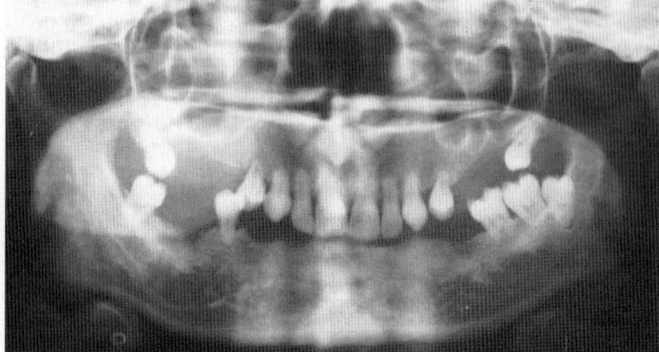

Figure 19.23 Dentin dysplasia (Type 1): Panoramic radiograph shows pathological drifting of the upper third molars. All the teeth have short roots, obliterated pulp chambers and root canals

Management

- *Type I*: Prosthetic replacement is about the only treatment.
- *Type II*: Crowns may be prepared to prevent abrasion.
- Esthetics of discolored teeth may be attended to.

Regional Odontodysplasia (Odontogenesis Imperfecta)

It is rare condition in which the enamel and dentine are hypoplastic and hypocalcified which results in the localized arrest in tooth development. It may affect only a few adjacent teeth in a quadrant, usually if the primary teeth are affected, their successors are also involved.

Clinical Features

- The affected teeth are small and mottled brown due to staining of the hypocalcified hypoplastic enamel.
- They are susceptible to caries and are brittle and subject to fractures and pulpal infections.
- Central incisors followed by laterals and canines are commonly affected (more maxillary than mandibular), and the eruption of the affected teeth is delayed or they may not erupt at all.

Radiographic Features

- They have a 'ghost like' appearance.
- The pulp chambers are large and root canals wide because of the hypoplastic dentine, which just outlines the root, which are also very short.
- The enamel is also thin, less dense and poorly mineralized that it may not be apparent on the radiograph.
- The tooth appears like a thin shell, and those which do not erupt appear to be resorbing.

Differential Diagnosis

Dentinogenesis imperfecta: This usually carries a history of familial involvement, and involves all the primary teeth, whereas in regional odontoplasia enamel is hypoplastic, only a few teeth are involved and it has no hereditary history.

Management

As far as possible the teeth should be retained with the help of the newer restorative materials available.

Severely damaged permanent teeth that become pulpally involved may require removal and replacement.

Turner's Hypoplasia (Turner's Tooth) (Fig. 19.24)

This is used to describe a permanent tooth with a local hypoplastic defect in the crown. The defect may be caused by the extension of the periapical infection from its deciduous predecessor or mechanical trauma, when the crown is forming which adversely affect the ameloblasts of the developing tooth and result in some degree of hypoplasis or hypermineralization.

Clinical Features

- It usually affects the mandibular premolars
- The hypomineralized area may get stained and develop a brownish spot
- In case of hypoplasia, the morphology of the crown may show pitting or a more pronounced defect.

Radiographic Features

- The affected area of hypoplasia of the crown may appear as an ill-defined radiolucent region.
- In case of hypomineralization it may not be apparent due to insufficient difference in the degree of radiopacity between the spot and the crown of the tooth. Hypomineralized area may become mineralized by continued contact with saliva.

Differential Diagnosis

Radiation caries usually has history of radiation treatment, and many teeth will be involved.

Management

Esthetics and function of the tooth may be restored in the root support is good.

Congenital Syphilis

Thirty percent of affected people develop dental hypoplasia of the permanent incisors (Hutchinson's teeth) and first molars (Mulberry molars or moon's molar), the primary teeth are rarely affected. The changes are a result of direct

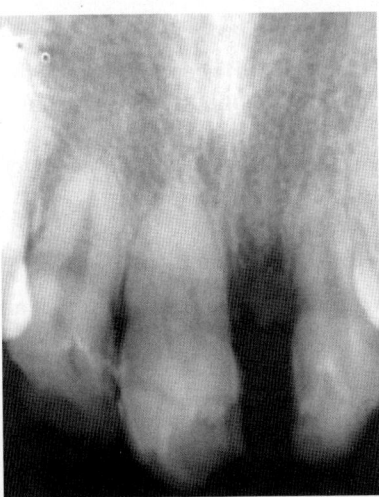

Figure 19.24 Turner's hypoplasia affecting the central incisor which also has a pulp stone

infection of the developing tooth as spirochete of syphilis has been identified in the tooth germ.

Clinical Features

- The affected tooth has a 'screw-driver' shaped crown, with the mesial and distal surfaces tapering from the middle of the crown to the incisal edge, which is often notched. The maxillary central incisor, followed by the maxillary lateral and mandibular central demonstrate these changes.
- The crowns of the affected first molars are characteristically smaller, constricted occlusal third, cusps are of reduced size and poorly formed. The enamel over the occlusal surface is hypoplastic, formed in uneven globules, like a 'mulberry' surface.

Radiographic Features

- The characteristic changes in shape of the affected teeth can be observed on the radiograph.
- As the crowns of these teeth form at about 1 year of age, radiographs may reveal the dental features of congenital syphilis 4 to 5 years before the teeth erupt.

Management

Esthetic treatment may be done to correct the hypoplastic defects.

ACQUIRED ANOMALIES OF THE TEETH

Attrition (Fig. 19.25)

It is the physiological wearing away of the dentition resulting from occlusal contacts between the maxillary and mandibular teeth. It occurs on the incisal, occlusal and interproximal surfaces. It depends on the abrasiveness of the diet, salivary factors, mineralization of the teeth and emotional tension. Physiologic attrition is a component of the aging process. When loss of dental tissue becomes excessive, however, as from bruxism, the attrition becomes pathological.

Clinical Features

- Occurs in 99% of young adults and is more in males than females.
- Wear facets appear on the cusps and marginal, oblique and transverse ridges.
- The incisal edges show broadening.
- The lingual cusps of the maxillary teeth and the buccal cusps of the mandibular teeth show more pronounced facets.
- The dentine is exposed and becomes stained.
- The incisal edges of the mandibular incisors tend to become pitted.
- In case of pathologic attrition the wear facets are generally not as uniformly progressive and develop at a faster rate.

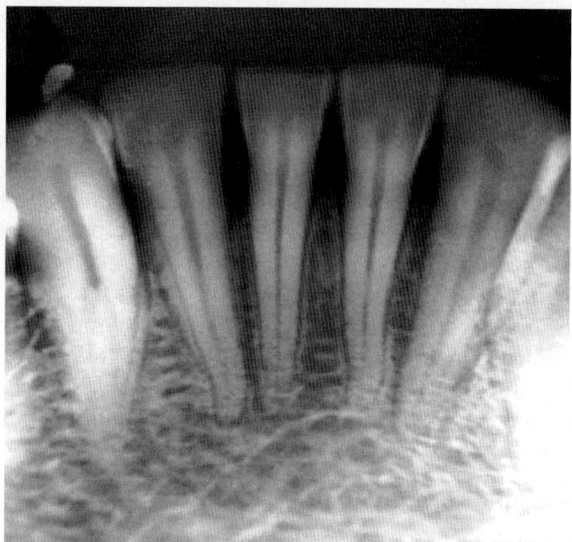

Figure 19.25 Attrition of the lower incisors

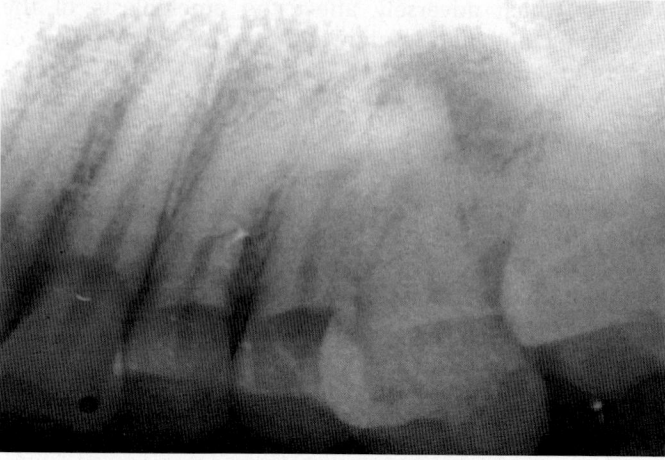

Figure 19.26 Abrasion cavities in relation to maxillary canine and premolars

Radiographic Features

- There is a change in the normal outline of the tooth structure, altering the normal curves into flat planes.
- The crown is shortened and is bereft of the incisal or occlusal surface enamel.
- Number of adjacent teeth in the arch may show the same wear pattern.
- Reduction in the size of the pulp chamber and root canals may be seen due to stimulation of deposition of the secondary dentin, which may lead to the complete obliteration of the pulp chamber and the root canal.
- Widening of the periodontal ligament space is seen if the tooth is mobile.
- Alveolar bone loss may be seen
- Occasionally there may be evidence of hypercementosis.

Differential Diagnosis

Clinically differentiated on the basis of history, location and extent.

Management

Pathologic attrition may be treated by giving a mouth guard.

Abrasion (Fig. 19.26)

This is the nonphysiological wearing of teeth by the contact with foreign substances. It results from friction induced by habits or occupational hazards. It may occur due to improper toothbrushing or tooth flossing, pipe smoking, opening hair pins with teeth, improper use of toothpicks, denture clasps and cutting thread with teeth.

Toothbrush Injury

Clinical Features

- The back and forth movement of the brush with heavy pressure caused a 'V' shaped groove in the cervical area, at the cementoenamel junction on the labial and buccal surfaces of maxillary premolars, canines and incisors, usually involving enamel and the softer root surface.
- Teeth become sensitive as the dentine is exposed.
- The lesions are more common on the left side for a right-handed person and vice versa. The premolars in the upper arch are usually the first to be affected.
- Deposition of secondary dentine keeps pace with the abrasion thus pulpal exposure is rarely a complication.

Radiographic Features

- Radiolucent defect at the cervical level of the teeth.
- The defect has well defined semilunar shape with borders of increasing radiopacity.
- The pulp chamber of the severely affected teeth is partially or completely obliterated.

Management

Treatment includes modification of the habit and restoration if required.

Dental Floss Injury

Clinical Features

Excessive and improper use of floss, results in abrasion of the dentition, the most frequent site being the cervical portion of the proximal surfaces just above the gingival.

Radiographic Features

- The lesion is seen as a narrow semilunar radiolucency in the interproximal surfaces of the cervical area.
- The radiolucent groove on the distal surface is deeper than that on the mesial surface, as it is easier to exert more pressure in a forward direction by pulling than by pushing the floss backward into the mouth.

Differential Diagnosis

It may simulate carious lesion located at the cervical region of the tooth, and should be differentiated by clinical inspection.

Management

Treatment consists of elimination of the habit and restoration of the abraded area.

Erosion

It is a result of chemical action not involving bacteria. The acid source may be from chronic vomiting or acid reflux from gastrointestinal disorders (involves lingual surfaces), a diet which contains large amounts of acidic food, citrus fruits or carbonated beverages (Involves demineralization of labial surfaces).

Clinical Features

- Involves multiple teeth, incisors more prone.
- The lesions are seen as smooth glistening depressions in the enamel surface, frequently near the gingival.
- There may be so much loss of enamel that a pink spot may show through the remaining enamel.

Radiographic Features

Areas of erosion appear as radiolucent defects on the crown. The margins may be well-defined or diffuse.

Differential Diagnosis

- Edges of lesions caused by erosion are usually more rounded off than those caused by abrasion.
- The margins of a restoration may project above the remaining tooth surface.

Management

Treatment includes removal of the causative agent and restoration of the defect to prevent additional damage, possible pulp exposure and objectionable esthetic appearance.

Abfraction (Stress Lesion)

It is the loss of tooth surface at the cervical areas due to tensile and compressive forces on the natural dentition.

Clinical Features

- It usually affects buccal/labial cervical areas, of single teeth which are subjected to excursive interferences or eccentric occlusal load.
- It appears as a V-shaped notch.

Radiographic Features

- Radiolucent defect at the cervical level of the teeth.
- The defect has well defined semilunar shape with borders of increasing radiopacity.
- The pulp chamber of the severely affected teeth is partially or completely obliterated.

Differential Diagnosis

Abrasion which involves more teeth and gives history of a faulty brushing habit.

Resorption

It is the removal of tooth structure by osteoclasts (odontoclasts). It may be classified as internal or external depending on the surface of the tooth involved. The resorption discussed here is not that associated with the normal loss of deciduous teeth. It may be sequelae of chronic infection (inflammation), excessive pressure and function, or factors associated with local tumors and cysts.

Internal Resorption (Figs 19.27A to C)

It occurs within the pulp chamber or canal and involves the resorption of the surrounding dentin, resulting in the enlargement of the pulp space at the cost of tooth structure. The condition may be transient, self-limiting or progressive. It may be initiated by acute trauma to the tooth, direct and indirect pulp capping, pulpotomy and enamel invagination.

Clinical Features

- It may affect primary or secondary dentition. More frequently in the permanent teeth, usually central incisors and the first and second molars
- It is seen more often in males in the fourth and fifth decades
- In the pulp chamber, it may enlarge until the crown has a dark shadow, or it may perforate the dentine and involve the enamel, and is seen as a 'pink spot'. It may further progress to perforate the crown causing infectious pulpitis.
- In the root, the progress is clinically silent, it weakens the root leading to a fracture. The pulp may expand into the periodontal ligament space and communicate with a deep periodontal pocket or the gingival sulcus, leading to pulpal infection.

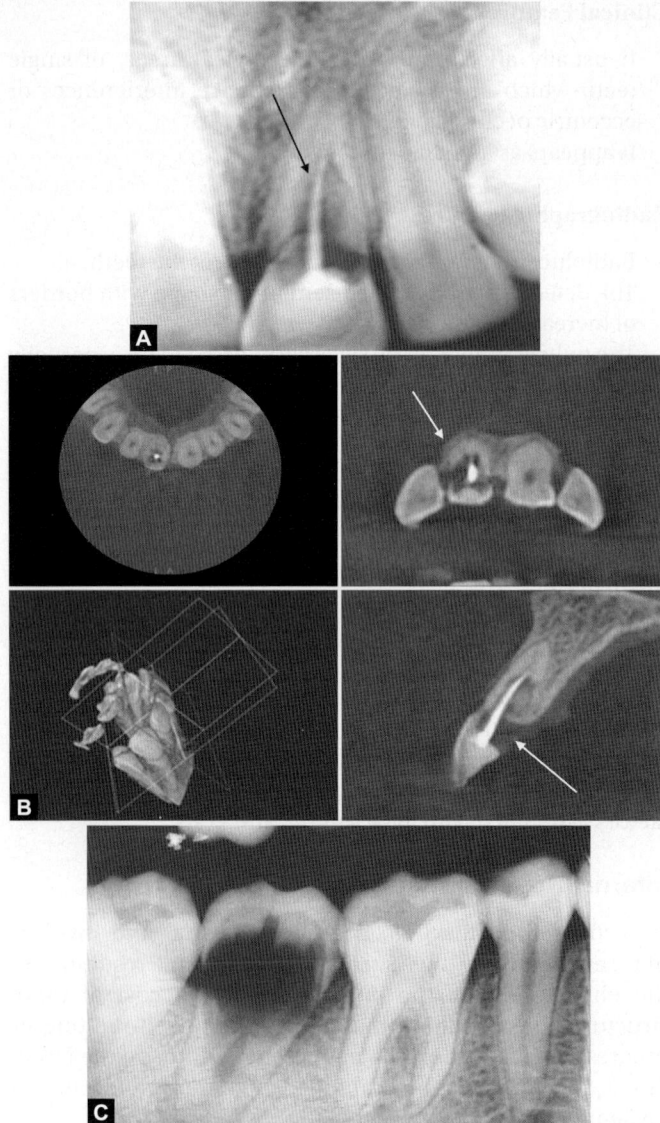

Figures 19.27A to C Internal resorption: (A) Periapical radiograph showing internal resorption in upper central incisor; (B) CBCT axial/coronal/3D/sagittal sections showing the same tooth with the extent of internal resorption seen on the lingual aspect which is camoflaged on the conventional radiograph; (C) Internal resorption in mandibular second molar

Radiographic Features

- Radiographs reveal symptom less early lesions of internal resorption.
- They appear as radiolucency round, oval or elongated within the root or crown and continuous with the image of the pulp chamber or canal.
- The outline is sharply defined and smooth or slightly scalloped.
- It is characteristically homogeneously radiolucent, without bony trabeculation or pulp stones.

Differential Diagnosis

- Carious lesion on the buccal or lingual surface of the tooth; these have more diffuse margins, the mesial and distal surfaces of the pulp chamber and canal can be separated from the borders of the carious lesion. It can be clinically verified.
- External root resorption.

Management

Depending on the stage of the disease the tooth root canal treatment or extraction may be advised.

External Resorption (Figs 19.28A to C)

The odontoclasts that resorb the outer surface of the tooth, usually involving the root surface, or the crowns of unerupted teeth. It may involve a single tooth, multiple teeth or in rare cases the entire dentition. The cause is attributed to localized inflammatory lesions, reimplanted teeth, tumors and cysts, excessive mechanical (orthodontic) and occlusal forces, and impacted teeth.

Clinical Features

- It is not clinically recognized as it is symptom free, and may show a sign only after considerable loss of tooth structure has occurred.
- It may occur at the apex or on the lateral root surface.
- It is more prevalent in the mandibular teeth, involving mostly the central incisors, canines and premolars.

Radiographic Features

- Blunting of the root apex, the bone and lamina dura follow the resorption and present a normal appearance around a shortened structure.
- If the resorption is due to periapical inflammatory lesion the lamina dura is lost.
- The pulp canal appears wide at the apex.
- Lateral resorption tends to be irregular, involving one side more than the other. An unerupted adjacent tooth may be a common cause.
- External resorption of an entire tooth may occur when the tooth is unerupted and completely embedded in bone (maxillary canine, third molar).

Differential Diagnosis

External resorption on the apex and lateral surface of the root is radiographically self-evident.

Management

Treatment includes removal of the underlying cause in the early stage.

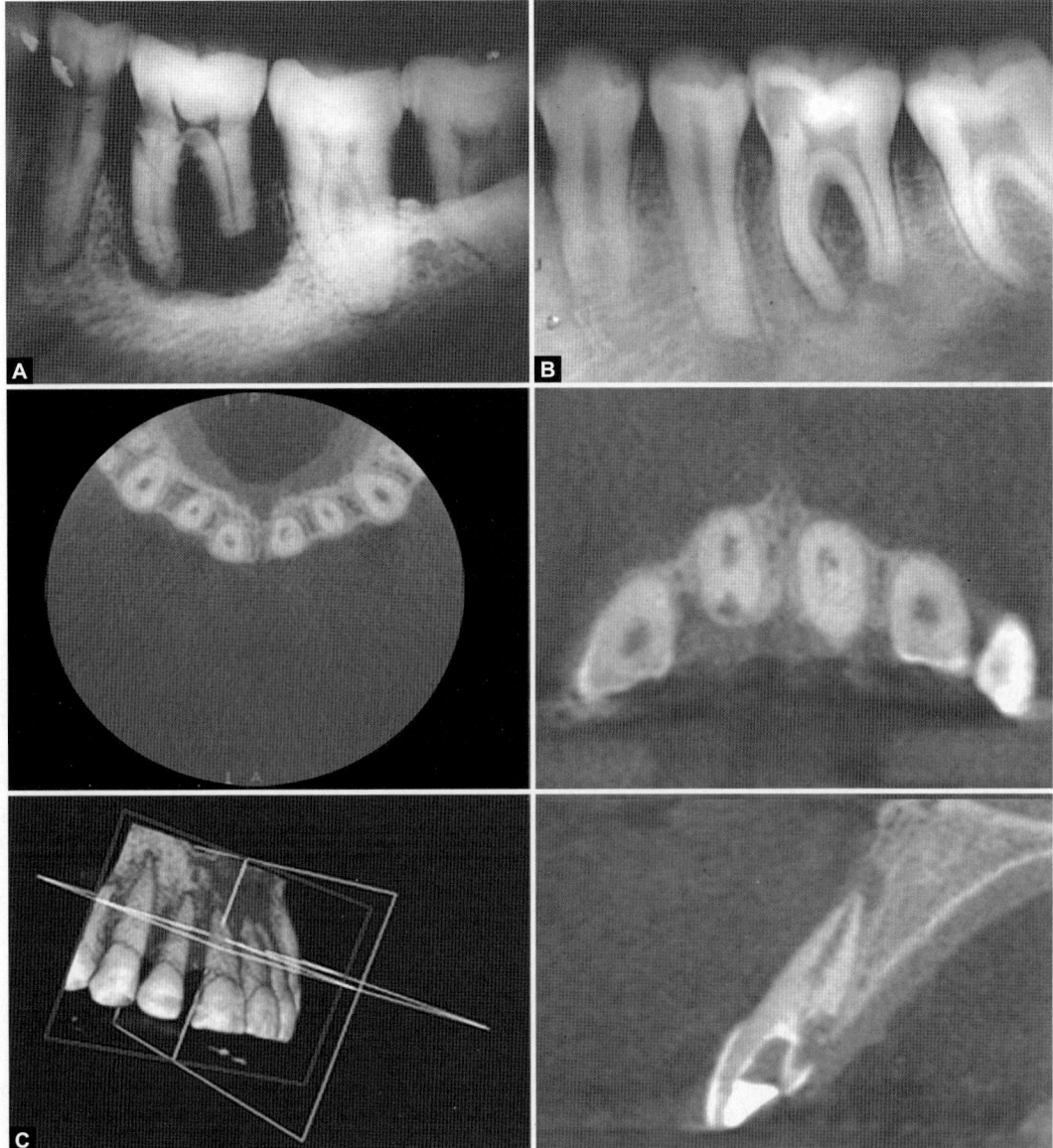

Figures 19.28A to C External resoption: (A and B) Periapical radiographs showing resorption of roots of mandibular molars; (C) CBCT axial/coronal/3D/sagittal views showing external resoption of an incisor tooth from the palatal aspect. Clinically the tooth appeared healthy and no abnormality was detected on the conventional intra oral radiograph

Dentinal Sclerosis

Also called transparent dentine, it is a regressive alteration in the tooth substance that is characterized by the calcification of the dentinal tubules, due to injury and/or aging process.

Clinical Features

- It is more calcified and harder than normal dentine.
- When examined under transmitted light, a translucent zone is observed.

Secondary Dentin

It is that which is deposited in the pulp chamber after the formation of primary dentin has been completed, and is a normal aging process (stimulated due to chewing or mild trauma). It may also occur due to chronic trauma from pathological conditions like progressive caries, trauma, erosion, abrasion, attrition or a dental restorative procedure. 'Tertiary dentin' has been coined to identify dentin initiated by stimuli other than the normal aging process and biologic function.

Clinical Features

It reduces sensitivity.

Radiographic Features

- It is indistinguishable from primary dentine.
- It may be seen as a reduction in size of the pulp chamber and canals.
- When the cause is normal aging process the result is generalized even reduction, in case of a more specific stimuli, the secondary dentine formation begins in the region adjacent to the source of stimuli and alters the normal shape of the pulp chamber.
- A small trace of pulp tissue remains even if the pulp chamber and canal appears to be completely obliterated.

Differential Diagnosis

Pulp stone, this occupies the chamber or canal space and has a round or oval shape.

Management

No treatment required.

Pulp Stones (Figs 19.29A and B)

These are foci of calcification in the dental pulp.

Clinical Features

These are not clinically discernible.

Radiographic Features

- Only the larger stones, which comprise 15–25% of pulpal calcifications are seen on the radiographs.
- They are seen as radiopaque structures within the pulp chamber or canal. They may be round or oval, and some may conform to the shape of the chamber or canal.
- They may occur as a single dense mass or as several small radiopacities.
- They occur in all tooth types, but are more common in molars.

Differential Diagnosis

Pulpal sclerosis.

Management

No treatment required.

Pulpal Sclerosis

It is another form of calcification, which is a diffuse process, of unknown origin. The 66% of all teeth in individuals between the ages of 10–20 years, as well as 90% of all teeth in individuals between the ages of 50–70 years, show histological evidence of pulpal sclerosis.

Clinical Features

It is a clinically silent process.

Radiographic Features

Diffuse pulpal sclerosis produces a generalized, ill-defined collection of fine radiopacities throughout large areas of the pulp chamber and pulp canals.

Differential Diagnosis

Small pulp stones.

Management

No treatment required, but like in pulp stones they may cause difficulty in endodontic treatment.

Hypercementosis (Fig. 19.30)

It is the excessive deposition of cementum on the tooth roots. It may be seen in a supraerupted tooth, reaction to an inflammatory process, in teeth that are in hyperocclusion or have been fractured. It is also related in patients with systemic disorders like; Paget's disease or hyperpituitarism (gigantism and acromegaly).

Clinical Features

No clinical signs or symptoms seen.

Radiographic Features

- It is seen as an excessive build up of cementum around all or part of a root, with thickening and blunting of the root
- The outline is usually smooth, or sometimes may be seen as an irregular enlargement of the root, with a bulbous apex
- This cementum is slightly more radiolucent than dentin
- The lamina dura and PDL space encompass the extra cementum
- If the cementum is distributed eccentrically there is a localized protuberance.

Differential Diagnosis

- Any radiopaque structure that is seen in the vicinity of the root, like; enostosis, mature cemental dysplasia
- Multirooted teeth and dilacerated root
- Fused root
- The main differentiating characteristics is the presence of the periodontal membrane space around the hypercementosis.

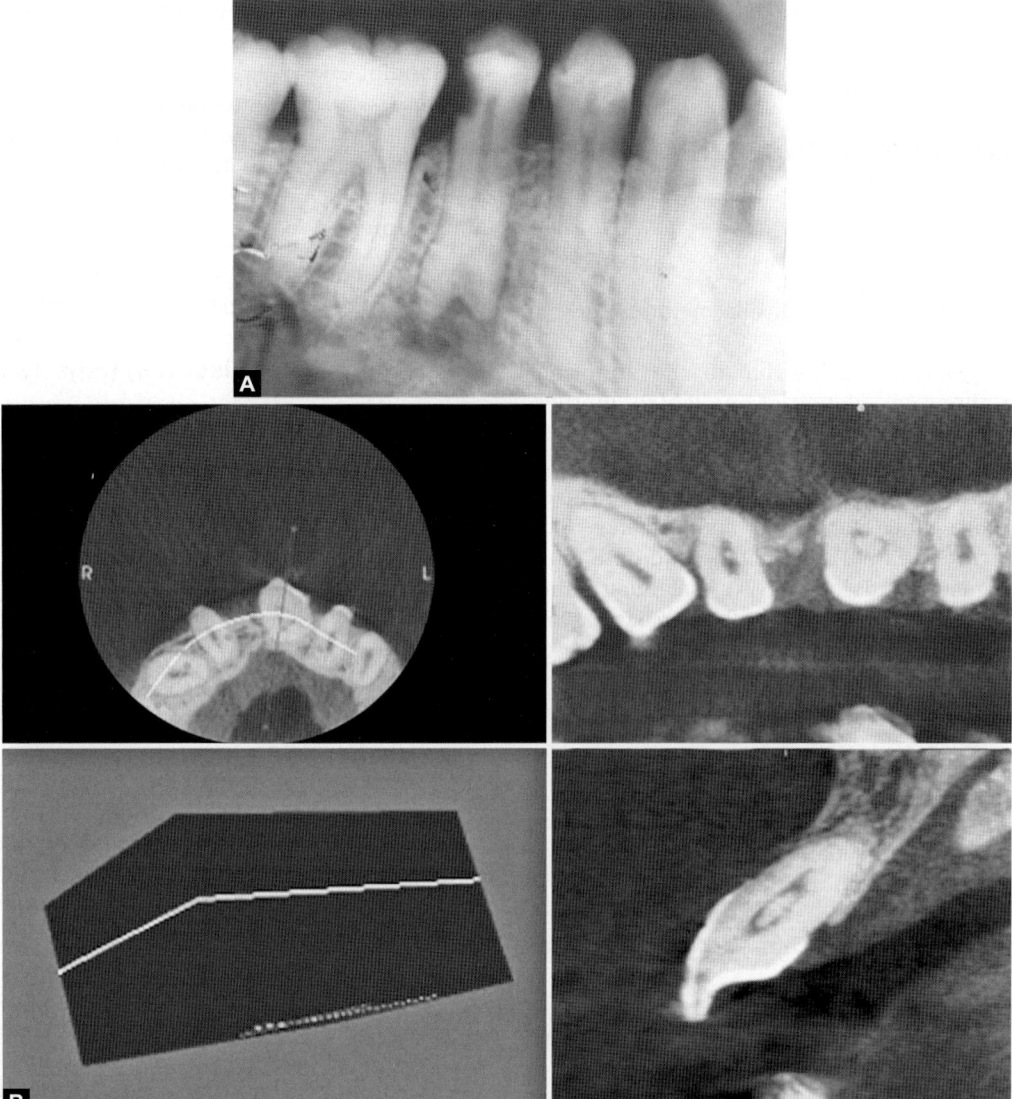

Figures 19.29A and B (A) Pulp stone in lower first premolar, the second premolar exhibits bifid roots; (B) CBCT axial/panoramic/3D sagittal view showing a well delineated pulp stone in the maxillary canine. 3D view appears as a box if there is incompatibility with the computer software

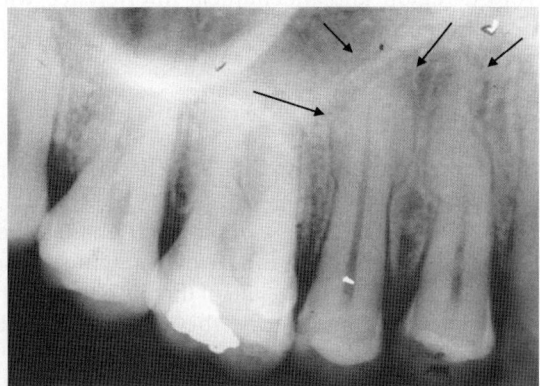

Figure 19.30 Hypercementosis

Management

No treatment required, it may pose difficulty in tooth extraction.

Cementicles

These are small, spherical particles of cementum that may lie free in the periodontal ligament adjacent to the cementum surface. They may be free, attached or sessile or embedded.

Clinical Features

No signs or symptoms.

Radiographic Features

Will appear as radiopaque opacities along the root surface, size ranging from 0.2–0.3 inches in diameter.

DEVELOPMENTAL DISTURBANCES OF THE JAWS

Micrognathia

Definition

This means small jaws, either the maxilla or the mandible may be affected. There are two types:
- *Apparent micrognathia*: This is due to the abnormal positioning or abnormal relation of one jaw to another, which produces an illusion of micrognathia.
- *True micrognathia*: It is due to small jaws. This may be:
  - *Congenital*: The exact etiology is not known. It is usually associated with other congenital abnormalities like, congenital heart disease, Pierre-Robin Syndrome (cleft palate, micrognathia and glossoptosis), Hallerman-Streiff syndrome, Trisomy 13, Trisomy 18, Turners syndrome, Treacher Collin's syndrome, Marfan's syndrome.
  - *Acquired*: This is usually a result of disturbances in the area of the TMJ and/or ankylosis.

Clinical Features

- Micrognathia of the maxilla is due to deficiency of the premaxillary area and the patient with this deformity appears to have the middle third of the face retracted.
- True mandibular micrognathia is rare. The patient is seen to have severe retrusion of the chin, a steep mandibular angle and a deficient chin button.
- There will be associated malocclusion.
- In infants it will cause difficulty in respiration and interfere with the feeding.

Management

The abnormality may be corrected with surgery and orthodontic treatment.

Macrognathia (Megagnathia)

Definition

This refers to a condition of abnormally large jaws. This may be hereditary, associated with pituitary gigantism, Paget's disease, acromegaly, leontiasis ossea.

Clinical Features

- Mandibular protusion or prognathism is common, due to disparity in the size of the maxilla to the mandible, posterior positioning of the maxilla in relation to the cranium or excessive condylar growth and anterior positioning of the glenoid fossa.

- The mandibular body length is increased.
- The ramus forms a steep angle with the body of the mandible.
- There is a prominent chin button.
- In some patients there may be an elongation of the maxilla, which produces a 'Gummy' smile.

Management

Treatment consists of osteotomy, resection of a part of the mandible, followed by orthodontic treatment.

Facial Clefts (Oral Fissures) (Figs 19.31A to C)

Definition

A failure of fusion of the developmental process of the face during fetal development may result in a variety of facial clefts.
- Cleft lip
- Double lip
- Cleft palate
- Mandibular clefts.

Cleft lip with or without cleft palate (CL/P) and cleft palate (CP) are two different conditions with different etiologies. Cleft of the lower lip is very rare.

CL results from a failure of fusion of the medial nasal process and the maxillary process. This may range in severity from a unilateral cleft lip to bilateral complete clefting through the lip, alveolus, hard and soft palate.

CP develops from a failure of fusion of the lateral palatal shelves.

There are various components attributed to the formation of CL/P, but the exact etiology is not completely understood. It may be an associated abnormality as part of a genetic malformation syndrome (e.g. Velocardiofacial syndrome (del 22q.11 syndrome) cleft palate, facial and cardiac abnormalities, Van der Woude syndrome; cleft lip and/or cleft palate and lip pits), nutritional disturbances (prenatal folate deficiency), environmental teratogenic agents, stress, defects of vascular supply to the involved region and mechanical interference with the closure of the embryonic processes (cleft palate in Pierre Robin syndrome).

Clinical Features

- CL/P is more common in males and CP is more common in females.
- The severity of CL/P varies from a notch in the upper lips to a cleft involving only the lip to extension into the nostril, resulting in deformity of the ala of the nose.
- As CL/P increases in severity, the cleft will include the alveolar process and palate.
- Bilateral cleft lip is more frequently associated with cleft palate.

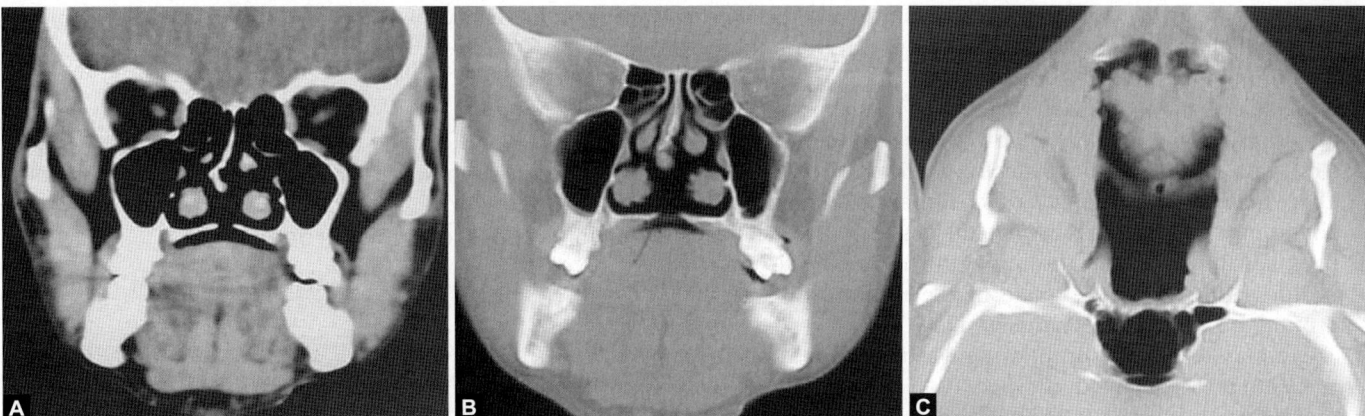

Figures 19.31A to C Cleft palate: (A and B) CT coronal section, bone and soft tissue window shows small vertical defect in the midline in the posterior part of the hard palate. The bone window showed thickening of the mucosa of both the maxillary sinuses. The soft tissue window showed a 'C' shaped deviation of the nasal septum; (C) CT axial section shows a midline defect in the soft palate

- The least manifestation of cleft palate is a submucous cleft, where the palate appears intact except for notching of the uvula (bifid uvula) or notching in the posterior border of the hard palate.
- The most severe presentation is complete clefting of the hard and soft palate. It may range from only the involvement of the uvula or soft palate to extension all the way through the palate to include the alveolar process in the region of the lateral incisor on one or both sides.
- With the involvement of the alveolar process, there is an increase in the incidence of dental anomalies in the region of the cleft including missing, hypoplastic and supernumerary teeth.
- The palatal defect in CL/P and CP interfere with speech and swallowing.
- These patients are more prone to ear infections because of the abnormal anatomy of the Eustachian tube.

Radiographic Features

- There is a well-defined vertical radiolucent defect in the alveolar bone.
- Numerous associated dental anomalies; absence of maxillary lateral incisor and presence of supernumerary teeth. The involved teeth may be malformed and poorly positioned.
- There may be a delay in the development of maxillary and mandibular teeth and an increased incidence of hypodontia in both arches.
- The osseous defect may be extended to include the floor of the nasal cavity.
- In cases of repaired clefts, a well-defined osseous defect may not be apparent, but only a vertically short alveolar process may be seen at the site of the cleft.

Management

Treatment should be carried out under the guidance of the cleft palate team.

Facial Hemiatrophy (Parry-Romberg Syndrome, Romberg Hemifacial Atrophy, Hemifacial Microstomia, Progressive Facial Hemiatrophy)

Definition

This is a rare disorder characterized by slowly progressive wasting (atrophy) of the soft tissues of half of the face (hemifacial atrophy).

Clinical Features

- The onset is noted in the first or second decade of life as a white line furrow or mark on one side of the face or brow near the midline.
- There is a predilection for the left side.
- The progressive tissue wasting continues for three to five years and then ceases.
- The affected side demonstrates shrinkage and atrophy of the tissue beneath the skin (subcutaneous tissue), in the layer of fat under the skin (subcutaneous fat) and in underlying cartilage, muscle and bone.
- The affected skin becomes darkly pigmented or depigmented (vitiligo).
- There may be hollowing of cheek and eyes may appear depressed in the orbits.
- There may be graying of the hair with bald patches with loss of eyelashes and eyebrows.
- There is underdevelopment of the base of the skull.

- The malar bone is small on the affected side and the face appears flat or in case of absence of the malar bone there is a depression inferior to the orbit.
- The patient may complain of severe headaches, visual abnormalities, involvement of the trigeminal nerve may cause facial pain. The patient may suffer from Jacksonian epilepsy.
- There may be atrophy of half of the upper lip and tongue.
- The initial facial changes involve the tissue of the maxilla, between the nose and the upper corner of the lip and progress to involve the angle of the mouth and areas around the eye, brow, ear and/or neck.
- There may be delayed eruption or wasting of the roots of the teeth on the affected side.
- The reduced growth of the jaws and delayed eruption of teeth leads to malocclusion on the affected side.

Radiographic Features

- Reduction in size of the bone on the affected side.
- Reduction in size of the condyle, coronoid process or overall dimension of the body and ramus of the mandible.
- The affected side of the face is smaller in all dimensions than the opposite side.

Differential Diagnosis

Mandibular dysostosis: Here there is an hereditary pattern and cleft palate is also present.

Management

Orthodontic treatment with plastic surgery.

Hyperplasia of Maxillary Tuberosity (Fig. 19.32)

Clinical Features

- There may be bilateral enlargement of the maxillary tuberosity
- This is usually seen in adults
- There is difficulty in normal mastication and wearing of dentures.

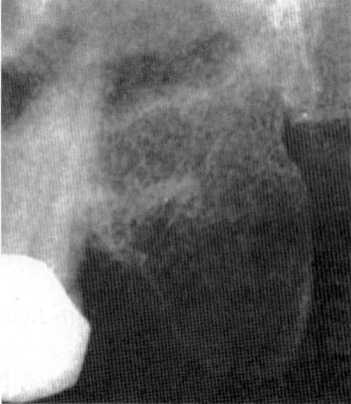

Figure 19.32 Hypertrophy of the maxillary tuberosity

Radiographic Features

The bone in the affected region appears more opaque.

Management

Treatment consists of surgical remodeling of the affected bone.

Hyperplasia of Coronoid Process

Refer Chapter 25—Temporomandibular Joint Disorders (Page 443).

Cleidocranial Dysostosis (Marie and Sainton Disease, Cleidocranial Dysplasia (CCD), Cranio-cleido-dysostosis) (Figs 19.33A to E)

Definition

This is an autosomal dominant malformation syndrome affecting bones and teeth. It is caused by mutation in the RUNX2 gene on chromosome 6.

Clinical Features

- Both sexes are equally affected.
- The affected individuals show a shorter stature. (This has recently been correlated due to the presence of supernumerary teeth, in a study)
- The face appears small in contrast to the cranium because of:
  - Hypoplasia of the maxilla.
  - Brachycephalic skull (reduced anteroposterior dimension with increased skull width)
  - Presence of frontal and parietal bossing.
- The paranasal sinuses may be underdeveloped
- There is delayed closure of the cranial sutures and the fontanels may remain patent for many years.
- The bridge of the nose may be broad and depressed.
- There is hypertelorism (excessive distance between the eyes)
- There is complete absence (aplasia) or reduced size (hypoplasia) of the clavicles, which allows excessive mobility of the shoulder girdle.
- There is prolonged retention of the primary dentition and delayed eruption of the permanent dentition. Extraction of primary teeth does not stimulate eruption of the permanent teeth.
- There is absence or paucity of cellular cementum on both erupted and unerupted teeth.
- There are multiple unerupted supernumerary teeth, leading to considerable crowding and disorganization of the developing permanent dentition.

Radiographic Features

- The characteristic skull findings are:
  - Brachycephaly
  - A widened cranium

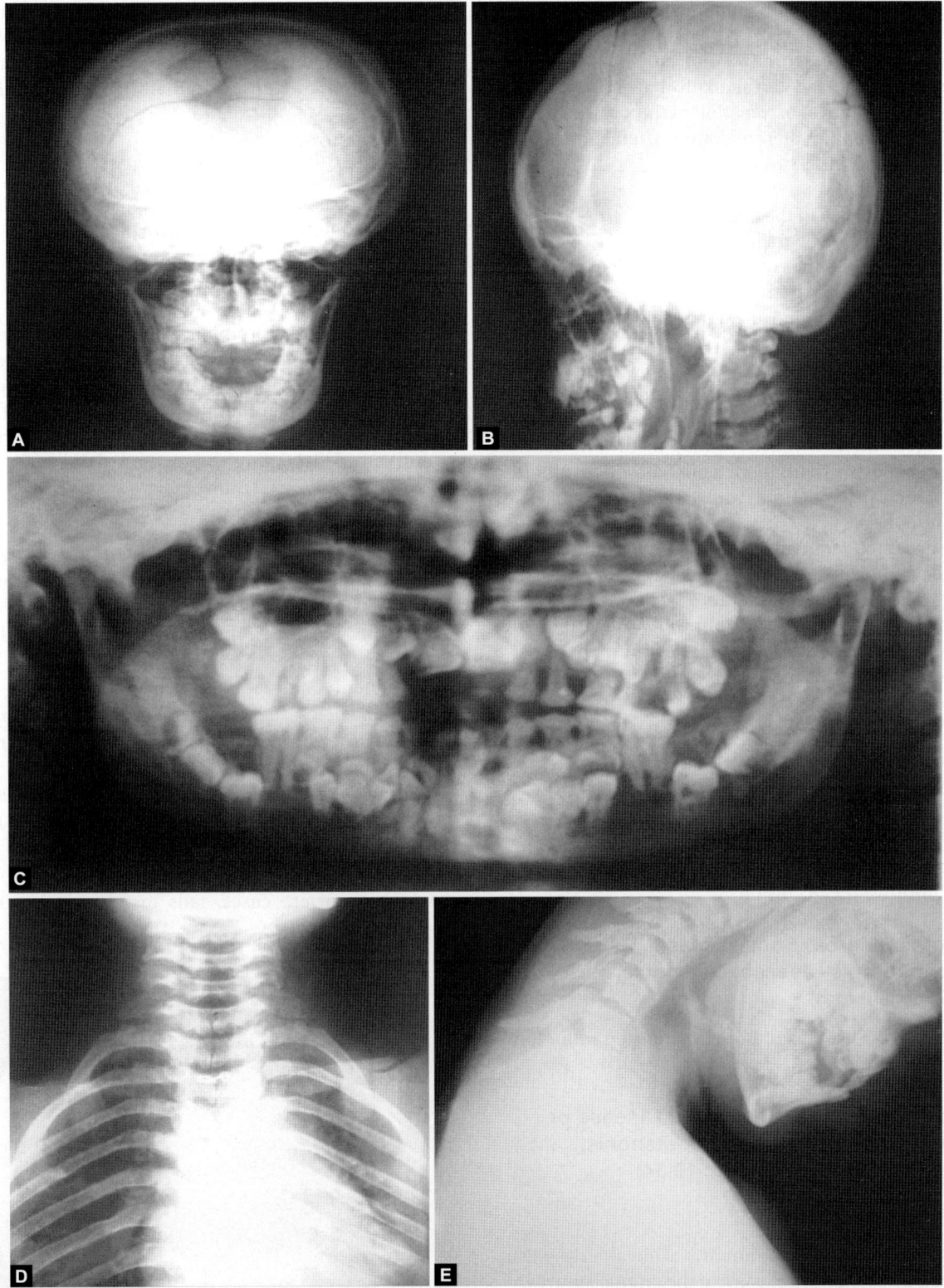

Figures 19.33A to E Cleidocranial dysostosis: (A) PA skull; (B) Lateral skull showing 'bulb sign'; (C) Panoramic radiograph showing multiple unerupted and supernumerary teeth; (D) Chest radiograph showing abscence of clavicles; (E) Lateral radiograph showing hyper flexion of the neck

- Delayed ossification of the fontanelles
- Opened skull sutures
- Large number of wormian bones (small, irregular bones in the sutures of the skull that are formed by secondary centers of ossification in the suture lines)
- Very little formation of frontal and parietal bones
- Frontal and occipital bossing
- Basilar invagination
• Aplasia or hypoplasia of the clavicles
• Other bones affected include long bones, vertebral column, pelvis and bones of the hands and feet.
• Radiographic evidence in the jaws:
  - Small, underdeveloped maxillae (micrognathia) and paranasal sinuses
  - Mandible is usually normal in size
  - The alveolar bone overlying unerupted teeth is more dense, with coarse trabecular pattern in the mandible.
  - Prolonged retention of deciduous teeth and delayed eruption of many permanent teeth and supernumerary teeth which are sometimes with associated dentigerous cyst formation.
  - The unerupted teeth are most common in the anterior maxilla and bicuspid region of the jaws.
  - The multiple supernumerary teeth are believed to develop on an average four years later than the corresponding normal teeth, and thus there is a proposed theory that these represent the third dentition.

Differential Diagnosis

• Gardners syndrome
• Pyknodysostosis.

Management

No specific treatment, removal of unwanted teeth may be planned to improve the occlusion.

Osteopetrosis (Marble Bone Disease, Albers-Schonberg's Disease, Osteosclerosis Fragilis Generalisata)

Refer Chapter 24—Diseases of Bone Manifested in the Jaws (Page 419).

Craniofacial Dysostosis (Crouzon's Disease or Syndrome (CS), Syndromic Craniostenosis, Premature Craniostenosis) (Fig. 19.34)

Definition

This is an autosomal-dominant skeletal dysplasia, characterized by premature closure of the cranial sutures.

CS is caused by mutation in fibroblast growth factor receptor II on chromosome 10. Mutations at this site are also responsible for other craniosynostosis syndromes with similar facial features but clinically visible limb abnormalities.

In patients with CS the coronal suture usually closes first, and eventually all cranial sutures close early. Premature fusion of the synchondroses and cranial coronal sutures produce the characteristic cranial shape and facial features.

Clinical Features

• The patients have:
  - Brachycephaly (short anteroposterior skull length)
  - Hypertelorism (increased distance between the eyes)
  - Orbital proptosis (protruding eyes)
• Patients may become blind due to increased intracranial pressure.
• The nose appears prominent and pointed as the maxilla is narrow and short in a vertical and anteroposterior dimension.
• The anterior nasal spine is hypoplastic and retruded, failing to provide adequate support to the soft tissue of the nose.
• The palatal vault is high and the maxillary arch narrow and retruded, leading to crowding of the teeth.

Radiographic Features

• The earliest signs of cranial suture synostosis are sclerosis and overlapping edges. Sutures that normally appear radiolucent may not be detectable or show sclerotic changes.
• Premature fusion of the cranial base leads to diminished facial growth.
• Prominent cranial markings appear as multiple radiolucencies (depressions) called digital impressions on the inner surface of the cranial vault, which results in a beaten metal appearance.
• The lack of growth in the anteroposterior direction at the cranial base results in maxillary hypoplasia, creating a class III malocclusion.
• The maxillary hypoplasia also creates orbital proptosis, which in severe cases, fails to adequately support the orbital contents.

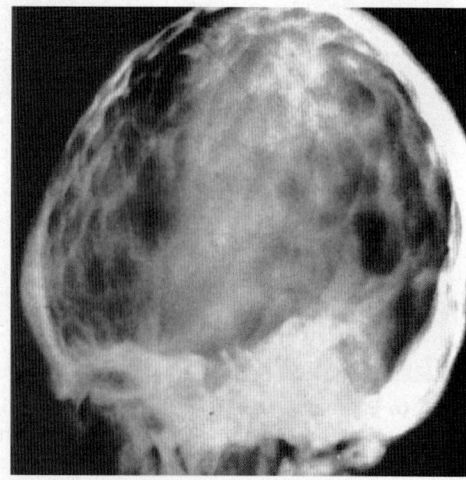

Figure 19.34 Copper beaten appearance—craniofacial dysostosis

- The mandible is smaller than normal but appears prognathic in relation to the severely hypoplastic maxilla.

Differential Diagnosis

- Other causes of craniosynostosis must be differentiated from CS, including other syndromic forms of craniosynostosis and nonsyndromic coronal craniosynostosis. The characteristic facial features must be present to suggest CS.
- *Apert's syndrome*: The cranial features of Apert's Syndrome are quite similar to those of Crouzon's disease, but in addition to these are anomalies of the extremities.

Management

Treatment objective in cases of early diagnosis is to allow normal brain growth and development by preventing increased intracranial pressure.

Mandibulofacial Dysostosis (Treacher Collins Syndrome (TCH), Franceschetti Syndrome) (Figs 19.35A and B)

Definition

This is an autosomal dominant disorder of craniofacial development. More than half the cases are a result of sporadic mutation, the rest are familial. It results from retardation or failure of differentiation of maxillary mesoderm at and after the 50 mm stage of the embryo.

Clinical Features

- There is relative underdevelopment or absence of the zygomatic bones resulting in a narrow face, downward inclination of the palpebral fissures.
- Underdevelopment of the mandible resulting in a down turned wide mouth.
- Malformation (hypoplasia or atresia) of the external ears, with or without the absence of the external auditory canal and ossicles of the middle ear may result in partial or complete deafness.
- Occasional facial clefts may be seen.
- Theses patients have a high arched or cleft palate.
- Hypoplasia of the mandible and a steep mandibular angle results in angle class II, with anterior open bite malocclusion.
- The patient has a typical fish or bird appearance.

Radiographic Features

- Hypoplastic or missing zygomatic bones and hypoplasia of the lateral aspects of the orbits.
- The auditory canal, mastoid air cells and articular eminence are smaller than normal or absent.
- The maxilla and especially the mandible are hypoplastic with an accentuated antegonial notch and a steep mandibular angle, which gives the impression that the body of the mandible is bending in an inferior and posterior direction.
- The ramus is usually short and the condyles are positioned posteriorly and inferiorly.
- The maxillary sinuses may be underdeveloped or absent.
- There may be partial anodontia and/or malformation of the teeth.

Differential Diagnosis

Other disorders that result in severe hypoplasia of the entire mandible includes: condylar agenesis, Hallermann-Streiff syndrome. Nager syndrome and Pierre-Robin syndrome which may be a part of several other genetic syndromes.

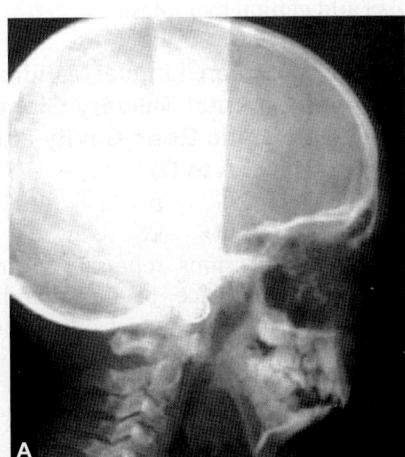 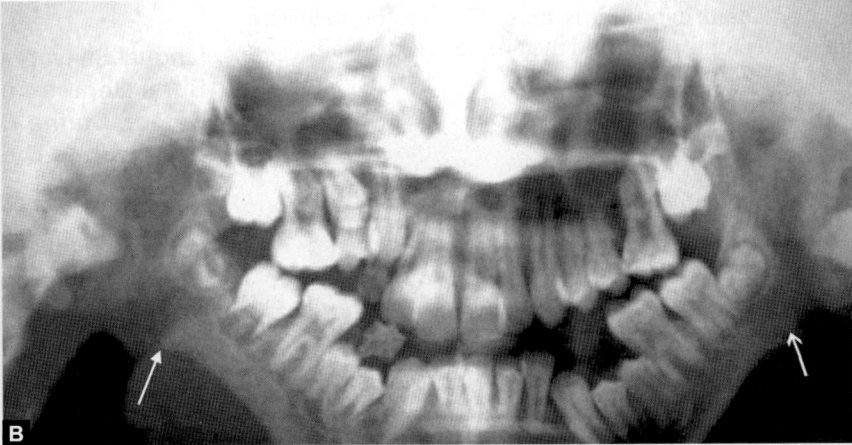

Figures 19.35A and B Mandibulofacial dysostosis [Treacher Collins syndrome (TCH), Franceschetti syndrome]. (A) Lateral cephalometric view (B) Panoramic view (Arrow shows accentuated antegonial notch)

Management

Comprehensive treatment of the patient is provided by a multidisciplinary craniofacial team.

Chondroectodermal Dysplasia (Ellis-van Creveld Syndrome) (Fig. 19.36)

Definition

This is a congenital disease with evidence of chondrodysplasia, ectodermal dysplasia, polydactylism and congenital morbus cordis.

Clinical Features

- The patients have an extra finger lateral to the normal fifth finger (post axial polydactyly) in the hands, this is a rare finding in the feet.
- There is relative shortening of the distal (acromelic) and middle (mesomelic) segments (bone dysplasia characterized by acromesomelic), which may interfere with the ability to make a tight fist.
- There may be a progressive deformity of the knees.
- The finger and toe nails are dysplastic or absent.
- The patient may have congenital heart defects which may include hypoplasia of aorta, atria and ventricular septal defects and a single atrium.
- The patient has the trunk of normal length but the long bones are short.
- Hair tends to be fine and sparse.
- There are less number of teeth, and those that are present are small, rudimentary, conical, spaced and irregular in position. Hypodontia (usually involving maxillary and mandibular incisors) abnormally formed teeth (conical incisors) malocclusion, enamel defects, mesiodens, taurodontism and premolar invagination, pulp stones in most teeth].
- The teeth erupt early at birth or shortly thereafter.
- The deciduous molars present a crenate occlusal surface.
- The permanent dentition is more likely to be defective than the deciduous one and the eruption is delayed.

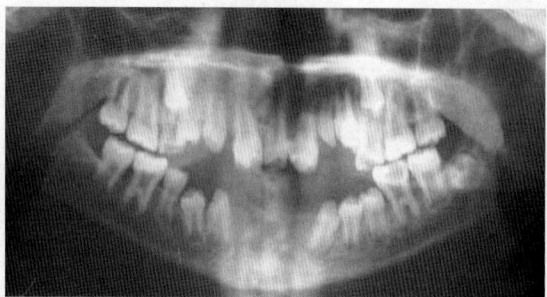

Figure 19.36 Panoramic view shows mandibular incisors were congenitally missing. Bulbous roots as compared to crowns were suggestive of taurodontism

- There may be a partial hair lip due to an abnormally short lip which may be sunken secondary to hypoplasia of the maxilla.
- Broad labial frenum obliterating maxillary labial vestibule.
- Mandibular labial vestibule often shows abnormal frenum attachments.
- Natal and neonatal teeth which were lost spontaneously.
- High caries rate.
- Bilateral partial clefts or notching of alveolar bone in maxillary and mandibular lateral incisor.

Radiographic Features

- There are shorter distal and middle phalangeal segments, in relation to the proximal phalangeal segments.
- Deciduous molar has a characteristic typical shape.

Differential Diagnosis

- It may be difficult to differentiate radiographically Ellis-van Creveld syndrome from asphyxiating thoracic dystrophy. Both syndromes may present identical changes in hands, pelvis and long bones. Differential diagnosis is based upon the following clinical changes present in Ellis-van Creveld syndrome: cardiac anomalies, nail hypoplasia, fusion of upper lip and gingiva, and when present the neonatal teeth. Later in life, the presence of genu valgum in chondroectodermal dysplasia and renal failure with hypertension in asphyxiating thoracic dystrophy will help to establish a more positive diagnosis.
- Ellis-van Creveld syndrome may be differentiated from other chondrodystrophies such as achondroplasia, chondrodysplasia punctata, the Morquio syndrome, and cartilage-hair hypoplasia by its distinctive radiographic features.
- Acrofacialdysostosis of Weyers and Trisomy 13 where polydactyly and hypodontia is also seen.
- *Bardet-Biedl syndrome*: It has polydactyly with adiposity, retinitis pigmentosa and genital hypoplasia.

Lingual Salivary Gland Depression (Lingual Mandibular Bone Depression, Developmental Salivary Gland Defect, Stafne Bone Cyst, Static Bone Cavity and Latent Bone Cyst) (Figs 19.37A to D)

Definition

Lingual mandibular bone depressions represent a group of concavities in the lingual surface of the mandible, where the depression is lined with an intact outer cortex. It is not a true cyst because there is no epithelial lining present.

Clinical Features

- It is more often found in males.
- The most common location is within the submandibular gland fossa and often close to the inferior of the mandible.

- The lingual posterior variant is a well-defined deep depression which is thought to result from or be associated with growth of the salivary gland adjacent to the lingual surface of the mandible.
- Similar defects have also been described in the anterior region near the apical region of the bicuspids, associated with sublingual glands (lingual anterior variant—LA).

- Very rarely on the medial surface of the ascending ramus, associated with the parotid gland (medial ramus variant—MR)
- The concavities are asymptomatic and almost impossible to palpate.
- They are generally discovered only incidentally during radiographic examination of the area.

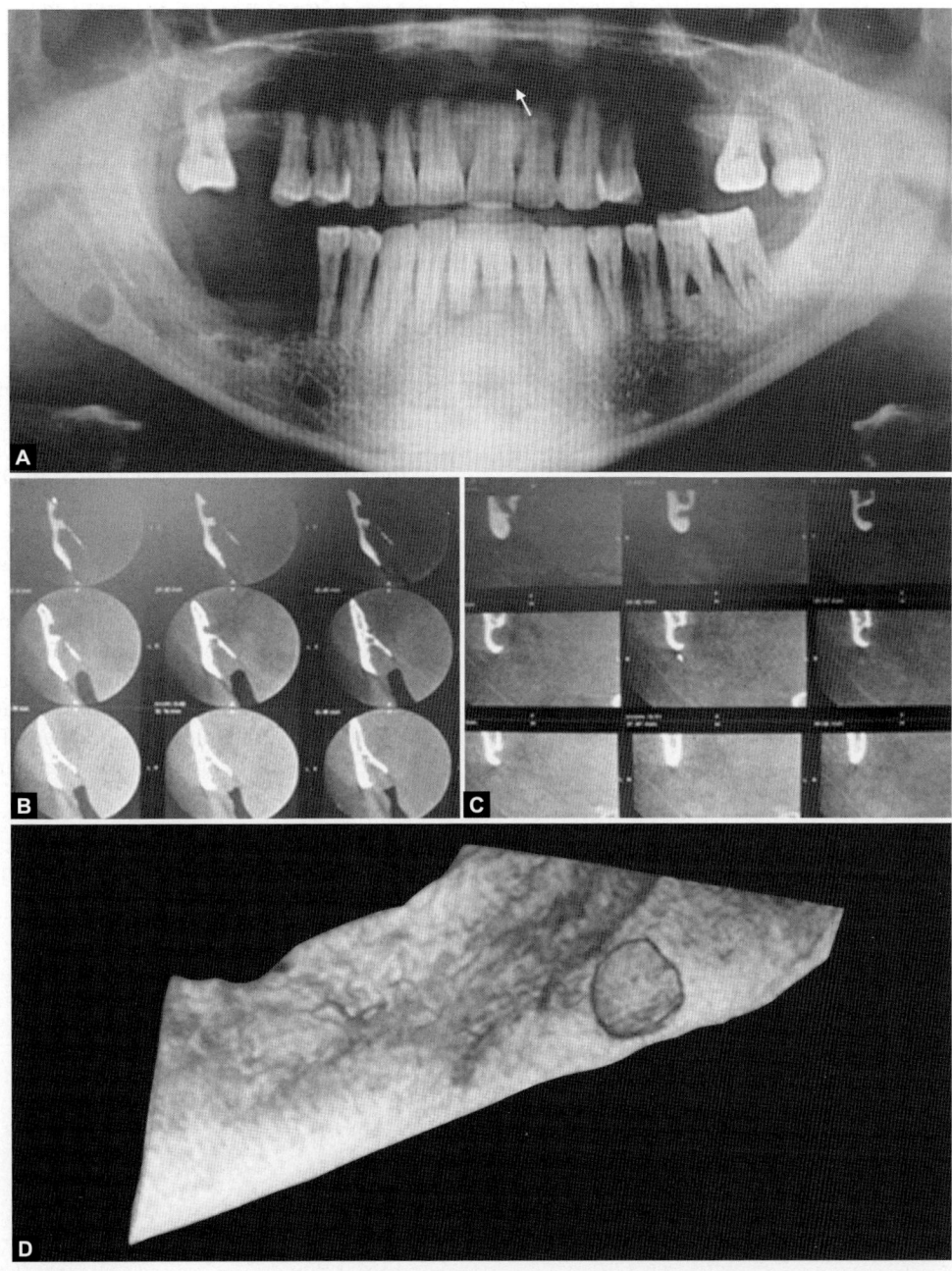

Figures 19.37A to D Stafne's cyst: (A) Panoramic radiograph shows a well-defined oval single radiolucent lesion below inferior alveolar canal right angle of mandible. CBCT; (B) Axial views; (C) Sagittal views; (D) 3D view shows a well-defined radiolucent lesion on the lingual side of the angle of the mandible below the inferior alveolar canal. The lesion is well corticated and oval in shape. Discontinuity of the lingual cortex at angle of mandible. No break in the continuity of inferior border of mandible. Cortical lining of inferior alveolar canal is intact

Radiographic Features

- The lingual mandibular bone depression appears as a round, ovoid or occasionally lobulated radiolucency that ranges in diameter from 1–3 cms.
- The LP defect is located below the inferior alveolar nerve canal and anterior to the angle of the mandible, in the region of the antegonial notch and submandibular gland fossa.
- Rarely LA examples may be found in the apical region of the mandibular premolars or cuspids and are related to the sublingual gland fossa, above the mylohyoid gland muscle.
- The margins of the radiolucent defects are well defined by a dense sclerotic radiopaque margin of variable width, which is usually thicker on the superior aspect. This is due to the fact that the X-rays pass tangentially through the relatively thick walls of the depression.
- The cortical outline is often less distinct in the LA variant.
- The LP defect may involve the inferior border of the mandible.
- CT imaging of these defects reveal tissue with the same density as fat tissue and no evidence of gland, or in some cases, there is continuity of the tissue within the defect with the adjacent salivary gland.

Differential Diagnosis

- Odontogenic cysts the epicenter of the cysts is located above the inferior alveolar canal and are thus easily differentiated from lingual mandibular bone lesions.
- Odontogenic lesions should be considered in the differential diagnosis when the defect is related to the sublingual gland and appears above the canal.

Management

No treatment necessary.

BIBLIOGRAPHY

1. Goaz PW, White SC. Principles and Interpretation. In: Oral Radiology, 3rd edition. St. Louis: Mosby Year Book; 1994.
2. Goodman RM, Gorlin RJ. Atlas of the face in genetic disorders, 2nd edition. St. Louis: Mosby; 1977.
3. Karjodkar FR, Mali S, Sontakke S, et al. Five Developmental Anomalies in a Single Patient. A rare case report. J Clin Diag Res. 2012;6(9):1603-5.
4. Mali S, Karjodkar FR, Sontakke S, et al. Supernumerary teeth in non-syndromic patients. J Imag Sci Dent. 2012;42:41-5.
5. Miles DA, Van Dis MJ, Jensen CW, et al. Interpretation normal versus abnormal and common radiographic presentations of lesions. In: Radiographic and Imaging for Dental Auxillaries, 3rd edition. Philadelphia: WB Saunders; 1999.pp.231-80.
6. Pinborg JJ. Pathology of the dental hard tissues. N Engl J Med. 1979;301:13.
7. Rohini Salvi, Karjodkar FR, Gadda RB, et al. Bhatia Cleidocranial Dysplasia—A report of 2 cases. JIDA. 2011; 5(12):1222-4.
8. Shafer WG, et al. A Text Book of Oral Pathology. Philadelphia: WB Saunders; 1983.
9. Stafne EC, Lovestealdt SA. Congenital hemihypertrophy of the face (facial gigantism). Oral Surg Oral Med Oral Path. 1962;15:184-9.
10. Winter GB. Hereditary and idiopathic anomalies of the tooth number, structure and form. Dent Clin North Am. 1969;13:355.
11. Wood NK, Goaz PW. Differential Diagnosis of Oral Lesions, 4th edition. CV Mosby: St. Louis; 1991.
12. Wood RE. Handbook of signs in dental and maxillofacial radiology. Warthog Publications, Toronto; 1988.
13. Worth HM. Principles and practice of oral radiographic interpretation. Year Book Medical Publishers, Chicago; 1963.

Infections and Inflammatory Lesions and Systemic Diseases Affecting the Jaws | 20

INFECTIONS AND INFLAMMATORY LESIONS

A common source of infection of the jaws and facial bones is inflammatory disease of the pulp. The inflammatory agents gain access into these bones by way of the root canals of the involved teeth, and hence the primary pathogenesis of many infections are initiated in the periapical connective tissue. Other sources of infection are extraction wounds, infections from the periodontal ligament, compound fractures and occasionally from hematogenous infections (**Table 20.1**).

Conventional radiographic views form the preliminary mode of investigation for maxillofacial infections. However CT scans with its excellent ability to detect the extent and pathway of spread of infection, help the clinician to map out the severity of the infection and thereby render an appropriate treatment.

INFECTIONS OF PERIAPICAL TISSUES (FIGS 20.1A TO F)

Infection products from the diseased pulp may be released from the tooth into the oral cavity and/or the peri apex. If it continues to drain into the oral cavity, the tooth will remain asymptomatic, if however, the degradation products reach the periapical connective tissue, the response produced will depend on the nature and amount of infection and the resistance of the host.

If the degradation products overcome the host's defense, a lesion may develop within the bone.

Conventional imaging gives adequate information, but when the clinical information does not correlate with the radiographic findings CBCT helps give added and better diagnostic information in case of periapical lesions and location of additional canals which help improve treatment plan and prognosis of the case (**Figs 20.1G and H**).

ACUTE INFECTIONS OF PERIAPICAL TISSUES

Acute Apical Periodontitis (Fig. 20.2)

When small amounts of noxious products are produced and are rapidly diluted as they diffuse through the apical periodontal membrane, there is a resulting minimal inflammatory reaction like edema, localized in the apical periodontal ligament. The inflammation is restricted to the periodontal membrane.

Clinical Features

- Tooth is nonvital
- It may or may not be sensitive to hot, cold, sweet or sour food
- Due to apical edema the tooth is elevated in the socket and sensitive to pressure and percussion
- Pain may develop spontaneously and is throbbing in nature.

Table 20.1 Summary of the effects of different inflammatory processes on the periapical tissues and the resultant radiographic appearances

State of inflammation	Underlying inflammatory changes	Radiographic appearances
Initial acute inflammation	Inflammatory exudate accumulates in the apical periodontal ligament space—acute apical periodontilis	Widening of the radiolucent periodontal ligamant space or No apparent changes evident
Initial spread of inflammation	Resorption and destruction of the apical bony socket-periapical abscess	Loss of the radiopaque line of the lamina dura at the apex
Further spread of inflammation	Further resorption and destruction of the apical alveolar bone	Area of bone loss at the tooth apex
Initial low-grade chronic inflammation	Minimal destruction of the apical bone. The body's defence systems lay down dense bone in the apical region	No apparent bone destruction but dense sclerotic bone evident around the tooth apex (Sclerosing osteitis)
Later stages of chronic inflammation	Apical bone is resorbed and destroyed and dense bone is laid down around the area of resorption-periapical granuloma or radicular cyst	Circumscribed, well-defined radiolucent area of bone loss at the apex, surrounded by dense sclerotic bone

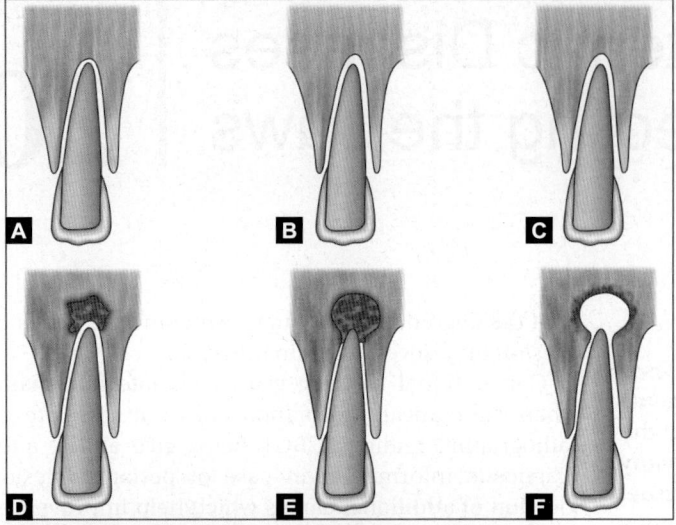

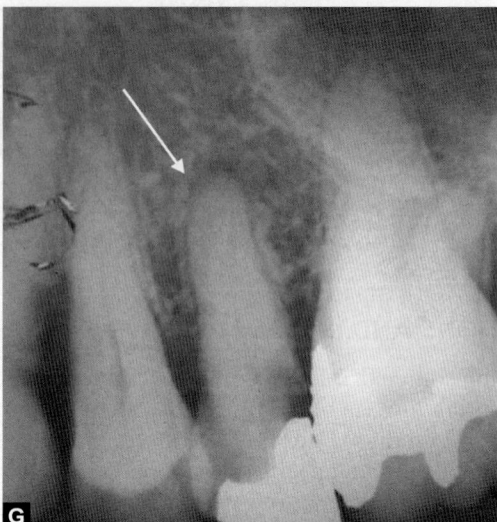

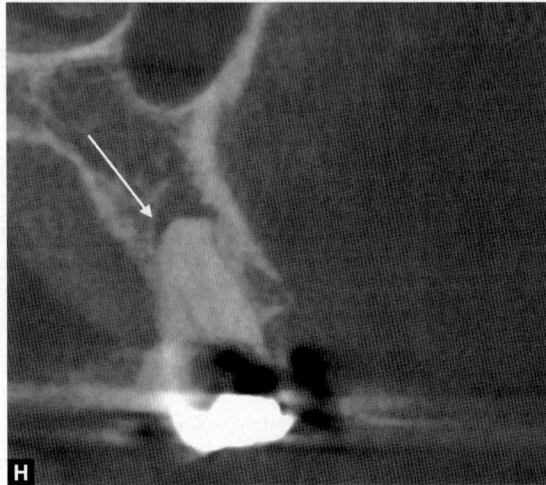

Figures 20.1A to H Various radiographic appearances of infection and inflammation in the apical tissues: (A) Normal; (B) Early apical change—widening of the radiolucent periodontal ligament space (acute apical periodontitis) (Arrowed); (C) Early apical change—loss of the radiopaque lamina dura (Early periapical abscess) (Arrowed); (D) Extensive destructive acute inflammation—diffuse ill-defined area of radiolucency at the apex (Periapical abscess); (E) Low grade chronic inflammation—diffuse radiopaque area at the apex (Sclerosing osteitis); (F) Longstanding chronic inflammation—well-defined area of radiolucency surrounded by dense sclerotic bone (periapical granuloma or radicular cyst); (G) Conventional radiograph shows widening of the periodontal space around upper premolar (Arrow); (H) CBCT coronal section of the same tooth shows a periapical radiolucency of a much larger size

Radiographic Features

Slight widening of the periodontal ligament space is seen.

Management

Relieving the cause and treating the tooth endodontically.

Acute Apical Abscess (Fig. 20.3)

If the exudates from the infected pulp continues to pass into the periapex it may cause tissue death with the development of pus.

Clinical Features

- The features are the same as those in acute apical periodontitis but the degree of intensity of pain and duration is more
- Patient may have slight fever

- Lymphadenopathy may be present
- Swelling may be seen in the adjacent tissues.

Radiographic Features

- Slight widening of the periodontal ligament space is seen
- After some period slight unsharpness of the trabeculae may be seen at the apex
- In case of infection of a deciduous tooth, damage to the permanent successor may be observed by the presence of rarefaction produced by the destruction of the cortex of the follicle.

Differential Diagnosis

Periodontal abscess; usually associated with a vital tooth with an associated periodontal pocket and lateral abscess. Radiographically apical rarefaction will not be present.

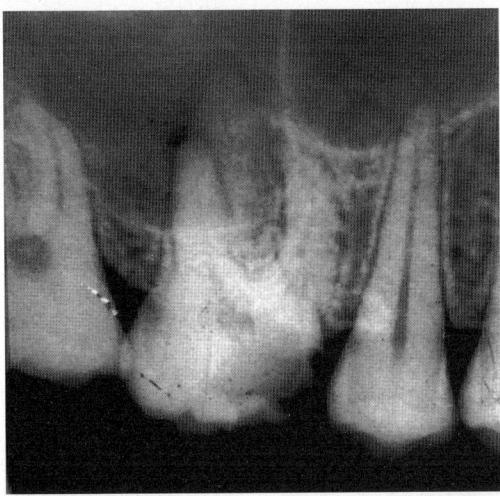

Figure 20.2 Apical periodontitis related to first premolar and periapical abscess in relation to carious first molar

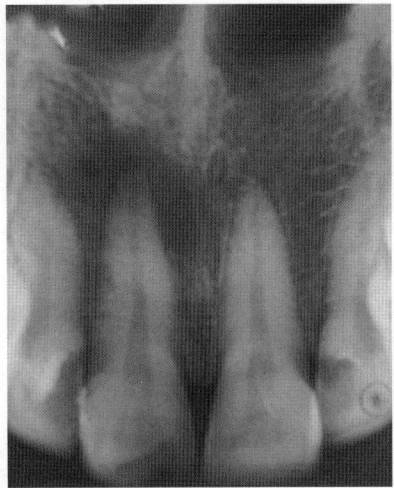

Figure 20.4 Dentoalveolar abscess

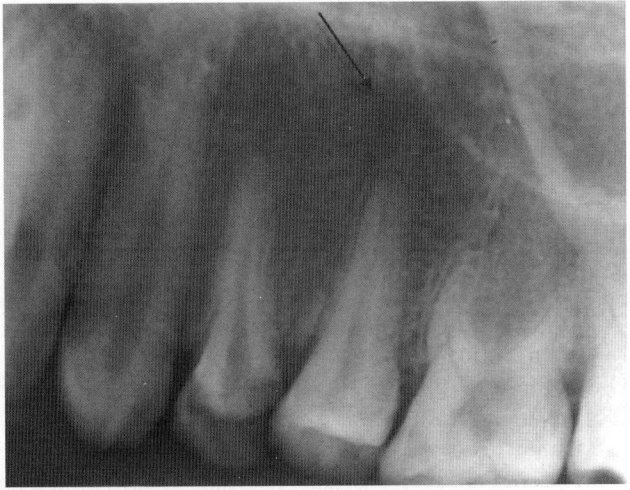

Figure 20.3 Acute periapical abscess

Management

Establish drainage under antibiotic cover.

Acute Dentoalveolar Abscess (Fig. 20.4)

When the exudates is increased in amount or the resistance capacity of the host is decreased, the inflammation initiates necrosis of the periapical tissues and diffuse rarefaction of the bone, leading to the formation of a periapical abscess.

Clinical Features

- The tooth becomes tender
- Patient may experience pain and pressure at the same region

- The abscess may extend towards the surface with redness and swelling of the soft tissues
- Periapical cellulitis may develop.

Radiographic Features

- The dento alveolar abscess developes so rapidly that many a times there may be no radiographic evidence other than widening of the periodontal ligament space
- In some cases demineralization of the bone in the periapical area may be seen, after a number of days
- When the acute phase subsides the radiographic appearance of most of the demineralized bone returns to normal.

Management

Extraction of the affected tooth or root canal treatment.

Cellulitis (Phlegmon) (Figs 20.5A and B)

The infectious process progresses out of the bone either in the vestibular region or extraorally. It is defined as a nonsuppurative inflammation of the subcutaneous tissues extending along the connective tissue planes and across intercellular spaces.

Clinical Features

- Wide spread swelling, redness and pain without definite localization
- Tenderness on palpation
- Tissues are grossly edematous and indurated and firm on palpation
- The discharge/pus may spread to adjacent structure depending on their location, proximity and anatomy,

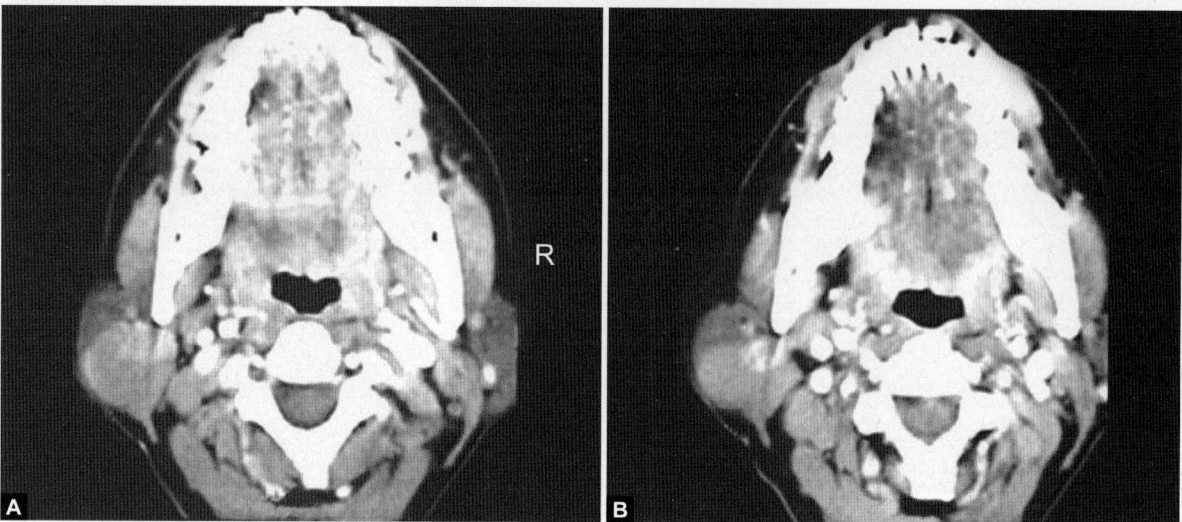

Figures 20.5A and B Axial CT depicting cellulitis

to the nose, maxillary sinus, oral vestibule, floor of the mouth, infratemporal fossa and into facial spaces

- Infections arising in the maxilla usually perforate the outer cortical layer of bone, above the buccinator attachment and cause swelling of the upper half of the face
- Infections arising in the mandible perforate the outer cortical plate below the buccinator attachment and cause swelling of the lower half of the face, which may spread superiorly and/or cervically
- If a maxillary tooth is involved there will be redness of the eye.

Management

Surgical incision and drainage under antibiotic cover.

Ludwig's Angina (Figs 20.6A to C)

The word angina means sensation of choking or suffocation, it is one of the most commonly encountered neck space infection. It may be defined as a rapidly spreading, septic cellulitis involving submandibular, submental and sublingual spaces. It is caused by extension of odontogenic infection, trauma, sialadenitis, calculi, osteomyelitis.

Clinical Features

There are three different appearances:
1. *First*:
   - Brawny induration
   - Tissue may become gangrenous
   - Sharp delineation is present between infected and normal tissues.

2. *Second*: Three facial spaces are involved bilaterally; submandibular, submental and sublingual.
3. *Third*:
   - The mouth is open and the tongue is lifted upwards and backwards, so that it is pushed against the roof of the mouth and the posterior pharyngeal wall causing acute respiratory obstruction
   - The swelling is firm, painful and diffuse
   - Floor of the mouth is erythematous and edematous
   - Stiffness and decreased movement of the tongue
   - Larynx and glottis become edematous
   - As the condition progresses the swelling starts involving the neck
   - Patient develops a toxic condition and speech is impaired
   - Patient has fever, is unable to swallow, dehydrated and may develop confusion and mental changes
   - If prompt treatment is not given, patient may develop:
     - Respiratory obstruction
     - Generalized septicemia
     - Erosion of the carotid artery
     - Cavernous sinus thrombosis
     - Other fatal complications.

Radiographic Features

Radiographic features will be similar as that of dentoalveolar abscess showing periapical rarefaction in relation to offending tooth (which is the source of infection).

Additional Imaging

CT demonstrates ill-defined infiltrative process with low attenuation areas reflecting abscess or localized areas of phlegmon.

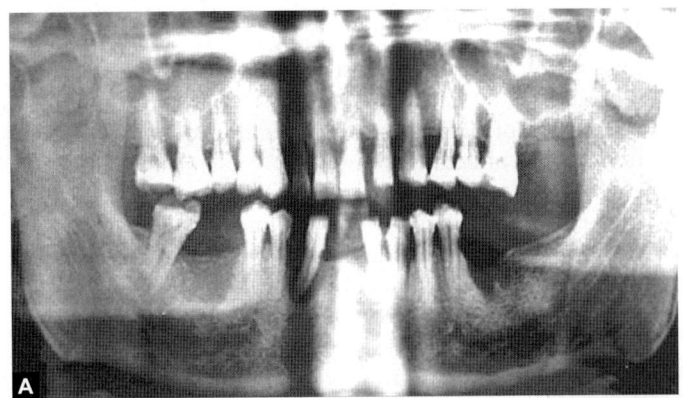

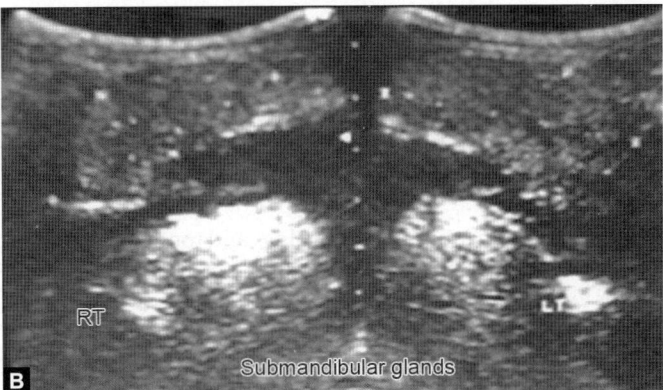

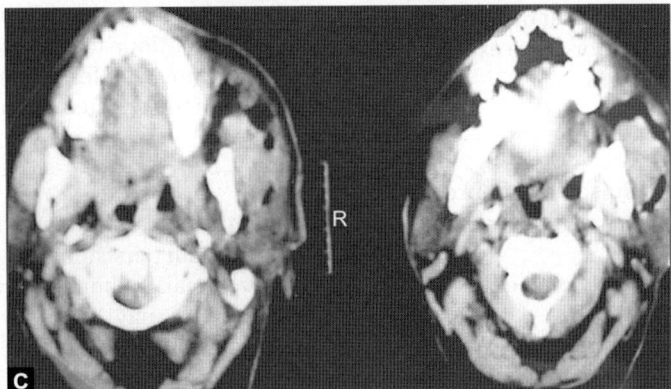

Figures 20.6A to C Ludwig's angina—a patient came in a febrile condition with a painful swelling in the neck and difficulty in opening the mouth since the last 5-6 days. Extraoral examination revealed a large bilateral swelling in the submandibular and submental region, which was tender, warm, firm, nonfluctuant, fixed diffuse swelling with erythematous overlying skin. Cervical lymph nodes were palpable and tender. Intraorally the floor of the mouth was elevated, indurated and tender: (A) Panoramic view revealed a generalized alveolar bone loss, with extensive loss around 42 and 35; (B) Ultrasound examination revealed a horseshoe shaped hypoechoic area in the submental region measuring 3.9 x 5 x 1.5 cm extending on either side towards the submandibular glands; (C) CT scan reveal generalized swelling of skin, soft tissue with air specks seen in submandibular, submental, buccal and masticator space. The left masseter shows heterogeneous enhancement of air and fluid collections within it

Management

Incision, drainage under high parental antibiotic cover and establishment and maintenance of and adequate airway.

CHRONIC INFECTIONS OF PERIAPICAL TISSUES

This may be a sequel of an acute episode or a low grade reaction to infection or inflammatory products of long duration and low virulence.

Chronic Apical Periodontitis (Fig. 20.7)

It is the result of a low virulent infection and high host resistance. Usually there are no signs or symptoms and the lesion is detected on a routine radiograph.

Clinical Features

Will range from dull aching pain to symptomless.

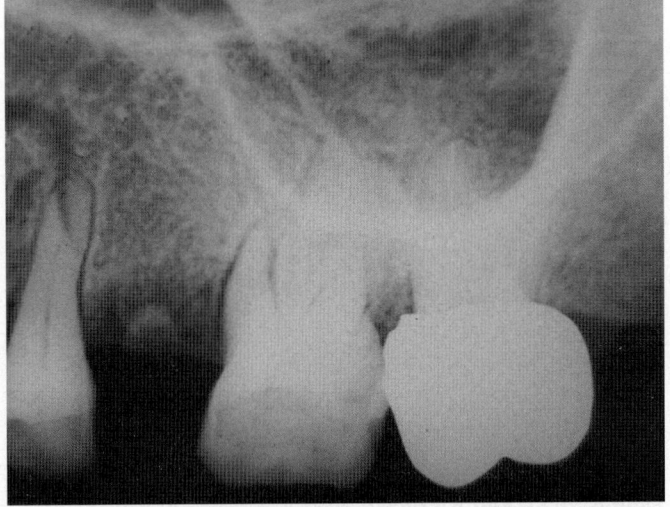

Figure 20.7 Chronic apical periodontitis in relation to upper second premolar and molar

Radiographic Features

It is seen as a widened periodontal space with a band of radiopaque sclerotic (dense, thick) trabeculae, which is the mark of chronicity.

Management

Depending upon amount of bone loss and tooth involvement the treatment will either be extraction or root canal treatment under antibiotic and anti-inflammatory drug cover.

Chronic Alveolar Abscess (Figs 20.8A and B)

This is a long standing low grade infection of the periradicular tissues. It may result due to the direct result of acute pulpitis or acute nonsuppurative periodontitis or acute exacerbation of periapical granuloma, cyst or abscess.

Clinical Features

- History of pain that started as a dull ache and progressed to severe throbbing type; decrease results in pain signals and formation of sinus
- Tooth is tender to percussion, and gives a negative vitality test
- Draining fistulas are often present. Majority of the time the fistula opens on the buccal and labial aspect of the alveolus. Sometimes the roots of the maxillary lateral and molars may be close to the palatal cortical plate, and so the sinus may appear on the palate. Most of the root tips lie below the mylohyoid muscle, so the pus drains into the submandibular space
- Lymphadenopathy may be present.

Radiographic Features

- Loss of thickness and density of the apical portion of the lamina dura
- Wide area of diffuse demineralization of the periapical bone, of the affected tooth
- The margins of the lesion vary from well-defined with hyperostotic borders to poorly defined, in chronic cases
- In some cases radiolucency may involve the adjacent teeth, with loss of lamina dura of the same
- Sometimes the lesion may appear at the side of the root, especially in cases where the infection has spread from the adjacent tooth or from perforation of the root or from an aberrant canal opening
- In cases of maxillary molars, destruction of a portion of the antral floor may be seen with the destruction at the apex, along with loss of lamina dura
- Roots of the affected teeth may show resorption.

Differential Diagnosis

- *Periapical osteofibrosis*: This is associated with a vital tooth, with persistence of the lamina dura in the presence of well marked bone destruction
- Foramens may be superimposed on the root, another radiograph with a different angulation will help to differentiate
- Inferior dental canal may be superimposed on the roots of the lower molars. The continuity of the lamina dura which will not be lost should be noted
- Large bone marrow space may be superimposed on the root and should be differentiated by the presence of an intact lamina dura.

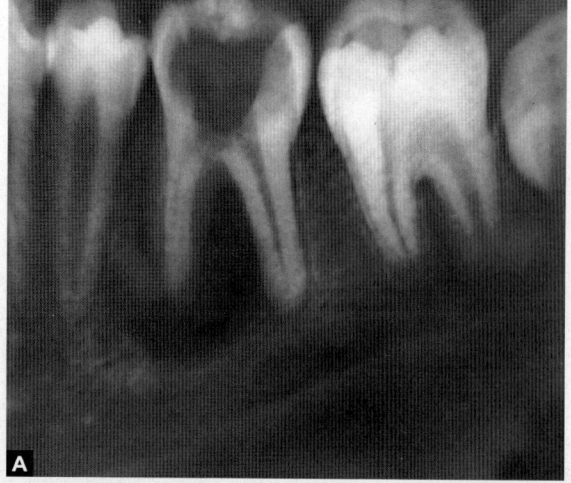 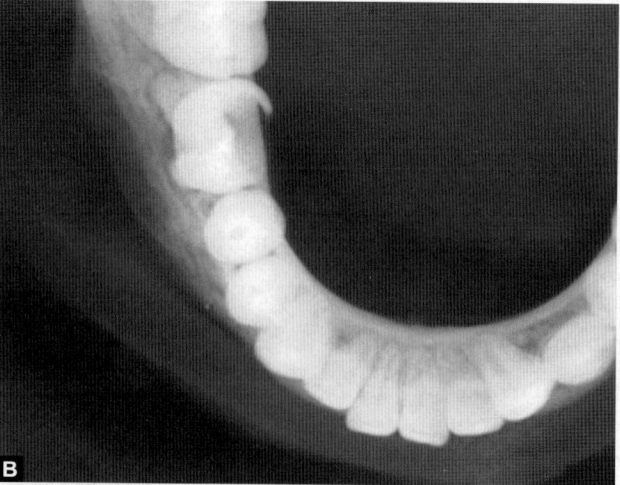

Figures 20.8A and B Chronic alveolar abscess: (A) Radiograph shows occlusal radiolucency involving enamel and dentin involving pulp chamber of mandibular molar with a well-defined oval periapical radiolucency not surrounded by corticated borders; (B) Mandibular occlusal view of the same patient shows a break in the buccal plate, surrounded by the radiolucency in the soft tissue space

Management

Endodontic treatment.

Periapical Granuloma (Figs 20.9A to C)

It is the result of a more intense or prolonged irritation from an infected root canal or a resolution of an acute alveolar abscess. It may be defined as a growth of granulation tissue continuous with the periodontal ligament resulting from the death of the pulp and diffusion of bacterial toxins from the root canals into the surrounding periradicular tissues through the apical and lateral foramina.

Clinical Features

- The associated tooth is usually nonvital and does not respond to thermal or electric pulp test
- The tooth may be of a darker color, because of the blood pigments that diffuse into the dentinal tubules
- Mild pain may be experienced while biting or chewing on solid foods
- Sensitivity may be present due to hyperemia, edema and inflammation of the apical periodontal ligament
- There is seldom any swelling or expansion of the overlying cortical bone
- The tooth may feel slightly elongated in the socket.

Radiographic Features

- Periapical area is radiolucent with loss of lamina dura
- The radiolucency may be of variable size at the apex of the tooth, usually of a diameter less than 1.5 cm
- The lesion may or may not have a well-defined border, which may or may not be hyperostotic
- There is loss of lamina dura and periapical bone, which is called 'periapical rarifying osteitis'
- Involved tooth may show a deep restoration, extensive caries, fracture or a narrow pulp canal with nonvital pulp.

Differential Diagnosis

- If the tooth is vital, possibility of a dental granuloma or cyst is ruled out
- If the tooth has a root canal filling, the radiolucency may be a periapical scar or surgical defect
- Surgical defect is further confirmed if the root apex shows evidence of modification
- Surgical defect is more radiolucent than a scar as one or both cortical plates may be missing
- *Osteolytic stage of cementoma*: In dental granuloma the tooth is nonvital.

Management

Root canal therapy or extraction depending on the dental surgeons discretion.

Periapical Scar (Figs 20.10A to C)

This is the possible end point of healing. It is composed of dense fibrous tissue and is situated at the periapex of the pulpless tooth, in which a root canal may have been successfully filled.

Clinical Features

It occurs after endodontic treatment and in patients treated by periapical curettage or root resection.

Radiographic Features

- A well-circumscribed radiolucency, that is smaller than granuloma and cyst
- Scar is constant in size.

Differential Diagnosis

- Chronic periapical abscess
- Periapical granuloma
- Periapical cyst
- Healing periapical lesion.

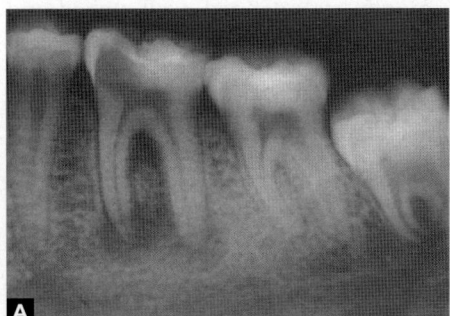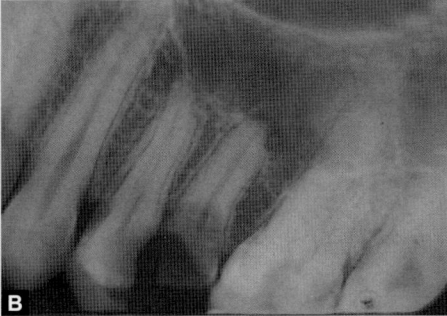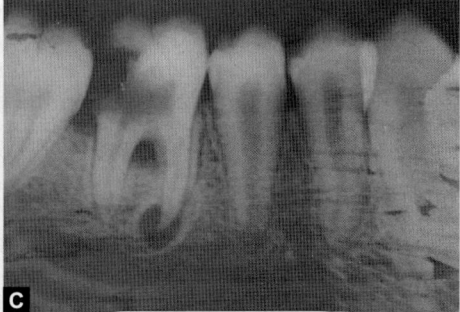

Figures 20.9A to C Periapical granuloma: (A) Well-defined radiolucency involving roots of 2nd mandibular molar; (B) Noncorticated, defined radiolucency involving roots of maxillary premolars; (C) Root of mandibular molar

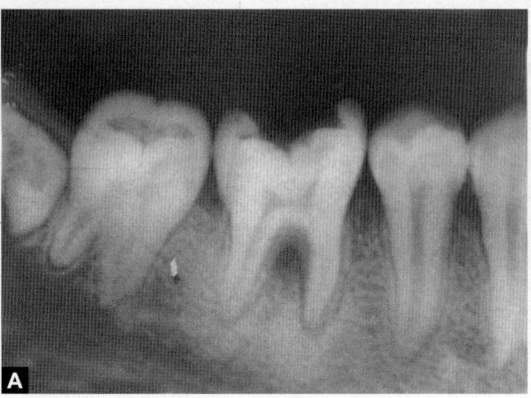 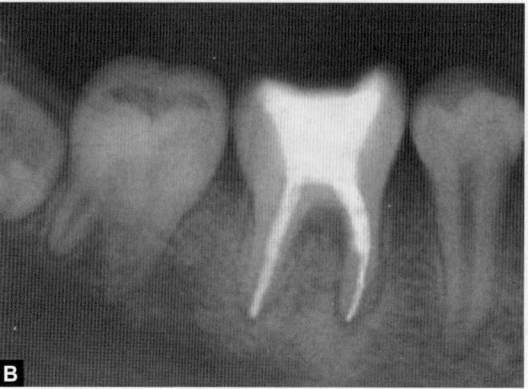 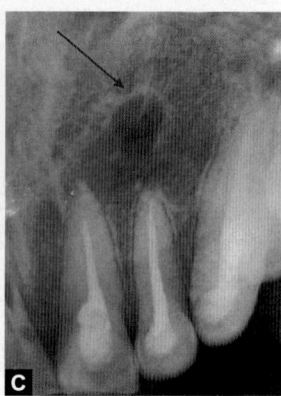

Figures 20.10A to C Dentoalveolar abscess/healing scar/condensing osteitis: (A) Well-defined saucer shaped radiolucency seen approaching the pulp in relation to mandibular first molar with an ill-defined radiolucency around the apical 1/3rd of root of 46 and furcation region (dentoalveolar abscess). There is loss of lamina dura in apical 1/3rd with an Ill-defined radiopacity suggestive of condensing osteitis around the roots; (B) The same patient after root canal treatment shows a healing scar with condensing osteitis; (C) Healing scar with typical spokes wheel appearance

Management

The tooth is usually asymptomatic and needs no treatment.

Periapical Cyst (Dental Root End Cyst, Apical Periodontal Cyst, or Radicular Cyst) (Figs 20.11A and B)

This is the stage subsequent to granuloma due to the progressive changes associated with bacterial invasion and death of the dental pulp. It is classified under inflammatory odontogenic cyst.

Clinical Features

- Usually seen in the third decade of life, more in males than females
- More common in the maxillary anterior teeth
- It is usually asymptomatic and associated with a non-vital tooth. Tooth not sensitive to percussion
- Does not cause expansion of the adjacent bone
- Swelling when present is usually bony hard or crepitations may be present if the overlying bone is thinned out or it may be rubbery or fluctuant, if the bone is completely destroyed
- Ameloblastoma, epidermoid carcinoma and mucoepidermoid carcinoma may arise in the epithelial lining of the periapical cyst.

Radiographic Features

- It appears as a round or pear shaped radiolucency at the apex of a nonvital tooth
- The radiolucency is more than 1.5 cm, but less than 3 cm in diameter, with a well-defined hyperostotic border

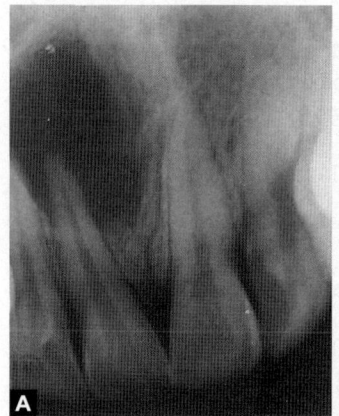 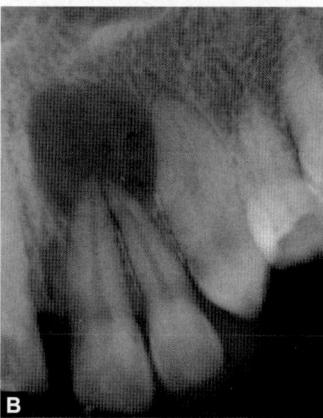

Figures 20.11A and B Periapical cyst: (A) A large radiolucency involving the root of maxillary central incisor causing displacement of the adjacent teeth; (B) Well-defined corticated radiolucent lesion associated with roots of central and lateral maxillary incisor

- The margins are smooth, well defined, well etched and continuous. A radiopaque line of corticated bone is seen surrounding the radiolucency
- The radiopaque border is continuous with the lamina dura around the associated teeth. Infection may cause the borders to appear diffuse and less distinct
- Radicular cyst of long duration may cause resorption of the roots
- The adjacent teeth are usually displaced. But, rarely resorbed. There may be buccal expansion and in the maxillary area there may be displacement of the antrum.

Differential Diagnosis

- *Periapical granuloma*: It is smaller, less than 1.5 cm in diameter. There is no presence of straw colored fluid on aspiration.
- *Periapical scar*: It is eliminated on the basis of history and location.
- *Surgical defect*: It is eliminated on the basis of history.
- *Periapical cementoma (early stage)*: Here the tooth is vital. This mostly involves the lower incisors.
- *Traumatic bone cyst*: Pulp of associated teeth is vital, and 90% of these cysts occur in the mandible (involving molars and/or premolars), whereas periapical cyst has no predilection for occurrence.
- *Periodontal abscess*: May show crestal bone loss, and tooth is vital.
- *Mandibular infected buccal cyst*: More common in young patients, involving the first molar. Tooth is vital with intact lamina dura.
- *Benign tumor*: Presence of septum in the cavity.

Management

Root canal treatment is usually sufficient. Alternately extraction with enucleation and marsupialization is recommended.

Condensing (Sclerosing) Osteitis (Figs 20.12A to H)

If the exudates from the infected pulp is of low toxicity and long standing, the resulting mild irritation may lead to a circumscribed proliferation of the periapical bone which may appear as condensing osteitis or focal sclerosing osteomyelitis. This is because of the deposition of new bone along the existing trabeculae, leading to an increase in their size and decrease in size or total elimination of the marrow space.

Clinical Features

- This is associated with a nonvital tooth or teeth whose pulps are in the process of degeneration
- The patient usually presents with an asymptomatic large carious lesion of long standing.

Radiographic Features

- The lesion is of variable size with margins which may be well-defined or diffuse
- At the diffuse margins the thickened trabeculae can be seen in continuation with the normal adjacent trabeculae
- The image of condensing osteitis is seen outside the lamina dura and periodontal spaces outlining the root, except when the density of the sclerotic bone is so great that details of the root are obscured.

Differential Diagnosis

- *Resolved acute apical periodontitis*: Thickened periodontal ligament space will persist within the image of sclerotic bone
- *Hypercementosis*: It is usually seen as an integral part of the malformed root and associated with an intact lamina dura and periodontal ligament space. The associated tooth is vital
- *Periapical cemental dysplasia*: It is usually associated with vital teeth and the lesion is separated from the surrounding bone by a radiolucent border
- *Osteosclerosis*: It is usually associated with an edentulous area.

Management

This includes either root canal treatment or extraction.

Osteosclerosis

It is believed to be a reparative process or a compensatory response to stress.

Clinical Features

No associated signs and symptoms.

Radiographic Features

- It is seen as areas of dense bone in jaws of individuals in the third decade of life and beyond
- They may be solitary, multiple which may be unilateral or bilateral, varying in size from 2 mm to 2 cm, in diameter and may have a round or irregular shape
- The border may be distinct to indistinct, ragged or blending with the adjacent bone
- Commonly seen in the mandible in the premolar-molar region, associated with healthy vital teeth. It is also seen in edentulous areas
- It is believed to occur around roots of teeth subjected to masticatory stresses, heavy occlusal forces or forces applied in abnormal direction
- Sometimes deciduous molar roots are resorbed and replaced by sclerotic bone
- Occasionally the tooth socket may be repaired by sclerotic bone called 'socket sclerosis'. When healing is almost complete a thin radiolucent line may be observed in the middle, running the length of the socket, which may resemble a root canal
- The sclerosing may be so dense that the trabecular pattern is not radiographically apparent and thus may be mistaken for a root, but this can be distinguished on close examination of the radiograph which may reveal the persistence of lamina dura but no periodontal membrane space.

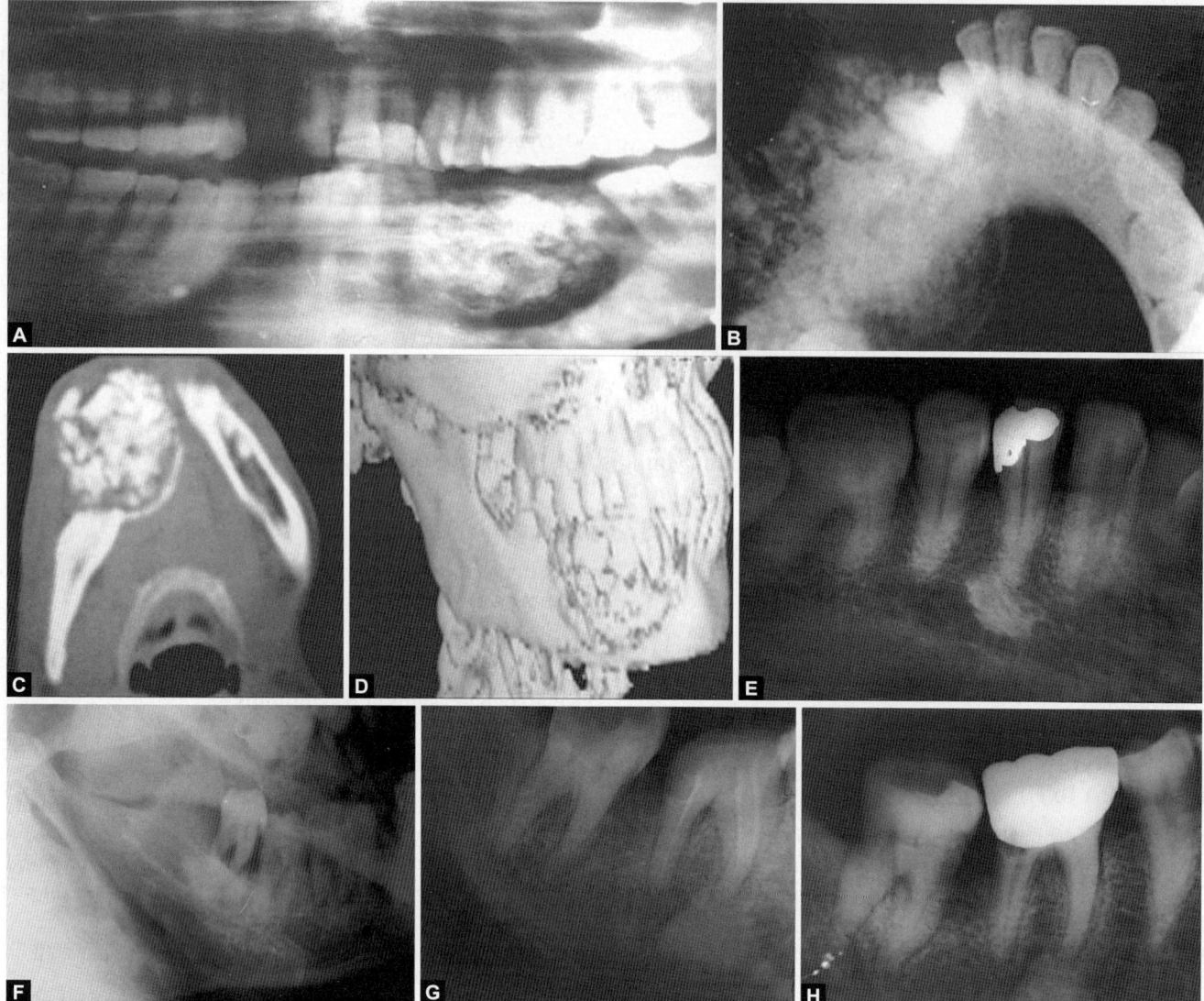

Figures 20.12A to H (A and B) A panoramic view and occlusal view showing condensing osteitis, as a well-defined solitary, diffuse radiopacity, a spherical shaped, corticated radiolucency in the right mandible 42 to 47, with expansion and discontinuity of the lower border of the mandible; (C) Axial CT shows an expansile lesion with heterogeneous radiopacity within it, measuring about 4 x 3.5 cm in size, seen in the body of the right hemimandible extending in the premolar molar region; (D) 3-DCT shows perforation of the buccal cortex both anterior and posterior; (E) Condensing osteitis at the apex of mandibular first molar; (F) Lateral oblique view showing condensing osteitis at the apex of mandibular molars; (G and H) Idiopathic condensing osteosclerosis

Differential Diagnosis

- Condensing osteitis is associated with a nonvital tooth, and infection in the intraosseous region from the infected pulp
- *Periapical cemental dysplasia or other fibro-osseous lesions*: At the apex of a vital tooth may be distinguished by the presence of a periapical radiolucent zone and a well defined border
- Hypercementosis has a bulbous shaped root apex and is separated from the surrounding bone by the radiolucent space of the periodontal membrane space

- Other radiographic entities that occur in the jaws such as retained roots, mature odontomas and unerupted teeth have distinctive and recognizable shapes and densities and can be distinguished from areas of osteosclerosis
- Shadows of exostosis, tori and peripheral osteoma can be distinguished as they are clinically palpable
- *Sclerosing osteomyelitis*: It is a mild bone infection, having symptoms of chronic infection and radiographically the sclerotic areas in this case are intermingled with radiolucent zones

- The symptoms and clinical findings associated with osteoblastic malignancy in the jaws and its mixed radiopaque-radiolucent radiographic appearance, helps to distinguish them from the symptomless lesions of osteosclerosis.

OSTEOMYELITIS (FIGS 20.13 TO 20.21)

This is an inflammation of the bone marrow that produces clinically apparent pus and secondarily affects the calcified components, (periosteum, cortex and marrow).

It may be caused due to an odontogenic infection from the root canal, infection from the periodontal ligament space, from an extraction wound, trauma or metastasis from a remote area of infection from any other part of the body.

The predisposing factors are those which lower the hosts resistance making them more susceptible to the infectious agent; like malnutrition, diabetes, leukemia, anemia, diseases that produce avascular bone, like osteopetrosis, Paget's disease, diffuse cementosis, postirradiation states and fluorosis.

The mandible is more prone than the maxilla for various reasons; the dense cortical plates of the mandible, especially in the posterior region, delays sinus formation and discharge of pus and therefore the infection is directed towards the spongia. Bone around the mandibular posterior teeth is more dense and makes extraction difficult, resulting in greater damage to the bone and greater probability of portions of infected teeth being left behind in the socket. Mandible is less vascular than the maxilla.

Infantile osteomyelitis is more common in the maxilla, as it spreads by hematogenous route and maxilla has more blood supply than the mandible.

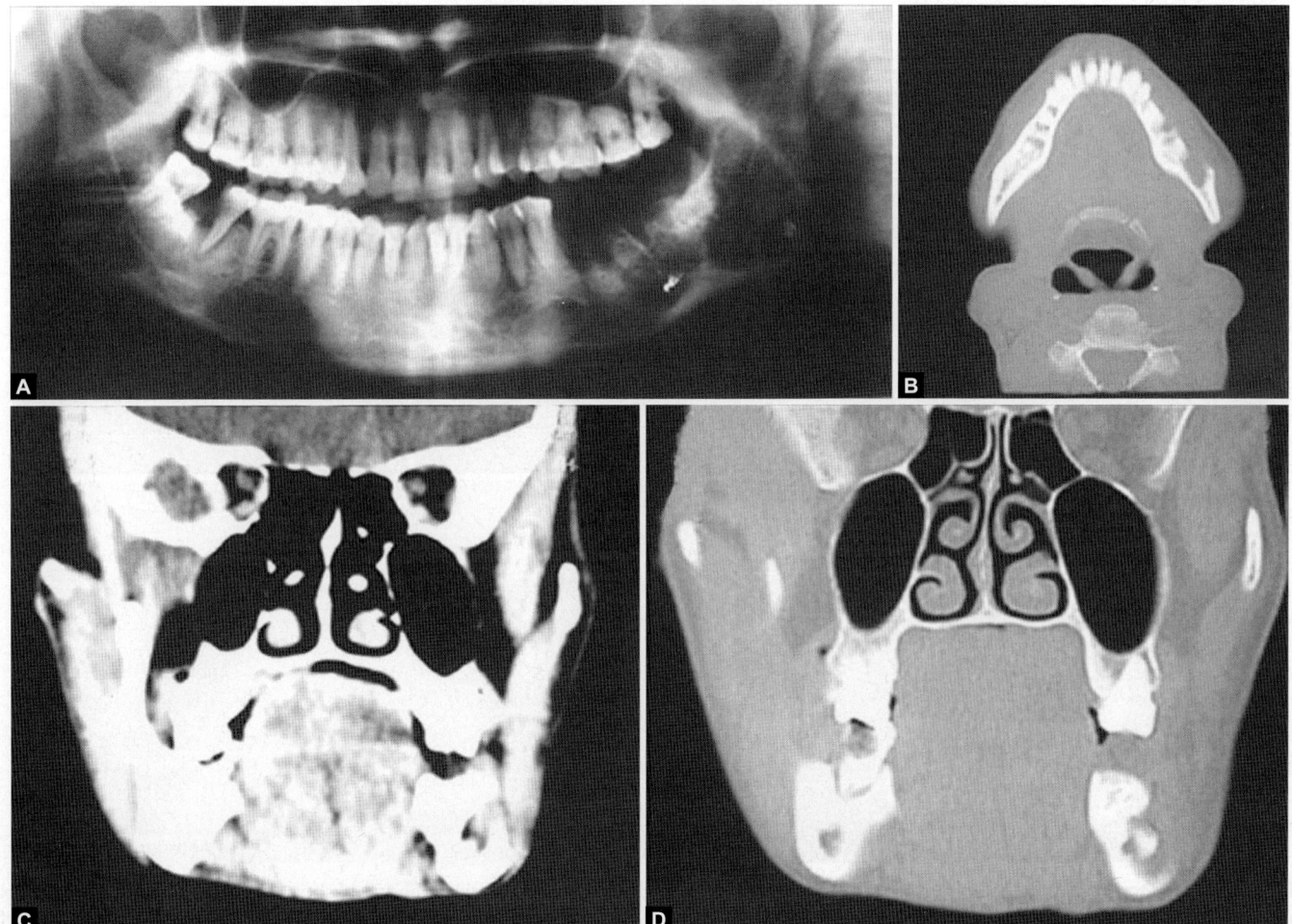

Figures 20.13A to D Osteomyelitis with draining sinus present since 3 months: (A) A panoramic view shows extraction sockets in relation to 36-37, diffuse radiolucency in the left ramus of the mandible, posteroiinferior border of the ramus is discontinuous, moth-eaten appearance. With hyperostosis on the left postalveolar ridge; (B) Axial section shows cortical break involving the left body of the mandible; (C and D) Coronal section shows destructive lesion with adjacent sclerosis. Sequestrum seen in the central cavity of the lesion

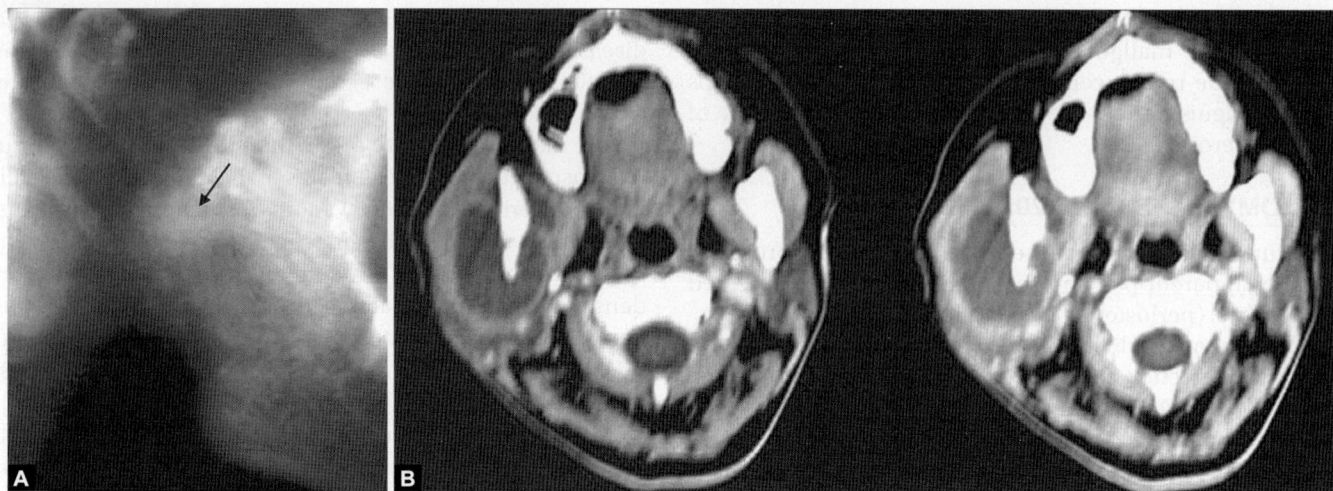

Figures 20.14A and B (A) Panoramic radiograph showing an ill-defined radiolucency, moth-eaten appearance, in the right posterior ramus, angle of the mandible and condyle of chronic osteomyelitis; (B) Axial CT hypodense peripherally enhancing lesion with erosion of the bone

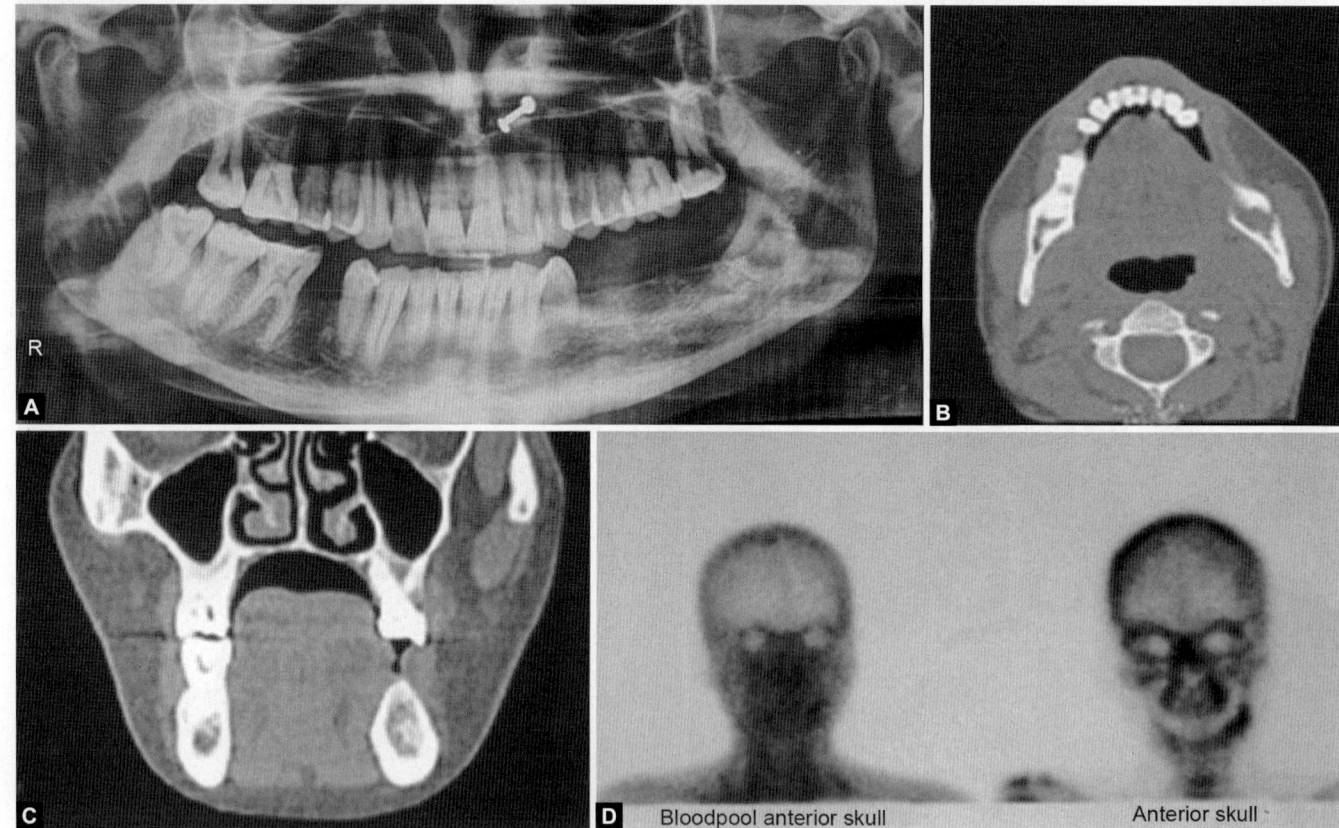

Figures 20.15A to D Chronic osteomyelitis of the body of the mandible: (A) Panoramic radiograph showed a ill-defined saucer shaped radiolucency over the left mandibular alveolar crest region; (B and C) Axial and coronal CT scan showed well defined lytic lesion in the left mandible causing thinning of the buccal and lingual cortices. Periosteal reaction also seen in the left hemimandible but is minimal; (D) Bone scintigraphy showed increased radiotracer ^{99m}Tc-MDP uptake in left mandible

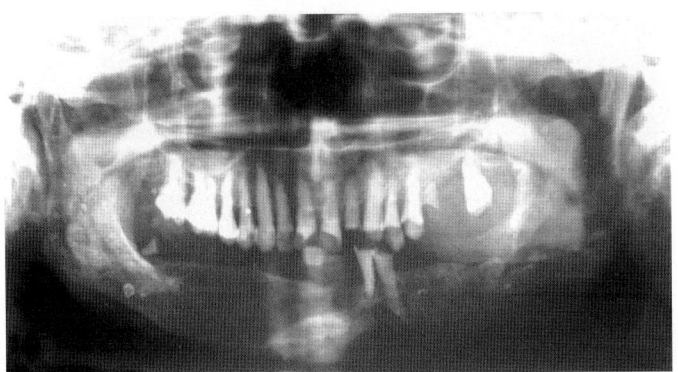

Figure 20.16 Pathologic fracture with osteomyelitis: Panoramic radiograph shows an ill-defined area of osteolysis seen in the left mandibular body extending in the canine to the third molar and involving the angle of the mandible. The lesion is extending from the half the height of alveolar crest till the inferior cortex of the mandible. An irregular oblique fracture line seen at the angle of the mandible on the left side

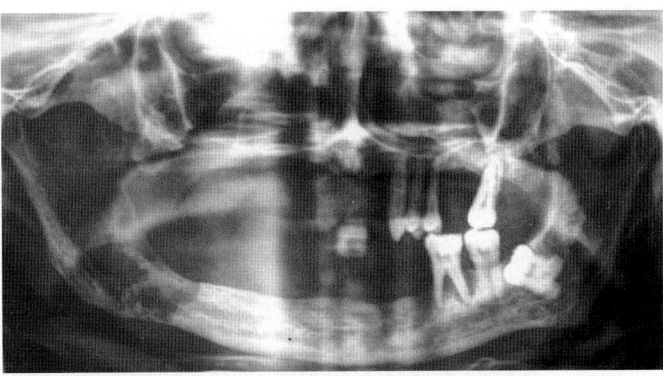

Figure 20.18 Osteomyelitis; panoramic radiograph showing: An ill-defined radiolucency extending from sigmoid notch involving it and the coronoid processs upto the first molar region over the right side of mandible. The borders of the lesion are irregular. The inferior alveolar canal is undisplaced. There are diffuse areas of radiopacities within the radiolucency. The inferior border of the mandible is continuous throughout. There is generalized crestal bone loss. Radiographic differential diagnosis is malignancy of the jaw

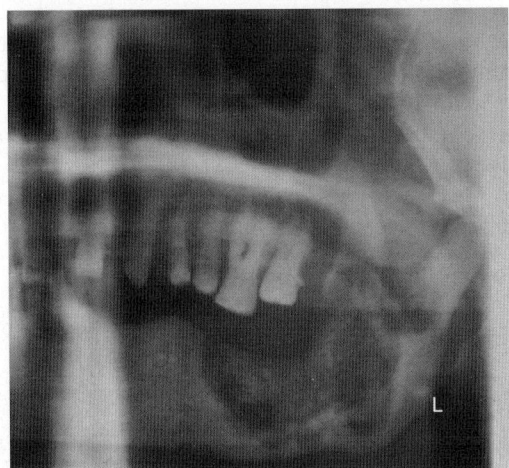

Figure 20.17 Chronic osteomyelitis: Cropped panoramic radiograph shows mixed radiolucent-opaque shadow involving left body, ramus, the condylar and coronoid process. Breach in the continuity of inferior border of body and posterior border of ramus and fractured coronoid process

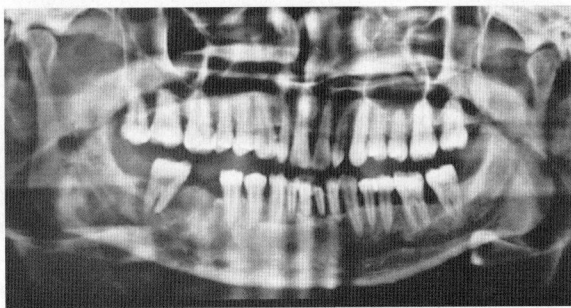

Figure 20.19 Osteomyelitis extending from lower right premolar posteriorly to the right ramus region, having a typical mottled moth-eaten appearance

It is seen more often in males than females.
Osteomyelitis can be broadly classified into:

According to location:

- Intramedullary
- Superosteal
- Periosteal.

According to duration:

- Acute
- Chronic.

According to the presence or absence of suppuration:

- Suppurative
  - Acute suppurative osteomyelitis
  - Chronic suppurative osteomyelitis
    - Primary
    - Secondary
  - Infantile osteomyelitis.
- Nonsuppurative
  - Chronic nonsuppurative
    - Focal sclerosing
    - Diffuse sclerosing
  - Radiation osteomyelitis
  - Garre's osteomyelitis
  - Osteomyelitis due to specific infection
    - Actinomycosis
    - Tuberculosis
    - Syphilis.

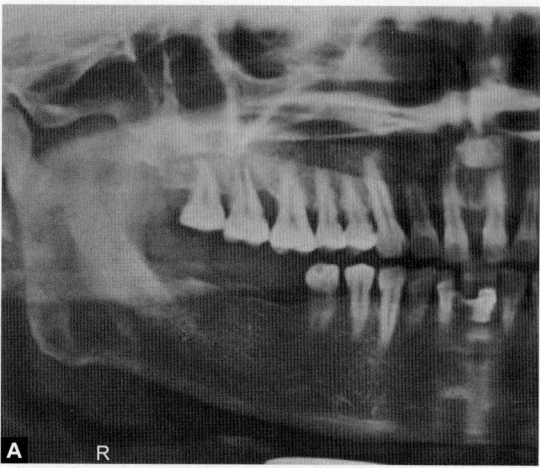 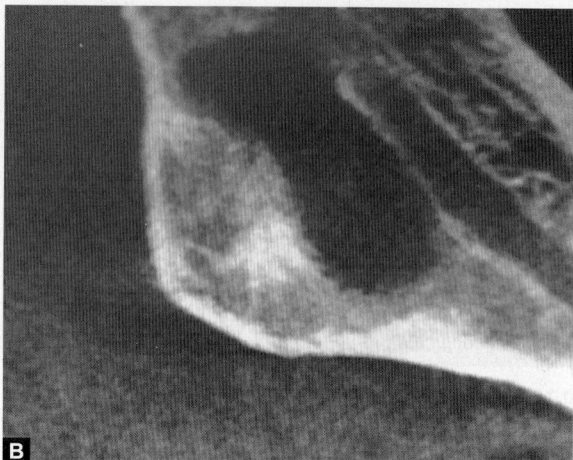

Figure 20.20A and B Tuberculous osteomyelitis of the mandible: (A) Cropped panoramic radiograph; (B) CBCT showing destruction of bone with sclerotic borders at the angle of the mandible below the inferior alveolar nerve canal mandible

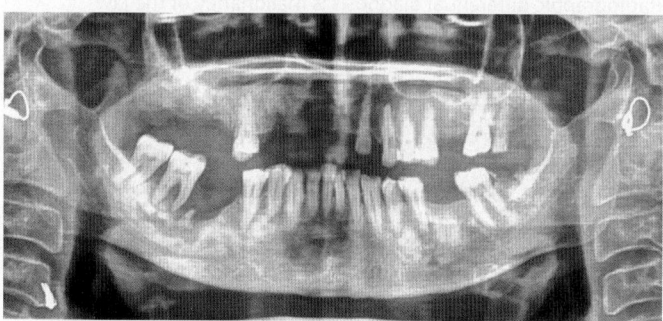

Figure 20.21 Radiographic impression-Fibro-osscous lesion w.r.t. 44 45, and osteomyelitis w.r.t. 37: Periapical well defined mixed lesion predominantly radiopaque w.r.t. 44 45, appears to be surrounded by the radiopaque borders. Missing 46, Floating teeth 37 surrounded by radiopaque band in wavy fashion, which in turn is surrounded by the wavy band of the radiolucency

According to clinical staging:

- *Initial stage*: Spontaneous localized pain
- *Acute stage (suppurative stage)*: There is severe pain, soreness and looseness of the involved teeth
  - *Early acute stage*: Progressive sensitivity of adjacent teeth to percussion and pain
  - *Late acute stage*: Paresthesia or anesthesia of the lip region supplied by the mental nerve
- *Osteonectrotic stage*: Diminished spontaneous pain, abscess formation and pus discharge
- *Sequestrum stage*: No symptoms, sequestrum formation is visible on the radiograph.

Acute Suppurative Osteomyelitis

It is a sequelae of periapical infection which spreads diffusely through the medullary spaces, with subsequent necrosis of bone.

Early Acute Suppurative Osteomyelitis

Clinical Features

- It has a rapid onset, the patient reports with severe pain, lymphadenopathy, paresthesia, soreness and tenderness of the involved teeth
- There may be no swelling, teeth are not mobile and no fistulae present.

Radiographic Features

No radiographic changes observed.

Established Suppurative Osteomyelitis

Clinical Features

- Deep intense pain, anorexia, malaise, fever, regional lymphadenopathy
- Soreness of the involved teeth which may become loose within 10–14 days
- Pus may exudate from the gingival sulcus or through mucosal or cutaneous fistula
- Firm cellulites of the cheek with abscess formation which is warm and tender to palpation.
- The patient may feel toxic, dehydrated and has a fetid oral odor.

Radiographic Features

- Radiographic changes can be observed only after about 10 days after the initiation of an acute bone infection, after structural alterations have occurred
- The density of the involved bone is decreased and there the trabeculae is loss of sharpness of the trabeculae and their outline becomes blurred or fuzzy

- Gradually solitary or multiple radiolucent areas may be seen on the radiograph, representing enlarged trabecular spaces due to foci of necrosis and frank bone destruction
- In some cases saucer shaped area of destruction with irregular margins, with teeth and some supporting bone is seen
- It may either stimulate bone resorption or formation. Inflammatory exudates may lift the periosteum, stimulating bone formation, which may be seen as a thin faint radiopaque line, adjacent to and almost parallel or slightly convex to the surface of the bone (proliferative periostitis)
- There is loss of continuity of lamina dura around the involved teeth
- *In children*: There is absence of trabeculae in the tooth bearing area, loss of density of part or whole of the cortical layer of one or more tooth follicle is seen sometimes. Follicular cortex may be lost or fragmented in that area. Once the wall of the tooth follicle is destroyed, there may be some evidence of the involved teeth moving.

Special Investigation

Technetium bone scan followed by gallium citrate scan, will help to confirm the diagnosis. In an inflammatory lesion, appositive result on the ^{99}Tc scan indicates increased bone activity and a positive result of gallium scan in the same location indicates an inflammatory lesion.

Differential Diagnosis

- Fibrous dysplasia, especially in children. The new bone that enlarges the jaws in osteomyelitis is laid down by the periosteum and therefore is on the outside of the outer cortical plate, in fibrous dysplasia the new bone is manufactured on the inside of the mandible, thus the outer cortex may be thinned and contains the lesion. This is important because the histological appearance of a biopsy of a new periosteal bone in osteomyelitis may be similar to that of fibrous dysplasia, and the condition may be reported as such.
- *Malignant neoplasia (osteosarcoma, squamous cell carcinoma)*: It invades the mandible, may be difficult to differentiate from the acute phase of osteomyelitis, especially if the malignancy is secondarily infected via an oral ulcer, giving mixed inflammatory and malignant radiographic characteristics. If part of the inflammatory periosteal bone has been destroyed, the possibility of a malignant lesion is more probable.
- Lesions which cause bone destruction and simulate a periosteal reaction as that seen in inflammatory lesions:
  - *Langerhans' cell histiocytosis*: This causes lytic, ill defined bone destruction with formation of periosteal reactive new bone, but a sclerotic bone reaction as that seen in osteomyelitis is not seen in this case.
  - Leukemia and lymphoma may stimulate a similar periosteal reaction.

Management

Antimicrobial therapy with drainage and/or extraction/ endodontic treatment of the causative tooth.

Acute Subperiosteal Osteomyelitis

Sometimes the periapical abscess develops close to and rapidly ruptures through the cortex and the exudates invades the subperiosteal spaces, the periosteum is stripped off the bone and as the exudates increases the pressure increases leading to local necrosis and resorption of the cortical plate. This also interrupts the blood supply to the cortex. Eventually multiple draining sinuses are formed.

Clinical Features

- The patient complains of severe pain, swelling and lymphadenopathy
- Involved teeth are sensitive to percussion
- As the sinuses form the symptoms start easing.

Radiographic Features

An occlusal radiograph will show an area of erosion of the cortex.

Osteomyelitis in Infants

This is a rare type of osteomyelitis, seen in infants few weeks after birth, which spreads by the hematogenous route, thus commonly involving the maxilla. It may be caused by trauma to oral mucosa from obstetrician's finger, infection from the mucous bulb used to clear the airway, infected human or artificial nipple.

Clinical Features

- It is more common in the maxilla
- The patient develops fever, redness, edema, development of intra or extra oral draining sinuses
- Intracanthal swelling, palpebral edema, conjunctivitis, and proptosis may result
- Complications of the TMJ and devitalization of the adjacent tooth germs may occur.

Radiographic Features

No changes are seen for at least three weeks, after which irregular demineralization and other changes as those seen in acute osteomyelitis may be observed.

Management

This includes extraction of the tooth with curettage and sequestrosectomy of the sequestrum.

Chronic Suppurative Osteomyelitis

This is a persistent abscess of the bone which is characterized by the usual complex of inflammatory processes, including necrosis of mineralized and marrow tissues, suppuration, resorption sclerosis and hyperplasia.

Chronic, Primary Type of Suppurative Osteomyelitis

The infection is localized, but persistent because it is isolated from the host's defense reactions. The lesion may be single or multiple.

Clinical Features

- This is not preceded by an episode of acute symptoms
- The patient may complain of local tenderness and swelling over the bone, lymphadenopathy, intra and extraoral intermittently draining sinuses
- Pain is experienced only in case of acute or subacute exacerbation.

Chronic, Secondary Type of Suppurative Osteomyelitis

It is secondary to incompletely treated acute osteomyelitis.

Clinical Features

- The symptoms are similar to that in acute infection, however, the symptoms are milder, bone destruction slower and the patient is comparatively more comfortable
- There is formation of fistulas which open intermittently and then stop draining and close
- There is induration of soft tissues, thickened and wooden character of the bone with pain and tenderness on palpation
- Regional lymphadenopathy is usually present.

Radiographic Features

- Multiple radiolucencies of variable size with irregular outline and poorly defined borders are seen
- The bone gradually develops 'a moth-eaten' appearance, as radiolucent areas enlarge and are separated by islands of normal bone. This is due to the enlargement of medullary spaces and widening of Volkmann's canals, secondary to lysis of bone and replacement with granulation tissue
- Segments of the necrotic bone become detached and calcified and are called 'sequestra'. Sequestra are more dense and better defined because of the sclerosis which was induced before the bone became necrotic, dead bone has affinity for absorbing calcium, inflammation of the surrounding vital bone stimulates its demineralization, thus enhancing the contrast. CT is superior for revealing the internal structure and sequestra, especially those with very dense sclerotic bone

- Chronic osteomyelitis often stimulates the formation of periosteal new bone, which is seen on the radiograph as a single radiopaque or a series of radiopaque lines (similar to onion peel) parallel to the surface of the cortical bone. Gradually, the radiolucent strip that separates the new bone from the outer cortical bone may be filled with sclerotic bone, making it difficult to differentiate the two. Subsequently the outer contour of the bone (mandible) may be altered, assuming an abnormal shape and the girth of the affected side will be more than that of the normal side
- Roots of the involved teeth may undergo external resorption and the lamina dura may become less apparent as it blends with surrounding granular sclerotic bone
- The fistula tracts may appear on the radiograph as radiolucent bands transversing the body of the jaw and penetrating the cortical plates
- In case of extensive spread, the mandibular condyle and joint may be affected, resulting in septic arthritis. Further it may spread to the inner ear and mastoid air cells.

Special Investigation

Computed tomography is more useful in revealing the internal structure and sequestra more readily than conventional radiography.

Differential Diagnosis

- Fibrous dysplasia
- *Paget's disease*: This affects the entire bone (mandible), which is rare in osteomyelitis. The presence of sequestra indicates osteomyelitis
- *Osteosarcoma*: This shows evidence of bone destruction with a characteristic speculated (sun ray) periosteal response
- Langerhans' cell histiocytosis
- Leukemia
- Lymphoma.

Management

Surgical intervention with hyperbaric oxygen.

Sclerosing Osteomyelitis

It is the result of a balanced equilibrium between the virulence of the infection and resistance of the host, the primary reaction being reactive proliferation of the bone.

Focal Sclerosing Osteomyelitis (Condensing Osteitis)

Clinical Features

It is a nonsuppurative inflammatory condition, caused due to high resistance of the alveolar bone to odontogenic infection or the virulence of the organism is low, or a chronic condition characterized by formation of focal areas of sclerosis around the tooth, especially roots of molars with large carious lesions in young persons.

Radiographic Features

- There is a well circumscribed radiopaque apical mass often mimicking benign cementoblastoma
- The root outline is always visible on the radiograph.

Management

Endodontic treatment or extraction.

Diffuse Sclerosing Osteomyelitis

There is a low grade infection of the bone involving a relatively large segment of the jaw.

Clinical Features

- It is more common in older female patients, in the edentulous mandibular jaw
- The patient may complain no symptoms or of mild pain and tenderness, during the period of growth which may last from few weeks to years
- Jaw may be slightly enlarged on the affected side.

Radiographic Features

- The early radiographic changes mimic osteomyelitis with ill-defined osteolytic and osteosclerotic zones. There is an increase in size of the involved part. Though a large part of the jaw is involved, the lesion usually does not cross the midline and the surface of the new bone is smooth
- Stripped or granular densification of bone, caused by subperiosteal deposition of new bone, obscures the intrinsic bone structure or deposition of new bone on the surface of marrow spaces. The deposition is more on the buccal and inferior surface of the jaw
- Shortening of the roots of the involved teeth is seen.

Special Investigation

Scintigraphy shows uptake of ^{99m}Tc polyphosphate or ^{99m}Tc diphosphonate in the diseased area, suggesting active bone deposition.

Differential Diagnosis

Osteomyelitis should be differentiated from:
- Malignancies like osteosarcoma, metastatic osteoblastic carcinoma and chondrosarcoma. Though the radiographic appearance is very similar, the presence of infection and frequency of occurrence tilts the diagnosis for osteomyelitis

- Lesions of intermediate stage of Paget's disease, mimic osteomyelitis, but Paget's disease usually affects multiple bones and there is complete involvement of the individual bones. Paget's disease may be complicated with osteosarcoma, which may be radiographically confused for osteomyelitis
- Lesions of Eosinophilic granuloma may be confused for osteomyelitis on the radiograph and can be distinguished by taking biopsy. Usually the bone lesions of Eosinophilic granuloma are better defined and show no evidence of bone sclerosis.

Chronic Subperiosteal Osteomyelitis

After the acute stage of the infection as soon as drainage for the pus is established by formation of intra and/or extraoral sinuses, the chronic phase of the infection begins. A portion of the cortical plate from which the periosteum has been stripped off becomes necrotic due to lack of blood supply, and multiple small sequestra are formed. These sequestra act as foreign bodies and perpetuate the suppurative process and are eventually discharged through the sinus, following which healing may occur if the odontogenic infection is controlled.

Clinical Features

- Patient may feel pain of low intensity
- Regional lymph nodes may be enlarged.

Radiographic Features

- Lateral radiographs will show 'moth-eaten' appearance
- The cortical sequestra appear as multiple small radiopaque flakes in the occlusal projection
- Some mottling of the adjacent trabecular bone is seen in both the radiographs.

Differential Diagnosis

- Mixed radiopaque and radiolucent lesions with ill-defined border should be considered
- Paget's disease. But this affects multiple bones and the involvement is complete of individual bone
- *Eosinophilic granuloma granulome*: Here the margins are better than in osteomyelitis and there is no evidence of bone sclerosis.

Garré's Osteomyelitis (Proliferative Periostitis)

This is a nonsuppurating sclerosing osteomyelitis, characterized by formation of hard, bony swelling at the periphery of the jaw. It is induced by a mild infection below the periosteum from the cancellous portion of the jaw that penetrates the cortex. For the lesion to develop the following conditions should be satisfied; the periosteum must possess a high potential for osteoblastic activity, mild infection should be present to serve as a stimulus, affine balance has to be maintained between the resistance of the host and number and virulence of the organism.

Clinical Features

- It occurs more often in males, below 30 years of age
- Mandible is more affected than the maxilla, especially inferior border of the mandible and in the first molar region
- It presents as a hard nontender swelling with medial and lateral expansion of jaw
- The size may vary from 1–2 cm to the involvement of the entire length of the affected side. The cortex may become 2–3 cm thick
- If it becomes secondarily infected it causes considerable discomfort
- *Other associated symptoms are*: Lymphadenopathy, hyperpyrexia and leukocytosis.

Radiographic Features

- An intraoral periapical radiograph will show a carious tooth opposite the hard bony mass
- Shadow of a thin convex shell of bone over the cortex, with radiolucent space between the two is seen
- As infection persists the cortex thickens and becomes laminated with alternating radiopaque-radiolucent layers (Onion peel appearance)
- Adjacent cancellous bone may remain normal, become sclerotic or show some areas of osteolytic changes within the scleroses spongiosa
- Following removal of the irritation, the cortical bone may remodel to a normal appearance.

Differential Diagnosis

- *Ewing's sarcoma*: The bony enlargement is very rapid and the tumor frequently produces osteophytes with 'sun ray' appearance. Facial neuralgia and lip paresthesia are a frequent complication
- *Caffey's disease (infantile cortical hyperostosis)*: This is more common at the angle or in the ramus of the mandible, more commonly seen in early age, before 2 years. Generalized expansion of cortices of several bones. Other bones besides the mandible may be involved, especially the clavicle
- *Fibrous dysplasia*: It is usually not associated with any dental infection and is more common in the maxilla. Here the cortex is thinned or completely replaced by the altered bone tissue depending to the very limit of the bone. The density is uniform, having a 'ground glass appearance'.
- *Osteosarcoma*: May produce a bony hard mass, but has the typical 'sun ray appearance', on the radiograph
- Hard, nodular or pendunculated growths like peripheral osteomas, tori, and exostoses, should be clinically

distinguished. Radiographically they appear as dense, uniformly radiopaque masses on the jaw, protruding from the cortex, depending on the manner of the exposure
- *Ossifying subperiosteal hematoma*: It may have a similar clinical appearance, however, it is not uniformly radiopaque having either a mottled appearance or an uneven trabeculae pattern. A history of trauma to the area may establish the diagnosis.

SPECIFIC CHRONIC INFECTIONS OF THE JAWS

A number of agents that produce granulomatous inflammations are occasionally found to be the cause of chronic osteomyelitis of the jaw bones; like tuberculosis, syphilis, brucellosis, actinomycosis, blastomycosis and coccidiodomycosis. From the radiographic point of view there is nothing characteristic about the appearances of the bony changes induced by these entities, all have a radiographic appearance of a chronic bone infection caused by pyogenic micro-organisms. The recognition of these diseases depends on their systemic symptoms and/or immunologic evidence.

Actinomycotic Osteomyelitis

This is a chronic infection which manifests both granulomatous and suppurative features that usually involve the soft tissues and sometimes the bone of cervicofacial, abdominal and thoracic region.

Clinical Features

- Patient presents with soft tissue masses of skin which have a purplish, dark red, oily areas with an occasional zone of flatulence. There may be spontaneous drainage of serous fluid, containing granular material (sulfur granules), which represent colonies of bacteria. The soft tissues harbor organisms and reduce the blood supply to the affected side
- Regional lymphadenopathy is present.

Radiographic Features

Actinomycosis produces dense bone and scarring of soft tissue which has been described as 'lumpy jaw'. This is common in cattle.

Management

Treatment consists of incision and drainage of the flatulent areas under antibiotic cover. Penicillin is the drug of choice, 10–20 million units for 3–4 months.

Tuberculous Osteomyelitis

- Tuberculosis of the bone and joints is hematogenous in origin
- The primary focus is related to the lungs or gastrointestinal tract

- The disease starts within the synovial membrane or intra-articular bone. Tuberculous osteomyelitis of the maxilla, mandible or TMJ is rare.

Radiation Osteomyelitis (Osteoradionecrosis) (Fig. 20.22)

Following exposure to intense radiation (40–80 Gy), bone undergoes a marked decrease in vascularity, leading to degenerative changes in the osteocytes and bone marrow, and thus bone becomes very susceptible to trauma and infections. The lesions that develop in such altered bone are similar to the usual chronic suppurative osteomyelitis, the only difference being that in osteoradionecrosis that inflammatory response is decreased or absent as a result of altered vascular bed. Due to reduced resistance there is minimal localization of the infection and the spread though slow is relatively diffuse with sequestration. The organisms most commonly found are *Staphylococcus aureus* and *Staphylococcus epidermidis*.

Clinical Features

- It occurs with a triad of radiation, trauma and infection
- More common in the mandible as the irradiation is often directed to it
- The patient has intense pain with inflammation, swelling and drainage (facial fistulas develop from the subperiosteal tissues)
- The involved teeth give a positive vitality test
- The spread is diffuse and throughout with signs of inflammation and swelling.

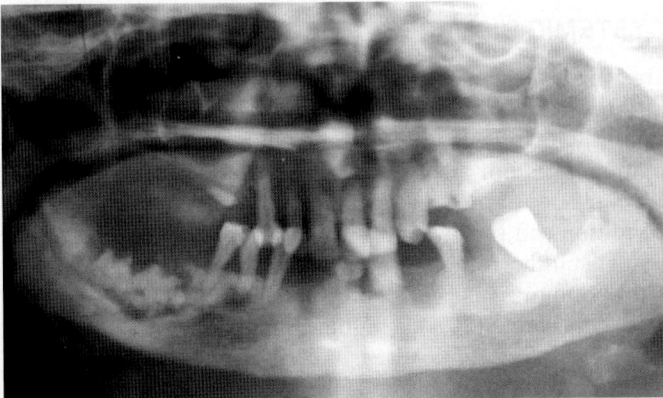

Figure 20.22 Osteoradionecrosis of the mandible: Panoramic radiograph shows mild to moderate generalized horizontal alveolar bone loss. A radiopaque mass with irregular borders surrounded by radiolucent band in lower right region extending from premolar to the angle of the mandible having moth-eaten appearance in some areas

Radiographic Features

- Areas of increased density interspaced with osteolytic regions and late forming sequestra are seen
- It resembles osteomyelitis, but this is more widespread.

Differential Diagnosis

- Chronic osteomyelitis can be differentiated by the history of radiation treatment
- Recurrence of malignant neoplasm (usually squamous cell carcinoma). CT scan and MRI imaging may be used to detect an associated soft tissue mass.

Management

Treatment consists of control of infection with antibiotics (penicillin).

PERICORONAL INFECTIONS

Pericoronitis (Operculitis, Pericoronal Abscess)

This is infection surrounding the crown of a partially erupted tooth, causing inflammation, and patient discomfort.

Clinical Features

- Operculum may get traumatized by the opposing teeth during mastication
- Edema may be visible in both submandibular area and peritonsillar region
- There is extreme tenderness on palpation of the abscess
- The patient may complain of pain, malaise and swelling of the peritonsillar region
- The involvement may become localized in the form of pericoronal abscess or spread posteriorly into the oropharynx area and medially to the base of the tongue, causing peritonsillar abscess, cellulitis or Ludwig's angina
- Pericoronal infection of infancy:
  - It is associated with the supradental tissues, involving the superior portion of the follicle and the overlying periosteum, which may become inflamed
  - It forms a small fluctuant abscess
  - Repeated infected folliculitis may develop a chronic pericoronal abscess that involves the bony crypt
  - It may result in cellulites and muscular trismus
  - There may be regional lymphadenopathy, submaxillary and pharyngeal abscess.

Radiographic Features

- Infection of short duration does not show any radiographic changes
- In cases of the lower third molar, there is a bony defect due to circumferential bone resorption.

- The defect may be of the mesial or distal aspect of the involved tooth and here it appears as a step like distortion of the crypt wall distal to the crown
- The periphery of pericoronitis is ill-defined with a gradual transition of the normal trabecular pattern into a sclerotic region
- The existing follicular margins may show sclerosing osteitis and generalized thickening of the crypt wall (indicating low grade infection)
- Mesially tipped impaction display semilunar shaped bone resorption mesial to the crown and in cases of distally placed impaction, it is distal to the crown
- The inflammatory process may also resorb the roots of the adjacent tooth
- The internal structure of the bone adjacent to the pericoronitis is often sclerotic with thick trabeculae. An area of bone loss or radiolucency immediately adjacent to the crown may be seen that enlarges the follicular space. If this lesion spreads considerably the internal pattern may become consistent with osteomyelitis
- The surrounding bone may show sclerosis with rarefaction. In extensive cases evidence of periosteal new bone formation may be seen at the inferior cortex, the posterior border of the ramus and along the coronoid notch of the mandible.

Differential Diagnosis

- Mixed density or sclerotic lesions that can exist adjacent to the crow of a partially erupted third molar; enostosis, fibrous dysplasia. The clinical symptoms indicative of an inflammatory lesion help exclude these conditions
- *Neoplasms*: Sclerotic form of osteosarcoma and in older patients, squamous cell carcinoma. The profound cortical bone destruction and invasion, which are characteristic of malignant neoplasia, aid in the diagnosis, but squamous cell carcinoma in midst of a pre-existing inflammatory lesion may be difficult to identify.

Management

Antibiotics (phenoxylmethyl penicillin 250 mg, 4 times a day/metronidazole 200 mg, 3 times a day for seven days) with drainage and/or extraction of the involved tooth or the opposing tooth, as in the case of a upper maxillary third molar which is impinging on the lower partially erupted tooth or operculectomy.

Folliculitis

Follicles of developing succedaneous teeth may become infected when the primary predecessors develop chronic periapical abscess. This may damage the ameloblasts resulting in hypoplastic defect called Turner's hypoplasia.

If the infection extends into the developing end it may kill the pulp of the unerupted tooth and terminate further development, the eruption is not affected and it will erupt into the oral cavity but is shed within a short period.

Clinical Features

- It may be acute or chronic involving deciduous or permanent dentition. (mandibular premolars are most commonly affected)
- The swelling of the mucosa in the vestibule, adjacent to the offending tooth appears red and tender
- Parulis may open opposite the primary tooth after the swelling subsides
- In some cases the infection from the infected follicle may extend to the buccal surface of the bone where it meets the periosteum and cause it to become inflamed, resulting in periostitis
- Regional lymphadenopathy and fever may be present.

Radiographic Features

- Because of the relationship of the developing permanent tooth, the radiographic picture of this condition does not show the sharp delineation of the infectious process in the periapex of the deciduous tooth
- There may be slight loss of density of the cortex that lines the follicle, followed by definite discontinuity of some part of the cortex
- In some cases, the cortical border surrounding the tooth is destroyed and the tooth appears to be infected.

Management

Treatment is same as that for pericoronitis.

SYSTEMIC DISEASES AFFECTING THE JAWS

The various systemic diseases have a major effect on the form and function of bone and teeth. The function of the bone not only includes support, protection and environment for hemopoiesis but also serves as a major reserve of calcium for the body. When considering the influence of systemic conditions on the jaws, it is important to note that the bone is constantly remodeling. Approximately 5–10% of the total bone mass is replaced each year. The turnover rate of trabecular bone (20%) is higher than for cortical bone (5%). The effects of systemic diseases of bone are brought about by changes in the number and activity of osteoclasts, osteoblasts and osteocytes.

General radiographic features of systemic disease manifested in the jaws:
- The bones of the entire skeleton are affected
- There may be a change in the size and shape of the bone

- There may be a change in the number, size and orientation of the trabeculae
- There may be an alteration in the thickness and density of the cortical structures
- There may be an increase or decrease in the overall bone density:
  - Systemic conditions that result in a decrease in bone density do not affect the teeth. Therefore the image of the teeth may stand out with normal density against a generally radiolucent jaw. Sometimes the teeth appear to be without any bony support. The cortical structures will appear thin, less defined and on occasions may not be seen.
  - A true increase in bone density may be detected by a loss of contrast of the inferior cortex of the mandible as the radiopacity of the cancellous bone approaches that of the cortical bone. The inferior alveolar canal may appear more distinct in contrast to the surrounding dense bone.
- Systemic diseases that occur during tooth formation may result in dental alteration:
  - Acclerated or delayed eruption
  - Hypoplasia
  - Hypocalcification
  - Loss of a distinct lamina dura.

Many a times there may be no detectable radiographic changes associated with systemic diseases, but the first symptom may present as a dental problem.

The systemic diseases that are manifested in the jaws may be broadly divided into:

- Endocrinal disorders
- Metabolic bone diseases due to nutritional deficiency
- Blood disorders.

ENDOCRINAL DISORDERS (TABLE 20.2)

The condition of the oral tissues reflects the nutritional and hormonal status of an individual. Some changes in the oral tissues are common to several hormonal disturbances and others are produced characteristically by a single endocrinal dysfunction. The problem is further complicated in man as usually multiple deficiencies or excesses frequently occur together.

The glands of the endocrine system regulate and co-ordinate the activities of the organism by secreting specific chemical substances called hormones into the blood stream. After dispersal throughout the tissue fluids these hormones act as catalysts to chemical reactions occurring in specific cells of the body.

Both external and internal environment can stimulate alterations in the level of hormone secretion. The stimuli may be transmitted by humoral or neural means or a combination of the two systems. Alteration in the secretion of one gland usually affects the secretions of the other glands, and in this way the scattered glands of the endocrine system act as a coordinated entity. The supreme control of the endocrinal system resides in the central nervous system and is expressed via the secretions of a mediator substance from the nuclei of the hypothalamus.

Hyperpituitarism

Definition

This results from hyper function of the anterior pituitary gland, usually with the increased secretion of the growth

Table 20.2 Classification of endocrinal disorders

- Disease of the pituitary gland
  - Hyperpituitarism
    - Gigantism
    - Acromegaly
  - Hypopituitarism
    - Dwarfism
    - Simmond's disease
  - Progeria
- Disease of the thyroid gland
  - Hyperthyroidism
  - Hypothyroidism
    - Cretinism
    - Juvenile myxedema
    - Myxedema
- Disease of the parathyroid gland
  - Hyperparathyroidism
    - Primary
    - Secondary
    - Tertiary
    - Ectopic
  - Hypoparathyroidism
    - DiGeorge's syndrome
    - Postoperative hypoparathyroidism
    - Idiopathic hypoparathyroidism
    - Pseudohypoparathyroidism
- Disease of the pancreatic gland
  - Diabetes mellitus
    - Type I
    - Type II
- Disease of the adrenal gland
  - Hypofunction of the adrenal gland
    - Acute insufficiency of the adrenal cortex (Water-House-friderichsen syndrome)
    - Chronic insufficiency of the adrenal cortex (Addison's disease)
  - Hyperfunction of the adrenal gland
    - Adrenogenital syndrome
    - Cushing's syndrome
    - Adrenal insufficiency
- Disease of the gonads
  - Hypergonadism
  - Hypogonadism
- Physiological causes
  - Puberty
  - Pregnancy
  - Menopause
- Oral contraceptives

hormone. An excess of growth hormone causes overgrowth of all tissues in the body still capable of growth. The most common cause being a benign, functioning tumor of the acidophilic cells in the anterior lobe of the pituitary gland.

When it occurs in childhood it is termed *Gigantism*, which is manifested as a generalized symmetrical overgrowth, with genital underdevelopment.

When it occurs in adults, (usually, due to eosinophilic tumors), it is called *Acromegaly*. Most adults are incapable of increased growth due to the fusion of the epiphysis with the shaft of the endochondral bone and the fusion of the sutures of the craniofacial bones.

Clinical Features

Gigantism

- Generalized excessive skeletal growth, patient may attain a height of 7–8 feet or more and yet exhibit remarkably normal proportions
- The eyes and other parts of the central nervous system do not enlarge, except in rare cases in which the condition is manifested in infancy
- It may induce hypogonadism causing decreased libido and menstrual problems in women
- There may be increased perspiration, headaches, lassitude, fatigue, hot flashes, muscle and joint pain
- There may be an increase in size of the calvarium
- As the jaws are enlarged, but the tooth size does not change, this may lead to diastema formation
- The crown size is normal but the roots of the posterior teeth are often enlarged because of secondary cemental hyperplasia
- Eruption of teeth is normal.

Acromegaly

- More common in males, in the third decade
- The terminal phalanges of the hands and feet may enlarge leading to clubbing of the toes and fingers. The ribs also enlarge in size
- The patient may experience photophobia, temporal headaches, reduction in vision
- There is bone overgrowth and thickening of the soft tissues which gives a characteristic coarsening of the facial features termed acromegaly. The lips become thick and negroid
- The supraorbital ridges and the underlying frontal sinus may be enlarged
- The tongue is enlarged and shows indentations. The anterior teeth are pushed forward and appear fan shaped.
- The palatal vault may be flattened due to the enlarged tongue
- In the mandible, the articular surface of the condyle which is covered with growth potential cartilage may

be stimulated to produce further endochondral bone, which produces a lengthening of the condylar process, lengthening of the ramus and body of the mandible, producing a Class III skeletal relationship and mandibular prognathism

- The vertical depth of the jaws may also be increased due to new bone laid at the crests of the alveolus as the teeth erupt. Over growth of the jaws, especially in the posterior region of the alveolus results in an anterior open bite.

Radiographic Features

- There is enlargement and ballooning of the sella turcica, as seen on the lateral radiograph
- There is enlargement of the paranasal sinuses and excessive pneumatization of the temporal bone squamous and petrous ridges. This is more so in acromegaly than in gigantism because the growth in the latter tends to be more in step with generalized enlargement of the facial bones
- In adults there is a diffuse thickening of the outer table of the skull
- In acromegaly there is an increase in the angle between the ramus and the body of the mandible
- Supra eruption of the posterior teeth may occur in an attempt to compensate for the growth of the mandible
- Hypercementosis is noted, especially in the posterior teeth.

Differential Diagnosis

- *Inherited prognathism*: Mandibular prognathism with incisal flaring helps to differentiate acromegaly prognathism from inherited prognathism.
- Hyperpituitarism can be diagnosed from the characteristic clinical and radiographic findings, and by doing a radioimmunoassay to study the concentration of the growth hormone.

Management

Medical therapy, surgery and radiotherapy.

Hypopituitarism

Definition

This is a result of decreased secretion of the pituitary hormone, which may be due to a congenital or destructive disease of the gland, space occupying lesions or pituitary adenomas.

If it occurs before puberty it is called *Dwarfism* and is manifested as an individual with a diminutive but well proportional body with fine sparse silky hair, wrinkled atrophic skin and hypogonadism.

When it occurs in adults or after puberty it is called *Simmond's Disease* or *Pituitary Cachexia*.

Total absence of pituitary secretions is known as *Panhypopituitarism*.

Clinical Features

Dwarfism

- Underdevelopment is symmetrical, with the growth retarded to a greater degree than the bone and dental development
- Hypocalcemia occurs due to the deficiency of growth hormone and cortisol. Lack of gonadotrophin delays puberty
- Marked failure of the development of the maxilla and the mandible, lack of condylar growth leading to a short ramus. The dental arches are smaller than normal and thus cannot accommodate all the teeth and may result in severe malocclusion and crowding of the teeth
- Osseous development of the maxilla is not as retarded as that of the mandible, leading to retrusion of the chin
- There is delayed eruption and shedding of the teeth
- Clinical crowns appear smaller than the normal, sometimes this may be due to the fact that the eruption is not complete
- Roots of the teeth are also shorter than the normal and the supporting structures show retarded growth.

Simmond's Disease

- Deficient secretion of vasopressin may induce diabetic insipidus
- Decreased secretion of the luteinizing hormone (LH) may cause loss of libido and impotence in men with gynecomastia and the skin becomes fair and wrinkled, in women it induces oligomenorrhea or amenorrhea
- There will be loss of weight, diminished sexual function, lowered basal metabolic rate, skin will show atrophic alterations
- There will be thinning of the lips, loss of eyelashes, thin eye brows, sharp features with an immobile expression
- Loss of alveolar bone due to marked resorption and loss of teeth has been seen but no specific dental changes have been described.

Radiographic Features

- The skull and facial bones are small (the dimensions of these bones in the adults are approximately the same as those of a normal children 5–7 years of age) and there is delay in the maturation of the skeleton and epiphysis may remain un-united through the life
- Eruption of the deciduous teeth is normal but the exfoliation may be delayed by several years.

- The crowns of the permanent teeth form normally but their eruption is delayed by several years
- Roots of the teeth are short, with wide open apices
- The third molar buds may be completely absent.

Differential Diagnosis

Sheehan's syndrome: This is a form of hypopituitarism caused by the infarction of the pituitary associated with postpartum hemorrhage.

Management

Removal of the cause or replacement of the pituitary hormones or those of its target gland.

Progeria

Definition

This is transmitted as an autosomal dominant trait, which results in pituitary dysfunction, presented as premature senility in an individual of infantile proportions.

Clinical Features

- The infants at birth appear normal, but the typical features are manifested within the first few years
- The patient exhibits alopecia, pigmented areas on the trunk, prominent veins, loss of subcutaneous fat and joint deformities
- The patient will have a pointed face, with a beak like nose, large head with a small mandible. There may be exophthalmus, and thin lips
- The patient at an early age behaves like an older person, intelligence may be normal or above normal, and the patient may have a high pitched squeaky voice
- There will be delayed eruption of teeth and accelerated formation of irregular dentin.

Radiographic Features

- There will be osteoporosis of the long bones
- There may be overdevelopment of the frontal and parietal bones, while the ossification may be delayed and deficient
- The mandible and maxilla are small, the mandible being more underdeveloped producing an underhung chin.

Management

There is no particular treatment; the individual usually dies in the second or third decade.

Hyperthyroidism (Fig. 20.23)

Definition

It is a condition in which there is excessive production of thyroxine in the thyroid gland. It is most commonly associated

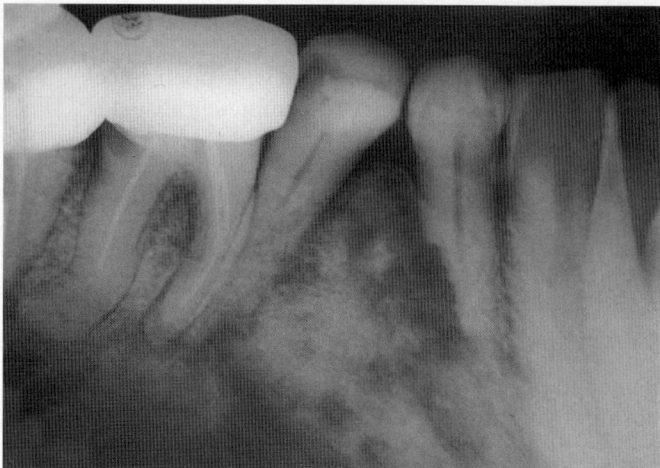

Figure 20.23 Hyperthyroidism: A change in the normal trabecular pattern gives a ground glass appearance of numerous, small, randomly oriented trabeculae

with diffuse toxic goiter (*Grave's disease*), or alternately, a toxic adenoma or benign tumor of the thyroid gland. Increase in thyroxin production, increases the metabolic activity of the tissues, and there is an increased basal metabolic rate. In patients with thyrotoxicosis, dental treatment can precipitate an acute emergency like thyroid crisis or thyroid storm.

Clinical Features

- It is more common in women, between the ages of 20–40 years
- There may be a symmetrical, diffuse nodular or smooth enlargement of the thyroid. It may be tender and a thrill may be present
- Abdomen, liver and spleen may be enlarged
- The patient may have weight loss in spite of normal appetite, diarrhea, bowel alterations, vomiting, anorexia and hyperdefecation
- Patients may have amenorrhea, oligomenorrhea, infertility, spontaneous abortion and libido impotence
- Due to increased metabolic rate, the patient develops tachycardia, increased blood pressure, sensitivity to heat and increased irritability
- Patient develops exophthalmus, partial paralysis of the ocular muscles, corneal ulcerations, optic neuritis, ocular muscle weakness, papilledema, loss of visual acuity
- There may be increased sweating, pruritus, digital clubbing, early fatigue, lymphadenopathy, thirst and osteoporosis
- The patient is usually highly emotional and has a facial expression of constant surprise
- Patient is sensitive to epinephrine
- There is increase in serum bound iodine concentration. Urinary iodine concentration is decreased due to increased iodine uptake by the thyroid gland.

- Plasma levels of T3 and T4 are increased, free thyroxin index is raised, thyroid-stimulating hormone (TSH) is decreased
- Hypochromic type of anemia may be present.

Radiographic Features

- There may be generalized osteoporosis
- There may be generalized decreased bone density or loss of some areas of edentulous alveolar bone. In some cases there may be greater density of the trabeculae
- There is advanced rate of dental development with early eruption and premature loss of primary teeth.

Differential Diagnosis

- Hyperparathyroidism
- Osteoporosis.

Management

Patient may be given antithyroid drugs, radioactive iodine or β-adrenoreceptor antagonist drugs, or a subtotal thyroidectomy may be advised.

Hypothyroidism (Figs 20.24A to C)

Definition

This result due to insufficient secretion of thyroxin by the thyroid gland, may be due to thyroiditis, insufficient thyroid replacement, post-thyroidectomy, postradioactive iodine therapy. When it occurs in infancy it is called cretinism, in childhood, it is called Juvenile myxedema, and in adults it is known as myxedema, and is associated with subcutaneous deposition of hydrophilic mucopolysaccharides.

Clinical Features

Cretinism and Juvenile Myxedema

- It may be present at birth or become evident within the first few months after birth
- It is characterized by mental retardation, generalized edema and retarded somatic growth. The hair is sparse and brittle, nails are brittle and sweat glands are atrophic
- There is delayed fusion of all the bony epiphysis
- The base of the skull shows delayed ossification and there is partial pneumatization of the paranasal sinuses
- As the base of the skull is shortened, there is retraction of the bridge of the nose with flaring
- The face appears wide and fails to develop in the horizontal direction. The mandible is underdeveloped and maxilla overdeveloped
- Retarded condylar growth leads to characteristic micrognathia and an open bite
- The lips are puffy, thickened and protruding.

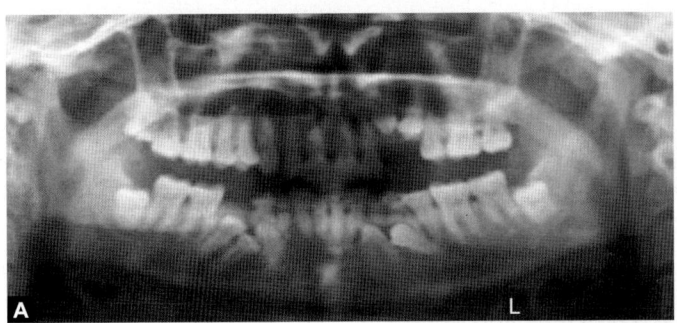
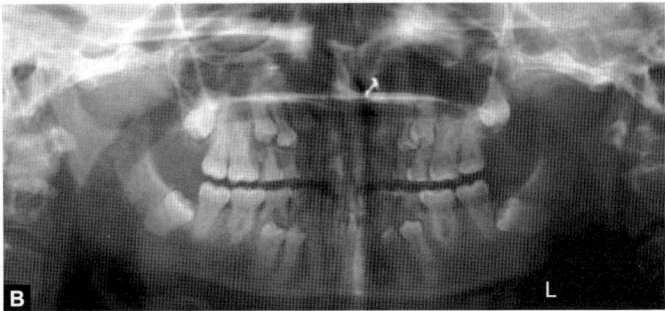
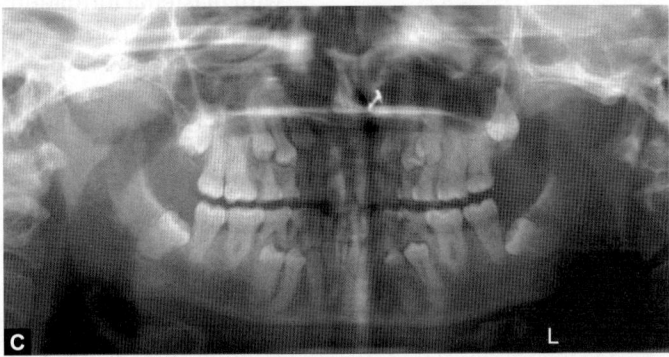

Figures 20.24A to C Hypothyroidism: (A and B) Panoramic radiographs showing multiple unerupted, over-retained and impacted teeth. Panoramic radiograph revealed erupted 11 12 16 17 21 22 26 27 36 37 46 47; (C) Hypothyroidism; radiographical panoramic radiograph revealed erupted 11 12 16 17 21 22 26 27 36 37 46 47, over-retained 51 53 54 55 63 64 65 71 72 73 74 75 81 82 83 84 85, impacted 13 14 15 18 23 24 25 28 31 32 33 34 35 38 41 42 43 44 45 48, periodontal ligament space not evident in relation to impacted 31 32 33 34 35 41 42 43 44 45, trabecular pattern, architecture and density was normal

- In juvenile myxedema, the tongue is enlarged due to fluid retention and may protrude leading to malocclusion
- Eruption of teeth is delayed and deciduous teeth are over retained
- There may be enamel hypoplasia and abnormal dentin formation with enlarged pulp chambers
- Dental caries is more prevalent in these patients.

Myxedema

- This occurs due to atrophy of the thyroid gland and results in a lowered basal metabolic rate, lethargy, poor memory, inability to concentrate, constipation, cold intolerance and a dull and expressionless face
- The soft tissues of the face and mouth, especially the lips, nose, eyelids and suborbital tissues become edematous and swollen
- The tongue is swollen and enlarged, which may cause separation of teeth and affect the patient's speech
- The patient usually presents with periodontal disease, with alveolar destruction and loosening of teeth. External root resorption in a common finding

- The laboratory findings in hyperthyroidism are increased thyroid stimulating hormone (TSH) and decreased T3 and T4. There may be raised cholesterol and triglyceride levels and low serum sodium. The ECG may show a classical sinus bradycardia with low voltage complexes and ST/T wave abnormalities.

In dentistry the use of sedatives and analgesics are dangerous, as they precipitate coma in these patients.

Radiographic Features

Cretinism and Juvenile Myxedema

- Delayed closing of epiphyses and skull sutures with production of numerous wormian bones (accessory bones in the sutures)
- There is delayed eruption, short roots and thinning of the lamina dura
- The alveolar processes are relatively large as compared to the body of the bone which is smaller than in normal individuals
- The maxilla and the mandible are relatively small.

Myxedema

- Presence of periodontal disease, with alveolar destruction
- Loss of lamina dura and external root resorption.

Differential Diagnosis

Clinical signs and symptoms and radiographic features along with laboratory tests with show reduction in serum T3 and T4 levels are confirmatory.

Management

Patients are given thyroid preparations like levothyroxine.

Hyperparathyroidism

Definition

This is a condition where excess parathyroid hormone is secreted, leading increase to in bone remodeling activity, in preference of osteoclastic resorption, which mobilizes calcium from the skeleton and also increases renal tubular reabsorption of calcium and renal production of active vitamin D metabolite [1,25(OH)$_2$D]. The net result is an increase in serum calcium levels.

Types

Primary Hyperparathyroidism

This is caused by autonomous secretion of the parathyroid hormone (PTH) due to hyperplasia, or benign (adenoma) of one or more of the four parathyroid glands. The incidence is 1%, and the combination of elevated serum levels of PTH and hypercalcemia is diagnostic of primary hyperparathyroidism.

Secondary Hyperparathyroidism

This results from a compensatory increase in the output of PTH in response to hypocalcemia. The underlying hypocalcemia may result from an inadequate dietary intake or poor absorption of vitamin D or from deficient metabolism of vitamin D in the liver or kidneys. The condition produces clinical and radiographic effects similar to those of primary hyperthyroidism.

Tertiary Hyperparathyroidism

Occasionally, the parathyroid tumor after long standing secondary hyperparathyroidism may develop a condition called tertiary hyperparathyroidism. The increased parathyroid levels produce increased bone resorption and a resultant hypercalcemia.

Ectopic Hyperparathyroidism

This is caused due to excessive parathyroid hormone synthesis in a patient with malignant disease.

Clinical Features

- It is more common in females, between the ages of 30–69 years
- The clinical symptoms are more related to hypercalcemia; the patients are prone to renal calculi, peptic ulcers, psychiatric problems, or bone and joint pains
- Bone deformities may occur, such as bending of long bones, occasional pathological fractures, collapse of vertebrae and formation of pigeon chest
- Loosening and drifting of teeth, leading to malocclusion with diastema formation
- In primary hyperparathyroidism the serum calcium level is increased and serum phosphorus levels decreased. The serum alkaline phosphatase level is increased. (Rarely, multiple myeloma and metastatic tumors may produce the same serum alterations)
- In secondary hyperparathyroidism the serum calcium level is decreased whereas the serum phosphorus and alkaline phosphatase levels are increased.

Radiographic Features

- Radiographically observable changes may be seen in 1 out of 5 patients with hyperparathyroidism.
- The earliest changes are subtle erosions of the bone from the subperiosteal surfaces of the phalanges of the hands.
- Overall demineralization of the skeleton, resulting in overall grayness and lack of normal contrast on the radiograph.
- There may be generalized osteoporosis, with abortive attempts at repair and new bone formation, this new bone is again resorbed, eventually leading to pseudocyst formation.
- In prominent hyperparathyroidism, the entire calvarium has a *granular appearance* of the bone, caused by loss of central (diploic) trabeculae and thinning of the cortical tables.
- *Osteitis fibrosa cystica* or *Osteitis fibrosa generalisata* are localized regions of bone loss produced by osteoclastic activity, resulting in a loss of all apparent bone structure. These appear cyst like on the radiograph.
- *Browns tumors* occur late in the disease (in about 10% of the cases). These peripheral or central tumors of bone are radiolucent. The gross specimen has a brown or reddish color.
- *Pathological calcifications* in soft tissues have punctate or nodular appearance and occur in the kidneys and joints.
- The density of the jaws is decreased, resulting in a radiolucent appearance and the teeth stand out in contrast. Demineralization and thinning of the cortical boundaries may occur, such as cortical borders of the inferior alveolar canal and that of the maxillary sinuses. A change in the normal trabecular pattern gives a *ground glass appearance* of numerous, small, randomly oriented trabeculae.

- Browns tumor is common in the facial bones and jaw bones, particularly in long standing cases. The lesions may be multiple within a single bone. They have variably defined margins and cause cortical expansion. If solitary the tumor resembles a central cell granuloma or an aneurysmal bone cyst.
- Following treatment the radiographic picture returns to normal, sometimes the healed browns tumor has a more sclerotic appearance.
- Periapical radiographs reveal loss of lamina dura (in 10% of the cases). Depending on the severity and duration of the disease loss of lamina dura complete or partial, may occur around one tooth or be generalized. The tooth root may have a tapered appearance due to the lamina loss causing decreased image contrast.
- Although PTH mobilizes minerals from the skeleton, mature teeth are immune to this systemic demineralization process.

Differential Diagnosis

Unilocular

- *Postextraction socket*: History of extraction.
- *Primordial bone cyst, traumatic bone cyst, odontogenic cyst*: Usually occur in younger individuals and the serum chemistry is normal.

Multilocular

- *Paget's disease*: Calcium metabolism is normal and bone formation exceeds the bone resorption resulting in an elevated blood alkaline phosphatase level.
- *Ameloblastoma*: It usually shows a honey comb appearance accompanied with paresthesia and normal serum chemistry.
- *Central giant cell granuloma*: The histological appearance is identical as that of Browns tumor, if it is seen in the second decade, the patient should be screened for an increase in serum calcium, PTH and alkaline phosphatase.
- *Cherubism*: These lesions are bilateral, and seen in children where there is a familial involvement.
- *Aneurysmal bone cyst, central hemangioma*: These occur in the younger age group.
- *Osteomalacia*: Here the blood calcium levels are decreased.
- *Fibrous dysplasia*: The osseous changes are usually localized and loss of lamina dura is less common.
- *Multiple myeloma*: The lesions are punched out, and in hyperparathyroidism there is generalized bone demineralization, which helps in distinguishing.

Management

After successful surgical removal of the causative factor, almost all radiographic changes revert to normal, except for Browns tumor which heals with bone that is radiographically more sclerotic than normal.

Hypoparathyroidism and Pseudohypoparathyroidism

Definition

This is an uncommon condition in which insufficient secretion of PTH occurs. The most common cause is surgical damage to the glands or their vascular supply during the thyroid gland procedures, (parathyroid damage from radioactive iodine-131 treatment for hyperthyroidism), autoimmune destruction of the parathyroid glands and developmental familial hypoparathyroidism.

Pseudohypoparathyroidism is a condition in which there is a defect in the response of the tissue target cells to normal levels of parathyroid hormone.

Clinical Features

- Both hypoparathyroidism and pseudohypoparathyroidism produce hypocalcemia which has a variety of clinical manifestations like:
  - Sharp flexion (tetany) of the wrist and ankle joints (carpopedal spasm: which can be induced by occluding the blood flow to the forearm for 3 minutes with the sphygmomanometer cuff applied to the arm and raising the pressure above systolic level. This is called *Trousseau's sign*).
  - Some patients have sensory abnormalities consisting of paresthesia of the hands, feet, or area around the mouth.
  - Neurological changes may include anxiety, depression, epilepsy, Parkinsonism and chorea.
  - Chronic forms may produce reduction in intellectual capacity, due to calcifications in the brain.
  - Some patients show no change at all.
- Patients with pseudohypoparathyroidism have early closure of certain bony epiphyses and thus manifest short stature or extremity disproportions, like short fingers due to shortening of the metacarpal bones and rounding of the face
- When hypoparathyroidism occurs in children, it may cause dental defects like, enamel hypoplasia, delayed eruption, external root resorption, root dilacerations, abnormal calcifications and large pulp chambers.
- There may be ectopic calcifications in subcutaneous tissues, pitted and brittle bones and thickening of the skull bones may be seen.
- *Positive Chvostek's sign*: A sharp tap over the facial nerve in front of the ear causes twitching of the facial muscle around the mouth.
- Chronic candidiasis is usually present.
- The serum calcium level is decreased (below 7 mg/dL), serum phosphate level is correspondingly increased. Urinary calcium may be low or absent.

Radiographic Features

- Calcification of the basal ganglia, which appears flocculent and paired within the cerebral hemisphere on the posteroanterior skull radiograph
- Radiographic examination of the jaws reveal enamel hypoplasia, external root resorption, root dilacerations, abnormal calcifications and large pulp chambers, there may be blunting of the molar roots.

Management

This condition may be controlled with oral administration of calcium and vitamin D.

Diabetes Mellitus

Definition

This is a metabolic disorder which causes inappropriate hypoglycemia due to tissue resistance to insulin action, reduced insulin secretion or both. A shortage of insulin adversely affects the carbohydrate metabolism, which causes a complex biochemical imbalance between the tissue demand for glucose and the release of this nutrient by the liver. The different forms are:

Primary

- *Type I*: Insulin dependent (IDDM), juvenile-onset diabetes which results from an absence or insufficiency of insulin, a hormone normally produced by the beta cells of the islets of Langerhans in the pancreas.
- *Type II*: Noninsulin dependent (NIDDM), this results from insulin resistance, the patients normally have half the number of beta cells, and is believed to be an autoimmune response in association with a virus. It is further divided in to:
  - Nonobese
  - Obese
  - Maturity onset diabetes of the young (MODY).

Secondary

- Pancreatic disease (pancreatitis, hemochromatosis, neoplastic disease, pancreatectomy, cystic fibrosis)
- Endocrine disease—excess endogenous production of hormonal antagonists to insulin, e.g. growth hormone in acromegaly
- Drug-induced like corticosteroid, thiazide diuretics and phenytoin
- Genetic syndromes like Down's syndrome, Klinefelter's syndrome and Turner's syndrome
- Impaired glucose tolerance
- Gestational diabetes.

Clinical Features

- The patient usually complains of weight loss and fatigue, with hyperglycemia and glycosuria
- There is presence of the classical symptoms of the 3P's polydipsia (excessive thirst), polyuria (excessive urination), polyphagia (excessive hunger)
- Presence of acetone breath and presence of acetone in the urine
- Visual impairment and color blindness
- Marked diabetic neuropathy, the trigeminal nerve may be involved
- There is a marked lowering of the body's resistance to infection, which demonstrates a number of adverse effects in the oral cavity
- The patient also complains of xerostomia, due to reduced salivary flow
- Both the above-mentioned symptoms and signs may be the aggravating factor for the presence of persistent gingivitis, periodontitis, dry burning tongue, increased caries activity (especially in children) and attrition of teeth
- The gingival appears spongy, purplish and bleeds, persistent gingivitis leads to resorption of the alveolar bone with periodontal pocket and abscess formation and eventual loss of teeth
- As such diabetes does not cause periodontal disease directly, but it alters the response of the periodontal lesion to local irritants, hastening bone loss and retarding postsurgical healing of periodontal lesions
- Vascular changes in the dental pulp, gingiva and periodontal ligament have been reported
- These patients are more prone to develop localized osteitis and dry socket due to delayed healing (decreased polymorphonuclear chemotaxis) and impaired immunological balance
- Oral candidiasis is commonly seen in these patients, with angular cheilitis, altered taste sensation, lichen planus and diffuse enlargement of the parotid gland
- Diabetes is considered to be one of the factors for median rhomboid glossitis
- Elevation in plasma glucose concentration levels.

Radiographic Features

- There are no characteristic distinct changes seen in the jaws or teeth
- A slight discontinuity or blurring of the cortex of alveolar crest to wide destruction of the lamina dura and intradental bone may be seen in uncontrolled diabetes
- There may be presence of horizontal and vertical bone loss.

Differential Diagnosis

- Periodontal disease associated with diabetes is indistinguishable from periodontal disease in patients without diabetes.

- *Diabetes insipidus*: This occurs due to insufficiency of the posterior pituitary hormone, there is decreased vasopressin production due to damage to the neurohypophyseal mechanism, or presence of tumors (craniopharyngioma), syphilis or basal meningitis.

Management

Diet control, with oral hypoglycemic drugs (sulfonylurea, biguanides, alfa-glucoside inhibitors) or insulin.

During any dental treatment care should be taken to give an adequate antibiotic cover and postpone any dental procedures except emergencies till the blood glucose level is stabilized. Use atraumatic procedures and short duration appointments. Use local anesthetics without epinephrine.

Addison's Disease (Chronic Adrenal Insufficiency of the Adrenal Cortex)

Definition

The deficiency may be caused due to autoimmune causes, drugs, bilateral destruction of the suprarenal glands. It may be associated with tuberculosis, metastatic carcinoma, intradermal hemorrhage, amyloidosis, hemochromatosis, adrenal infarction and congenital adrenal hypoplasia.

Clinical Features

- It is more common in males in the 3rd and 4th decades
- It is characterized by the bronzing of the skin, pigmentation of the mucous membrane, feeble heart action (low blood pressure), general debility, vomiting, diarrhea and severe anemia
- Decrease in cortisol levels interferes with the manufacture of carbohydrates from proteins, causing hypoglycemia and diminished glycogen storage in the liver
- The neuromuscular junction is inhibited, producing muscle weakness
- There is resistance to infection, trauma and stress
- Pale brown to deep chocolate pigmentation of the oral mucosa spreading over the buccal mucosa from the angle of the mouth and/or developing on the gingiva, tongue and lips, may be the first sign of the disease
- Histopathology shows acanthosis with silver positive granules in the cells of the stratum germinativum
- There is normocytic anemia, elevated level of blood urea nitrogen and potassium and low blood concentrations of sodium and chloride.

Radiographic Features

No radiographic changes seen.

Management

Supplementation of corticosteroids.

Cushing's Syndrome

Definition

This arises due to excess of secretion of glucocorticoids by the adrenal glands, due to any of the following reasons adrenal adenoma, adrenal carcinoma, adrenal hyperplasia (usually bilateral), basophilic adenoma of the anterior lobe of the pituitary gland (Cushing's disease) which produces excess of adrenocorticotrophic hormone (ACTH), medical therapy with exogenous corticosteroids, which causes catabolism of the proteins.

The increased level of glucocorticoid results in a loss of bone mass due to reduced osteoblastic function and either direct or indirect osteoclastic activity.

Clinical Features

- Females in the 3rd and 4th decades are more commonly affected
- Obesity, which is rapidly acquired around the upper portion of the body and rounded moon face. The extremities are spared
- The patient may complain of weakness, weight loss, hypertension, muscular weakness, menstrual irregularities, backaches, hirsutism, alterations in hair distribution, dusky plethoric appearances with formation of purple striae on the abdomen and/or overt diabetes
- There may be kyphosis of the thoracic spine. (Buffalo hump: Deposition of excess fat in lower midcervical and upper thoracic area of the back)
- In children growth and development, including skeletal and dental may be retarded
- Cases of children with cleft palate, born to mothers on steroid therapy in the first three months of pregnancy have been reported.

Radiographic Features

- *Generalized osteoporosis*: The vertebrae, ribs, long bones are most commonly affected.
- Osseous demineralization with pathological fractures superimposed, are common.
- The skull shows diffuse thinning and has a mottled appearance.
- The jaw shows loss of lamina dura in some areas.

Management

It may be treated with combination of surgery and radiotherapy. Sometimes drugs (metyrapone, aminoglute-thimide) may be prescribed.

Hypergonadism

Clinical Features

- When it occurs in children it causes precocious puberty. The long bones develop quickly and the child may initially turn towards tallness, but this is offset by the early fusion of the epiphyses so that the adult person is short
- The teeth may erupt early, compared with the normal, but the eruption is in harmony with the skeletal age.

Hypogonadism

Clinical Features

- It occurs with equal frequency in males and females
- The long bones are slender and the epiphyses fuse late
- The supraciliary ridges, malar bone and the mandible all show greater development
- The chin is pointed, high arched palate with irregularities of the teeth is a common finding
- The mandible tends to become enlarged and sometimes even massive, with short rami in case of male hypogonadism.

Radiographic Features

The skull is small and there is marked enlargement of the frontal and sphenoid sinuses, especially the mastoid air sinuses.

Pregnancy

The alteration in the circulating female sex hormones (estrogens and progesterone) modifies the response of the periodontium, producing pregnancy gingivitis and diffuse gingival enlargement. Pregnancy tumors are exuberant growth of granulation tissue that develops in the interdental papillary region.

Before the menstrual cycle and if the patient is taking oral contraceptive drugs the same hormone produces gingival enlargement, bleeding, pulpal hyperemia (due to capillary dilatation) and mucosal ulcerations.

Menopause

This begins when the menstrual function ceases, between 40 to 55 years of age, and there is a deficiency of estrogen. The patient will complain of irritability, insomnia, nervousness, osteoporosis, backache and joint pain. She may also complain of burning mouth and tongue, taste abnormalities and dryness of the mucosa.

The patient presents with desquamative gingivitis with atrophy and ulceration of the gingival tissue and bleeding.

In all the three conditions no radiographic changes are seen.

METABOLIC BONE DISEASES DUE TO NUTRITIONAL DEFICIENCY (TABLE 20.3)

Nutrition is a multidisciplinary integrated life science which deals with growth and development, reproduction and maintenance of life by the provision of energy building tissues and preservation of a relatively constant environment. Nutritional science has attained great importance in the last few decades. The diet of the individual is of extreme importance in maintaining health and preventing disease.

Nutritional deficiencies may be broadly divided into:
- *Primary nutritional deficiencies*: Caused due to inadequate intake.
- *Secondary nutritional deficiencies*: Caused due to a number of predisposing factors and conditions, such as:
  - Increased metabolic rate
  - Malabsorption
  - Functional or organic GI tract disorders
  - Increased excretion of essential factors.

Metabolism may be defined as the sum total of tissue activity as considered in terms of physiochemical changes associated with and regulated by availability, utilization and disposal of proteins, carbohydrates, fats, vitamins, minerals, and water with the influence that the endocrinal system exerts on these processes. Alteration from this normal metabolic process constitutes the disturbances of metabolism.

The severity of clinical and oral symptoms depends upon the intensity and duration of nutritional deficiency. An alert dentist may detect the early changes before they become irreversible.

Langerhan's Cell Histiocytosis (Histiocytosis X, Idiopathic Histiocytosis, Langerhan's Cell Disease)

Definition

The disorders included in the category of Langerhan's cell histiocytosis (LCH) are abnormalities that result from the abnormal proliferation of Langerhan's cells or their precursors. These cells are specialized cells of the histiocytic cell line that are normally found in the skin. The abnormal proliferation of Langerhan's cells and eosinophils results in a spectrum of clinical diseases.

Historically, it was believed to be a disturbance in the lipid metabolism and histiocytosis-X was classified into three distinct clinical forms:
1. Eosinophilic granuloma (solitary)
2. Hand-Schüller-Christian disease (chronic disseminated)
3. Letterer-Siwe disease (acute disseminated).

A newly proposed LCH classification creates two categories:
1. Nonmalignant disorders such as unifocal or multifocal eosinophilic granuloma
2. Malignant disorders, including Letterer-Siwe disease and its variants of histiocytic lymphoma.

Recent research has shown that all forms of LCH are clonal and thus may represent a form of malignancy.

Table 20.3 Classification of nutritional disturbances

- Disturbances in carbohydrate metabolism
  - Hurler's syndrome
  - Lipoid proteinosis
  - Hereditary fructose intolerance
  - Hypoglycemia
- Disturbances in protein metabolism
  - Protein deficiency (marasmus, kwashiorkor disease)
  - Amyloidosis
    - Type A (secondary)
    - Type B (primary)
    - Type C
  - Porphyria
    - Erythropoietic porphyria
      - i. Uroporphyria
      - ii. Protoporphyria
    - Hepatic porphyria
      - i. Acute intermittent porphyria
      - ii. Porphyria variegate
      - iii. Porphyria cutaneous tarda
      - iv. Hereditary coproporphyria
- Disturbances in lipid metabolism
  - Nonlipid reticuloendotheliosis
    - Hand-Schüller-Christian disease
    - Letterer-Siwe disease (acute disseminated histiocytosis X)
    - Eosinophilic granuloma (chronic disseminated histiocytosis X)
  - Lipid reticuloendotheliosis
    - Gaucher's disease
    - Niemann-Pick disease (sphingomyelin lipidosis)
- Disturbances in vitamin metabolism
  - Water-soluble vitamins
    - Vitamin B complex
      - i. Vitamin B_1 (thiamine), beriberi, Wernicke's encephalopathy Korsakoff's psychosis
      - ii. Vitamin B_2 (riboflavin)
      - iii. Vitamin B_3 (niacin), pellagra
      - iv. Vitamin B_5 (pantothenic acid)
      - v. Vitamin B_6 (pyridoxine)
      - vi. Vitamin B_8 (biotin)
      - vii. Vitamin B_9 (folic acid), macrocytic anemia
      - viii. Vitamin B_{12} (cyanocobalamin), pernicious anemia
    - Vitamin C (ascorbic acid), scurvy
    - Choline
    - Inositol
  - Fat-soluble vitamins
    - Vitamin A (Retinol), vitamin A deficiency, hypervitaminosis A carotenemia
    - Vitamin D, rickets, osteomalacia, vitamin D resistant rickets
    - Vitamin E (Tocopherol)
    - Vitamin K (phylloquinone)

Contd...

Contd...

- Disturbances in mineral metabolism
  - Zinc
    - Acrodermatitis enteropathica (zinc deficiency syndrome)
  - Calcium
  - Phosphorus, hypophosphatasia, pseudohypophosphatasia
  - Magnesium
  - Sodium
  - Potassium, hyperkalemia
  - Iron, iron deficiency anemia, Plummer Vinson syndrome
  - Fluorides
  - Iodine
- Water
- Others
  - Malabsorption syndrome, (Sprue, idiopathic steatorrhea, celiac disease)

Clinical Features

The early lesions are usually seen in the head and neck region, and approximately 10% of all patients with LCH have oral lesions, which many a times may be the first clinical signs of the disease.

Eosinophilic Granuloma

- This is more common in males, older children and young adults are more affected
- It usually involves the skeleton (ribs, pelvis, long bones, skull and jaws) and in rare cases it involves soft tissue (such as lymph nodes, skin, lungs, gingiva and palate)
- The lesions develop quickly and may be painful. It is usually destructive, well-demarcated, roughly round or oval in shape. The destroyed area is replaced by soft tissue (soft and brown) which eventually becomes fibrous and grayish
- In the jaws there is evidence of bony swelling, loosening and sloughing of teeth due to destruction of the alveolar bone by one or more foci of EG
- There may be superficial loss of alveolar bone, often mimicking juvenile periodontitis
- The patient may have a soft tissue mass, gingivitis, bleeding gingiva, pain and ulceration
- The sockets of teeth lost to the disease generally do not heal normally
- EG may have a single focus or may develop into a multifocal, aggressive, disseminated form which involves multiple bones, diabetes insipidus and exophthalmus, a condition previously defined as Hand-Schüller-Christian disease (multifocal eosinophilic granuloma, chronic disseminated histiocytosis X, xanthomatosis).

Hand-Schüller-Christian Disease

- This usually begins in childhood, but sometimes may not develop until the third decade. Males are more commonly affected
- The patient may have otitis media and papular or nodular lesions on the skin
- The facial bone is commonly affected with associated soft tissue swelling, tenderness and facial asymmetry
- The patient shows a triad of single or multiple areas of punched out bone destruction in the skull, unilateral or bilateral exophthalmus and diabetes insipidus
- Oral manifestations include sore mouth with or without ulcerative lesions, halitosis, gingivitis, loose or sore teeth, failure of extraction socket to heal, loss of alveolar bone
- Many cases end fatally.

Letterer-Siwe Disease

- This is a malignant form of LCH, which is a fulminating condition, often occurs in infants below 3 years of age
- The initial onset is manifested as skin rash involving the trunk, scalp and extremities. The rash may be erythematous, purpuric and ecchymotic sometimes it may be ulcerative
- Soft tissue and bony granulomatous lesions are disseminated throughout the body, and the condition is marked by intermittent fever with splenohepatomegaly, lymphadenopathy, anemia, hemorrhage and failure to thrive
- The oral cavity is affected with multiple ulcers and enlargement of the gingival tissues. There is diffuse destruction of the maxilla and mandible leading to loosening and premature loss of teeth
- Death usually follows, and sometimes so quickly that no manifestations are seen.

Radiographic Features

Eosinophilic Granuloma

- The mandible is a more common site than the maxilla, and the posterior regions are more involved than the anterior regions. The mandibular ramus is a more common site of intraosseous lesions
- The lesions may be solitary or multiple. The solitary lesions may be accompanied by lesions in other bones
- The lesions are circular or elliptical, well-defined radiolucency with discrete borders that are rarely hyperostotic. They have a *punched out appearance*
- The alveolar lesions commonly start in the mid root region of the teeth, the bone destruction progresses in a circular shape, and after it includes a portion of the superior border of the alveolar process, it may give the impression that a section of the alveolar process has been *scooped out*.

- The alveolar bone around the teeth, including the lamina dura is destroyed, giving a *floating teeth appearance*
- Displacement of erupted teeth and follicle are common. Only minor root resorption has been reported
- In some cases there may be complete loss of continuity of the mandible, so that there may be a pathological fracture
- The lesions have an ability to stimulate new bone formation, this occurs commonly with the intraosseous type of lesions. The new periosteal bone formation is indistinguishable from the appearance seen in inflammatory jaw lesions.

Additional Imaging

- CT examination may disclose how the lesion can destroy the outer cortical plate and in rare cases extend into the surrounding soft tissues
- Nuclear imaging—to detect other possible bone lesions.

Differential Diagnosis

- *Oral carcinoma*: Found in the older age group, the borders are more irregular.
- *Periodontal disease*: The epicenter of bone destruction in LCH is approximately at the mid-root region, resulting in a scooped out appearance. In contrast, the bone destruction in periodontal disease starts at the alveolar crest and extends apically down the root surface and it usually has condensing osteitis around the lesion.
- *Primordial cyst, dentigerous cyst*: These are more round with cortication.
- *Benign giant cell tumor*: These contain more bone within the cavity and cause expansion of bone.
- *Traumatic bone cyst*: They have a more well-defined border.
- *Fibrous dysplasia*: These lesions have a clearly marked, corticated border.
- *Apical infection*: It is associated with an infected tooth and dead pulp.
- *Cherubism*: The lesions are bilateral and limited to the jaws.
- *Metastatic carcinoma*: The incidence is less in children, there will be history of the primary lesion.
- *Leukemia*: The jaw bone lesions of LCH are more common at the crest of the alveolar ridge, by contrast those of leukemia originate in the deeper medullary portion.
- *Multiple myeloma*: This has to be differentiated by laboratory tests. In multiple myeloma the ratio of albumin to globulin is reversed and Bence-Jones proteins are present in the urine.

Management

Surgical curettage or limited radiation therapy. Disseminated disease is usually treated with chemotherapy.

Gaucher's Disease

Definition

This is a familial derangement of lipid metabolism. Death usually occurs before 3 years of age. There are three types:
1. *Type I (Chronic non-neuronopathic)*: There is no cerebral involvement.
2. *Type II (Infantile neuropathic acute neuropathic)*: This is characterized by hepatosplenomegaly and central nervous system disorders.
3. *Type III (Subacute neuronopathic)*: This resembles type II but has a later onset and a more protracted clinical course.

Clinical Features

- There may be bone pain due to involvement of the bone marrow
- The skin may be pigmented and the conjunctival fibrous tissue may be thickened and has a brownish discoloration, called Pinguela
- Bleeding from the nose and gums
- The bone changes occur due to destructive infiltration of the cerebrosidic reticulosis of the bone marrow. As a result of the proliferation of the Gaucher's cells the bone undergoes rarefaction.

Radiographic Features

- There is generalized porosity of the mandible and maxilla, with loss of trabeculae structure and thinning of the mandibular cortex
- Large areas of rarefactions have a cyst like appearance especially in the molar premolar region (mental region) of the mandible and premolar region of the maxilla
- The large bones of the body have pseudocystic radiolucent areas which have a *worm eaten appearance.*

Management

The prognosis of infantile form is very poor. The less virulent form can be treated with purified glucocerebrosidase which decreases hepatic accumulation of glucocerebroside. Enzyme replacement therapy with recombinant enzymes is also available.

Hurler's Syndrome

Definition

This is caused by deficiency of mucopolysaccharides and is usually apparent in the first two years of life. The disease usually terminates in death as the patient attains puberty.

Clinical Features

- The head is large with a prominent forehead, broad saddle nose and wide nostrils. The patient has hypertelorism, puffy eyelids with coarse bushy eyebrows, thick lips, large tongue, open mouth, nasal congestion with noisy breathing
- There is hepatosplenomegaly, resulting in the protuberance of the abdomen
- The patient has a typical short neck, spinal abnormalities with typical flexion contractures which result in a *claw hand*
- The patient is usually mentally challenged
- There is shortening and broadening of the mandible with prominent gonions and wide intergonial distance
- The teeth are small, with a changed morphology and with typical spacing between them
- Gingival hyperplasia may occur due to poor oral hygiene.

Radiographic Features

Localized areas of bone destruction in the jaws are found, which may represent hyperplastic dental follicles.

Differential Diagnosis

Dentigerous cyst.

Management

There is no treatment for the disease.

Calcium Metabolism Disorders (Table 20.4)

Definition

The 99% of the body calcium is present in bones and teeth, the remaining 1% is found in soft tissue and fluids. Daily recommended dose of calcium intake is 360 mg for new born and infants and 800 mg for children and adults.

Deficiency may lead to internal hemorrhage due to derangement of blood coagulation and the integrity of the capillaries, tetany, and pathologic calcification.

Deficiency of calcium during the formative period leads to enamel hypoplasia and large amounts of interglobular dentine.

Alveolar bone is very sensitive to calcium deficiency and becomes hemorrhagic and filled with calcified fibro-osteoid tissue.

Teeth become loose: There is generalized loss of lamina dura.

Hypophosphatasia

Definition

This is a rare inherited disorder that is caused by either a reduced production or a defective function of alkaline phosphatase. This enzyme is required for normal mineralization of osteoid, its deficiency results in formation of defective bone matrix. These patients have a low level of

Table 20.4 Disorders of calcium metabolism

- Disturbances in calcium homeostasis with resultant effect upon bone mineralization
  - Dietary deficient calcium
  - Vitamin D deficiency
    - Rickets
    - Osteomalacia
  - Vitamin D excess
  - Abnormal vitamin D metabolism due to liver and renal tubular disease
  - Hyperparathyroidism
  - Hypoparathyroidism
  - Uremia
- Osteoporosis
  - Steroid hormones
  - Pituitary hormone
  - Thyroid hormone
  - Senile osteoporosis
- Disease causing bone destruction
  - Carcinomatosis
  - Myelomatosis
- Disorders of unknown etiology
  - Paget's disease of the bone
- Acidosis
- Hypercalcemia

serum alkaline phosphatase activity and elevated urinary excretion of phosphoethanolamine.

There are three types:

1. Infantile type (begins *in utero*, severe hypocalcemia, poor survival)
2. Juvenile type (after 6 months of age, increased infection, growth retardation, costochondral junction enlargement (rohitic rosary), pulmonary, gastrointestinal and renal disorders.
3. Adult type (which is mild, prior history of rickets and osseous radiolucency).

Clinical Features

- In individuals with homozygous involvement, it begins *in utero*, and the patient usually dies within the first year. These infants demonstrate bowed legs and a marked deficiency of skull ossification
- Individuals with heterozygous disease show the biochemical defects but a milder disease clinically. They show poor growth, delayed walking, fractures and deformities similar to rickets. The skull suture close early resulting in bulging sutures and gyral marking on the internal surface of the skull. The skull has a brachycephalic shape
- Often the first clinical sign of hypophosphatasia may be premature loss of primary teeth, particularly incisors and delayed eruption of the permanent dentition
- There may be inflammation of the gingiva.

Radiographic Features

- The long bones show irregular defects in the epiphysis, with spotty, streaky or irregular ossification
- The skull is poorly calcified. In older children with premature closure of the sutures, multiple radiolucent areas of the calvarium may exist, called *gyral* or *convolutional* markings. These resemble a *beaten copper appearance*
- There is a generalized reduction in bone density in adults
- There is a generalized radiolucency of the mandible and the maxilla. The cortical bone and the lamina dura are thinned. The alveolar bone is poorly calcified and may appear deficient
- There is almost total absence of cementum and normally attached periodontal fibers
- Teeth are hypoplastic. The pulp chamber and root canals are larger than normal
- The roots may fail to develop fully or undergo early resorption of the apices.

Management

Vitamin D in high doses has resulted in partial improvement in some cases, but it may lead to deposition of calcium in many tissues. Administration of high oral dose of phosphate results in moderate improvement in bone calcification as judged radiographically.

Pseudohypophosphatasia

This disease resembles hypophosphatasia, but has normal serum alkaline phosphatase levels. There is osteopathy of the long bones and skull. There is premature loss of deciduous teeth.

Vitamin A Deficiency

Definition

Carotene is a yellow pigment found in vegetable foods which is converted into vitamin A in the body. Vitamin A or retinol is also found in foods of animal origin. The daily requirement of vitamin A is 420 mg to 800–1000 mg.

Clinical Features

- Causes failure of growth in the young and collagenous tissue is affected
- Keratinizing metaplasia of the epithelial cells
- Deficiency causes night blindness, dry conjunctiva, Bitot's spot, corneal xerosis, corneal ulcerations or keratomalacia. There may be xerophthalmia due to decrease in lacrimal secretion
- There is an imbalance between the osteoblasts and osteoclasts causing aberrations in the shape of the bone

- Alveolar bone formation is retarded, there is delayed eruption of the teeth
- The teeth have defective enamel formation with distorted morphology, enamel hypoplasia, and atypical dentin. There is increased susceptibility to caries, hyperplastic gingival and periodontal disease with abscess formation
- There is crowding of the teeth and the roots may be stunted and thickened
- The salivary glands undergo typical keratinizing metaplasia.

Radiographic Features

Widening of the periodontal membrane is seen, and at times the loss of periodontal space is so severe that roots are seen in direct contact with the alveolar bone.

Hypervitaminosis A

Definition

If more than 30,000 mcg is taken daily it can produce toxic effects in adults if continued for many months.

Clinical Features

Painful joints, thickening of long bones, anorexia, low grade fever, loss of hair, hepatosplenomegaly, blurred vision, rashes, irregular menstruation, fatigue and headache.

Radiographic Features

Long bones show fragmentation of the distal fibular epiphysis and pronounced periosteal thickening.

Vitamin D

Definition

It is also known as sunshine vitamin, and is found in fish liver oils, animal fats and sunlight. The daily requirement is 0.01 mg or 400 iu. It helps to regulate the parathyroid glands, maintaining the plasma levels of calcium and phosphorus. It is also very important for the proper formation of teeth and bones and plays an important part in caries prevention.

Deficiency in children and infants is called *Rickets* and in adults it is called *Osteomalacia*. Deficiency of Vitamin D tends to cause hypocalcemia.

Rickets and *osteomalacia* result from a defect in the normal activity of the metabolites of vitamin D, especially 1,25-dihydroxycholecalciferol, which is required for resorption of calcium in the intestine, which leads to failure of normal mineralization of the bone.

Failure of the normal activity of vitamin D may occur as a result of the following:
- Lack of vitamin D in the diet
- Lack of absorption of vitamin D resulting from various gastrointestinal malabsorption problems
- Lack of metabolism of the active metabolite $1,25(OH)_2D$ that is required for intestinal absorption of calcium.

Interference may occur anywhere along the metabolic pathway for $1,25(OH)_2D$:
- Lack of exposure to ultraviolet light required for conversion of provitamin D_3
- Lack of conversion of D_3 to $25(OH)D$ in the liver because of liver disease
- Lack of metabolism of $25(OH)D$ to $1,25(OH)_2D$ by the kidney because of kidney diseases
- A defect in the intestinal target cell response to $1.25(OH)_2D$ or inadequate calcium supply.

Clinical Features

Rickets

- It occurs in infants and children
- In the first 6 months of life, tetany and convulsions are the clinical problems resulting due to hypercalcemia
- This may be followed with swelling of the wrist and ankles. The bone changes are seen in the epiphyseal plates, metaphysis and the shaft
- Many a times *craniotabes* or softening of the posterior of the parietal bones is the initial sign of the disease
- The patient has:
  - Short stature with deformed extremities
  - Rickety rosary due to over growth of cartilage or osteoid bone at the costochondral junction
  - Pigeon breast, the weakened metaphyseal areas of the ribs are subject to pull of the respiratory muscles and thus bend inwards creating anterior protrusion of the sternum.
  - Harrison grooves, the inward pull at the margins of the diaphragm creates these grooves, girdling the thoracic cavity at the lower margins of the rib cage.
  - Lumbar lordosis, when an ambulatory child develops rickets deformities are likely to affect the spine, pelvis and the long bones causing lumbar lordosis
  - Frontal bossing and squared appearance of the head.
- The development of the dentition is delayed and the eruption rate is retarded
- The osteoid of the jaws is soft, so that the teeth are displaced leading to malocclusion
- There are developmental anomalies of the enamel and dentin. Enamel hypoplasia with mottled yellow gray color of the teeth.

Osteomalacia

- This is seen in adults and the pelvic deformities are more common in females
- Remodeling of the bone occurs in the absence of adequate calcium resulting in softening and distortion of the skeleton

- Patient will have bone pain and muscle weakness
- They have a peculiar waddling or *penguin gait*, tetany and *green stick* (incomplete) bone fractures
- Dental abnormalities are rarely seen, though there may be some incidences of severe periodontitis.

Radiographic Features

Rickets

- Widening and fraying of the epiphysis of the long bones
- The soft weight-bearing bones such as the femur and tibia undergo characteristic bowing
- Changes in the jaws generally occur after changes in the ribs and long bones
- The jaws cortical structures, such as the inferior mandibular border or the walls of the mandibular canal the follicular walls of developing teeth and lamina dura are thinned or missing
- Within the cancellous portion of the bone, the trabeculae become reduced in density, number and thickness. Many a times the jaws become so radiolucent that the teeth appear to be bereft of bony support
- Enamel hypoplasia, thinning of the dentinal layer, grossly enlarged pulp chambers of deciduous teeth, and narrowing of the periodontal ligament space is seen
- There may be unerupted teeth seen on the radiographs due to delayed eruption.

Osteomalacia

- The cortex of the bone may be thinned
- Pseudofractures which may be poorly calcified, ribbon like zones extending into the bone at approximate right angles to the margin of the bone, may also be present. These fractures usually common in the ribs. Pelvis, weight bearing bones are rarely seen in the mandible
- There may be osteoid formed in the defect of actual fractures, but due to lack of calcium the healing is not complete and thus the fracture remains apparent radiographically, called *Looser's zone*
- Many a times, there are no radiographic manifestation in the jaws. However, an overall radiolucent appearance of the jaws may be seen on a panoramic projection, and sparse and coarse bony trabeculae are apparent on a periapical radiograph
- The lamina dura may be thinned in cases of long standing osteomalacia, and these cases should be differentiated from hyperparathyroidism
- Teeth are not affected as they are fully developed before the onset of the disease.

Differential Diagnosis

Osteomalacia should be differentiated from hyperparathyroidism, rheumatoid arthritis and muscle strain.

Management

Dietary enrichment of vitamin D and calcium.

Vitamin D Resistant Rickets (Hypophosphatemia, Hypophosphatemic Rickets, Familial Hypophosphatemia, Refractory Rickets)

Definition

This represents a group of inherited conditions that produce renal tubular disorders, resulting in excessive loss of phosphorus. There is failure to reabsorb phosphorus in the proximal renal tubules, which results in decrease in serum phosphorus (hypophosphatemia). For normal calcification of the osseous structures, the correct amount and ratio of serum calcium and phosphorus is required. Multiple myeloma may induce hypophosphatemia as a result of secondary damage to the kidneys.

Clinical Features

- It is recognized in children when they start to walk
- They show reduced growth and ricket-like bony changes, which include bowing of legs, enlarged epiphysis, skull changes. Bony outgrowths at the site of muscular attachments and around the joints may limit the movements
- Adults have bone pain, muscle weakness and vertebral fractures.

Radiographic Features

- In children, the radiographic findings are indistinguishable from those of rickets
- In adults, the long bones may show persistent deformity, fractures or pseudofractures
- The jaws are osteoporotic and remarkably radiolucent. Cortical boundaries are also not apparent
- There is no evidence of the normal cortical layer of bone around the follicle of developing teeth, as a result they appear unsupported by solid tissue
- There is a marked effect on the teeth and supporting structures
  - The enamel cap is thinned, the pulp horns are elongated and extend right up to the dentoenamel junction and enlarged root canals
  - The lamina dura may be lost or appears indistinct
  - There is a high incidence of periapical and periodontal abscess. When periodontal infections occur in these patients the lesions tend to spread diffusely through bone. Periapical rarifying osteitis involving teeth which are caries free are often seen, in these cases. This may be attributed to the enlarged pulp horns and hypoplastic enamel and defects in the dentin formation, which allows the ingress of oral microorganisms, leading

to pulp necrosis, before clinical signs of caries can be seen. Another hypothesis is that these apical lesions are primarily periodontal in nature owing to the presence of defective cementum

- If the disease is severe, there is premature loss of teeth.

Management

Decreased dosages of vitamin D (15,000–50,000 Iu/day) combined with supplemented oral phosphates have been used successfully.

Renal Osteodystrophy (Renal Rickets)

Definition

In this case the bone changes result from chronic renal failure. The kidney disease interferes with the hydroxylation of 25(OH)D into 1,25(OH)$_2$D, which normally occurs in the kidney. The vitamin D metabolite 1,25(OH)$_2$D is responsible for the active transport of calcium in the duodenum and upper jejunum. Affected patients suffer from hypocalcemia as a result of impaired calcium absorption and hyperphosphatemia resulting from reduction in renal phosphorus excretion. Prolonged low serum calcium stimulates the parathyroid glands to produce PTH and this results in, secondary hyperparathyroidism and systemic metabolic acidosis.

Clinical Features

- The clinical features are similar to those of chronic renal failure
- In children, growth retardation and frequent bone fractures may occur
- In adults, there will be a gradual softening and bowing of the bones.

Radiographic Features

- Changes of the skeleton resemble those seen in rickets and hyperparathyroidism
- Generalized loss of bone density and thinning of the cortices
- Occasionally there may be increased bone density: Brown tumors may occasionally be seen
- The density of the mandible and maxilla varies sometimes being more and sometimes less dense, with a coordinated increase and decrease in the number of internal trabeculae, which appear granular
- The cortical boundaries may be thinner or less apparent
- There may be hypoplasia and hypocalcification of the teeth, resulting in loss of any radiographic evidence of enamel
- The lamina dura may be absent or less apparent in instances of bone sclerosis.

Differential Diagnosis

- *Osteoporosis*: Refer Chapter 24 Diseases of Bone Manifested in the Jaws (Page 419).
- *Osteopetrosis*: (Albers-Schönberg, marble bone disease, osteosclerosis fragilis generalisata); refer Chapter 24 Diseases of Bones Manifested in the Jaws (Page 419).
- It is important to note that the bone changes in renal osteodystrophy may persist even after a successful renal transplant because of the hyperplasia of the parathyroid glands, resulting in continued elevation of PTH.

BLOOD DISORDERS (TABLE 20.5)

Erythroblastosis Fetalis (Hereditary Disease of the Newborn)

Definition

This occurs due to isoimmune antibodies. Congenital hemolytic anemia results due to Rh incompatibility which results in destruction of fetal blood brought about by the reaction between maternal and fetal blood factors.

Clinical Features

- Some infants are stillborn
- Others have anemia with pallor, jaundice, compensatory erythropoiesis (both medullary and extramedullary) and edema resulting in fetal hydrops
- Presence of Kernicterus. It may manifest itself as apathy and poor breastfeeding and later by mental retardation, irritability and cranial nerve palsies
- There is deposition of blood pigment in enamel and dentin of developing teeth giving them a green, brown or blue hue
- Enamel hypoplasia, which involves the incisal edges of anterior teeth and the middle portion of the deciduous cuspid and first molar crown. It presents as a ring like defect called as *Rh hump*
- The red cell count at birth may vary from less than 1,000,000 cells per cubic millimeter to a near normal level. The peripheral smear shows large number of immature RBCs
- The icterus index is very high and may reach a level of 100 units.

Radiographic Features

- Transverse lines of increased and decreased radiolucency, occurs at the ends of some long bones in some cases
- There is increased thickness of the cranial bone which also includes the maxilla and the mandible
- The bones of the vault are thickened as a result of increased thickness of diploe, radiating spicules may be present.

Table 20.5 Blood disorders

- Disorders of RBC
  - Quantitative
    - Increase in number
    - Polycythemia vera
    - Secondary polycythemia
    - Apparent polycythemia
  - Decrease in number
    - Iron deficiency anemia
      i. Plummer-Vinson syndrome (Paterson-Brown-Kelly syndrome)
    - Pernicious anemia (Addisonian anemia, Biermer's anemia)
    - Normocytic anemia
    - Aplastic anemia
    - Hemolytic anemia
    - Extracorpuscular causes
      i. Infection and toxin
      ii. Hypersplenism
      iii. Rh factor incompatibility (hemolytic disease of the new born, erythroblastosis fetalis)
      iv. Chronic liver disease
      v. Autoimmune disease
      vi. Transfusion reaction, intracorpuscular causes, abnormal size and shape
      vii. Hereditary spherocytosis
      viii. Sickle cell anemia, abnormal hemoglobin
      ix. Thalassemia (Cooley's anemia), erythrocyte enzyme deficiency
      x. Glucose-6 phosphate dehydrogenase deficiency
      xi. Pyruvate kinase deficiency
      xii. Folic acid and vitamin B_{12} deficiency
  - Qualitative
- Disorders of WBC
  - Quantitative
    - Increase in number
      i. Granulocytosis
      ii. Neutrophilia
      iii. Basophilic leukocytosis
      iv. Eosinophilic leukocytosis
      v. Lymphocytosis
      vi. Monocytosis
  - Decrease in number
    - Granulocytopenia
    - Neutropenia
      i. Cyclic neutropenia
      ii. Primary splenic neutropenia
      iii. Chronic hypoplastic neutropenia
      iv. Chronic granulocytopenia in childhood
      v. Familial neutropenia
      vi. Transitory neonatal neutropenia
  - Qualitative
    i. Lazy leukocyte syndrome
    ii. Chédiak-Higashi syndrome
    iii. Leukemia, acute lymphocytic, acute myelocytic, chronic granulocytic, chronic lymphocytic, infectious mononucleosis, lymphoma, Hodgkin's disease, non-Hodgkin's disease, Burkitt's lymphoma

Contd...

Contd...

- - Multiple myeloma
  - Plasmacytosis
- Disorders of platelet
  - Quantitative
    - Increase in number
      i. Thrombocytosis
    - Decrease in number
      i. Purpura
        1. Idiopathic thrombocytopenic purpura
        2. Secondary thrombocytopenic purpura, drugs, infection, autoimmune disorders, radiation, lymphomas
        3. Congenital purpura
        4. Thrombocytopathic purpura, Glanzmann's thrombasthenia, Von Willebrand's disease, Bernard-Soulier syndrome, Wiskott-Aldrich syndrome
- Disorders of coagulation
  - Hemophilia A
  - Hemophilia B (Christmas disease)
  - Factor V deficiency (parahemophilia)
  - Factor XI deficiency
  - Factor X deficiency
  - Hypoprothrombinemia
  - Hypofibrinogenemia
  - Macroglobulinemia
  - Fibrin stabilizing factor deficiency
  - Hereditary hemorrhagic telangiectasia (Osler-Rendu-Weber syndrome)
  - Disseminated intravascular coagulation
  - Hemangiomata
  - Hemorrhage of iatrogenic causes

Sickle Cell Anemia

Definition

This is an autosomal recessive chronic, hemolytic blood disorder, characterized by abnormal hemoglobin (deoxygenated hemoglobin, substitution of amino acid, glutamic acid on position 6 present in the chain of the HbA, by valine giving rise to abnormal hemoglobin), which under low oxygen tension results in sickle shaped red blood cells, with decreased oxygen carrying capacity to the tissues. Because of damage to the membrane lipids and proteins, RBC's adhere to vascular endothelium and obstruct capillaries. The spleen traps and destroys these abnormal cells. The hematopoietic system responds to the resultant anemia by increasing the production of red blood cells, which produces compensatory hyperplasia of the bone marrow.

There are two types:
1. *Homozygous type*: Here the whole of HbA is replaced by HbS and is called sickle cell disease.
2. *Heterozygous type*: Only 50% of the HbA is replaced by HbS and is known as *sickle cell trait*. They do not show related clinical findings.

Clinical Features

- This is more common in females, children and adolescents
- There are long spells of hemolytic *latency*, occasionally *punctated* by exacerbations known as sickle cell crises
- The patient may experience severe abdominal, muscle and joint pain, high temperature and may even undergo circulatory collapse
- During the milder periods the patient may complain of fatigability, weakness, shortness of breath, muscle and joint pain
- There is generalized retardation of bone growth
- Infarction of the bone and spleen and thrombosis may also occur
- The heart is usually enlarged and a murmur may be present. It is compatible with a normal life span but, many patients are known to die of the complications of the disease before the age of 40 years
- The patient may have mongoloid facies with high cheek bones and bimaxillary prognathism. This is due to marrow hyperplasia which results in the increase in hard palate length and the maxillary alveolar ridge angle
- The patient may present with paresthesia of the mental nerve, secondary to compression of the nerve and the blood vessels
- The oral mucosa shows pallor, with delayed eruption and hypoplasia of the teeth
- Patient is more prone to develop osteomyelitis, due to hypovascularity of the bone due to thrombosis
- Bone changes of sickle cell anemia are more in children because there is apparently less circulatory adaptation to the disease, a higher ratio of hematopoietic elements in the marrow of children and a greater incidence of sickle cell crisis. Most of the affected children show osteoporosis and alveolar bone loss. The feasibility of using dental X-rays as a screen test for detection of sickle cell anemia has been recommended
- The peripheral smear will show atypical sickle shaped RBCs, a decreased hemoglobin level (5–12 gm/dL). RBC count may reach the level of 10 lakh cells or less per cu mm.

Radiographic Features

- The radiographic manifestations of sickle cell anemia in the various bones are principally due to the expansion of the bone marrow at the expense of the spongy bone. The extent of the bone changes depends on the degree of hyperplasia present
- There is thinning of the individual trabeculae and cortices in the vertebral bodies, long bones, skull and jaws
- The skull may have a widening of the diploe space with thinning of the inner and outer tables. In extreme cases, the outer table is not visible with perpendicular trabeculation radiating outwards giving a *hair on end* appearance

- Small areas of bone infarction due to blockage of the microvasculature produce areas of localized bone sclerosis
- In the jaws, there is generalized osteoporosis, due to decrease in the volume of trabeculae which becomes coarser (*ground glass appearance*) and thinning of the cortical plates (inferior border of the mandible)
- The lamina dura appears more prominent against the background of increased radiolucency
- Deep in the spongy portion of the bone, there are delicate trabeculae which are particularly prone to pressure resorption with the heavy internal bony architecture relatively less affected
- In inter dental portions of the jaws, the trabeculae are coarser and appear as horizontal rows creating a *step ladder effect*
- Rarely bone marrow hyperplasia may cause enlargement and protrusion of the maxillary alveolar ridge.

Differential Diagnosis

- Hypophosphatasia
- Hyperparathyroidism
- Osteoporosis.

Management

Patients should avoid precipitating factors. They should be given regular supplements of folic acid, prophylactic antibiotics, and analgesics to control pain. Blood transfusion may be given during a crisis.

Thalassemia (Cooley's Anemia, Mediterranean Anemia, Erythroblastic Anemia)

Definition

This is a hereditary disorder that results in a defect in hemoglobin synthesis. The defect may involve either the alpha or the beta globin genes. The resultant red blood cells have reduced hemoglobin content, are thin and have shortened life span. The different types are:

- *Alpha thalassemia*: Reduction or absence of α chain synthesis.
- Beta thalassemia—reduction or absence of β chains.
- Thalassemia major or homozygous β-thalassemia or Cooley's anemia:
  - *Hemoglobin H disease*: This is a very mild form of the disease in which the patient may live a relatively normal life.
  - *Hemoglobin Bart disease*: In which infants are still born or die shortly after birth.
  - Thalassemia minor or thalassemia trait or heterozygous form of the disease

Clinical Features

In the severe form the onset is in infancy and the survival time is short. The face develops prominent cheek bones and protrusive maxilla, resulting in a *rodent-like face.*

- The milder form of the disease occurs in children
- The patient may show saddle nose, prominent malar bone and decreased pneumatization of the maxillary sinus—As a result of these skeletal defects the upper lip is retracted giving the child a chip-munk facies
- The maxillary teeth are protruded with spacing, and there may be discoloration of the teeth due to high levels of iron concentrations in the body
- The patient has microcytic and hypochromic anemia. Peripheral blood smear shows abnormal RBCs, reticulocyte count is increased and the bone marrow shows increased erythropoietic activity
- Serum bilirubin and fecal and urinary urobilinogen are elevated due to hemolysis and an elevated fetal hemoglobin is present.

Radiographic Features

- The radiographic features result from hyperplasia of the ineffective bone marrow and its subsequent failure to produce normal red cells
- There is a generalized radiolucency of the long bones with cortical thinning
- In the skull the diploic space exhibits marked thickening, especially in the frontal region. The skull shows generalized granular appearance and occasionally a hair-on-end effect may develop
- Severe bone marrow hyperplasia prevents pneumatization of the paranasal sinuses, especially the maxillary sinus, and causes expansion of the sinus that results in malocclusion
- The jaws appear radiolucent with thinning of the cortical borders and enlargement of the marrow spaces. The trabeculae are blurred but in some areas they are large and coarse and referred to as compensatory lamellar striation.

A circular radiolucency may be seen in the lower anterior region and there may be thinning of the crypt of developing teeth.

The lamina dura is thinned and the roots of the teeth may be short. The roots of the mandibular first molar and central incisors may be spike shaped.

Differential Diagnosis

Sickle cell anemia.

Management

Repeated blood transfusions, splenectomy may be advised. Use of chelating agents to reduce the overload of iron. Folic acid supplements.

Hereditary Spherocytosis

Definition

It is a disorder in which the red blood cells are excessively permeable to sodium ions. The osmotic fragility of the cells is abnormal which leads to loss of cell membrane and the cell gradually becomes spherical in shape and is destroyed in the spleen, giving rise to hemolytic anemia.

Clinical Features

- Usually seen in childhood
- There may be moderate hepatosplenomegaly, jaundice and anemia
- The peripheral smear shows presence of spherocytes, reticulocyte count is increased and the hemoglobin count ranges from 5 to 12 gm/mL.

Radiographic Features

- The bone of the vault are thickened as a result of increase of the amount of diploe
- Radiating spicules may be present, although less widely distributed.

Differential Diagnosis

- Sickle cell anemia
- Thalassemia.

Management

Splenectomy is the treatment of choice, with folic acid supplementations.

Agranulocytopenia (Granulocytopenia, Agranulocytic Angina)

Definition

This is characterized by marked leucopenia with reduction and absence of neutrophilic leukocytes. The different types are:

- *Primary agranulocytosis*: This is of unknown etiology.
- *Secondary agranulocytosis*: This may be secondary to deficiencies, infections, autoimmune diseases, hemodialysis, irradiation, allergic reactions and indiscriminate use of drugs.
- *Mild neutropenia*: When $1000/mm^3$ to $2000/mm^3$ neutrophils are present.
- *Moderate neutropenia*: When $500/mm^3$ to $1000/mm^3$ neutrophils are present.
- *Severe neutropenia*: When fewer than $500/mm^3$ neutrophils are present.
- *Agranulocytosis*: When no neutrophils are seen in the peripheral smear.

Clinical Features

- It may occur at any age, but is more common in adult females. It is more common in people who have easy access to offending drugs (hospital staff)
- It may have a gradual onset, with sore throat, high fever and rigors. The skin appears pale, anemic or jaundiced
- There may be rapidly advancing necrotic ulcerations of the mouth with little evidence of pus formation
- The patient may dies within 3–5 days due to toxemia and septicemia
- The most common oral sites involved are gingiva, palate, tonsil and pharynx
- There are necrotizing ulcerations with a gray/black membrane with no inflammation at the margins of the lesions. There may be associated pain, excessive salivation and spontaneous hemorrhage
- The lesion spreads quickly to the supporting structures, destroying them with the inevitable loss of deciduous and permanent teeth
- There is a reduced leukocyte count below 2000 cells/cu mm and—granulocyte count below 100 cells per cu mm. Hemoglobin and platelet counts are below normal.

Radiographic Features

- Supporting alveolar bone is rapidly destroyed so that the teeth are denuded of bone and are supported by soft tissue only
- Sometimes the infection may spread to the marrow to cause osteomyelitis.

Differential Diagnosis

- *Leukemia, anemia, purpura*: Leukocyte count is above 1,000,000/mm^3 with prolonged bleeding and clotting time.
- *Cyclic neutropenia*: Marked cyclic appearance every 20 to 25 days.
- *Wegener's granulomatosis*: There is kidney and lung involvement.
- *ANUG*: Necrosis starts on the papilla tips, not necessarily associated with leukopenia.
- *Necrotizing sialometaplasia*: There are large ulcerations with indurations on the hard and soft palate, with flat borders and is painless. The general condition of the patient is not affected.
- *Erythema multiforme*: There are target lesions and no specific blood picture.

Management

Removal of the cause, blood transfusion, and antibiotic cover.

Cyclic Neutropenia (Periodic Neutropenia)

Definition

This is a rare disorder characterized by periodic or cyclic diminution in circulating neutrophils due to failure of the stem cells of the bone marrow. It may be inherited or may appear spontaneously during the first few years of life. The patient is healthy between the neutropenic periods.

Clinical Features

- It appears in infancy and childhood and both the sexes are equally affected
- The episodes vary from once in 2–4 weeks and last for 3–5 days
- The patient manifests fever, sore throat, stomatitis and regional lymphadenopathy
- He may also have headaches, arthritis, cutaneous infections and conjunctivitis
- Less frequently the patient experiences lung, urinary tract infections and rectal and vaginal ulcers
- There may be amyloidosis, due to repeated increased antigenic stimulating neutropenic episodes
- There may be severe gingivitis painful ragged ulcers with a core like center found on the lips, tongue, palate, gums, buccal mucosa, which heal with scarring after two weeks
- Isolated painful ulcers may occur which correspond to the period of neutropenia
- The normal blood count will over a period of 4–5 days begin to show a decline in the neutrophil count, compensated by an increase in the monocytes and lymphocytes. At the peak of the disease the neutrophils completely disappear for a day or two.

Radiographic Features

- There may be a mild or severe loss of superficial alveolar bone advancing to periodontitis
- In children this loss of bone around multiple teeth is called prepubertal periodontitis.

Management

There is no specific treatment. Corticosteroids may be given. The oral hygiene needs to be maintained.

- *Multiple myeloma*: Refer Chapter 23—Malignant Diseases of the Jaws (Page 393).
- *Lymphoma*: Refer Chapter 23—Malignant Diseases of the Jaws (Page 393).
- *Leukemia*: Refer Chapter 23—Malignant Diseases of the Jaws (Page 393).

BIBLIOGRAPHY

1. Baer PN, Brown NC, Hamner JE. Hypophosphatasia: Report of two cases with dental findings. Periodontics. 1964;2:209-15.

2. Goaz PW, White SC, Principles and Interpretation, In: Oral Radiology, 3rd edition. St. Louis: Mosby Year Book, 1994.

3. Karjodjkar FR, Saxena VS, Maideo A, et al. Osteomyelitis affecting mandible in tuberculosis patients. J Cli Exp Dent. 2012;4(1):e72-6.

4. Miles DA, Van Dis MJ, Jensen CW, et al. Interpretation normal versus abnormal and common radiographic presentations of lesions. In: Radiographic and Imaging for Dental Auxillaries, 3rd edition. Philadelphia: WB Saunders, 1990.pp.231-80.

5. Sansare K, Gupta A, Khanna V, et al. Oral Tuberculosis: Unusual radiographic findings. DMFR (2011) 40, 251-256. Doi: 10.1259/dmfr/75047143.

6. Shafer WG, et al. A text book of oral pathology. Philadelphia: WB Saunders; 1983.

7. Trapnell DH, Bowerman JE. Dental manifestations of systemic disease. Butterworth Scientific, Oxford; 1973.

9. Wood NK, Goaz PW. Differential diagnosis of oral lesions. 4th edition. CV Mosby: St. Louis; 1991.

10. Wood RE. Handbook of signs in dental and maxillofacial radiology. Warthog Publications, Toronto; 1988.

11. Worth HM. Principles and practice of oral radiographic interpretation. Year Book Medical Publishers, Chicago; 1963.

A cyst is a pathological cavity in the hard or soft tissues filled with fluid, semifluid or gas not always lined by epithelium, and surrounded by a definite connective tissue wall. The cystic fluid either is secreted by the cells lining the cavity or derived from the surrounding tissue fluid.

Cysts occur more in the jaws than in any other bone because cysts originate from the numerous rests of odontogenic epithelium that remain after tooth formation.

Cysts have a clinical importance for the fact, that they not only attain a large size, produce facial asymmetry, disturbance of the dentition, neurological symptoms, predisposes the jaws to fractures, but also often they have a high frequency of occurrence.

CLASSIFICATION OF CYSTS OF THE JAWS (TABLE 21.1)

General Characteristics

- A small cyst is unlikely to be diagnosed on routine examination.
- As the cyst grows larger, expansion of the alveolar bone occurs. Usually, the labial or the buccal side is expanded (odontogenic cyst), in some cases the lingual expansion may occur (cysts of the ramus and third molar areas). Expansion of both inner and outer bony wall is not indicative of a cyst.
- As the cyst increases in size the periosteum is stimulated to form a layer of new bone (subperiosteal) deposition.
- The lateral expansion causes a smooth, hard, painless prominence, but as the cyst enlarges further, the bone covering the center of the convexity becomes thinned (elastic) and can be indented with pressure.
- Eventually the periosteum is unable to maintain the new bone formation, forming a 'window' at the summit of the convexity.
- Eventually the outer shell becomes fragmented giving a 'egg shell crackling' feel on palpation.
- In advanced cases, the cystic lining lies immediately below the mucosa and 'fluctuation' can be elicited.
- Sometimes there is eventual discharge of the fluid into the mouth (usually seen with progressive enlargement of periodontal and dentigerous cysts).
- *Diagnostic features varying as per the site of the cyst*: Periodontal cysts occur anywhere in the dental arch, dentigerous cysts are usually associated with impacted

Table 21.1 Classification of cysts of the jaws

- Odontogenic
  - Developmental
    - Primordial cyst
    - Keratocyst (basal cell nevus syndrome)
    - Gingival cyst of infant
    - Gingival cyst of adult
    - Lateral periodontal cyst
    - Dentigerous cyst (follicular)
    - Eruption cyst
    - Calcifying epithelial odontogenic cyst
    - Botryoid cyst
  - Inflammatory
    - Periodontal cyst
      - i. Radicular (dental root apex) cyst
      - ii. Lateral cyst
      - iii. Residual cyst
    - Paradental cysts (inflammatory collateral cyst, mandibular infected buccal cyst)
- Nonodontogenic
  - Nasopalatine (incisive canal, median anterior maxillary) cyst
  - Median cyst
  - Median alveolar cyst
  - Median mandibular cyst
  - Globulomaxillary cyst (premaxilla maxillary cyst)
  - Nasoalveolar cyst (nasolabial klestadt's cyst)
  - Palatal cyst of new born infants
- Cysts associated with maxillary sinus
  - Benign mucosal cysts of the maxillary sinus
    - Mucocele (mucous retention cyst)
    - Serous cyst (serous nonsecretary cyst)
    - Cyst of McGregor (mesothelial cyst)
    - Lymphangiectatic cyst
  - Surgical ciliated cyst of the maxilla
- Cysts of the soft tissues of the face and neck
  - Dermoid cyst
  - Epidermoid cyst
  - Branchial cleft (lymphoepithelial cyst)
  - Thyroglossal duct cyst
  - Anterior median lingual cyst
  - Oral cysts with gastric or intestinal epithelium (gastromucosal cyst)
  - Cystic hygroma
  - Parasitic cysts (hyatid cysts and cysticerous cellulose)

Contd...

Contd...

- Cysts of the salivary glands
  - Mucocele
  i. Mucous retention cyst
  ii. Mucous extravasation
     - Ranula
- Pseudocysts
  - Static (developmental latent) bone cyst
  - Simple (traumatic,hemorrhagic solitary) bone cyst
  - Idiopathic bone cyst
  - Aneurysmal bone cyst

teeth (molars and canines), fissural cysts are mostly seen in the maxilla, solitary is found only in the mandible till date, odontogenic keratocysts are mostly seen in the lower third molar region extending into the ramus.

- Unless they become extremely large, cysts rarely cause loosening of adjacent teeth. A missing tooth without history of extraction may indicate: dentigerous cyst, odontogenic keratocyst, primordial cyst.
- As cysts are usually slow growing it exerts very slight pressure on the neurovascular bundle, thus it is unusal to find symptom of anesthesia associated. However, in case of acute infection due to accumulation of pus, there may be sudden increase in pressure which may cause neuropraxia of the nerve, causing paresthesia or anesthesia.
- The adjoining teeth may be vital (odontogenic keratocyst, fissural cyst, solitary cyst, lateral periodontal cyst) or nonvital (apical periodontal cyst).
- *Effect of the growth of the cyst will differ as the associated structure*: Distortion of the nostril-nasolabial cyst, involvement of the antrum by an infected cyst will produce sinusitis, a large expanding cyst in the jaw will cause the roots of the involved teeth to diverge and the crowns to converge.

General Symptoms

- Pain, swelling and sometimes a salty discharge (infected cyst)
- Lump in the sulcus
- Edentulous patient may complain of dislodgement of denture.

General Radiographic Features

- Oral cysts are usually central (within bone), they may also arise in the soft tissues peripheral to the bone but only central cysts can be well delineated on the radiograph.
- Central cysts are usually painless and slow growing with a well defined radiolucent image. This may be modified in case of infection.
- The cyst may have a unilocular or a multilocular architecture.

- They usually present either as a well defined or moderately unilocular or multilocular radiolucency with or without cortication.
- The shape is usually round or oval (radicular, dentigerous cyst), heart shaped (incisive canal cyst), inverted pear-shaped (globulomaxillary cyst) or scalloped (traumatic bone cyst).
- It may cause cortical bulging or expansion of the overlying bone, which may sometimes progress to cortical erosion and pathological fracture of the involved bone.
- It may lead to displacement or distortion of the adjacent vital structures (teeth, inferior alveolar canal, maxillary sinus).
- Internal calcifications may sometimes be seen. Some cysts also have presence of septa.
- *Suppurating cysts*: The thin white line that represents the cortex of the cyst becomes less dense and thinner and may be entirely lost. Instead a broad band of sclerosed bone which is less dense but wider than a normal cortex and has a granular appearance is seen.
- *Healing cysts*: The cyst caused by an infected tooth, usually heals after the extraction of that tooth. There is a gradual loss of the cortical layer of bone (unless the cyst is infected, then the bone in the immediate vicinity becomes radiolucent due to hyperemia). As the healing progresses there is gradual lessening of radiolucency of the cavity, the dark shadow is slowly replaced by a gray one with a gradual return of the surrounding bone to the normal density. A large cyst may fail to heal completely, resulting in a smaller cyst.

Radiographic Features

- *Odontogenic cysts*:
  - It is always associated with the tooth forming apparatus.
  - It may either be attached or in relation to a tooth (erupted, impacted, supernumerary) or in place of a tooth (normal or supernumerary).
  - It may cause external root resorption (radicular cyst) of the attached tooth or displace it (dentigerous cyst, odotogenic keratocyst)
- *Nonodontogenic cysts*:
  - The origin may be fissural, developmental or traumatic.
  - It is mostly seen along lines of fusion of various bones or embryonic process of oral or adjacent soft tissue structures or at the site of trauma.
  - It may cause divergence of the adjoining teeth with the lamina dura intact (incisive canal cyst, globulomaxillary cyst).

CT scan plays a vital role in detecting the extent of the lesions and its effect on the adjacent structures. The CT examination must include:

- Bone and soft tissue window settings.
- 2–5 mm axial sections parallel to the inferior bony margin of the mandible from the level of the TM joint to the hyoid bone.

4 mm coronal scans from the external auditory meatus to the anterior margins of the symphysis of the mandible (perpendicular to the orbitomeatal line).

Axial sections are especially useful in demonstrating the curved buccal and lingual surfaces of the symphysis, body and ascending ramus of the mandible. The coronal sections are valuable in demonstrating lesions in the maxilla and palate, especially within the maxillary sinus.

ODONTOGENIC DEVELOPMENTAL CYSTS

Primordial Cyst (Fig. 21.1)

Definition

This develops due to cystic changes in the stellate reticulum of a tooth germ before it mineralizes. Therefore, the tooth does not develop.

The term 'primordial cyst' is considered an outdated term and should be avoided. Most 'primordial cysts' are actually keratocyst odontogenic tumors (KOT's).

Clinical Features

- If the primordial cyst develops in a supernumerary tooth bud or from remnants of the lamina dura then the number of teeth present will be complete (i.e. 32). Otherwise the affected tooth will be missing.
- It can arise in any portion of the jaw, but is commonly seen in the ascending ramus of the mandible and the third molar area.
- It may be associated with an erupted over retained deciduous tooth.
- It is more common in children and young adults, in the third molar region.
- It enlarges slowly and painlessly causing expansion of the cortical plates.
- It becomes painful only if infected.
- On aspiration it reveals a thick, granular, yellowish material.

- Histological findings are similar to any other odontogenic cyst, the epithelial cells are arranged in a 'picket fence' or 'tombstone pattern' and showing no retepeg formation.

Radiographic Features

- It appears as a well defined radiolucency, usually unilocular sometimes having scalloped outline, which gives a multilocular appearance.
- The borders are hyperostotic
- The involved tooth is usually missing. The adjacent teeth may be displaced, diverged or deflected.
- Primordial cysts in the maxilla are smaller than their mandibular counterparts.

Differential Diagnosis

Absence of a tooth without the history of extraction favors primordial cyst diagnosis.
- Kerato odontogenic tumor
- Residual cyst
- Traumatic bone cyst
- Early ameloblastoma
- Myxoma.

Management

Treatment consists of surgical enucleation, with regular check up, because of the high rate of recurrence.

Odontogenic Keratocyst (Figs 21.1 to 21.7)

Definition

Many people believe that these cysts are the same as primordial cysts, but this view is not universally accepted.

This cyst arises from the dental lamina. Unlike other cysts which are thought to grow solely by osmotic pressure, the epithelium in odontogenic keratocyst (OKC) appears to

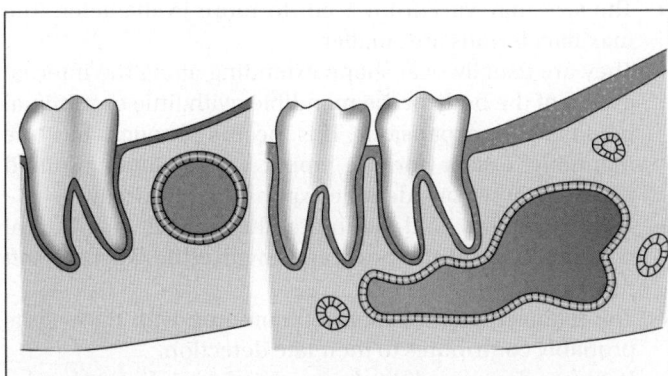

Figure 21.1 Diagram of primordial and keratocystic odontogenic tumor

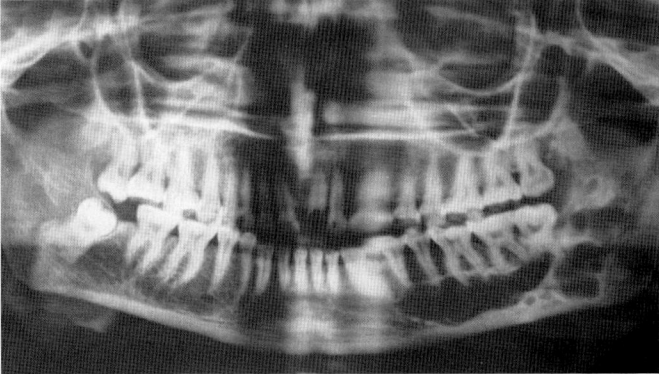

Figure 21.2 A multilocular KCOT seen in relation to the mandibular premolar and molars, on a panoramic radiograph

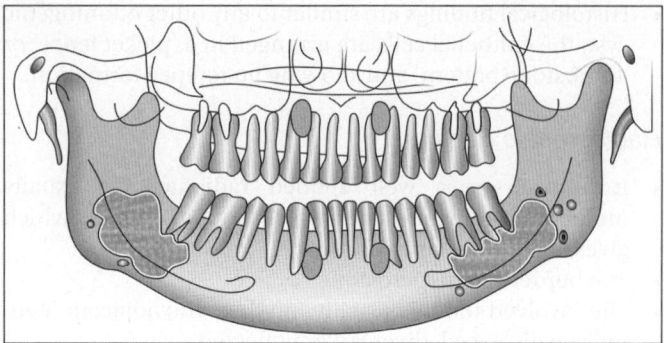

Figure 21.3 A diagrammatical representation of the most likely sites of the KCOT of the jaws

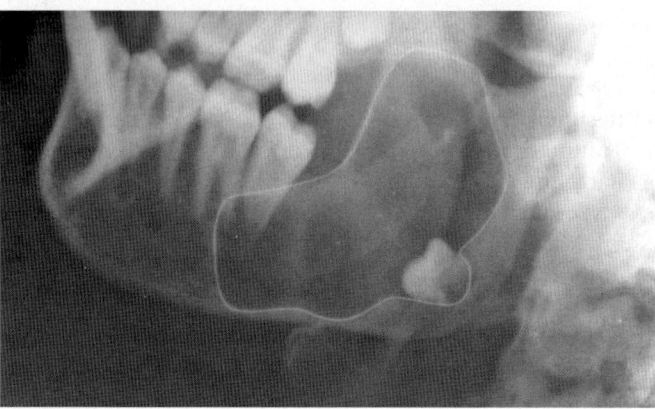

Figure 21.4 A KCOT, seen as an unilocular radiolucency extending from lower right first molar into the ramus, with sclerotic borders and showing displacement of the third molar

have an innate growth potential, similar to a benign tumor. This difference in growth mechanism gives OKC a different radiographic appearance.

The epithelial lining is distinctive because it is keratinized and thin. In some cases, bud like proliferation from the basal cell layer into adjacent connective wall or proliferation of islands of odontogenic epithelium that may be present in the wall giving rise to satellite microcysts which support the fact that OKC's have a high recurrence rate. Five percent of dentigerous and radicular cysts are keratocysts and a variety of many primordial, gingival, lateral periodontal and residual cysts are of keratocysts variety. Thus, many believe that OKC is not a clinical diagnosis but a designation for a group of cysts of possibly diverse origin having a number of highly characteristic microscopic and clinical features in common.

Odontogenic keratocyst: The odontogenic keratocyst is now designated by the World Health Organization (WHO) as a keratocystic odontogenic tumor (KCOT) and is defined as 'a benign uni- or multicystic, intraosseous tumor of odontogenic

origin, with a characteristic lining of parakeratinized stratified squamous epithelium and potential for aggressive, infiltrative behavior'. WHO 'recommends the term keratocystic odontogenic tumor as it better reflects its neoplastic nature'.

Clinical Features

- Approximately 11% of all jaw cysts are KCOT's and they have a very high recurrence rate.
- It occurs in a wide age range, more common in teenagers, young adults, especially males.
- More common in the mandible near the angle, extending into the ramus and forward into the body. The canine region of the maxilla and mandible, and the mandibular molar region are the preferred sites.
- In the maxilla it causes buccal expansion.
- It is usually symptomless unless infected. Occasionally there may be paraesthesia of the lower lip and/or teeth, or a pathological fracture may also occur.
- They sometimes forms around unerupted tooth, sometimes the adjacent teeth may be displaced.
- Aspiration may reveal a thick, yellow, cheesy material (keratin).
- Multiple KCOT's are found in the following syndromes:
  - Gorlin goltz syndrome
  - Marfan syndrome
  - Ehlers-danlos syndrome
  - Noonan's syndrome.

Radiographic Features

- Ninety percent are seen posterior to the canines in the mandible and more than 50% at the angle. The epicenter is located superior to the inferior alveolar nerve. It may have the same pericoronal position as that of a dentigerous cyst.
- Radiographically it shows aggressive growth with undulating borders, cloudy interiors, and presence of internal septas which may give a multilocular appearance. The margins are hyperostotic.
- The size may vary from 5 cm to more in diameter. The maxillary lesions are smaller.
- They are usually oval shape extending along the internal aspect of the body of the mandible, with little or minimal mediolateral expansion. This occurs through out the mandible except for the upper ramus and coronoid process where considerable expansion may occur.
- It may expand and perforate the lingual and buccal cortical plates of the bone and involve the adjacent soft tissue.
- The relatively slight expansion common with these cysts probably contributes to their late detection.
- It causes downward displacement of the inferior alveolar anal and resorption of the lower cortical plate of the mandible causing a perforation or a pathological fracture.

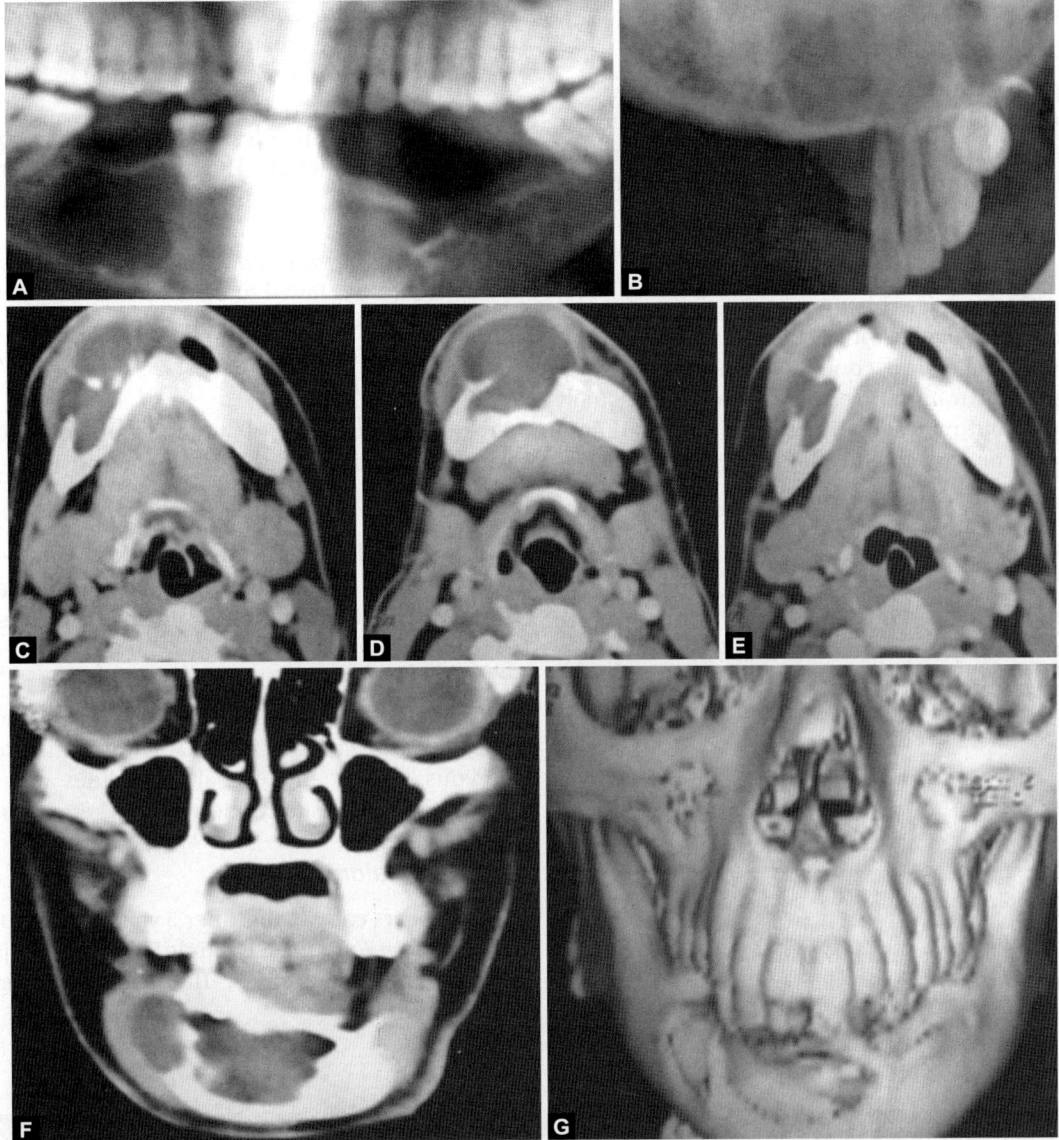

Figures 21.5A to G KCOT, radiographs showed a multilocular, extensive radiolucency extending from the right mandible, crossing the midline up to the left mandible, closely approaching the lower border as seen on the (A) Panoramic; (B) An occlusal view; (C, D and E) Axial CT scan revealed a large well-defined cystic lesion, with septae, measuring 5.5 × 3.5 cm. The lesion extends more towards the right side of the mandible as compared to the left and is extending and indenting the overlying soft tissue structures. The outer cortex of the mandible is eroded where as the inner cortex is preserved; (F) Coronal CT shows a large well-defined cystic lesion, with septae; (G) 3D CT shows labial perforation

- As it enlarges it may produce deflection of the unerupted teeth mostly in the region of the angle of the mandible or the ascending ramus and towards the orbital floor. In some cases root resorption may be seen.
- Radiological types of KCOT:
  - Envelopmental type, this embraces an adjacent unerupted tooth
  - Replacement type, this forms in the place of normal teeth
  - Extraneous type, these are in the ascending ramus away from the teeth
  - Collateral type, those adjacent to the roots of teeth which are indistinguishable radiologically from the lateral periodontal cyst.

Additional Imaging

On CT scan KCOT's appear as minimally expanding lesions with a thick sclerotic margin and a cloudy lumen. The interior of the lesion may show as water like density.

Differential Diagnosis

- *Dentigerous cyst*: In OKC the cyst is connected to the tooth at a point apical to the cementoenamel junction.
- *Ameloblastoma*: It is usually seen in the older age group, usually multilocular, causes paraesthesia, resorption of adjacent teeth, no amber or straw colored fluid on aspiration.
- *Primordial cyst*: Absence of tooth without history of extraction.
- *Residual cyst*: Patient gives history of extraction.
- *Traumatic cyst*: Unilocular with scalloped margins, rarely shows cortical expansion, if it does occur then buccal only, positive history of trauma. Needle aspiration is usually nonproductive, but may sometimes yield a few milliliter of straw colored or serosangious fluid.

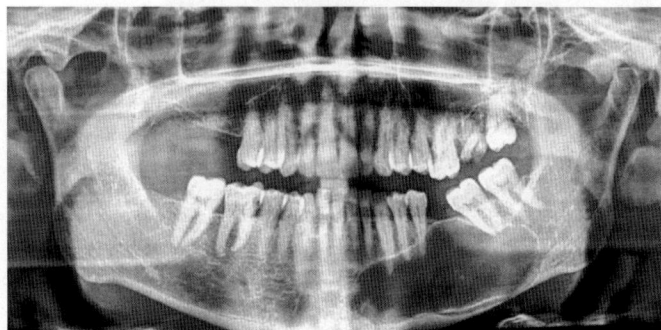

Figure 21.6 Panoramic radiograph shows a multilocular radiolucent lesion (KCOT) in lower left third molar region, extending superiorly from the external oblique ridge, inferiorly up to the mandibular canal, which is displaced. Anteriorly it starts from posterior to the second molar up to the ramus

- *Benign odontogenic tumor and cementifying or ossifying fibroma*: These are not common lesions.
- *Giant cell granuloma*: Usually found in the anterior region of the jaw.
- *Tooth crypt*: This is less likely as calcification of the tooth starts in the 8th year. The halo has a thin outer radiopaque border which is continuous with the lamina dura in the area of cementoenamel junction.
- *Odontogenic myxoma*: It is rare but must be considerd if the tooth has failed to develop and may be seen as a cyst like radiolucency.

Management

Treatment consists of enucleation of the entire cyst with vigorous curettage of the cystic wall with periodic post-treatment examination.

Basal Cell Nevus Syndrome (Jaw Cyst—Basal Cell Nevus Bifid Rib Syndrome, Nevoid Basal Cell Carcinoma, Gorlin-Goltz Syndrome) (Figs 21.8A to E)

Definition

This is an inherited abnormality which includes multiple nevoid basal cell carcinoma of the skin, skeletal, central nervous system and eye abnormalities and multiple jaw cysts, which are usually odontogenic keratocysts.

Clinical Features

- It appears early in life, after 5 years and before 30 years.
- *Oral manifestations*: Multiple KCOT's of the jaw, appearing in multiple quadrants. There may be mild mandibular prognathism.

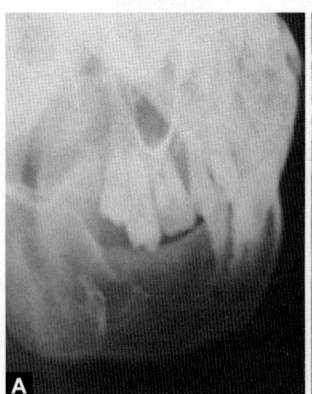
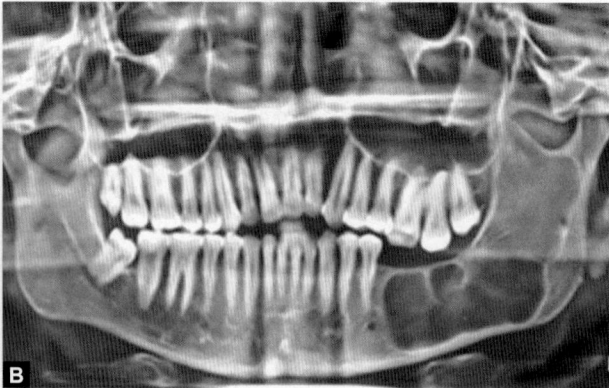
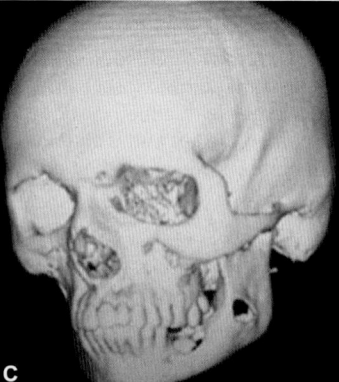

Figures 21.7A to C KCOT: (A) Left lateral oblique shows ill-defined radiolucency in the region of the alveolar ridge in relation to lower molars; (B) Panoramic radiograph shows well defined radiolucency extending from coronoid process to the region of the molars and from the crest of the alveolar ridge to the inferior border of mandible. The radiolucency encompasses the entire width of the ramus. The continuity of the posterior border of the ramus and inferior border of mandible is maintained. The lower border appears scalloped. An arc shaped radiopacity seen lying at the crest of the ridge suggestive of remnants of dental follicle; (C) CT scan shows a well circumscribed expansile lytic lesion involving left half of body, perforating the ramus of the mandible

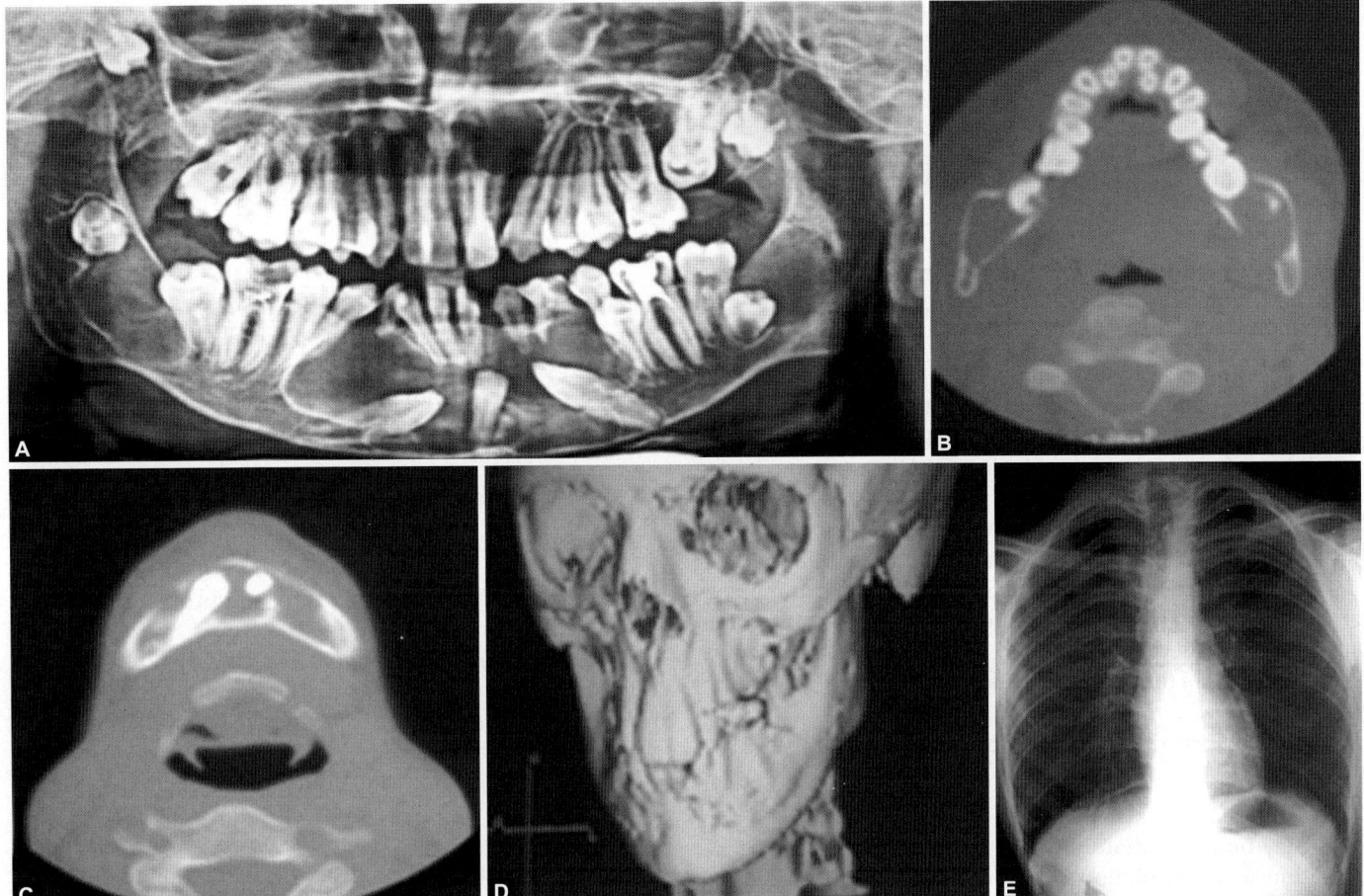

Figures 21.8A to E Gorlin Goltz syndrome: (A) Panoramic view shows multiple well corticated radiolucencies in the bilateral parasymphyseal region of mandible and angle of mandible with minimal expansion. Bilateral displaced lower canine to the lower border of mandible. An impacted tooth is noted in right maxillary region with increased follicular space around it. CT scan (B and C) axial view shows multiple nonenhancing, expansile well corticated lesion in the bilateral angle of mandible and bilateral parasymphseal region. Loss of cortication on the left side lingually; (D) 3D reconstruction shows expansile lesion bilaterally; (E) Chest X-ray shows bifid right 4th and left 3rd rib

- *Cutaneous abnormalities*: Basal cell carcinoma, dermal cyst and tumors, palmar pitting, palmar and plantar keratosis and dermal calcinosis. Nevoid basal cell carcinoma is seen as brownish colored papules, predominantly on the skin, neck and trunk. The skin lesions are small, flattened, flesh colored or brownish papules occurring anywhere in the body, but more prominent on the face and trunk. Basal cell carcinoma is less aggressive in this syndrome than in solitary cell carcinoma.
- *Skeletal abnormalities*: Rib anomalies and brachymetacarpalism, bifid rib, agenesis, deformity and synostosis of rib, kyphoscoliosis, vertebral fusion, poldactyly and shortening of metacarpals.
- *Ophthalmic abnormalities*: Hypertelorism with wide nasal bridge, dystopia canthorum, congenital blindness and internal strabismus.
- *Neurological abnormalities*: Mental retardation, calcification of falx cereberi and other parts of dura,

agenesis of corpus callosum, congenital hydrocephalus and occurrence of medulloblastomas.
- *Sexual abnormalities*: Hypogonadism in males and ovarian tumors.

Radiographic Features

- Multiple radiolucencies of variable size from few millimeter to several centimeters may be seen in multiple quadrants, more common in the premolar-molar region.
- Radiopaque lines of falx cerebri are seen on PA projection, sometimes this calcification may appear laminated.

Differential Diagnosis

- *Multiple myeloma*: Presence of Bence Jones protein in the urine
- *Metastatic carcinoma*: History of primary tumor
- *Histiocytosis X*: It does not have hyperostotic borders

- *Cherubism*: It is a bilateral lesion with jaw expansion. The posterior teeth are pushed in the anterior direction
- *Dentegerous cyst*: These cysts are more expansile.

Management

Complete enucleation with regular screening with an OPG. Genetic counseling is advised.

Lateral Periodontal Cyst (Developmental)

Definition

Lateral periodontal cysts are thought to arise from epithelial rests in the periodontium lateral to the tooth root. The condition is usually unicystic, but may appear as a cluster of small cysts, a condition referred to as botryoid odontogenic cysts. It has been postulated that the lateral periodontal cyst which arises from the periodontium and located in the interproximal bone, between the apex and the alveolar crest, is the intrabony counterpart of the gingival cyst of the adult, which occurs as a dome shaped swelling in the attached gingival. There histological features are so similar that they are believed to the intra and extraosseous manifestations of the same pathosis.

Lateral Periodontal Cyst (Inflammatory) (Fig. 21.9)

Definition

This may be inflammatory (near the alveolar crest, due to irritation and stimulation of the cell rests of malassez) or developmental (associated with the developing tooth germ).

Clinical Features

- It is asymptomatic and less than 1 cm in diameter occurs chiefly in adults between the age of 22 to 85 years, more seen in males.
- It is usually found on the lateral surfaces of vital teeth, most often the mandibular canine and premolar region,

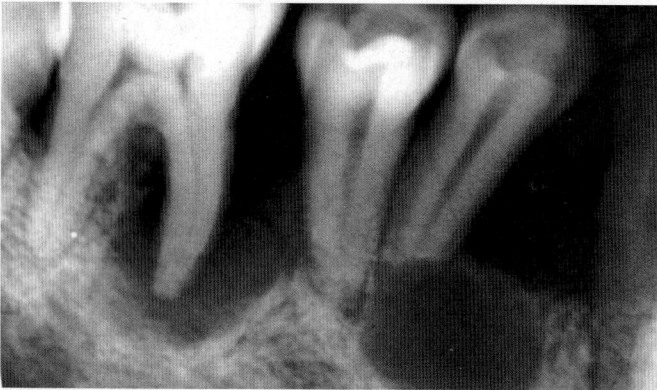

Figure 21.9 Lateral periodontal cyst

followed by the anterior region of the maxilla. When observed on the labial surface it appears as a slight obvious mass.
- It appears as a dome shaped fluctuant selling of the interdental papilla.
- If the cyst becomes infected it resembles a periodontal abscess.

Radiographic Features

- It is seen as a round to ovoid radiolucency with hyperostotic margins, located between the cervical margin and apex of the root surface, less than 1 cm in diameter.
- Small cysts efface the lamina dura of the adjacent root. Large cysts can displace adjacent teeth and cause expansion.

Differential Diagnosis

- *Gingival cyst of adult*: The overlying mucosa is blue.
- *Botryoid cyst*: Histopathological the lumen of this cyst is shows focal thickened plaque of the proliferating lining cell which is more prominent.
- *Lateral radicular cyst*: This is associated with a nonvital tooth, pulpal infection and a discontinuous lamina dura.
- *Lateral periodontal abscess*: If the size is less than 1.5 cm, it is considered an abscess.
- *Lateral dentigerous cyst*: Usually associated with an impacted tooth.
- *Residual cyst arising from the primary or permanent dentition*: There will be a history of extraction of the tooth.
- *Primordial cyst*: This is more common in the younger age group. If the primordial cyst arising from a supernumerary is superimposed on the adjacent tooth surface, then it may be considered in differential diagnosis. Radiographic examination with different angulations should be carried out.
- *Globulomaxillary cyst*: This is pear shaped seen typically between the maxillary lateral and canine region and more common in the younger age group.
- *Median mandibular cyst*: This occurs in the midline of the mandible.
- Small KCOT
- Mental Foramen
- Small neurofibroma
- Radicular cyst at the foramen of a lateral (accessory) canal.

Management

Treatment consists of surgical excision. Recurrence rate is very low or not at all.

Gingival Cyst of the Adult

Definition

It is an uncommon cyst occurring either on free or attached gingival, from the degenerative changes in the epithelium or from the remnants of dental lamina, enamel organ or epithelial islands of periodontal membrane, traumatic implantation of epithelium or from postfunctional rests of dental lamina.

Clinical Features

- It occurs at any age, but more common in adults in the 5th and 6th decade of life, more so in males.
- Mostly found in the mandibular canine and premolar region, associated with vital teeth.
- Slowly growing, soft, fluctuant painless swelling, less than 1 cm in diameter in the attached gingival or interdental papilla.
- It may appear smooth, bluish red, when filled with blood as a result of trauma.

Radiographic Features

- No radiological changes.
- Sometimes a faint round shadow which is indicative of superficial bone erosion with extension into the periodontium may be seen.

Management

Treatment consists of surgical excision.

Botryoid Odontogenic Cyst

Refers to multilocular periodontal cyst which resembles a cluster of lateral periodontal cysts. These are multilocular with thin fibrous connective tissue septa. It has a high rate of recurrence and needs to be carefully excised.

Glandular Odontogenic Cyst (Sialo-odontogenic Cyst, Mucoepidermoid Cyst)

It occurs over a wide age range in either jaws and has the propensity to grow to a very large size and to recur. Radiologically, it is an intrabony, unilocular or multilocular radiolucency with either smooth or scalloped margins. It has the presence of both secretary elements (mucinous material) and stratified squamous epithelium.

Dental Lamina Cyst (Epstein's Pearls, Bohn's Nodules)

Definition

These are multiple, occasionally solitary nodules on the alveolar ridge of the new born originating from remnants of dental lamina.

Epstein's pearls are cystic keratin filled nodules found along the midpalatine raphe, may be derived from entrapped epithelial remnants along the line of fusion.

Bohn's nodules are keratin filled cysts, scattered over the palate most numerous along the junction of the hard and soft palate and may be derived from palatal salivary gland structure.

Dental lamina cyst of newborn is derived from the remnants of the dental lamina, and is found on the crest of the maxillary and mandibular dental ridges.

Clinical Features

- These are rarely seen after 3 months of age.
- They tend to cluster along the junction of the hard and soft palate in a linear fashion or are scattered over the hard palate. Sometimes they may be large enough to be clinically obvious as small discrete white swellings on the alveolar ridge.
- They appear as small whitish projections, measuring a fraction of a millimeter to 2–3 mm in diameter, on the alveolar ridge of the jaws of infants, which may be mistaken for a tooth. Sometimes it may appear blanched.

Differential Diagnosis

These cysts probably correspond to the predeciduous dentition in older literature.

Management

These disappear by opening onto the surface of the mucosa or through disruption by erupting teeth, this most of the time no treatment is required.

Dentigerous Cyst (Follicular, Pericoronal) (Figs 21.10 to 21.16)

Definition

This forms around the crown of an unerupted tooth. It begins when fluid accumulates in the layers of reduced enamel epithelium or between the epithelium and crown of the unerupted tooth, or may be due to cystic changes of the enamel organ after the formation of the crown. An eruption cyst is the soft tissue counterpart of a dentigerous cyst.

Clinical Features

- This is the second most common type of cyst of the jaws, but most of the times it is asymptomatic and discovered on routine radiographs, taken for children and young adults.
- Its incidence is equal in both sexes.
- It is most commonly associated with mandibular third molar and maxillary canines which are often impacted. It may also be found enclosing a complex compound odontome or a supernumerary tooth.

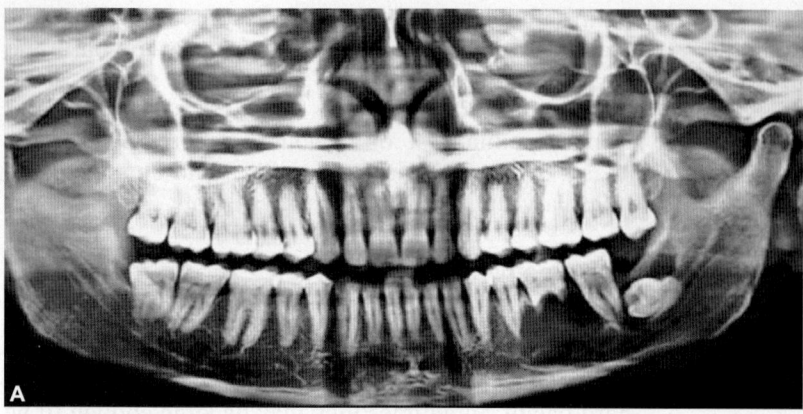
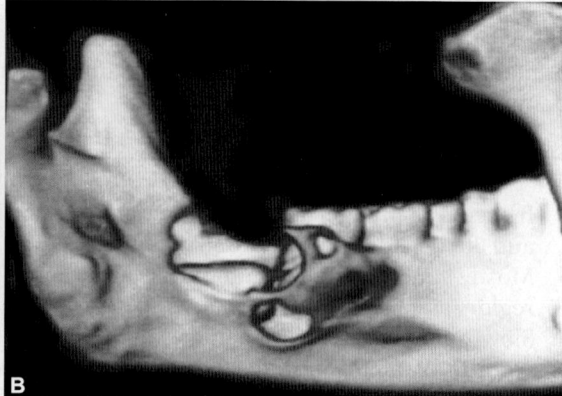

Figures 21.10A and B (A) Panoramic radiograph showing a dentigerous cyst in relation to lower left third molar. On the panoramic radiograph a second lesion appears to be involving the lower premolar and first molar resorbing the involved teeth. The two radiolucencies seen on the radiograph were actually continuous on the lingual aspect of 37 sparing the tooth supporting bone and buccal cortex of 37; (B) 3D CT of the dentigerous cyst lesion seen in A, from the lingual aspect it can be seen that the radiolucent lesion is continuous showing a dentigerous cyst in relation to lower third molar

- It may vary in size from a little more than the diameter of the involved crown or an expansion that causes painless enlargement of the jaws and facial asymmetry.
- The teeth adjacent to the developing cyst and involved teeth may be severely displaced and resorbed. Sometimes the displacement of the third molars is to the extent that it comes to lie compressed against the lower border of the mandible.
- When it expands rapidly it may compress sensory nerve and produce pain which is referred to other sites and described as headache.
- It can become an aggressive lesion with expansion of the bone, asymmetry and pathological fracture.
- The expansion can be so aggressive, in the third molar, so as to hollow out the entire ramus extending to the coronoid process and condyle as well as the body. In the maxillary cuspids, expansion of the anterior maxilla occurs which may superficially resemble acute sinusitis or cellulitis.
- Bilateral dentigerous cysts are found in association with basal cell nevus syndrome, cleidocranial dysplasia and a rare form of amelogenesis imperfecta.
- When it contains blood it is called 'Blue domed cyst'.
- It has the potential to transform to ameloblastoma (mural ameloblastoma), squamous cell carcinoma or mucoepidermoid tumor.

Radiographic Features

- Radiographically it appears as a well defined radiolucency, usually with a hyperostotic border, unless secondarily infected, associated with the crown of unerupted teeth.
- It is usually unilocular but sometimes may appear multilocular, due to the ridges in the bony wall and not the appearance of septa.

- It may envelope the crown symmetrically or may expand laterally from the crown. But the roots of the same may be located in the bone outside the lesion.
- The associated tooth may be displaced in any direction apically, to the coronoid process, high up above the tooth bearing area of the maxilla, into the sinus, adjacent nasal fossa or even in the floor of the orbit.
- It is usual for unerupted teeth which become surrounded by the growing cyst to retain their follicle, which indicates that the tooth is actually outside the cyst.
- Large cysts are always confined to the mandible. The outline may expand from the ramus into the coronoid process or the condyle.
- There may be resorption of the adjacent teeth.

Many authors have classified this cyst into radiographic types.

- *According to Thomas:*
  - *Central variety:* Here the crown is enveloped symmetrically. The pressure is applied to the crown of the tooth and may push it away from its direction of eruption. Thus, the mandibular third molar may be found at the lower border of the mandible and in the ascending ramus and a maxillary canine in the sinus as far as the floor of the orbit. The maxillary incisors may be found below the floor of the nose.
  - *Lateral type:* In this type the dentigerous cyst is a radiographic appearance which results from the dilatation of the follicle on one aspect of the crown. The type is commonly seen when an impacted molar is partially erupted so that its superior aspect is exposed.
  - *Circumferential type:* In this the entire tooth appears to be enveloped by the cyst. The entire enamel organ around the neck of the tooth becomes cystic often allowing the tooth to erupt through the cyst.

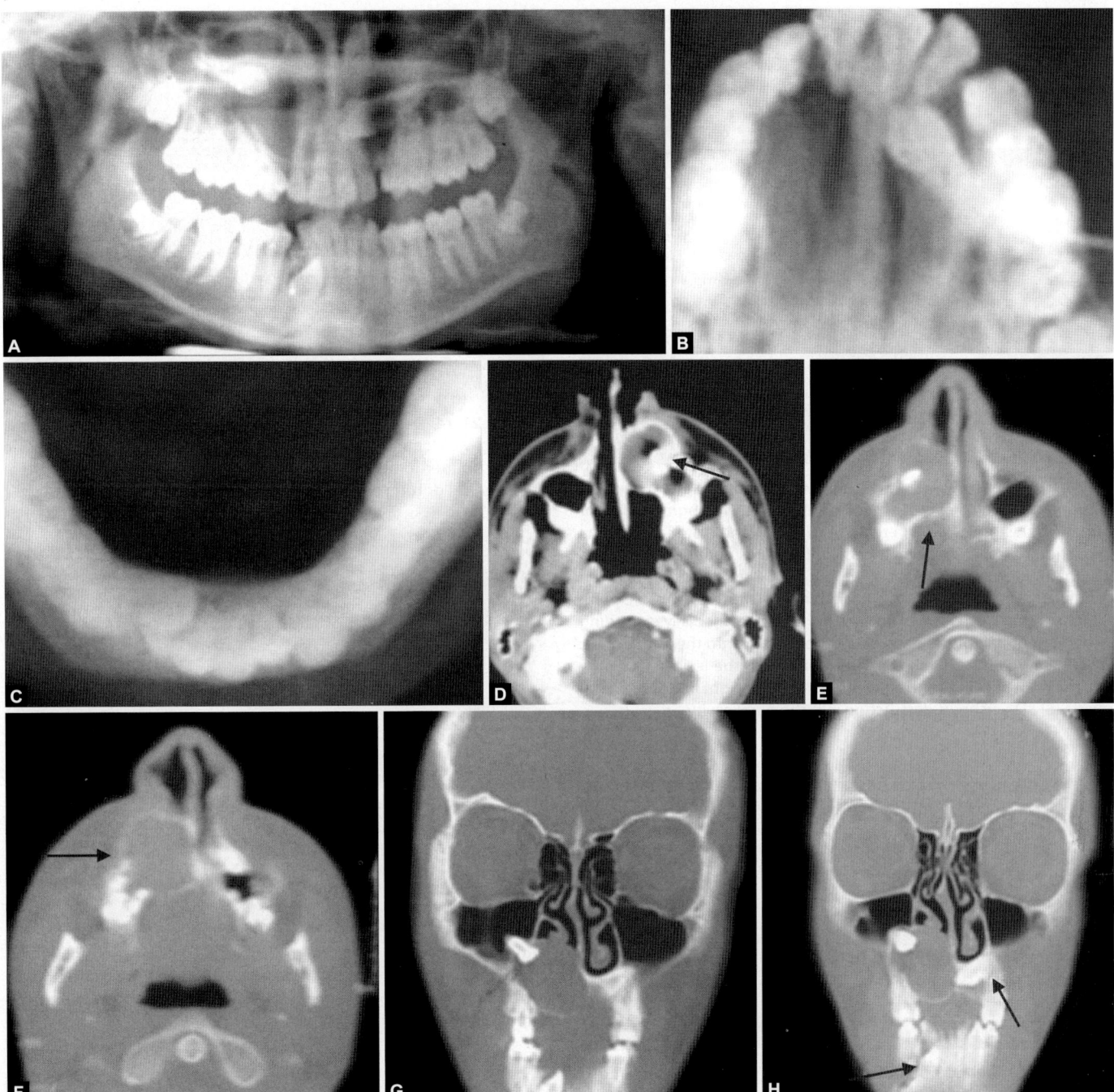

Figures 21.11A to H Dentigerous cysts: (A) Panoramic radiograph shows impacted 13 surrounded by a well-defined radiolucency, displaced into the sinus, 23 surrounded by a well-defined radiolucency, displaced above the apex of 24, 25, impacted 43 surrounded by a comparatively small radiolucency; (B and C) The occlusal radiographs did not add any further information; (D, E and F) The CT, axial section showed a well-defined cystic lesion with thinned out cortex with an impacted tooth in the right side extending anteriorly into the right labial fold, posteriorly into the right half of the hard palate; (G and H) CT, coronal section shows a well-defined cystic lesion with thinned out cortex with a single impacted tooth within the right alveolar process of the right maxilla, extending superiorly into the right maxillary antrum and right half of the nasal cavity, inferiorly into the oral cavity. There are also small cystic lesions with impacted tooth within it in the alveolar process of the left maxilla just across the midline and in the right hemi mandible

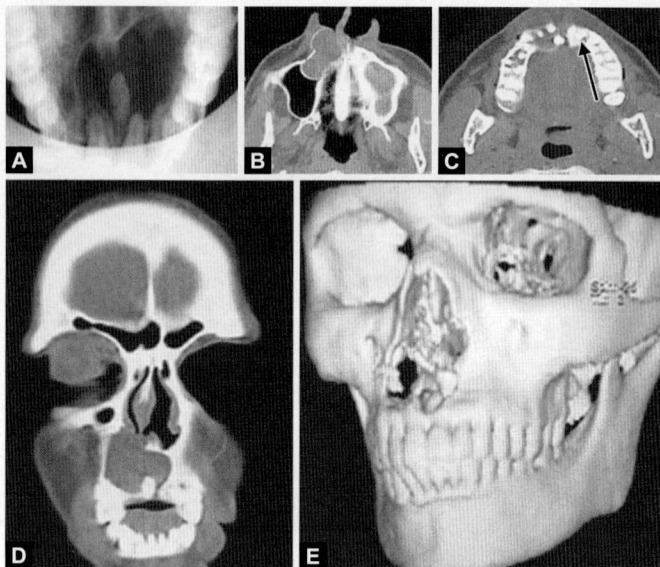

Figures 21.12A to E (A) Dentigerous cyst associated with an inverted mesiodens or radicular cyst as seen on an occlusal radiograph. Patient came with history of pain in relation to 11, 21 and history of trauma in relation to upper anterior. It was confirmed as dentigerous cyst on histopathological examination; (B and C) CT axial section showed radiolucency (4 × 3 × 2 cm) in relation to the crown of 13 with thinning of the cortex, involving the right maxilla, medially extending into the right half of the nasal cavity, posteriorly into the hard palate; (D) The coronal section shows the extension of the lesion superiorly into the right maxillary antrum, medially into the right half of the nasal cavity; (E) 3D CT shows destruction into the nasal cavity

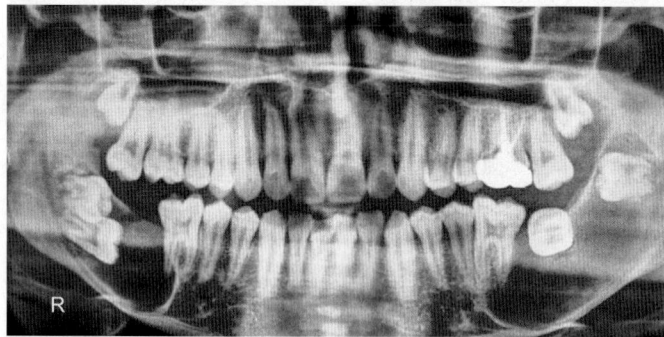

Figure 21.13 Dentigerous cyst: Panoramic radiograph showing a well-defined round radiolucency seen with corticated border in the region of 46, 36, region involving impacted crown of 47, 48, 37, 38

- *According to Mourshed:*
  - Class I dentigerous cyst associated with completely unerupted teeth.
  - Dentigerous cyst associated with unerupted teeth, who fail to erupt due to lack of space in the dental arch.
  - Dentigerous cyst associated with unerupted teeth, who fail to erupt due to malpositioning of the tooth germ.

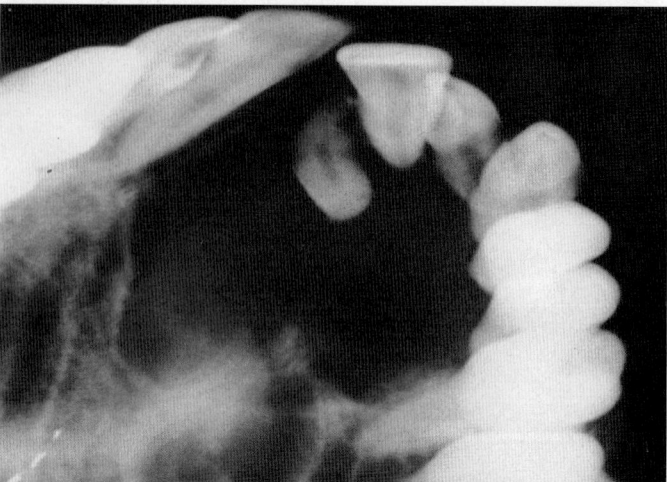

Figure 21.14 Dentigerous cyst: Maxillary occlusal projection was showing well-defined radiolucent area surrounded by thin sclerotic border. A supernumery tooth (mesiodens) was seen within the lesion. Pathological drifting of the roots of central incisors is seen

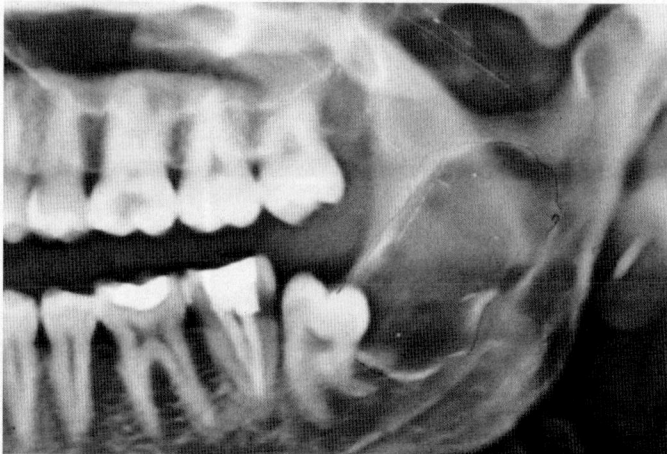

Figure 21.15 Cropped panoramic shows a well-defined radiolucent lesion with sclerotic margin in relation to impacted and developing lower left third molar, attached to CEJ. The lesion extends into the ramus almost up to the sigmoid notch

  - Dentigerous cyst associated with unerupted supernumerary teeth.
  - Class II dentigerous cyst associated with partially erupted teeth.

Differential Diagnosis

- *Ameloblastoma and ameloblastic fibroma:* These are multilocular, not associated with crown of unerupted tooth. They will grow laterally away from the tooth in comparison to dentigerous cyst, which envelop the tooth symmetrically and is more common in the premolar-molar area.

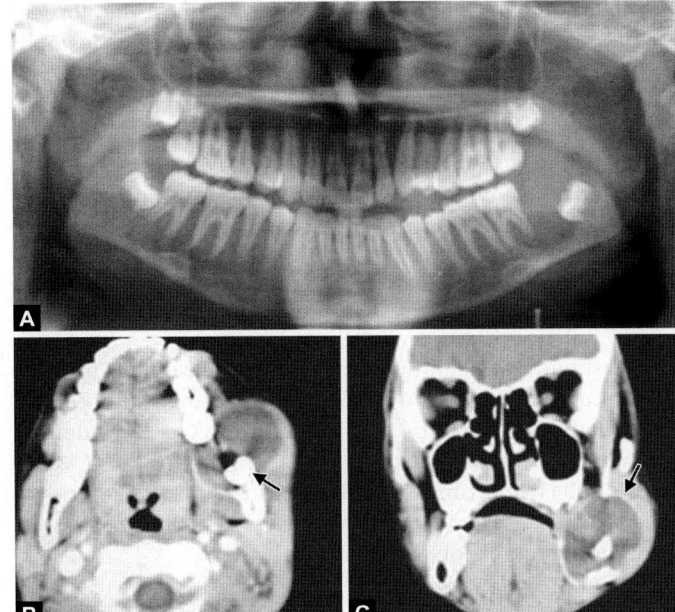

Figures 21.16A to C Dentigerous cyst: (A) Panoramic radiograph showed a large well-circumscribed radiolucency in left angle of mandible extending from lower left second molar up to half the height of ramus, in relation to developing mesioangularly placed third mandibular molar. CT scan: (B) Contrast enhanced axial; (C) Coronal section revealed a 5 × 4 × 3 cm well-defined expansile cystic lesion involving left half of mandible extending to middle of ramus, in relation to crown of unerupted third molar. Buccolingual expansion was noted, laterally it indented and displaced the masseter muscle and caused cortical thinning

- *Adenomatoid odontogenic tumor*: These are rare and usually occur in the maxillary anterior region.
- *Calcifying odontogenic cyst*: It may occur as a pericoronal radiolucency and may contain evidences of calcification.
- *Developmental primordial and follicular primordial cyst*: This occurs in close proximity to the crown of unerupted teeth and the superimposition of the image may cause the cyst like radiolucency to appear as dentigerous cyst on the radiograph. In primordial cyst the cystic lining surrounds the crown whereas in dentigerous cyst, it is attached to the neck of the tooth. A radiograph with a changed angulation will help in the diagnosis.
- *KCOT*: It does not expand the bone to the same extent, is less likely to resorb teeth and may attach further apically on the root instead of at the cementoenamel junction.
- *Cystic ameloblastoma.*
- *Radicular cyst*: At the apex of a primary tooth, surrounds the crown of the developing permanent tooth positioned apical to it, giving a false impression of a dentigerous cyst. Especially in the mandibular deciduous molars and developing bicuspids. The clinician should look for deep caries or extensive restorations in the primary tooth which would indicate a radicular cyst.

- *Hyperplastic follicle*: If the follicular space is more than 5 mm (normal is 2–3 mm) a dentigerous cyst is suspected. The region may be re-examined 4–6 monthly to detect any increase in size or changes in the surrounding structures.

Additional Imaging

- Reverse townes projection with maximum jaw opening, is an ideal view if the mandibular third molar is impacted in the ascending ramus, the cystic expansion can thus be depicted in the frontal plane.
- Axial CT is required to localize large cysts in the body of the mandible or at the angle, especially before surgery.
- It has been found that malignant tumors especially squamous cell carcinoma and mucoepidermoid carcinoma, may arise in the lining of the dentigerous cyst. CT examination aids in delineating the extent of the malignant lesions and discloses the invasion of adjacent anatomic regions.

Management

Treatment consists of surgery or decompression depending on the size of the lesion.

Eruption Cyst (Eruption Hematoma)

Definition

This is a form of dentigerous cyst associated with the erupting deciduous or permanent teeth in children. It occurs when a tooth is embedded in its eruption within the soft tissue overlying the bone.

Clinical Features

- It appears as a circumscribed, fluctuant often translucent swelling of the alveolar ridge over the site of eruption of the tooth.
- When the circumscribed cystic cavity contains blood the swelling appears purple or deep blue, hence it is called eruption hematoma.

Radiographic Features

- There is the expansion of the normal follicular space of the erupting tooth crown.
- In some cases there is a saucer shaped excavation of bone projecting very slightly into the cavity.

Calcifying Epithelial Odontogenic Cyst (CEOC) (Calcifying Odontogenic, Gorlin's Cyst) (Fig. 21.17)

Definition

This is an unusual lesion with features suggestive of a cyst and characteristics of a solid neoplasm. The World Health

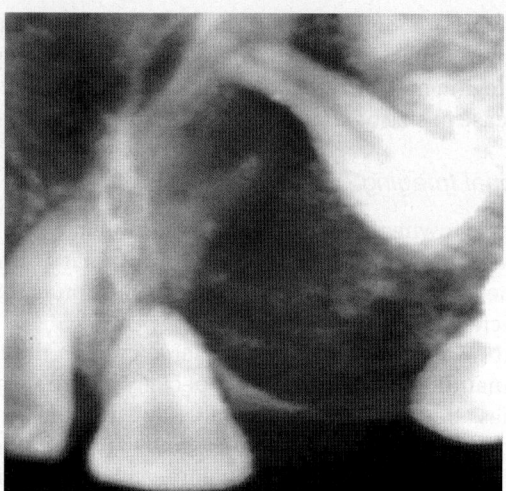

Figure 21.17 Radiograph showing a well-defined, unilocular radiolucency with sclerotic border associated with an unerupted 22 in the center, extending anteroposteriorly from the periapex of 11 to mesial root apex of 26, medially extending from the periapex of 11 to nasal septum causing obliteration of left nasal cavity and superiorly causing displacement of the floor of the maxillary antrum in the upward direction. There was dense cluster of radiopacity seen close to the crown of 22 and radiopaque foci dispersed throughout the radiolucency. Displacement of 21 and 23 was seen

Organization has now categorized calcifying odontogenic cysts as benign tumors. It usually arises centrally within the bone, but it may occur peripherally in the soft tissue. It is also known as intraosseous odontogenic cyst.

It is divided into three stages: Simple unicystic, unicystic odontome producing type, unicystic ameloblastomatous proliferating type.

Clinical Features

- It is more common in women, with a wide age range that peaks at 10 to 19 years, with a mean age of 36 years and the second peak occurs during the seventh decade.
- 3/4th of the lesions occur centrally, 75% occurring anterior to the first molar. It is equally affecting both the jaws.
- It is a slow growing. Painless, nontender swelling, which may cause expansion and/or destruction of the cortical plates. The cystic mass may become palpable and discharging.
- Adjacent teeth may be displaced.
- It may be associated with an odontoma, and may have calcified material identified as dysplastic dentine.
- Aspiration yields a viscous, granular, yellow fluid.

Radiographic Features

- The radiographic picture is variable.
- The central lesion may appear as a cyst like radiolucency with variable margins which may be smooth well defined or irregular in shape with poorly defined borders. It may

be unilocular or multilocular. Perforation of the cortical plate can be seen radiographically with enlarging lesions.
- It may be associated with unerupted teeth (usually a cuspid) and in some cases as a pericoronal radiolucency.
- It may resorb roots of adjacent teeth.
- The radiolucency may contain small foci of calcified material, seen as white flecks or smooth pebbles (radiopacities). At times the entire lesion may be occupied by the calcific body and thus appear radiopaque.

Additional Imaging

The desquamated keratin creates an increased attenuation area in a cyst. By varying the window setting, both keratin and calcifications can be identified on the CT. By widening the window settings, desquamated keratin with a CT value of 100–200 HU becomes less distinct due to less of soft tissue details, whereas calcifications with HU value of 800–1600 HU remains detectable on the CT.

Differential Diagnosis

- *Fibrous dysplasia (initial stage)*: It appears as mottled or has smoky defined borders, more common in the maxilla.
- *Partially calcified odontoma*: This is surrounded by a capsule.
- *AOT*: In the intermediate stage of development AOT appears like a CEOC.
- *Ossifying fibroma (initial stage)*: This fibro-osseous lesion is situated in a more inferior position in the mandible. It may show root resorption. Histologically, it shows Chinese letter shaped islands of bone or calcifications distributed throughout the connective tissue.
- *Odontogenic fibroma*: Histologically, it shows odontogenic tissue like cementum.
- *Cementoblastoma*: The radiographic image is well defined and attached to the root of the tooth.
- Dentigerous cyst
- *Ameloblastic fibroadenoma*: The location is different.
- *Calcifying epithelial odontogenic tumor*: The location is different.
- Long standing cysts with dystrophic calcifications.

Management

Enucleation with curettage, with regular follow-up as malignant transformation has been reported.

ODONTOGENIC INFLAMMATORY CYSTS

Radicular Cyst (Apical Periodontal Cyst, Periapical Cyst or Dental Cyst) (Figs 21.18 to 21.23)

Definition

This is most likely the results when rests of epithelial cells (Malassez) in the periodontal ligament are stimulated to

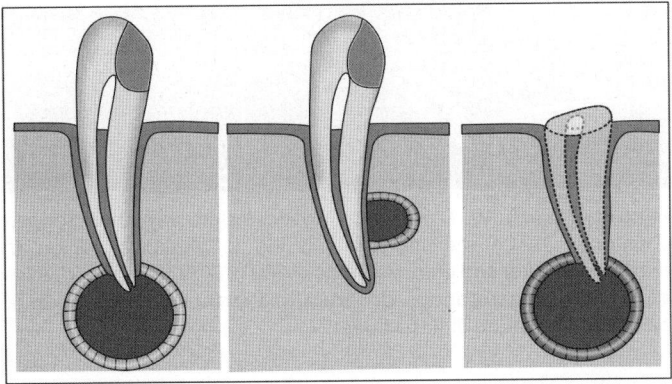

Figure 21.18 Schematic representation of apical, lateral and residual radicular cysts

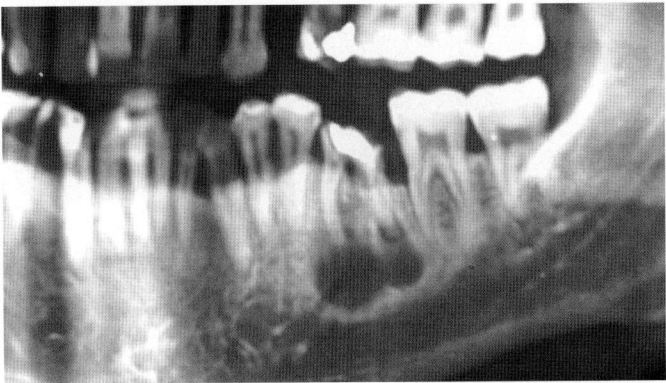

Figure 21.19 Cropped panoramic showing a well-defined radiolucency associated with lower first molar with corticated margins and loss of lamina dura, infected radicular cyst

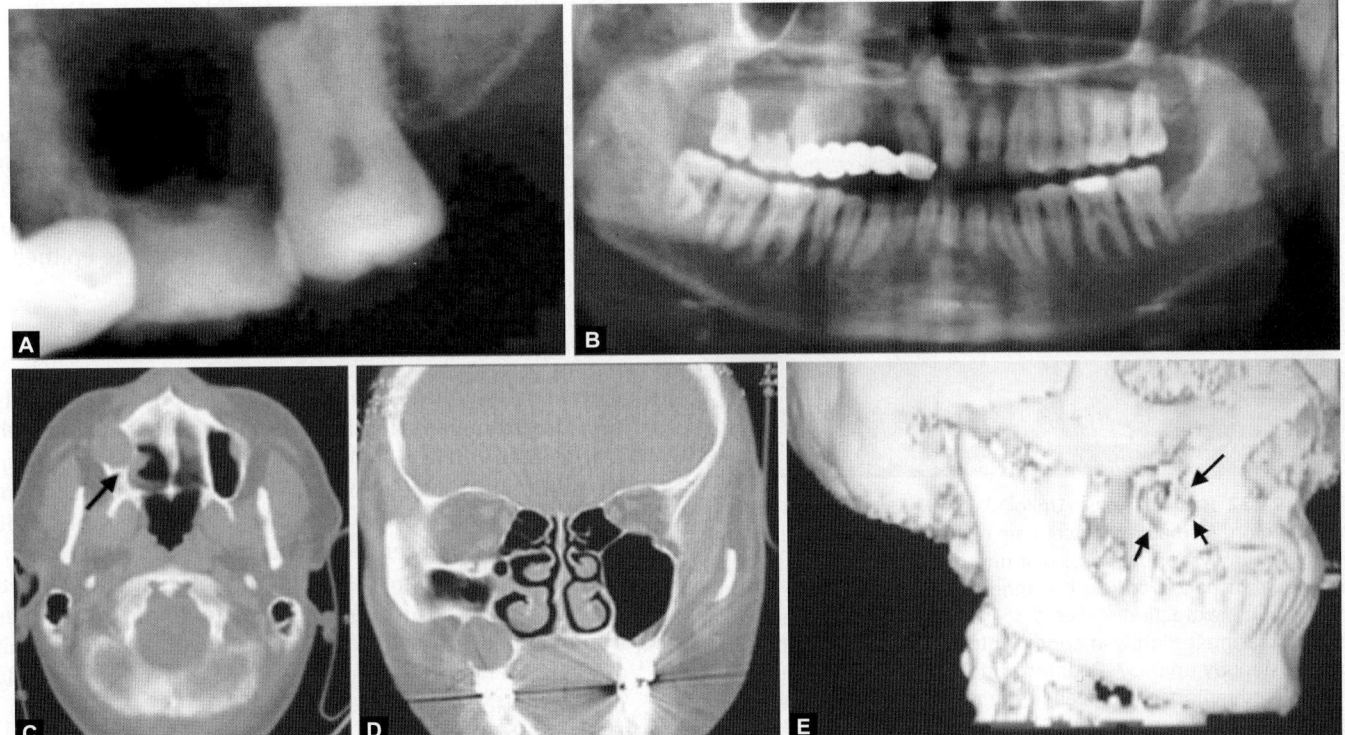

Figures 21.20A to E Radicular cyst: (A) IOPA shows complete resorption of roots of maxillary right first molar; (B) Panoramic radiograph showed a well-demarcated cystic lesion, involving maxillary right second premolar and first and second molar; (C) CT showed the expansion and resorption of the buccal cortical plate in 16 region, and thinning of the lingual cortical plate; (D) Coronal section also shows the buccal expansion and resorption, superiorly, displacing the floor of the maxillary sinus; (E) Defect seen on 3D CT

proliferate and undergo cystic degeneration by inflammatory products which are a common sequela in the progressive changes associated with bacterial invasion of the pulp and death of the dental pulp.

Clinical Features

• One of the most common types of cyst seen in the oral cavity

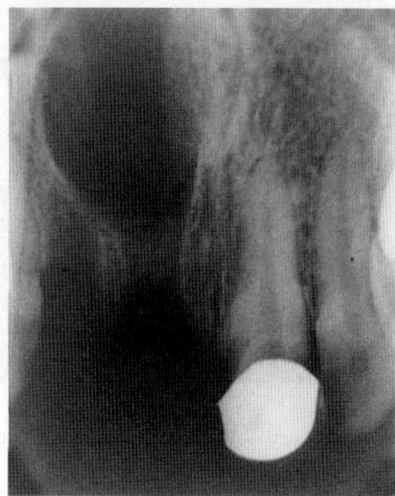

Figure 21.21 Residual radicular cyst with a well-defined circular radiolucency with sclerotic border is seen in relation to missing 11, 12. The radiolucency extends from the sockets of 11,12 and extends posteriorly

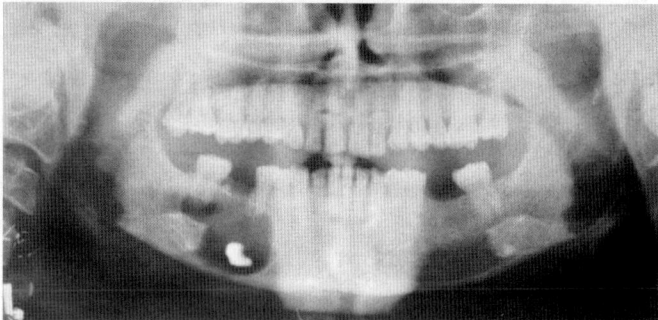

Figure 21.22 Radicular cyst: Unilocular radiolucent lesion seen in the 36 region. A small radiolucent area within the radiolucency seen giving cyst in cyst appearance pointing out towards break in either the lingual or buccal cortex. It extends superiorly from the alveolar crest from the extraction socket of 36 inferiorly up to the mandibular canal displacing it slightly inferiorly. Anteriorly it starts from posterior to 34 posteriorly up to 37. Root resorption in relation to 35 and 37. A well-defined radiopacity is seen in the radiolucent lesion suggestive of a restoration or a crown

- It most frequently occurs in the third decade of life, but a large number of cases are also seen from the third to sixth decades. Although dental caries is the most common in deciduous teeth, in the first decade, radicular cysts are not commonly found, may be because these teeth tend to drain more readily than permanent teeth and the antigenic stimuli that evoke the changes leading to the formation of radicular cyst may be different.
- There tends to be a male dominance, with the maxillary anterior teeth most commonly affected.
- They are usually associated with nonvital teeth.

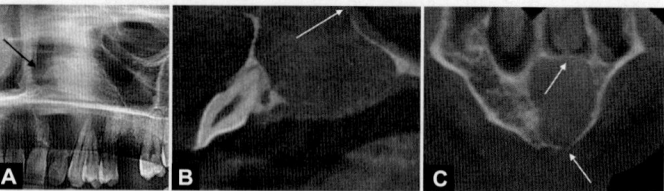

Figures 21.23A to C Periapical cystic lesion: (A) The cropped panaromic image showing cystic lesion in periapical region of maxillary anterior and premolar region. CBCT; (B) Sagittal and (C) Axial section showing expansion of cortical plates causing perforation of palate and elevation of nasal floor

- It represents an asymptomatic phase in periapical inflammatory process following death of dental pulp. It tends to remain small, if it grows, it may cause a nontender expansion of the overlying cortical bone; usually palatal in the maxilla and buccal in the mandible.
- The swelling may be bony hard or crepitations may be present as bone is thinned or it may be rubbery or fluctuant, if the bone is completely resorbed.
- Histologically, hyaline bodies or rushton bodies are found in great numbers. Straw colored fluid is obtained on aspiration.
- Ameloblastoma, epidermoid carcinoma and/or muccoepidermoid carcinoma may arise in the epithelial lining of periapical cyst.

Radiographic Features

- It appears as a round or pear shaped radiolucency, usually resulting from dental caries or trauma, in association with a nonvital tooth (a nonvital tooth may have a larger pulp chamber than the neighboring teeth because of the lack of secondary dentin, which normally forms with time in the pulp chamber and canal of a vital tooth.
- The epicenter of the radicular cyst is usually located approximately at the apex of a nonvital tooth. Sometimes it may appear on the mesial or distal surface of the root apex, at the opening of an accessory canal or infrequently in deep periodontal pockets.
- The radiolucency is usually more than 1.5 cm, but less than 3 cm in diameter. It has a well defined outline with hyperostotic borders. The margins are smooth, corticated and well-defined unless there is infection.
- The radiopaque border is continuous with the lamina dura around the associated teeth. Infection may cause it to become indistinct.
- Adjacent teeth are usually displaced. The cyst may invaginate the antrum, but usually an evidence of cortical boundary between the contents of the cyst and the internal structure of the antrum. Cysts may displace the mandibular alveolar nerve canal in an inferior direction. Radicular cysts formed in relation to nonvital deciduous molars may be positioned buccal to the developing cuspid.

- Radicular cyst of long duration may cause resorption of the tooth. The resorption pattern may have a curved outline. Dystrophic calcification may also develop in long standing cysts appearing as sparsely distributed, small particulate radiopacities.

Differential Diagnosis

- *Periapical granuloma*: It is less than 1.5 cm in diameter. Morse's method to differentiate, using alkaline copper tartrate with aspirate of root canal fluid from patients. If there is a cyst it will show an intense albumin pattern and definite pattern in globular zones on polyacryalamide gel electrophoresis and the fluid associated with periapical granuloma will show only faint to moderate pattern in the albumin zone.
- *Periapical scar*: It can be differentiated on the basis of history and location.
- *Surgical defect*: It can be differentiated on the basis of history and location.
- *Periapical cementoma (early stage)*: Here the involved tooth is vital and this usually and more commonly involves the lower incisors.
- *Traumatic bone cyst*: Associated with vital teeth and more often found in the mandibular premolar-molar region.
- *Periodontal abscess*: Tooth is vital, may show moderate to severe crestal bone loss, lesion appears more diffuse with hazy margins.
- *Mandibular infected buccal cyst*: It is more common in young patients, tooth is vital, with intact lamina dura, most commonly the first molar is involved.
- *Benign tumor*: Presence of septa in the cavity, radiopaque band (capsule) and resorption of the involved teeth.
- *KCOT*: It should be differentiated from radicular cysts that originate from the maxillary lateral incisor and are positioned between the roots of the maxillary lateral incisor and cuspid. The associated tooth is usually vital.
- *Ossifying fibroma or fibro-osseous lesion*: A large radicular cyst that has invaginated the antrum may collapse and star filling in with new bone. Radiographically new bone always forms first at the periphery of the cyst wall as the cyst shrinks and not in the center, which is different from the pattern of bone formation that is seen in fibro-osseous lesions. Biopsy and histological analysis may result in erroneous diagnosis of ossifying fibroma or fibro-osseous lesion.

Management

Treatment consists of root canal therapy, apical surgery, extraction, enucleation and/or marsuperization.

Residual Cyst

Definition

This is that which remains after incomplete removal of the original cyst or one that has either remained after the associated tooth was extracted or formed in the residual epithelial cell rests from the periodontal ligament of the lost tooth.

Clinical Features

- Usually asymptomatic and found on routine radiographic examinations. Seldom more than 5 to 10 mm in diameter.
- More common in older patients, males with higher incidence in the maxilla. It is found in the tooth bearing areas like, the alveolar process or the body of the tooth bearing area and sometimes lower ramus of the mandible.
- Patient may give history of a previous painful tooth.

Radiographic Features

- Pre-extraction radiograph will show tooth with evidence of deep caries or fracture with pulpal involvement and/or an associated cyst.
- It is seen as a round to ovoid, well circumscribed unilocular radiolucency with thin radiopaque margins. In cases of infection it loses its well defined margins.
- They may cause root displacement or resorption. The cyst enlarges in an elliptical shape leading to expansion of the outercortical plates of the jaws. The cyst may invaginate the maxillary antrum or depress the alveolar nerve canal.
- Dystrophic changes may be seen in long standing cysts.

Differential Diagnosis

- *Primordial cyst*: Here the tooth is missing without history of extraction, more common in the mandibular posterior region, younger age group and on aspiration shows straw colored fluid.
- *KCOT*: It is more common in mandibular posterior region, younger age group, may appear multilocular and is larger than a residual cyst.
- *Traumatic cyst*: Usually in the mandible, associated with the apical region of a tooth, having a scalloped outline, more common in the younger age group and aspiration is nonproductive.
- *Ameloblastoma (initial stages/unilocular)*: Usually the lesion appears larger with no history of tooth extraction.
- *Stafne developmental salivary gland defect*: The epicenter is located below the mandibular canal and is thus less likely to be odontogenic in nature.

Management

Treatment consists of enucleation or marsuparization.

Buccal Bifurcation Cyst (Mandibular Infected Buccal, Paradental, Inflammatory Collateral Dental Cyst)

Definition

The source of epithelium probably is the epithelial cell rests in the periodontal membrane of the buccal bifurcation of mandibular molars. It is proposed the inflammation may be the stimulus. It is unclear whether the paradental cyst of the third molar and the buccal bifurcation cyst of the first and second molars is the same entity.

Clinical Features

- Usually detected in the younger age group, in the first two decades.
- Delay in the eruption of the mandibular first and second molar. The first molar is more frequently involved than the second molar.
- On clinical examination the molar may be missing or the lingual cusp tips may be abnormally protruding through the mucosa, higher than the position of the buccal cusps.
- The teeth are vital.
- A hard swelling may be present, buccal to the involved molar, pain is present only in case of secondary infection.

Radiographic Features

- On the periapical and panaromic films the lesion may appear to be centered a little distal to the furcation of the involved tooth.
- Located in the buccal furcation of the mandibular first molar, followed by the second molar. The entire interradicular bone may be lost.
- The cyst is usually bilateral.
- The lesion is seen as a circular shaped with well defined radiolucency with cortical borders, which may be superimposed over the image of the roots of the molar. The lamina dura is intact.
- The cyst may become quite large before it is detected on the radiograph.
- It causes tipping of the involved molar so that the root tips are pushed into the lingual cortical plate of the mandible and the occlusal surface is tipped towards the buccal aspect of the mandible. The best diagnostic film is the cross-sectional (standard) mandibular occlusal projection, which demonstrates the abnormal position of the root apex.
- If the cyst is large it may displace or resorb the adjacent teeth and cause smooth expansion of the buccal cortical plate.
- If the cyst is secondarily infected, periosteal new bone formation is seen on the buccal cortex adjacent to the involved tooth. The new bone may be laid down either as a single linear band or laminated, if there are more than two layers. Sometimes the new bone may be homogeneous.

Differential Diagnosis

- *Periodontal abscess*: This also elicits an inflammatory periosteal response on the buccal side of the mandible, but there is no tilting of the involved teeth.
- *Langerhan's cell histiocytosis*: This also elicits an inflammatory periosteal response on the buccal side of the mandible, but there is no tilting of the involved teeth.
- *Dentigerous cyst*: The epicenter is different, the buccal bifurcation cyst sarts near the bifurcation region of the tooth and does not surround the crown, as does the dentigerous cyst.

Management

Removal by conservative curettage, extraction of the involved molar, or sometimes the lesion may resolve on its own.

Paradental Cyst

Definition

This is an inflammatory cyst occurring on the lateral aspect of the third molar with an associated history of pericoronitis.

Clinical Features

- Usually detected in the younger age group, in the third decade, with predilection for males.
- It is usually associated with the third molar on the buccal surface and covers the bifurcation. The tooth is usually vital.
- It may occur bilaterally.

Radiographic Features

- It is a well demarcated radiolucency occurring distal to the partially erupted tooth with buccal superimposition.
- The radiolucency may sometimes extend apically, but an intact periodontal ligament space confirms that the lesion did not originate at the apex.

Differential Diagnosis

- *Periodontal abscess*: This also elicits an inflammatory periosteal response on the buccal side of the mandible, but there is no tilting of the involved teeth.
- *Langerhan's cell histiocytosis*: This also elicits an inflammatory periosteal response on the buccal side of the mandible, but there is no tilting of the involved teeth.
- *Dentigerous cyst*: The epicenter is different, the buccal bifurcation cyst sarts near the bifurcation region of the tooth and does not surround the crown, as does the dentigerous cyst.

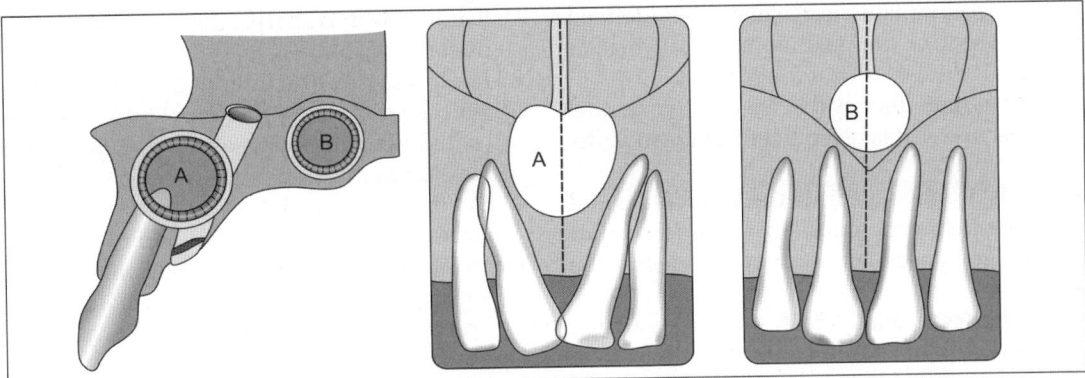

Figure 21.24 Schematic representation of: (A) Nasopalatine cyst; (B) Median fissural cyst

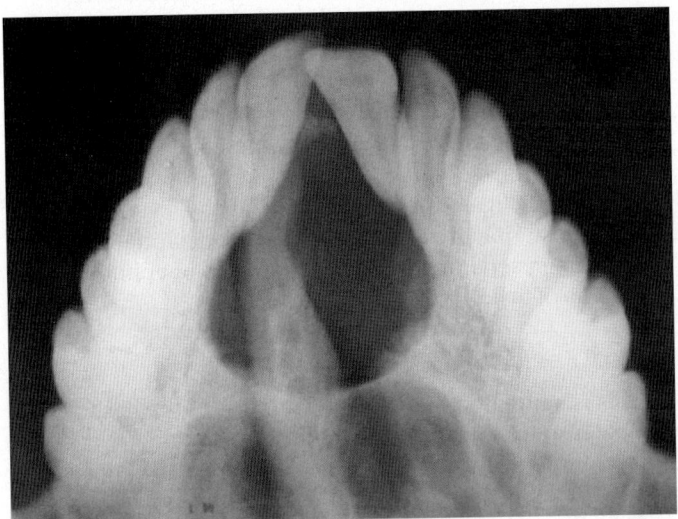

Figure 21.25 Maxillary occlusal shows a nasopalatine cyst with a well circumscribed unilocular cystic radiolucency in anterior maxilla between central incisors. The lesion is round and has corticated margins. Superiorly it extends into the palatal vault causing expansion and resorption of nasal floor

Management

Treatment consists of surgical enucleation.

NONODONTOGENIC CYSTS

Nasopalatine Canal Cyst (Nasopalatine Duct Cyst, Incisive Canal Cyst, Nasopalatine Cyst, Median Anterior Maxillary Cyst) (Figs 21.24 to 21.26)

Definition

This is developmental in origin and arises in the nasopalatine canal when embryonic epithelial remnants of the nasopalatine duct undergo proliferation and cystic degeneration.

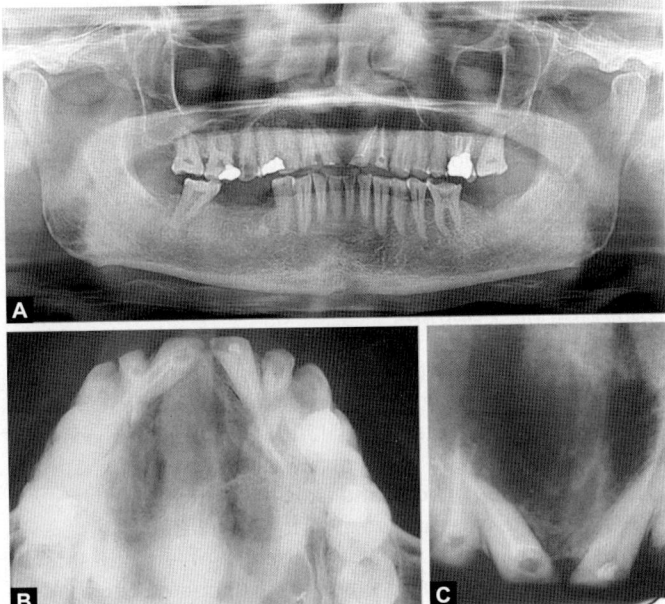

Figures 21.26A to C Nasopalatine cyst: (A) Panoramic radiograph shows well-defined corticated radiolucent lesion in anterior maxilla. The lesion is roughly heart shaped. It extends from root of lateral incisor crossing the midline to mesial aspect of roots of left premolar. The lesion has caused the distal displacement of the roots of the central incisors; (B) Maxillary occlusal radiograph shows well-defined corticated radiolucent lesion. The lesion was roughty heart shaped; (C) Periapical radiograph shows a well-defined radiolucent corticated lesion extending from the mesial aspect of the root of central incisor crossing the midline up to the crestal bone between the two centrals

Clinical Features

- It accounts for 10% of the jaw cysts, common in the 4th and 6th decade of life, more frequent in edentulous patients with a greater tendency for males.
- Most of these cysts are asymptomatic.

- The most frequent complaint is a small well defined swelling, just posterior to the palatine papilla, which is fluctuant and blue if the cyst is near the surface.
- The deeper nasopalatine duct cyst is covered by normal appearing mucosa unless it is ulcerated from masticatory trauma.
- If the cyst expands. It may penetrate the labial plate and produce a swelling below the maxillary labial frenum or to one side, or bulge into the nasal cavity and distort the nasal septum.
- Pressure from the cyst may affect the nasopalatine nerve, causing a sensation or numbness over the palatal mucosa.
- In some cases the cystic fluid may drain into the oral cavity through a sinus tract or a remnant of the nasopalatine duct, which the patients reports as a salty taste.
- The roots of the central incisors may diverge.
- Sometimes a variety of the cyst may be seen formed in the palatine papillae. This is evidenced by an elevation or a round soft swelling of the palatine papillae which extends posteriorly along the midline of the palate and is not usually radiographically apparent, as it does not cause sufficient pressure on the bone to cause discernible bone resorption, but sometimes it may cause bony erosion.

Radiographic Features

- This is found in the nasopalatine foramen or canal. If it extends posteriorly to involve the hard palate it may be referred to as a median palatine cyst; and if it extends anteriorly between the centrals, destroying or expanding the labial plate of bone and causing the teeth to diverge, it is referred to as a median anterior maxillary cyst.
- It is well defined corticated, circular or oval in shaped radiolucency. 6 mm to several cm in diameter. The shadow of the nasal spine is superimposed on the cyst giving it a heart shape.
- Two separate radiolucencies may develop in the two canals and cause 'a paired cyst' like radiolucency.
- If the cyst is formed in one of the branches of the canal, the image will be displaced on one side of the midline.
- The adjacent teeth show distal displacement but are rarely resorbed. Sometimes there is divergence of the central incisor roots with external root resorption.
- When seen laterally, the cyst may expand the labial as well as palatal cortex. The floor of the nasal fossa may be displaced in a superior direction.
- In some cysts internal dystrophic calcifications may be seen which appear as ill-defined amorphous scattered radiopacities.

Differential Diagnosis

- *Incisive fossa*: The shape varies from round/triangular/diamond/funnel shaped. The radiolucency is less than 6 mm wide. It is sharply defined at the lateral margins and no fluid is aspirated.
- *Radicular cyst*: The pulp of the involved tooth is nonvital with loss of lamina dura. Slob rule may be applied to differentiate between a periapical lesion and the developmental cyst.
- *Dentigerous cyst with mesodents*: Radiographic evidence of association with supernumerary teeth.
- *Median palatine cyst*: Radiolucent lesion is behind the incisive canal in the premolar region.
- *Primordial cyst from supernumerary*: More common in posterior teeth. .

Management

Treatment consists of enucleation or marsupalization.

Median Palatine Cyst

Definition

Some people believe that this cyst is actually a nasopalatine cyst that has developed posteriorly.

Some investigators now believe that this cyst represents a more posterior presentation of a nasopalatine duct cyst, rather than a separate cystic degeneration of epithelial rests at the line of fusion of the palatine shelves.

Clinical Features

- This is a rare cyst, found in the midline of the hard palate, posterior to the roof of the mouth
- As it enlarges it produces a swelling on the roof of the mouth
- It is fluctuant, nontender and the overlying mucosa is normal
- As the cyst enlarges there is perforation of the cortical plate, if the cyst is displaced superiorly there may be erosion of the floor of the nasal fossa
- The maxillary teeth are vital
- On aspiration, amber colored fluid is obtained.

Radiographic Features

A radiolucent lesion with well defined hyperostotic borders is seen behind the incisive canal in the premolar-molar region.

Differential Diagnosis

- *Nasopalatines cyst*: Location is more anterior
- *Radicular cyst*: Tooth involved is nonvital with a discontinuous lamina dura and widened periodontal ligament
- *Plexiform neurofibroma*: Aspiration is nonproductive
- *Palatal space abscess*: Adjacent teeth will be nonvital, swelling will be soft, fluctuant and pus will be aspirated
- *Incisive canal cyst*: This occurs in the canal above the palatine papillae whereas the midpalatine occurs in midline of palate posterior to palate

- *Retention phenomenon*: It is seen laterally and not in the midline. Aspiration will yield viscous, clear sticky liquid
- *Malignant and benign tumors of the salivary gland*: These are usually placed laterally and not in the midline.

Management

Treatment is surgical excision.

Globulomaxillary Cyst (Intra-alveolar Cyst, Premaxillary Maxillary Cyst) (Figs 21.27 and 21.28)

Definition

It occurs in the globulomaxillary region and is considered to be an inclusion or developmental cyst that arises from entrapped nonodontogenic epithelium in globulomaxillary suture (at the junction of the globular portion of the medial nasal process and maxillary process).

The developmental origin has been disputed. Today, most literature agree based on overwhelming evidence that the cyst is predominantly of tooth origin (odontogenic), demonstrating findings consistent with periapical cysts, odontogenic keratocysts or lateral periodontal cysts.

Clinical Features

- It is asymptomatic and usually discovered on routine radiological examination.
- If the cyst becomes infected, the patient may complain of pain or local discomfort in that area.
- As it enlarges it expands the buccal plates between the maxillary lateral and canine, and also diverges the roots causing rotation of the crowns with their contact point moving incisally. Adjacent teeth are usually vital.
- The mucosa over the expanding cortex remains normal in color, and if there is erosion of the cortical plate, then a fluctuant swelling develops, which on palpation produces crepitus.
- It may get secondarily infected and mimic a lateral periodontal abscess.
- Aspiration produces a typical amber straw colored fluid.

Radiographic Features

- It appears as a 'inverted pear shaped' or 'inverted tear shaped' radiolucency between the roots of the maxillary lateral incisor and canine. The small end of the pear is directed towards the crest of the alveolar ridge. The upper borders may invaginate the floor of the nasal fossa or antrum.
- The size may vary from small to a maximum diameter of 3–4 cm.
- Displacement of the teeth is common, with divergence of the adjacent roots. The lamina dura of the teeth is well-defined and intact.
- There may be root resorption.

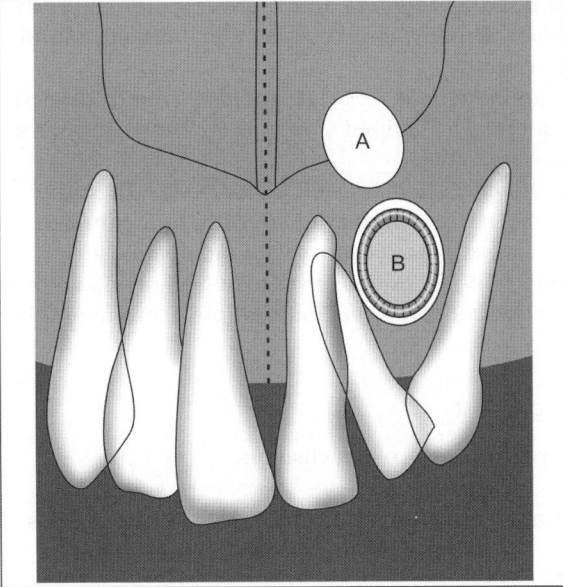

Figure 21.27 Schematic representation of nasoalveolar (A) and globulomaxillary cysts (B)

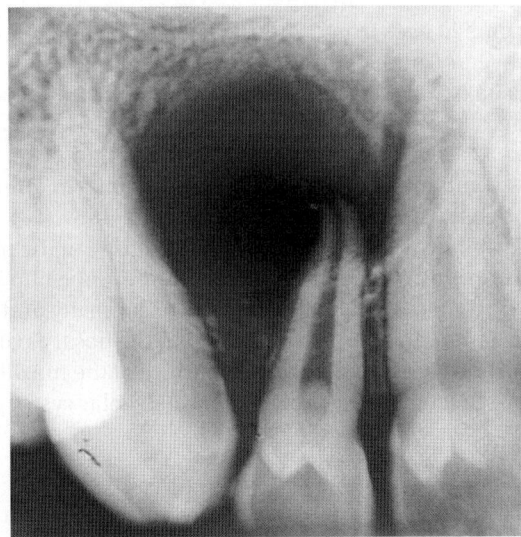

Figure 21.28 Globulomaxillary cyst as seen on a cropped panoramic radiograph between the maxillary lateral and canine

Differential Diagnosis

- *Lateral periodontal cyst*: It appears as a dome shaped radiolucency commonly seen in the mandibular lateral incisor and first premolar region, in the older age group.
- *Lateral dentigerous cyst*: It is associated with impacted teeth, especially the radiolucency is associated with the crown (attached to the neck of the tooth).
- *Primordial cyst (KCOT)*: It is more common in the mandibular posterior region.

- *Giant cell granuloma*: It is more common in the anterior region. Usually, it appears as a mandibular multilocular radiolucency.
- *Traumatic bone cyst*: It appears round shaped with moderately defined outline. Needle aspiration is nonproductive.
- *Adenomatoid odontogenic tumor (AOC)*: The radiolucency is associated with unerupted teeth. In the mature stage it appears as a radiolucency with radiopaque foci.
- *Surgical defect*: Patient gives history of previous surgery.
- *Anatomical variation*: For example, a prominent incisive fossa.

Management

Treatment consists of enucleation.

Nasoalveolar Cyst (Nasolabial Cyst, Klestadt's Cyst)

Definition

This is a soft tissue cyst which may involve the bone secondarily.

Clinical Features

- It occurs in ages from 12 to 75 years, with a mean average of 41 years, more common in women.
- It usually occurs unilaterally, but on rare occasions bilateral occurrence has also been seen.
- There is a swelling of the nasolabial fold and nose, which may sometimes cause pain and difficulty in breathing through the nose.
- The swelling is fluctuant, and causes flaring of the ala and distortion of the nostril, fullness of the upper lip below the vestibule. It may bulge into the nasal cavity and cause obstruction. Infection may drain into the nasal cavity.
- Superficial erosion of the outer surface of the maxilla may be produced by pressure of the nasoalveolar cyst.

Radiographic Features

- This is primarily a soft tissue lesion located adjacent to the alveolar process above the apices of the incisors. Thus, plain radiographs may not show any detectable changes. CT or MRI will provide an image of the soft tissues.
- An increased radiolucency of the alveolar bone beneath the cyst and above the apices of the incisors, sometimes causing erosion of the underlying bone, and an outline of the inferior border of the nasal fossa is distorted resulting in posterior convergence of the margins.
- A tangential view will demonstrate a kidney shaped lesion below the margin of the nasal fossa and above the apices of the incisors, if the cystic fluid is aspirated and replaced with a radiocontrast material.

- A thin axial CT image using a soft tissue algorithm with contrast reveals a circular, oval lesion with slight soft tissue enhancement of the periphery. The internal aspect appears homogeneous and relatively radiolucent compared to the surrounding soft tissues.

Differential Diagnosis

- *Acute dentoalveolar abscess*: Teeth involved or adjacent are nonvital
- Nasal furuncle
- Mucus extravasation cyst
- Cystic salivary adenoma.

Management

Treatment consists of surgical excision.

Median Mandibular Cyst (Fig. 21.29)

Definition

This is a rare cyst of the symphyseal region of the mandible. Some believe that it may not be a distinct entity but a primordial cyst from a supernumerary tooth, a lateral periodontal cyst or a radicular cyst.

A true median mandibular cyst would therefore be classified as a non-odontogenic, fissural cyst. The existence of this lesion as a unique clinical entity is controversial, and some reported cases may have represented misdiagnosed odontogenic cysts, which are by far the most common type of

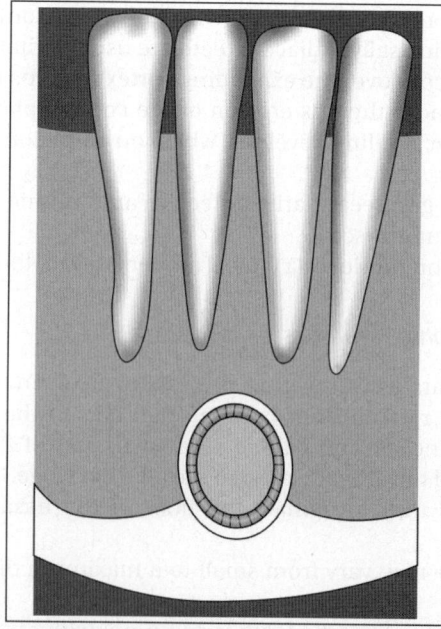

Figure 21.29 Schematic representation of a median mandibular cyst

intrabony cyst occurring in the jaws. It has also been suggested that the mandible develops as a bilobed proliferation of mesenchyme connected with a central isthmus. Therefore it is unlikely that epithelial tissue would become trapped as there is no ectoderm separating the lobes in the first instance.

Clinical Features

- It has a predilection for the inferior part of the mandible, thus it does not come in close relation with the roots of the lower incisors.
- These are usually clinically asymptomatic and are discovered on routine roentogenographic examination.

Radiographic Features

It appears as a unilocular, well circumscribed, well-defined round or ovoid radiolucency that may be regular or irregular in shape. It might have a multilocular appearance. As it expands it may separate the roots of the mandibular incisors, but the lamina dura remains intact. Sometimes the associated teeth may be nonvital. It seldom produces obvious expansion of the cortical plate of the bone.

Management

Treatment consists of surgical excision.

Anterior Alveolar Cyst (Median Alveolar Cyst)

Definition

This cyst appears in the intermaxillary suture anterior to the site of anterior palatine cyst.

Clinical Features

- It arises near the labial surface of the premaxilla between the two incisors.
- It may produce a swelling.

Radiographic Features

- It appears as an area of radiolucency in the midline in a position more close to the shadow of the crowns of the incisors than the root.
- The margins may or may not be sharply defined, with or without a thin layer of cortical bone at the periphery of the cavity.
- In some cases the cyst may come in contact with the roots and may cause symmetrical resorption of the teeth.

Management

Treatment consists of surgical excision.

CYSTS OF THE SOFT TISSUES OF THE FACE AND NECK

Dermoid Cyst

Definition

These are a rare developmental anomaly which may be found anywhere in the body. It is a cystic form of a teratoma, which is believed to be derived from trapped embryonic cells that are totipotent. In the oral cavity they are found in the floor of the mouth and tongue, usually in the midline or lateral to it. The resulting cysts are lined with epidermis and cutaneous appendages and filled with keratin (epidermoid cyst) or sebaceous material (dermoid cyst), (and in rare cases with bone, teeth, muscle or hair, called teratomas).

Types

Median variety:
- Supramylohyoid variety
- Inframylohyoid variety.

Lateral variety:
- Supramylohyoid variety
- Inframylohyoid variety.

Clinical Features

- It develops in the soft tissues at any time from birth, but usually becomes clinically evident between 12–25 years of age, about equally distributed between the sexes.
- It is a slow growing painless swelling, which can grow to several centimeters in diameter, and when located in the neck or tongue, it may interfere with breathing, speaking or eating. Depending on how deep the cyst is positioned in the neck, it can deform the submental area.
- If superficial, it appears yellow to white and the surface is smooth and nonulcerated until traumatized.
- Inframylohyoid variety, causes swelling in the submental area and gives rise to a double chin appearance.
  - On palpation it is soft to firm, rubbery or cheesy, fluctuant or doughy, usually sharply delineated with straw colored fluid. Teeth are not affected as it lies in the midline.
- It does not move with the protrusion of the tongue.
- Transillumination test is usually negative.

Radiographic Features

- It appears radiolucent except in cases where teeth or bones are present which appears radiopaque.
- If the extent of the cyst has to be defined, then some of its contents need to be removed to enable introduction of an opaque substance such as lipiodol, after which a

radiographs are taken from various positions to enable the opaque material to find its way by gravity to each portion of the cyst.

- Diagnostic imaging is best accomplished by CT or MRI.
- On the CT the periphery of the lesion is well defined by more radiopaque soft tissue of the cyst compared with surrounding soft tissue. They seldom have any mineralized structures especially when they occur in the oral cavity. It may show a soft tissue multilocular appearance.

Differential Diagnosis

- *Ranula*: This is not in the midline, appears bluish, with transillumination test positive.
- *Unilateral or bilateral blockage of the Wharton's duct*: Complain of pain associated with eating.
- *Thyroglossal duct cyst*: It lifts when the patient swallows or protrudes the tongue.
- *Cellulitis*: The swelling is diffuse and wide spread.
- *Submandibular lymph node swelling*: This is solid.
- *Cystic hygroma*: Painless compressible swelling, bluish in color and transillumination is positive.
- *Branchial cleft cyst (lymphoepithelial cyst)*: The swelling varies in size from small to large (10 cm in diameter), which may be progressive or intermittent and pain is also a prominent sign.
- *Tumors*: Lipoma, liposarcoma.
- Normal fat masses in the submental areas.

Management

Treatment consists of surgical removal.

PSEUDO BONE CYSTS

Simple bone cyst (traumatic bone cyst, hemorrhagic bone cyst, extravasation cyst, progressive bone cyst, solitary bone cyst, unicameral bone cyst, idiopathic bone cavity) (**Figs 21.30 to 21.32**).

Definition

This is a cavity within the bone that is lined with connective tissue. It may be empty or it may contain fluid, but it has no epithelial lining. It may be caused due to a localized aberration in normal bone remodeling or metabolism, this is supported by the fact that the bone cavities often occur inside lesions of cemento-osseous dysplasia and fibrous dysplasia. No evidence exists to support the traumatic cause.

As there is no epithelium present in this cavity, traumatic bone cyst is now named 'Idiopathic bone cavity'.

Clinical Features

- These are common lesions, which occur in the first two decades of life. The lesion shows male predominance.

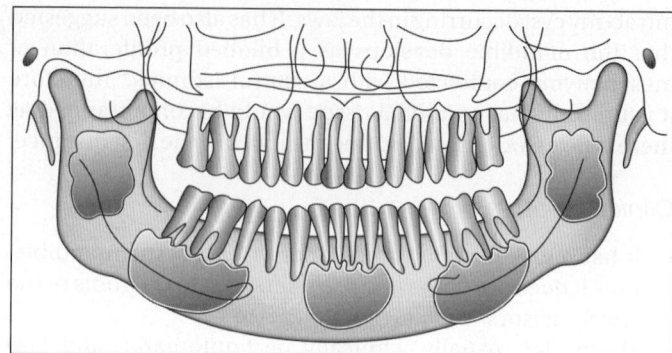

Figure 21.30 Schematic representation of typical sites of solitary bone cysts. The aneurysmal bone cyst is also commonly seen in the horizontal ramus of the mandible in 10 to 15 year old patients

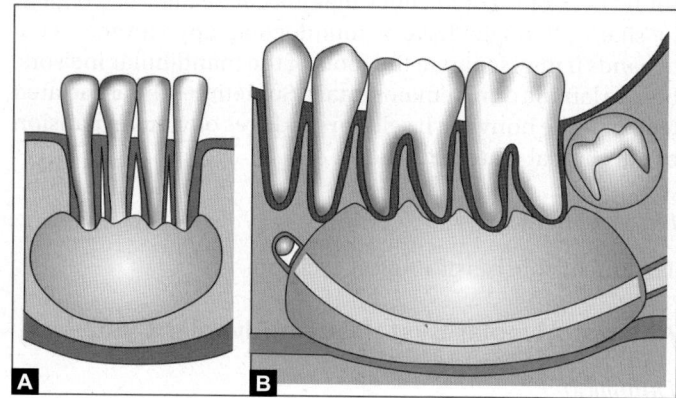

Figures 21.31A and B A schematic representation of solitary bone cyst in the mandible. Typical localization of traumatic bone cyst is seen in the figure on the left

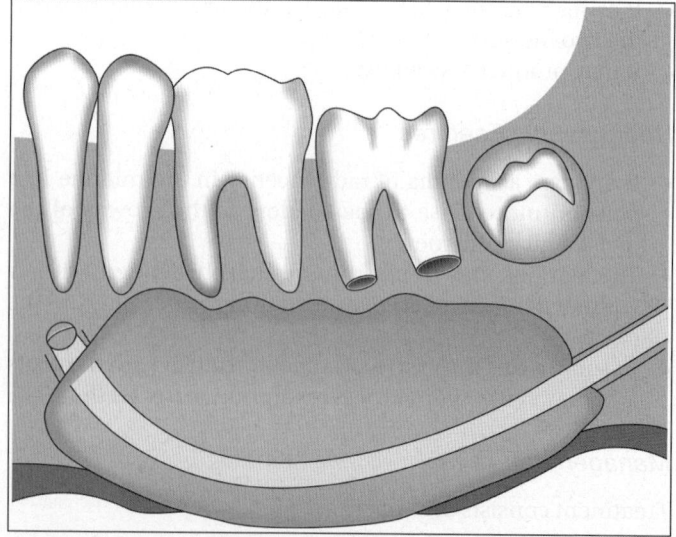

Figure 21.32 Schematic representation of an aneurysmal bone cyst

- Multiple simple bone cysts may develop when the disorder occurs with cemento-osseous dysplasia. This is more often seen in the older population with a female predominance.
- These are usually asymptomatic but occasionally pain or tenderness may be present, especially if it is secondarily infected. Usually, it is discovered on routine radiographic examination.
- They are usually found in the mandible anywhere from the symphysis to the ramus, but 1/3rd are found in the maxilla, usually in the anterior region.
- Expansion of the mandible or tooth movement may be observed.
- There is no significant incidence of pathologic fracture.
- When and if aspiration is productive, usually only a few milliliters of straw-colored or serosanguineous fluid is obtained.

Radiographic Features

- It appears as a radiolucent lesion with a spectrum of well-defined to moderately defined border.
- The margin may vary from a well-defined, delicate cortex to an ill-defined border that blends into the surrounding bone. The boundary is usually better defined in the alveolar process around the teeth than in the inferior aspect of the body of the mandible. The most commonly seen appearance is smooth and curved cyst like, with an oval or scalloped border. The lesion often scallops between the roots of the teeth.
- It usually appears radiolucent, but occasionally it may appear multilocular, although the lesion has no septa, the appearance may be a result of pronounce scalloping of the endosteal surface of either the buccal or lingual plates. The ridges of the bone produced by the scalloping give the appearance of septa on a lateral view of the mandible.
- The cyst may only one centimeter in diameter to that involving most of the molar area of the body of the mandible as well as part of the ramus, and extend to involve the alveolar process. It may be found in the edentulous as well the dentulous arch.
- The lesion usually has no effect on the surrounding teeth, sometimes tooth displacement and resorption may be noted. Often the lesion involves all the bone around the roots of the teeth but leaves the lamina dura intact or only partly disrupted. Similarly, the sparing of the cortical boundary of the crypt around a developing tooth is characteristic.
- Solitary bone cysts have a tendency to grow along the long axis of the bone, causing minimal expansion, however, in larger lesions buccal expansion may occur. The surfaces of the cortical plates are not disrupted and pathological fracture does not result.

Differential Diagnosis

- *Radicular cyst*: The involved tooth is nonvital, and all true cysts have a more rounded appearance.
- *Odontogenic keratocyst*: It have a definite cortical boundary, resorb and displace teeth, and occur in the older age group.
- *Central giant cell granuloma*: It shows evidence of internal bony septa, and more often found in the mandibular anterior region.
- *Ameloblastoma and odontogenic myxoma*: These are usually multilocular.
- *Lesions of eosinophilic granuloma*: These lesions are not as well corticated.
- *Fibrous dysplasia*: These lesions are not as well corticated.
- *Malignant lesion*: Bone around teeth is lost, but in solitary bone cyst there is some maintenance of the lamina dura, lack of invasive periphery and bone destruction.
- These lesions heal spontaneously sometimes, and biopsy and analysis of a healing cyst may falsely indicate presence of an ossifying fibroma or fibrous dysplasia because of the formation of immature bone.

Management

Treatment consists of enucleation and curettage.

Aneurysmal Bone Cyst (Figs 21.33 and 21.34)

Definition

This is an uncommon hemorrhagic lesion of the bone. The name of this entity is misleading, in that, it does not contain vascular aneurysms and it is not a true bony cyst. It represents an exaggerated localized proliferative response of the vascular tissue.

Aneurysmal bone cyst, the term is a misnomer, as the lesion is neither an aneurysm nor a cyst. Today it is termed central giant cell tumor as CGCT have venous pressure bleeding quality. ABC has macroscopic blood filled spaces. The term aneurysmal is also false as blood filled spaces contain fibroblasts and not endothelium and also there is no cystic lining.

Clinical Features

- More common in individuals less than 30 years of age, with a predisposition for females.
- More often found in the mandibular molar region.
- There may be history of traumatic injury and of recent displacement of teeth which are vital.
- It produces a firm, painful and tender swelling which rapidly progresses and worsens the symptoms.
- The patient will have difficulty in opening the mouth (if there is impingement of the lesion on the capsule of the TMJ).

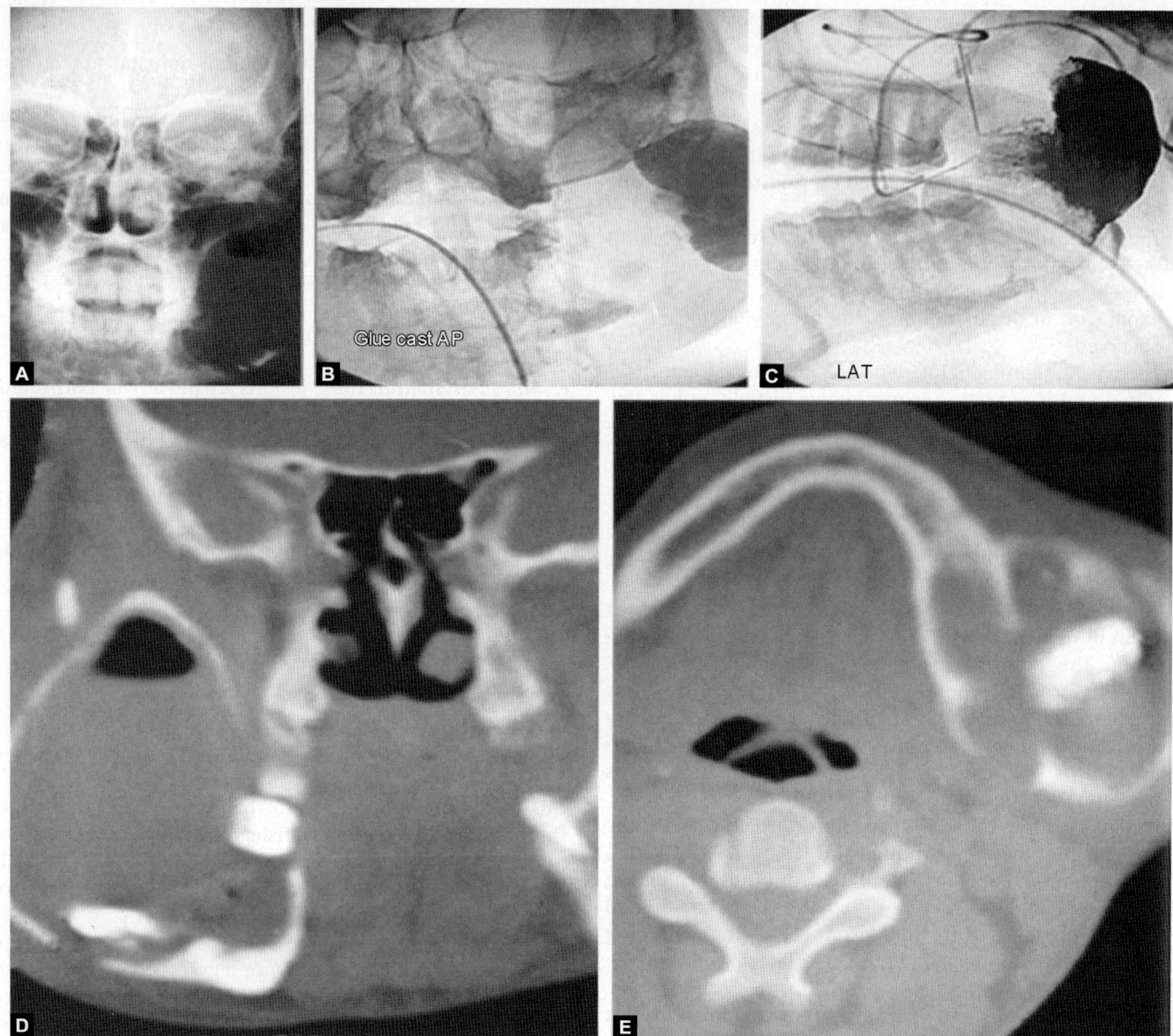

Figures 21.33A to E Aneurysmal bone cyst: (A) PA mandible revealed, a solitary, multilocular well-defined ovoid shaped corticated radiolucency in the left mandible. Expansion and bossing of the inferior and lateral margins of the mandible are seen; (B and C) Subtraction digital angiography revealed no vascularity in the lesion, but displaced branches could be seen due to the tumor effect; (D) CT scan (contrast) shows expansile lesion; (E) CT scan axial view shows expansile lesion

- There may be tilting or bodily displacement of the affected vital teeth.
- Excessive bleeding may occur.
- The lesion perforates the cortex and is covered by periosteum or only a thin shell of bone, it may exhibit springiness or egg-shell crackling, but is nonpulsatile. Bruit is not heard.

Radiographic Features

- This is an expansile osteolytic process within the affected bone and is seen as a definite radiolucency.
- As it enlarges in the anterior-posterior dimension, it produces expansion of the buccal and lingual cortical plates, which may be marked and described as ballooning or blowing out.

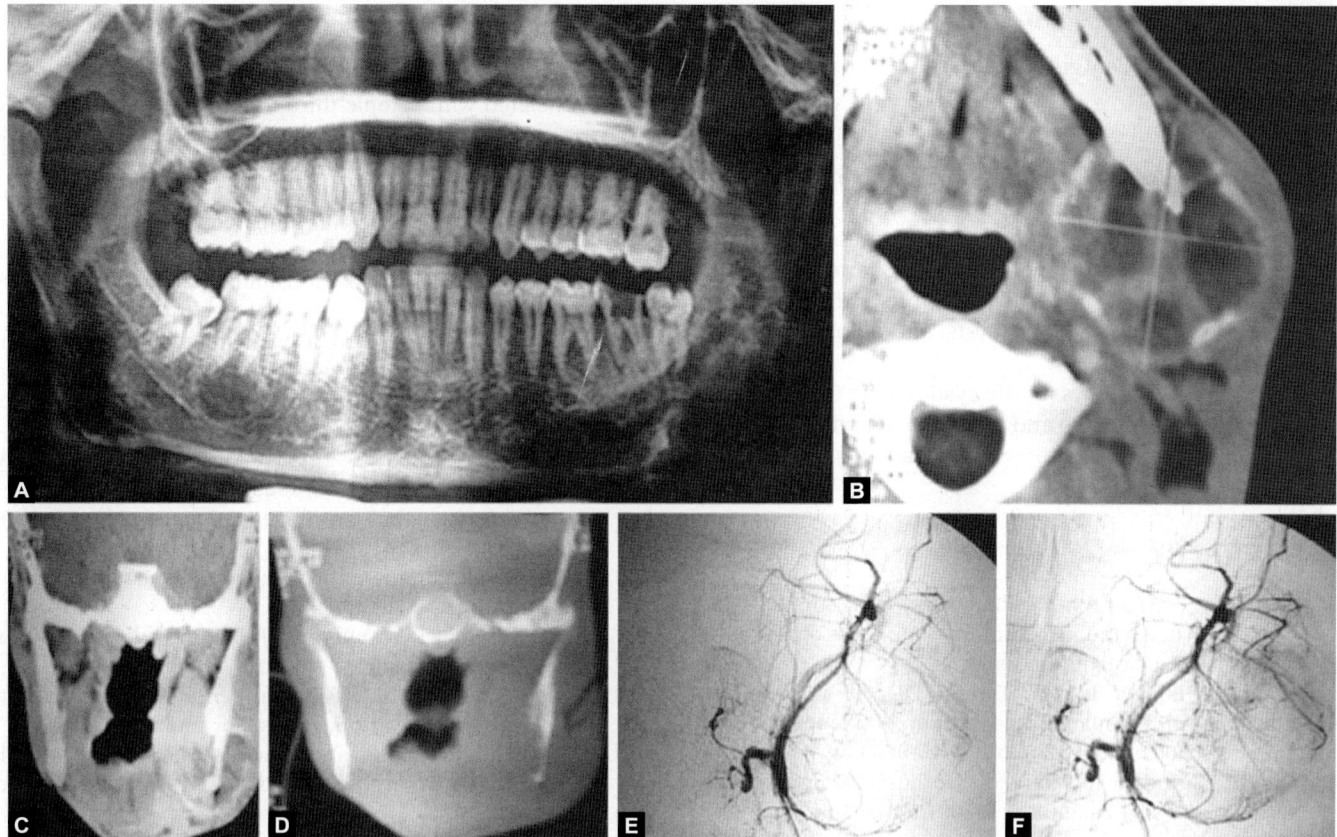

Figures 21.34A to F Aneurysmal bone cyst: (A) Panoramic radiograph revealed a multilocular radiolucency on the left side of mandible having a soap bubble appearance, extending anteroposteriorly from 38 region to middle of left ramus, with discontinuity of the outer cortical plate in left angle region. Grossly carious 36, 37. Vertically impacted 38, mesioangular impacted 48. Apical periodontal space widening in relation to 37. A well circumscribed area of rarefaction apical to 46; (B) Axial CT; (C and D) Coronal CT Scan: A multilocular well-circumscribed radiolucency with destruction of the lingual and inferior cortical plates of left angle and ramus of mandible was seen. Marked expansion of buccal and lingual cortices was pesent. There was heterogeneous enhancement of the lesion on contrast sections; (E and F) Angiogram of left carotid artery, revealed normal arterial phase, mild abnormal blush in capillary phase. The massetric branches of external carotid artery and jugular branches of right facial artery were stretched around the lesion

- Septa may be seen within the lesion. It has a soap bubble appearance, with regular margins.
- The involved teeth may be tilted, bodily displaced with some degree of external root resorption, though the tooth is not devitalized.

Differential Diagnosis

- *Ameloblastoma*: It is more in the older age group and in the mandibular posterior region.
- *Giant cell granuloma*: It is more common in the anterior region.
- *Central hemangioma*: It is more common in the mandible, it shows profuse hemorrahge if aspirated. Bruit is present.
- *Multilocular cyst*: It is more common in the mandibular posterior region and the borders are very well defined.
- *Odontogenic cyst*: The borders of aneurysmal bone cyst are less regular and distinct than that of an odontogenic cyst.
- *Odontogenic myxoma*: It is frequently associated with congenitally missing or unerupted teeth. It shows a typical honey comb appearance.
- *Cherubism*: It occurs in the younger age group and is usually bilateral.
- *Metastatic tumor*: It occurs in the older age group.
- *Giant cell lesion of hyperthyroidism*: More common in the older age group. Serum shows increased levels of alkaline phosphatase.
- *Central malignancy*: The borders of the aneurysmal bone cyst are much more discrete than that of central malignancy.

Management

Treatment consists of surgical curettage or cryosurgery.

General Treatment

- Regression of cysts without surgical treatment; this is usually true in cases of small radicular cysts.
- *Marsupialization of dental cysts*: It is also known as Partsch's operation. It involves making an opening into the cyst as large as practically possible and packing the cavity. This is useful for large cysts, and helps to preserve the remaining structures.
- *Enucleation*: This allows for the cystic cavity to be covered by a mucoperiosteal flap and the space fills with blood clot which will eventually become organized and form normal bone.

BIBLIOGRAPHY

1. Barnes L Eveson JW, Reichart P, et al. Pathology and genetics of head and neck tumors, Lyon: IARC Press; 2005. WHO classification of tumors series.
2. Bouquot JE, Neville BW, Damm DD, et al. Oral and maxillofacial pathology, 2nd edition. Philadelphia: WB Saunders; 2002.pp.30-1. ISBN 0-7216-9003-3.
3. Garg P, Karjodkar FK, Garg SK. Gorlin-Goltz Syndrome—Case Report. Clin Diagnos Res. 2001;5(2)393-5.
4. Goaz PW, White CS. Principles and Interpretation. In: Oral radiology, 3rd edition. St Louis: Mosby Year Book; 1994.
5. Kasad V, Karjodkar FR, Laddha R. Dentigerous Cyst Associated with ectopic third molar in maxillary sinus. A case report and review of literature. Contemparary Clinical Dentistry. 2012;3(3):373-6.
6. Miles DA, Van Dis MJ, Jensen CW, et al. Interpretation normal versus abnormal and common radiographic presentations of lesions. In: Radiographic and Imaging for Dental Auxillaries, 3rd edition. Philadelphia: WB Saunders; 1999.pp.231-80.
7. Neville BW, et al. (Eds). Developmental defects of the oral and maxillofacial region. In: Oral and Maxillofacial Pathology, 2nd edition. Philadelphia: WB Saunders; 2002.p.27.
8. Shafer WG, et al. A Text Book of Oral Pathology. Philadelphia: WB Saunders; 1983.
9. Shear M. Cysts of the Jaws: Recent advances. J Oral Pathol. 1985;14:43.
10. Shear M. Developmental odontogenic cysts: an update. J Oral Pathol. 1994;23:1.
11. Wood NK, Goaz PW. Differential Diagnosis of Oral Lesions. 4th edition. CV Mosby: St Louis; 1991.
12. Wood RE. Handbook of signs in dental and maxillofacial radiology. Warthog Publications, Toronto; 1988.
13. Worth HM. Principles and practice of oral radiographic interpretation. Year Book Medical Publishers, Chicago; 1963.

Benign Tumors of the Jaws

INTRODUCTION

A benign tumor is a new growth resembling the tissue of origin. It may be defined as a well differentiated structure which may be typical of tissue origin and shows progressive and slow rate of growth.

A growth disturbance that does not have the capacity for limitless proliferation is not a true neoplasm and is called *Hamartoma* or *Hyperplasia*.

Hamartoma are abnormal new growths (proliferation) of tissue in its usual location that cease growing along with the tissues of the associated parts (e.g. odontoma). Hamartomas are usually congenital and have a major period of growth at the time the rest of the body is growing. Once they have reached their adult dimensions, they do not extend to involve more tissue and rarely increase in size unless trauma, thrombosis, or infection complicates (e.g. hemangioma, lymphangioma, glomus tumor, granular cell myoblastoma of the tongue, fibrous dysplasia of bone (ossifying fibroma). They have a limited growth potential.

Hyperplasia is enlargement caused by an increase in the number of cells, and the tissue is in a normal arrangement. These are slow growing growths of new bone with normal architecture, on the bones of the skull and facial skeleton. It is believed to be a reaction to a stimulus such as inflammation. These growths have their limit and undergo spontaneous arrest, but are never seen to regress in size (e.g. exostosis, tori).

Neoplasm are tumors that continue to grow indefinitely. It is defined by sir Rupert Willis as an abnormal mass of tissue the growth of which exceeds and is unco-ordinated with that of normal tissues and persists in some excessive manner after cessation of stimulus which evoked the change.

Hypertrophy enlargement caused by an increase in the size of the cells.

Teratoma are neoplasms composed of a mixture of tissues, more than one of which exhibits neoplastic proliferation. They are congenitally acquired and usually found in the ovary.

CLASSIFICATION OF BENIGN TUMORS OF THE JAWS (TABLE 22.1)

General Characteristics

- Benign tumors are insidious in onset, are slow growing and spread by direct extension and not by metastases. They have an unlimited growth potential.

Table 22.1 Classification of benign tumors of the jaws

- Odontogenic tumors
  - Epithelial or ectodermal origin
    - Enameloma or enamel pearl
    - Ameloblastoma
      i. Follicular
      ii. Plexiform
    - Calcifying epithelial odontogenic tumor (CEOT, Pindborg's tumor)
    - Adenoameloblastoma (OAT, Odontogenic adenomatoid tumor)
    - Primary intra-alveolar epidermoid carcinoma (malignant variety is rare in odontomes)
  - Mesenchymal or mesodermal origin
    - Dentinoma
    - Cementoma (periapical cemental dysplasia)
    - Cementoblastoma (true cementoma)
    - Central cementifying fibroma
    - Florid osseous dysplasia (FOD)
    - Central odontogenic fibroma
    - Odontogenic fibrosarcoma (malignant variety is rare in odontomes)
    - Peripheral odontogenic fibroma
  - Mixed tissue origin
    - Ameloblastic fibroma
    - Ameloblastic fibrosarcoma (malignant variety is rare in odontomes)
    - Ameloblastic fibro-odontoma
    - Ameloblastic odontoma
    - Ameloblastic hemangioma
    - Ameloblastic neurinoma
    - Odontogenic fibroma
    - Odontogenic myxoma
    - Odontogenic myxofibroma
    - Odontoma
      i. Compound composite
      ii. Complex composite
    - Teratoma (non odontogenic)
    - Retinal enlarge tumor
  - Developmental malformation
    - Dens invaginatus (dilated odontome)
    - Dens evaginatus
- Nonodontogenic tumors
  - Epithelial tissue origin
    - Papiloma
    - Keratocanthoma

Contd...

Contd...

- Pigmented cellular nevus
- Adenoma
- Squamous acanthoma
– Connective tissue origin
- Fibroma of bone
    i. Central fibroma
    ii. Ossifying fibroma (fibro-osteoma)
    iii. Fibroid epulis
- Epulis
- Pregnancy tumor
- Benign giant cell tumor
    i. Central giant cell tumor
    ii. Peripheral giant cell tumor
    iii. Reparative giant cell granuloma
    iv. Giant cell tumor of bone
    v. Giant cell tumor of hyperparathyroidism
    vi. Giant cell epulis
- Fibrous hyperplasia
- Fibrous histocytoma
- Desmoplastic fibroma
- Myxoma
- Myxofibroma
- Xanthoma verruciform
- Aneurysmal bone cyst
– Adipose tissue origin
- Lipoma
- Angiolipoma
– Cartilage tissue origin
- Chondroma
    i. Central
    ii. Ecchondroma
- Benign chondroblastoma
- Chondromyxoid fibroma
- Osteochondroma
    i. Central
    ii. Peripheral
– Bone tissue origin
- Osteoma
    i. Ivory osteoma
    ii. Cancellous osteoma
    iii. Osteoid osteoma
- Benign osteoblastoma
- Torus
    i. Palatinus
    ii. Mandibularis
    iii. Exostosis
    iv. Enostoses
- Osteomatosis
– Vascular tissue origin
- Hemangioma
- Hemangioma of bone (cavernous haemangioma)
- Hereditary hemorrhagic telengiectasia (Rendu-Osler-Weber syndrome)
- Encephalo trigeminal angiofibroma

Contd...

Contd...

- Nasopharyngeal angiofibroma
- Glomus tumor
- Hemangiopericytoma
- Lymphangioma
- Arteriovenous fistula
– Neural tissue origin
- Traumatic neuroma
- Neurofibroma
- Neurofibromatosis (Von Recklinghausen's disease)
- Neurilemmoma (schwannoma, neurinoma)
- Neuropolyendocrine syndrome (Sipple's syndrome)
- Neuroblastoma
- Ganglioneuroma
- Melanotic neuroectodermal tumor of infancy
– Muscle tissue origin
- Leiomyoma
- Rhabdomyoma
- Granular cell myoblastoma
- Congenital epulis of the new bone
– Teratoma
– Salivary gland tumors
- Mixed tumor (Pleomorphic adenoma)
- Wartin's tumor (papillary cystadenoma lymphomatosis, adenolymphoma)
- Oncytoma
- Monomorphic tumor
    i. Basal cell adenoma
    ii. Clear cell adenoma
    iii. Membrane adenoma
    iv. Myoepithelioma
- Sebaceous tumor
    i. Adenoma
    ii. Lymphoadenoma
- Papillary ductal adenoma
- Benign lymphoepithelial lesion
- Sjögren's syndrome
- Canalicular adenoma
- Oxycytoma
- Oxyphilic or acidophilic adenoma

- It is a well-defined mass of regular, smooth outline with a fibrous capsule.
- They tend to resemble the tissue of origin histologically.
- These may be detected clinically by enlargement of jaws or are found during a radiographic examination.

General Symptoms

- These are painless and do not metastasize, and are not life-threatening unless they interfere with a vital organ by direct extension.
- Benign tumors usually produce symptoms due to swelling and pressure effect on the surrounding structures.

- Adjacent teeth may be bodily shifted.
- A slow growing benign lesion approaching the lower border of the mandible, causes the cortex to expand or bow outward. This expansion is due to resorption of the bone along the inner wall of the cortex with simultaneous bone formation along the outer cortical surface because of stimulation of the periosteum.
- Few benign tumors of the bone infiltrate or invade the adjacent normal bone (ameloblastoma). Although destructive, these are considered benign because they do not metastasize but are locally invasive and tend to reoccur as their complete removal is difficult.
- Roots of the involved teeth may be resorbed. (ameloblastoma, ossifying fibroma, central giant cell granuloma).

General Radiographic Features

- The tumors have a specific anatomic predilection.
  - Odontogenic tumors occur in the alveolar process, above the inferior alveolar nerve canal, where the tooth formation occurs.
  - Vascular and neural lesions may originate inside the mandibular canal, arising from the neurovascular tissues.
  - Cartilaginous tumors occur in jaw locations where residual cartilaginous cells lie, such as around the mandibular condyle.
- They enlarge slowly by formation of additional internal tissue, thus the borders are relatively smooth, well-defined or moderately defined and sometimes corticated or hyperostotic. They are usually sharply demarcated by a radiolucent band of soft tissue or capsule at the periphery which separates more mature internal radiopaque portion from the surrounding normal bone. The shape is usually round or oval, regularly shaped lesions.
- The internal structure may be completely radiolucent or radiopaque or mixture of radiopaque-radiolucent structures.
  - Radiolucent, unilocular, multilocular, cystic, honeycomb or soap bubble appearing lesion (ameloblastoma, myxoma, hemangioma, central giant cell granuloma).
  - Mixed radiopaque-radiolucent lesions:
    - Curved septae that are characteristic in ameloblastoma represent residual bone trapped into the tumor that has remodeled into curved septa, ameloblastoma does not produce bone.
    - Irregularly thickened trabeculae are typically seen in central giant cell granuloma.
    - Numerous scattered radiopaque foci of varying size and density imparting a driven snow (CEOT) or mottled (AOT, odontome).
  - Predominantly radiopaque, these structures usually represent either residual bone or a calcified material that is being produced by the tumor.

- Osteoblastoma has an internal granular radiopaque pattern produced by abnormal bone that is actually being manufactured by the tumor.
    - Others are tori, osteoma, cementoblastoma.
- The adjacent structures are affected differently depending on the behavior of the benign lesion:
  - It may exert pressure on the neighboring structures resulting in the displacement of teeth or bony cortices. It may bodily displace adjacent teeth, this movement is slow due to the slow growth of the lesion. Displacement of vital structures, like the inferior dental canal.
  - If the growth is slow, there will be remodeling of the outer cortex, resulting in an appearance that the cortex has been displaced by the tumor. This is caused by simultaneous resorption of bone along the inner surface (endosteal) of the cortex and deposition of bone along the outer surface by the periosteum. The integrity of the cortex is maintained and it can thus resist perforation.
  - Sometimes, the extent of erosion, pathological fracture and infiltration or invasion of the adjacent normal bone may before considerable distance beyond the radiographically apparent margin (ameloblastoma, central giant cell granuloma).
  - The roots of the teeth are usually resorbed, in a smooth fashion (ameloblastoma, ossifying fibroma, central giant cell granuloma). Bone dysplasias (fibrous dysplasia), does not resorb teeth. Root resorption associated with malignancy is different, in that the resorption is less and causes thinning of the root into a 'spiked' shape.

ODONTOGENIC TUMORS

Those that arise from the tissue of odontogenic apparatus and these may further be ectodermal, mesodermal or mixed (ecto-mesodermal).

Odontogenic Epithelial Tumors

Enameloma (Enamel Nodule)

Refer to Chapter 19 on Dental Anomalies and Developmental Disturbances of the Jaws (Page 252, Fig. 19.18).

Ameloblastoma (Adamantinoma, Adamantoblastoma, Adotomes Embryolastiques, Epithelial Odontoma) (Figs 22.1 to 22.7) (Table 22.2)

Definition

It is a true neoplasm of odontogenic epithelium, (remnants of the dental lamina or dental organs) it is slow growing, which sometimes turns aggressive, and tends to recur if not thoroughly eradicated and is therefore considered locally malignant.

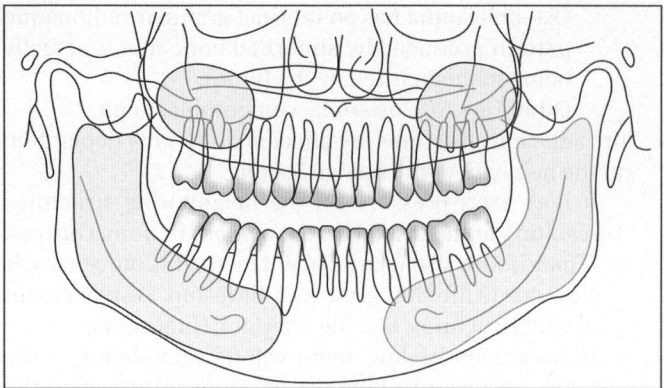

Figure 22.1 Schematic diagram showing most common ameloblastoma sites. Eighty percent of ameloblastoma is in the mandible and 20 percent in the maxilla

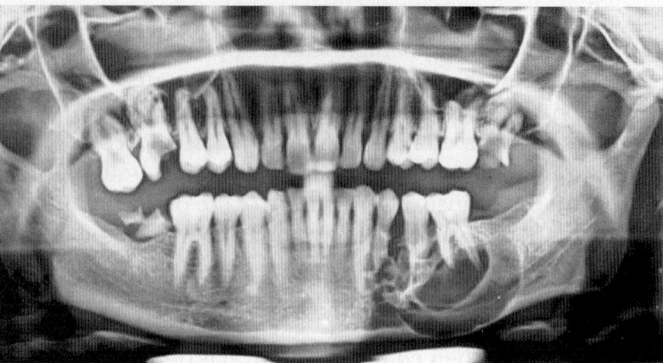

Figure 22.3 Ameloblastoma: Panoramic radiograph shows a well-defined multilocular lesion with sclerotic borders in relation to left mandibular body apical to the premolars and molars. Two large locules with sclerotic borders seen in relation to second premolar and first molar with multiple small locules more mesial in the lesion. The radiolucency extends inferiorly to involve the lower border of mandible. The inferior alveolar canal does not seem to be displaced. Differential diagnosis includes CEOT, giant cell lesions

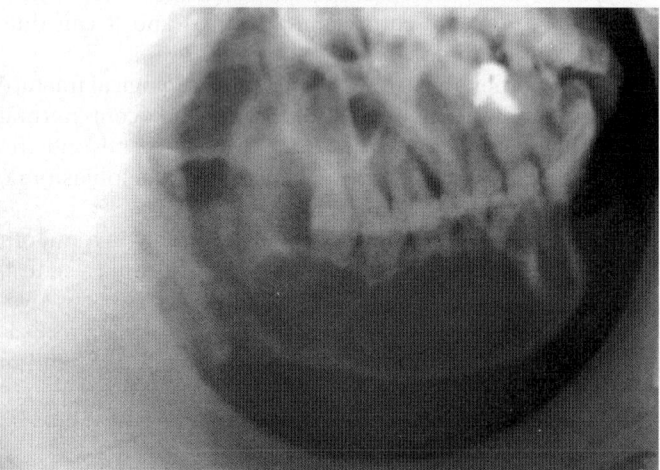

Figure 22.2 Lateral oblique shows multilocular well-defined radiolucency with well corticated borders extending from symphyseal area beyond the lower right third molar also involving some part of ramus of mandible. There is evidence of expansion of inferior cortex of mandible. Root resorption of premolar and molars is observed. Inferior alveolar canal is displaced downwards

- More common in molar ramus region of the mandible. May occur in the maxilla, especially in the 3rd molar area, and may involve the maxillary sinus and the floor of the nasal cavity. The right side of the mandible is affected slightly more as compared to the left side .
- It begins as a central lesion of the bone which is slowly destructive but tends to expand bone rather than perforate it. The overlying mucosa appears normal. It is frequently discovered during routine dental examination.
- There is gradual facial asymmetry, with mobility and displacement of the involved teeth.
- Pain and paraesthesia may occur if the lesion is pressing upon a nerve or is secondarily infected.
- In later stages the lesion becomes hard, non tender and show ovoid or fusiform enlargement. Surrounding bone may become thin so that fluctuation and egg shell crackling may be elicited.
- As it grows, it may cause bony expansion and sometimes erosion through the adjacent cortical plate with subsequent invasion of the adjacent soft tissues.
- If left untreated for many years the expansion may be very disfiguring, fungating and an ulcerative type of growth characteristic of that of carcinoma may be seen.
- Maxillary lesions are more dangerous than mandibular lesions due to the tendency for the former lesion to spread more extensively in the more porous maxillary bone and the possibility of the involvement of the vital structures at the cranial base. It may extend into the paranasal sinuses, orbit or the nasopharynx.
- Ameloblastoma may form from the epithelial lining of dentigerous cyst and is then called mural ameloblastoma.

Robinson defines ameloblastoma as a tumor that is usually unicentric, nonfunctional, intermittent in growth, anatomically benign and clinically persistant.

The probable etiological factors are; chronic irritation, infection with history of traumatic injury or extraction, dietary deficiencies. Polyoma viruses have shown to produce ameloblastoma like lesions in animals.

Clinical Features

- It accounts for 1 percent of all oral tumors and 11 percent of all odontogenic tumors
- More common in males (black), between 20 to 50 years of age

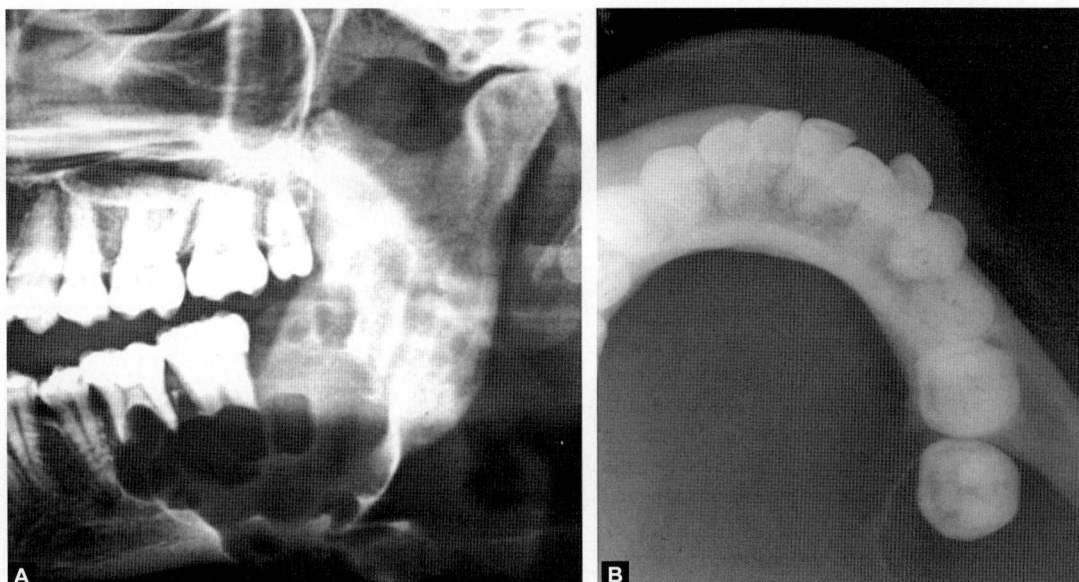

Figures 22.4A and B Multilocular ameloblastoma: (A) Part of a panoramic view (left side) showing an ameloblastoma with the typical multilocular appearance of a large ameloblastoma at the angle of the mandible, with extensive expansion and resorption of adjacent teeth; (B) Occlusal view shows displacement of the adjacent teeth showing the buccolingual extent of the lesion

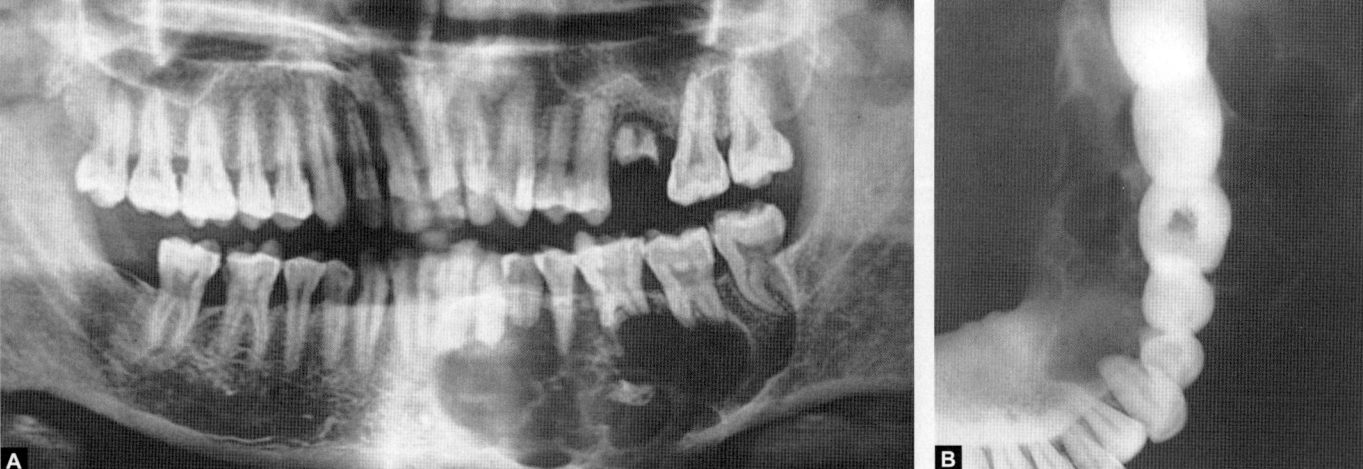

Figures 22.5A and B Multilocular ameloblastoma: (A) Panoramic view showing an ameloblastoma in a more unusual anterior position causing resorption of the adjacent teeth and extending downwards causing thinning of the lower border; (B) Lower occlusal shows well-defined multilocular radiolucent lesion perforating the buccal cortical plate

Radiographic Features

- Eighty percent develop in the molar-ramus region of the mandible, but may extend to the symphyseal area. In the maxilla, it is more common in the third molar region and may extend into the maxillary sinus and nasal floor. In either jaw the tumor usually originates in an occlusal position to a developing tooth.

- In caries free young individuals, the exclusive use of bitewing radiographs will not give adequate overview of the jaws and the diagnosis of a silent ameloblastoma may be missed.
- It usually has a well-defined corticated border, which is curved and in small lesions the border and shape may be indistinguable from a cyst. The periphery of the lesion in the maxilla is more ill-defined.

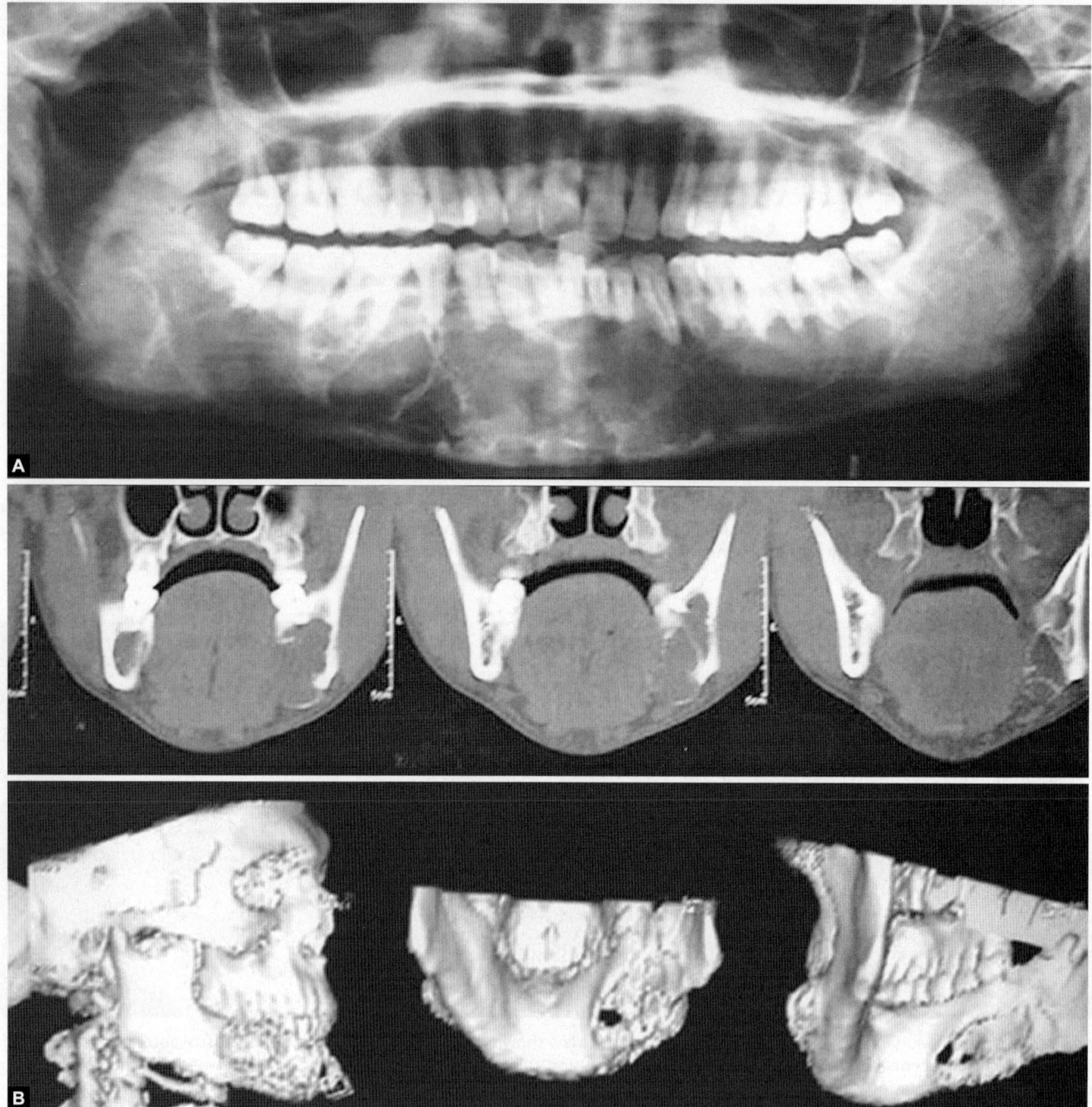

Figures 22.6A and B (A) Ameloblastoma seen on a panoramic view as a multilocular lesion with a soap bubble appearance, involving the entire mandible from left second molar to right third molar also involving the right angle of mandible; root resorption of all the teeth in the affected area was noted; (B) Coronal views and 3D CT of the same patient with ameloblastoma showing destruction of the buccal and lingual plates

- The internal structure varies from totally radiolucent to mixed with presence of bony septa:
  - Unilocular cyst like appearance with a hyperostotic border. Usually present in the ascending ramus. If the lesion extends even for a short distance into the horizontal portion of the mandible and/or presence of septa of the bone within the cavity adds to the probability that it is an ameloblastoma.
  - Area of bone destruction having smooth curved margins, which are well-defined, corticated and

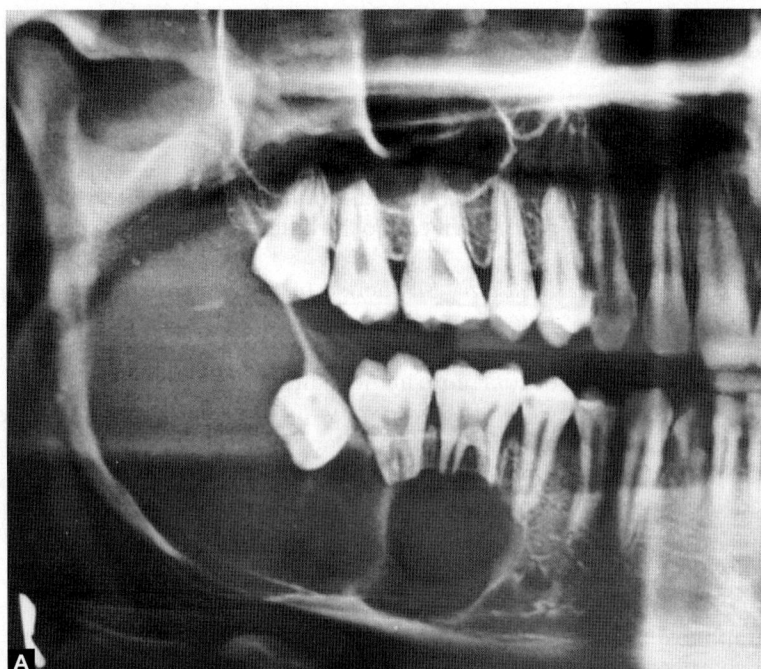 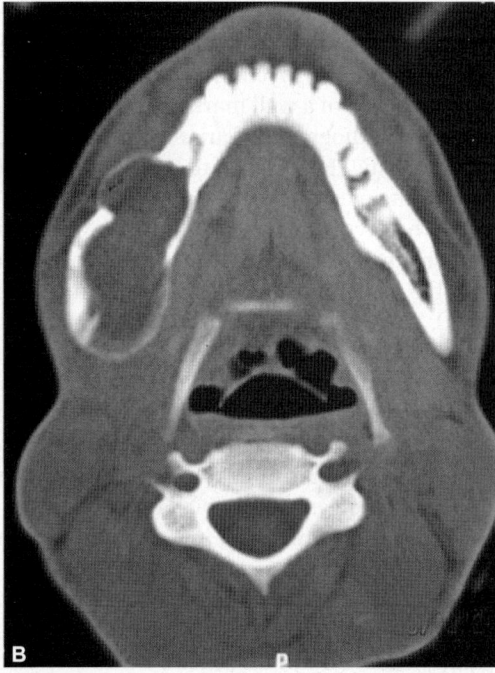

Figures 22.7A and B Ameloblastoma: (A) Panoramic radiograph shows an incompletely developed third molar. Large multilocular lesion surrounding the molar extending from the body of the mandible in to the ramus and right coronoid process of the mandible. Cortication present, radiopaque septa present in the region of second molar. Root resorption of involved teeth; (B) CT axial image slice shows bicortical expansion

Table 22.2 Classification of ameloblastoma

- On pathological basis
  - Peripheral ameloblastoma (extraosseous ameloblastoma)
  - Pituitary ameloblastoma (craniopharyngioma, Rathke's pouch tumor)
  - Adamantinoma of long bones.
- On histological type
  - Follicular ameloblastoma
  - Plexiform ameloblastoma
  - Acanthomatus ameloblastoma
  - Basal cell ameloblastoma
  - Unicystic ameloblastoma
  - Plexiform unicystic ameloblastoma
  - Granular cell ameloblastoma
  - Papilleferous ameloblastoma
  - Hemangio ameloblastoma
  - Desmoplastic ameloblastoma
  - Clear cell ameloblastoma
  - Dentino ameloblastoma
  - Melano ameloblastoma
  - Kerato ameloblastoma.

situated within the cavity in an arrangement of coarse trabaculae. The thickness of the trabaculae vary from delicate to coarse strands of more than 2 mm width. A gross caricature of a spider may be seen.

– In some large tumors it is found that there is almost complete loss of bony margins of the jaws, but usually this is in the anterior part of the ramus and the superior border of the body of the jaw that is affected. Extension may also be seen in the condyle and posterior border of the ramus which presents a concave anterior border. The inferior aspect of the mandible may be ballooned out with a marked smooth downwards convexity and in the center there may be trabeculae.

– Multilocular cyst like appearance, which shows multiple cystic cavities, with thin septae separating them. Usually there is a loss of continuity of one of the walls.

– A common variation of the multilocular type is the presence of many cysts bunched together and compromising cavities which vary in size, enlargement of the lower border and expansion of the posterior aspect of the ramus, leading to lateral expansion of the jaws. The septa within the tumor are well-developed and relatively coarse giving a gross honey-comb appearance. An unerupted tooth may be lying horizontally in the inferior and posterior aspect of the tumor.

– Any cystic cavities in the jaws whose borders are undulating or made up of small arcs of small circles suggest the possibility of a more serious lesion.

- Variations of the above may appear as a large cystic cavity with one or more daughter cysts adjacent, may be mistaken for Myeloma, the distinguishing point is the presence of a well marked cortex in the tumor.
- Another radiographic variation is associated with the solid variety. Here the soft tissue has not yet been broken down into a cyst. The normal bone structure is replaced by a honeycomb appearance (in which the cavities are relatively small and fairly uniform in size) or soap bubble appearance (larger compartments of variable size). The walls of the cavity are coarse and the margins of the tumor are lobulated. The margins separating normal bone from the tumor are denser than the normal bone but less well corticated than seen in other cysts and tumors. The jaw may be expanded laterally and inferiorly. An unerupted tooth may be present.
- The multilocular type is rare in the maxilla, but when present the antrum may be invaginated and/or obliterated, but the antrum *per se* is not involved. That is the tumor remains separated by a bony wall from the air sinus.
- A subclinical lesion, usually presents in radiographs as many small rounded cavities in bone having sharply defined and sometimes corticated borders. In some cases there are two rounded and well-defined small cavities having good bony cortex; in the center of which there is a small white dot.
- There is a pronounced tendency of the ameloblastoma to cause extensive root resorption, though root displacement is also seen. As the common point of origin is occlusal to the tooth, the displacement is of the tooth is apically.
- An occlusal radiograph may demonstrate cyst like expansion and thinning of an adjacent cortical plate, leaving a thin egg-shell of bone.
- Actual perforation of bone into the surrounding tissues or anatomical spaces is a late feature of ameloblastoma.
- Unicystic types may cause extreme expansion of the mandibular ramus and often the anterior border of the ramus is not visible in the panaromic radiograph.
- Recurrent ameloblastoma (inadequate resection) has a characteristic appearance of multiple small cyst like structures with very coarse sclerotic cortical margins, sometimes separated by normal bone.

Additional Imaging

- CT not only helps to confirm the diagnosis but also accurately demonstrates the anatomical extent of the tumor. It helps to detect perforation of the outer cortex and invasion into the surrounding soft tissues. It is also important for the post surgical follow-up assessement.
- CT findings in ameloblastoma consist of low attenuation cystic areas intermixed with isodense areas reflecting the solid component of the lesions. The size of the low attenuation cyst may vary from small to large. The expanding lesion may cause a thin bony rim at the periphery.

- MRI provides superior images of the nature and extent of invasion in the soft tissues.

Differential Diagnosis

- *Small and unilocular ameloblastoma*:
  - These are located around the crown of an unerupted tooth often cannot be differentiated from a dentigerous cyst.
  - *Residual cyst*: There is history of extraction of the tooth.
  - *Lateral periodontal cyst*: It is found in incisor, canine and premolar area in the maxilla, ameloblastoma occurs more in the mandibular molar area.
  - *Giant cell granuloma*: It is found more often in areas anterior to the molars, younger age group and have more granular and ill-defined septae.
  - *Traumatic bone cyst*: This occurs in the mid twenties, whereas ameloblastoma is more common in the 3rd and 4th decades.
- *Primordial cyst*: Same as traumatic bone cyst:
  - *Multilocular ameloblastoma*.
  - *Odontogenic keratocyst*: Contains curved septae but tends to grow along the bone without marked expansion.
  - *Odontogenic myxoma*: There is history of missing tooth and has a presence of septa that divide the image into much finer coarse than those in ameloblastoma. Myxoma has one or two thin, sharp, straight septa which are characteristic of it. Myxomas are not expansile and tend to grow along the bone.
  - *Ossifying fibroma*: The septa are usually wide, granular and ill-defined. Small irregular trabeculae are seen.

Management

- Complete removal with resection
- Intraoral block excision
- Extraoral enbloc resection
- Peripheral osteotomy
- Radiation therapy may be used for inoperable tumors especially those in the posterior maxilla.

Malignant Ameloblastoma

Refer Chapter 23, Malignant Diseases of the Jaws (Page 395).

Calcifying Epithelial Odontogenic Tumor (CEOT) (Pindborgs Tumor, Ameloblastoma of Unusual Type with Calcification) (Figs 22.8A to D)

Definition

It is a rare tumor of distinctive microscopic appearance, that appears to arise from the reduced enamel epithelium or dental epithelium. The tumors are usually located within the bone and produce a mineralized substance within amyloid-like material.

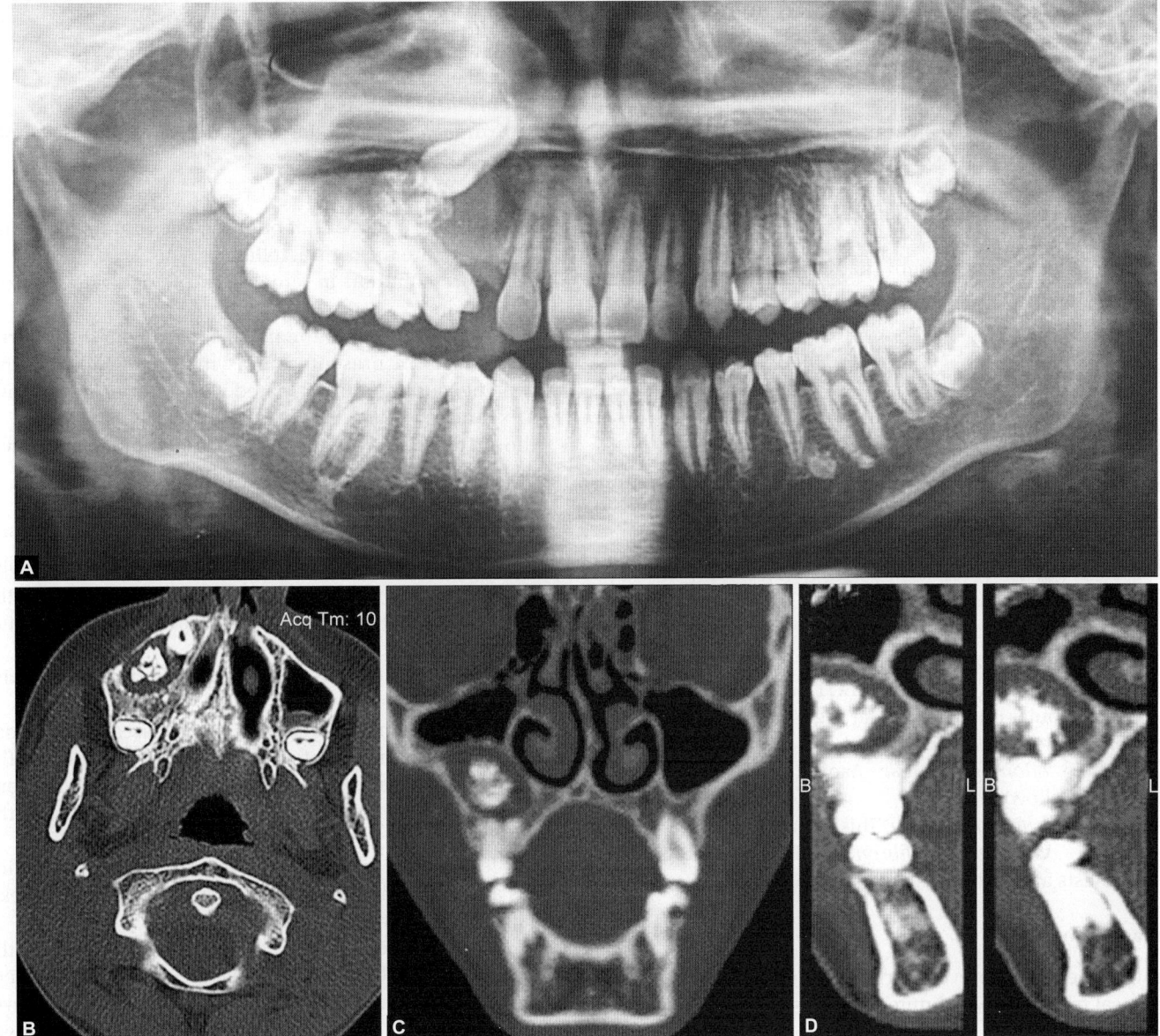

Figures 22.8A to D Calcifying epithelial odontogenic tumor (CEOT): (A) Panoramic view shows well-defined noncorticated, uniloculated, expansile, and irregular shaped radiolucency in upper right side in relation to maxillary right lateral incisor to first molar. Superiorly it is extending up to middle of nasal septum, inferiorly till crestal bone and eroding the crestal bone medially till lateral surface of the central incisor and laterally distal surface of molar. Cortication is lost in crestal aspect of the involved teeth. An impacted canine is seen associated with a radiolucency and an irregular radiopaque mass is seen in proximity. CT Scan: (B) Axial; (C) Coronal; (D) Sagittal shows a well circumscribed osteolytic lesion in the right maxilla of soft tissue density with hyperdense foci of calcification. Thinning of the cortices with breech of the buccal wall. Extension into the anterior portion of sinus. Root resorption and lateral displacement of the premolar, medial displacement of lateral incisor is seen

Clinical Features

- It accounts for 1 percent of odontogenic tumors
- It is more common in men with an age range of 8 – 92 years
- The mandible is more commonly affected than the maxilla, and more so in the premolar-molar region. Rarely this tumor may have an extraosseous location

- It is usually asymptomatic, presenting as a painless swelling. It may be associated with paresthesia
- It is usually associated with unerupted teeth
- Cortical expansion is a regular feature
- Palpation indicates a hard swelling with well-defined or diffuse borders

- It behaves like an ameloblastoma, less aggressive but is locally invasive with a high rate of recurrence

Radiographic Features

- It appears as a radiolucent area surrounding the crown of an unerupted or impacted tooth.
- The boundary on the lesion may from well-defined to diffuse to irregular and ill-defined.
- As the lesion matures it may appear unilocular or multilocular (honeycomb pattern) with numerous scattered radiopaque foci (produced by mineralization of amorphorous proteinaceous material generated by the tumor cells), found close to the crown of the embedded tooth. In addition, small thin, opaque trabeculae may cross the radiolucency in many directions. This gives a driven snow appearance.
- The lesion may displace the developing tooth or prevent its eruption. Expanded cortices may be visualized in the buccal and lingual dimension.

Differential Diagnosis

- *Dentigerous cyst.*
- *Ameloblastoma.*
- *Adenomatoid odontogenic tumor*: This is more common in anterior maxilla as compared CEOT, which is common in the mandibular molar-premolar region.
- *Ameloblastic fibro-odontoma.*
- *Calcifying odontogenic cyst*: Aspiration yields viscous granular yellow fluid.
- *Partially calcified odontoma*: This has a capsule.
- *Central odontogenic fibroma*: Histopathologically, fibroblasts are prominent and abundant.

Management

The treatment is more conservative than ameloblastoma, with local resection, with limited margins.

Adenomatoid Odontogenic Tumor (AOT) (Adenoameloblastoma, Ameloblastic Adenomatoid Tumor) (Figs 22.9 to 22.13)

Definition

This is an uncommon, nonaggressive tumor of odontogenic epithelium, with a duct like structure and varying degree of inductive changes in the connective tissue. The tumor may be partly cystic and in some cases the solid lesion may be present only as masses in the wall of a large cyst. It was first reported by Stafne.

Many authors believe it to be a hamartoma and not a tumor.

It is now known histopathologically that in adenomatoid odontogenic cyst the proliferation that fills the lumen is arising from the epithelial lining and the calcifications present are dentinoid materials derived from root sheath epithelium.

Classification

- Peripheral adenomatoid odontogenic tumor
- Central adenomatoid odontogenic tumor
  - *Follicular type*: Associated with embedded tooth
  - *Extrafollicular type*: Not associated with embedded tooth.

Clinical Features

- It represents 3 percent of odontogenic tumors. Of which 73 percent are the central follicular type.
- It is more common in females, in the age ranging from 5 – 50 years.
- It is more common in the maxilla, usually in the anterior cuspid region. It presents as an asymptomatic slow growing swelling, commonly associated with an unerupted tooth. It expands the cortices, but is noninvasive.
- The extraosseous tumor is very uncommon, and when seen it is usually located on the gingiva.

Radiographic Features

- The tumor may have a follicular relationship with the impacted tooth; however it does not attach at the cementoenamel junction but surrounds a greater part of the tooth, most often a canine.
- It appears as a well-defined, unilocular radiolucency, with sclerotic borders.
- Radiopacities may develop in some cases, which may show dense clusters of ill-defined radiolucencies. The calcifications are usually small, with well-defined borders, like a cluster of pebbles. These are best seen on the intraoral radiographs.
- The lesion may give a typical target appearance; which has a radiolucent circumferential halo which envelopes a dense, central and radiopaque mass.
- As the tumor enlarges it causes displacement of the adjacent teeth. Root resorption is rare. It may also prevent the eruption of the associated impacted tooth. Expansion of the cortices may occur, but the outer cortex is maintained.
- When the tumor occurs independently of unerupted teeth it is often encapsulated.

Differential Diagnosis

- *Follicular cyst*: It may be discounted if the attachment of the radiolucent lesion is more apical than the cementoenamel junction.
- *Pericoronal odontogenic cyst.*
- *Calcifying odontogenic cyst*: It is difficult to differentiate from the extrafollicular type of AOT. It occurs in the older age group and usually in the premolar area.
- *Ameloblastic fibro-odontoma*: It is found more commonly in the posterior mandibular region. It is multilocular and radiopacities of enamel and dentine are seen inside the radiolucency, whereas in AOT the snow flakes are seen at the periphery.

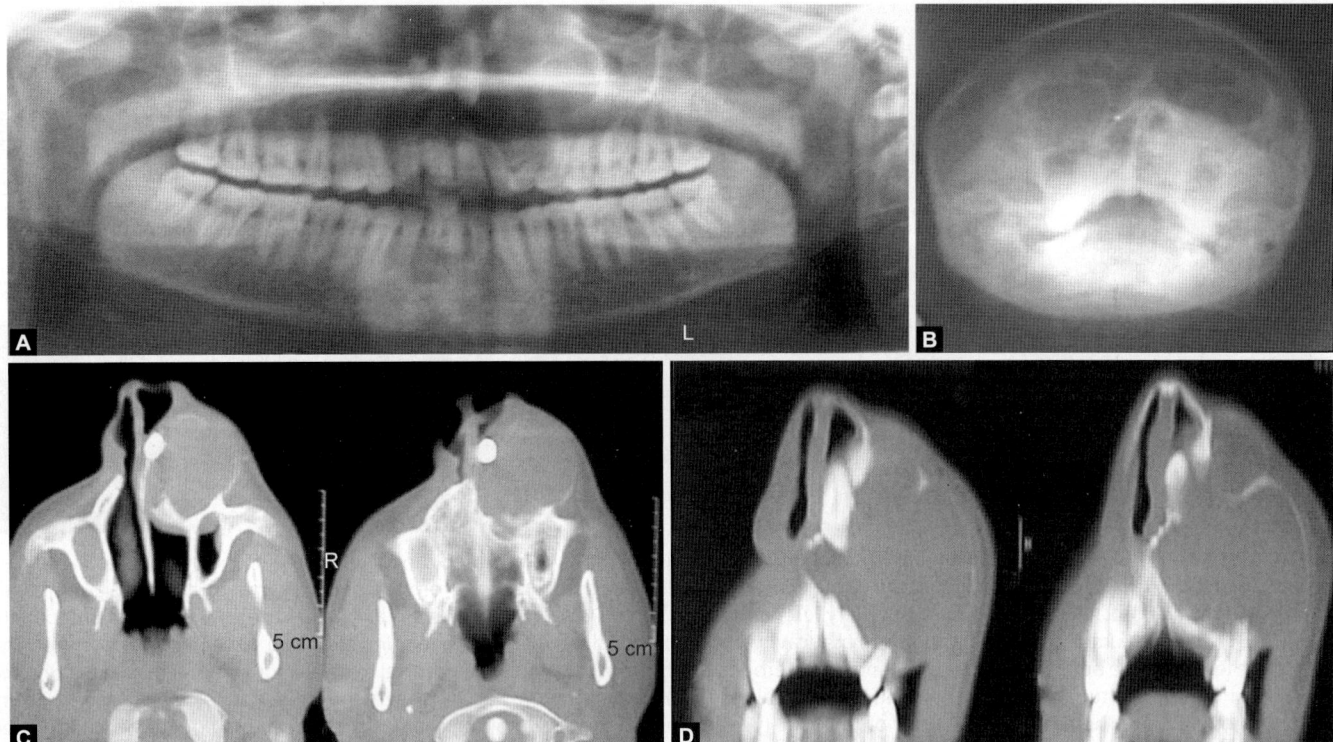

Figures 22.9A to D Adenomatoid odontogenic tumor (AOT): (A) Panoramic view shows presence of a well-defined radiolucency in left maxillary region extending from right central to molar region in relation to impacted canine at the superior and medial aspect of the lesion. Floor of maxillary sinus was not traceable on left side. Roots of lateral and premolar were displaced. Over-retained deciduous canine; (B) Posteroanterior (PA) Water's view shows a well-defined radiopaque shadow seen superimposed over the left maxillary sinus with an impacted tooth near the medial wall. CT scan: (C) Axial; (D) Coronal view shows presence of isodense nonenhancing mass lesion in left maxilla with destruction of anterior portion of hard palate and lateral nasal wall. The mass extended into the lateral portion of the nasal cavity, causing deviation of septum to right side. Impacted tooth was seen at the superomedial aspect of the lesion. Mucosal thickening of bilateral maxillary sinus was seen

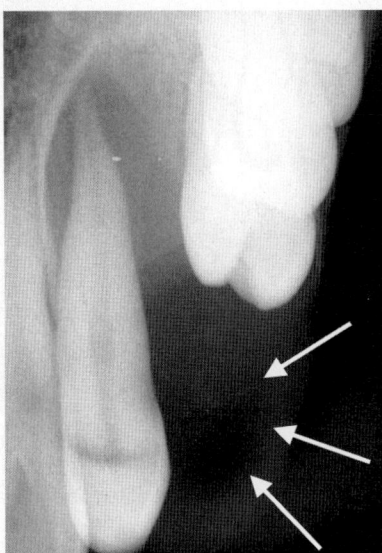

Figure 22.10 AOT: Cropped occlusal view showing a well-defined corticated radiolucent lesion in the left maxilla in relation with the lateral and canine. The radiograph shows the soft tissue shadow and small radiopaque mass within the soft tissue delineations

- *Calcifying epithelial odontogenic tumor*: It is found more commonly in the posterior mandibular region.
- *Dentigerous cyst*: This is seen in the 2nd to 4th decade as compared AOT which is seen in the younger age group. It is found more commonly in the posterior mandibular region. AOT has the tendency to surround more than just the crown of the unerupted tooth.
- *Ameloblastoma*: It is more common in the older age group, posterior region. It is most often multilocular.
- *Odontogenic fibroma or myxoma*: This has the tennis racket appearance.

Management

Conservative surgical excision with curettage is effective.

Squamous Odontogenic Tumor

Definition

It is a well differentiated odontogenic tumor composed of islands or sheets of squamous epithelium that lack recognizable features of the enamel organ. It is believed to arise from the cell rests of malassez.

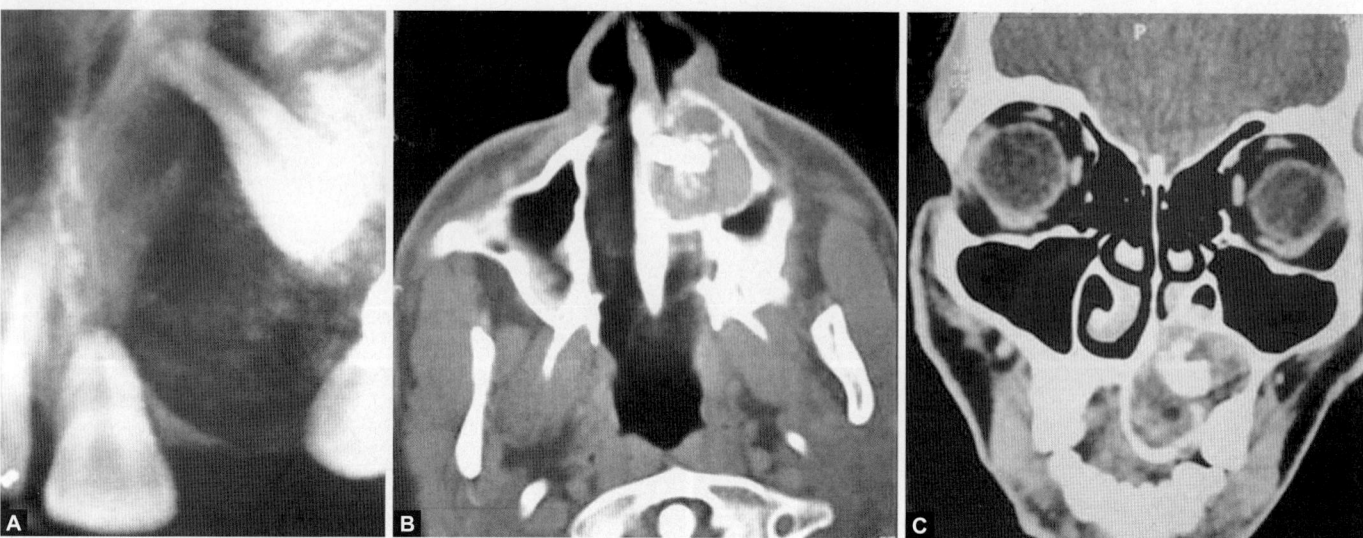

Figures 22.11A to C AOT: (A) AOT seen on an intraoral periapical radiograph. A well-defined, unilocular radiolucency with sclerotic border associated with an unerupted maxillary left lateral in the center, extending anteroposteriorly from the periapex of central to mesial root apex of maxillary right first molar. Displacement of maxillary left central and canine is seen; (B and C) An axial and coronal CT of the same patient showing AOT with the tumor mass displacing the nasal cavity and maxillary sinus medially extending from the periapex of the central. The extent of the lesion can be better appreciated, extending anteroposteriorly from the periapex of central to mesial root apex of maxillary right first molar, incisor to nasal septum causing obliteration of left nasal cavity and superiorly causing displacement of the floor of the maxillary antrum in the upward direction. There is a dense cluster of radiopacity seen close to the crown of maxillary left lateral and radiopaque foci dispersed throughout the radiolucency

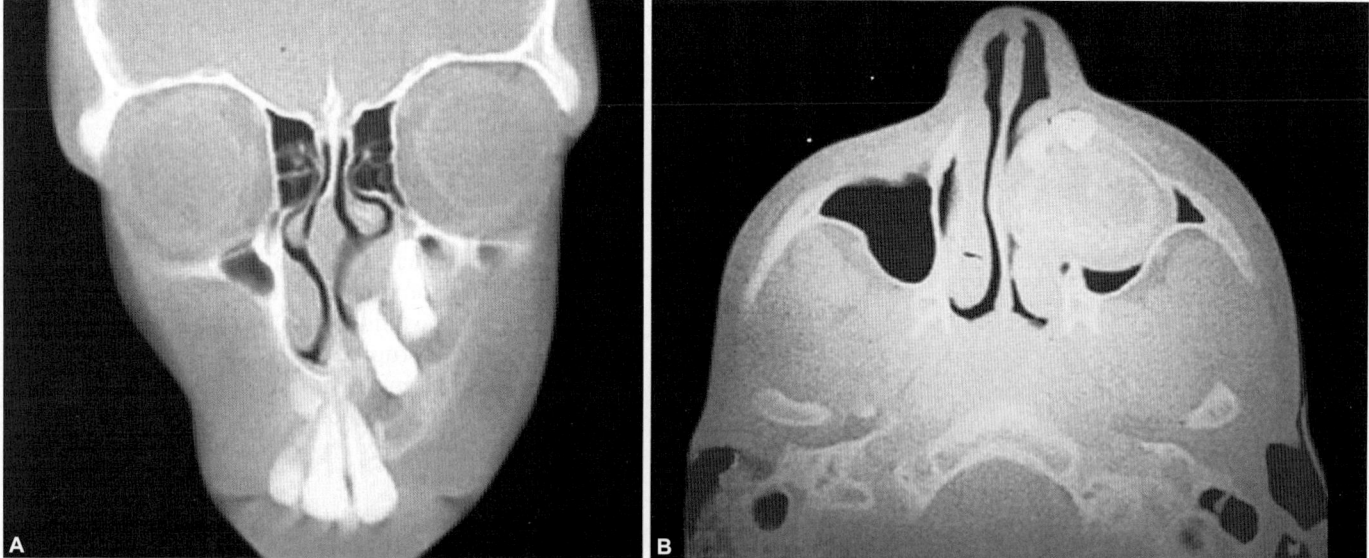

Figures 22.12A and B A coronal and axial CT showing AOT in association with unerupted teeth and presence of scattered radiopaque foci. There is displacement of the nasal septum and floor of the maxillary sinus. CT scan showed unilocular radiolucent lesion with faint demarcation at some places associated with unerupted tooth with scattered radiopaque foci and causing gross displacement of left lateral wall of nose and elevation of floor of maxillary antrum and almost completely filling the maxillary antrum

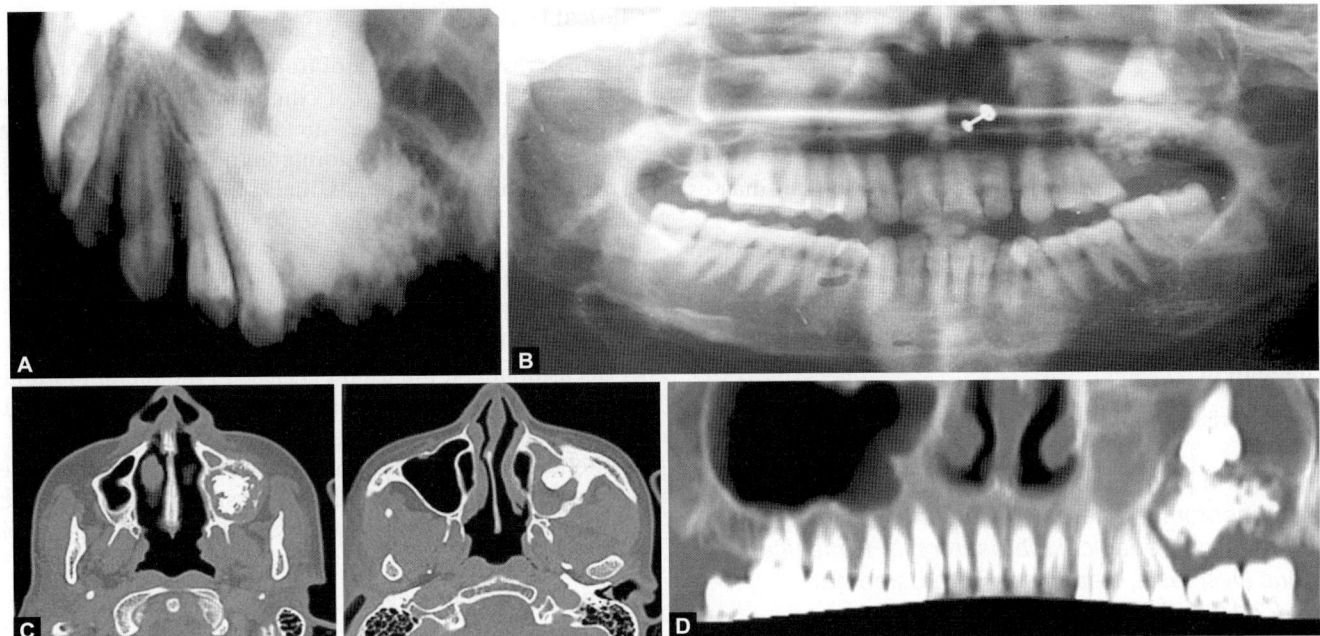

Figures 22.13A to D AOT: (A and B) Occlusal and panoramic radiograph shows a well delineated irregular dense radiopaque shadow involving the pericoronal area of impacted maxillary second molar, surrounded by a radiolucent halo, extending from first premolar region to posterior wall of maxilla and up to the alveolar crest. CT Scan: (C) Axial views; (D) Reformatted panoramic view revealed a well-defined cystic lesion in relation to superiorly displaced and impacted maxillary left second molar in left maxillary sinus. Irregular calcification was seen in the lesion. Expansion of buccal cortical plate in premolar to maxillary tuberosity region. Perforation of cortex in certain areas and reactive bone formation seen in anterolateral portion of left maxilla and left zygomatic bone

Clinical Features

- It is a very rare lesion.
- Females are more commonly affected, in the age range of 11 to 67 years.
- More often found in the maxilla, in the incisor cuspid region, and when occasionally seen in the mandible, it has a predilection for the bicuspid molar area.
- It is asymptomatic, slow growing, with mobility, pain, tenderness to percussion and occasionally abnormal sensation of the involved teeth.

Radiographic Features

- It is seen as a well circumscribed, semicircular or triangular, radiolucent area in association with the cervical portion of the tooth.
- The borders may or may not be sclerotic.

Differential Diagnosis

- If one discovers a solid fleshy lesion which is associated with a vital tooth root on the cervical portion then squamous odontogenic tumor is the most likely diagnosis.

- It is a very rare lesion and thus should not be considered high on the differential diagnostic list when considering radiolucent lesions of the jaws.

Management

It has a low recurrence rate and conservative enucleation and curettage is usually sufficient.

Odontogenic Mesenchymal Tumors (Odontogenic Ectomesenchyme)

Dentinoma

Definition

This is a rare tumor of odontogenic origin composed of immature connective tissue, odontogenic epithelium and irregular dysplastic dentin.

Clinical Features

- It has no sex predilection, and is more common in the younger age group.
- It is most commonly seen in the mandible, associated with the crown of an unerupted (third molar) tooth.

- It presents as a painful swelling, with perforation of the overlying mucosa, discharge and may get secondarily infected.

Radiographic Features

- It appears as a radiopaque mass or several masses associated with the crown of an unerupted tooth.
- The calcified mass is usually surrounded by a radiolucent area.
- It may cause local destruction of bone.

Management

Surgical excision with through curettage of the area.

Cementoma (Periapical Cemental Dysplasia, Fibrocementoma, Sclerosing Cementum, Periapical Osteofibrosis, Periapical Fibrosarcoma, Periapical Fibrous Dysplasia, Periapical Fibro-osteoma) (Figs 22.14 and 22.15)

Definition

It is a reactive fibro-osseous lesion derived from the odontogenic cells in the periodontal ligament. It is located at the apex of the tooth.

The term cementoma is no longer used as it is now recognized as periapical cemental osseous dysplasia, which is a disorganized product of bone periodontal membrane cementum complex.

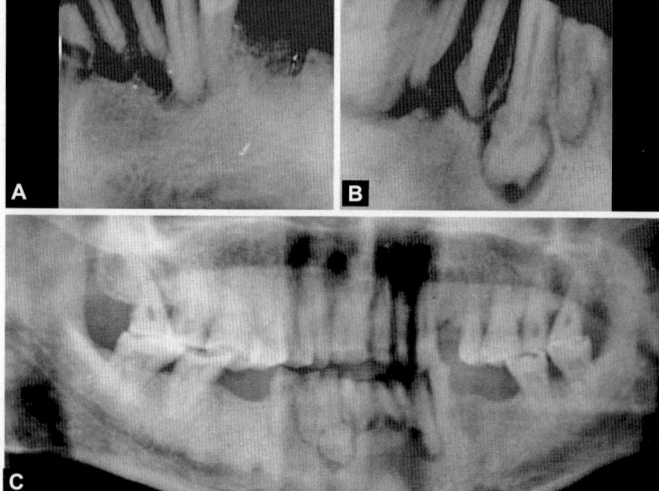

Figures 22.14A to C Periapical cemental dysplasia: Periapical and panoramic view shows; radiopacity at the apex of the involved teeth. The epicenter of the lesion involving the mandibular canine appears to be high, over the apical third of the root. There are multiple lesions, the margins are well-defined, with a radiolucent border of varying width, surrounded by a band of sclerotic bone

Clinical Features

- It may result as a result of trauma, endocrinal imbalance (abnormal secretion of the female sex hormone), nutritional deficiency, metabolic disturbances, past history of syphilis and anomalous development.
- More common in females, blacks and in the middle age.
- The mandibular anterior region is the most commonly affected site.
- It is usually asymptomatic and the involved teeth are vital. It is usually discovered as an incidental finding on routine radiographic surveys.
- Occasionally, if the lesion is close to the mental foramen and impinges on the mental nerve, it may produce pain, paresthesia or even paraethesia.
- The lesions are usually small less than 1 cm in diameter, but it may become quite large, causing notable expansion of the alveolar process, and may continue to enlarge slowly.

Radiographic Features

- It usually lies at the apex of the tooth. In rare cases if the epicenter is high, it may lie over the apical third of the root.
- The lesion is usually multiple and bilateral.
- The margins are well-defined, with a radiolucent border of varying width, surrounded by a band of sclerotic bone.
- If the involved teeth have been extracted, this lesion may still develop, but the periapical location is less evident (the term cemental dysplasia would be more appropriate here).
- The radiographic appearance changes as the lesion matures:
  - *Stage I*: Radiolucent (fibrous)
    - The lesion appears as a circumscribed radiolucency, accompanied by localizes bone destruction. This is due to loss of bony substance which is replaced by connective tissue, within the lesion.
    - The margins of the lesion vary from well-defined but not corticated, poorly defined, or partly well and partly ill-defined.
    - Loss of lamina dura around the involved tooth.
  - *Stage II*: Mixed stage
    - Radiopaque tissue appears in the radiolucent structure. The material is amorphous; has a round, oval or irregular shape; and is composed of cementum and abnormal bone. These structures are called cemeticles.
    - Sometimes the radiopaque material resembles the abnormal trabeculae pattern seen in fibrous dysplasia.
  - *Stage III*: Radiopaque
    - Complete opacification of the lesion occurs.
    - It appears as a well-defined radiopacity usually bordered by a radiolucent capsule separating it from the adjacent bone.

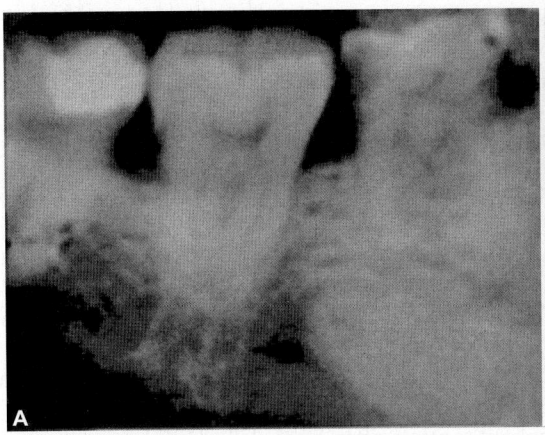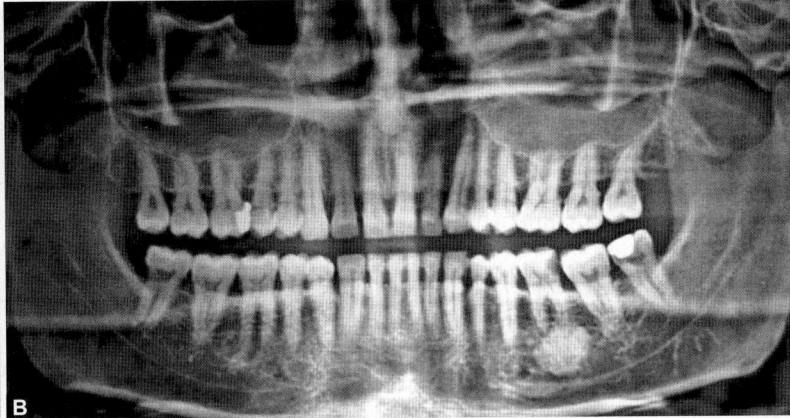

Figures 22.15A and B Periapical cemental dysplasia: Intraoral and panoramic view showing radiopaque lesion in relation to the roots mandibular left first molar, the margins are well-defined, with a radiolucent border, surrounded by a band of sclerotic bone

- The margins vary from well-defined to poorly defined. The lamina dura of the adjacent teeth is discontinuous.
- The internal structure may appear dramatically radiolucent if cavities resembling simple bone cysts form within the cemental lesion.
- The normal lamina dura is lost, but the tooth structure is not affected. There is no root resorption.
- Occasionally hypercementosis occurs on the root of the tooth positioned within the lesion.
- Some lesions stimulate a sclerosing bone reaction from the surrounding bone.
- Small lesions do not cause expansion of the involved jaw. But, in case of larger lesions, expansion of the jaws may occur but it is always bordered by a thin, intact outer cortex similar to that seen in fibrous dysplasis. In the maxilla the lesion may elevate the floor of the maxillary sinus.

Differential Diagnosis

- *Stage I*: Radiolucent (fibrous)
  - *Pulpoperiapical lesions (periapical rarefying osteitis)*: These are associated with pulpal disease and the associated tooth is sensitive to percussion.
  - *Traumatic bone cyst cavity*: This is usually much larger and found in the younger age group.
  - *Cementifying and ossifying fibroma in early stage*: This affects a younger age group, has a potential to become a very large lesion, and is more commonly found in the premolar region.
  - *Cementoblastoma*: May be confused in the early stages, but this is a rare lesion and is usually associated at the apex of mandibular molars. It extends higher on the root and is connected to the root surface.

- *Stage II*: Mixed Stage
  - *Malignant osteoblastic carcinoma*: This is rapidly growing with borders that are irregular and ill-defined.
  - *Odontoma (intermediate stage)*: This is located above the crown of an unerupted tooth, sometimes between the teeth but rarely at the apex. The internal structure shows orderly relationship of radiopaque enamel, dentin and pulp space in compound odontoma, whereas in complex odontoma, more radiopaque component of enamel is seen. The peripheral cortex and soft tissue capsule of an odontoma are more uniform in width and better defined.
  - *Calcifying crown*: This is seen in the first and second decade and can be identified by the location in the jaw and presence of a similar picture in the contralateral jaw.
  - *Fibrous dysplasia*: It occurs in the younger age group, more often in the maxilla and the margins are poorly defined.
  - *Periapical rarefying osteitis*: It is associated with nonvital teeth, there may be presence of pain, tenderness on palpation, inflammation and regional lymphadenopathy.
  - *Cementifying and ossifying fibroma in late stage*: This affects a younger age group, has a potential to become a very large lesion (more than 2–4 cm in diameter), and is more commonly found in the premolar region.
  - *Benign cementoblastoma*: This tumor is usually solitary and attached to the surface of the root, which may be partially resorbed. There is presence of clinical symptoms.
- *Stage III*: Radiopaque
  - *Hypercementosis*: This involves anterior teeth, but is attached to a part of the root and is separated from the periapical bone by the radiolucent periodontal ligament space which surrounds the entire root.

- *Condensing osteitis*: This occurs at the apex of nonvital teeth, and it does not have a radiolucent border.
- *Periapical idiopathic osteosclerosis*: This occurs at the apex of healthy, vital teeth but this has an irregular shape and there is an absence of the radiolucent border.
- *Paget's disease and osteoblastic metastatic carcinoma*: It can be ruled out if there is absence of systemic symptoms.
- *Benign cementoblastoma*: This tumor is usually solitary and attached to the surface of the root, which may be partially resorbed. There is presence of clinical symptoms.

Management

It requires periodic radiographic evaluation.

Surgical enucleation is indicated only in cases of larger lesions which cause expansion of the cortical plates or in cases where the clinician is unsure of the working diagnosis.

Benign Cementoblastoma (Cementoblastoma, True Cementoma) (Figs 22.16 to 22.19)

Definition

This is a slow growing, mesenchymal neoplasm composed principally of cementum. It manifests as a large bulbous mass of cementum or cementum like tissue on the roots of teeth.

The term true cementoma is now recognized as cementoblastoma, which is a slow growing neoplastic proliferation of cementoblasts.

Clinical Features

- It is more common in males, between the ages of 12–65 years.
- The tumor most often develops with permanent teeth but in rare cases occurs in primary teeth.
- It occurs more often in the mandible, in the premolar and first molar region.
- The tumor is usually solitary, slow growing and may displace teeth.
- The involved tooth is often vital and painful.

Radiographic Features

- It is seen as a well-defined radiopacity with a cortical border surrounded by a well-defined radiolucent band just inside the cortical border. (This indicates that the tumor is maturing from the central portion to the periphery).
- They appear as mixed radiolucent radiopaque lesions that may have an amorphous or a wheel spoke pattern.
- The density of the cemental mass usually obscures the outline of the enveloped root. If the root outline is apparent, then in most cases external resorption can be seen.
- If large enough the tumor may cause expansion of the mandible, with intact outer cortex, which may be well demonstrated on an occlusal radiograph.

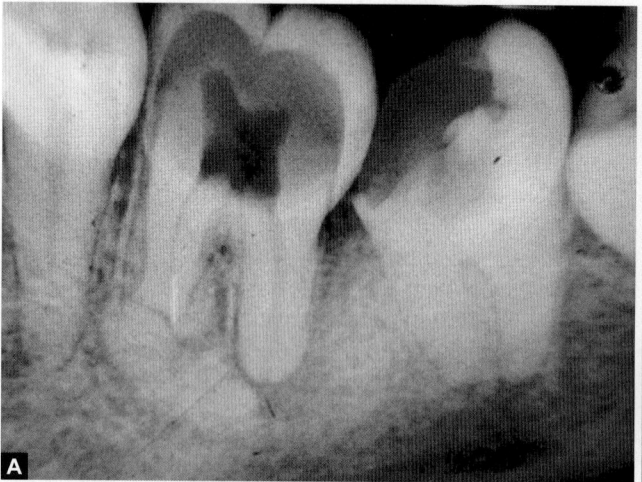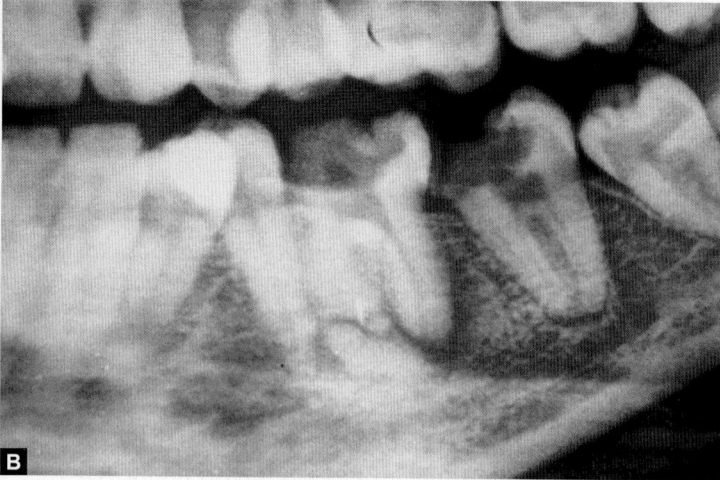

Figures 22.16A and B Cementoblastoma: (A) The periapical view showed well-defined radiopaque mass covering the apical portion of the mesial root extending near the distal root. The mass was surrounded by a radiolucent halo; (B) Cropped panoramic image showed gross coronal radiolucency with molars suggestive of caries. Periapical region of first molar revealed a radiopaque mass which was well-defined, surrounded by a radiolucent halo

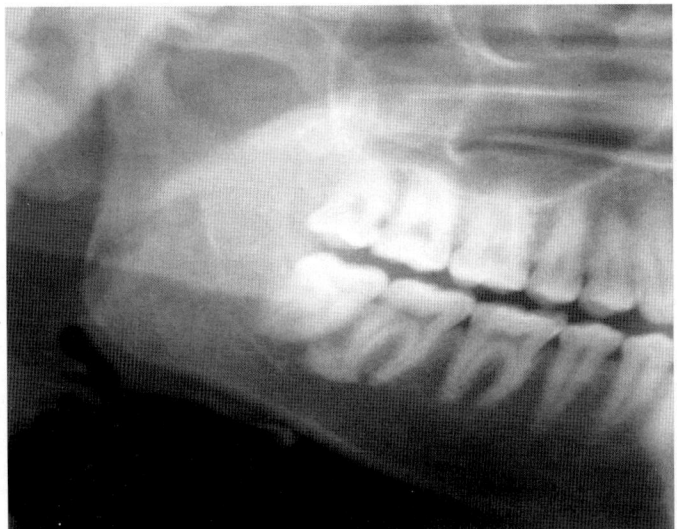

Figure 22.17 Cementoblastoma: Cropped panoramic view showing a well-defined radiopacity seen in relation to apical portion of the distal root of mandibular left second molar. The radiopacity is attached to the root. Differential diagnosis—condensing osteitis, focal sclerosing osteomyelitis, osteosclerosis

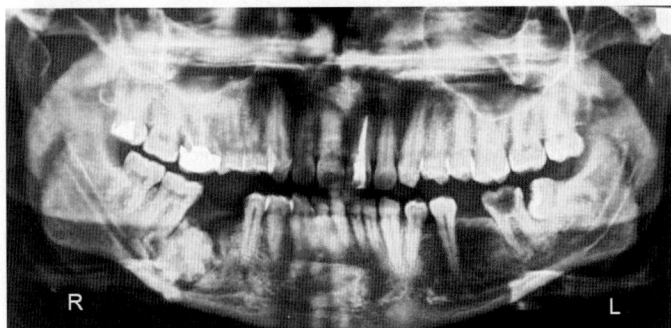

Figure 22.18 Radiopaque clustered irregular mass in the region of mandibular right molar, highly suggestive of cementoblastoma

Differential Diagnosis

- *Periapical cemental dysplasia*: There is no expansion of the jaws, females are more commonly affected, the radiolucent band is less uniform, in the first molar region cementoblastoma has a more rounded shape than cemental dysplasia.
- *Periapical sclerosing osteitis*: It does not have a soft tissue capsule.
- *Enostosis*: It does not have a soft tissue capsule.
- *Hypercementosis*: It does not have a soft tissue capsule, but is surrounded by the periodontal ligament space which is much thinner than the soft tissue capsule of cementoblastoma. There is no root resorption or jaw expansion.

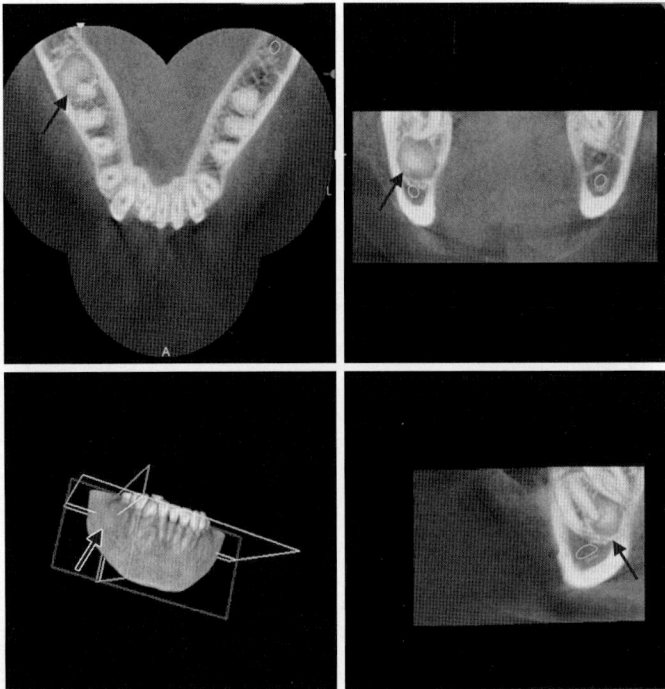

Figure 22.19 Benign cementoblastoma: CBCT; axial, coronal, 3D and sagittal sections showing innocuous periapical radiopacity surrounded by a radiolucent capsule in relation to the maxillary first molar which would not be detected on the panoramic radiograph

- *Chronic focal sclerosing osteomyelitis*: It does not have a soft tissue capsule, therefore no radiolucent halo present.

Management

It is self-limiting. Excision with extraction of the associated tooth or tumor may be amputated from the tooth which is then endodontically treated.

Cemento-ossifying Fibroma (Ossifying Fibroma, Cementifying Fibroma) (Figs 22.20 to 22.23)

Definition

This is considered as a type of fibro-osseous lesion. In the past it was classified as two different entities depending upon whether the bone (ossifying fibroma) or cementum (cementifying fibroma) was the predominant calcified product.

Ossifying fibroma may also be classified as:
- Osssifying form
- Cementifying, psammomatoid forms
- Aggressive (juvenile) form
- Multiple ossifying fibromas
- Familial giganiform cementoma.

Gigantiform cementoma is now recognized as ossifying fibroma, as this lesion is usually a large ossifying fibroma with mature ossification.

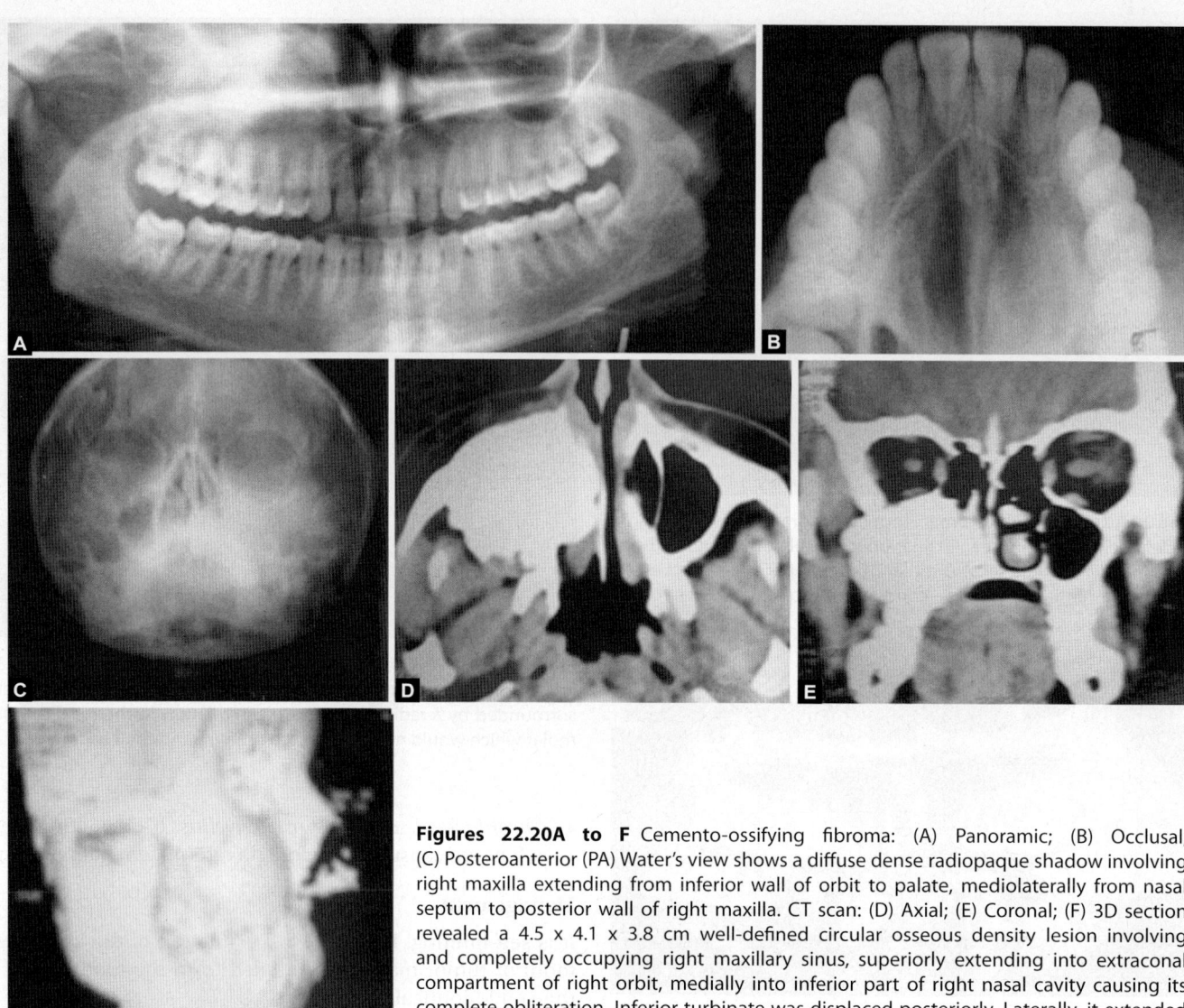

Figures 22.20A to F Cemento-ossifying fibroma: (A) Panoramic; (B) Occlusal; (C) Posteroanterior (PA) Water's view shows a diffuse dense radiopaque shadow involving right maxilla extending from inferior wall of orbit to palate, mediolaterally from nasal septum to posterior wall of right maxilla. CT scan: (D) Axial; (E) Coronal; (F) 3D section revealed a 4.5 x 4.1 x 3.8 cm well-defined circular osseous density lesion involving and completely occupying right maxillary sinus, superiorly extending into extraconal compartment of right orbit, medially into inferior part of right nasal cavity causing its complete obliteration. Inferior turbinate was displaced posteriorly. Laterally, it extended into right buccal space and inferiorly up to alveolar margin of maxilla and hard palate in region of premolars and molars. Posteriorly, it extends up to anterior margin of pterygopalatine fossa

Clinical Features

- It may occur at any age, more often in young adults and females are affected more than males.
- It occurs exclusively in the facial bones. Mandible is more often involved, with the lesion usually typically involving the areas inferior to the premolars and molars and superior to the inferior alveolar canal. In the maxilla it is often seen in the canine fossa and the zygomatic arch region.
- The lesion is asymptomatic and discovered on routine radiographic examination.
- The patient may develop facial asymmetry, with displacement of the associated teeth.

- Juvenile ossifying fibroma is a more aggressive form of COF, seen in the first two decades, the rapid growth may result in severe deformity of the involved jaw.

Radiographic Features

- Initially it is seen as a radiolucent defect within bone (medullary part), which enlarges concentrically. There is a tendency of bone destruction beneath the periosteum. A thin radiolucent line, represents a fibrous capsule which separates it from the surrounding bone. Sometimes hyperostotic borders may separate the lesion.
- Subsequent calcifications results in the appearance of radiopaque foci. The pattern may be similar to that seen in

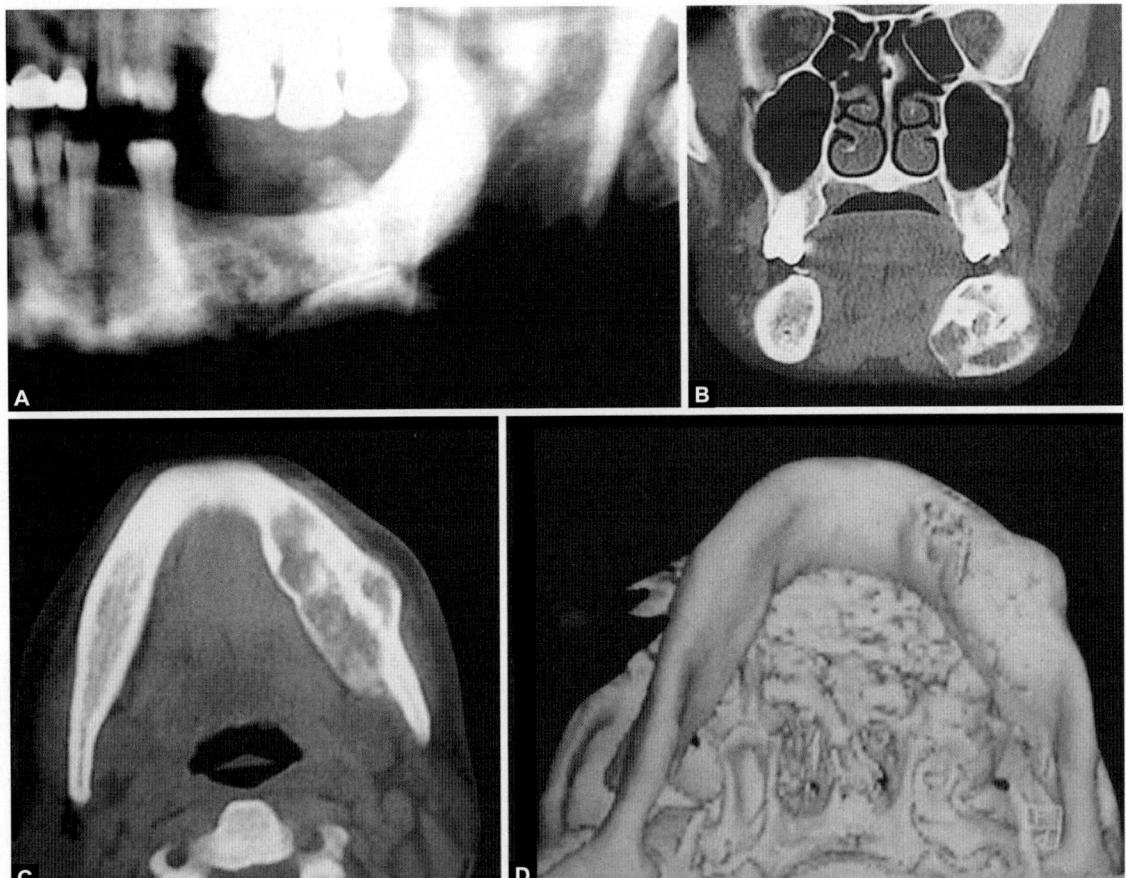

Figures 22.21A to D Cemento-ossifying fibroma: (A) A cropped panoramic radiograph shows a solitary well-defined ovoid, corticated radiolucency in the left mandible extending superiorly-inferiorly from the superior alveolar margin of 34 region to the inferior cortex of the mandible and anterioposteriorly from mandibular left first premolar to angle region, causing expansion of the inferior margin of the mandible at the body and angle with no discontinuity and inferiorly displaced inferior alveolar canal—ossifying fibroma; (B and C) CT scan shows a heterogeneous, radiolucent, radiopaque, expansile lesion, with a well-defined periphery, extending from the left para symphysis region to the angle of the mandible; (D) 3D CT shows perforation of the lingual plate

fibrous dysplasia, or wispy (tufts of cotton), or flocculent pattern (heavy snowflakes). Lesions that produce more cementum like material may contain solid, amorphous radiopacities (cementicles) as seen in cemental dysplasia.

- The radiopaque calcified masses tend to coalesce and the tumor may become radiopaque after some years.
- The tumor grows concentrically within the medullary part of the bone, with outward expansion approximately equal in all directions. It causes displacement of teeth and inferior alveolar canal, with expansion of the outer cortical plates, which may be displaced and thinned but remain in tact.
- Lamina dura of the involved teeth is missing with resorption of the teeth.
- In the maxilla the tumor produces a unique growth pattern in which there is dissolution of neighboring bones, without displacement by pressure. The COF may grow entirely into the maxillary sinus, expanding its walls outward, but a bony partition remains between the internal aspect of the remaining sinus and the tumor.

Additional Imaging

Large lesions require a detailed determination of the extent of the lesion, which can be obtained with CT imaging.

Differential Diagnosis

- *Early radiolucent stage*:
  - *Postextraction socket and residual cyst*: History of extraction and/or surgery.
  - *Primordial cyst*: It is always associated with a missing permanent tooth.
  - *Ameloblastoma*: It occurs in the posterior part of the mandible, multilocular appearance is more common and may cause paresthesia of the lip.

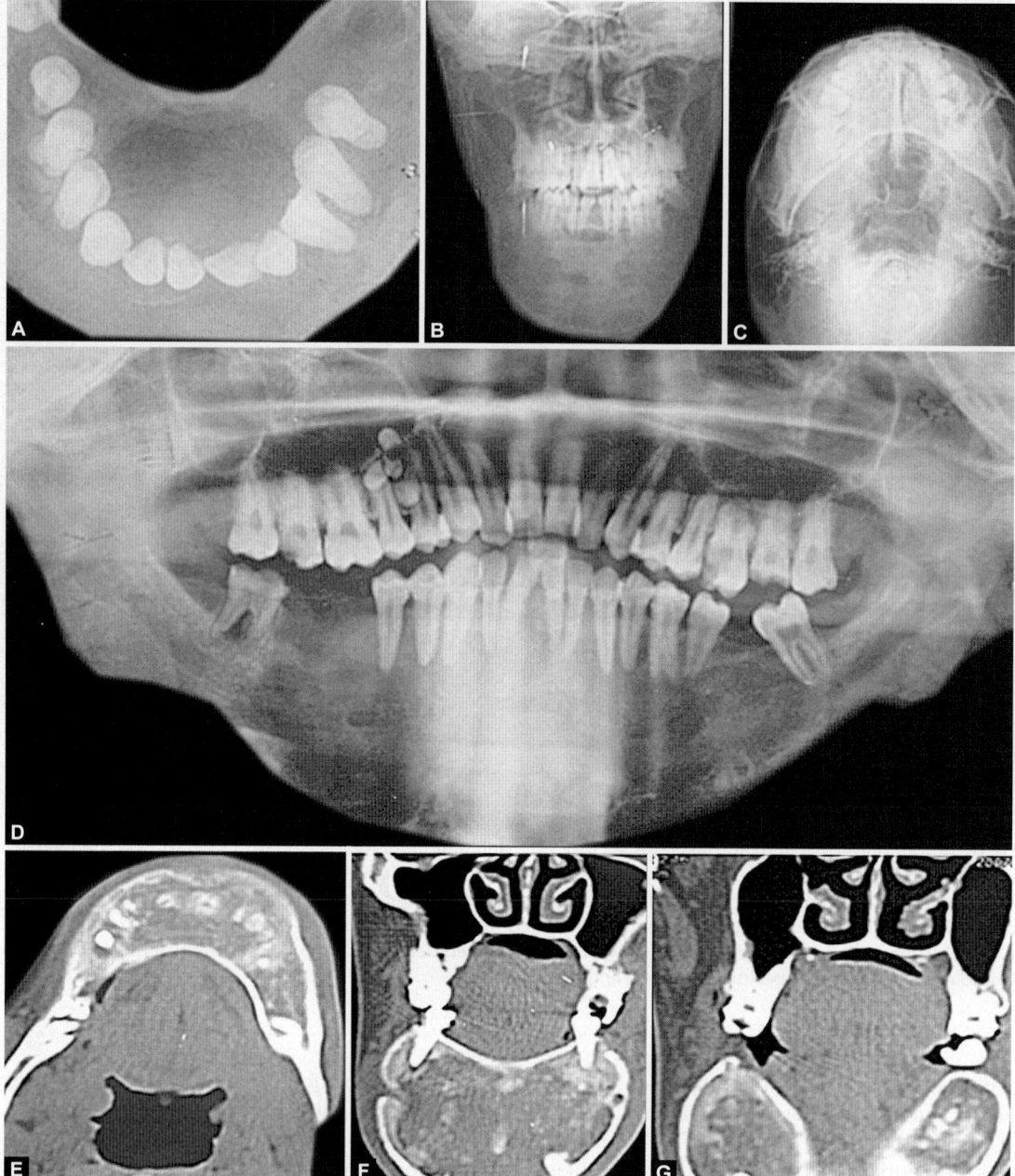

Figures 22.22A to G Cemento-ossifying fibroma: (A) Mandibular occlusal topical view: Revealed a mixed radiopaque radioucent lesion causing expansion of buccal and lingual cortical plates. Greater expansion on the lingual aspect; (B) PA mandible: Well-defined mixed lesion seen extending from the left to right mandibular third molars and involving the entire height of the mandible. Margins are well corticated in the superior and inferior borders. Thinning of the inferior border of the mandible with expansion in the downward direction. Ill-defined calcifications seen within the lesion. Flaring of mandibular incisors seen; (C) Submentovertex view: Well-defined mixed lesion seen extending from the anterior border of ramus on one side till the ramus of other side and involving the entire width of the mandible. Margins are well corticated in the buccal and lingual borders. Ill-defined calcifications seen within the lesion. Buccolingual expansion seen, greater on the lingual aspect; (D) Panoramic view showed a mixed radiopaque-radiolucent lesion of the mandibular body extending from right mandibular third molar to left mandibular third molar. Increase in the height of the mandible from molar-to-molar regions. Margins are well corticated in the superior and inferior borders. Thinning of the inferior border of the mandible with expansion in the downward direction. Ill-defined calcifications seen within the lesion. Flaring of mandibular incisors seen. Multiple well-defined radiopacities seen in the right maxillary premolar region suggestive of odontome. Supernumerary premolar in the left mandibular premolar region. CT Scan: (E) Axial view; (F and G) Coronal view show expansion and sclerosis in relation to the body of the mandible from molar-to-molar region with a regular outline and diffuse calcifications. Supernumerary premolar in the left mandibular premolar region, mandibular canal was inferiorly displaced to the lower border of the mandible

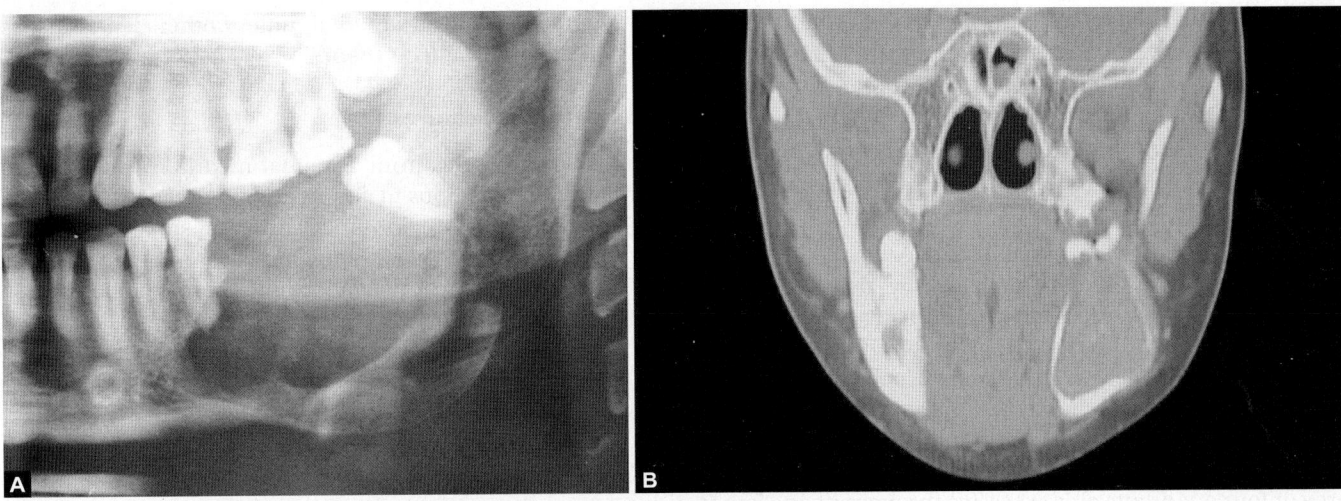

Figures 22.23A and B Cemento-ossifying fibroma: (A) Cropped panoramic image showed large well-defined circular radiolucent lesion extending from apical region in respect to right premolar to third molar involving the left angle of mandible; (B) CT scan coronal view shows 4.2 x 2.5 cm sized expansile, unilocular lytic lesion involving body of left mandible perforating the buccal cortex

- *Periapical cemental dysplasia*: It is associated with vital teeth, usually in the lower anterior region, and affect an older age group.
- *Adenomatoid odontogenic tumor*: It is found in younger individuals, usually associated with an impacted maxillary canine and has regular borders.
- Mixed radiopaque radiolucent lesion:
  - *Calcifying odontogenic cysts.*
  - *Calcifying epithelial odontogenic tumor*: It occurs in the posterior body and ramus of the mandible.
  - *Osteoblastoma and osteoid osteoma*: These are located at the inferior aspect of the mandible, and osteoblastoma is a larger and more aggressive tumor.
  - *Osteogenic sarcoma, metastatic osteoblastic carcinoma and chondromasarcoma*: These have ill-defined borders with periosteal bone formation. These are rapidly growing and do not have a fibrous capsule.
  - *Periapical cemental dysplasia*: It is a more common lesion, with a predilection for lower incisors, with no displacement, in a younger age group and seldom attains a diameter above 1 cm, whereas COF usually attains a diameter more than 2-4 cm. It has a wide sclerotic border. This is usually multifocal whereas COF is not. There may presence of a simple bone cyst.
  - *Paget's disease*: This shows cotton wool appearance with enlargement of the affected bone.
  - *Fibrous dysplasia*: It is more commonly found in the mandible with equal sex distribution. It appears as a homogeneous radiopaque area with an internal structure that is evenly granular and obliterates normal bone marrow space. The borders are ill-

defined and gradually blending into the surrounding normal bone. Root resorption is rare. Both can displace teeth but COF displaces from a specific point or epicenter. In fibrous dysplasia, the expanded bone resembles normal morphology, whereas the expansion of bone with COF is more concentric about a definite epicenter.
  - It is difficult to differentiate fibrous dysplasia from juvenile ossifying fibroma when the lesion involves the maxillary sinus. Fibrous dysplasia usually displaces the lateral wall of the maxilla into the maxillary sinus, maintaining the outer shape of the wall whereas ossifying fibroma has a more convex shape as it extends into the maxillary sinus.
- Mature stage
  - *Periapical spherical type of hypercementosis*: This is attached to a part of the root and is separated from the periapical bone by a radiolucent periodontal ligament space which surrounds the entire root.
  - Condensing osteitis; it occurs at the periapex of nonvital teeth, and does not have a radiolucent band around the lesion.
  - Periapical idiopathic osteosclerosis; this is usually irregular in shape, without a radiolucent rim, and is associated in the periapical region of vital teeth.
  - Complex odontoma; its density is not uniform and it seldom occurs periapically.

Management

Conservative enucleation. Recurrence is rare.

Florid Osseous Dysplasia (Gigantiform Cementoma, Florid Cemeto-osseous Dysplasia, Familial Multiple Cementomas, Chronic Sclerosing Osteomyelitis, Sclerosing Osteitis, Multiple Enostosis, Sclerotic Cemental Masses) (Figs 22.24 to 22.26)

Definition

FOD appears to be a widespread form of cemental dysplasia. Normal cancellous bone is replaced by dense acellular cemento-osseous tissue in a background of fibrous connective tissue. It is derived from the cells in or near the periodontal ligament space. The lesion has a poor vascular supply and is susceptible to infections. It may be inherited as an autosomal dominant trait. No clear definition indicates when multiple regions of PCD should be termed FOD. If PCD is identified in three or four quadrants or is excessive throughout one jaw, it is usually considered to be FOD.

Clinical Features

- Most of the patients are middle-aged females.
- The lesions are restricted to the jaw bones, usually bilateral with the mandible more commonly affected. The epicenter is apical to the teeth, within the alveolar process and usually posterior to the cuspid. In the mandible the lesions occur above the inferior alveolar canal.
- It is asymptomatic, painless expansion of the alveolar process of the mandible and is usually discovered on routine radiographic examinations.
- Patient may complain of intermittent, poorly localized pain in the affected bone, especially when a simple bone cyst has developed within the lesion.
- If the lesion becomes secondarily infected it may develop mucosal ulcerations, fistulous tracts with suppuration and pain.

- The teeth involved are vital, unless other dental disease coincidentally affects them.

Radiographic Features

- The lesion varies from an equal mixture of radiolucent-radiopaque regions to almost complete radiopacity.
- The radiopaque regions may vary from small oval circular regions (cotton wool appearance) to large, irregular, amorphous areas of calcification. These calcified masses appear similar to those seen in mature PCD lesions.
- The periphery is usually well-defined and has a sclerotic border that may vary in width. The soft tissue capsule may not be apparent in mature lesions.

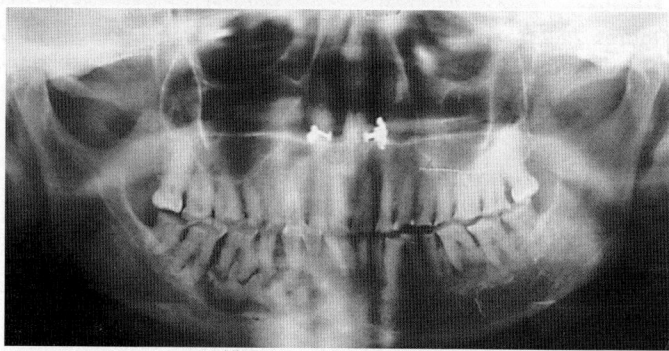

Figure 22.24 Florid osseous dysplasia: Panoramic radiograph showing involvement of mandible bilaterally above the inferior alveolar canal, radiolucent-radiopaque lesions with well-defined sclerotic border surrounded by a soft tissue capsule which may not be apparent in mature lesions. Cotton wool appearance to amorphous areas of calcification. Roots of associated teeth show hypercementosis which may fuse with the lesion. Displacement of inferior dental canal inferiorly and floor of the maxillary sinus superiorly is normally observed

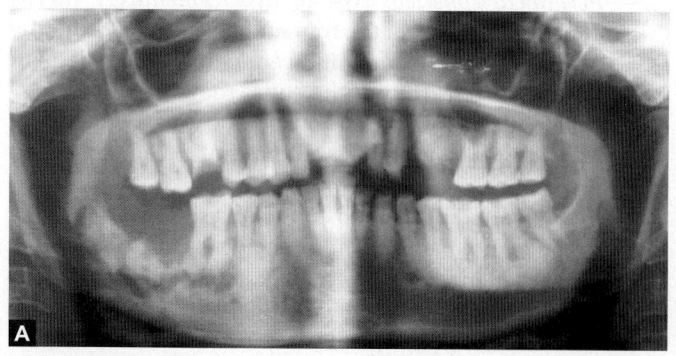

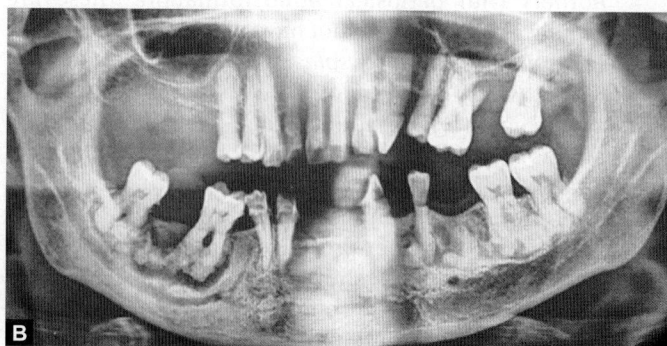

Figures 22.25A and B Florid osseous dysplasia: (A) Panoramic view shows an ill-defined area of mixed radiolucent radiopaque lesion seen in the right mandibular body extending in the right premolar to molar region from the alveolar crest till the inferior cortex of mandibular canal. Area of dense bone structure seen in the periapical regions of the involved teeth. Another area of dense bone structure seen in the periapical regions of left premolar-molar region above the mandibular canal; (B) Florid osseous dysplasia: Panoramic view shows multiple mixed radiopacity surrounded by radiolucency, in the region mandibular molars, which appears to be close to the root apex not attached to it. Generalized mild bone loss

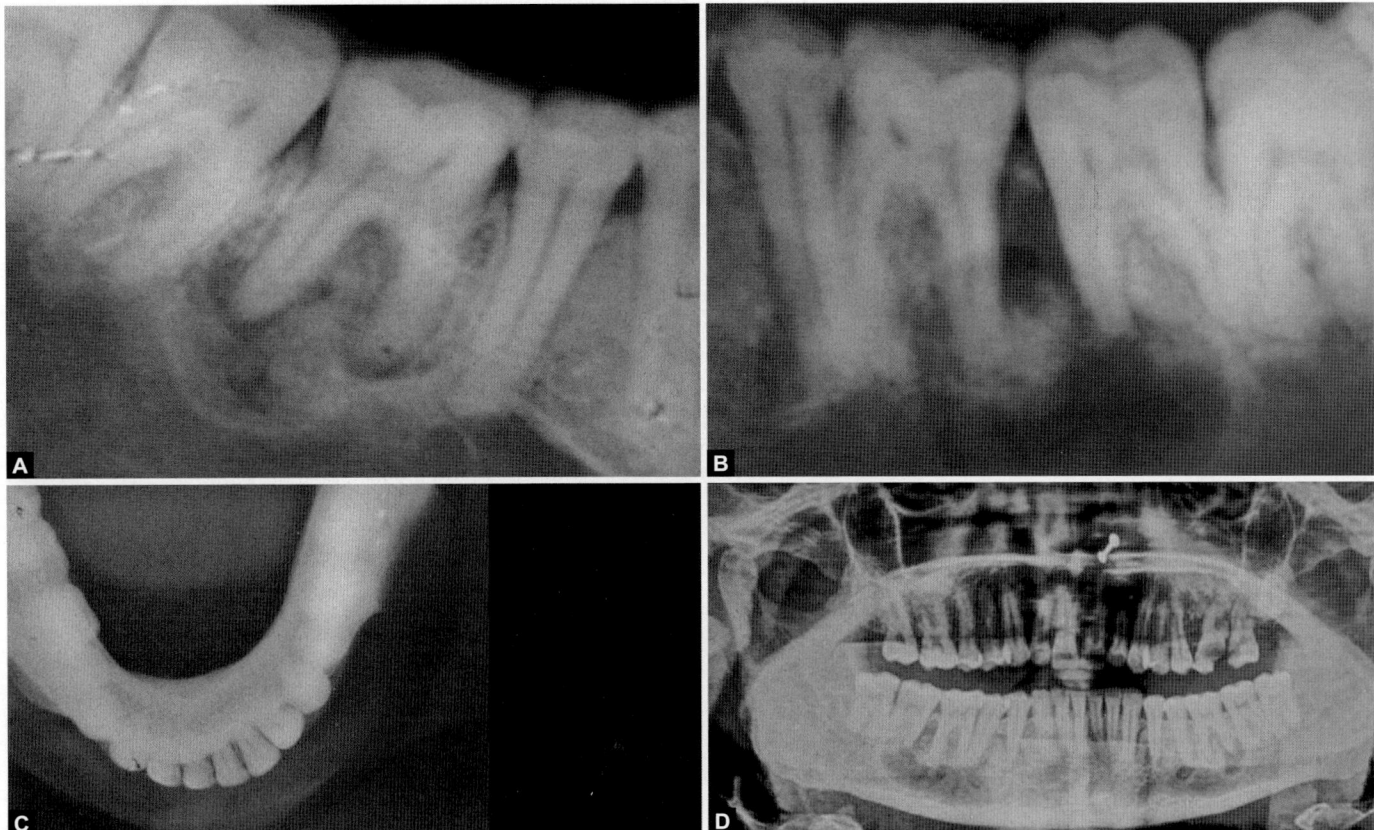

Figures 22.26A to D Florid osseous dysplasia: (A and B) Periapical views of mandibular right and left molar region shows oval, 1 cm in diameter, well-defined radiolucency surrounded by the thin corticated margins in the periapical; (C) Mandibular occlusal view: Expansion of the cortex in right and left molar region; (D) Panoramic view shows oval, 1 cm in diameter, well-defined radiolucency surrounded by the thin corticated margins in the periapical region of mandibular molars

- Some prominent radiolucent regions may be present which may be due to the development of a simple bone cyst. These cysts may enlarge with time beyond the boundary of the lesion into the surrounding normal bone or may fill in with abnormal dysplastic cemento-osseous tissue.
- Large lesions may displace the inferior alveolar canal in the inferior direction, and the floor of the antrum in the superior direction. It can cause enlargement of the alveolar bone by displacement of the buccal and lingual cortical plates.
- The roots of the associated teeth may show hypercementosis, which may fuse with the abnormal surrounding cemental tissue of the lesion. Extraction of these teeth is difficult.

Differential Diagnosis

- *Paget's disease*: No radiolucent capsule. Increased serum alkaline phosphatase levels. This affects nearly all the bones of the skeleton (polyostotic). In the mandible it involves and affects the entire mandible whereas FOD is centered above the inferior alveolar canal.

- *Osteopetrosis*: There is profuse thickening of the skull base or calvarium and diffuse bony radiopacities. It will cause enlargement of bone, which is not a feature of FOD.
- *Chronic sclerosing osteomyelitis*: Regions of cementum may appear similar to that of sequestrum, CT imaging can aid in differentiating.

Management

No treatment is required, regular check ups with maintenance of oral hygiene to prevent secondary infection. In denture wearers, the pressure may cause dehiscence in the mucosa, resulting in osteomyelitis.

Central Odontogenic Fibroma (Simple Odontogenic Fibroma, Odontogenic Fibroma) (Figs 22.27A to I)

Definition

This is a rare neoplasm, which may occur centrally or in the periphery (where it mimics fibroma). They are divided into

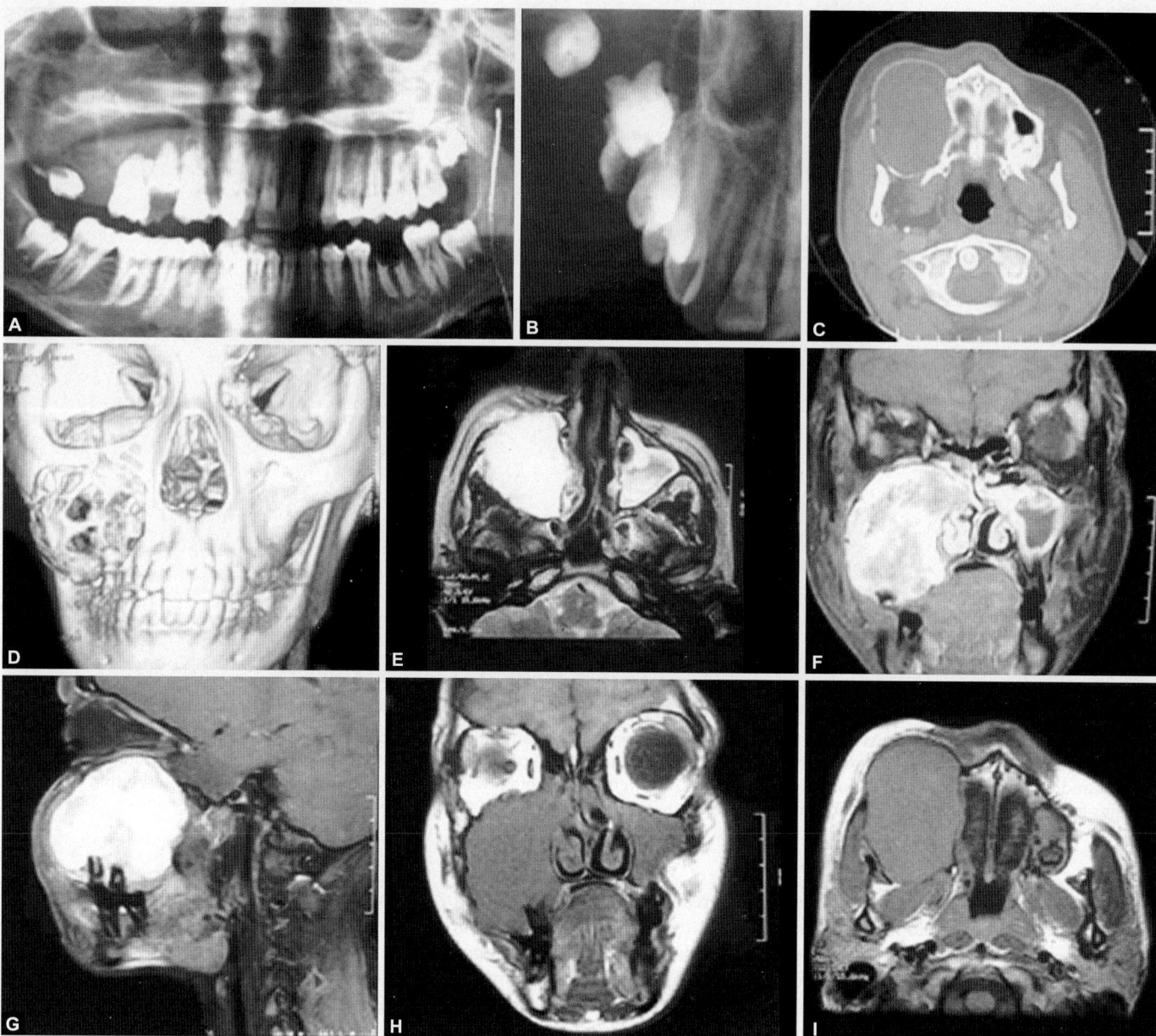

Figures 22.27A to I Central odontogenic fibroma: Central odontogenic fibroma related to maxillary right molar area: (A) Showing a large well-defined multilocular lesion in right maxilla, extending from right canine to the tuberosity, and superiorly to the inferior margin of the orbit, completely obliterating the sinus, extending up to the right middle and inferior meatus; (B) Occlusal radiograph showing central odontogenic fibroma in the same patient, seen as a multilocular radiolucency with ballooning of the cortex extending palatally. Impacted third molar present; (C) CT (Bone window) axial view shows lesion occupying the right maxillary sinus, with thinning of the walls, the floor of the orbit is indented by the expansile lesion. Here the lesion appears heterogeneously hyper intense. Discontinuity of the buccal cortex; (D) 3D CT showing a multilocular lesion, with well-defined septae, dividing the lesion into locules. Central fibroma in the same patient. MRI -T_2 Scan, central odontogenic fibroma in the same patient; (E) Axial section; (F) Coronal section; (G) Sagittal section, showing lesion occupying the right maxillary sinus, with thinning of the walls, the floor of the orbit is indented by the expansile lesion. Here the lesion appears heterogeneously hyper intense,—central odontogenic fibroma instead of central fibroma in the same patient. MRI Scan T_1 images shows; (H and I) Lesion occupying the right maxillary sinus, with thinning of the walls, the floor of the orbit is indented by the expansile lesion. Here the lesion appears homogeneously panoramic view to muscle

two types according to histological appearance; the simple type which contains mature fibrous tissue with sparsely scattered odontogenic epithelial rests and the granular cell or WHO type, which is more cellular, has more epithelial rests and may contain calcifications, which resemble dyplastic dentine, cementum or osteoid.

Clinical Features

- It is more common in females, between 11–39 years of age.
- It is more common in the mandible in the molar-premolar region and in the maxilla and in the region anterior to the first molar.
- It is usually asymptomatic or the patient may complain of a swelling with mobility of teeth.

Radiographic Features

- The smaller lesions are unilocular and larger lesions are multilocular.
- The internal septa may be fine and straight (as in myxoma) or granular (as in giant cell granuloma). Some lesions are totally radiolucent whereas unorganized internal calcifications may be seen in others.
- The margins are well-defined and sclerotic.
- It may cause expansion with maintenance of a thin cortical boundary or may grow along the bone with minimum expansion.
- Tooth displacement and root resorption is commonly seen.

Differential Diagnosis

- *Central desmoplastic fibroma*: Histological findings are similar, but, desmoplastic fibromas are more aggressive and tend to break through the peripheral cortex and invade the surrounding tissue. The septa are very thick, straight and angular.
- *Odontogenic myoma.*
- *Giant cell granuloma.*

Management

Simple excision. They have a very low recurrence rate.

Peripheral Odontogenic Fibroma (Peripheral Ossifying Fibroma, Peripheral Ameloblastic Fibro-dentinoma, Calcifying Fibrous Epulis, Peripheral Fibroma with Calcification) (Figs 22.28A to C)

Definition

It is believed to be associated with irritation like over extended margin of faulty restoration or deposits of calculus. It involves the periodontal ligament superficially and contains odontogenic epithelium rests and deposits of cementum, bone and dystrophic calcifications scattered through the background of fibrous tissue.

Clinical Features

- It is more common in females, between the age 5–25 years.
- It occurs on the free margin of the gingival and involves the interdental papillae, more often in the mandible.
- It is asymptomatic and slow growing, but some lesions may grow large enough to cause facial asymmetry.
- They are solid, sessile or pedunculated mass, firmly attached to the gingival mass, and may displace teeth when positioned in between them.
- Early lesions are soft, vascular and bleed readily. Mature lesions are firm, fibrous and pale pink.

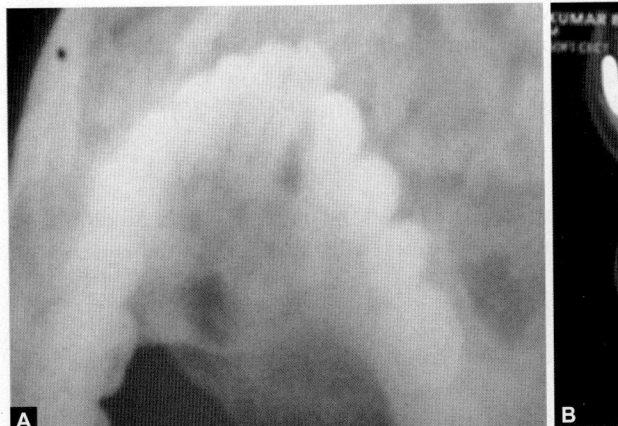 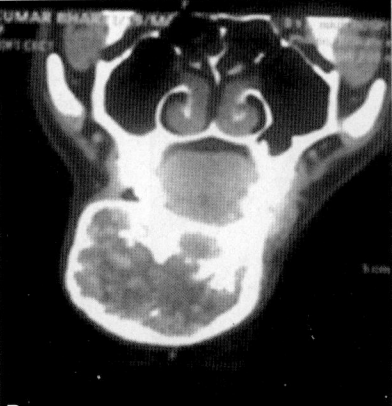 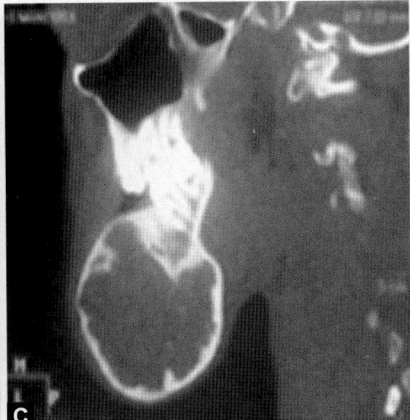

Figures 22.28A to C Peripheral ossifying fibroma: (A) Occlusal view showing and expansile lesion. CT: (B) Coronal; (C) Sagittal view showing Large 7 × 5.5 × 5 cm, mixed expansile lesion in the right hemimandible is seen with involvement of the menti, left parasymphysis up to premolar region. Involvement of the mandibular canal is seen. Calcific/ossific foci are seen within the lesion

Radiographic Features

- Superficial erosion may be seen.
- Presence of radiopaque foci within the tumor mass, due to calcifications within the tumor may be on the radiograph.

Differential Diagnosis

- *Chondrosarcoma and osteogenic sarcoma*: These are less likely to be gingival lesions, severe bony changes are seen, asymptomatic widening of the periodontal ligament space may be seen.
- *Inflammatory hyperplasia*: No displacement and separation of teeth seen.

Management

Simple surgical excision.

Mixed Tumors of Odontogenic Epithelium and Odontogenic Ectomesenchyme

Ameloblastic Fibroma (Soft Odontoma, Soft Mixed Odontoma, Mixed Odontogenic Tumor, Fibroadamantoblastoma, Granular Cell Ameloblastic Fibroma) (Figs 22.29A and B)

Definition

It is characterized by neoplastic proliferation of maturing and early functional ameloblasts and the primitive mesenchymal components of the dental papilla. Enamel, dentine and cementum are not formed in this tumor.

Clinical Features

- There is no sex predilection, they occur between 5–20 years of age, during the period of tooth formation.

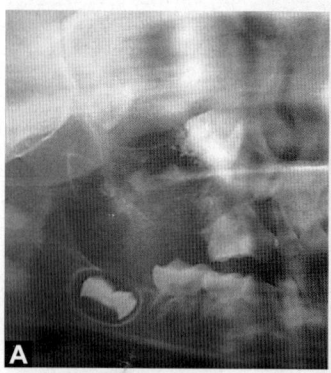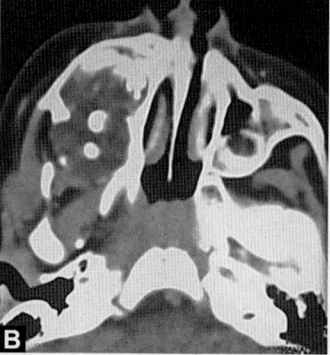

Figures 22.29A and B Ameloblastic fibroma: (A) Cropped panoramic radiograph; (B) CT axial view, showing well-defined uniformly smooth corticated expansile radiolucency which contains solitary radiopaque masses or multiple small doughnut shaped radiopacities. Usually associated with an impacted tooth

- It is more common in the premolar-molar region of the mandible, and may involve the ramus and extend forward to the molar-premolar region. It may be located near the crest of the alveolar process or in follicular relationship with an unerupted tooth (is located occlusal to the tooth), or it may arise in an area where a tooth has failed to develop.
- It produces a painless, slow growing expansion, and displacement of the involved teeth. It may at times be asymptomatic and discovered on routine radiographic survey, especially when associated with a missing tooth.

Radiographic Features

- It is usually seen as an unilocular radiolucency but may sometimes appear multilocular with indistinct curved septa
- The borders are well-defined and corticated
- If the lesion is large, there may be expansion with an intact cortical plate. The associated tooth may be prohibited from normal eruption or may be displaced in an apical direction.

Differential Diagnosis

- *Small dentigerous cyst.*
- *Hyperplastic follicle.*
- *Ameloblastoma*: It occurs in a later age and the septa are more defined and coarse
- *Giant cell granuloma*: These are multilocular and have the epicenter anterior to the first molar and the septa are granular and ill-defined
- *Odontogenic myxoma*: It occur in the older age group, these are multilocular and usually have a few sharp straight septa.

Management

A conservative surgical enucleation with mechanical curettage of the surrounding bone is sufficient.

Ameloblastic Fibro-odontoma (Fig. 22.30)

Definition

It is a mixed tumor with all the elements of an ameloblastic fibroma but with scattered collections of enamel and dentin.

Clinical Features

- Males are more commonly affected, in the younger age group
- More common in the posterior aspect of the mandible in the molar region and in the maxilla it involves the maxillary sinus. The epicenter is usually occlusal to the developing tooth or towards the alveolar crest.

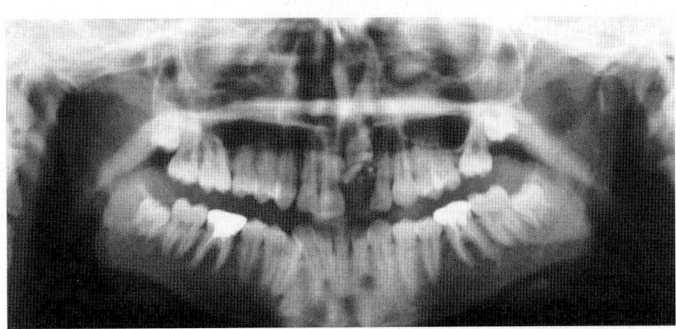

Figure 22.30 Ameloblastic fibrodontoma: Ameloblastic fibrodontoma with respect to impacted upper central incisor which is surrounded by the heterogeneous masses encircling the crown of same density as of the dentin. Not surrounded by the capsule, should be differentiated from odontome

- The most common complaint is a swelling and failure of tooth eruption. The maxillary tumor if large may interfere with nasal respiration, eating and speech.
- It consists of elements of ameloblastic odontoma but is more aggressive than a common odontoma.

Radiographic Features

- It presents as a well-defined, uniformly smooth and corticated expansile radiolucency containing either a solitary radiopaque mass or multiple small radiopacities (small doughnut shaped) representing the odontoma portion of the lesion.
- Some lesions may be relatively small (1–2 cm) while others may involve a considerable portion of the body of the mandible and extending into the ramus.
- Most often an associated impacted tooth is present.

Differential Diagnosis

- *Ameloblastic fibroma*: It usually has no calcifications.
- *Developing odontoma*: The ameloblastic fibro-odontoma has greater soft tissue component (radiolucency) than an odontoma. Even when the amount of hard tissue increases the complex odontoma has one mass of disorganized tissue in the center, whereas the ameloblastic fibro-odontoma will have multiple scattered mature pieces of dental hard tissue, in case of the compound odontome, it has multiple denticles, the posterior part of the mandible is a rare location and the organization of tooth material in ameloblastic fibro-odontome is never organized to resemble a tooth.

Management

Conservative enucleation.

Ameloblastic Odontoma (Odonto-ameloblastoma)

Definition

It is an extremely rare odontogenic tumor characterized by simultaneous occurrence of an ameloblastoma and a composite odontoma.

Clinical Features

- It is more common in children in the second decade of life
- More often found in the mandible
- It is a slowly expanding lesion of bone which may produce considerable facial deformity or asymmetry if left untreated
- It may also cause bony expansion and destruction of the cortex with displacement of the associated teeth
- There will be delayed eruption of teeth and the patient may complain of mild pain.

Radiographic Features

- The radiographic density is similar to that of complex odontoma
- The radiopaque masses that are present may or may not bear resemblance to miniature teeth. Sometimes a single irregular radiopaque mass of calcified tissue may be present
- The margins are well-defined, uniformly smooth and even
- The central destruction of bone with expansion of the cortical plates is seen
- Tooth displacement may occur.

Management

Should be treated similar to ameloblastoma.

Odontogenic Myxoma (Myxoma, Myxofibroma, Fibromyxoma, Odontogenic Fibromyxoma)
(Figs 22.31 to 22.33)

Definition

It is a benign, intraosseous neoplasm that arises from odontogenic ectomesenchyme and resembles the mesenchymal portion of the dental papilla. These develop only in the facial bones. It is occasionally related to a tooth that failed to erupt or is missing, and in some cases odontogenic epithelium can be detected microscopically.

Clinical Features

- It accounts for 3–6 percent of odontogenic tumors.
- It is more common in females, with an age range of 10 to 30 years.

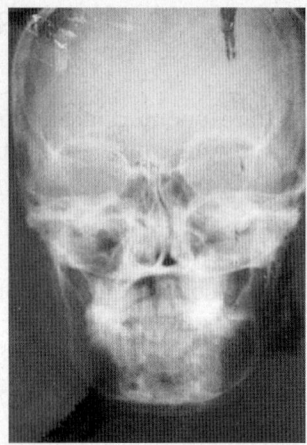

Figure 22.31 Odontogenic myxoma: Posteroanterior (PA) mandible showing ill defined, multilocular, osteolytic radiolucent lesion of right mandible with irregular borders, with cortical expansion

- It is more common in the mandible in the premolar-molar area and in the maxilla in the alveolar process in premolar-molar area and the zygoma
- It is usually associated with congenitally missing tooth/teeth
- It is a slow growing hard fusiform swelling which may cause facial asymmetry and pain
- It may perforate the cortical plate producing a bosselated surface (several small nodules on the surface).
- The involved teeth may be displaced and loosened but resorption is rare.
- If it invades the maxillary sinus it may cause exophthalmus.

Radiographic Features

- The lesion is usually well-defined with a corticated margin. In the maxilla it may be poorly defined. It may be scalloped between roots of adjacent teeth.
- If it occurs pericoronally with an impacted tooth it may appear cyst like, with an unilocular outline.
- Most of the time it appears multilocular having a mixed radiolucent-radiopaque internal pattern.
- There is presence of septa which give it the multilocular appearance, there may be straight, thin-etched septa (tennis racket like or step ladder pattern) or septa that are curved and coarse with two or three straight septa.
- The tumor has a tendency to grow along the involved bone without the same amount of expansion seen in other benign tumors.

Addition Imaging

- *CT*: Help in establishing the intraosseous extent of the tumor and guide in planning the resection margins. The scan also shows small trabeculae within the lesion, with a characteristic straight or angular arrangement.

- *MRI*: Help in establishing the intraosseous extent of the tumor and guide in planning the resection margins. The high tissue signal characteristic of the tumor in T2 weighted MR images is particularly useful in establishing tumor extent and presence of a recurrent tumor.

Differential Diagnosis

- *Central giant cell granuloma*: It has a preferred anterior location in the mandible.
- *Ameloblastoma*: This occurs in older patients.
- *Cherubism*: This occurs in the younger age group and has a bilateral involvement.
- *Giant cell lesion of hyperthyroidism*: History of kidney disease and abnormal serum chemistry.
- *Metastatic carcinoma*: In the older age group and there will be presence of the primary tumor.
- *Aneurysmal bone cyst*: This is tender and painful.
- *Central hemangioma*: This is not associated with a missing tooth. Pumping tooth syndrome may be seen, and aspiration is diagnostic.
- *Osteogenic sarcoma*: This also has a spiculated appearance but the outer cortex is lost in osteogenic sarcoma which is not so in odontogenic myxoma.

Management

Surgical excision with generous amount of surrounding bone, to ensure removal of myomatous tumor infiltrates from the adjacent marrow spaces.

Odontoma (Compound Odontoma, Compound Composite Odontoma, Complex Odontoma, Complex Composite Odontoma, Odontogenic Hamartoma, Calcified Mixed Odontoma, Cystic Odontoma) (Figs 22.34 to 22.37)

This is a hamartoma of odontogenic origin in which both epithelial and mesenchymal cells exhibit complete differentiation with enamel and dentine laid down in abnormal position. It may result from the extraneous buds of odontogenic epithelial cells from the lamina dura, from any of the three dental tissues, enamel, dentine or cementum. The cause may be trauma, infection or genetic transmission.

Classification

- Ectodermal origin
  - Enameloma (enamel pearl, enamel nodule)
- Mesodermal origin
  - Dentinoma
  - Cementoma
- Mixed
  - Complex composite odontoma—non discrete masses of dental tissue

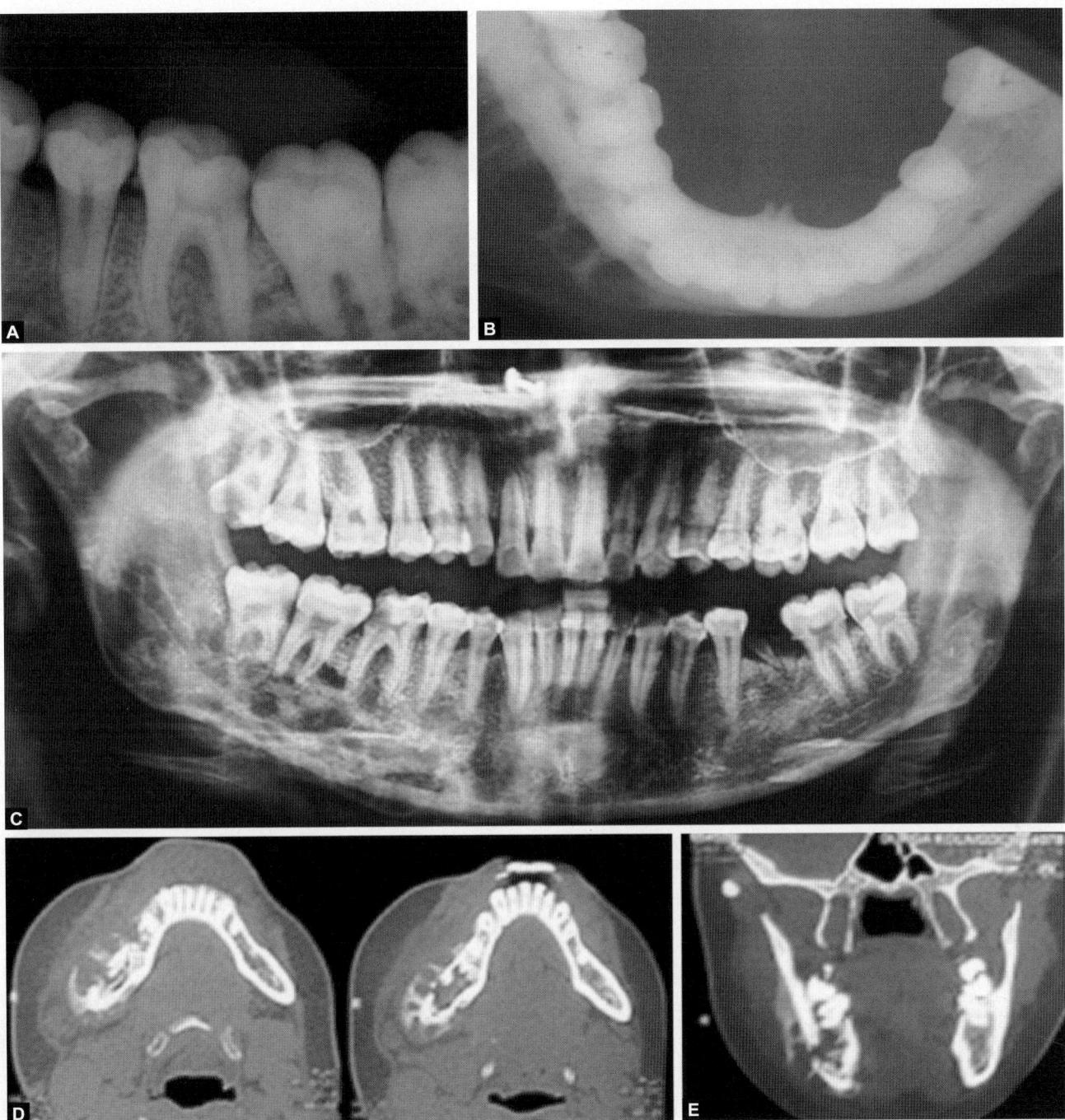

Figures 22.32A to E Odontogenic myxoma: (A) Periapical radiograph showing mandibular first premolar and molar with distal radiolucency approaching the pulp of first molar with apical loss of lamira dura of the distal root of 46. Small radiolucencies seen in the alveolar bone between teeth; (B) Mandibular occlusal radiograph shows expansion of the buccal cortex with multiple small radiolucencies with coarse radiopaque angular septae extending from region of premolar to molar region; (C) Panoramic view shows a mixed radiopaque-radiolucent lesion extending from mesial of first premolar to the angle of mandible and from alveolar crest to inferior border of the mandible. Margins are ill-defined. Lesion is also extending between the roots. Some trabeculae can be traced within the posterior portion of the lesion. Superior cortical lining of the mandibular canal cannot be traced. Raised area of periosteum seen under the inferior cortical border of mandible right side. CT scan: (D) Axial; (E) Coronal section shows irregular destructive lesion seen on the right side of the mandible involving the body, angle and lower half of the ramus extending from canine to the mandibular angle. Heterogenously enhancing soft tissue extension of the lesion present .Thick irregular periosteal reaction predominantly on the buccal surface of cortical plate with multiple radiolucencies which may be located in the ramus, angle and body of right mandible. Subcentimetric right level 1, bilateral level II lymph nodes visualized

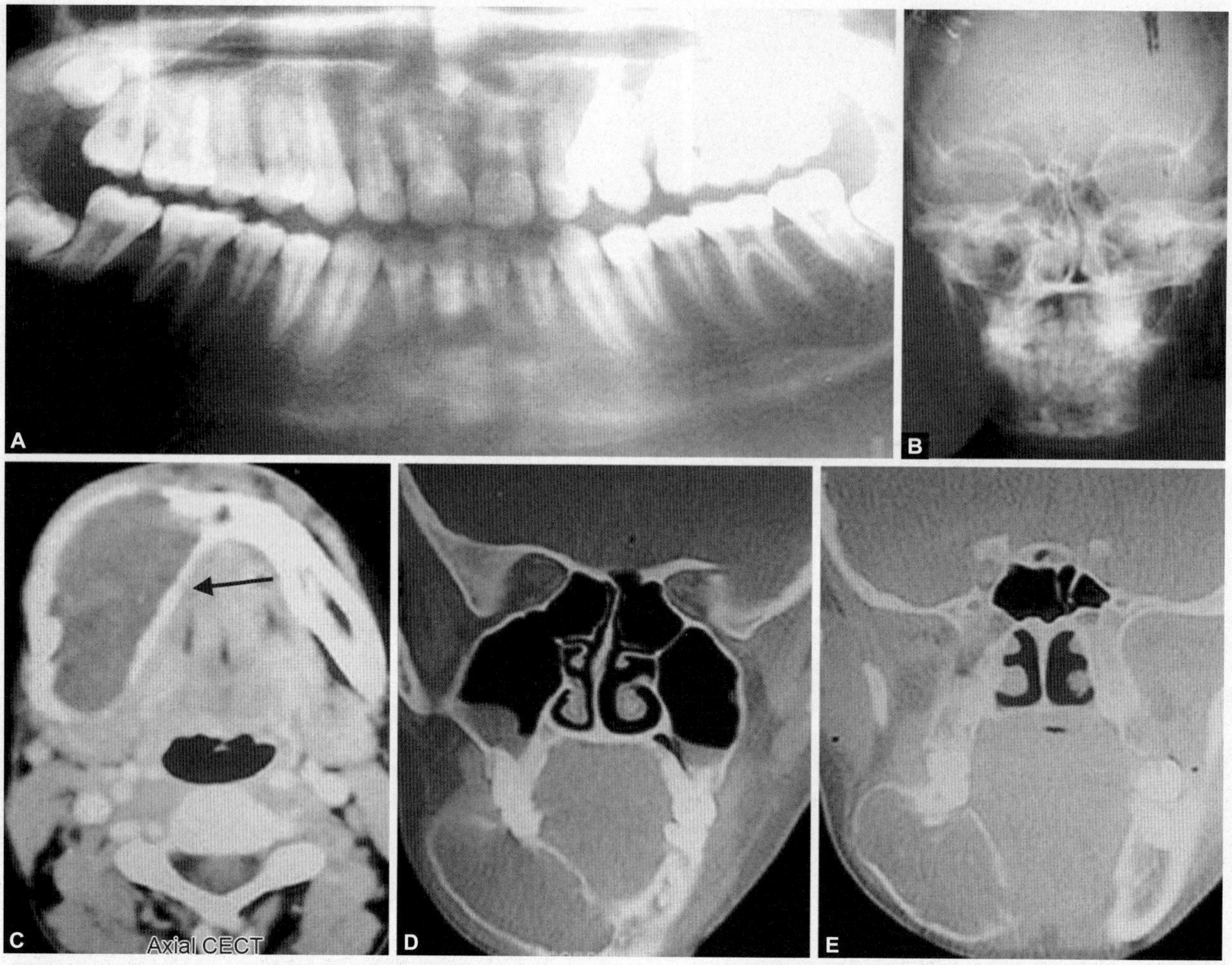

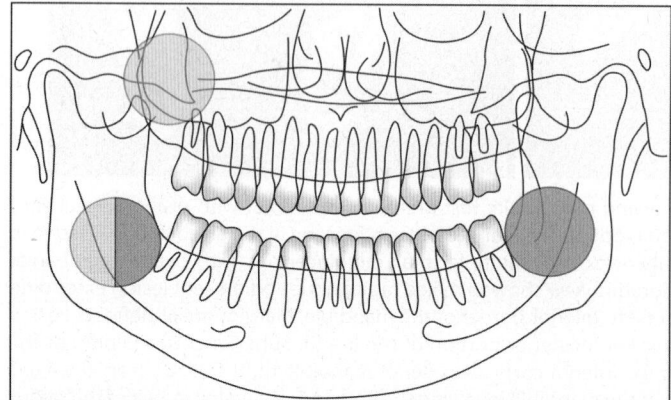

Figures 22.33A to E Odontogenic myxoma: (A and B) Panoramic and PA mandible revealed an ill-defined, multilocular, osteolytic radiolucent lesion of right mandible with irregular borders, with cortical expansion; (C to E) CT scan showed a minimally enhancing well-circumscribed cystic lesion extending from the left of the symphysis menti to the angle causing expansion of the bony cortex. Malalignment of the overlying teeth is present

Figure 22.34 Schematic diagram showing sites of odontomas. The most frequent sites are shown for males (dark) and for females (light)

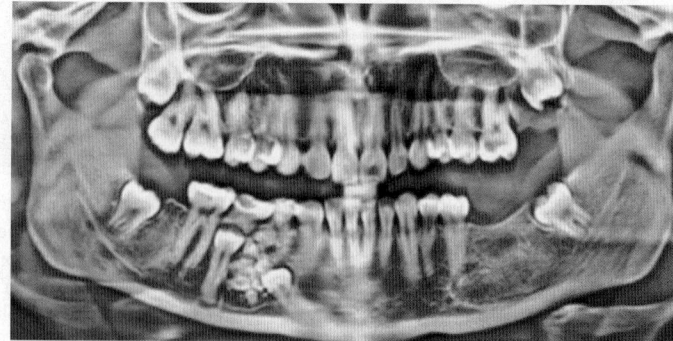

Figure 22.35 Odontoma: Panoramic view showing compound composite odontome, circumcoronal, heterogeneous, mixed radiopaque and radiolucent mass w.r.t. impacted mandibular right premolar, surrounded by radiolucent capsule at places. The premolar is pushed near the lower border of mandible. No root resorption seen

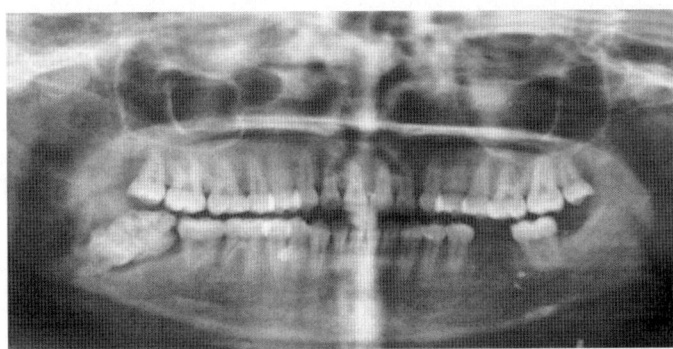

Figure 22.36 Odontoma: Panoramic view showing irregular mass of calcified tissue with radiolucent band at the periphery in mandibular right third molar region suggestive of odontome of complex variety

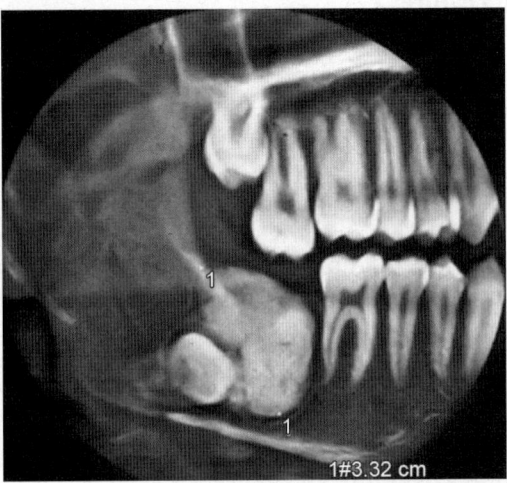

Figure 22.37 Odontoma: Cropped panoramic view showing compound complex odontome, circumcoronal homogenous radiopacity with respect to impacted mandibular right second molar surrounded by the radiolucent halo (capsule), which in turn is surrounded by corticated border. Impacted molar is pushed close to lower border of mandible, mandibular canal appears to be displaced in inferior direction. No root resorption is seen. Supraerupted maxillary right second molar is seen

- Compound composite odontoma—multiple well formed teeth
- Compound complex odontoma—tumors not only contain multiple teeth like structures but also calcified masses of dental tissue in a haphazard manner.
- Geminated odontoma
- Dilated odontoma with dens in dente.

Complex and Compound Odontoma

Clinical Features

- These are the most common odontogenic tumors. Compound is twice as common than complex.

- It has no gender predilection (60 percent of complex odontoms occur in women), and occur in the second decade of life. They develop and mature while the corresponding teeth are forming and cease development when the associated teeth complete development. In rare cases odontomas form from primary teeth.
- The compound variety (62 percent) occur in the anterior maxilla in association with the crown of the unerupted canine. Seventy percent of the complex odontomas are found in the mandibular first and second molar area. Unusual situations include maxillary sinus, inferior border of the mandible, ramus and condylar region.
- The compound odontoma is usually between 1–3 cm in diameter in size and may sometimes increase to the size of the tooth.
- They are usually detected during investigation of delayed eruption of adjacent teeth or retained primary teeth. If untreated they persist but do not increase in size.
- Tooth or teeth are usually missing from the arch in the presence of an odontoma.
- It may produce expansion of bone with facial asymmetry, with swelling and infection.
- In 70 percent of the cases the adjacent teeth are; impacted, malpositioned, have diastema, aplasia, malformed or deviated, devitalization of adjacent teeth.
- A cyst may develop in relation to complex or compound odontoma.

Radiographic Features

- Appear as irregular masses of calcified material surrounded by narrow radiolucent bands (soft tissue capsule) with a small outer periphery, the borders are corticated, well-defined and may be smooth or irregular.
- They usually situated between the roots of teeth.
- Large odontomas may cause expansion of the jaws with maintenance of the cortical boundary.
  - Compound
    - Shows a number of teeth like structures or denticles that look like deformed teeth, mostly in the region of the canine.
    - Each tooth like structure has radiopaque with a dark line surrounding it.
    - The radiopaque mass is surrounded by a radiolucent line that separates the pericoronal space of the unerupted teeth.
  - Complex
    - This appears as a dense radiopaque object, density greater than that of bone and equivalent to that of teeth.
    - It is associated with unerupted teeth.
  - Cystic odontoma
    - It shows a solid mass of the odontoma but without any associated unerupted tooth. There is a dark shadow of the cystic cavity and has well-defined corticated margins except in the cases of infection.

– Cystic compound odontoma
  - There is an area of bone destruction which appears as a dark shadow having well-defined margins lined by a thin white layer of cortical border. Within the cystic cavity there are numerous white radiopacities which vary in size and shape. In some cases there are small amorphous granular densities scattered through out the cavity and in some cases there are small denticles with enamel caps or without distinction of the compound mass.
– Dilated odontoma
  - Has a single calcified structure with more radiolucent central portion that has an overall form of a doughnut.

Differential Diagnosis

- *Difference between the compound and complex type*: Compound has more than one fragment and is more commonly seen in the maxillary canine region, while complex has one solid mass and is commonly seen in the mandibular molar area.
- *Cementifying or ossifying fibroma*: Odontoma is associated with unerupted molar teeth and is more radiopaque than fibroma. It also occurs at a much younger age than a fibroma
- *Adenomatoid odontogenic tumor*: Rarely as opaque as the complex type and found in association with maxillary canines
- *Periapical cemental dysplasia*: Smaller than the complex type and is limited to the mandibular anterior region. Periapical cemental dysplasia are usually multiple lesions and it has a wider uneven sclerotic border, whereas odontomas have a well-defined cortical border and usually the soft tissue capsule is more uniform and better defined. But if the cemental dysplasia is solitary and located in an edentulous region of the jaws, the differential diagnosis may be more difficult.
- *Calcifying epithelial odontogenic tumor*: Rare, less opaque and develops in the midline.
- *Fibrous dysplasia*: Mottled or smoky pattern with poorly defined borders.
- *Enostosis*: Areas of enostosis although radiopaque do not have a soft tissue capsule, as seen with odontomes.

Management

Removal by simple excision.

NONODONTOGENIC TUMORS

Those that are the intrinsic primary bone tumors that arise from the components of bone other than the odontogenic tissue (fibrous, osteoid, condral, vascular, neural or mixed).

Bony hyperplasia are not considered to be tumors because of the normal arrangement of the tissue, limited growth potential and in some cases the fact that the growth is in response to a stimulus. In dentistry the word hyperostosis and exostosis are both used to describe a bony growth that occurs on the surface of normal bone.

Torus Palatinus (Palatine Torus) (Fig. 22.38)

Definition

This is a bony out growth on the lingual surface of the palate. The base of the nodule extends along the central portion of the hard palate, and the bulk reaches downwards into the oral cavity.

Clinical Features

- This is the most common of all the exostoses, more common in women than men, and the patient is usually unaware of this hyperplasia, and those who discover it may insist that it occurred suddenly and has been growing rapidly.
- It is rare in children, and usually begins developing in young adults before thirty years of age. It is believed to be due to an interplay of genetic and environmental factors.
- It may appear single, multiple, unilateral or bilateral.
- The size and shape varies, from flat, lobulated, nodular or mushroom like. The normal mucosa covers the bony mass, and it may appear pale or sometimes become ulcerated if traumatized.
- Clinical significance is only apparent when the patient requires a denture.

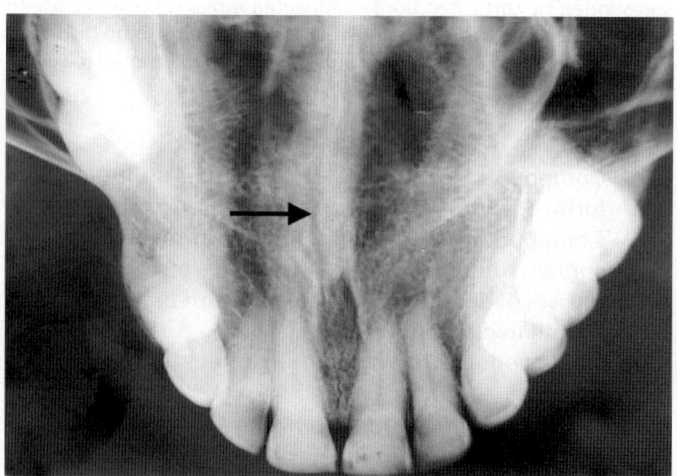

Figure 22.38 Torus palatinus

Radiographic Features

- On the maxillary periapical or panoramic radiographs, it is seen as a dense radiopaque shadow below and attached to the hard palate. It may be superimposed over the apical areas of the maxillary premolar or molar teeth, but this shadow will usually move in its position relative to the roots of the teeth if another film is taken with a different horizontal angulation of the central ray.
- The border of the radiopaque shadow is usually well-defined and may have a cortex or a lobulated out line.
- The internal aspect is homogeneously radiopaque.
- This lesion is well appreciated on the maxillary occlusal radiograph.

Differential Diagnosis

It may be differentiated from periapical radiopacity by taking another radiograph with a different horizontal angulation of the central ray.

Management

No treatment required, unless it causes obstruction in the path of denture insertion, where surgical removal may be necessitated.

Torus Mandibularis (Mandibular Torus) (Fig. 22.39)

Definition

This is a bony out growth on the lingual surface of the mandibular alveolar process.

Clinical Features

- This is the less common of all the exostoses, more common in women (and the occurrence may correlate with that of torus palatinus, which is not the case with men), the patient is usually unaware of this hyperplasia, and those who discover it may insist that it occurred suddenly and has been growing rapidly.
- It is rare in children, and usually begins developing in middle aged adults.
- It is believed to be due to an interplay of genetic and environmental factors. Masticatory stress is reported to be an essential factor.
- It may appear single, multiple, unilateral or bilateral, more often in the premolar region.
- The size and shape varies, from an outgrowth that is just palpable to one that contacts a torus on the opposite side. The normal mucosa covers the bony mass, and it may appear pale or sometimes become ulcerated if traumatized.
- Clinical significance is only apparent when the patient requires a denture.

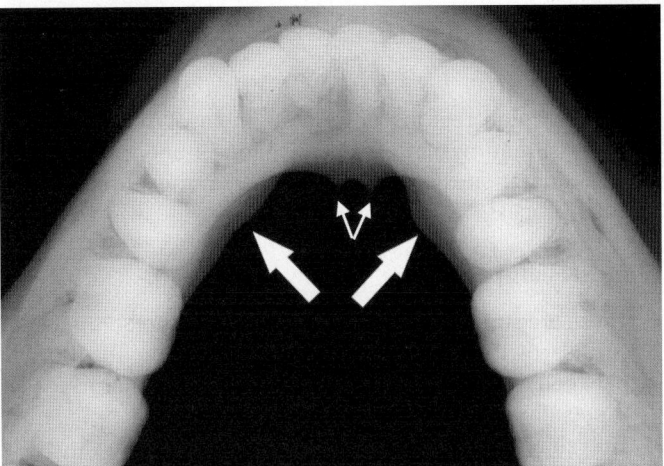

Figure 22.39 Mandibular torus: Thick arrow—mandibular tori; thin arrow—genial tubercles

Radiographic Features

- On the mandibular periapical, it is seen as a dense radiopaque shadow superimposed over the apical areas of the mandibular premolar or molar teeth and occasionally over a canine or an incisor. The shadow usually superimposes over three teeth, but this shadow will usually move in its position relative to the roots of the teeth if another film is taken with a different horizontal angulation of the central ray.
- The border of the radiopaque shadow is usually sharply demarcated anteriorly on periapical films and are less dense and less defined as they extend posteriorly. There is no margin between the periphery of the torus and the surface of the mandible as the torus is continuous with the mandibular cortex.
- The internal aspect is homogeneously radiopaque.
- On the occlusal radiograph the tori appears as a radiopaque knobbly protruberance from the lingual surface of the mandible. Here too the border is not sharp but somewhat continuous, suggesting that the exostosis is not a growth on the bone but a part of the bone.

Differential Diagnosis

It may be differentiated from periapical radiopacity by taking another radiograph with a different horizontal angulation of the central ray.

Management

No treatment required, unless it causes obstruction in the path of denture insertion, where surgical removal may be necessitated.

Exostosis (Hyperostosis) (Figs 22.40A and B)

Definition

These are small regions of osseous hyperplasia of cortical bone or sometimes internal cancellous bone, which may occur on other sites of the jaw, usually on the surface of the alveolar process.

Clinical Features

- These are small exostosis which may develop on the facial surface of the maxillary alveolar process at the border between the attached gingival and the vestibular mucosa, especially in the canine and molar areas.
- They may also occur on the palatal surface or crest and less common on the mandibular alveolar process. Rarely they may grow on the crest under a pontic of a fixed bridge.
- These are less common than mandibular or palatal tori, have no known gender predilection, may attain a large size, and may be solitary or multiple.
- They are nodular, pedunculated or flat prominences on the surface of the bone, covered with a normal mucosa and are bony hard on palpation.

Radiographic Features

- The radiopaque image overlaps the roots of adjacent teeth.
- The periphery of the exostosis is usually, well-defined, smoothly contoured, with a curved border. Sometimes it may have poorly defined borders that blend radiographically into the surrounding normal bone.
- Large exostosis may have an internal cancellous bone pattern; they usually consist of cortical bone, which appears homogeneous and radiopaque.

Differential Diagnosis

It may be differentiated from periapical radiopacity by taking another radiograph with a different horizontal angulation of the central ray.

Management

This tumor requires no treatment.

Enostosis (Dense Bone Island, Periapical Idiopathic Osteosclerosis)

Definition

These are internal counterparts of exostoses. They are localized growths of compact bone that extend from the inner (endosteal) surface of the cortical bone into the cancellous bone.

Clinical Features

- More common in the mandible than maxilla, more in the premolar molar area.
- Usually asymptomatic.

Radiographic Features

- The periphery is well-defined but occasionally blends with the trabeculae of the surrounding bone.
- There is no radiolucent margin or capsule as the radiopaque dense bone abuts directly against the normal bone.
- It is uniformly radiopaque without any characteristic pattern, occasionally depending on its form and thickness it may show patches of more radiolucent areas.
- In rare instances an area of enostosis is located periapical to a tooth root and may be associated with external root resorption. The tooth most often involved is the

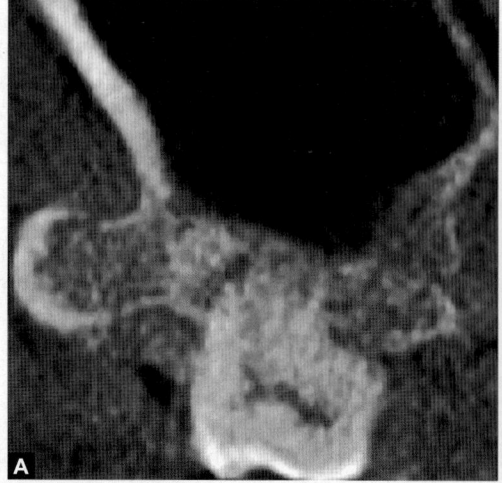
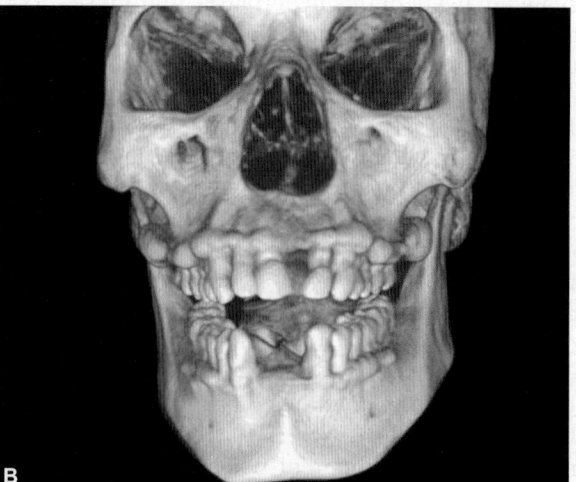

Figures 22.40A and B Exostosis seen on cone beam computed tomography (CBCT): (A) Maxillary cross-sectional; (B) 3D view

mandibular first molar. The tooth is usually vital and the root resorption appears to be self-limiting.

- Enostosis, in rare cases may inhibit the eruption of a tooth and/or even displace a tooth.
- These are often static, but in rare cases may increase in size, especially when there is active growth of the jaws.
- If several areas of enostosis, (five or more) are present, multiple polyposis syndromes (e.g. Gardener's syndrome) should be considered.

Differential Diagnosis

- *Periapical cemental dysplasia*: This has a radiolucent periphery.
- *Periapical sclerosing osteitis*: Here there is associated widening of the periapical portion of the periodontal membrane space. This lesion is more centered on the root apex and extends in a more symmetrical form in every direction. It usually associated with a large restoration or a carious lesion.
- *Hypercementosis*: Presence of a soft tissue radiolucent capsule at the periphery.
- *Benign cementoblastoma*: Presence of a soft tissue radiolucent capsule at the periphery.

Management

- Does not require treatment.
- If multiple are present, then the patient's family history should be reviewed for incidence of cancer of the intestine.

Desmoplastic Fibroma of the Bone (Aggressive Fibromatosis)

Definition

It is an aggressive infiltrative neoplasm that produces abundant collagen fibers. It is composed of fibroblast like cells that have ovoid or elongated nuclei in abundant collagen fibers. The lack of pleomorphism of the cells is important.

Clinical Features

- There is no sex predilection and it usually occurs in the second decade of life.
- The mandible, molar-ramus-angle area is more commonly involved.
- The patient usually presents with a swelling which may be painful and tender, and dysfunction, if the lesion is close to the joint.
- Although it originates in the bone the tumor may invade the surrounding soft tissue.
- It may occur as a part of Gardener's syndrome.

Radiographic Features

- If the lesion is small it appears as a well-defined, unilocular, radiolucency, larger lesions appear multilocular with very coarse, thick septa. The septa may are wide and may be straight or irregular in shape.
- The margins are poorly defined and have an invasive characteristic commonly seen in malignant tumors.
- This tumor may expand and often breaks through the outer cortex, invading the surrounding soft tissue.
- Divergence of contiguous teeth with resorption may be seen.

Additional Imaging

- *MRI*: In T_1 weighted scans the internal structure has a low signal, which helps in determining intraosseous extent because of the contrast with the high signal from the bone marrow.
- *CT*: It also helps to delineate the exact extent of the lesion.

Differential Diagnosis

- *Fibrosarcoma*: Presence of coarse, irregular and sometimes straight septa are seen in desmoplastic fibroma of the bone.
- *Multilocular tumors*: Presence of coarse, irregular and sometimes straight septa is seen in desmoplastic fibroma of the bone.
- *Simple bone cysts*: It may be confused with the very small lesions of desmoplastic fibroma of the bone.
- *Nonossifying fibroma*.

Management

Local excision with extraction of the involved teeth. Regular radiographic check-ups are recommended due to the recurrence rate.

Chondroma

Definition

The mandible and maxilla are membranous bones. They sometimes contain vestigial rests of cartilage.

There are two types:
1. *Enchondroma or central*: This is more commonly seen and develops deep into the bone.
2. *Ecchondroma*: This develops on the surface.

Clinical Features

- It is seen more in the males, in the 5th and 6th decade of life
- It is seen more in the maxilla, in the anterior region (the maxilla develops in close association with the

chondrocranium. The maxillary sinus develops as an out growth from the lateral walls of the nasal capsule. As it grows into the maxilla it may take with it remnants of cartilage from the capsule. Sometimes the remnants of the paraseptal cartilage may persist within the maxilla). In the mandible it occurs in the premolar-molar region, symphysis, condyle and coronoid process. It usually occurs in the phalanges and metacarples.

- It may present as a painless, slow growing, and locally invasive swelling. The overlying mucosa is usually not ulcerated.
- Associated teeth may become mobile and exfoliate.
- It may be associated with Ollier's syndrome, in which there are multiple enchondromatosis.

Radiographic Features

Enchondroma

- The radiographic appearance is variable and quite unspecific
- There may be a well-defined area of bone destruction, which may be place either centrally or near one of the borders. The margins may be well demarcated or corticated or both or none.
- It may develop radiopacities in the osteolytic areas, which produce mottled or blurry appearance.
- The jaw is sometimes expanded by the tumor or the lesion, as there is no new bone formation on the surface of the tumors it may cause destruction of the lateral margins.
- Resorption of the involved teeth occurs.
- Some of the central chondromas may appear loculated, may be due to the surface strands of bone.

Ecchondroma

- It is usually situated in the mandibular notch, giving the notch and abnormal shape. Radiographically it appears shallow.
- When the coronoid is involved it is directed forward and upward at a much less steep angle although its length and girth are normal, the density of the adjacent bone is increased.

Differential Diagnosis

- *Chondrosarcoma*: There is presence of pain.
- *Osteogenic sarcoma*: It has a typical sun ray appearance.
- *Osteoblastic metastatic carcinoma*: There will be presence of a primary tumor.
- *Ossifying sub-periosteal hemangioma*: Aspiration should be done.
- *Fibrous dysplasia*: This can be differentiated histologically and radiographically it has a ground glass appearance.
- *Hemangioma*: May contain phleboliths.

- From the radiographic point of view it is not possible to identify chondroma in the jaws. An area of bone destruction without the characteristics of a cyst, occurring in the region of the condyle or the coronoid process, should be considered as possible of being cartilaginous origin.

Management

Should be carefully excised, as recurrence is very common.

Chondroblastoma (Codman's Tumor)

Definition

It usually involves the long bones, femur or tibia, but there are reports that it may also occur in the condyle of the mandible. Benign cartilaginous tumors are a rare entity in jaw bones

Osteoma (Figs 22.41 to 22.43)

Definition

These form from the membranous bones of the skull and face. It may arise from the cartilage or embryonal periosteum or periosteum. Structurally they are divided into:

- *Ivory osteoma*: It consists of compact bone, which has dense lamellae of bone.
- *Cancellous osteoma*: It is composed of cancellous, trabaculae of bone.
- *Combination*: It is a combination of the compact and cancellous bone.

Clinical Features

- Cortical type is more common in males, where as women have a high incidence of the cancellous type. They are found in the older age group the mandible is more affected, especially the posterior aspect of the mandible, lingual side of the ramus or inferior border below the molars. The condyle and the coronoid may also be involved. The mandibular lesions may be exophytic.
- Osteomas that originate from the periosteum may occur either externally or within the paranasal sinuses. It is more common in the frontal and ethmoid than in the maxillary sinus.
- It may produce a painless, hard swelling of the jaws causing asymmetry. The overlying mucosa is normal in color and freely movable. It is painless until the size interferes with function.
- The osteomas are attached to the cortex of the jaw by a pedicle or along a wide base.
- Mandibular lesions may be exophytic extending outwards into the soft tissue.
- Most osteomas are small, but some may become large and cause severe damage, especially those in the frontoethmoidal region.

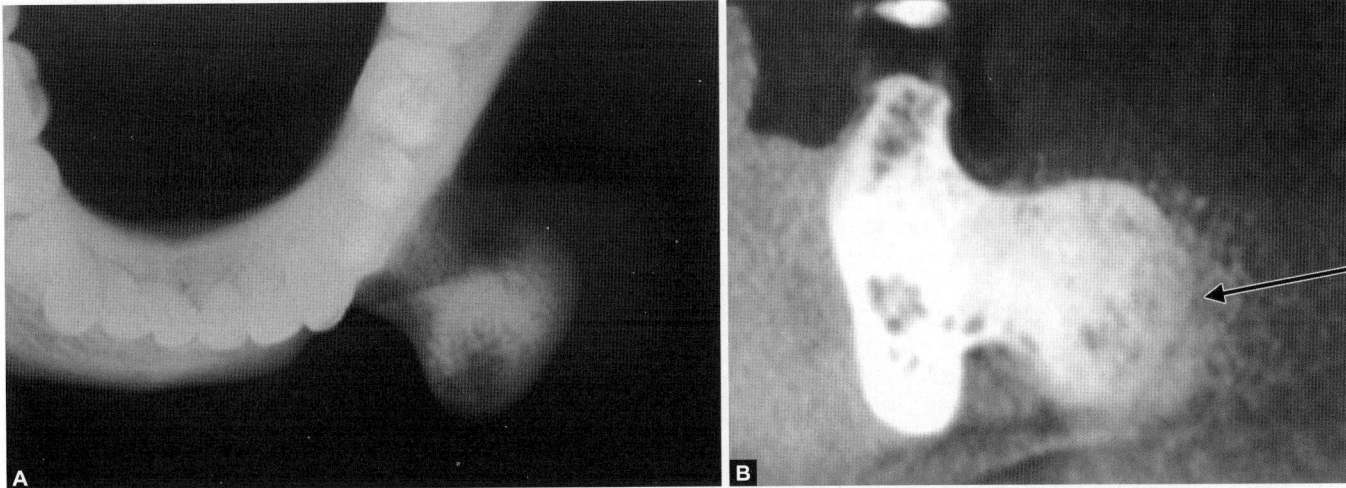

Figures 22.41A and B Osteoma: (A) Occlusal view showing bony growth on the buccal aspect of the mandible opposite the premolar region; Compact osteoma; (B) Coronal CBCT image showing bony out growth, osteoid osteoma

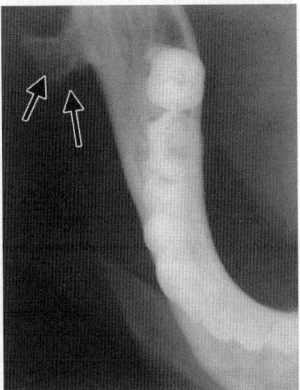

Figure 22.42 Osteoma of mandible: Occlusal radiograph showed radiopaque outgrowth on mandibular right molar region on buccal side, which appears to be pedunculated. Normal trabeculae pattern was noticed in the radiopacity. Some part of the radiopacity shows hyperostotic border

- *Osteomatosis*: Multiple osteoma occur in the absence of other abnormalities, in the mandible, frontal and maxillary sinus. This feature is also seen in Gardener's syndrome.

Radiographic Features

- It appears as a well-defined uniform radiopacity, few centimeters in diameter near the level of the root of the lower molar or paranasal sinus (ivory osteoma).
- Or it may appear as a well-defined radiopacity with evidence of internal trabeculae structure. This may or may not be in the superficial layer of cortical bone. Bone structures within the tumor are continuous with that of parent bone (cancellous osteoma).

- Large lesions may displace adjacent soft tissue, such as muscles and cause dysfunction.

Differential Diagnosis

- *Solid odontome*: Presence of the soft tissue capsule.
- *Fibrous dysplasia*: Border are not clearly defined, and does not reveal the same homogeneous density as in osteoma.
- *Osteochondroma*: It has a cartilaginous capsule and may associate with irregularity on the surface of the tumor.
- *Sclerosing osteitis*: The margins are ill-defined. This lesion usually has an easily identifiable cause, like retained root or infected tooth.
- *Enostosis*: There is absence of any mass on the surface of bone in enostosis.
- *Osteosarcoma*: There is bony enlargement with typical sun ray appearance.
- *Chondrosarcoma*.
- *Ossifying fibroma*: There is a bony enlargement with a dense radiopaque mass.
- Osteoma of the condylar head is difficult to differentiate from osteochondroma, osteophyte or condylar hyperplasia, those involving coronoid like osteochondroma.

Management

Resection, in case it interferes with normal function or presents a cosmetic problem.

Gardener's Syndrome (Familial Multiple Polyposis)

Definition

This is a type of familial multiple polyposis, in which there is an associated neoplasm.

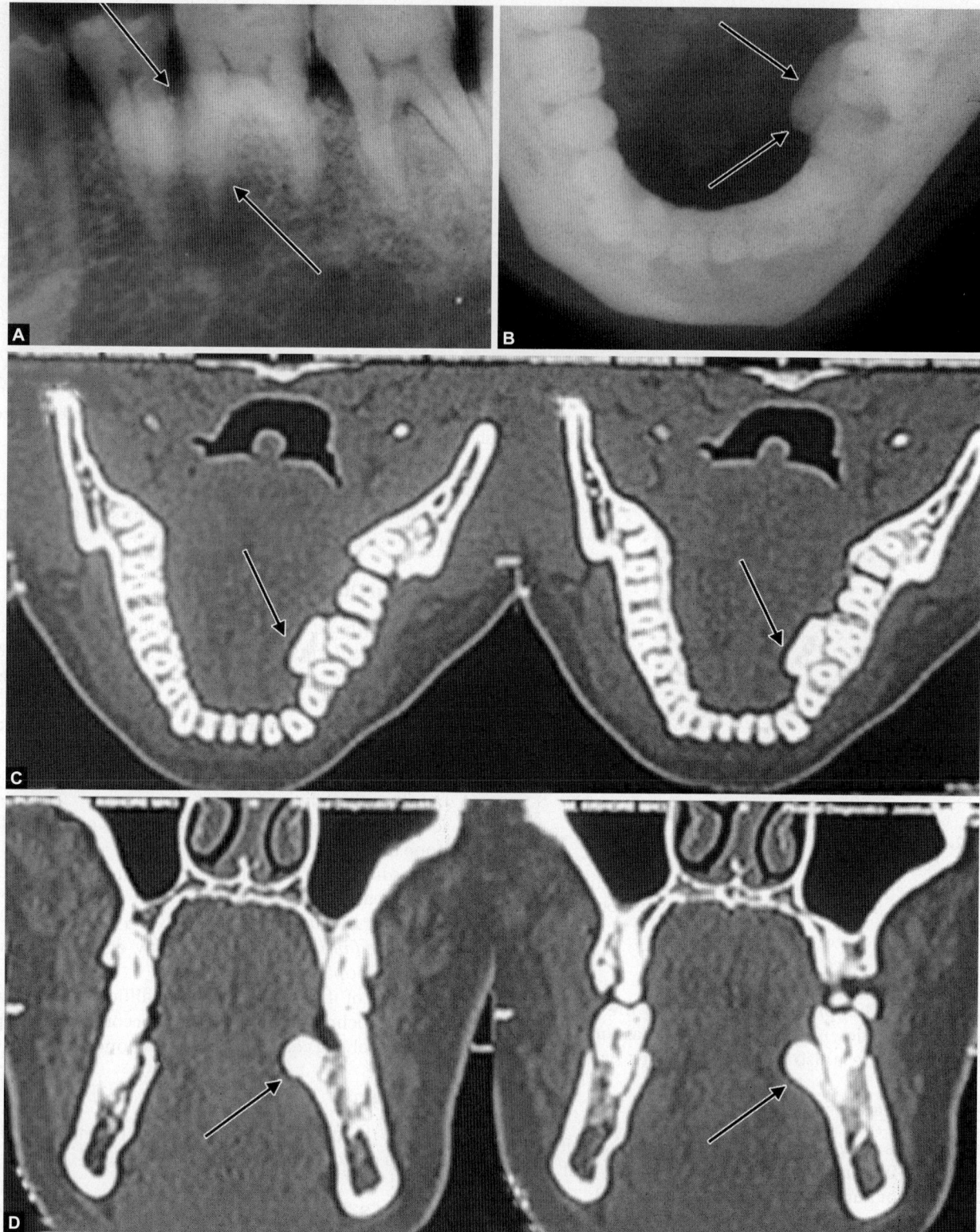

Figures 22.43A to D Osteoma: (A) IOPA of 35, 36—Well-defined radiopaque lesion seen in the 35, 36 region near the crest of the bone; (B) Mandibular occlusal view shows well-defined radiopaque lesion seen in the 35, 36 region on the lingual surface. The internal structure showed dense trabecular pattern. CT scan: (C) Axial view; (D) Coronal view showed well-defined radiopaque lesion seen in the 35, 36 region on the lingual surface. The lesion was sessile and arising from the cortex of the mandible. Differential diagnosis—mandibular tori

Clinical Features

- It is a hereditary condition characterized by multiple osteomas, multiple enostosis(dense bone islands), cutaneous sebaceous cysts, subcutaneous fibromas and multiple polyps of the small and large intestines.
- The associated osteomas appear in the second decade.
- The osteomas are most commonly found in the frontal bone, mandible, maxilla and sphenoid bones.
- The osteomas and enostosis develop before intestinal polyps which tend to undergo malignant change, early recognition of the syndrome may be life saving.
- Multiple unerupted supernumerary and permanent teeth are present in both jaws.

Management

Early recognition of the syndrome is important so the patient may be referred to the required specialist.

Osteoid Osteoma

Definition

It is a small oval or rounded tumor like nidus which is composed of osteoid and trabeculae of newly formed bone deposited within the substratum of highly vascularised osteogenic connective tumor.

Clinical Features

- It is more common in males, between the age of 10 to 15 years
- Any part of the skeleton may be involved, though the skull and the jaws are rarely involved. It has a greater predilection for the mandible, especially the body
- It may be oval or round, with a core of 1 cm in diameter. It produces a marked reaction in the adjacent tissue, which may extend for a considerable distance from the tumor itself. The soft tissue over the involved bone may be swollen and tender
- In spite of the small size this tumor is very painful. It pain occurs more at night time.

Radiographic Features

- It appears as a small well-defined, corticated oval or round radiolucency
- Central radiolucency may exhibit some calcifications which are seen as radiopaque foci
- The revealation of a nidus, with a small central opaque spot within the nidus is most indicative of an osteoid osteoma
- The inferior dental canal may be displaced
- In the occlusal view the overlying cortex is seen to be thickened, a varying region from narrow zone to an extensive area of several centimeters of dense sclerosis may be seen around the tumor.

Differential Diagnosis

- *Sclerotic osteitis*: There is no central radiolucency.
- *Ossifying fibroma*: Root resorption is present. Osteoid osteoma is present more on the inferior aspect.
- *Monostotic fibrous dysplasis*: This is more common in the maxilla, and there is no central radiolucency.
- *Benign cementoblastoma*: This is surrounded by a radiolucent halo.
- *Periapical cemental dysplasia*: This is more often exclusively found in females.
- *Osteoblastoma*: This is less painful than osteoid osteoma.
- *Small cortical abscess.*
- *Osteogenic sarcoma and Garre's osteomyelitis.*

Management

Complete excision is recommended.

Osteoblastoma (Giant Osteoid Osteoma)

Definition

This is a rare benign tumor of the osteoblasts with areas of osteoid and calcified tissue.

Clinical Features

- It is more common in males, between the 2nd and 3rd decade of life.
- It is more common in the vertebral column and sacrum, rarely found in jaws. If it occurs, it is found more often in the mandibular teeth bearing areas, and temporomandibular joint.
- Here is localized expansion of bone with pain and swelling of the affected area, which may be of a few weeks to a year in duration.

Radiographic Features

- It may be seen as a radiolucent lesion or may show varying degrees of calcification, with borders that are diffuse or show some signs of cortication. The mandibular lesion may have a radiolucent halo with outer cortical boundaries.
- The internal calcification may appear as sun-ray or fine granular bone trabeculae.

Differential Diagnosis

- *Osteoid osteoma*: This is a more eccentric radiolucency with sclerotic borders. This is much more painful.
- *Osteogenic sarcoma*: The borders are irregular and the lesion does not appears benign as in osteoblastoma.

Management

Curettage and conservative surgical excision. There is a tendency for the tumor to reoccur.

Osteochondroma (Figs 22.44A and B)

Definition

This may represent choristoma rather than a neoplasm. There is an intermingling of two lesions. It is developmental in origin.

There are two types:
1. Central.
2. Peripheral.

Clinical Features

- The central type is very rare in the jaws and has no sex, age or site predilection.
- The peripheral variety is seen to occur more often in women between the age of 20–39 years.
- The tongue and the coronoid are most commonly affected.
- On the tongue it appears as a pedunculated swelling about 1–2 cm in the posterior dorsum, near foramen caecum, with abroad base. It may cause dysphagia.
- When the coronoid is involved there is difficulty in opening and closing, which becomes very painful, and there may be a deviation of the mandible to one side.

Radiographic Features

- The central type appears as a spherical or round radiolucency, with sharp localized borders and is corticated. The presence of bone in the lesion is seen in the form of trabecular or irregularly shaped amorphous mass.
- The peripheral type appears as a protrusion of bone from the surface of bone. The base is wide, with a narrow stalk which may end in an expansion of considerable size. There is continuity of the cancellous and cortex of the parent bone into the base of the tumor.

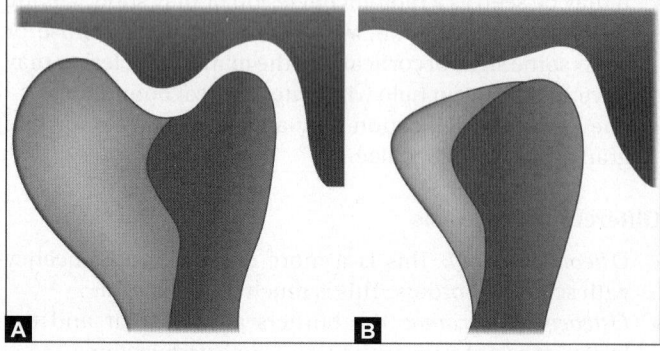

Figures 22.44A and B Schematic diagram which depicts two typical shapes of the osteochondroma as they appear from lateral view on the panoramic film

- The coronoid process is enlarged, giving a drum stick appearance. No trabecular is seen in this bone which appears of uniform density. Islands of cartilage may be seen at the terminal end.
- The malar bone may show destruction of bone on its deep and inferior surface, while the superficial surface of the maxilla is indented to receive the additional size of the coronoid process.
Management: Surgical removal.

Hemangioma (Vascular Nevus) (Figs 22.45A to D)

Definition

It is a proliferation of blood vessels creating a mass, connected to the main vascular system, that resembles a neoplasm, although some believe it to be a hamartoma. These can occur anywhere in the body but are frequently noticed in the skin and subcutaneous tissues. There are different types:
- *Central*: It occurs in bone.
- *Capillary*: It is a mass of intercommunicating capillary vessels of more or less normal size and structure.
  - Strawberry angioma
  - Port wine stain
  - Salmon's patch
- *Cavernous*: This consists of dilated blood containing spaces, lined with endothelium.
  - Arterial or plexiform hemangioma; this arises from the arteries.

Clinical Features

Central Hemangioma

- More common in females in the first to third decade.
- It is more common in the mandible, ramus and body, especially within the inferior alveolar canal.
- The lesion may originate from the periosteum and resorb the underlying bone or it may occur as an anomaly of blood vessels in the marrow spaces.
- There will be a nontender, hard swelling with expansion.
- Pain if present will be of the throbbing type.
- Some tumors may be compressible with bruit on auscultation.
- Anesthesia of the skin supplied by the mental nerve may occur.
- The lesion may cause loosening and migration of the involved teeth. Bleeding may occur from the gingiva around the neck of the affected teeth. The teeth may exhibit, pumping tooth syndrome (tooth when depressed into the socket will rebound into its original position within a few minutes).
- Aspiration of the lesion will produce blood.

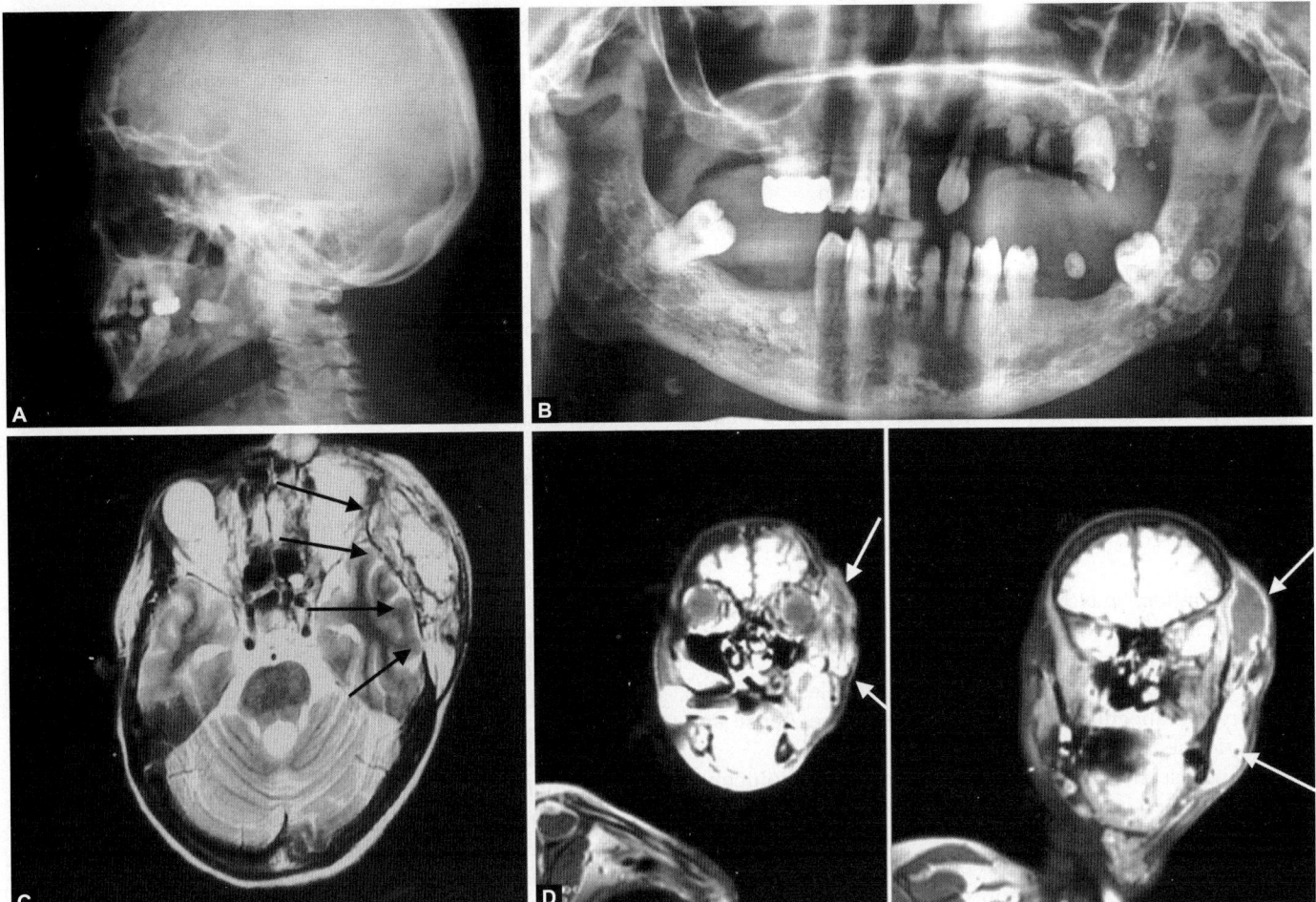

Figures 22.45A to D Hemangioma: (A) Lateral skull view showing calcification foci in pharynx and neck region; (B) Panoramic view shows multiple missing teeth. Calcification foci seen on the left side over body and angle of mandible and one on the right side in submandibular region. MRI: (C) Transverse section shows hyperintense area seen on the lateral surface of temporal bone on the left side involving anteriorly orbit space; (D) Coronal section shows well-defined hyperintense area seen over the temporal region on the left side

Strawberry Angioma

- This is a red patch which is noticed at birth and usually regresses in size and the involution is usually completed by 7–8 years.
- It involves the subcutaneous tissues and skin. It is dark red or strawberry colored, compressible and protrudes from the skin surface as a sessile hemisphere. Small areas of ulceration with scabs may be present.

Port-wine Stain

These are reddish-deep purple colored, not more than 5 mm in diameter which occurs at birth and darkens as the child grows. It is usually found on the face, shoulders, neck and buttock. The color blanches readily on pressure.

Salmon's Patch

is present at birth, over the forehead, or occiput or anywhere in the midline of the body, and usually disappears before the first birthday.

Cavernous Hemangioma

- More common in females in the first to third decade of life, commonly seen on the lip, tongue, buccal mucosa and palate. The swelling will show positive compressibility test (continued pressure will drive the blood out of the lesion, the swelling crumbles, on release of pressure the swelling reappears due to refilling).
- Superficial lesion are lobulated and blanch on pressure, deeper lesions are dome-shaped and do not blanch.

- The swelling may increase in size and burry the involved teeth causing disfigurement, the overlying mucosa may appear pebbly.
- The mucosal hemangioma is usually soft and well circumscribed. Larger lesions are warm may be pulsatile.
- The tumor if traumatized bleeds profusely and may undergo ulceration with secondary infection.
- In case of hemangioma of the tongue, there may be loss of mobility of the tongue.

Arterial or Plexiform Hemangioma

This is a congenital arteriovenous fistula, with pulsatile swelling of the arteries, veins become tortuous and thick walled and the lesion is pulsatile and feels like a bag of pulsating earthworms.

Radiographic Features

Central

- The periphery may be well-defined and corticated or it may be ill-defined and even simulate the appearance of a malignant tumor.
- When present in the maxilla, the locules resemble enlarged trabecular spaces which are coarse, dense and well-defined.
- It may be seen as a moderately well defined radiolucency within which trabecular spaces get enlarged and the trabeculae become coarse and thick. These internal trabeculae produce a pattern composed of small circular radiolucent spaces that represent blood vessels oriented in the same direction of the X-ray beam. This is seen as a multicystic, soap bubble or honeycomb appearance.
- The larger lesions may cause cortical expansion with radiating spicules at the expanding periphery producing a sun ray or sun burst appearance.
- Sometimes the structure of the bone is changed in the affected area so that the trabeculae are arranged in a manner which has a rough resemblance to the spokes of a wheel.
- Some lesions are totally radiolucent.
- When the inferior alveolar canal is involved, the whole canal is increased in width and often the normal path of the canal is altered into a serpiginous shape, with a multilocular appearance.
- When hemangiomas involve soft tissue the formation of phleboliths may occur within the surrounding soft tissues. These develop from thrombi that become organized and mineralized and consist of calcium phosphate and calcium carbonate.
- The roots of the involved are resorbed or displaced
- The mandibular canal, mandibular and mental foramen may be enlarged.

- Hemangiomas may influence the growth of bone and teeth. The involved bone may be enlarged and have coarse, internal trabeculae. The developing teeth may be larger and erupt earlier.

Additional Imaging

- *Ultrasound*: It will show heterogeneous hypoechoic lesions in which calcified phleboliths may be identified.
- *CT*: It shows similar appearance with enhanced quality. Hemangiomas appear as enhancing masses, often lobular in contour with phleboliths within the tumor masses.
- *MRI*: It shows the lesions to have a low to intermediate, non-homogeneous T_1 weighted signal intensity and high T_2 weighted signal intensity.

Differential Diagnosis

- *Central giant cell granuloma*: This crosses the midline.
- *Giant cell lesions of hyperparathyroidism*: May be differentiated by biochemical investigations.
- *Aneurysmal bone cyst*: Hemangioma will show profuse hemorrhage, if aspirated.
- *Ameloblastic fibroma*: No local gingival bleeding or pumping action of the involved tooth seen.
- *Odontogenic myxoma*: It shows a typical tennis racket appearance.
- *Ameloblastoma*: It occurs in older age group.
- *Metastaic tumor*: In it, the history of primary tumor is present.
- *Cherubism*: It is usually seen in children, with a typical facial appearance and is bilateral.
- *Traumatic bone cyst*: It is a well-defined entity.
- *Odontogenic keratocyst*: It is a well-defined entity.
- *Sarcoma*: The margins are irregular whereas in any benign tumor the margins are usually well- corticated.
- *Hereditary hemorrhagic telangiectasia (Rendu-Osler-Weber syndrome)*: Hemangioma that is characterized by numerous telangiectasia (permenantly enlarged capillaries that are localized superficially, just under the skin and mucosa) or angiomatous areas which are widely distributed on the skin or mucosa of the oral cavity.
- *Sturge-weber syndrome*: Hemangioma of the face that is sometimes associated with gross calcification in the walls of the vessels on the surface of the brain in the occipital region.

Management

Central hemangiomas should be treated without delay because it may result in lethal exsanguinations. It may be treated by en bloc resection, laser surgery, cryo surgery, intralesional sclerosing or corticosteroid injections, radiation therapy, and embolization.

Arteriovenous Fistula (A-V Defect, A-V Shunt, A-V Aneurysm, A-V Malformation) (Figs 22.46A to D)

Definition

An A-V fistula is an uncommon lesion, where there is a direct communication between an artery and a vein that bypass the intervening capillary bed. It may be congenital or acquired. (A lesion with a thrill or bruit, or one that is obviously warmer is most likely to be a special vascular malformation called arteriovenous malformation with direct flow of blood from the venous to the arterial system, by passing the capillary beds).

The different types are.
- *Cirsoid aneurysm*: It is a tortuous mass of small arteries and veins linking a larger artery and vein.
- *Varicose aneurysm*: This consists of an endothelium lined sac connecting an artery and vein.
- *Aneurysmal varix*: This is a direct connection between artery and vein.

Clinical Features

- The lesions may develop in the ramus, retromolar area of the mandible and involve the mandibular canal.
- It may expand the bone, and a mass may be present in the extraosseous soft tissue. This soft tissue swelling may have a purple discoloration. Palpation or auscultation of the swelling may reveal pulse.
- Sometimes, neither the bone nor the soft tissue is expanded and no pulse is clinically apparent.
- Aspiration produces blood.
- An innocent extraction may be followed by life-threatening bleeding.

Radiographic Features

- The lesion is usually seen as a resorptive radiolucent, well defined corticated margin.
- A tortuous path of an enlarged vessel may give a multilocular appearance.

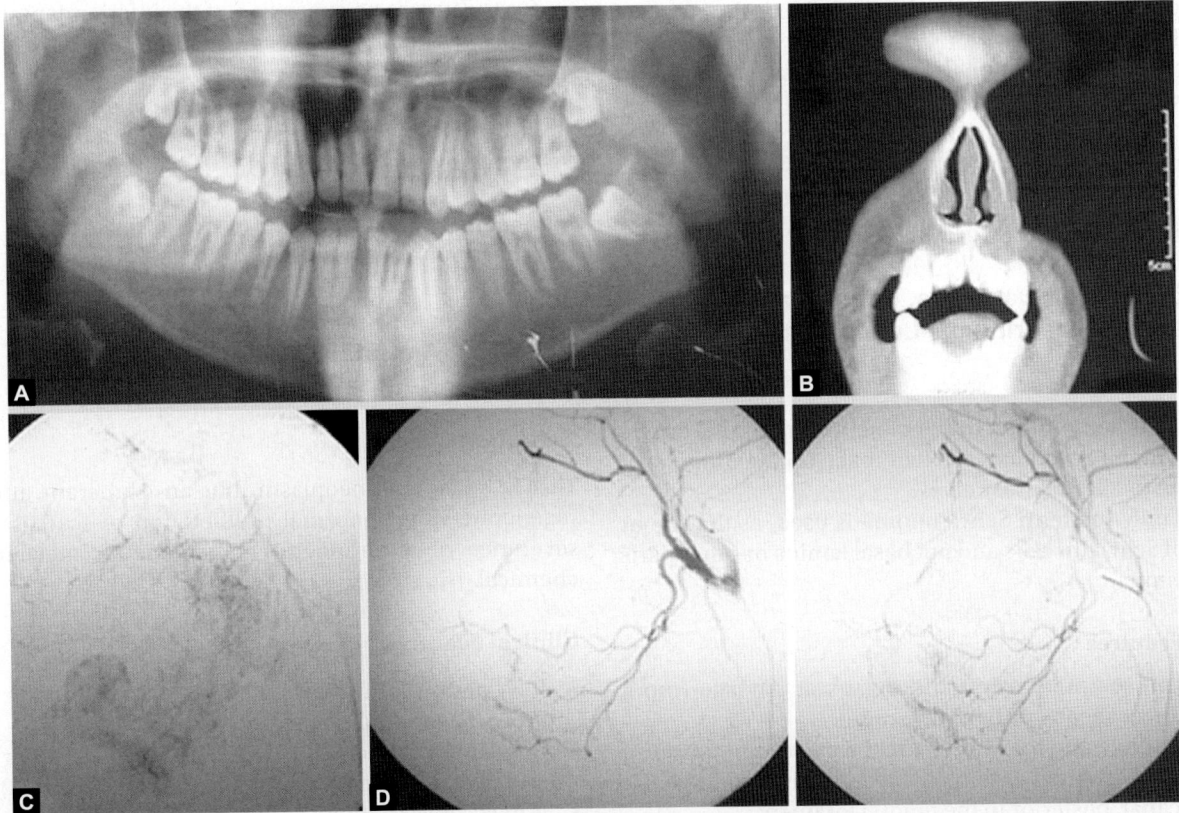

Figures 22.46A to D (A) Panoramic view of a patient with arteriovenous malformation, revealed horizontal alveolar bone loss in 31, 41 region, with displacement. Developing 18, 28, 38, 48; (B) CT scan, cornal section of the same patient showed an ill-defined moderately enhancing soft tissue lesion in lower anterior region extending to the floor of mouth. There was no evidence of bone erosion or calcification within the growth; (C and D) Arteriography of the same patient showing left external carotid artery angiogram which revealed tortuosity at the end of lingual and deep lingual veins

- The central lesions and those in the adjacent soft tissue can erode bone, resulting in well-defined (cyst like) lesions in the bone.
- When the inferior alveolar canal is involved, the whole canal is increased in width and often the normal path of the canal is altered into a serpiginous shape, with a multilocular appearance.

Additional Imaging

- *Angiography*: It is used when interventional therapy is planned.
- *CT with contrast injection*: It aids in differentiating from other vascular lesions and neoplasms.
- *MR angiography*: It helps to document the size, extent and vessels involved with the vascular lesion.

Differential Diagnosis

- *Hemangioma*: Soft tissue hemangioma does not involve bone.
- *Ameloblastoma*: Aspiration will not produce blood.
- *Radicular cyst*: This is associated with a nonvital tooth.
- *Dentigerous cyst*: The radiolucency surrounds the crown of a tooth.
- Other multilocular lesions, especially those involved with the alveolar canal.

Management

Surgical treatment or embolization with arteriography and the excision of the external growth if present.

Neurilemoma (Schwannoma, Perineural Fibroblastoma, Neurinoma, Lemmonma)

Definition

A central neurilemoma is a tumor of neuroectodermal origin, arising from the Schwann cells that make up the inner layer covering of the peripheral nerves.

Today only the term Schwannoma is used, as the tumor consists of Schwann cells and not basal lamina or other parts of neurilemma.

Clinical Features

- It has no sex predilection and occurs at any age (more common in second and third decade).
- The mandible and the sacrum are the most common sites. It is usually located within an expanded inferior alveolar nerve canal, posterior to the mental foramen.
- It causes few symptoms like swelling, pain, paresthesia, as related to the location and size of the tumor.
- It is a slow growing tumor.

Radiographic Features

- The tumor is uniformly radiolucent with well- defined and corticated margins.
- Small lesions may appear cyst like, but as the tumor expands the canal it becomes fusiform in shape.
- Sometimes the lesion may have a scalloping outline, which gives a false multilocular appearance.
- It may cause enlargement of the mandibular and/or mental foramen.
- Expansion of the inferior alveolar canal is slow and thus the outer cortex of the canal is maintained and the expansion of the canal is usually localized with a definite epicenter unless the lesion is large.
- Root resorption of the adjacent teeth may occur.

Additional Imaging

On CT it appears as heterogeneous hypodense areas. It may also show cystic areas within the lumen.

Differential Diagnosis

- *Cysts*: There is no expansion of the inferior dental canal
- *Ameloblastoma*: This occurs above the inferior dental canal
- *Vascular lesion*: This increases the girth of the canal down the entire length and often alters the shape into a serpiginous form.

Management

Surgical excision.

Neuroma (Amputation Neuroma, Traumatic Neuroma)

Definition

This is not a true neoplasm, but an exuberant attempt to regenerate with abnormal proliferation of scar tissue after severance of a peripheral nerve, due to mechanical or chemical irritation.

Clinical Features

- It is a slow growing; reactive hyperplasia that seldom grows beyond 1 cm in diameter.
- It is usually found in the mental foramen, anterior maxilla and posterior mandible (in the mandibular canal).
- It may cause a variety of symptoms like; extreme pain due to increased pressure as the tangled mass increases in its bony cavity. The patient may have reflex neuralgia with the pain referred to the eyes, face and head.

Radiographic Features

- It is seen as a radiolucent lesion with well-defined corticated borders.
- The shape may vary depending upon the amount of resistance to expansion.
- Expansion of the inferior dental canal is seen.

Differential Diagnosis

- *Odontogenis cyst*: Not as painful and no history of trauma, fracture or surgery.
- *Other benign neural tumors*: It is difficult to differentiate from neuroma.

Management

Simple excision of the nodule, along with proximal portion of the involved nerve.

Neurofibroma (Neurinoma)

Definition

These are moderately firm, benign, well-circumscribed tumors caused by proliferation of Schwann cells in a disorderly pattern that includes portions of nerve fibers, such as peripheral nerves, axons and connective tissue sheath of Schwann. As neurofibromas grow, they incorporate the axons. In contrast, neurilemomas are composed entirely of Schwann cells and grow by displacing axons.

Clinical Features

- These may occur at any age but are usually found in young patients.
- Central neurofibromas may occur in the mandibular canal, in the cancellous bone, and below the periosteum.
- It may expand and perforate the cortex, causing a swelling that is hard or firm to palpation.
- Those associated with the mandibular nerve may produce pain or paresthesia.

Radiographic Features

- It appears as a unilocular radiolucency with sharply defined and corticated borders.
- Some times it may appear multilocular and/or have indistinct margins.
- Neurofibroma of the inferior dental anal shows a fusiform enlargement of the canal.

Differential Diagnosis

- *Vascular lesions*: These enlarge the whole canal and alter its path.

- *Other neural lesions*: It is difficult to differentiate from neurofibroma.

Management

Excision.

Neurofibromatosis (von Recklinghausen's Disease)

Definition

This is a syndrome consisting of Café au lait spots on the skin, multiple peripheral nerve tumors and a variety of other dysplastic abnormalities of the skin, nervous system, bones, endocrine organs and blood vessels.

There are two major types:
1. *Neurofibromatosis 1*: This is a generalized form (a desmo dermal dysplasia may be apart of the spectrum of changes that are observed in these lesions).
2. *Neurofibromatosis 2*: This is a central form.
   Oral lesions may occur as apart of NF-1 or may be solitary and are called segmental or form first manifestations.

Clinical Features

- It is a genetic disease, which occurs 1 in every 3000 births. It is manifested gradually during childhood and adult life.
- The peripheral nerve tumors are of two types, Schwannomas and neurofibromas.
- Café au lait spots become larger and more numerous with age, usually there will be more than 6 spots larger than 1.5 cm in diameter.
- Other skin lesions include freckless, soft pendunculated, cutaneous neurofibromas; and firm, subcutaneous neurofibromas.
- Central neurofibromas are rare.

Radiographic Features

- Alterations in the shape of the mandible:
  - Enlargement of the coronoid notch in either or both the horizontal and vertical dimension
  - An obtuse angle between the body and ramus
  - Deformity of the condylar head
  - Lengthening of the condylar neck
  - Lateral bowing and thinning of the ramus (seen in basal skull view).
- Enlargement of the mandibular canal and mental and mandibular foramina.
- An increased incidence of branched mandibular canal.
- Erosive changes to the outer contour of the mandible.
- Interference with the normal eruption of molars.

Addition Imaging

CT: Abnormal collection of fatty tissue within deformities of the mandible have been observed.

Management

Most patients live a normal life with few or no symptoms. Some neurofibroma may be removed if painful. Malignant conversions of these lesions have occurred.

Melanotic Neuroectodermal Tumor of Infancy (Pigmented Ameloblastoma, Melano Ameloblastoma, Retinal Anlage Tumor, Melanotic Progonoma)

Definition

This tumor is of the neural crest origin, having both pigmented and nonpigmented cells.

Clinical Features

- It occurs in infants under the age of 6 months, with equal sex distribution.
- Maxilla is more affected.
- It is a rapidly growing, non-ulcerated, darkly pigmented lesion.
- The tumor forms a mass that expands the bone without pain and tenderness.

Radiographic Features

It appears as a radiolucency whose borders may be well-defined (like a cyst), or it may have irregular margins.

Management

Conservative surgical excision.

Giant Cell Tumor

Definition

This term is applied to lesions containing giant cells. It is usually seen in the long bones, occurring at the epiphyseal end involving the adjacent metaphysis. It is rare in the head and neck region.

Clinical Features

- It is seen in the third or fourth decade. The jaw lesions are seen much before the age of 20 and may undergo complete spontaneous regression which terminates in complete healing. The jaw lesions usually maintain a bony covering despite a large size.
- The patient may present with pain, swelling, tenderness and egg shell crackling may be seen in case of large tumors

Radiographic Features

It may appear as a radiolucent area, with soap bubble or honey comb appearance, with thinning and expansion of the cortex, with little or no periosteal bone formation.

Differential Diagnosis

Central giant cell granuloma: It occurs in children, commonly seen in the mandibular anterior region, anterior to the first molar. It is usually preceded with history of trauma. Foci of osteoid and new bone are frequently present.

Management

Curettage, but recurrence rate is very high.

Giant Cell Granuloma

Are of two types:
1. *Peripheral giant cell granuloma*: This involves gingival and alveolar mucosa.
2. *Central giant cell granuloma*: It occurs as an endosteal lesion in the jaw bones.

Peripheral Giant Cell Granuloma (Giant Cell Epulis, Osteoclastoma) (Figs 22.47 to 22.49)

Definition

This is 5 times more common than the central type. It seems to originate from the periodontal ligament or mucoperiosteum, due to trauma, chronic infection or hormonal changes.

Clinical Features

- Females are more affected than males, in the above 20 age group
- It commonly occurs on the gingival and alveolar mucosa, most frequently anterior to the molars, more in the mandible than maxilla

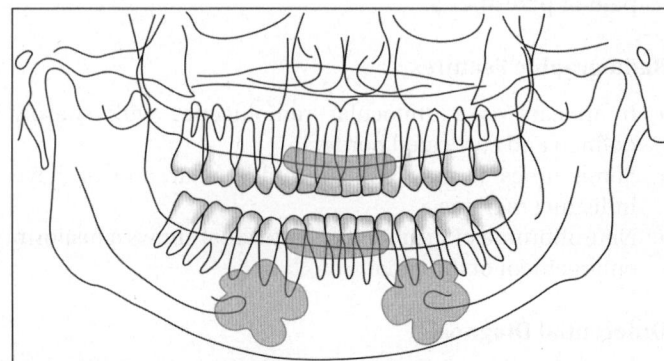

Figure 22.47 Schematic diagram showing the most common sites for central (dark) and peripheral (light) reparative giant cell granulomas

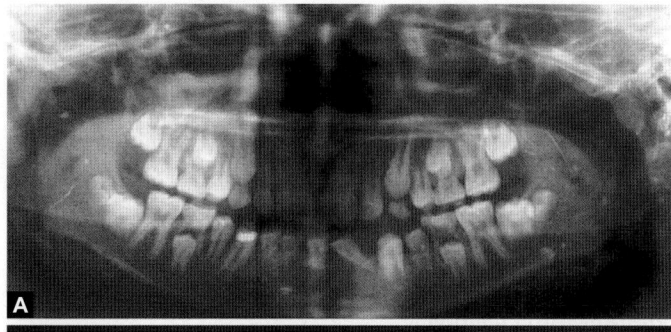

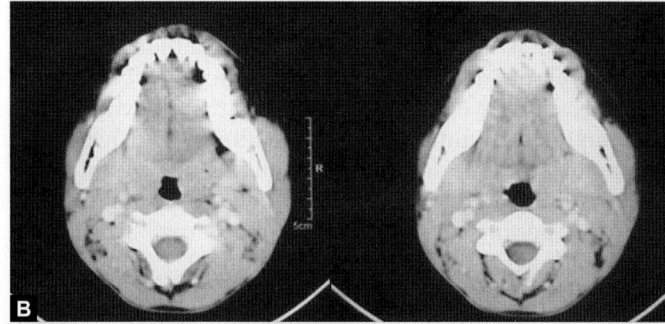

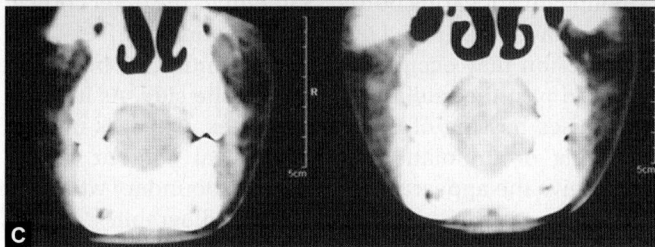

Figures 22.48A to C Peripheral giant cell granuloma: (A) Panoramic view revealed mild horizontal alveolar bone loss in 32 region, with displacement of 32. CT scan: (B) Axial; (C) Coronal view showed: An ill-defined isodence, enhancing lesion of size 1.9 x 2.5 cm was noted involving the floor of mouth in left anterior part. There was no evidence of bone erosion or calcification within the growth

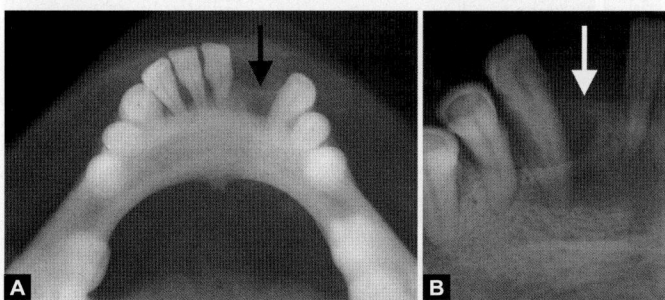

Figures 22.49A and B Peripheral giant cell granuloma: Mandibular occlusal view and IOPA showing (arrow) peripheral cuffing of bone in peripheral giant cell granuloma

- It initially appears as a discoloration on the gingival and slowly increases in size and becomes pedunculated or round. The size varies from 0.5–1 cm in diameter. It may be dark red or maroon, sometimes bluish or pink in color or if it has more fibrous tissue it may appear paler. It may feel soft to hard
- It may sometimes have an hour glass shape, with the waist of the lesion between the two teeth and the globular extremities presenting buccally and lingually
- The lesion may be vascular or hemorrhagic, with ulcerations and tenderness
- In edentulous cases, it may present as a vascular, ovoid or fusiform swelling on the crest of the ridge, little more than 1–2 cm in diameter. Or it may appear as a granular mass of tissue growing from the tissue covering the ridge.

Radiographic Features

- In dentulous cases there may be superficial destruction of the alveolar margins or crest of the interdental bone
- In the edentulous area, it characteristically exhibits superficial erosion of bone with peripheral cuffing of the bone.

Differential Diagnosis

- *Hemangioma*: It usually present at birth and seldom occurs on the gingival.
- *Lymphangioma*: The color of the lesion is usually the same as that of the tissue involved, and it is rarely found on the gingival.
- *Metastic carcinoma*: There will be history of a primary tumor.
- *Oral nevi, nodular melanoma*: These are darker in color and usually firm on palpation.

Management

Excision.

Central Giant Cell Granuloma (Osteoclastoma, Myeloid Sarcoma, Chronic Hemorrhagic Osteomyelitis, Giant Cell Reparative Granuloma, Giant Cell Tumor) (Figs 22.50 to 22.54)

Definition

It is believed to be a non-neoplastic bone lesion, reactive to some unknown stimulus. However, radiologically the characteristics are similar to that of a benign tumor. The relationship of the benign giant cell tumor to giant cell granuloma is controversial and unclear.

There are two types:

1. *Nonaggressive*: This exhibits slow growing benign behavior
2. *Aggressive*: It shows typical features of rapidly growing, destructive lesion.

Clinical Features

- More often seen in adolescent and young adults
- The mandible is more commonly involved, with a high percentage crossing the midline (symphysis), the epicenter of the lesion is usually anterior to the first molar region, (anterior and bicuspid region). In the maxilla, the canine fossa and ethmoid region are more prone

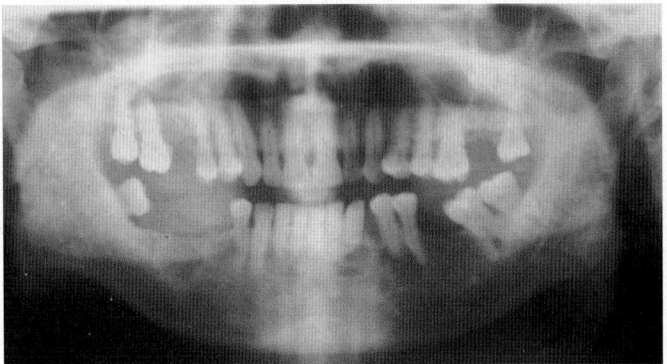

Figure 22.50 Central giant cell granuloma: Panoramic view shows well-defined noncorticated, multiloculated, expansile, and irregular in shaped with scalloped margins radiolucency in relation to parasymphyseal region of left mandible. Superiorly it is extending up to periapical area of canine and premolar and inferiorly till mental foramen of mandible. Anteriorly till mesial surface of canine, posteriorly till second premolar

- Some lesions cause no symptoms and may be found on routine examination
- The patient may present with a painless swelling which is tender on palpation and purplish red in color
- There may be expansion of bone, with facial asymmetry and premature loosening and shedding of deciduous teeth
- The involved teeth may become mobile but maintain their vitality till they are exfoliated.

Radiographic Features

- It is seen as a solitary unilocular or multilocular lesion, with well-defined margins but no cortication.
- It may show no evidence of internal structure when small; sometimes a stubble granular pattern of calcification may be seen. These may be organized into wispy septa. Sometimes the septa are better defined, at right angles to the periphery and divide the internal aspect into compartments (honeycomb appearance).
- Lesions in the maxilla may have an ill-defined, almost malignant appearing border. Sometimes the outer cortical plate may be destroyed instead of expanded.
- The lesion may occupy the entire mandibular body and extend past the midline to the opposite side. As it grows it causes bossing of the buccal cortex, which is uneven bulging or undulation of the cortical contour, which may give the appearance of a double boundary when the expansion is viewed on the occlusal radiograph.
- Displacement of adjacent teeth, tooth buds and resorption may occur. The lamina dura of teeth within the lesion are usually missing. The inferior alveolar canal is displaced in the inferior direction.

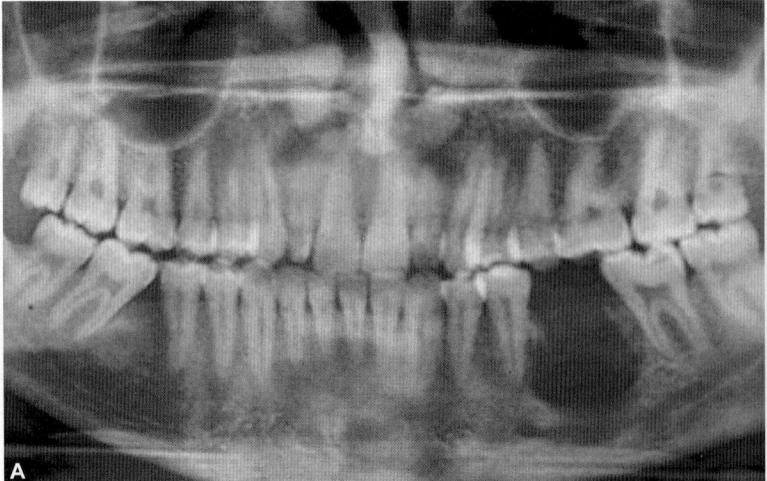
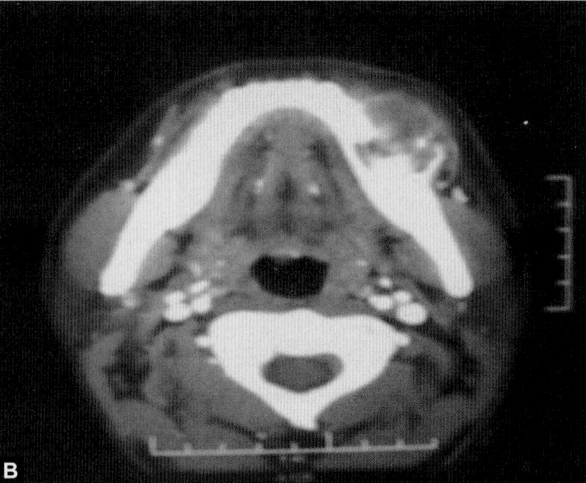

Figures 22.51A and B Central giant cell granuloma: (A) Panoramic radiograph shows well-defined radiolucency in the region of mandibular left molar with no cortication present surrounding the radiolucency; (B) CT axial view shows an expansile lytic lesion in the body of mandible on left side. Lesion has soap bubble appearance

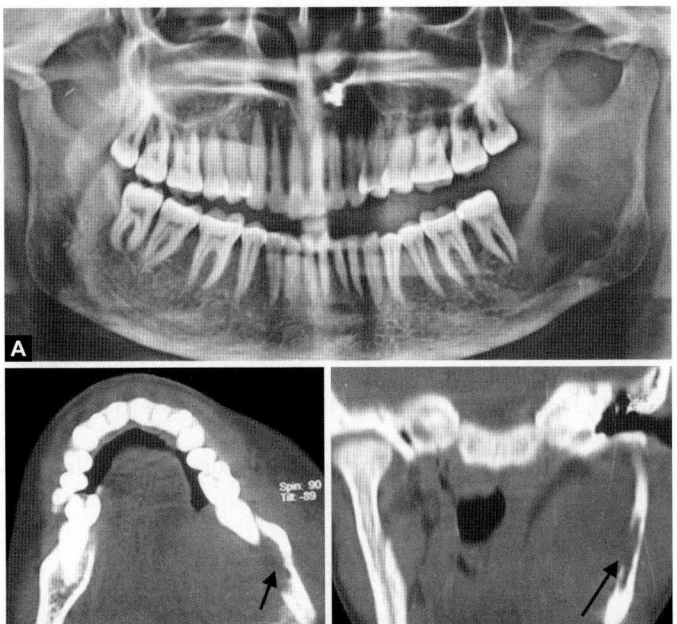

Figures 22.52A to C Central giant cell granuloma: Panoramic view revealed single radiolucent lesion extending from distal of mandibular left second molar to the sigmoid notch. Margins are ill-defined. Lesion is also extending between the roots leading to scalloped margins. Some trabeculae can be traced within the posterior portion of the lesion. Erosion of the superior cortical lining of the mandibular canal. CT scan: Axial and coronal view. There was a osteolytic lesion seen on the left side of the mandible extending from mandibular molar to the sigmoid notch. Soft tissue extension of the lesion present both buccally and lingually with erosion of the ramus on the lingual aspect. Loss of the cortical lining of the canal. Subcentimetric left level 1, bilateral level II lymph nodes visualized

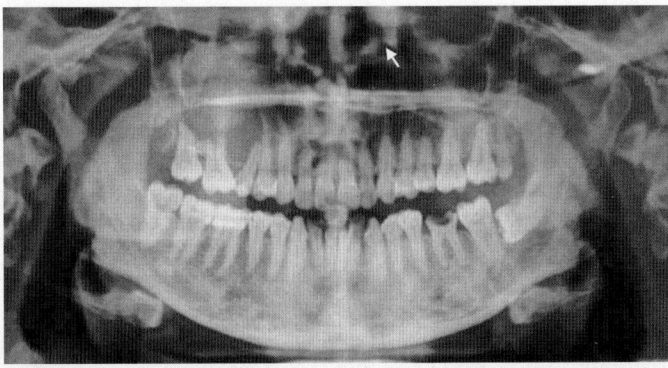

Figure 22.53 Central giant cell granuloma: Panoramic view showing a well-defined, multilocular radiolucency surrounded by corticated borders in right maxillary sinus region extending from maxillary right premolar to second molar region, with displacement of the premolar root mesially and first molar distally. Root resorption is seen in apical 1/3rd of all affected teeth

Addition Imaging

CT scan will give the exact extent and involvement of the surrounding structures, especially in the maxilla, such as maxillary antrum or nasal cavity. It is also advised in case of larger lesions where there is a possibility of destruction of the outer cortical bone. CT helps to determine whether the adjacent soft tissue has been invaded.

Differential Diagnosis

- *Ameloblastoma*: This is found in the older age group, seen in the posterior part of the mandible. This demonstrates internal hard curved arch like septa and is usually multiloculated.
- *Aneurysmal bone cyst*: It is comparatively rare, does not occur in the anterior segment of the mandible and usually causes profound expansion. Aspiration produces blood.
- *Odontogenic myxoma*: It is usually associated with a missing or impacted tooth. Has a multilocular and typical honeycomb appearance, with sharper and straighter septa, and do not have the same propensity to expand as giant cell granuloma.
- *Giant cell tumor*: It is more common in the third or fourth decade, rare in the jaws, more common in the femur and tibia. This is not preceded with history of trauma. No new bone formation is present.
- *Traumatic bone cyst, simple bone cyst*: No expansion of the overlying bone, no bodily movement of the teeth present.
- *Odontogenic cyst*: No internal septa, no bony spicules protruding from the radiographic margins. Regular smooth bony expansion of the cortical plates with scalloped undulating bulging of the cortex.
- *Browns tumor of hyperparathyroidism*: It is seen after the second decade of life, serum calcium levels are elevated. Investigation for parathormone or full body technetium scans should be done.
- *Cherubism*: Lesions are multiple, bilateral with epicenters located more in the posterior aspect of the mandible and maxilla. There is a history of familial involvement.
- *Metastatic tumor*: History of primary tumor, seen in older age groups, with multilocular lesions.
- *Central hemangioma*: This shows localized bleeding around the necks of involved teeth which may also show pumping action.
- *Post extraction socket, surgical defect, residual cyst*: There will be history of extraction in case of post extraction socket and residual cyst, history of some surgery in case of surgical defect.
- *Malignant tumor of the maxilla*: In case of giant cell granuloma a bony partition separates the air sinuses or nasal fossa from the tumor, unlike a malignant tumor, which extends into the said cavities.

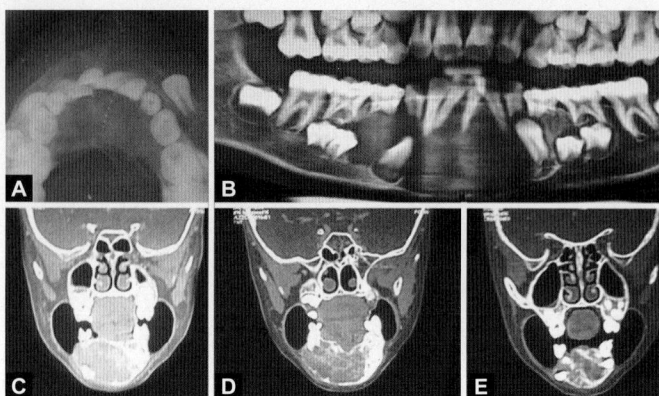

Figures 22.54A to E Central giant cell lesion: (A) Occlusal radiograph shows labial and lingual expansion with left canine transposed labially. (B) Panoramic view showed radiolucent lesion extending from lower deciduous second molar from right to left side crossing the midline, with displacement of the lower permanent anteriors; (C) CT coronal views showed expansile lytic lesion involving body of the mandible, crossing the midline. This lesion should be differentiated from central giant cell granuloma (CGCG), ameloblastoma, aneurysmal bone cyst, fibrous dysplasia

Management

Enucleation, curettage or partial resection.

Reparative Giant Cell Granuloma

This is now called central giant cell tumor, as it is associated more with a destructive than a reparative process, and it is not a granuloma and but a proliferative reaction.

Clinical Features

It occurs in the younger patients, more often seen in the region anterior to the first molar in the jaws.

Most of the lesions are single, though multiple lesions may occur. Spontaneous regression of the lesion is seen in many cases, which is not seen in benign giant cell lesions of other bones.

Radiographic Features

- The lesion may vary from small to that involving the greater part of the bone.
- The margins are poorly defined and undulating and there is no cortication.
- The outer and inner cortical plates may become involved in the extension of the tumor and are sometimes destroyed, but the periosteum lays down new bone leading to expansion of the lesion.
- One single indentation of the bony covering may suggest the nature of the lesion.

- The internal structure is variable, there are no visible trabeculae, yet the grayness suggests that bone may be present. Wispy or delicate trabeculae may be seen or sometimes coarse trabeculae giving a honeycomb appearance may also be seen.
- External resorption of the involved teeth may be seen.

Differential Diagnosis

- *Ameloblastoma*: This is found in the older age group, seen in the posterior part of the mandible. This demonstrates internal hard curved arch like septa and is usually multiloculated.
- *Cyst*: Displacement of teeth is seen and it is well corticated, with smooth margins.
- *Hyperparathyroidism*: There is generalized loss of lamina dura.

Giant Cell Tumor of Hyperparathyroidism

Refer Chapter 20, Infections and Inflammatory Lesions and Systemic Diseases Affecting the Jaws (Page 298).

BIBLIOGRAPHY

1. Daley TD, et al. Relative incidence of odontogenic tumors and oral jaw cysts in a Canadian population. Oral Surg Oral Med Oral pathol. 1994;77:276.
2. Goaz PW, White SC. Principles and Interpretation. In: Oral Radiology, 3rd edition. Mosby Year Book, St Louis; 1994.
3. Kshar A, John A, Umarji A. Adenomatoid Odontogenic Tumor—Report of three cases. JIAOMR. 2005;17(2):61.
4. Miles DA, Van Dis MJ, Jensen CW, et al. Interpretation normal versus abnormal and common radiographic presentations of lesions. In: Radiographic and Imaging for Dental Auxillaries, 3rd edition. Philadelphia: WB Saunders; 1999.pp.231-80.
5. Patil D, Gandhi A, Karjodkar FR, et al. An Amelanotic melanoma of the Oral Cavity—A rare entity: a case report. J Clin Diag Res. 2011;5(6):1314-7.
6. Regezi JA, et al. Odontogenic tumors: an analysis of 706 cases. J Oral Surg. 1978;36:771.
7. Sansare, Raghav R, Mupparapu M, Mandada, Karjodkar FR, Bansal S, et al. Keratocystic odontogenic tumor: Systematic review with analysis of 72 additional cases from Mumbai, India, Triple O. 2011;115(1):128-39.
8. Shafer WG, et al. A textbook of oral pathology. Philadelphia: WB Saunders; 1983.
9. Wood NK, Goaz PW. Differential diagnosis of oral lesions. 4th edition. CV Mosby, St Louis; 1991.
10. Wood RE. Handbook of signs in dental and maxillofacial radiology. Warthog Publications, Toronto; 1988.
11. Worth HM, Principles and practice of oral radiographic interpretation. Year Book Medical Publishers, Chicago; 1963.

Malignant Diseases of the Jaws | 23

Malignant tumors represent uncontrolled growth of tissue which exceeds and is uncoordinated with the normal tissue and persists in the same excessive manner even after the cessation of stimuli which evoked the changes. They are more locally invasive, have a greater degree of anaplasia, and have the ability to metastasize regionally to lymph nodes or distant other sites. They may be defined as tumors with lack of differentiation which have slow to rapid rate of growth with invasion without encapsulation. They may be broadly classified into:

- *Primary tumors*: These arise *de novo*, and may be:
  - Central
  - Peripheral
- *Secondary or metastatic malignancy*: That which originates from distant primary tumors.

Cancer is a commonly used term for all malignant lesions. They may be caused by:
- Infections (e.g. viruses, syphilis)
- Actinic and ionizing radiations
- Genetic defects caused by exposure to pollution and carcinogenic chemicals (like use of tobacco, alcohol, etc.)
- Chronic infections
- Intraoral lesions (chronic ulcers and fissures, lichen planus, candidiasis, leukoplakia, median rhomboid glossitis, Plummer Vinson syndrome, submucous fibrosis, oral melanosis, discoid lupus erythromatosus, epidermolysis bullosa)
- Orodental factors
- Immunity, trauma
- Dietary and other deficiency states.

CLASSIFICATION OF MALIGNANT TUMORS OF THE JAWS (TABLE 23.1)

General Characteristics

- It may occur at any age in either gender, but oral cancers are seen to occur more in men aged 50 years and older.
- Primary carcinomas are more commonly seen in the tongue, floor of the mouth, tonsillar area, lip, soft palate or gingiva and may invade the jaws from these sites.
- Sarcomas are more common in the mandible and in the posterior region of both the jaws.

Table 23.1 Classification of malignant tumors of the jaws

- Odontogenic
  - Odontogenic carcinoma
    - Malignant ameloblastoma
    - Primary intraosseous carcinoma
    - Malignant variant of other odontogenic epithelial tumors
    - Malignant changes in odontogenic cysts
  - Odontogenic sarcoma
    - Ameloblastic fibrosarcoma
    - Ameloblastic fibrodentinosarcoma
    - Odontogenic fibrosarcoma
- Nonodontogenic
  - Epithelial
    - Squamous cell carcinoma
    - Metastatic carcinoma
    - Basal cell carcinoma
    - Transitional cell carcinoma
    - Malignant melanoma
    - Verrucous carcinoma
    - Spindle cell carcinoma
    - Primary intra-alveolar carcinoma
    - Intra epidermoid carcinoma
    - Adenoid squamous cell carcinoma
  - Fibrous connective tissue
    - Fibrosarcoma
    - Malignant fibrous histiocytomas
    - Miscellaneous locally aggressive fibrous lesions
  - Adipose tissue
    - Liposarcoma
  - Cartilage
    - Chondrosarcoma
  - Bone
    - Osteosarcoma
    - Osteochondrosarcoma
    - Ewing's sarcoma
  - Vascular tissue
    - Hemangioendothelioma
    - Hemangiopericytoma
    - Angiosarcoma
  - Neural tissue
    - Neurosarcoma
    - Neurofibrosarcoma (malignant schwannoma)
    - Neuroblastoma
    - Ganglioneuroma

Contd...

Contd...

- Muscle
  - Leiomyosarcoma
  - Rhabdomyosarcoma
  - Malignant granular cell myoblastoma
- Lymphoid tissue, R-E system
  - Hodgkin's lymphoma
  - Non-Hodgkin's lymphoma
  - Primary reticular cell sarcoma
  - Burkitt's lymphoma
  - Leukemia
  - Lymphosarcoma
  - Giant cell follicle lymphoma
  - Multiple idiopathic hemorrhagic sarcoma of Kaposi
- Myeloma
  - Multiple myeloma
  - Plasmacytoma
- Tumors of salivary gland
  - Mucoepidermoid carcinoma
  - Adenocystic carcinoma (cylindroma)
  - Adenocarcinoma
  - Acinic cell adenocarcinoma
  - Malignant pleomorphic adenoma
  - Central mucoepidermoid carcinoma of the jaws
  - Adenocarcinoma of miscellaneous form
  - Epidermoid carcinoma
  - Stromal salivary gland tumor

- Metastatic tumors are most common in the posterior mandible and maxilla. Some lesions may grow at the apices of teeth or in the follicles of developing teeth.
- Pain and rapid swelling with no demonstrable dental cause.
- Displaced or loosened teeth over a short period of time.
- Foul smell, ulceration, presence of an indurated border, exposure of the underlying bone.
- Sensory or motor neural deficits.
- Lymphadenopathy.
- Weight loss, dysgeusia, dysphagia, dysphonia, hemorrhage and/or lack of normal healing.
- They always metastasize by direct spread by lymphatics or through the blood stream.
- Patient may give positive history of any of the above mentioned causes.

General Radiographic Features

The absence of visible radiographic signs does not preclude malignancy; it only implies that no visible radiographic signs exist.

Primary Lesions

- It is seen as an ill-defined osteolytic lesion with lack of cortication and absence of encapsulation (a soft tissue or radiolucent periphery). The infilterative border has uneven extensions of bone destruction.
- Finger like extensions of the tumor occurs in many directions; this extension is followed by osseous destruction producing a region of radiolucency.
- Evidence of osseous destruction with adjacent soft tissue mass is highly suggestive of malignancy. Such a mass may exhibit a smooth or ulcerated peripheral border if cast against a radiolucent background.
- The shape of the malignant tumor of the jaw is irregular.
- Most malignancies do not produce bone or simulate formation of reactive bone and thus they are seen as radiolucent lesions.
- Occasionally, residual islands of bone are present, giving an appearance of patchy destruction. With some scattered residual internal osseous structure.
- Osteogenic sarcomas produce abnormal bone giving the involved bone a sclerotic (radiopaque) appearance.
- Peripheral lesions present a cupped out appearance with ragged borders on the alveolar crest.
- Rapidly growing malignant lesions generally destroy supporting alveolar bone so that the teeth appear to be floating in space.
- Occasionally root resorption is present, more so in sarcomas.
- Internal trabecular bone is destroyed, as are cortical boundaries such as sinus floor, inferior border of the mandible, follicular cortices and cortex of the inferior alveolar nerve.
- They infiltrate along the path of least resistance, such as through the maxillary sinus, along the periodontal ligament space around the teeth, resulting in irregular widening and destruction of the lamina dura, along the inferior alveolar canal, which is widened.
- When the outer cortex of the bone is destroyed, there is no stimulation of new periosteal bone formation, except in the case of osteosarcoma, which may stimulate the formation of thin straight spicules of bone giving a hair-on-end or sun burst appearance.
- If there is a secondary inflammatory lesion coexsisting with the malignancy, a periosteal reaction associated with the inflammatory lesion (onion-skin appearance) may be seen.

Metastatic Carcinoma

- These are not uniformly or concentrically destructive and may have a multicentric appearance.
- It may present as a well-defined radiolucency, mimicking a benign lesion, or may exhibit unilateral widening of the periodontal space in the absence of periodontal disease or local factors.
- Metastatic lesion from the prostrate, thyroid and breast may produce a radiopaque or mixed lucent dense bone lesion in the jaws.

- Metastatic prostrate or breast lesions, can induce bone formation, resulting in an abnormal appearing, internal osseous architecture.
- Metastatic tumors may also give a hair-on-end or sun burst appearance.

GENERAL COMPUTED TOMOGRAPHY FEATURES

Malignant diseases frequently affect the oropharyngeal region. Out of these, the oral squamous cell carcinoma is the most common. These neoplastic diseases are characterized by sudden rapid growth causing extensive destruction of the adjacent hard and soft tissues. Computed tomography (CT) can be reformatted in various planes and the gray scale can be adjusted for viewing the hard and soft tissues. CT images can be enhanced with contrast to detect the exact extent of the lesion precisely. The common CT findings associated with oropharyngeal neoplasms are:

- Palatal perforation
- Asymmetry and/or thickening of the tonsillar pillars
- Exophytic masses
- Ulcerations
- Deep infilteration with thickening of the adjacent soft tissues and/or loss of facial planes
- Asymmetric or symmetric narrowing of the oropharyngeal airway
- Tumor extension into the adjacent para pharyngeal airway
- Tumor extension superiorly into the nasopharynx, inferiorly into the base of the tongue and hypopharynx and anteriorly into the oral cavity
- Adenopathy in the draining lymph node chains.

Note: Global examination as performed with a 2 mL/kg dose of intravenous contrast material injected at 2 mL/sec and a scanning delay of 50–70 seconds. No additional contrast material is used for the dynamic maneuvers.

Malignant Ameloblastoma

Definition

This is a rare type of tumor, with typical benign histological features and the diagnosis depends upon the presence of metastases, which in some cases is seen in the lymph nodes and lungs.

Clinical Features

- Males are more commonly affected, between the 1st to 6th decades of life.
- It mostly involves the mandible, premolar-molar area.
- It manifests as a swelling with pain which rapidly enlarges, with loosening and displacement of teeth and tenderness of the overlying soft tissue.
- It may locally extend into the adjacent bone, connective tissue or salivary gland. It may metastasize to the cervical lymph nodes, lungs, spleen, kidney, spine and ileum.

Radiographic Features

- It has a well-defined border with cortication with presence of crenations or scalloping in the perimeter. There may be loss of the cortical boundary, with spread into the adjacent soft tissue.
- It may be unilocular or multilocular, having robust, thick septae which gives a honeycomb or soap bubble appearance.
- The involved teeth may be displaced, may exhibit root resorption with loss of lamina dura.
- The bony borders may be effaced or breached, and displace normal anatomical structures such as floor of the nose and maxillary sinus.
- The mandibular neurovascular canal may be displaced or eroded.

Differential Diagnosis

- *Benign ameloblastoma*: There is no evidence of metastasis.
- *Central giant cell granuloma*: This lesion is more often found in the region anterior to the premolars, in young patients.
- *Malignant changes in odontogenic cysts*: These lesions are locally invasive and this is apparent on the radiograph.
- *Odontogenic myxoma*: It is associated with a missing tooth.
- *Odontogenic keratocyst*: Aspiration should be done.
- *Central mucoepidermoid tumor*.

Management

En bloc resection, followed by radiation and chemotherapy as necessary.

Squamous Cell Carcinoma Originating in Bone (Primary Intraosseous Carcinoma, Intra-alveolar Carcinoma, Primary Intra-alveolar Epidermoid Carcinoma, Primary Epithelial Tumor of the Jaw, Central Squamous Cell Carcinoma, Odontogenic Carcinoma, Central Mandibular Carcinoma)

Definition

This is a squamous cell carcinoma arising within the jaw that has no original connection with the surface epithelium of the oral mucosa. It is presumed to arise from the intraosseous remnants of odontogenic epithelium. They may be classified as:

- Those originating from odontogenic cysts.
- Those arising from ameloblastoma
  - Well-differentiated (malignant ameloblastoma)
  - Poorly differentiated (ameloblastic carcinoma)
- Those arising *de novo* from odontogenic epithelium residues, either keratinizing or nonkeratinizing.

Clinical Features

- This is a rare tumor and may remain silent until it has reached a fairly large size.
- It is more common in males, in the fourth to eighth decade.
- The mandible is more commonly involved than the maxilla; and the first molar region more involved, followed by the anterior aspect of the jaws. It originates only in the tooth bearing parts of the jaws.
- Pain, pathological fracture, sensory nerve abnormalities such as lip paresthesia and lymphadenopathy may occur. The surface epithelium invariably remains normal.
- Occasionally the pulp of the teeth may be invaded by the neoplasm.
- Extraction of teeth result in nonhealing socket and the tumor may protrude from the nonhealing socket.

Radiographic Features

- It presents as a diffuse radiolucency, with ill-defined to well-defined periphery. It may be rounded or irregular in shape with borders that demonstrate osseous destruction. The degree of raggedness of the border reflects the aggressiveness of the lesion.
- The internal structure is wholly radiolucent with no evidence of bone production and very little residual bone. If the lesion is small, overlying buccal or lingual plates may cast a shadow that may mimic the appearance of internal trabecular bone.
- If it grows sufficiently in size it may cause expansion, distortion and/or a pathological fracture, with associated step defects, thinned cortical borders and subsequent soft tissue mass.
- It may cause destruction of the antral or nasal floors, loss of cortical outline of the dentoalveolar canal.
- It causes effacement of the lamina dura. The teeth lose both lamina dura and supporting bone, to have a floating teeth appearance. Root resorption is unusual.

Differential Diagnosis

- *Periapical cysts or granulomas*: These lesions are not aggressive, are radiolucent with a smooth border. In case of periapical cyst the involved tooth is nonvital.
- *Odontogenic tumors*: Margins are usually well-defined.
- *Metastatic carcinoma, multiple myeloma, fibrosarcoma, carcinoma arising in dental cyst*: The margins are not infiltrative and there is no extensive bone destruction.
- *Peripheral squamous cell carcinoma*: The surface epithelium is involved.

Management

En bloc resection, along with chemotherapy and radiation.

Squamous Cell Carcinoma Originating in a Cyst (Epidermoid Cell Carcinoma, Carcinoma Ex-odontogenic Cyst)

Definition

This condition may arise from inflammatory periapical, residual, dentigerous and odontogenic keratocysts. Invasion from surface epithelial carcinomas, metastatic tumors, and primary intraosseous tumors is ruled out. Histologically the lining of sqamous epithelium of the cyst gives rise to the malignant neoplasm.

Clinical Features

- The tumor is more common in the mandible, and can be found anywhere an odontogenic cyst is found, namely the tooth bearing areas of the jaws.
- The common complain is pain which is dull and of several months duration.
- Swelling is occasional.
- Pathological fracture may occur, as may fistula formation and regional lymphadenopathy.
- If the upper jaw is involved, sinus pain may or swelling may be present.

Radiographic Features

- Initially it appears as a small radiolucency, with the shape of the cyst from which it arises, i.e. round or oval. The periphery is smooth and corticated.
- As the lesion progresses, the malignant tissue replaces the cyst lining and the border becomes ill-defined.
- The advanced lesion has an ill-defined, infiltrative periphery that lacks cortication. The shape becomes less 'hydraulic' and more diffuse.
- The lesion remains wholly radiolucent, more so than the invasive surface carcinoma owing to prior osteolysis by the cyst and no ability to produce bone.
- It causes thinning and loss of lamina dura around the involved teeth.
- Thinning and destruction of the adjacent cortical boundaries such as inferior border of the jaw or floor of the nasal cavity.
- It may produce complete destruction of the alveolar process.

Differential Diagnosis

- *Infected dental cyst*: This usually shows a reactive peripheral sclerosis because of the inflammatory products present in the cyst lumen. Histological examination will help verify.
- *Metastatic tumor*: This is multifocal and will have history of the primary lesion.
- *Multiple myeloma*: Multiple separate radiolucencies may be seen. In case there is a solitary lesion it becomes difficult to distinguish.

Management

En bloc resection, along with chemotherapy and radiation.

Clear Cell Odontogenic Tumor or Carcinoma

Definition

This is a rare odontogenic tumor with potential for lymphatic or pulmonary metastasis. Its origin is unknown. Some consider this tumor to be a clear cell variant of the ameloblastoma.

Clinical Features

- It is more common in women, over 60 years of age. The maxilla and mandible are equally involved.
- It may present as an asymptomatic or painful bony swelling.

Radiographic Features

It appears as a unilocular or multilocular radiolucency with ill-defined margins.

Management

Extensive resection with chemo and radiotherapy.

Squamous Cell Carcinoma Arising in Soft Tissue (Epidermoid Carcinoma) (Figs 23.1 to 23.13)

Definition

This represents 90% of all malignant tumors occurring in the mouth and jaws. It is defined as a malignant tumor

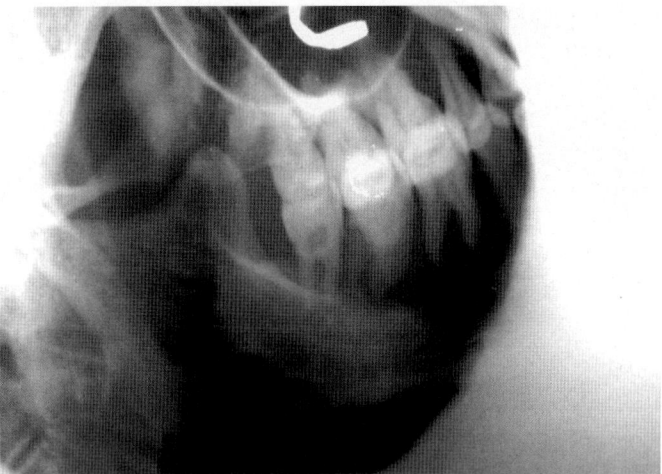

Figure 23.2 Invasive carcinoma of the mucosa of the floor of the mouth, the left side mandibular premolar-molar region exhibits an osseous defect with spotty osteolysis in the body of the mandible

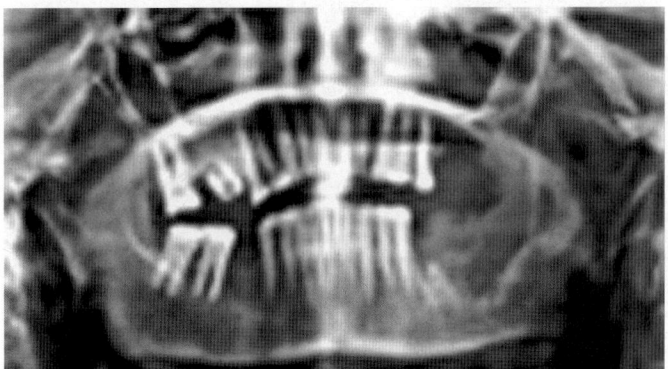

Figure 23.3 The radiograph shows two areas of poorly defined radiolucency with a ragged or moth-eaten appearance

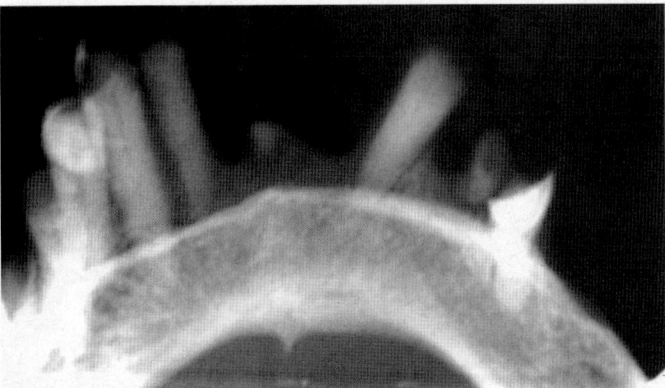

Figure 23.1 Invasive carcinoma of the alveolar ridge as seen in an occlusal radiograph. The tumor has destroyed nearly all the normal anatomical structures. The incisor teeth appear to 'hang' within the region of osteolysis, maintaining their normal position even in case of an aggressively proliferating malignant tumor, in contrast to benign lesions which displace teeth (with an exception of eosinophillic granuloma)

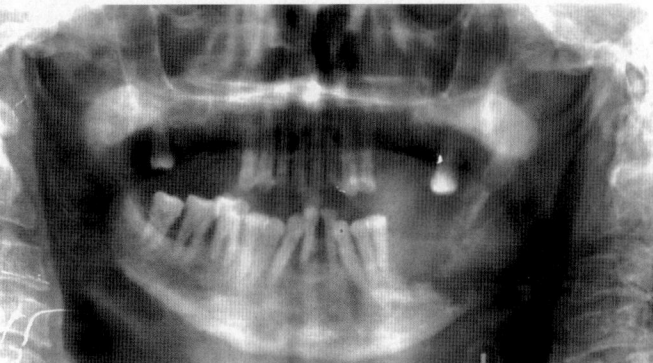

Figure 23.4 A panoramic radiograph of a patient who presented with a very large squamous cell carcinoma of the floor of the mouth that had penetrated through the mandible causing a pathological fracture

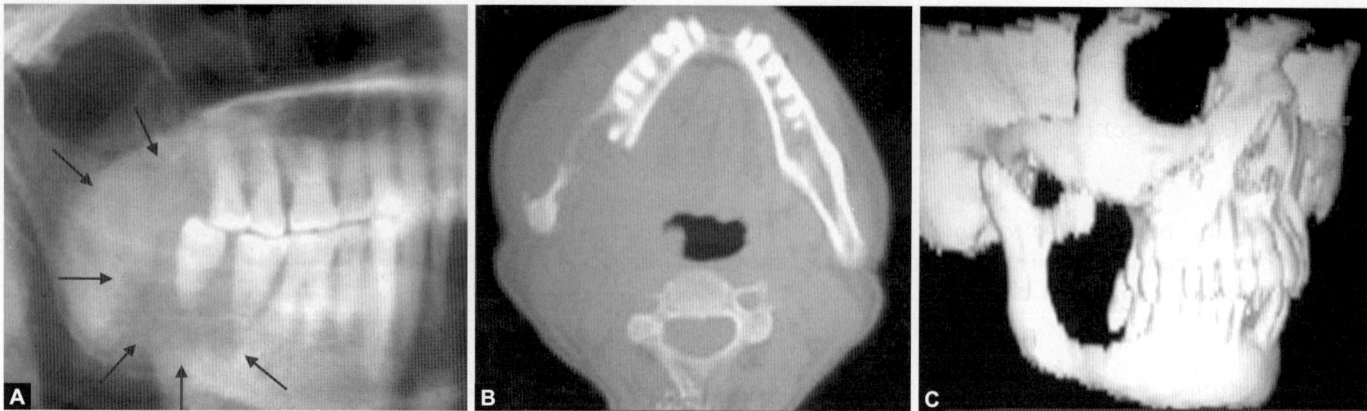

Figures 23.5A to C (A) Part of a panoramic radiograph showing an extensive destructive lesion—ill-defined radiolucency near the angle of the mandible. The patient was a known case of carcinoma of the tongue, this was an accidental finding on taking the radiograph; (B) Axial CT of the same patient showing destruction of the ramus and posterior body of the mandible; (C) 3D-CT of the same patient showing gross destruction of the ramus and body of the mandible

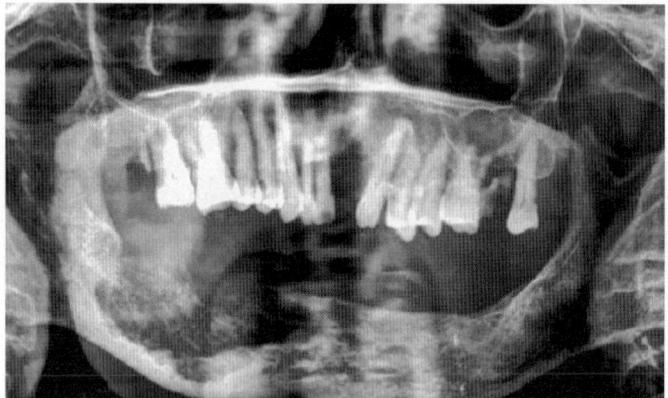

Figure 23.6 Carcinoma of the alveolar ridge: Panoramic radiograph showing extensive infiltrative lesion

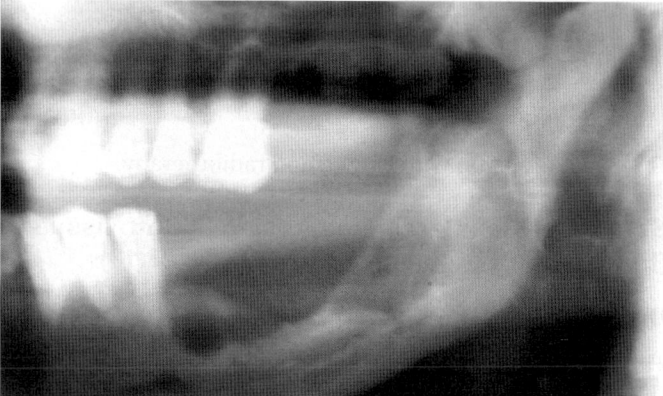

Figure 23.7 A section from an panoramic radiograph showing destruction of the mandibular canal

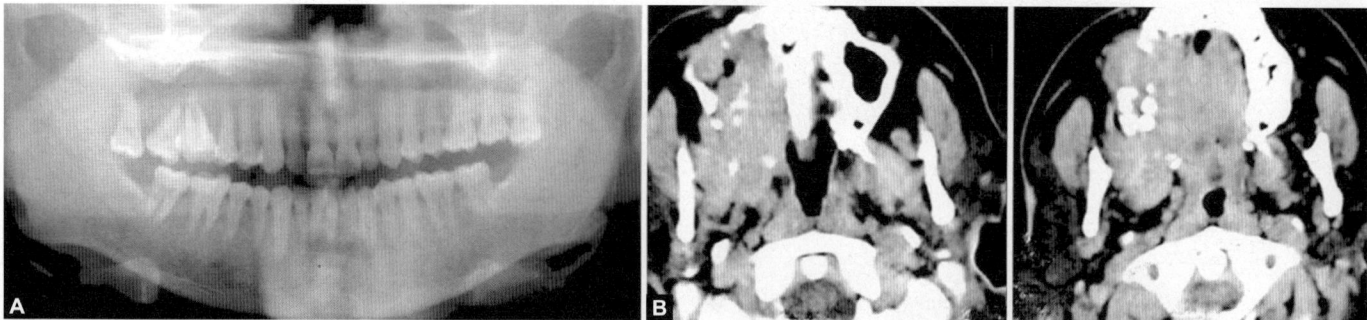

Figures 23.8A and B (A) Carcinoma of the right maxilla, the panoramic view shows an ill-defined radiolucency with permeating borders; (B) Axial CT showing the lesion of the same patient as an hypodense heterogenous enhancing growth in the right vestibule of the mouth and destruction of the right half of the hard palate and alveolar process, with involvement of the right maxillary sinus

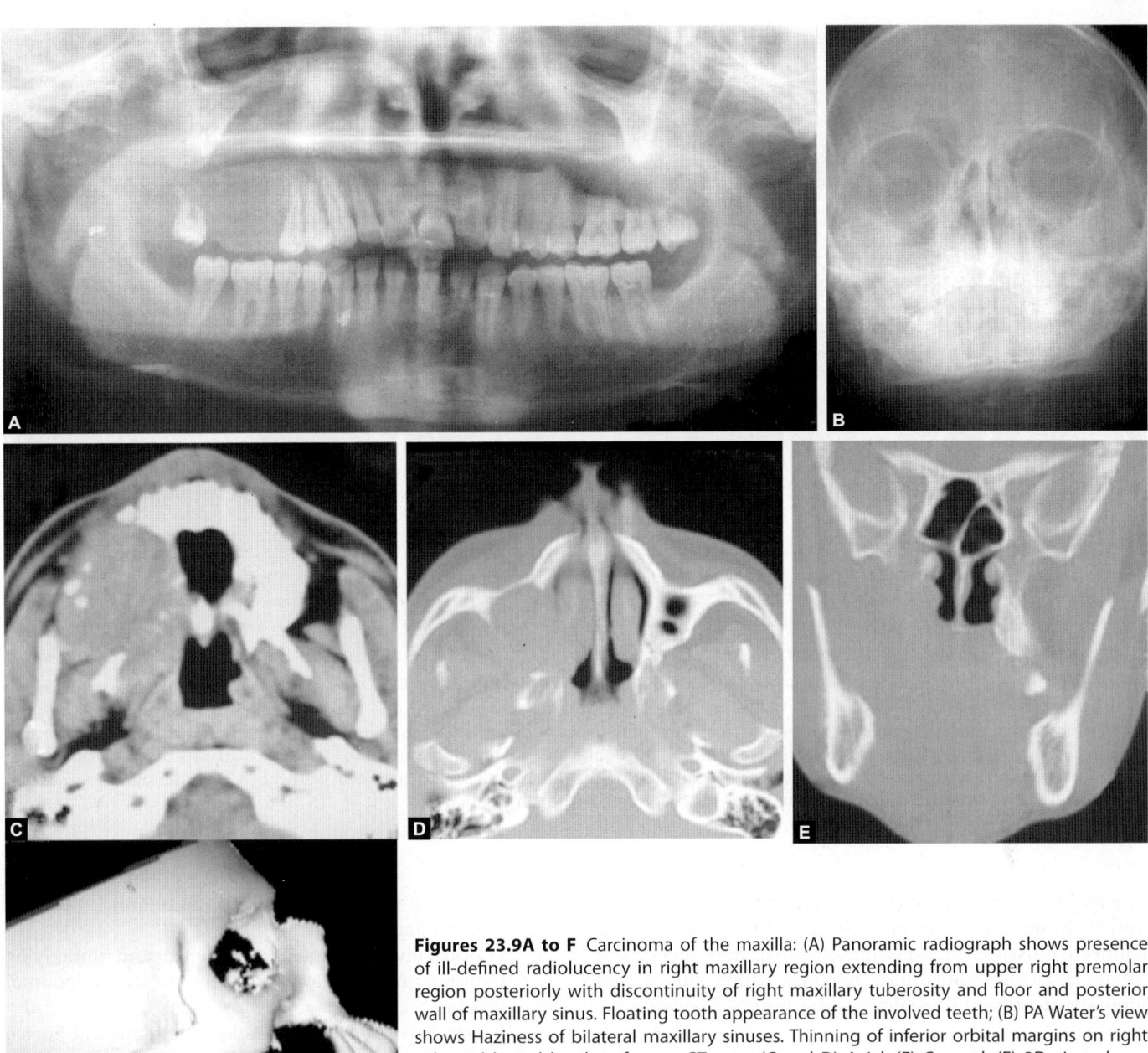

Figures 23.9A to F Carcinoma of the maxilla: (A) Panoramic radiograph shows presence of ill-defined radiolucency in right maxillary region extending from upper right premolar region posteriorly with discontinuity of right maxillary tuberosity and floor and posterior wall of maxillary sinus. Floating tooth appearance of the involved teeth; (B) PA Water's view shows Haziness of bilateral maxillary sinuses. Thinning of inferior orbital margins on right side and lateral border of nose. CT scan: (C and D) Axial; (E) Coronal; (F) 3D view shows presence of isodense moderately enhancing soft tissue filling the right maxillary sinus, with erosion of its inferior and lateral walls and adjacent alveolar process of maxilla and lateral part of hard palate on right side. Mass extended posterolaterally effacing the right antral fat, anterolaterally into the buccal space and medially involved the right half of nasal cavity and inferiorly it extended into superior part of oral cavity. 18 was seen suspended from this mass. Erosion of medial pterygoid plate on right side is also seen

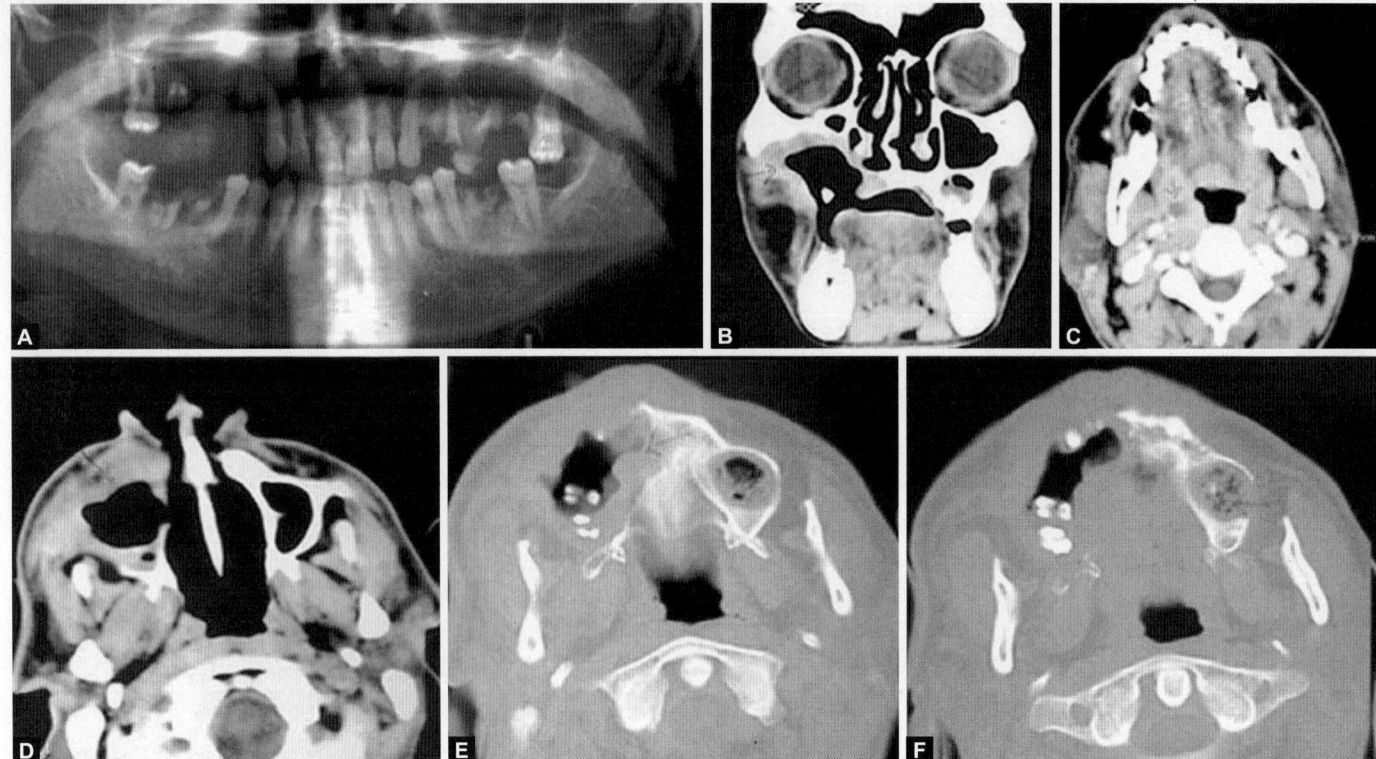

Figures 23.10A to F Carcinoma maxilla: (A) Panoramic radiograph shows that the right side floor, lateral and mesial wall not traceable. Floating tooth appearance in relation to 11, 12, 13, 17, 18. The maxillary tuberosity could not be traced; (B) CT scan coronal shows destruction of the bony, anterior, postlateral, medial and the floor of the right maxillary sinus, the bony defect is seen communicating with the oral cavity; (C) CT scan axial view shows a hypodense peripherally enhancing collection in the right parapharyngeal space; (D and E) CT scan axial view shows, destruction of the sinus walls, with a isodense heterogeneously enhancing mass in the right maxilla; (F) CT scan axial view shows, an expansile lesion was also detected on the left side involving the floor of the left maxillary sinus in the same patient

originating from the surface epithelium, characterized initially by invasion of the epithelial cells into the underlying connective tissue with subsequent spread into deeper soft tissue, adjacent bone, local regional lymph nodes and ultimately to distant sites such as lung, liver and skeleton.

Clinical Features

- Males, more than 50 years are more affected. The condition is fatal if untreated.
- It may initially appear as a white/red/mixed irregular patch, with a broad base (dome like or nodular), with surface that may be granular to pebbly to deeply creviced, which gradually exhibits central ulceration, rolled or indurated border which represent peripheral invasion of malignant cells; and palpable infiltration into adjacent muscle or bone.
- It commonly involves:
  - The lateral border of the tongue from where it tends to invade the posterior portion of the mandible.
  - Lesions of the lip and floor of the mouth invade the anterior part of the mandible.
  - Lesions involving attached gingival and underlying bone may mimic inflammatory disease, like periodontal disease.
  - It may also involve the tonsils, soft palate and buccal vestibule.
  - It is uncommon on the hard palate, except in cases where there is history of reverse smoking.
- Pain may be variable with regional lymphadenopathy characterized by rubber-hard lymph nodes that are tethered or fixed to the underlying structures. They are usually nontender, unless secondarily infected.
- Soft tissue mass, paresthesia, anesthesia, dysesthesia, pain, foul smell, trismus, grossly loosened teeth with history of spontaneous exfoliation, hemorrhage may be seen.
- Large lesions may obstruct the airway, the opening of the eustachian tube (decreased hearing), or nasopharynx.
- Patient may complain of weight loss and general unwell feeling.

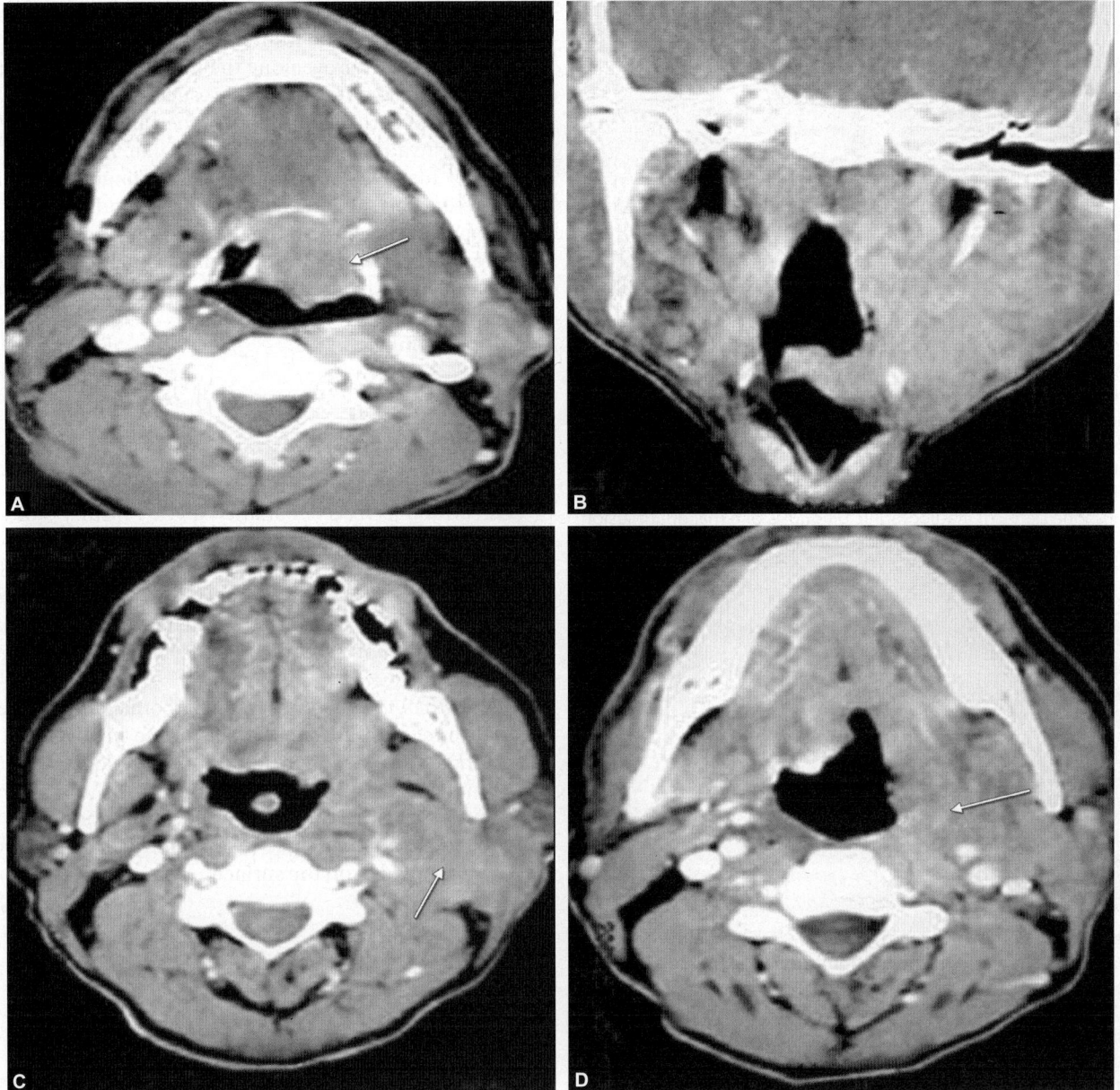

Figures 23.11A to D (A) Axial CT showing mass arising from the base of the tongue—carcinoma of the tongue; (B) Coronal CT shows the mass extending up to the left tonsillar fossa superiorly and the aryepiglottic fold inferiorly. Narrowing of the oropharynx; (C) Metastasis to the left parotid space; (D) Thrombosis of the internal jugular vein

Radiographic Features

- It may erode into the underlying bone in any direction, producing a radiolucency that is polymorphous and irregular in outline.
- Sclerosis in underlying osseous structures (likely from secondary inflammatory disease) may be seen in association with erosions from surface carcinoma. These erosions appear semicircular or saucer shaped. The border may appear smooth without a cortex, indicating erosion rather than invasion.
- Invasion occurs in more than 50% of the cases, and is characterized by an ill-defined, noncorticated border. The periphery will appear to have bays of bone destruction which extend into the bone appearing as finger like extensions preceding a zone of osseous destruction.
- If a pathological fracture occurs, the borders show sharpened thin bone ends with displacement of the segments.

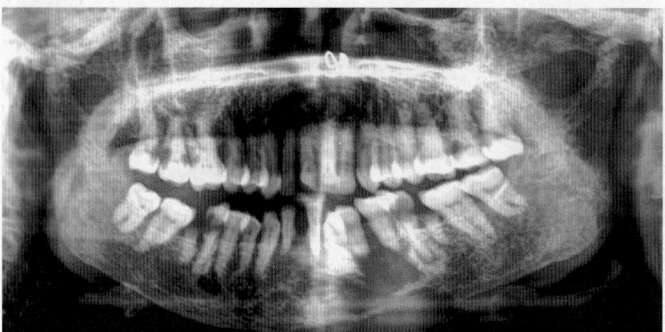

Figure 23.12 Panoramic radiograph showing A single lesion is seen in the left side of the mandibular parasymphyseal region and symphyseal region. The lesion is radiolucent extending from left central incisor to the molar region involving the inferior border of the mandible. Margins are ill-defined without cortication causing pathologic fracture in the region of canine and premolar. Resorption of roots seen interspersed within the radiolucency lie diffuse areas of radiopacity. There is generalized widening of trabecular spaces (Herring bone pattern). Radiographic diagnosis of a malignant lesion within the mandible with osteoporosis causing pathologic fracture

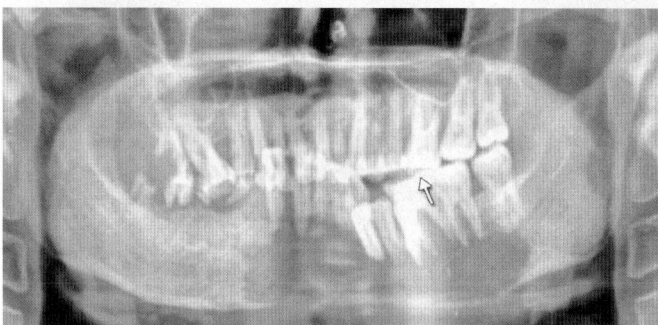

Figure 23.13 Central malignancy: Large, dark, radiolucency due to the bone destruction extending from the left mandibular molars to the right premolar region crossing the midline. Borders of the radiolucency are well-defined and irregular. There is complete destruction of the lower border of the mandible with resorption of the apical 1/3rd of roots of the involved teeth. Mandibular nerve canal is not traceable in the region of the radiolucency. Displacement of the teeth seen with anterior region having a floating tooth appearance

- The adjacent soft tissue mass may be seen as a faintly increased density in the radiograph, standing above the general level of the bone.
- The squamous cell carcinoma in jaw lesions appears totally radiolucent, with occasional small islands of residual normal trabecular bone.
- The periodontal ligament space is widened, with loss of lamina dura, which is evidence of invasion of bone around the involved teeth. The teeth appear to float in a mass of radiolucent soft tissue bereft of any bony support, floating or hanging teeth. In extensive tumors this soft tissue mass

may grow with the teeth in it as 'passengers', so the teeth are grossly displaced from their normal position.
- The tumor may grow along the inferior alveolar canal and through the mental foramen, resulting in increased width and loss of cortical boundary of the canal.
- It may invade adjacent structures like, floor of the nasal cavity, maxillary antrum, buccal or lingual mandibular plates by destruction of the cortical boundaries.
- The posterior aspect of the maxilla may also be effaced.
- Inferior border of the mandible may be thinned or destroyed, with occurrence of a pathological fracture.

Additional Image

Computed tomography.

Differential Diagnosis

- *Osteomyelitis*: This produces periosteal reaction.
- *Osteoradionecrosis*: Patient gives history of prior malignancy and radiation therapy.
- *Periodontitis*: The margins of the periodontal lesion are smooth and well-defined. The lesions are usually generalized and if localized it will have a specific cause.
- *Papillon-lefevre syndrome*: Other clinical findings are present.
- *Osteosarcoma (osteolytic type)*: Sarcoma originates within the bone, with absence of soft tissue involvement. This extends more deeply resulting in pathological fractures. Complete dissolution of continuity of the mandible occurs. Sarcoma produces bone destruction in a more concentric manner since it starts in the substance of the bone, instead of on the surface.

Management

Combination of surgery, chemotherapy and radiation therapy.

Metastatic Carcinoma (Metastatic Tumor, Secondary Malignancies) (Figs 23.14 to 23.16)

Definition

These represent the establishment of new foci of malignant disease from a distant tumor usually by way of blood vessels. Metastatic tumors of the jaws accounts for less than 1% of metastatic malignancies found elsewhere, and are usually believed to arise from sites that are anatomically inferior to the clavicle. Most frequently the tumor is a type of carcinoma, the most common primary sites being, the breast, kidneys, lung, colon, rectum, prostrate, thyroid, stomach, melanoma, testes, bladder, ovary and cervix. In children the tumors include neuroblastoma, retinoblastoma and Wilm's tumor.

Although the metastatic carcinoma of the jaws is uncommon, its recognition is important because the jaw

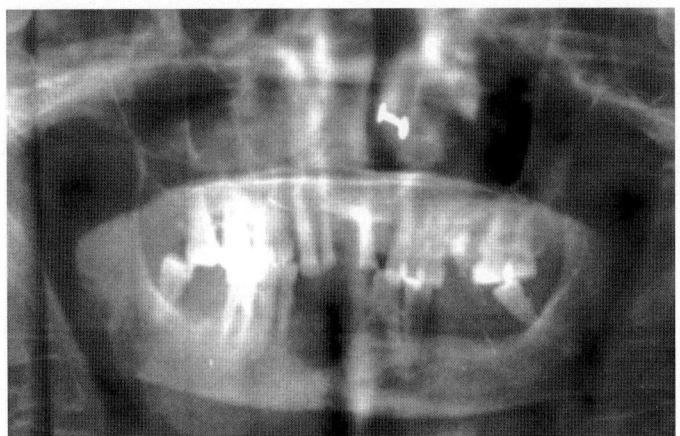

Figure 23.14 Metastasis from a mammary carcinoma, leading to destruction of the lamina dura and expansive osteolysis with indistinct boundaries

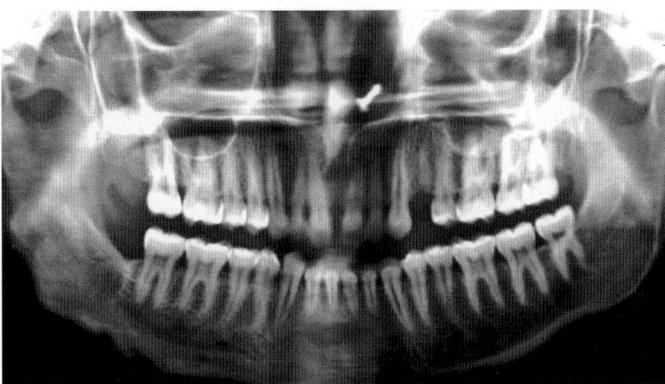

Figure 23.15 Panoramic radiograph showing a well-defined radiolucency (scalloping) at the inferior border of the mandible an posterior border of the ramus in the region of angle of mandible, there is loss of cortication along the inferior border of mandible and posterior border of ramus from lower right first molar up to the condyle. This was a case of metastatic lesion from a primary malignancy a differential diagnosis of osteomyelitis could be given if there is no clinical history

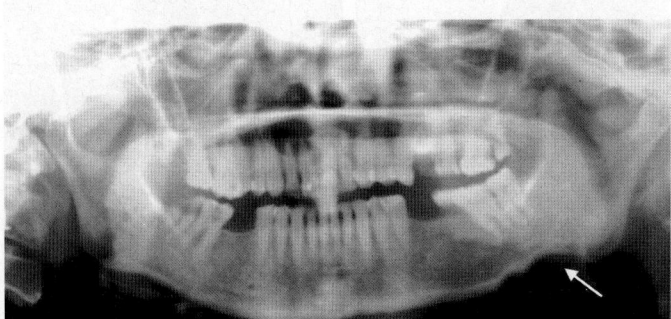

Figure 23.16 Panoramic radiograph showing resorption of the lower border of the mandible (arrows); case of metastatic carcinoma

tumors may be the first indication that the patient has a malignant disease.

Clinical Features

- It is common in the fifth to seventh decade of life, with history of a primary tumor. The posterior areas of the jaws are more commonly affected, as the tumor metastasizes to those bones that are rich in hemopoietic marrow, with the bilateral mandibular involvement more favored. The maxillary antrum, followed by anterior hard palate and mandibular condyle are the next most commonly affected sites. They may also be located in the periodontal ligament space (at the root apex), or in the papilla of a developing tooth.
- Patients may complain of dental pain, numbness or paresthesia of the third branch of the trigeminal nerve (lip or chin), pathological fracture of the jaw or hemorrhage from the tumor site.
- The tumor may breach the outer cortical plate of the jaws and extend directly into the surrounding soft tissue or presents as an intraoral mass.
- Loosening and exfoliation of teeth.
- Extraction sockets fail to heal. (All soft tissue curetted from extraction socket, even in the absence of clinical suspicion should be submitted for histological examination).

Radiographic Features

- They are generally seen as radiolucent (there is residual normal trabecular bone in association with areas of bone lysis), moderately well-demarcated lesion with no cortication or encapsulation. The lesions are usually not round but polymorphous in shape.
- If sclerotic metastases is present (i.e. prostrate and breast), the normally ragged radiolucent area may appear as areas of patchy sclerosis (which is the result of new bone formation by stimulating the surrounding bone), with ill-defined invasive margins.
- The tumor may begin as few zones of osseous destruction separated by normal bone, and if the tumor is multiseeded in multiple regions of the jaw, the result is a multifocal appearance (multiple small radiolucent lesions) with normal bone in between the foci (salt and pepper appearance). After sometime these small areas may coalesce into a larger, ill-defined mass and the jaws may become enlarged. Significant dissemination of the metastatic tumor may give the jaws a general radiolucent appearance occasionally mimicking osteopenia.
- It may stimulate a periosteal reaction that presents a spiculated pattern (prostrate and neuroblastoma).
- It effaces the lamina dura and causes an irregular increase in the width of the periodontal space. The teeth may be seen floating in soft tissue mass and may be in altered position due to loss of bony support.

- Resorption of teeth is rare.
- If the tumor is seeded in the papilla of a developing tooth, the cortices of the crypt may be totally or partially destroyed.
- The cortical bone of adjacent structures (such as: inferior alveolar canal, maxillary sinus, nasal fossa) are destroyed.
- The tumor may also breach the outer cortical plate.

Differential Diagnosis

- *Exophytic squamous cell carcinoma*: History of primary tumor which is clinically well-distinguishable.
- *Multiple myeloma*: The borders of the lesion are well-circumscribed and defined, it causes root resorption.
- *Periapical inflammatory lesion*: The periodontal ligament space widening in case of an inflammatory lesion is at its greatest width and centered about the apex of the root, in contrast the malignant tumor usually causes irregular widening, which may extent up to the side of the root.
- *Malignant salivary gland tumors*: These are not common in the mandible.
- *Secondarily infected odontogenic cys.*
- *Chondrosarcoma*: It causes root resorption.

Management

This has poor prognosis. Current trend is to add concomitant chemotherapy as an adjunct to either radiation or surgical treatment.

Malignant Melanoma (Figs 23.17A to C)

Definition

This is a neoplasm of epidermal melanocytes and is one of the biologically unpredictable and deadly of all human neoplasms. The different types are:
- Superficial spreading melanoma
- Nodular melanoma
- Lentigo maligna melanoma.

Clinical Features

- It is an uncommon neoplasm of the oral mucosa, more common in males, between the ages of 40–70 years.
- It has a definite predilection for the palate and maxillary gingival/alveolar ridge followed by buccal mucosa, mandibular mucosa, tongue, lips and floor of the mouth.

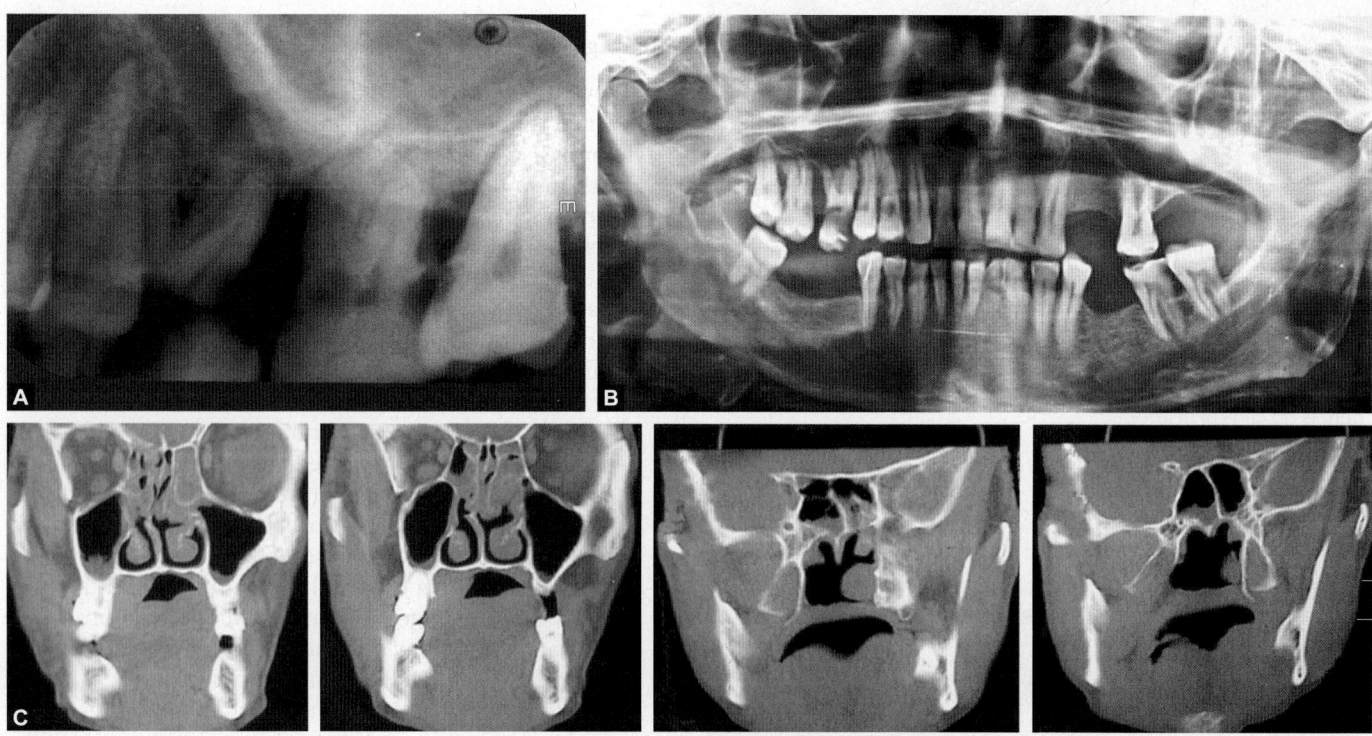

Figures 23.17A to C Malignant melanoma: (A) Intraoral radiograph showed grossly carious maxillary right molars with a well-defined periapical radiolucency and horizontal bone loss in this region; (B) Panoramic radiograph showed missing teeth, grossly carious maxillary right molar with a well-defined periapical radiolucency in relation to 16 and horizontal bone loss; (C) CT scan showed an ill-defined enhancing soft tissue mass on right side of hard palate, extending posteriorly up to the soft palate. There was no evidence of erosion or sclerosis of bone due to the soft tissue mass. Bilaterally enlarged level I, II, V lymph nodes were seen. Incisional biopsy findings were suggestive of malignant melanoma

- Focal pigmentation preceding the development of actual neoplasm usually occurs, several months to years before clinical symptoms appear.
- The lesions may present as painless soft darkish brown mass with nodular or papillary surface which may get ulcerated and hemorrhagic and tend to progressively increase in size.
- Loosening of the involved teeth is seen.

Radiographic Features

- The tumor causes extensive destruction of the underlying bone.
- These present a radiographic appearance which is indistinguishable from osteomyelitis.

Management

Combination of surgical irradiation, immunotherapy and/or chemotherapy.

Fibrosarcoma

Definition

This is a neoplasm composed of malignant fibroblasts that produce collagen and elastin. It may arise in the periosteal tissue, endosteally or it may arise secondarily in tissues that have received therapeutic levels of radiation.

Clinical Features

- It occurs equally in males and females, in the fourth decade. More common in the mandible, in the premolar-molar region.
- It may present as a painful slow to rapidly enlarging mass within the bone.
- Peripheral lesions or those exiting from the bone may invade the local soft tissues, causing bulky, clinically obvious lesions. Overlying mucosa may become erythematous or ulcerated.
- If the central or peripheral lesion attains a large size it may cause pathological fractures.
- If it involves the course of the peripheral nerves, sensory-neural abnormalities may occur.
- Involvement of the temporomandibular joint or paramandibular musculature is often accompanied by trismus.
- Involved teeth are displaced and mobile.

Radiographic Features

- It usually presents as an ill-defined, ragged, noncorticated radiolucency, with no capsule around it. The borders are infiltrative, and may be underestimated in defining the extent of the lesion. Sclerosis may occur in the normal adjacent bone.

- The tumors tend to be elongated in shape, which suggests that they may have grown along the bone, through the marrow space.
- Soft tissue lesions adjacent to the bone, may cause saucer like depressions in the underlying bone or invade it, as would squamous cell carcinoma.
- If the lesion has been present for sometime and is not overly aggressive, residual jawbone or reactive osseous bone formation may occur.
- There is massive destruction of the adjacent structures:
  - In the mandible, the alveolar process, inferior border of the jaw and cortices of the inferior alveolar canal are lost.
  - In the maxilla, the inferior floor of the maxillary sinus, posterior wall of the maxilla, and nasal floor are destroyed.
  - In either jaw, lamina dura and follicular cortices are obliterated.
  - Destruction of the outer cortical plate is accompanied by protruding soft tissue mass.
- Widening of the periodontal space, with gross displacement of the teeth due to loss of the supporting bone giving a floating tooth appearance. There is no resorption of the tooth.
- Periosteal reaction is uncommon, however, if the lesion disrupts the periosteum, a Codman's triangle or sunray spiculation may be seen.

Differential Diagnosis

- *Metastatic carcinoma, multiple myeloma, primary or secondary intraosseous carcinoma*: There is history of primary tumor and does not cause enlargement of the jaws.
- *Osteosarcoma*: There is typical sunray appearance.
- *Liposarcoma*: This is very rare in jaws.
- *Neurogenic sarcoma.*
- *Infected odontogenic cyst.*
- *Chondrosarcoma.*
- *Ewings sarcoma.*
- *Peripheral invasive squamous cell carcinoma*: Ulcerative surface features are clinically obvious.

Management

Surgery, with radiation and/or chemotherapy.

Malignant Fibrous Histiocytoma (Malignant Fibroxanthoma)

Definition

This exhibits both histiocytic and fibrocytic features. The different types are:
- Giant cell
- Inflammatory
- Myxoid

- Storiform
- Pleomorphic
- Angiomatoid.

Clinical Features

- It has a predilection for adult males.
- Common in the head and neck area, especially the paranasal sinuses and centrally within the jaws.
- It appears as an indurated swelling and usually metastasizes.

Radiographic Features

It appears as unilocular or multilocular radiolucent areas with ill-defined borders.

Management

Surgical excision followed with radiation.

Chondrosarcoma (Chondrogenic Sarcoma) (Fig. 23.18)

Definition

This is a malignant tumor of cartilaginous origin. It may develop centrally or on the periphery of bone, the most

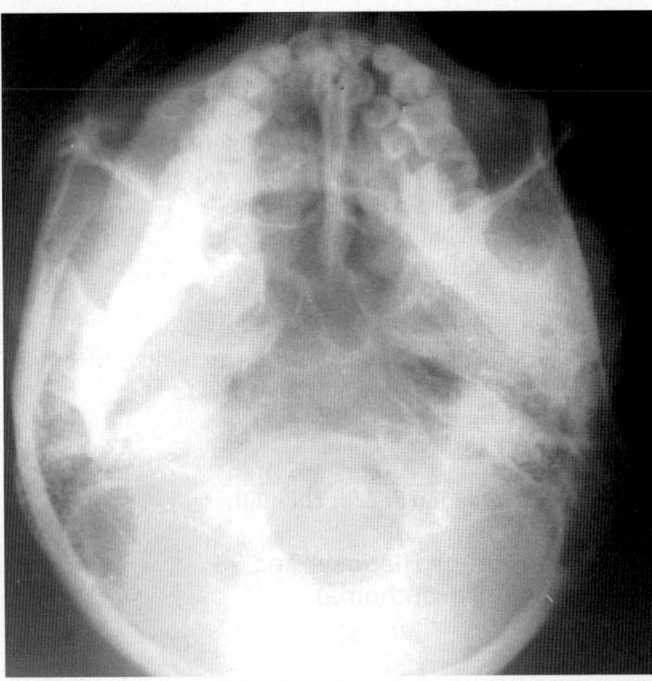

Figure 23.18 Chondrosarcoma: Submentovertex view shows a well-defined corticated homogenous radiopaque swelling attached to left side of condyle protruding on left side. Deviation of mandible towards right side. Radiographic diagnosis: Chondrosarcoma with a differential diagnosis of chondroma, osteoblastoma or osteoid osteoma

commonly occurring histologic sub types which develop in the craniofacial region are: the clear cell, dedifferentiated, myxoid and mesenchymal forms. They can also be classified as:

- *Primary*: Directly from the cartilage
- *Secondary*: This develops within pre-existing benign cartilaginous tumors.

Clinical Features

- It affects both sexes equally and may occur at any age, but primary type occurs in the younger age group as compared to the secondary type.
- These are unusual in the facial bones, they occur in mandible and maxilla with equal frequency, in areas where cartilaginous tissues may be present. In the mandible it occurs more often in the coronoid process, condylar head and neck, and occasionally in the symphyseal region. In the maxilla it occurs in the anterior region.
- The patient presents with a firm hard swelling of long duration. This on enlargement had started giving pain, headache and deformity.
- The overlying skin or mucosa is usually normal unless secondarily ulcerated.
- Less frequent signs and symptoms related with thus neoplasm are: hemorrhage from tumor or around the necks of the teeth, sensory nerve deficits, proptosis and visual disturbances.
- If it occurs near the temporomandibular joint region, trismus or abnormal joint function may result.
- The involved teeth may be displaced and resorbed.
- This metastases by vascular channel. Lung is the most common region of metastasis.

Radiographic Features

- These are slow growing tumors, and the radiologist signs may be misleading and benign in nature.
- The lesions are usually round, ovoid or lobulated with well-defined and corticated margins, sometimes they may merge with the surrounding bone. Sometimes the peripheral new bone may be present perpendicular to the original cortex, giving a sunray or hair-on-end appearance.
- Some aggressive lesions may have infiltrative, ill-defined and noncorticated borders.
- They usually exhibit some form of calcification within their center, giving a mixed radiopaque-radiolucent appearance.
  - It may take the form of moth eaten bone alternating with islands of residual bone unaffected by the tumor.
  - The central radiopaque structure may be defined as flocculent, implying snow like features.
  - The diffuse calcifications may be superimposed on a bony background that resembles granular or ground-glass appearing abnormal bone.

- It may also reveal areas of flocculence with a central radiolucent nidus, which may be cartilage surrounded by calcifications, giving a speckled appearance.
- This lesion is slow growing and thus usually expands normal cortical boundaries rather than destroying them.
  - In the mandible, the inferior border and the alveolar process are grossly expanded, maintaining the cortical covering.
  - Maxillary lesions may push the walls of the sinus or nasal fossa and/or impinge on the infratemporal fossa.
  - Lesions of the condyle may cause its expansion with remodeling of the corresponding articular fossa and eminence.
  - If present in the articular disk region, a widened joint space may be present with remodeling of the corresponding condylar neck. Erosion of the articular fossa may also occur.
  - If it occurs near the teeth, there will be widening of the periodontal ligament space, displacement and resorption of the involved teeth.

Differential Diagnosis

- *Osteosarcoma*: Though it is radiographically indistinguishable, the typical calcifications of chondrosarcoma are usually absent.
- *Fibrous dysplasia*: Its periphery is better defined. Here, the bone pattern is altered up to and including the lamina dura, leaving a normal or thin periodontal ligament space. (The radiopaque portion of fibrous dysplasia is abnormal bone and not calcifications).
- The benign characteristics of chondrosarcoma, are misleading and delay the correct diagnosis, thus endangering the patients life.

Management

Surgery.

Mesenchymal Chondrosarcoma

Definition

This contains mesenchymal cells. Most tumors arise in the bone and tend to metastasize of unusual locations, after long period of time.

Clinical Features

- It is commonly seen in the younger age group, more in the maxilla, skull, mandible and ribs. It may also occur in tubular bones and pelvis.
- There may be swelling, pain due to compression of nerve and/or pathological fracture.

Radiographic Features

Same as chondrosarcoma.

Management

The prognosis is poor as usually the patient dies due to metastasis.

Osteosarcoma (Osteogenic Sarcoma) (Figs 23.19 to 23.22)

Definition

This is a malignant neoplasm of the bone where osteoid is produced directly by malignant stroma as apposed to adjacent reactive bone formation. The cause is unknown, but mutation

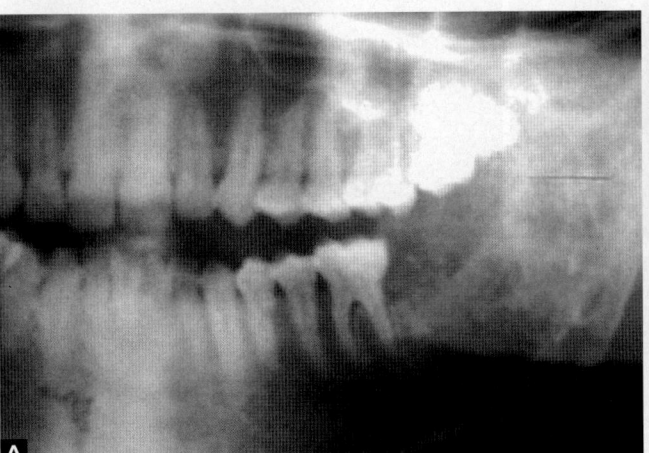
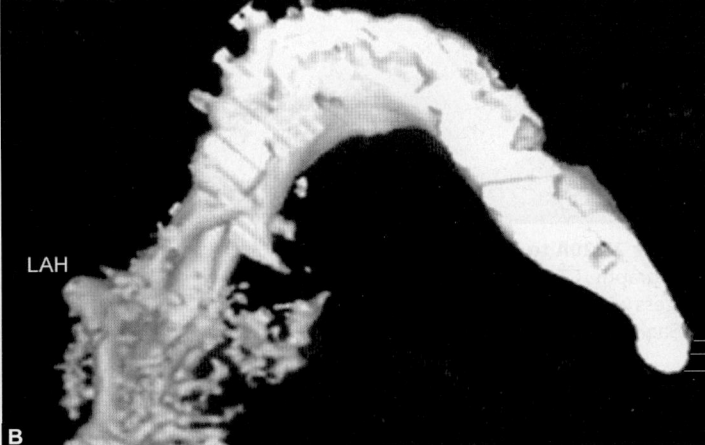

Figures 23.19A and B (A) Osteosarcoma seen on a panoramic radiograph as an ill-defined radiolucency with interspersed radiopacity; (B) 3D CT of the same patient showing a 6.5 × 6 × 6 cm lesion

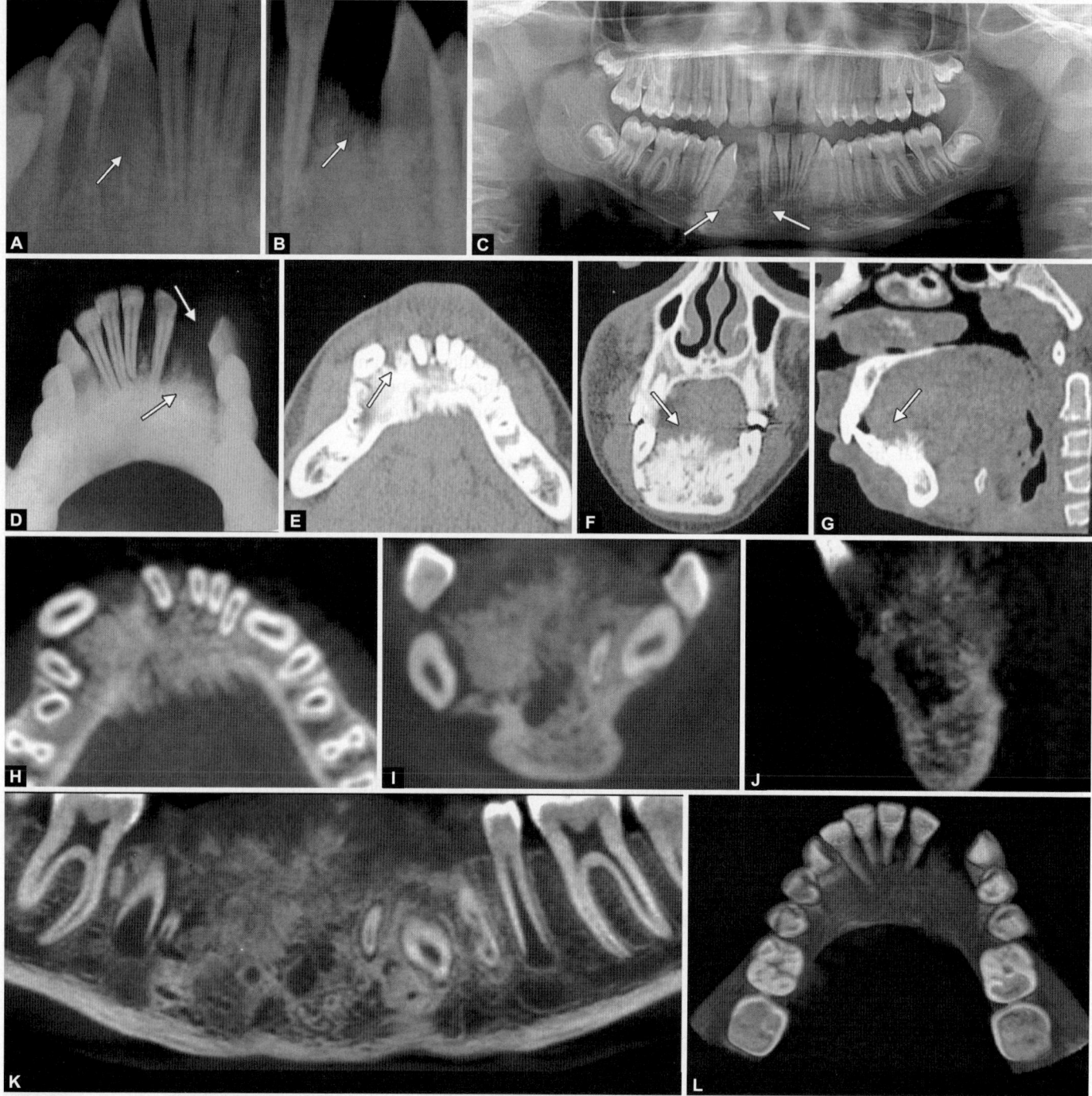

Figures 23.20A to L Osteosarcoma: (A and B) Intraoral; (C) Panoramic radiograph shows a similar appearance as appreciated in the intraoral radiographs. CT scan: (D) Occlusal radiographs showed typical sun burst appearance. (E) Axial; (F) Coronal; (G) Sagittal views shows sclerotic process with few lytic areas in the anterior part of the mandible. Aggressive sun burst periosteal reaction seen. CBCT images: (H) Axial; (I) Coronal; (J) Sagittal; (K) Reformatted panoramic; (L) 3D views. All sections show typical 'sun ray' appearance

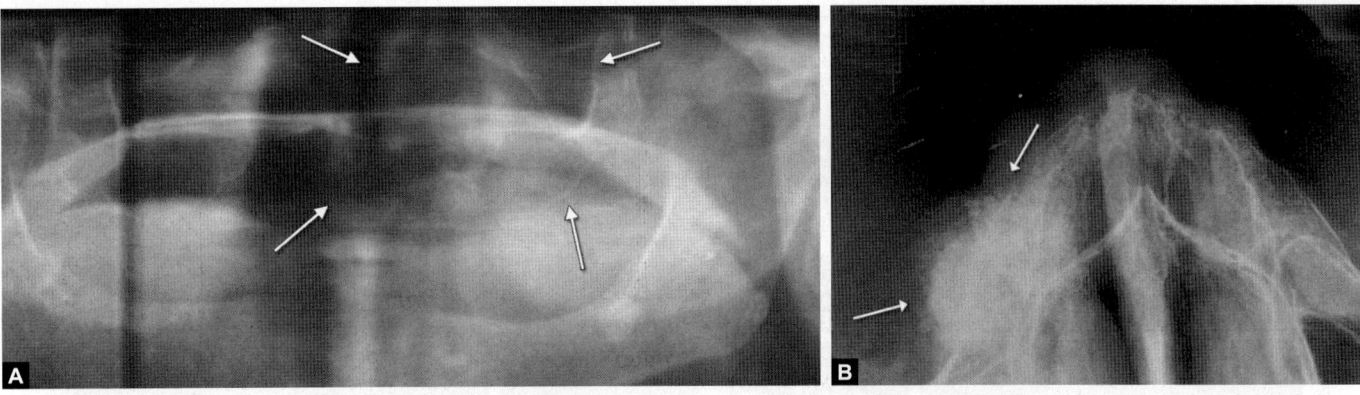

Figures 23.21A and B Osteosarcoma: (A) Panoramic radiograph showing radiopaque lesion in the left maxilla; (B) Occlusal radiograph showing expansion, perforation of the bony cortex with typical 'sun ray' appearance

and viral causes have been suggested. It is also known to occur in association with Paget's disease and fibrous dysplasia after therapeutic irradiation. Osteosarcoma of the jaws accounts for 7% of all osteosarcomas. The different types may be classified:

- Histological
  - Fibroblastic
  - Osteoblastic
  - Chondroblastic
  - Telangiectatic
- Radiological
  - Sclerosing
  - Mixed
  - Osteolytic
- Location
  - *Parosteal* (*juxta*): It is extremely rare in the jaws, more common in the femur. It grows on the external surface of the bone. It is slow growing and often metastasizes.
  - *Periosteal*: This is an aggressive variant of the parosteal osteosarcoma, but with a better prognosis than intramedullary osteosarcoma.
  - *Extraosseous*: This is a highly malignant osteosarcoma of the soft tissue, it occurs in the breast, liver and kidney.

Clinical Features

- It is more common in males, in the third and fourth decade. Although it may occur in any part of the jaws, the posterior mandible, including the tooth bearing region, angle and vertical ramus are more commonly affected. Posterior region of the maxilla may also be affected, the most frequent sites being, alveolar ridge, antrum and palate. The lesion may cross the midline.
- The patient may complain of a long standing rapidly growing swelling.
- Pain, tenderness, erythema of overlying mucosa, ulceration, loosening of the involved teeth, epitaxis, hemorrhage, nasal obstruction, exophthalmus, trismus and blindness are some of the other symptoms observed as the lesion progresses.

- Hypoesthesia (numbness of the lip and chin) has been reported in cases where the neurovascular canal has been involved.
- There may be history of tooth extraction followed by nodular or polypoid reddish granulomatous mass growing from the tooth socket.
- Serum alkaline phosphatase level is increased.

Radiographic Features

- There is symmetrical widening of the periodontal ligament space in the early stage of the disease.
- Osteosarcoma is usually a radiolucent lesion with an ill-defined border, there is no peripheral sclerosis or encapsulation. In the lesion involves the periosteum directly or by extension, one may see.
  - The typical *sun-ray spicules* or *hair-on-end trabeculae*, this occurs when the periosteum is displaced, partially destroyed and disorganized.
  - If the periosteum is elevated, but maintains its osteogenic potential, but it is breached in the center, a *Codman's triangle* is formed at the edge.
  - Sometimes subperiosteal bone is laid down in layers and it may give a laminated *onion peel appearance*.
  - In rare cases, extension is prominent and a soft tissue mass is visible radiographically.
  - There is no distortion of the alveolar ridge.
- Radiographic features differ as per the stage of the lesion:
  - *Frankly osteolytic type*: These lesions are unicentric, with ill-defined borders and a *moth eaten appearance*. There may be perforation and expansion of the cortical margins by extension into subperiosteal bone.
  - *Mixed type*: These lesions have presence of a small amount of new bone formation. The bone within the radiolucent area of destruction may take the form of strands, which may be few and intersecting, producing a *honey comb appearance*.

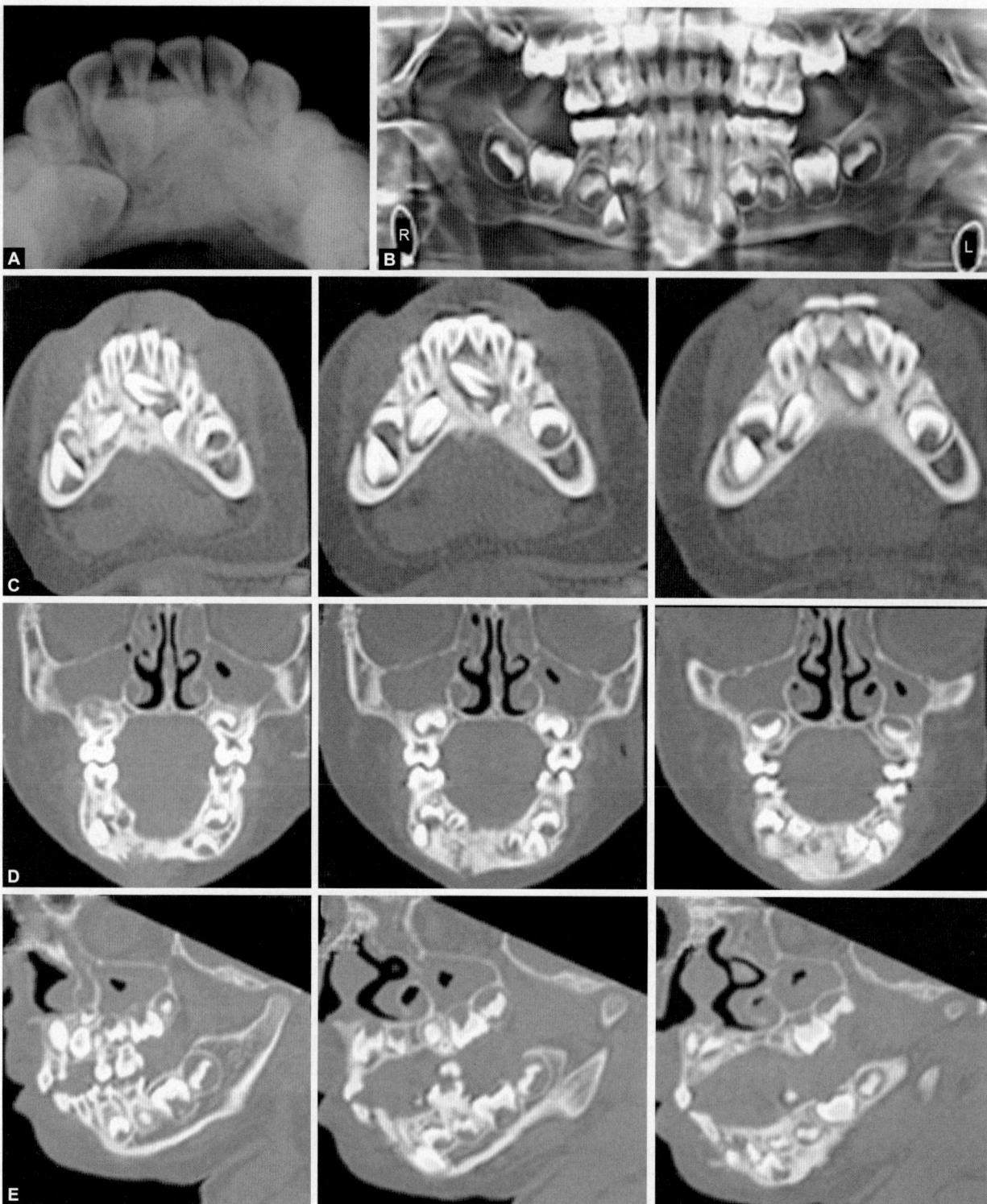

Figures 23.22A to E Osteosarcoma: (A) Occlusal; (B) Panoramic radiograph shows a mixed radiopaque-radiolucent lesion in lower mandibular region with peripheral sun ray appearance of the lesion. Breach in the inferior cortex of the mandible seen in right canine region seen in the panoramic radiograph. CT scan: (C) Axial; (D) Coronal; (E) Sagittal views show a diffuse expansion of symphysis menti region predominantly on the right side up to the canine region with multiple lytic areas extending on either side superolaterally involving the roots of the lateral incisor and canine. Breach in the lingual cortex in right canine region. Enhancing soft tissue mass seen surrounding the lesion. Areas of cortical erosion seen with areas of foci of periosteal reaction. Bilateral maxillary sinuses show mucosal thickening with focal fluid collection

– *Frankly osteoblastic (sclerotic osteogenic sarcoma) type*: The lesion has ragged, ill-defined borders and the radiographic pattern is the result of excessive bone production intermingled with radiolucent foci of bone destruction. The sclerotic portion of the lesion may show vertical obliteration of the trabecular pattern, giving a dense *granular appearance*.

- The mandibular lesions may destroy the cortex of the neurovascular bundles, or the canal of the inferior alveolar nerve may be symmetrically widened and enlarged.
- Pathological fractures occur more often in sarcomas as these extend more deeply into the bone.
- The sarcoma may develop near the floor of the maxillary antrum or nasal fossa, which may result in destruction of bone with no demarcation of the tumor and the air cavity.
- Lamina dura of involved teeth is completely destroyed.

Differential Diagnosis

- *Carcinoma*: May be confused with the frankly osteolytic stage, carcinoma usually has a tendency to extend along the surface of the bone, usually the overlying soft tissue involvement is clinically apparent, pathological fractures are rare, and complete dissolution of the continuity of the mandibular bone takes longer in case of carcinoma.
- *Metastatic carcinoma*: There will be history of a primary lesion.
- *Peripheral fibroma with calcification*: This is a benign and slow growth.
- *Ossifying subperiosteal hematoma*: Patient will history of recent trauma.
- *Chondrosarcoma*: This occurs in the older age group and the maxilla is more often involved.
- *Ossifying fibroma*: This is better demarcated and has a more uniform internal structure.
- *Fibrous dysplasia*: These lesions are well-demarcated and have a more uniform appearance as compared to lesions of osteosarcoma.
- *Osteomyelitis*: Here there are signs of infection.
- *Ewing's sarcoma*: It is difficult to distinguish radiographically from osteosarcoma, a histopathological investigation is conclusive.
- *Solitary plasmacytoma*.

Management

Radical resection with chemo and radiation therapy.

Ewing's Sarcoma (Endothelial Myeloma, Round Cell Sarcoma)

Definition

This is of intermediate histogenesis. It is relatively rare in the jaws and considered a tumor of the long bones. Lesions arise in the medullary portion of the bone and spread to the endosteal and periosteal surface.

Clinical Features

- It is more common in males in the second decade of life. Though this neoplasm rarely occurs in the jaws, it is more frequent in the posterior area of the jaws; the mandible is more affected than the maxilla. The lesions develop within the marrow spaces and then extend to involve overlying cortical plates.
- It is a rapidly growing highly invasive tumor with early, rapid and widespread metastases. It may have multicenteric lesions.
- Other signs and symptoms in descending frequency include: swelling, pain, loosening of teeth, paresthesia, exophthalmus, ptosis, epistaxis, ulceration, shifted teeth, trismus, sinusitis and cervical lymphadenopathy.
- The patient may also have febrile attacks, leukocytosis and facial neuralgia.

Radiographic Features

- It is seen as a poorly demarcated, noncorticated radiolucency, with ragged borders. The lesions are usually solitary and may be round or ovoid, but generally they do not have a typical shape.
- This is a destructive lesion with little induction of bone formation.
- It may stimulate the periosteum to produce new bone, leading to the appearance of Codman's triangle or hair-on-end appearance like speculation. Sometimes laminar periosteal new bone formation (onion skin appearance) has been reported.
- It may cause pathological fractures.
- Adjacent normal structures such as the inferior alveolar canal, inferior border of the mandible, the alveolar cortical plates may be effaced.
- If the lesion abuts teeth of tooth follicles, the cortices of the same are destroyed. It does not usually cause root resorption, but there is destruction of the lamina dura and the supporting bone.

Differential Diagnosis

- *Osteomyelitis*: There is presence of sequestra within the lesions. This being an inflammatory lesion, it may contain signs of reactive bone formation, resulting in some sclerosis internally or at the periphery, and differs in the associated periosteal bone formation.
- *Eosinophillic granuloma*: This is associated with laminar periosteal reaction, which is quite rare in Ewing's sarcoma.
- *Osteosarcoma, osteochondroma, fibrosarcoma*: These are difficult to distinguish radiographically from Ewing's sarcoma, a histopathological investigation is conclusive.

Management

This has poor prognosis. Surgery, radiotherapy and chemotherapy may be used alone or in combination.

Neurofibrosarcoma (Malignant Schwannoma)

Definition

It arises from nerve tissue (nerve sheath cells). It is rare in the oral cavity. Patients suffering from neurofibromatosis may undergo sarcomatous transformation in some cases, usually deep seated lesions.

Clinical Features

- It is common on the lips, gingival, palate and buccal mucosa. The central tumor affects the mandible more than the maxilla.
- The patients usually presents with the presence of a mass, which may be accompanied with pain or paresthesia.

Radiographic Features

- It appears as a diffuse radiolucency, with infiltrating borders.
- If the tumor originates in the inferior alveolar nerve, there may be dilatation of the mandibular canal.

Management

Surgery and radiation.

MALIGNANT LYMPHOMA

These are a group of lymphoproliferative disorders arising from the lymph nodes and from lymphoid components of various organs. It may be defined as a neoplastic proliferative process of the lymphopoietic portion of reticuloendothelial system that involves cells of either the lymphocytic or histiocytic series, in varying degrees of differentiation and occurs in an essentially homogeneous population of a single cell type.

There are of two types:
1. Hodgkin's lymphoma.
2. Non-Hodgkin's lymphoma.

Hodgkin's Lymphoma

Definition

This was first described by Thomas Hodgkin in 1832. It is characterized by painless enlargement of lymphoid tissue through out the body. The etiology has been presumably attributed to viruses (herpes and oncorna) or idiopathic. It has been further grouped and staged as under:

- Clinical staging (ANN Arbor staging):
  - *Stage I*: Involvement of single lymph node region or extra lymphatic sites.
  - *Stage II*: Involvement of two or more lymph node regions or an extra lymphatic site and lymph node region of the same side of diaphragm.
  - *Stage III*: Involvement of lymph node region on both sides or without extra lymphatic involvement or involvement of spleen or both.
  - *Stage IV*: Diffuse involvement of one or more extra lymphatic tissues (e.g. liver of bone marrow).

    Such stages are further divided into A and B categories depending on systemic symptoms.
- Histological types:
  - Lymphocyte predominant
  - Mixed cellularity
  - Nodular sclerosis
  - Lymphocyte depletion.

Clinical Features

- It does not have a sex predilection, and has a bimodal age incidence, in young adults and fifth to sixth decade of life.
- It starts with the enlargement of any group of superficial nodes; cervical lymph nodes are usually the first to be involved. They are usually painless, discrete and rubbery, with the overlying skin being freely mobile.
- There is characteristic Pel Ebstein fever; a cyclic spiking of high fever and generalized severe pruritus of unknown etiology (it may be due to sphenomegaly which is seen in the later stages).
- Generalized weakness, loss of weight, cough, anorexia, pressure of enlarged lymph nodes on adjacent structures may cause; dyspnea, dysphagia, venous obstruction, jaundice and paraplegia, pain in back and abdomen due to pressure of enlarged nodes or involvement of the vertebrae.
- Histologically it is characterized by the presence of Reed-Sternberg cells.

Radiographic Features

- Malignant lymphoma arising in the oral cavity spreads to the bone causing irregular bone loss. There are multiple radiolucent areas, with diffuse ill-defined borders, which are separated by normal appearing bone, which later confluence.
- An osteoblastic type of, well-defined lesion is rarely seen in the jaws, but it is seen in the vertebrae and pelvis.

Differential Diagnosis

Non-Hodgkin's lymphoma: There is no presence of Reed-Sternberg cells.

Management

Radiotherapy and/or chemotherapy.

Non-Hodgkin's Lymphoma (Malignant Lymphoma, Lymphosarcoma)

Definition

This is a neoplastic proliferation of the B-lymphocytes. The term Non-Hodgkin's lymphoma describes a family of heterogeneous tumors of varying type and severity. The etiology may be viral (herpes) or immunological. The classification of this disease is difficult.

The tumors are classified on their histological appearance as:
- Nodular
- Diffuse
Or
- Low grade
- Intermediate grade
- High grade.

Clinical Features

- It affects persons of all age groups from infants to elderly, more common in the middle age group.
- Most non-Hodgkin's lymphoma of the head and neck occur in the lymph nodes. Those that are extranodal are likely to affect the maxillary sinus, posterior mandible, palate and tonsillar area.
- There may be palpable painless lymph node enlargements of mediastinal and abdominal region, with cervical, axillary and inguinal lymph nodes being most often the first group to be affected.
- Patients may feel unwell; have night sweats, pruritus and weight loss, abdominal pain, nausea, diarrhea.
- Sensorineural deficits may accompany isolated lesions of the jaws.
- Pressure effect of the lymphoma may cause dysphagia, breathlessness, vomiting, intestinal obstruction, ascites or paraplegia.
- Hepatosplenomegaly may be present.
- Lesions present for sometime may cause pain and ulceration.
- The teeth involved in a lymphoma may become mobile as the supporting bone is lost.
- In the oral cavity, it usually arises from the tonsils.
- The palatal lesions are slow growing, bluish soft tissues masses which may be clinically mistaken for salivary gland tumors. The swelling may ulcerate, discolor and progressively cause necrotic proliferation of the palate.
- There may be pain and neuralgia associated with the 2nd and 3rd division of the trigeminal nerve and paresthesia of the mental nerve has been reported.
- Blood picture shows reduced WBC and RBC counts, reduced hemoglobin levels, reticulocytosis, increased lymphocytes and thrombocytes. High urate levels may be seen which may precipitate renal failure.

Radiographic Features

- They appear radiolucent round or multiloculated, with lack of defining outer cortex. The borders are ill-defined and invasive. There is no reactive bone formation. Occasionally patchy radiopacity may be seen.
- It usually takes the shape and form of the host bone. But if untreated it can cause destruction of the overlying cortex.
- They may occur as multiple areas of destruction, with finger like extensions in the buccal or lingual direction.
- Lesions in the maxillary sinus or nasopharynx may have a smooth periphery. Sometimes the antral walls may be effaced and a soft tissue mass may be visible radiographically, either internally within the sinus or external to the maxillary sinus. More clearly seen on CT.
- Lesions involving the mandible destroy the cortex of the inferior dental canal.
- The tumor has the propensity to grow in the periodontal ligament space of mature teeth. The cortex and crypts of developing teeth may be lost when the lymphoma is located in the developing papilla, and the involved teeth may be displaced in an occlusal direction and exfoliated.
- Periosteal reaction is not common, but may take the form or laminated or spiculated bone formation.

Additional Imaging

MRI: This distinctly shows how the tumor has a habit of growing along soft tissue spaces (fat layers) and along the surface of the bone.

Differential Diagnosis

- *Multiple myeloma*: Bence Jones proteins are present in urine, borders of the lesions are usually well-defined.
- *Metastatic carcinoma*: There will be history of a primary tumor.
- *Ewing's sarcoma*: It occurs in a younger age group.
- *Langerhan's histiocytosis*: A younger age group (this also displaces teeth in an occlusal direction).
- *Leukemia*: This also displaces teeth in an occlusal direction.
- *Osteosarcoma (osteolytic)*: It may be differentiated by the clinical findings.
- *Central squamous cell carcinoma.*
- *Apical rarefying osteitis*: It is well-defined radiolucency, with no destruction of the adjacent bone.

Management

Chemotherapy and/or radiotherapy with transplantation, if necessary.

Primary Reticular Cell Sarcoma (Primary Lymphoma of Bone)

Clinical Features

- More common in males and young adults. Mostly seen in the long bones (femur, tibia, and humerous). More associated with the mandible than the maxilla.
- It is usually asymptomatic except in the presence of localized swelling of the involved bone. Persistent pain and regional lymphadenopathy is usually present.
- The oral mucosa over the lesion is never ulcerated but may appear diffusely inflamed.
- The involved teeth are very mobile.
- When the lesion involves the maxilla, there may be evidence of expansion of the bone as well as symptoms of nasal obstruction due to superior growth of the tumor into the floor of the nasal cavity.

Radiographic Features

It is seen as a diffuse radiolucency involving the alveolar bone, the margins are infiltrative. There may be periosteal bone reaction, and new bone may be laid down in a linear or radiating spicule type.

Management

Surgical excision with radiotherapy.

Burkitt's Lymphoma (African Jaw Lymphoma)

Definition

This is a high grade B-cell lymphoma that differs from other B-cell lymphomas with respect to its histological appearance and clinical behavior.

There are two separate form of this disease:
1. The endemic African Burkitt's lymphoma.
2. The nonendemic American.

Clinical Features

- The endemic African Burkitt's lymphoma:
  - This affects young children, with no sex predilection.
  - Secondarily involves the extra nodal tissue.
  - This is a rapidly growing tumor mass of the jaws; it may involve one or both the jaws, especially the posterior part, and destroys and distends the alveolar bone with loosening of the teeth. It causes facial deformities, involves the maxillary, ethmoidal and sphenoidal sinuses, blocks the nasal passage, displaces orbital contents, and erodes through the skin.
  - There is derangement of the arch and occlusion.
  - Gingival and mucosa adjacent to the affected teeth become swollen, ulcerated and necrotic, as the tumor mass increases the teeth are pushed out of their sockets.
  - There may be a large quantity of mass protruding into the mouth, on the surface of which may be seen rootless, developing permanent teeth.
  - Once the tumor perforates the bone, and breaks through the periosteum it spreads rapidly to the soft tissues of the oral cavity and face and obliterates the same. The skin becomes tense and shiny.
  - The visceral organ involvement is less frequent.
  - Maxillary and mandibular nerves are not involved. But paresthesia of the inferior alveolar nerve and other sensory facial nerves may occur.
  - Antibody titer is negative.
- The nonendemic American:
  - This affects adolescents and young adults with a predilection for males
  - It involves the lymph nodes, lymphoid tissue and bone marrow
  - It is uncommon in the jaws, but usually involves visceral organs (abdominal viscera, testes)
  - Antibody titer is positive.

Radiographic Features

- It may be seen as multiple, ill-defined, noncorticated radiolucencies, which later coalesce into larger, ill-defined radiolucencies with an expansile periphery. They have no specific shape but as it expands rapidly it has been likened to a balloon.
- The expansion breaches its outer cortical limits, causing balloon-like expansion and thinning of adjacent structures and production of soft tissue tumor mass next to the osseous lesion.
- Lesions that abut on the maxillary sinus or the orbital contents may show a smooth surface tissue mass radiologically. Eventually the cortical boundaries of the maxillary sinus, nasal floor, orbital walls, inferior border of the mandible and inferior alveolar canal are destroyed. The orbital contents are displaced.
- Tumor cells within the crypt displace the developing tooth bud to one side of its crypt. If the tumor is located apical, the displacement may be seen as if the tooth is erupting. Root development ceases as soon as the tumor involves the developing dental structures.
- Erupted teeth in the area of the tumor are grossly displaced, and the lamina dura is destroyed.

Differential Diagnosis

- *Non-Hodgkin's lymphoma*: It occurs in the older age group.
- *Cherubism*: The lesion has more internal structure, does not breach the bony borders, is bilateral and grows much more slowly.

- *Osteosarcoma (osteolytic):* It is indistinguishable clinically, but on the radiographic osteoblastic activity is visible.
- *Metastatic neuroblastoma.*
- *Ewings tumor.*

Management

Chemotherapy.

Leukemia (Acute Myelogenous Leukemia, Acute Lymphoblastic Leukemia, Chronic Myelogenous Leukemia, Chronic Lymphocytic Leukemia, Leucosis)

Definition

It is a malignant tumor of the hematopoietic stem cells. The malignant cells displace the normal bone marrow constituents and spill out into the peripheral blood, with resultant anemia, granulocytopenia and thrombocytopenia. Most cases of leukemia are associated with nonrandom chromosomal abnormalities, viral infections, exposure to—radiations, chemical agents and/or anticancer drugs, immunodeficiency syndromes (Wiskott-Aldrich syndrome). It is a progressive fatal condition causing death from hemorrhage and infection. They may be divided into different types based on:

- *Cell types:*
  - *Stem or blast cell leukemia:* Cells are too immature to be classified to the cell type.
  - *Sub leukemia:* When the total WBC count is normal and leukemic cells are seen in the peripheral blood.
  - *Aleukemia:* When no abnormal leukocytes are found in the peripheral blood.
  - *Leukemoid reaction:* When the peripheral blood picture is nonleukemic, but patient give clinical signs of leukemia. The absolute neutrophil count remains above 30,000/mm^3.

Classification

- *Acute:*
  - Acute lymphoblastic leukemia:
    - L_1: Acute lymphoblastic (principally pediatric), in this small cells predominate and nuclei are generally round.
    - L_2: Acute lymphoblastic (principally adults), in this cells are heterogenous in size and sharp in features, nuclei often show cleft.
    - L_3: Burkitt's, here there is a homogeneous population of large cells. Nuclei are round to oval with prominent nucleoli.
  - Acute nonlymphoblastic or myeloid leukemia:
    - M_1: Myeloblastic (without maturation), myeloblasts predominate with distant nucleoli, few granules are present.

- M_2: Myeloblastic (with maturation), myeloblasts and promyelocytes predominate with distant nucleoli, Auer rods are seen.
- M_3: Promyelocytic, hypergranular promyelocytes often with Auer rods are seen.
- M_4: Myelomocytic, myelocytic and monocytic differentiation is evident, myeloid elements resemble peripheral monocytosis.
- M_5: Monocytic, promonocytes or undifferentiated blast.
- M_6: Erythroleukemia, bizarre, multinucleated, megaloblastoid erythroblasts predominate.
- M_7: Megakaryocytic, pleomorphic undifferentiated blast cells with anti-platelet antibodies, myelofibrosis is present.
- *Chronic:*
  - Chronic lymphatic leukemia (lymphogeneous, lymphocytic) involving lymphocytes series.
  - Chronic myeloid leukemia (myelogeneous, myelocytic) leukemia involving granulocyte series.

Clinical Features

- *Acute leukemia:*
  - More common in young and adult males.
  - The onset is usually abrupt, with pyrexia and enlargement of the spleen. The patient may complain of weakness, fever, headache, vomiting, generalized swelling of the lymph nodes, petechiae or hemorrhage in the skin and mucous membrane. Bone pain and tenderness, nerve palsies, dyspnea, epitaxis, melena.
  - There is recurrent infection of the lungs, urinary tract, skin, mouth, rectum and upper respiratory tract.
  - Localized tumors consisting of leukemic cells called chloroma, whose surface turns green when exposed to light (due to presence of myeloperoxidage) are seen.
  - The oral cavity shows pallor, ulceration with necrosis, petechiae, acchymosis and bleeding of the oral mucosa. Gingival appears boggy, hypertrophic (due to leukemic cell infiltration), with cyanotic discoloration. There may be paresthesia of the lower lip and chin with toothache due to leukemic cell infilteration of the dental pulp. The submental, cervical and pre- and post auricular lymph nodes may be enlarged and tender.
  - There may be associated normochromic anemia, thrombocytopenia and decrease in the normal functioning of the neutrophils.
- *Chronic leukemia:*
  - This usually occurs in the older age group.
  - There may be no presenting signs or complains and be discovered during routine examination, when splenomegaly or an elevated count is noted.
  - There may be complain of attacks of acute left upper abdominal pain, weakness, fatigue and dyspnea on

exertion (due to anemia), petechiae, ecchymosis and hemorrhage on the skin and mucous membrane (due to thrombocytopenia).

- Oral findings are—hypertrophy of the gingival, with ulceration, necrosis and dark gangrenous degeneration (a dark brown exudates and foul fetor oris are present). The tongue is frequently swollen. There is rapid loosening of the teeth due to necrosis of the periodontal ligament and sometimes destruction of the alveolar bone. There is regional lymphadenopathy.
- There is presence of normocytic and normochromic anemia. There is presence of large leukemic cells and differentiated WBCs in the bone marrow, peripheral blood and other tissues.

Radiographic Features

- Leukemia affects the entire body, because it is a malignancy of bone marrow, which discharges malignant cells into the circulating blood. Its manifestations in the jaws are seen more in the areas of developing teeth. It may be sometimes localized around the periapical region of a tooth, giving the appearance of rarefying osteitis.
- The lesions are seen as patchy areas of radiolucency which may later coalesce to form generalized areas of ill-defined radiolucency of the bone, the lesions are usually bilaterally present.
- Occasionally, foci of leukemic cells may be present as a mass (chloroma), which may behave like a localized malignant tumor. These are rare in the jaws.
- The teeth may appear to stand out conspicuously from their surrounding, osteopenic bone.
- Leukemia does not cause expansion of the bone, but a single layer of periosteal new bone may be seen in association with the disease.
- The developing teeth in their crypts and teeth undergoing eruption may be displaced in the occlusal direction or into the oral cavity before root development resulting in the premature loss of teeth, or they may be merely displace from their normal position. The lamina dura and cortical outlines of the follicles may be effaced, and if the lesion involves the periodontal structures, the crestal bone may also be lost.

Additional Imaging

Magnetic resonance imaging (MRI).

Differential Diagnosis

- *Metabolic disorders*: These cause generalized rarefaction of the bone. They may be differentiated on the basis of the blood picture.
- *Lymphoma, neuroblastoma*: The clinical presentation is different and it may be differentiated on the basis of the blood picture.

- *Rarefying osteitis*: Careful clinical and radiological examination will show no appearent cause for the same in case of leukemia.

Management

Leukemia is primarily treated with a combination of chemotherapy with or without allogenic or autologous bone marrow transplantation.

Multiple Myeloma (Myeloma, Plasma Cell Myeloma, Plasmacytoma, Myelomatosis)

Definition

It is a malignant neoplasm of plasma cells of the bone marrow with widespread involvement of the skeletal system, including the skull and jaws. It is a fatal systemic malignancy. Single lesions are called plasmacytoma, and multiple lesions are called multiple myeloma.

Clinical Features

- It is more common in men between the ages of 35 and 70 years. It involves the skull, clavicle, vertebrae, ribs, pelvis, femur and the jaws. The mandible is more commonly involved than the maxilla, particularly the ramus, angle and posterior body because of the greater marrow contents. Lesions have also been reported in the posterior aspect of the maxilla and the temperomandibular joints.
- The patient will complain of—fatigue, weight loss, fever, bone pain (lower back pain) and anemia. Hypercalcemia is commonly found in these patients.
- In the oral cavity, the patient may complain of pain, swelling and numbness of the jaw.
- Intraoral swelling is usually tender and may elicitate egg shell crackling, it tends to be ulcerated and bluish red, similar to peripheral giant cell granuloma. Sometimes the swelling may erode the buccal plate and produce a rubbery expansion of the jaw.
- Intraoral hemorrhage and susceptibility to infection may also be present. Excessive hemorrhage may cause thrombocytopenia, secondary to increased proliferation of plasma the plasma cells in marrow.
- Oral amyloidosis is a complication of this disease. The tongue, lips, cheeks and occasionally the gingiva may be enlarged with small garnet colored enlargements.
- Bone marrow examination will show increased number of plasma cells. There is associated anemia but the WBC and platelet count is normal. There is increased ESR, serum monoclonal immunoglobulin with reversal of the albumin globulin ratio and increased serum protein to a level of 8–16 gm% (hyperproteinemia due to increase in globulins). Bence jones proteins are present in the urine.

Radiographic Features

- The lesions are usually bilateral, well-defined but not corticated (no sign of bone reaction) radiolucencies, with an oval or a cystic shape, which are described as punched out. Sometimes it may appear ragged and even infiltrative.
- As the disease progresses aggressive areas of destruction may confluence giving the appearance of multilocularity.
- If the lesion is present in the periapical periodontal space, it may have a border similar to that seen in an inflammatory or infectious periapical disease. The lamina dura and follicle of impacted teeth loose its cortication similar to that seen in hyperparathyroidism. The teeth may appear to be too opaque and may stand out conspicuously from their osteopenic background.
- Soft tissue lesions in the jaws and nasopharynx appear as smooth-bordered soft tissues masses, due to underlying bone destruction.
- The inferior alveolar canal looses its cortical boundary. The mandibular lesions may cause thinning of the lower border of the mandible or endosteal scalloping.
- The lesion effaces any cortical boundary it encounters; periosteal reaction is uncommon, but is present appears as a single radiopaque line or more rarely a sunray appearance.

Differential Diagnosis

- *Metastatic carcinoma*: This is comparitinely less common. There is absence of definitive serum findings, history of treatment of earlier tumor.
- *Histiocytosis-X*: Incidence is more in children. The lesions have ragged and vague margins.
- *Cherubism*: This has multiple lesions scattered through out the jaws, commonly seen in the first or second decades of life. Radiolucent lesions may be multilocular or unilocular, elliptical without well circumscribed or hyperostotic borders.
- *Advanced osteomyelitis*: Shows the presence of a known cause. Inflammatory and infectious lesions cause sclerosis in adjacent bone.
- *Simple bone cyst*: It may be bilateral, but it is usually corticated and characteristically interdigitate between the roots of teeth of much younger population.
- *Hyperparathyroidism*: Causes generalized radiolucencies of the jaws but is differentiated on abnormal blood chemistry. Browns tumors appears very similar to lesions of multiple myeloma.
- *Thalessemia, Gaucher's disease or oxalosis (metabolic diseases)*: Show similar changes on the dental radiographs, but may be ruled out on the basis of medical history.

Management

Chemotherapy with or without autologous or allogenic bone marrow transplantation. Radiation therapy may be used when palliation is required.

Plasmacytoma (Plasma Cell Myeloma)

Definition

In the extramedullary location without bony involvement it may occur in the nasopharynx, nasal cavity, paranasal sinuses and rarely in the oral cavity.

Clinical Features

Males are more commonly affected in the fifth decade of life.

It is found in the nares, tonsils, palate, tongue, gingival and the floor of the mouth. Besides it may also be found in pleura, mediastinum, thyroid, ovary, intestine, kidney and skin.

It presents as a painful swelling, with pathological fractures and regional metastases occurring sometimes.

Bence jones proteins are found in the urine. Russell bodies may also be found. (Both are findings in multiple myeloma).

There is also hyperglobulinemia and anemia.

Radiographic Features

It occurs in two forms:
1. *Purely destructive, suggestive of metastatic carcinoma*:
   - There is no new bone formation at the margins or under the periosteum, it shows infiltrative margins.
   - In flat bones, it extends along the bone and produces a sausage shaped lesion with undulating margins.
2. *Expansile lesion, suggestive of a giant cell tumor*:
   - The area of bone destruction is well demarcated and sometimes corticated.
   - If expansion takes place, the subperiosteal new bone completely covers the tumor.
   - In the substance of the lesion the trabeculae may vary in number and thickness (from thin and delicate to thick and coarse).

Management

Surgery.

Central Mucoepidermoid Carcinoma (Mucoepidermoid Carcinoma) (Figs 23.23A and B)

Definition

It is an epithelial tumor originated in bone and is believed to be derived from salivary gland. It is likely to be derived from pluripotential odontogenic epithelium or from a cyst lining.

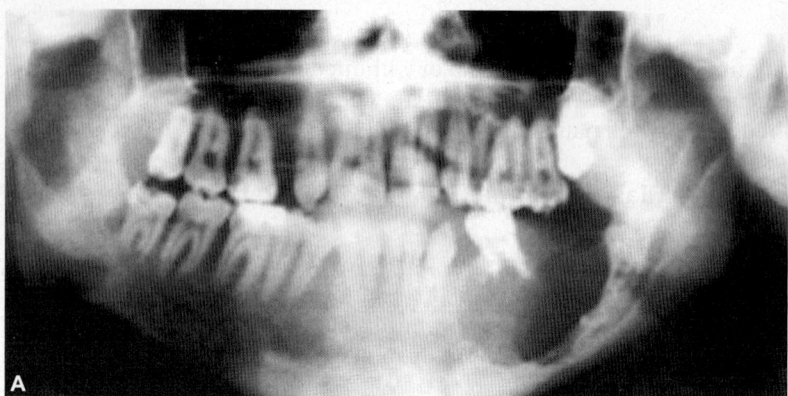 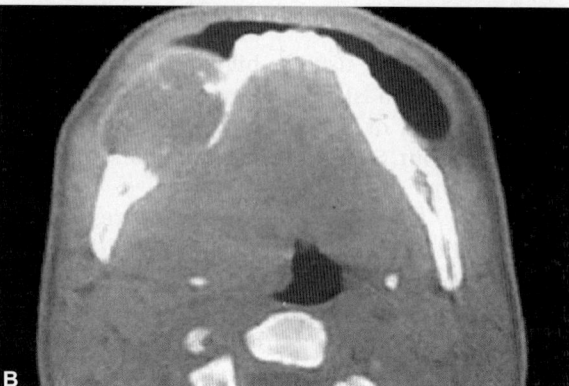

Figures 23.23A and B   (A) Mucoepidermoid tumor, having a radiographic appearance of a benign lesion—soap bubble like radiolucency, which may be mistaken for an ameloblastoma or a central giant cell granuloma; (B) Mucoepidermoid tumor of the same patient as seen in an axial CT with bone window. In this view it is clear that the cavity is filled with soft tissue

Clinical Features

- It is more common in females, in the premolar-molar region of the mandible, and is rarely seen in the anterior region. It commonly occurs above the mandibular canal.
- It presents as a painless swelling, which may have been present for several years, and caused facial asymmetry. Tenderness, paresthesia, involvement of regional lymph nodes and involved teeth feel as if they have moved or a denture may no longer fit.

Radiographic Features

- Its appearance is very similar to a benign lesion.
- It may appear as a unilocular or a multilocular expansile mass, with compartments created by thick or thin internal cortical septae, giving a honey comb or soap bubble appearance. The borders are well corticated and often crenated or undulating in nature.
- It causes expansion of adjacent bony walls, the buccal and lingual cortical plates, inferior border of the mandible; alveolar crests remain intact but may be thinned and grossly displaced.
- The mandibular canal may be depressed or pushed laterally or medially.
- Teeth are largely unaffected, except that adjacent lamina dura is lost.

Differential Diagnosis

- *Ameloblastoma*: Diagnosis to be confirmed on histopathological investigation.
- *Odontogenic myxoma*: There will be history of a missing tooth.
- *Central giant cell granuloma*: This lesion frequently crosses the midline.

Management

Surgical en bloc resection.

BIBLIOGRAPHY

1. Casiglia J. Woo SB. A comprehensive review of oral cancer. Gen Dent. 2001;49:72.
2. Dinkar A, Satoskar S. Diagnostic aids in early oral cancer detection—A review. JIAOMR. 2006;18:02,82-89.
3. Divya MR, Nagesh KS, Iyengar AR, et al. Recent advances in the treatment of oral cancer—an overview. JIAOMR. 2006;18(2);98-102.
4. Goaz PW, White SC. Principles and interpretation. In: Oral Radiology, 3rd edition. St Louis: Mosby Year Book, 1994.
5. Miles DA, Van Dis MJ, Jensen CW, et al. Interpretation normal versus abnormal and common radiographic presentations of lesions. In: Radiographic and Imaging for Dental Auxillaries, 3rd edition. Philadelphia: WD Saunders; 1999.pp.231-80.
6. Noyek AM, et al. The radiologic diagnosis of malignant tumors of the paranasal sinuses and related structures. J Otolaryngol. 1977;6:399.
7. Sciubba JJ. Computer-assisted analysis of the oral brush biopsy, improving detection of precancerous and cancerous oral lesions. J Am Dent Ass. 1999;130:1445-56.
8. Shafer WG, et al. A textbook of oral pathology, Philadelphia: WB Saunders; 1983.
9. Wood NK, Goaz PW. Differential diagnosis of oral lesions 4th edition. CV Mosby: St Louis; 1991.
10. Wood RE. Handbook of signs in dental and maxillofacial radiology. Warthog Publications, Toronto; 1988.
11. Worth HM. Principles and practice of oral radiographic interpretation. Year Book Medical Publishers, Chicago; 1963.

Fibrosseous lesions refer to those lesions wherein the bone is replaced by connective tissue fibers. The spongy bone is replaced by peculiar fibrous tissue, which may or may not show the presence of osteoid metaplasia. It results from the abnormality of development of bone forming mesenchyme. Varying amount of mineralized substances may be present.

It may be defined as "lesions in which there is replacement of normal bone by a tissue composed of the collagen fibers and fibroblasts that contain varying amounts of mineralized substance which may be bony or cementum like in appearance" (This definition does not include peripheral (extraosseous) lesions.

Bone dysplasias constitute a group of conditions in which normal bone is replaced with fibrous tissue containing abnormal bone or cementum.

FIBROSSEOUS DISEASES OF THE JAWS (TABLES 24.1 TO 24.3)

Fibrous Dysplasia

Fibrocystic disease, osteitis fibrosa localisata, focal osteitis fibrosa, fibrosteodystrophy, Jaffé-lichtenstein (**Figs 24.1 to 24.12**).

Definition

This is a fibrosseous condition involving one or more bones of the cranial and extra cranial skeleton, consisting of nonencapsulated lesions which have undergone localized change in normal bone metabolism and shows replacement of the normal cancellous bone by cellular fibrous tissues containing islands of metastatic bone. It may be attributed to developmental aberrations or endocrinal disturbances. It has been classified into:

Clinical Types

- *Monostotic fibrous dysplasia*: Only one bone is involved.
- *Polyostotic fibrous dysplasia*: More than one bone is involved:
  - *Jaffe type*: Fibrous dysplasia involving variable number of bones, accompanied by pigmented lesions of the skin or *café au lait spots*.

Table 24.1 Classification of the jaws

- Developmental
  - Solitary bone cyst
  - Cherubism
  - Choristomas
  - Gigantiform cementoma
- Reactive/Reparative
  - Central (intraosseous)
    - Traumatic periostitis
    - Garre's osteomyelitis
    - Sclerosing osteomyelitis
      - i. Focal
      - ii. Diffuse
  - Osseous keloid
  - Central giant cell granuloma
  - Periapical cemental dysplasia
  - Aneurysmal bone cyst
  - Peripheral (extraosseous)
    - Peripheral giant cell granuloma
    - Myositis ossificans
- Neoplasm
  - Compact and cancellous osteomas
  - Osteoid osteoma
  - Osteoblastoma
  - Benign cementoblastoma
  - Periodontoma (ossifying fibroma)
  - Aggressive periodontoma (Juvenile ossifying fibroma)
- Endocrinal/Metabolic
  - Brown's tumor of hyperparathyroidism
- Unknown etiology
  - Fibrous dysplasia (monostotic and polyostotic)
  - Paget's disease

- *McCune-Albright's syndrome*: This is a severe form of fibrous dysplasia involving nearly all the bones in the body, accompanied by pigmented lesions of the skin plus endocrinal disturbance of various types.
- *A craniofacial form*: Here the lesions are confined to the bones of the craniofacial complex.
- *Monomelic*: Where there is involvement of only one extremity. This is very rare.

Table 24.2 Classification of fibrosseous diseases of the jaws

- Fibrosseous lesions of the medullary bone origin
  - Fibrous dysplasia
  - Fibrosteoma
  - Cherubism
  - Juvenile ossifying fibroma
  - Giant cell tumor
  - Aneurysmal bone cyst
  - Jaw lesions in hyperparathyroidism
  - Paget's disease.
- Fibrosseous lesions of periodontal origin
  - Periapical cemental dysplasia
  - Florid osseous dysplasia
  - Cementossifying fibroma
  - Cementifying fibroma
  - Ossifying fibroma.

Table 24.3 Waldron's classification (oral and maxillofacial surgery CNA Vol 9, No. 4, Nov 1997) of fibrosseous disease of the jaws

- Fibrous dysplasia
- Reactive (dysplastic) lesions arising in the toothbearing areas—these are predominantly periodontal in origin.
  - Nonhereditary
    - Periapical cementosseous dysplasia
    - Focal cementosseous dysplasia
    - Florid cementosseous dysplasia
  - Hereditary
    - Familial gigantiform cementoma
- Fibrosseous neoplasm
  - Cementifying fibroma
  - Ossifying fibroma
  - Cementossifying fibroma
  - Juvenile ossifying fibroma
- Cherubism

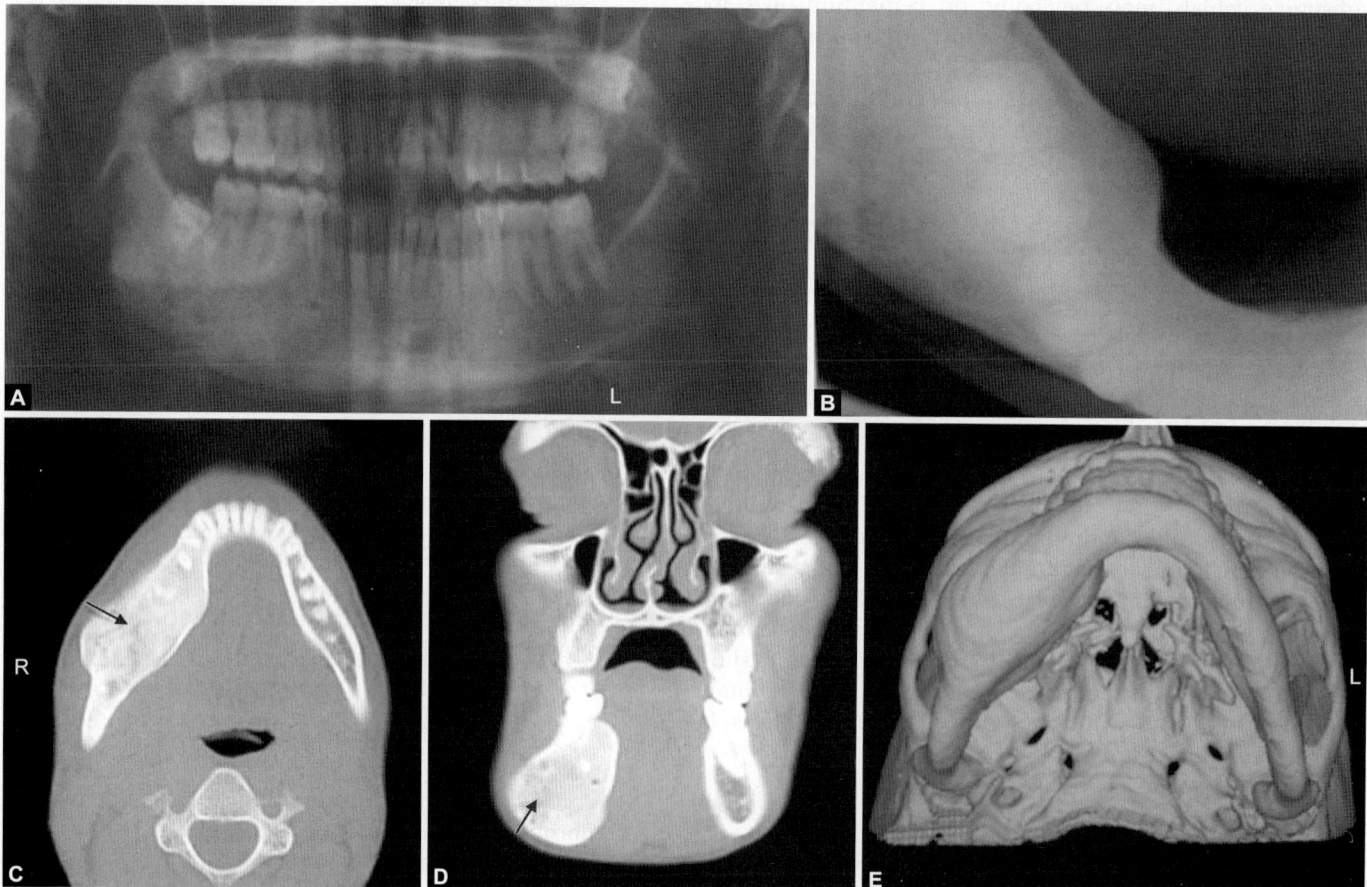

Figures 24.1A to E Fibrous dysplasia: (A) Panoramic radiograph revealed a ground glass appearance of trabeculae on right side of mandible, extending anteroposteriorly from 42–48 region with ill-defined diffuse margins, loss of corticated inferior border and superoinferior expansion of the body of mandible in 42–48 region. Displaced roots of 45 and 46; (B) Mandibular occlusal topical view: revealed marked expansion of buccal and lingual cortical plates in 43–48 region with ground glass appearance. CT Scan: (C) Axial view; (D) Coronal view; (E) 3D view revealed a 5 × 3 cm well-defined expansile lesion with ground glass appearance was seen involving right half of boby and ramus of mandible. Few calcified densities were seen within it. No abnormal soft tissue was noted

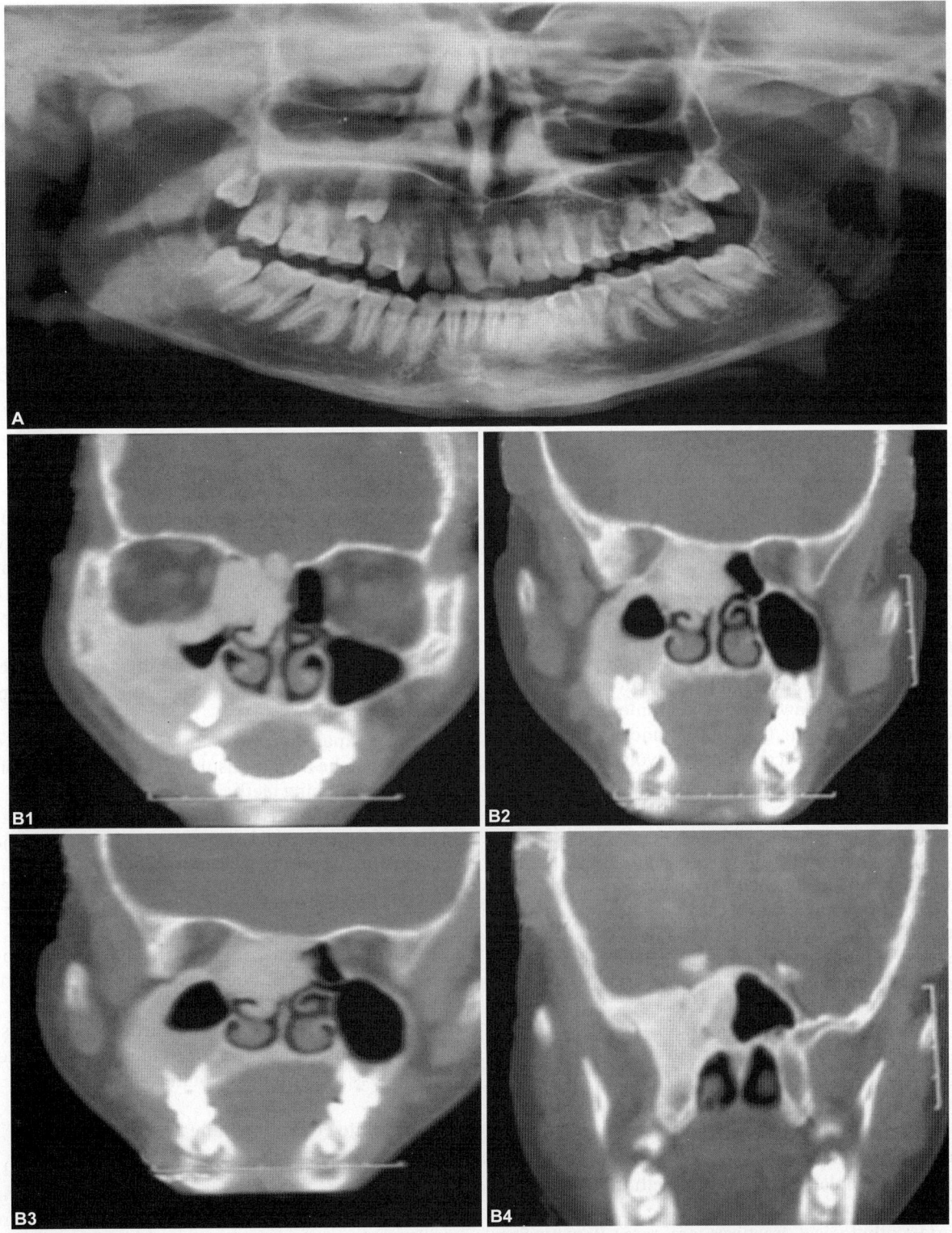

Figures 24.2A and B Fibrous dysplasia: (A) Panoramic view shows altered trabecular pattern with ground glass appearance impacted 15 extending throughout the height of the maxillary bone from region of 13 to 18 and involving the right maxillary sinus. Thinning of cortex noticed. No signs of erosion noticed. Unilateral haziness of maxillary sinus was seen. CT scan: (B1 to B4) Coronal sections shows diffuse expansion and ground glass attenuation noted involving the right maxillary alveolar processes, zygomatic bone, nasal process of maxilla, hard palate, right maxillary sinus, sphenoidal and ethmoidal sinus, greater and lesser wing of sphenoid

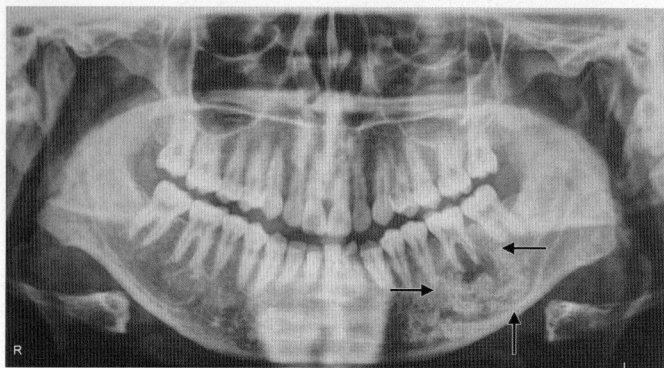

Figure 24.3 Fibrous dysplasia: Panoramic radiograph shows well defined mixed radiolucent—radiopaque lesion extending apically from the middle third of mandibular left 1st molar displacing the inferior alveolar canal to the lower border of mandible

- *Subclinical fibrous dysplasia*: Sometimes an unsuspected lesion of fibrous dysplasia may be discovered on routine radiographic examination, without any clinical evidence of the suspected disease, these may be termed as subclinical fibrous dysplasia.

Clinical Features

Monostotic

- This accounts for 70% of all cases, involves only one bone and most often involves the jaws. The most common sites in order of affection are ribs, femur, tibia, maxilla and mandible.
- The maxilla is more commonly involved than the mandible, more common in the premolar-molar region.
- This occurs in the older age group, there is no sex predilection.
- The lesions become static after skeletal growth stops, but these may become active in pregnant females or with the use of oral contraceptives.
- It is often discovered as an incidental radiographic finding.
- Patient may complain of a unilateral facial swelling or an enlarging deformity of the alveolar process, involving the buccal and labial cortical plates.
- In the mandible it causes protuberant excrescence of the inferior border of the mandible.
- The teeth involved are either malaligned, tipped or displaced. Presence of supernumerary teeth has been reported in monostotic type of fibrous dysplasia, which is commonly found in the mid line of the maxilla and mandibular premolar region. These teeth may affect the eruption of the normal teeth.
- Pain and pathological fractures are rare. If extensive craniofacial lesions have impinged on nerve foramina, neurologic symptoms such as anosmia (loss of sense of smell), deafness or blindness may develop.

Polyostotic (Jaffe's Type)

- This involves multiple bones, accompanied by pigmented lesions of the skin or *café au lait spots*.
- This is usually found in children less than 10 years of age.
- The lesion usually become static when skeletal growth stops, but proliferation may continue in some cases.
- There is expansion and deformity of the jaws, the eruption pattern of the teeth is disturbed because of loss of support of the developing teeth.
- There is asymmetry of the facial bones, with ballooning of the jaws which results in gross enlargement and deformity.
- The patient may complain of pain, in extensive cases it may cause fractures, deformity or blindness.
- The serum alkaline phosphatase levels which are usually within normal levels are sometimes elevated in the polyostotic type of fibrous dysplasia.

Polyostotic with Endocrinopathy (McCune-Albright's Syndrome)

- This is usually found in females and in addition shows endocrinal disturbances like precocious puberty, goiter, hyperthyroidism, Cushing's syndrome and acromegaly.
- Secondary sexual characteristics such as pubic hair and axillary hair and development of breasts are evident by the age of 5 years.
- It may result in crippling deformities and fractures.
- Bone and skin lesions are usually unilateral, long bones are frequently affected.
- There is expansion and deformity of the jaws, the eruption pattern of the teeth is disturbed because of loss of support of the developing teeth.
- There is asymmetry of the facial bones, with ballooning of the jaws which results in gross enlargement and deformity.

Polyostotic (Craniofacial Type)

- Here the dysplasia extends to involve the maxillary sinus, zygomatic process, floor of the orbit and sometimes the base of the skull.
- It results in severe facial deformity and malocclusion.
- The lesions may produce anosmia, deafness and blindness, with proptosis of the affected eye.

Radiographic Features (Table 24.4)

- The early lesions are radiolucent with ill-defined borders which blend into the surrounding bone. Surrounding the margins of the radiolucency is a wider band of increased density having a granular appearance.
- The defect is often unilocular, but presence of occasional bony septa may give a multilocular impression.

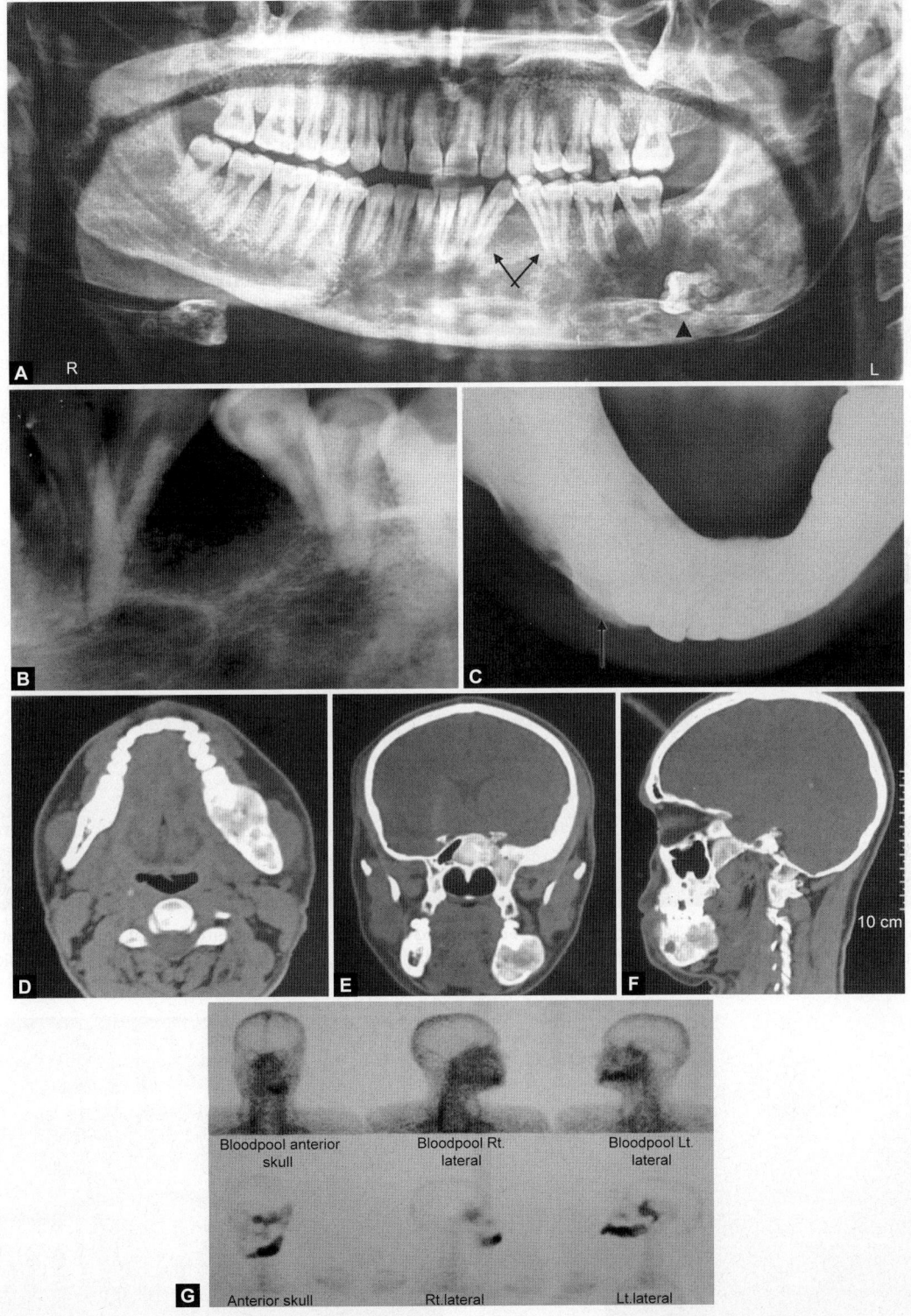

Figures 24.4A to G Fibrous dysplasia: (A) Panoramic radiograph shows mixed radiolucent radiopaque lesion extending from left condyle, coronoid process and ramus involving the body of mandible crossing midline to the right first premolar with horizontally impacted 38 (arrow head), and displacement of left canine and premolar (arrows); (B) Mandibular canine premolar region IOPA shows diffuse mixed radiolucent and radiopaque lesion in 33 and 34 region with displacement of the roots; (C) Mandibular occlusal view shows well-defined smooth expansion of the buccal cortex in 33, 34 region. CT Scan: (D) Axial; (E) Coronal; (F) Sagittal section shows diffuse expansion and ground glass attenuation; (G) Bone scan images reveal increased vascularity (blood pool) in the left mandibular body and ramus region

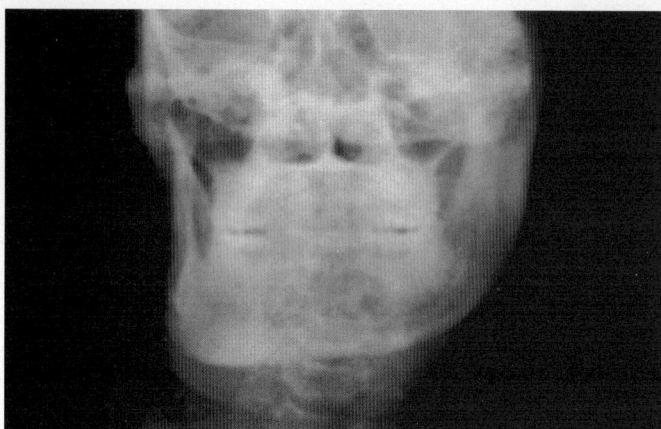

Figure 24.5 Fibrous dysplasia: Posteroanterior view of mandible showing radiopaque lesion in right angle and body mandible region with expansion of inferior border of mandible

- As the lesion matures, a mixed radiolucent radiopaque lesion appears, depending on the stage of maturity and the distribution of fibrous and osseous tissue. The new bone takes the form of very small radiopacities of poor density, which appear granular as they enlarge.
- The variation is more pronounced in the mandible and more homogenous in the maxilla. The internal density is more opaque in the maxilla and the base of the skull.
- Mature radiopaque lesions appear where the bone is predominant, it may have a varied appearance, because the abnormal trabeculae are usually shorter, thinner, irregularly shaped and more numerous than normal trabeculae. This creates a radiopaque pattern that can vary; it may have a granular appearance (ground glass appearance, resembling the small fragment of a shattered windshield), a pattern resembling the surface of an orange (peau d'orange), a wispy arrangement (cotton wool), or

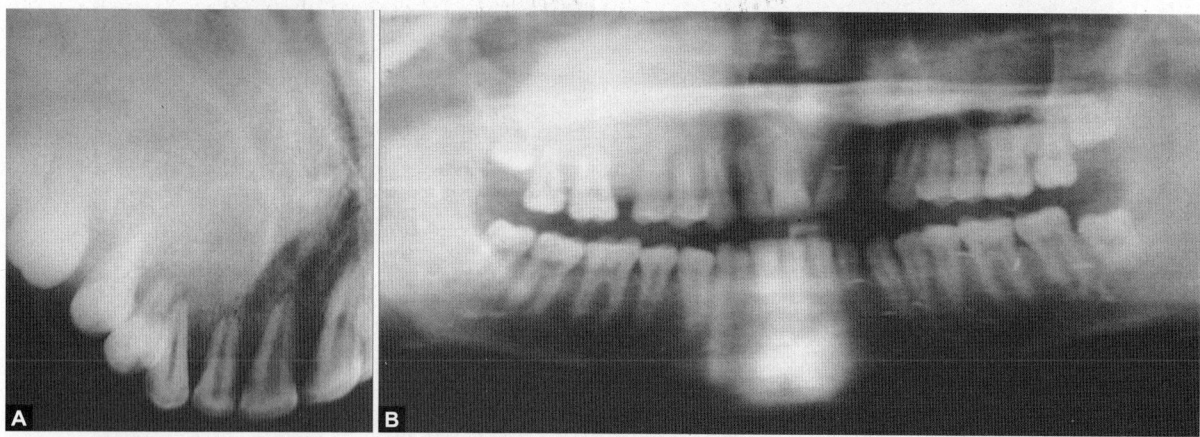

Figures 24.6A and B Fibrous dysplasia: (A) Upper occlusal view of showing homogenous radiopacity and palatal midline suture and incisive foramen deviated to left; (B) Panoramic radiograph showing homogenous radiopacities in the right maxilla region

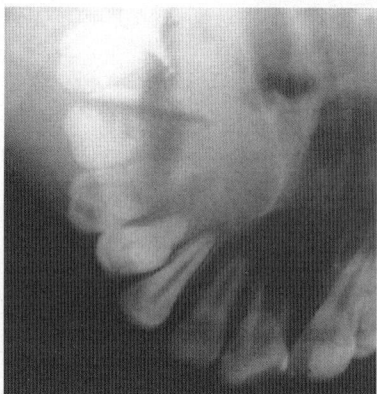

Figure 24.7 Fibrous dysplasia: Upper occlusal view showing buccal cortical plate expansion with ground glass appearance and periapical cyst with root resorption of upper left central incisor and incisal edge fracture

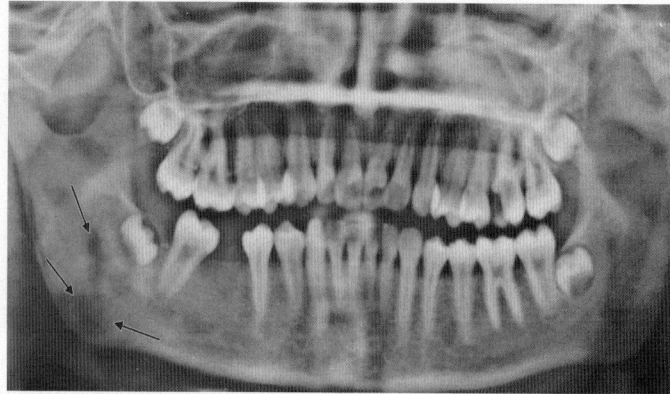

Figure 24.8 Fibrous dysplasia. Mild distension of the left mandible with milk glass shadowing and honeycomb like radiolucencies. This is difficult to radiographically, differentiate from osteomyelitis

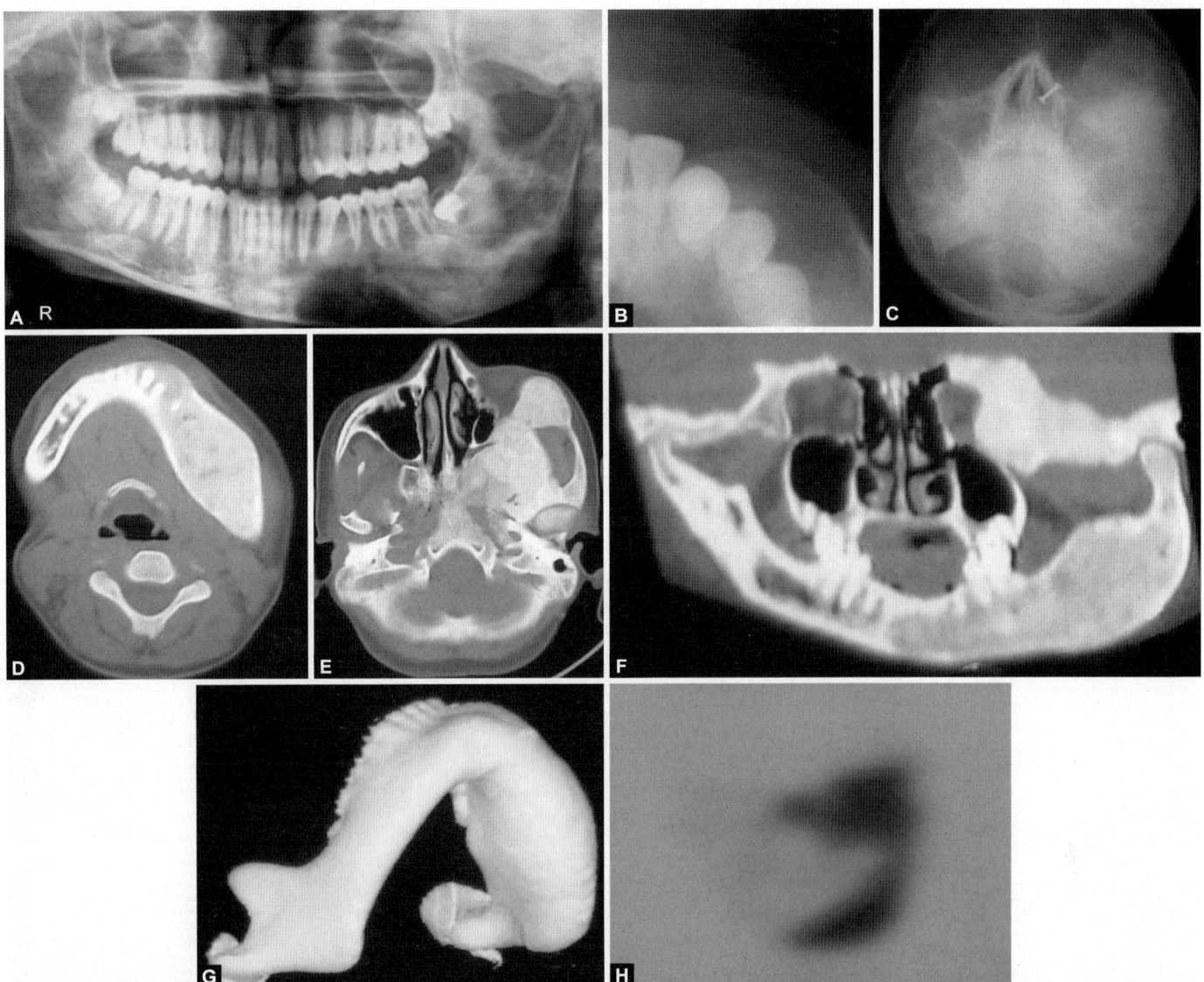

Figures 24.9A to H Polyostotic fibrous dyspalsia: (A) Panoramic radiograph shows distension of the left mandible with honeycomb like radiolucencies; (B) Occlusal radiograph revealed a mixed radiolucent-radiopaque lesion with ground glass appearance in periapical relation to 33 to 35; (C) PNS view shows increased density of the sinus region. CT Scan: (D and E) Axial soft tissue and bone window; (F) Denta scan; (G) 3D shows mixed radiolucent radiopaque lesion with ground glass appearance seen in the left body and ramus of mandible with peripheral enhancing soft tissue within and thickening of the cortex with areas of ground glass attenuation. Expansion of the outer cortex of the left mandible is seen. Involvement of the right maxillary sinus; (H) Bone scan shows an increased radiotracer uptake in left side of mandibular body and ramus and left orbital region. Rest of the skeleton was normal

an amorphous, dense pattern. A distinctive characteristic is the organization of the abnormal trabaculae into a swirling pattern similar to a finger print. Occasionally, the radiolucent regions resembling cysts may occur in the mature lesions, these are bone cavities analogous to simple bone cysts.

- The subclinical variety of fibrous dysplasia has no effect on the surrounding bone.
- The involved bone is expanded with thinning of the outer cortex.

- It may expand into the antrum by displacing its cortical boundary and subsequently occupying part or whole of the maxillary antrum. Extension into the antrum usually occurs from the lateral border, and the last section of the antrum to be involved is the most posterosuperior portion. The cortical boundaries of the floor of the antrum may be changed into abnormal bone pattern.
- There is loss of lamina dura of the involved teeth, as the surrounding bone is altered, the bone density increases and the periodontal space may appear very narrow.

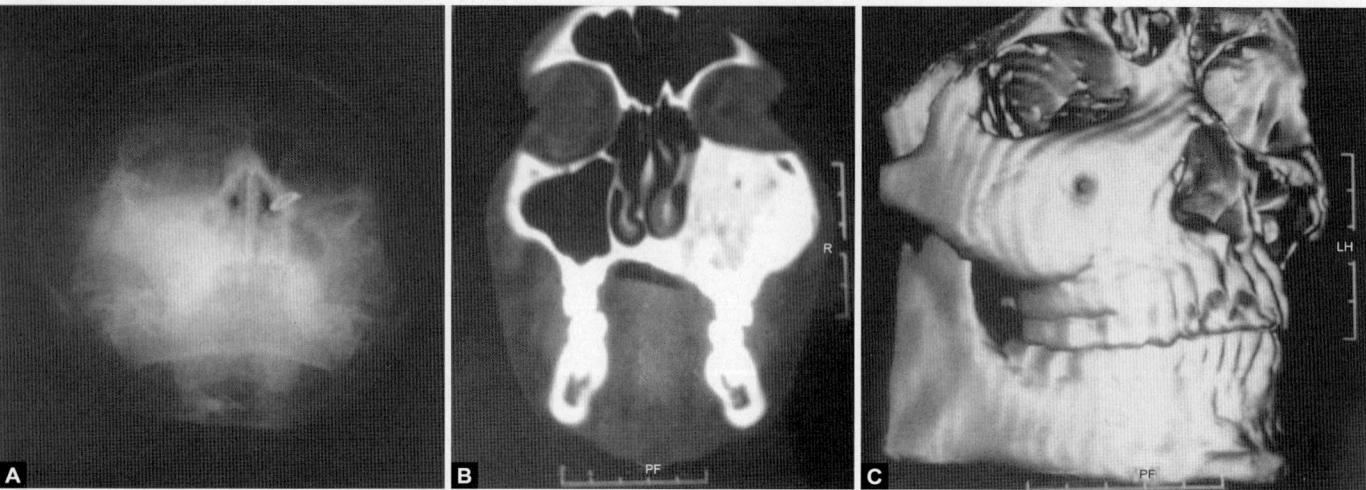

Figures 24.10A to C Fibrous dysplasia: (A) PNS view showing increased density of ground glass appearance in right maxillary sinus region; (B) CT coronal image showing thickening and expansion of right maxilla with obliteration of right maxillary sinus; (C) 3D reconstruction CT of facial bone suggestive of prominence of right maxilla

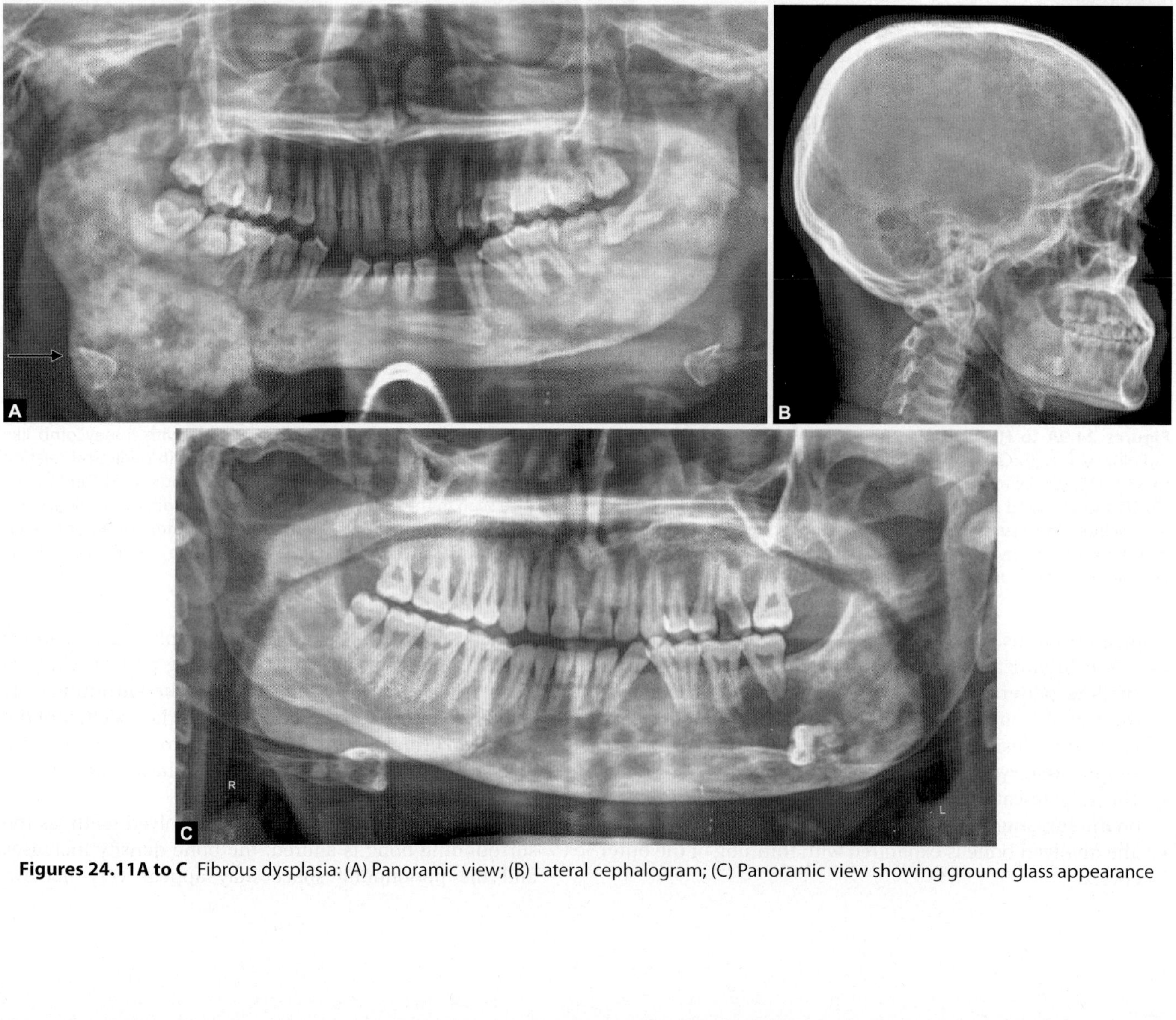

Figures 24.11A to C Fibrous dysplasia: (A) Panoramic view; (B) Lateral cephalogram; (C) Panoramic view showing ground glass appearance

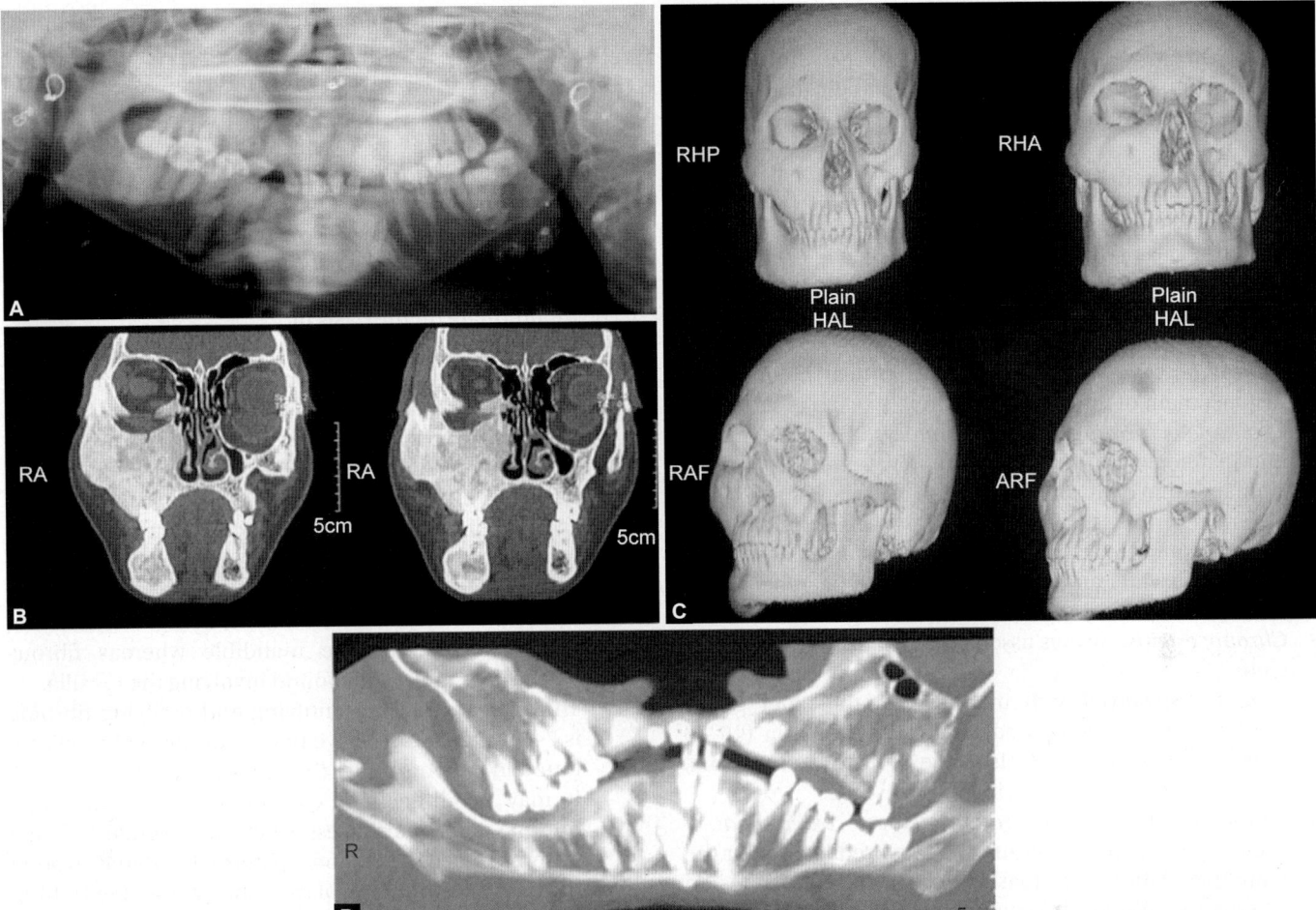

Figures 24.12A to D Fibrous dysplasia: (A) Panoramic radiograph; (B) CT scan coronal view; (C) CT 3D view, showing gross expansion of the maxilla and mandible; (D) Denta scan

Table 24.4 Obisesan et al. classification of radiographic appearances of fibrous dysplasia

- *Peau d'orange or orange peel:* In this type there are alternating areas of granular density and radiolucency giving a radiographic appearance resembling the peel of the orange.
- *Whorled plaque like type:* In this type, the matrix of the well-circumscribed lesion is composed of plaques of amorphous material of intermediate radiodensity, which on close examination are seen to be arranged in whorled finger print appearance.
- *Diffuse sclerotic type:* The lesions of this type are seen as homogenous dense areas, which gradually merge with normal bone.
- *Cyst like type:* In this type the lesion is radiolucent, unilocular or more often, multilocular with well-defined margins.
- *Pagetoid type:* In this type of lesion, the affected area of bone markedly expands and shows alternating areas of opacity and lucency, as seen in Paget's disease.
- *Chalky type:* It manifests as a well-circumscribed lesion consisting of an amorphous dense radiopaque material.

It may displace teeth or interfere with normal eruption, complicating orthodontic therapy. Roots of the involved teeth may be resorbed sometimes and there is destruction of the developing tooth bud.

- The inferior dental canal is displaced in a superior direction.

Craniofacial Fibrous Dysplasia

- Marked radiodensity is seen encroaching upon the orbit and antral cavity.
- Granular type of changes is seen in the base of the skull, where the affected bones are thickened and have greater density.
- The frontal bone is also thickened and appears homogenous and dense.
- The nasal septum is grossly thickened, dense and curved, so that it represents the gross caricature of the letter 'S'.

Additional Imaging

CT: It will give a more accurate, three dimensional representation of the extent of the lesion and can serve as a precise baseline study for future comparisons.

Differential Diagnosis

Lesions likely to be confused with the osteolytic stage of fibrous dysplasia:

- *Central giant cell granuloma*: This has faint wispy trabeculae, whereas fibrous dysplasia shows calcifications, and a stippled or granular appearance.
- *Traumatic bone cyst*: There is no cortical bulging and displacement of the involved teeth.
- *Spontaneous healing of a simple bone cyst*: The radiographic and histologic appearance of the new bone may be very similar to that of fibrous dysplasia.
- *Dental cyst*: This is thin walled with a well-defined cortex which is smooth, whereas in fibrous dysplasia, the cortex tends to be wider and more granular in appearance.
- *Aneurysmal bone cyst*: There is hemorrhagic aspirate.
- *Chronic osteitis*: Always associated with roots of pulp less teeth.
- *Chronic osteomyelitis*: It manifests in the older group (30–80 years) as compared to fibrous dysplasia (10–20 years). The patient will also give a history of trauma, fracture or any debilitating systemic disease.
- *Peripheral and central squamous cell carcinoma*: It occurs in the older age groups, with a predilection for the mandible. Fibrous dysplasia grows by slow expansion whereas peripheral and central squamous cell carcinoma spreads rapidly.
- *Metastatic tumor*: Seen in the older age group and shows a predilection for premolar-molar region of the mandible.
- *Reticular cell sarcoma, Ewing's sarcoma*: These are rarely seen in the maxilla.

Lesions likely to be confused with the mottled stage of fibrous dysplasia:

- *Lymphoma of the bone*: This is rare and poorly defined. The radiographic pattern is irregular and bizarre. In fibrous dysplasia a smooth, well contoured external bony borders are always maintained.
- *Chondrosarcoma*: This is an uncommon malignant tumor of the jaws which is often painful and affects a much older age group.
- *Osteoblastic metastatic carcinoma*: Seldom shows a monotonous pattern as seen in fibrous dysplasia. A history of either symptoms of treatment for a primary tumor elsewhere will be elicited during history taking. Osteoblastic metastatic carcinoma is found in the older age group.
- *Osteosarcoma*: This has a disorderly appearance with a sun burst pattern. Codman's triangle and asymmetrical band like widening of the periodontal ligament is seen. This shows more malignant radiological features.

- *Paget's disease*: This simultaneously affects several bones of the skeleton, bilaterally. It is a disease of the older age group and the serum alkaline phosphatase levels are elevated.
- *Periapical cemental dysplasia*: It may show similar bone pattern, but the distribution is often bilateral with the epicenter in the periapical region. This also occurs in the older age group.
- *Cementifying and ossifying fibroma*: This exhibits a similar mottled appearance to that of fibrous dysplasia, but can be differentiate on the basis of:
  - Cementifying and ossifying fibroma have a predominantly round shape, whereas fibrous dysplasia has a more rectangular shape.
  - Cementifying and ossifying fibroma usually causes a nodular or dome shaped jaw expansion, in fibrous dysplasia there is fusiform elongation.
  - Margins of fibrous dysplasia are indistinct and blending imperceptibly with normal bone while in cementifying and ossifying fibroma, the margins are well-defined.
  - Approximately 70% of the cementifying and ossifying fibromas occur in the mandible whereas fibrous dysplasia is more often found involving the maxilla.
  - The age range of cementifying and ossifying fibroma is 7–58 years. Most active fibrous dysplasia lesions are found in patients under the age of 20 years.
  - It may be difficult to differentiate cementossifying fibroma of the maxilla, especially the juvenile ossifying fibroma type. If the bone pattern is altered around the teeth without displacement of the teeth from one specific epicenter, the lesion probably is fibrous dysplasia. The shape of the bone expansion of fibrous dysplasia into the antrum reflects the original outer contour of the antral wall, which is different from the more convex expansion of a neoplasm.
- *Chronic osteomyelitis*: It may mimic the mottled appearance of fibrous dysplasia, but generally, there is associated purulent discharge and identification of sequestra. Osteomyelitis may result in the enlargement of the jaws, but the additional bone is generated by the periosteum, therefore the new bone is laid down on the surface of the outer cortex, with evidence of the original cortex within the expanded portion of the jaw. Fibrous dysplasia in contrast expands the internal aspect of the bone, displacing and thinning the outer cortex so that the remaining cortex maintains its position at the outer surface of the bone.

Lesions likely to be confused with the mature stage of fibrous dysplasia:

- *Paget's disease*: This also produce lesions with ground glass appearance, but the overall effect is of rarefaction and not radiopacities. This disease is polyostotic and bilateral. It may occasionally cause expansion. Paget's disease usually occurs in the older age group. When it involves the mandible the whole mandible is involved.

- *Giant cell lesion of hyperparathyroidism*: A change in the normal trabecular pattern may occur, resulting in a ground glass appearance of numerous small, randomly oriented trabeculae. There is demineralization and thinning of the cortical boundaries such as inferior border, mandibular canal, and cortical outlines of the maxillary sinuses. The density of the jaws is reduced, resulting in the teeth standing out in contrast. These may be generalized loss of lamina dura. Brown's tumors of hyperparathyroidism may also be seen in the facial bones and jaws. Serum alkaline phosphatase and serum calcium levels are raised, with decrease in serum phosphate levels.

Management

Orthodontic and cosmetic surgery may be done after the completion of skeletal growth.

Juvenile Ossifying Fibroma (Ossifying Fibroma, Aggressive Ossifying Fibroma, Trabecular Demosteoblastoma) (Figs 24.13A and B)

Definition

It is a controversial term that has been distinguished from the larger group of ossifying fibroma on the basis of age of the patient.

Clinical Features

- It is seen in young patients, under the age of 15 years. It may occur with equal frequency in both the jaws.
- The presenting clinical symptom is a swelling. This disease is neither fatal nor locally invasive.

Radiographic Features

It appears as a radiolucent or mixed lesion which may be unilocular or multilocular with a distinct radiopaque border.

Differential Diagnosis

Ossifying fibroma: This occurs in comparatively older individuals (mean age 26.4 years). It contains lamellar bone and cementicles as well as smoothly contoured cells. It also has curvilinear trabeculae. All these features are absent in juvenile ossifying fibroma.

Management

Clinical management and prognosis of juvenile ossifying fibroma are uncertain. Complete local excision or through curettage is the line of treatment.

Cherubism (Familial Fibrous Dysplasia of the Jaws, Disseminated Juvenile Fibrous Dysplasia, Familial Multilocular Cystic Disease of the Jaws, Hereditary Fibrous Dysplasia of the Jaws) (Figs 24.14)

Definition

This is a rare, inherited developmental abnormality that causes bilateral enlargement of the jaws, giving the child a cherubic facial appearance. It is not a bone dysplasia, and therefore the terms familial fibrous dysplasia, etc. are debatable. It is composed of giant cell granuloma like tissue and does not form a bone matrix. The lesion regresses with age.

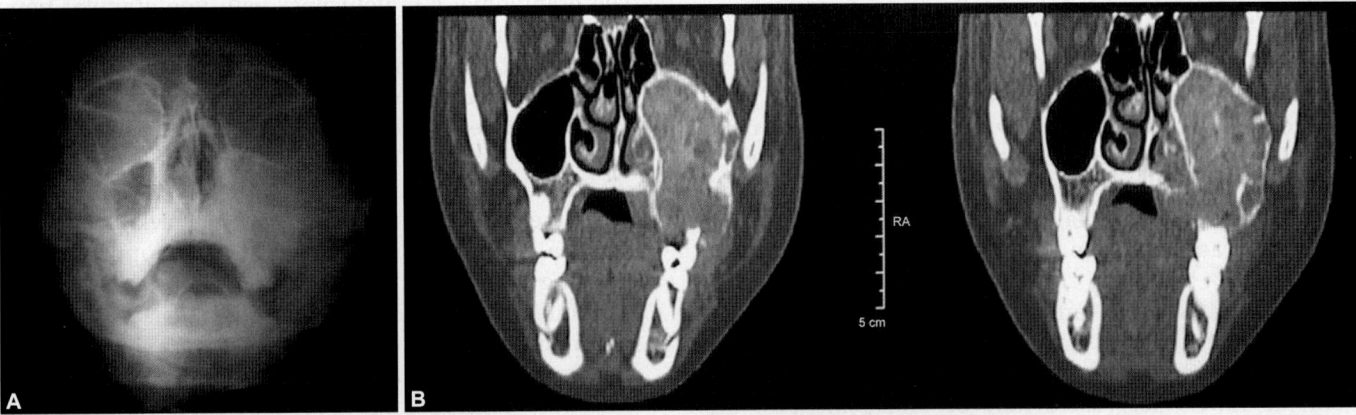

Figures 24.13A and B Juvenile ossifying fibroma: (A) PA Waters view shows a well-defined radiopaque mass in the maxillary sinus on the left side extending into the nasal cavity and causing mild displacement of lateral wall of nose; (B) CT scan coronal view shows a large expansile, circumscribed lesion involving maxillary alveolus in the left side and left half of hard palate. It had a multilocular appearance and caused expansion of the walls of the maxillary sinus. The lesion was slightly protruding into the nasal cavity. Left middle and inferior turbinates were deviated superolaterally. The medial wall of left maxillary sinus was bowed. Displacement of the inferior wall of orbit was seen

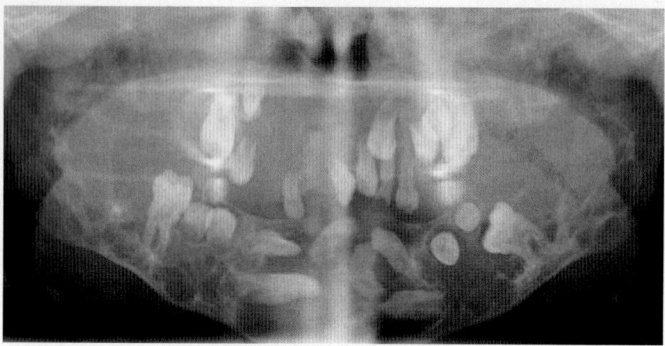

Figure 24.14 Cherubism: Panoramic radiograph shows bilateral involvement of the jaws. It is seen as a radiolucency with fine granular bone and wispy trabeculae forming a prominent multilocular pattern, which tend to coalesce as it enlarges. The margins are well-defined and corticated. There is expansion of buccal and lingual cortical plates. Inferior alveolar canal is displaced inferiorly and maxillary lesions enlarge at the expense of the sinus. Teeth appear to be hanging in air. Displacement of teeth. Erupted deciduous teeth are shed prematurely. Posterior tooth buds may be destroyed

Classification

This is based on the severity and location of the lesion and the extent to which jaws are affected.

- *Grade I*: The fibrosseous expansion tends to be bilateral and symmetrical. It is primarily in the ramus of the mandible.
- *Grade II*: In more severe cases the ramus and the body of the mandible are involved resulting in congenital absence of the third and occasionally the second mandibular molar teeth. In this group the tuberosity region of the maxilla may also be affected.
- *Grade III*: In these cases the lesions affect the mandible and maxilla entirely and may result in considerable facial deformities.

Clinical Features

- It develops in early childhood between 2 and 6 years of age. The lesion is bilateral and often affects both the jaws. When present in only one jaw, the mandible is the most common location. The epicenter is always in the posterior aspect of the jaws, in the ramus of the mandible or the tuberosity of the maxilla. The lesion grows in the anterior direction and in severe cases may extend almost to the midline.
- As children's faces are usually chubby, it may go undetected until the second decade.
- It presents as a painless, firm, bilateral enlargement of the lower face. There may be enlargement of the submandibular lymph nodes. Bilateral enlargement of the maxilla gradually follows.
- In the rapidly increasing stage, the child assumes a chubby, cherubic facial appearance, especially if combined with the involvement of the orbital floor with

upward displacement of the globe and exposure of the scleral rims.

- The patient may have difficulty in speech, deglutition, mastication, respiration and limited jaw movement.
- Profound swelling of the maxilla may result in stretching of the skin of cheeks, which depresses the lower eyelids, exposing a thin line of sclera and causing an eyes raised to heaven appearance.
- The swelling is nontender, firm and hard on palpation with an intact overlying mucosa.
- The alveolar processes are so wide, that they occupy almost the whole of the roof of the mouth; the actual palate being reduced to a narrow fissure between the two approximating alveolar processes.
- The fibrous replacement of bone displaces the deciduous dentition. The primary teeth may be irregularly spaced and sometimes may be absent. There is premature loss of primary teeth. The developing permanent teeth are also affected, and often displaced (as the epicenter is in the posterior aspect of the jaws, the teeth are displaced in the anterior direction), unerupted or absent, along with malocclusion.
- There is rapid increase in the size up to 7–8 years of age, after which the lesion becomes static or progresses very slowly up to puberty. After puberty the maxillary lesions tend to regress. The mandibular lesions progress slowly up to the age of 20 years and then regress. The facial expression almost returns to normal in the 4th and 5th decade of life.
- The calcium, phosphorous and alkaline phosphatase levels are within normal limits. But in active cases, serum alkaline phosphatase levels may be raised.

Radiographic Features

- The internal structure resembles that of a central giant cell granuloma; a radiolucency with fine granular bone and wispy trabeculae forming a prominent mutilocular pattern, which tends to coalesce as it enlarges. The margins are well defined and corticated.
- There may be initial destruction near the angle of the mandible with later expansion of the lesions posteriorly into the ramus and anteriorly into the body of the mandible.
- There is expansion of the buccal and lingual cortical plates.
- On the posteroanterior views the teeth appear to be hanging in air.
- The inferior alveolar canal may be displaced and the lesion may occupy alveolar process, angle and ramus. The thin cortex may eventually disappear.
- Maxillary lesions enlarge at the expense of the sinus.
- There is displacement of numerous teeth, prior to calcification. Erupted deciduous teeth in the area of bone development are shed prematurely. A few posterior teeth may be missing due to early developing mass which destroys the buds and follicle.

Differential Diagnosis

- *Fibrous dysplasia*: Cherubism is bilateral.
- *Giant cell granuloma*: It is more common in the anterior segment of the mandible.
- *ABC*: The lesions of ABC are tender.
- *Central hemangioma*: There is localized gingival bleeding and pumping tooth syndrome.
- *Giant cell lesion of hyperparathyroidism*: These are not bilateral and can be differentiated on abnormal blood chemistry levels.
- *Metastatic tumors*: These are seen in the older age group, and there will be history of a primary tumor elsewhere in the body.
- *Ameloblastoma*: This is usually unilateral and usually in the older age group.
- *Odontogenic myxoma*: This is of developmental origin and there will be history of a missing tooth.
- *Nevoid basal cell carcinoma*: There is no facial swelling. There are characteristic cutaneous abnormalities or rib abnormalities as seen on the chest radiograph.
- *Multiple dentigerous cyst*: Impacted teeth are present in and associated with the lesion.

Management

The surgical procedure may be delayed till the end of skeletal growth. If required conservative surgical procedures may be done for cosmetic problems, along with orthodontic treatment.

Aneurysmal Bone Cyst

Refer Chapter 21—Cysts of Jaws (Page 339).

Central Giant Cell Granuloma (Osteoclastoma, Myeloid Sarcoma, Chronic Hemorrhagic Osteomyelitis, Giant Cell Reparative Granuloma, Giant Cell Tumor)

Refer Chapter 22—Benign Tumors of the Jaws (**Figs 24.15A to F**) (Page 389).

Paget's Disease (Osteitis Deformans) (Figs 24.16 to 24.18)

Definition

This is a condition of resorption and apposition of osseous tissue in one or more than one bone simultaneously, but it is

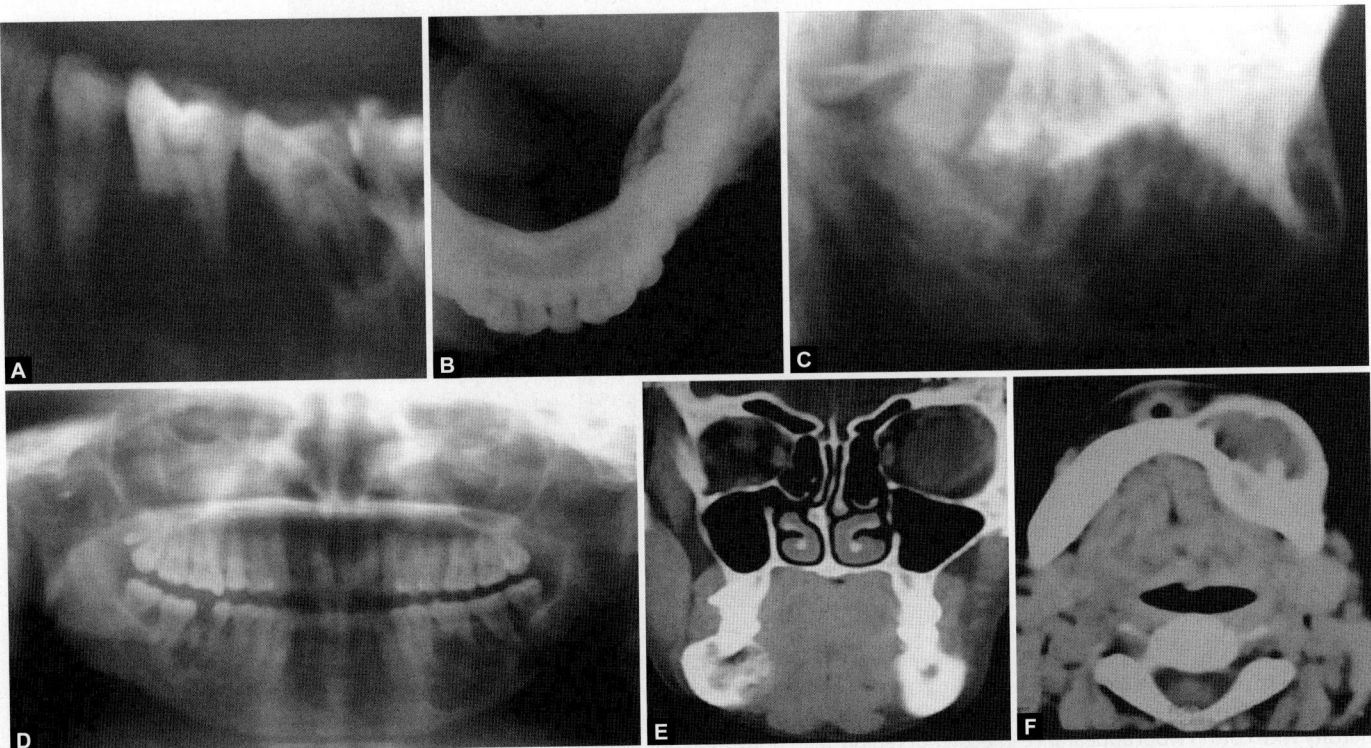

Figures 24.15A to F Central giant cell granuloma: (A to D) The various radiographs of the same patient showed a solitary, expansile mutilocular lesion with a corticated margin, and a few interdental septae, inferior border shows expansion, displacement of mandibular left second premolar and resorption of second premolar and first and second molar; (E and F) CT scan shows enhancing, expansile, bulky lesion, not affecting the cortical plates, with well marked extensions

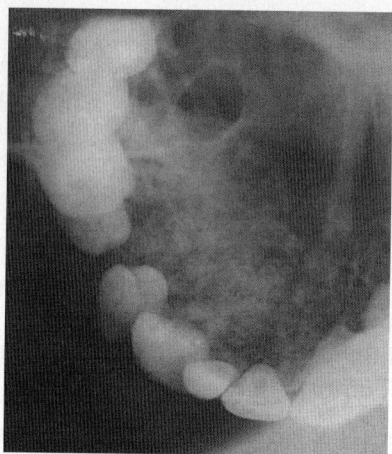

Figure 24:16 Paget's disease, upper occlusal view showing mixed radiolucent radiopaque (mottled appearance) and displacement of upper first and second premolar

not a generalized skeletal disease. It is initiated by an intense wave of osteoclastic activity, with resorption of the bone resulting in irregularly shaped resorption cavities. After some time, this is followed by osteoblastic activity, forming woven bone. The changes may be attributed to a slow virus theory, genetic and environmental factors, etc.

Clinical Features

- It is most frequently seen in Great Britain, Australia and less frequently in North America.
- It is a disease of later middle and old age, more in the males. It occurs more often in the pelvis, femur, skull and vertebrae and infrequently in the jaws. It affects the maxilla more often than the mandible, and the disease is bilateral.
- The affected bone is usually enlarged and commonly deformed, resulting in the bowing of the legs, curvature of the spine and enlargement of the skull.

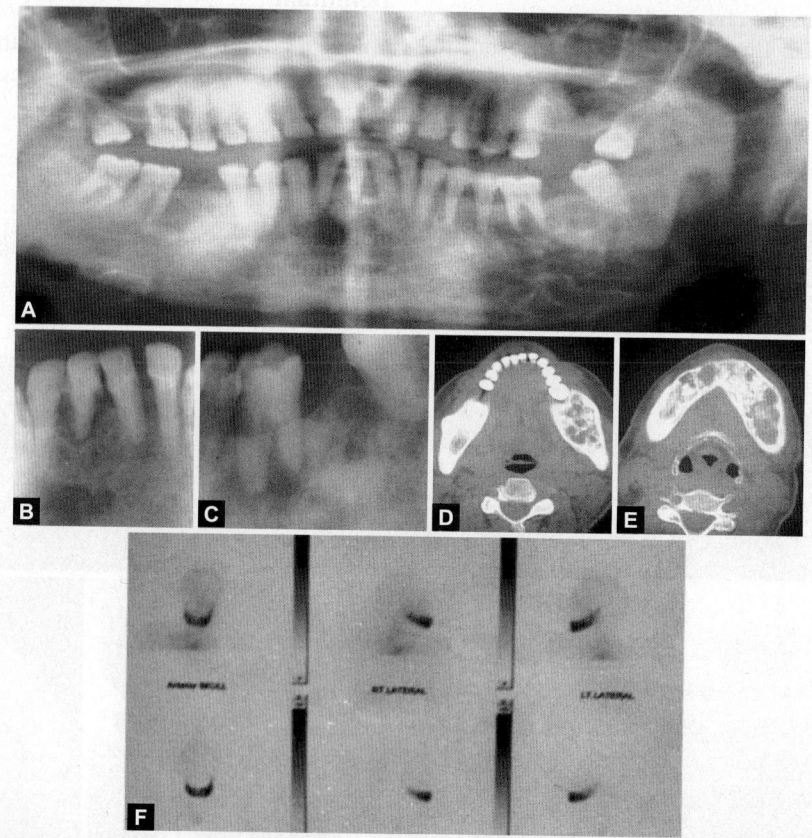

Figures 24.17A to F Paget's disease: (A) Panoramic radiograph shows a mixed radiolucent—radiopaque lesion extending from left angle of mandible to 47 region, extending downwards to the inferior border of mandible and upwards near the alveolar crest. It had a cotton wool appearance. Altered trabecular pattern near left angle of mandible, long linear arrangement was seen; (B and C) IOPA's shows increased bone density with cotton wool appearance in posterior region. Mild horizontal bone loss in anterior region. Increased bone density with narrowing of marrow spaces in anterior region; (D and E) CT scan report axial view shows cortical expansion with patchy areas of sclerosis, radiolucency and ground glass attenuation. Similar changes involving hard palate were noted. Retention cyst involving left maxillary sinus was evident; (F) Bone scan shows an intense increased radiotracer uptake was seen in entire mandible compatible with Paget's disease. Rest of the skeleton showed unremarkable tracer uptake

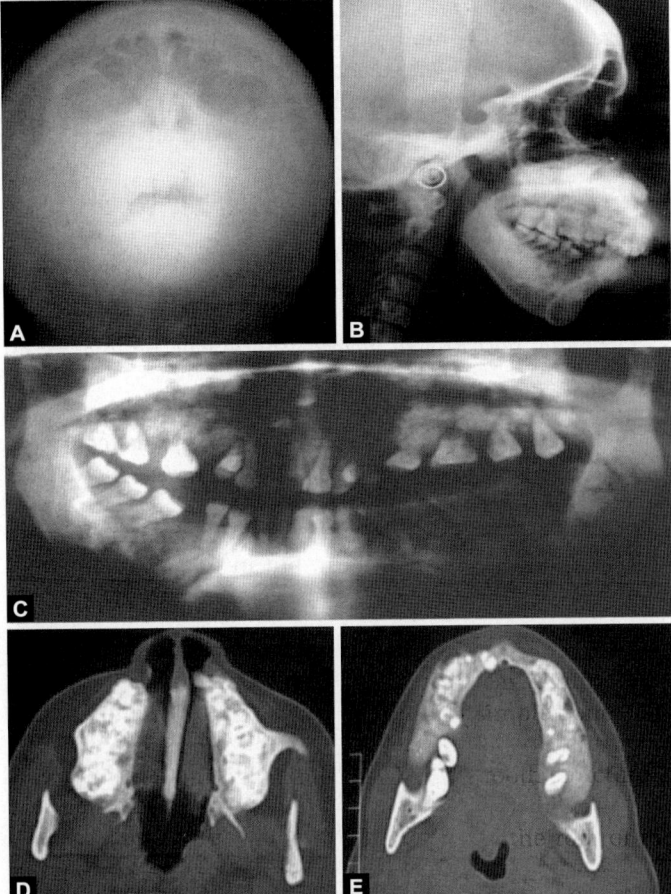

Figures 24.18A to E Paget's disease: (A) PA waters view showed increased trabecular pattern in the entire jaw with enlargement of the buccal and palatal/lingual cortices; (B) Lateral cephalogram showed dense trabecular pattern in the maxillary and mandibular alveolus causing severe prognathism and enlargement of the jaws; (C) Panoramic radiograph showed increased density of bone seen in relation to the maxillary and mandibular alveolar bone which had a cotton wool appearance. Spacing between the teeth with their displacement seen. Impacted 23. CT Scan: (D and E) Axial view of the maxilla and mandible-cortical expansion with areas of sclerosis, ground glass attenuation of the maxillary and mandibular alveolus. Similar changes involving hard palate were noted

- When affected the jaws also enlarge, with increase in the alveolar width, associated with the flattening of the palate when the maxilla is involved. There is movement and migration of the affected teeth, malocclusion and in edentulous cases poor fit of the denture.
- As the disease progresses the mouth may remain open exposing the teeth as the lips are too small to cover the enlarged jaws.
- Bone pain is an inconsistent symptom, more often in the weight bearing bones, and is uncommon in the facial and jaw bones. Patients may have ill-defined neurologic pain

as a result of bone impingement on the foramina and nerve canals.

- Extraction sites heal slowly and incidences of osteomyelitis is higher. Extraction may be further complicated by excessive bleeding from highly vascular abnormal bones in the lytic phase of the disease. Dry socket may also result.
- Complications associated with Paget's disease are osteogenic sarcoma, osteomyelitis, giant cell tumor, carcinoma of the overlying mucosa, carcinoma of the maxillary antrum, pathological fractures and facial paralysis. Occurrence of renal and salivary calculi and hypercalcemia is common.
- There may be severely elevated levels of serum alkaline phosphatase (greater than in any other disorder), during the osteoblastic phase of the disease. The patients will also have high levels of hydroxyproline in the urine.

Radiographic Features

The appearance of the internal structures depend on the developmental stage of the disease, it has three radiographic stages, although these may often overlap in the clinical setting, and are much less apparent in the jaws.

An early radiolucent resorptive stage:

- In the mandible, the inferior cortex appears osteoporotic and has a laminated structure, as the trabeculae may be altered in shape and decreased in number, and they may be long and align themselves in a horizontal linear pattern. This is more so in the posterior to bicuspid region. In the anterior region, the bony trabeculae are coarse and relatively straight and normal, but they intersect producing bone spaces that are larger than normal. Coarse and sparse trabeculae, sometimes tend to converge towards the midline of the mandible, which is highly suggestive of Paget's disease.
- Root resorption may be seen.
- In the skull the early lytic lesions may be seen as discrete radiolucent areas termed as osteoporosis circumscripta. The margins are somewhat irregular, with appearance of denser bone around the radiolucency.

A granular or ground glass second stage:

- As the disease progresses, the trabeculae become short, with random orientation, and have a granular pattern similar to fibrous dysplasia.
- There are rounded patches of abnormal bone of greater density (which may be a centimeter or a few millimeters in diameter), within the radiolucent bone, within which it is not possible to see any actual bone structure. This pattern is more common in the mandible than the maxilla.

A denser more radiopaque appositional stage:

- In the later stages, the trabeculae may be more organized into rounded radiopaque patches of abnormal bone, creating a cotton wool appearance.

- As the fully opacified areas becomes more numerous and enlarged, they tend to coalesce. The bone is denser and appears whiter on the radiograph.
- The bone is enlarged and appears nearly four times its normal thickness on the lateral radiographs. The outer cortex may be thinned but remains intact and appears laminated when seen on the occlusal radiograph.
- Sometimes, there is irregular enlargement of the alveolar process (which may appear radiolucent as compared to the increased density of the surrounding bone), which become prominent and bulge.
- The mandible becomes largely prognathic.
- Paget's disease in the maxilla may encroach the maxillary sinus, involving the floor which may appear more granular and less apparent as sharp boundaries. The air space is usually not diminished to a great extent.
- Hypercementosis is seen on the involved teeth and the lamina dura and periodontal ligament space is obliterated around the hypercementosed and normal roots resulting in ankylosis of the teeth.
- Development of osteogenic sarcoma may produce frank dissolution or destruction of bone. In some cases soft tissue shadow may be seen.

Differential Diagnosis

Early stage (radiolucent appearance):
- *Giant cell lesions of hyperparathyroidism*: Here there is overall radiolucency, the serum alkaline phosphatase and serum calcium levels are raised, with a decrease in serum phosphate levels.
- *Osteoporosis*: It may be confused with Paget's disease in the early stage, but if the area is pathologically enlarged with straight linear trabeculae seen aligned parallel to the long axis of the affected bone, osteoporosis is ruled out. Blood chemistry is normal.
- *Osteomalacia*: Pseudofractures are common in this case. The serum calcium and serum phosphorous levels are decreased in this case, whereas they are normal in Paget's disease.
- *Multiple myeloma*: Here there is a painful enlargement of the jaws and shows typical radiolucent punched out lesions on the skull radiograph. Bence-Jones protein test is positive.

Second stage (mixed radiolucent radiopaque appearance):
- *Osteogenic sarcoma*: This occurs in the younger age group, and shows a variety of radiographic appearances like, sunburst and Codman's triangle.
- *Cementifying and ossifying fibroma*: This is also seen in the younger age group, and shows well-defined margins in contrast to the diffuse border of the lesions of Paget's disease.

- *Fibrous dysplasia*: Seen in younger patients, Paget's disease spreads more diffusely, seen bilaterally and has linear trabeculae and a cotton wool appearance which is distinctive. In fibrous dysplasia the maxillary sinus size is reduced, whereas in Paget's disease the air space is not reduced.
- *Osteoblastic metastatic carcinoma*: There will be history of a primary tumor.
- *Ossifying subperiosteal hematoma*: It is seen in patients younger than 15 years of age, and the patient usually gives history of recent trauma.
- *Ossifying postsurgical defect*: There will be history of surgery.
- *Chronic osteomyelitis*: This is rare in the maxilla.
- *Chondroma and chondrosarcoma*: There is complain of intense pain which is usually not there in the case of Paget's disease.
- *Metabolic diseases*: Both conditions may be bilateral and have a similar bone pattern, but in Paget's disease the bone is enlarged, which is not seen in metabolic diseases.

Advanced stage (purely radiopaque appearance):
- *Florid osseous dysplasia*: Hypercementosis is present, but it is only confined to the jaw bones, in localized area only. In case of Paget's disease when the jaw bones are involved, it affects all of the jaw. This may have a cotton wool pattern, but these lesions are centered above the inferior alveolar canal and commonly have a radiolucent capsule.
- *Osteosclerosis*: The lesion is usually small and confined to the jaw bones.
- *Tori*: The lesion is usually small and confined to the jaw bones.
- *Osteoma*: The lesion is usually small and confined to the jaw bones.

Management

It may be managed medically by using either calcitonin (this suppresses bone resorption and also relieves pain) or sodium etidronate (retards bone resorption). Surgery may be required to correct deformities of the bone. The complications of the disease may be treated with radiotherapy.

Giant Cell Lesions of Hyperparathyroidism

Refer Chapter 20—Infections and Inflammatory Lesions and Systemic Diseases Affecting of the Jaws (Page 298).

Periapical Cemental Dysplasia (Cementoma, Fibrocementoma, Sclerosing Cementum, Periapical Osteofibrosis, Periapical Fibrosarcoma, Periapical Fibrous Dysplasia, Periapical Fibrosteoma)

Refer Chapter 22—Benign Tumors of the Jaws (Page 356).

Florid Osseous Dysplasia (Gigantiform Cementoma, Florid Cemetosseous Dysplasia, Familial Multiple Cementomas, Chronic Sclerosing Osteomyelitis, Sclerosing Osteitis, Multiple Enostosis, Sclerotic Cemental Masses)

Refer Chapter 22—Benign Tumors of the Jaws (**Figs 24.19 and 24.20**) (Page 364).

Ossifying Fibroma (Cementossifying Fibroma, Cementifying Fibroma)

Refer Chapter 22—Benign Tumors of the Jaws (**Fig. 24.21**) (Page 359).

OTHER BONE LESIONS

Osteoporosis (Figs 24.22 and 24.23)

Definition

It is a generalized decrease in the bone mass in which the histological appearance of the bone is normal. An imbalance occurs in the bone resorption and bone formation. Decrease in bone formation results in a lower trabecular bone volume and thinning of the cortical bone.

There are two types:
1. *Primary*: This is associated with the aging process. Bone mass normally increases from infancy to about 35–40 years of age, and then there begins a gradual and progressive decline. The loss of bone mass with age is so gradual that it is virtually imperceptible until it reaches significant proportions.
2. *Secondary*: May result from nutritional deficiencies (scurvy), hormonal imbalance, inactivity or corticosteroid or heparin therapy.

Clinical Features

- The population at most risk is the postmenopausal women
- The bones are fragile and susceptible to fractures, the fractures typically affect the forearm (Colle's fracture), spine (vertebral fracture), hip (femur fracture) and ribs.

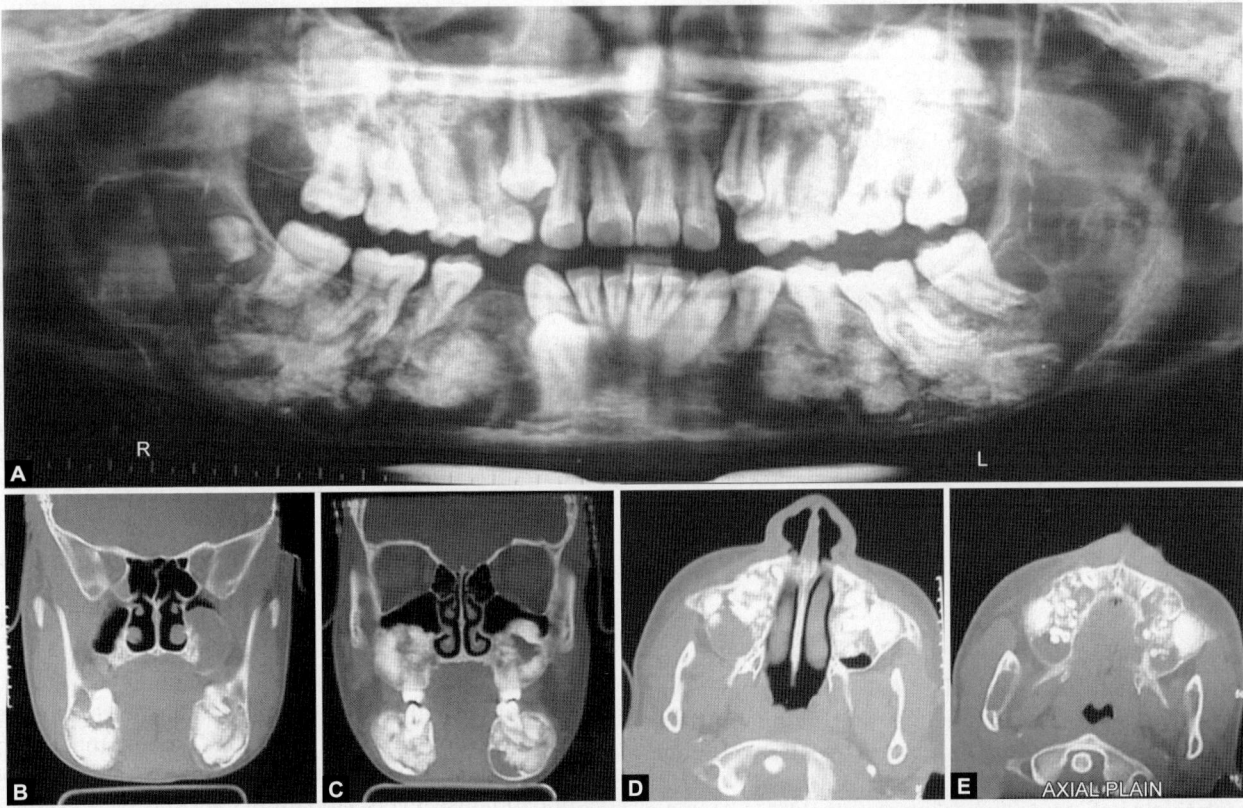

Figures 24.19A to E Florid osseous dysplasia: (A) Panoramic view showing multiple irregular radiopaque globular masses symmetrically involving all four quadrants surrounded by radiolucency in the upper and lower molar region with displacement of the inferior alveolar canal. CT scan confirmed the presence of mixed-density, expansile lesion with areas of sclerosis and ground-glass attenuation involving bilateral maxilla (extending into the maxillary sinuses), body and rami of mandible. The lesion consisted of dense lobulated masses with indistinct radiolucent borders; (B and C) Coronal CT scan showing showing extensive mixed radiopaque and radiolucent lesions involving both the maxilla and mandible; (D and E) Axial CT scan showing sclerotic masses causing bilateral bicortical expansion of mandible

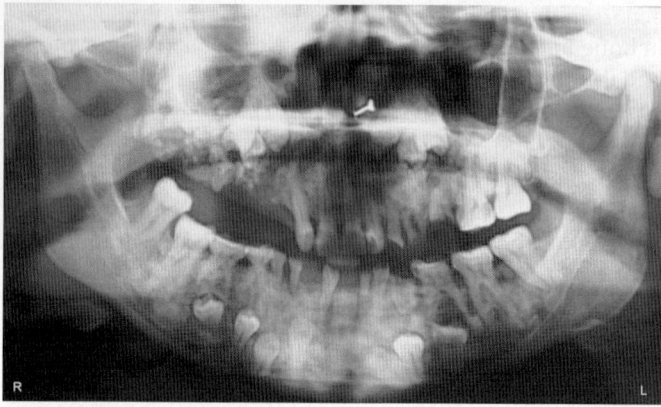

Figure 24.20 Cementosseous dysplasia: Bilateral expansion of the maxillary arch, and in the mandible mild expansion of the arch seen. Amorphorous calcifications (cotton wool appearance), inferior alveolar nerve displaced towards the lower border

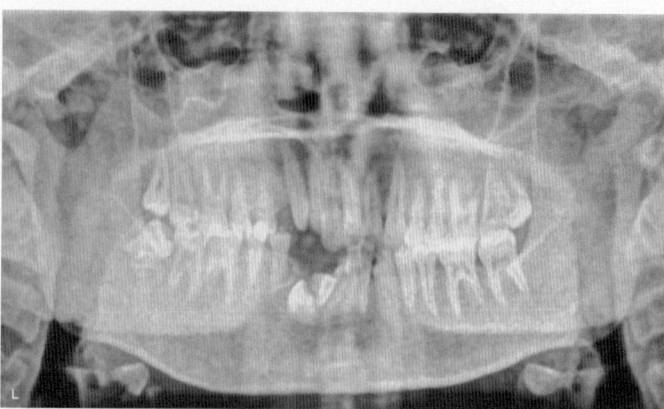

Figure 24.22 Osteoporosis: Panoramic view showing generalized granular appearance of the trabeculae involving entire maxilla and mandible vertebrae. Maxillae and mandibular appearing of the same size

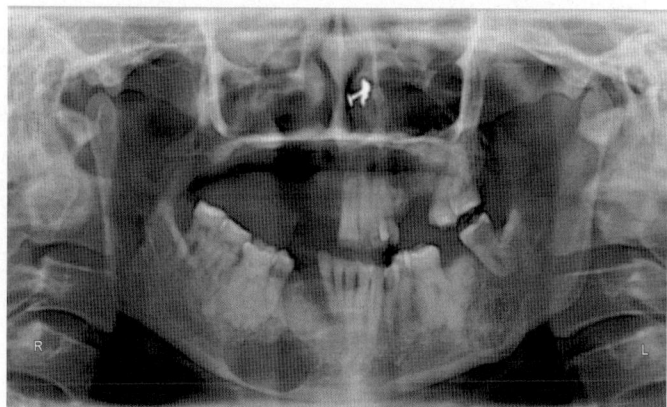

Figure 24.21 Ossifying fibroma: Panoramic radiograph showing lesion inferior to premolar, molars and superior to inferior alveolar canal. The radiolucency subsequently calcifies with radiopaque foci with a wispy or flocculent pattern or solid amorphorous radiopacities. The masses coalesce and grow concentrically in the medullary part of the bone with outward expansion. Lamina dura is lost and there is displacement of involved teeth and inferior alveolar canal. In the maxilla it causes unique growth pattern with dissolution of neighboring bones without displacement

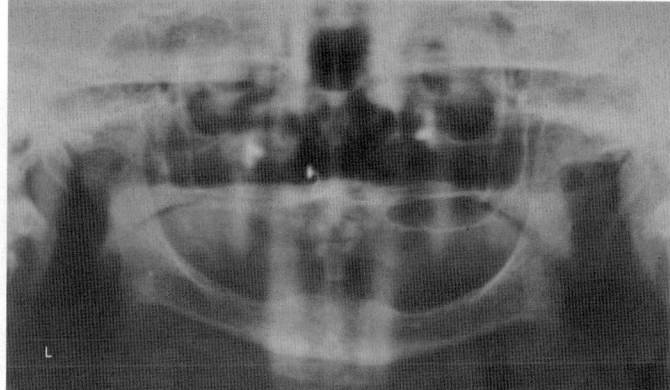

Figure 24.23 Osteoporosis: Advanced senile osteoporosis and atrophy, the panoramic view shows inferior border of left maxillary sinus not traceable, suggestive of ridge resorption. The mandible bone has thinned profile. Both the ascending rami exhibit spotty areas of osteoporosis as well as thinning of the compact bone, except for the oblique line which remains clearly visible

- Congenital form is inherited as an autosomal recessive disorder, which is invariably fatal in early life due to massive hemorrhage, anemia and rampant bone infections occurring due to progressive loss of bone marrow and their cellular products.
- Osteoporotic patients may notice a gradual loss of height due to shortening of trunk, which may be characterized by attacks of severe pain, which is aggravated by movements.
- Percussion over the affected vertebrae is painful.
- As the bone becomes relatively avascular, it is very susceptible to osteomyelitis.

- Fracture of the jaws is common during tooth extraction, with common occurrence of osteomyelitis.
- The teeth may show delayed eruption, early loss of teeth, arrested root formation, enamel hypoplasia, and are more prone to caries due to poor calcification.
- Patients usually have anemia due to the replacement of hemolytic marrow by bone. RBC count may be below 1,000,000 per cubic meter. There may be increased serum phosphatase levels. Hepatomegaly may be present.

Radiographic Features

- It results in overall reduction in the density of bone, which may be observed in the jaws by using the unaltered density of teeth as comparison.

- There may be reduced density and thinning of the cortical boundaries of the inferior mandibular cortex.
- Reduction in the volume of cancellous bone is more difficult to assess, due to the constant stress applied to the alveolar process by the teeth, reduction in the number of trabeculae is less evident.
- The lamina dura may appear thinner than normal.
- Anatomical shadows such as the nasal fossa and maxillary sinus are less distinct.
- There is a wedge-shaped appearance of the affected vertebrae on the lateral radiograph.

Additional Imaging

- *Dual energy X-ray absorptiometry (DEXA)*: This gives more accurate assessment of bone mineral density (BMD), than the routine radiograph.
- *Quantitative computed tomography (QCT)*: This also gives more accurate assessment of bone mineral density (BMD), than the routine radiograph.

Differential Diagnosis

Infantile cortical hyperostosis: There will be a positive history of highly specific soft tissue and bony abnormalities. Sites of involvement are limited to few bones. New bone is laid subperiosteally.

Management

Estrogens and calcium supplement after menopause helps to prevent further cortical and trabecular bone loss, exercise programs are also effective.

Infantile Cortical Hyperostosis (Caffey's Disease, Caffey-Silverman Syndrome)

Definition

It is characterized by unusual cortical thickening of certain bones.

It occurs in two forms:
1. Autosomal dominant.
2. Sporadic form.

Clinical Features

- It occurs before 6 months of age and has no sex predilection. The bones most commonly affected are mandible, clavicle, scapula, frontal bone and ulna. The involvement is usually bilateral.
- The infants will have fever and become hyperirritable. The onset is usually sudden and is manifested as a soft tissue swelling, which may be warm and tender. The swelling may subside and recur again in the same place or at a new involved site.

- Other features are pseudoparalysis, pleurisy and dysphagia.
- The mandible is the most commonly affected bone. The patient may present with, asymmetrical deformity of the mandible, especially in the angle and ramus area. There may be malocclusion and enamel hypoplasia.
- There may be anemia, leukocytosis, elevated erythrocyte sedimentation rate, monocytosis and increased serum alkaline phosphatase levels.

Radiographic Features

- The bone changes occur after the swelling has subsided and the area ceases to be tender.
- There is thickening of the inferior cortex due to formation of subperiosteal new bone. The new bone may be laid down in layers giving the cortex a laminated appearance. The surface of the new bone may be smooth or in some cases it may be irregular.
- There is overall enlargement of the body of the mandible with homogeneously increased density throughout.
- The lamina dura and cortices of the tooth follicle are normal.

Differential Diagnosis

- *Callus formation*: This is usually unilateral or asymmetrical when seen bilaterally.
- *Osteoma*: Rare at such a young age.
- *Cherubism*: Multilocular expansile radiolucency with no cortical thickening.
- *Osteoporosis*: The cancellous bone is affected.
- *Osteomyelitis*: This may be associated with laying down of subperiosteal bone, but it rarely occurs within the first 6 months of life. In osteomyelitis the whole mandible is not involved.
- *Periostitis of jaw*: This is usually unilateral and localized. It usually has a definite underlying cause. The laminated structure is visible only at the inferior margins as compared to that in infantile cortical hyperostosis, where it is visible all over the bony surface of the jaw.
- *Fibrous dysplasia*: This is an abnormality within the bone, whereas infantile cortical hyperostosis represents changes added to the bone.
- *Hypovitaminosis A*: This produces a condition called cortical hyperostosis, which usually affects the metacarpal bone and occurs over the age of one year. Infantile cortical hyperostosis occurs below 6 months of age and the mandible is usually affected.

Osteopetrosis (Albers-Schönberg, Marble Bone Disease, Osteosclerosis Fragilis Generalisata)

Definition

This is a disorder of the bone that results from a defect in the differentiation and function of the osteoclasts, leading to abnormal formation of the primary skeleton and a generalized increase in bone mass. This bone is dense, fragile and highly susceptible to fracture and infection. Obliteration of the marrow spaces comprises hematopoiesis and compresses the cranial nerves.

There are three types:

1. *Severe autosomal recessive type (osteopetrosis congenital)*: This is a malignant childhood condition with a severe form showing skeletal and neurological signs. Those affected rarely live beyond the age of two years.
2. *Mild autosomal recessive*: The adult is characterized by predominantly skeletal signs including unerupted teeth, mandibular prognathism, pathological fractures and osteomyelitis.
3. *Benign autosomal dominant (osteopetrosis tarda)*: This affects most of the bones. Osteomyelitis of the mandible is a common finding.

Clinical Features

- In the autosomal recessive type, there is progressive loss of bone marrow and its cellular products with severe increase in bone density. The narrowing of the bony canals results in hydrocephalus, blindness, deafness, vestibular nerve dysfunction, and facial nerve paralysis. Frontal bossing and obliteration of the maxillary and paranasal sinuses is also seen. The patient is usually mentally retarded.
- The benign dominant form is milder and may be totally asymptomatic, discovered any time between childhood and adulthood as an accidental finding or a pathological fracture of bone.
- In the chronic cases due to neural compression there may be bone pain and cranial nerve palsies.
- Osteomyelitis may complicate the disease due to lack of vascularity. This is more common in the mandible. Osteomyelitis may also be secondary to dental or periodontal disease.
- The teeth may show delayed eruption, early tooth loss, missing teeth, malformed roots and crowns, enamel hypoplasia, defective dentine, disturbed tooth development, small pulp chambers and tendency towards caries. The normal eruption pattern of the primary and secondary teeth may be delayed as a result of increased bone density or ankylosis.
- Due to displacement of hematopoietic bone marrow anemia ensues and the hematopoietic function is assumed by the liver, spleen and the lymph nodes, resulting in hyperplasia of lymphoid tissue and hepatosplenomegaly.
- The RBC count is below 1,000,000 cells per cu.mm.
- The serum calcium and phosphate levels are normal, but the serum acid phosphatase levels are elevated in patients with benign dominant osteopetrosis.

Radiographic Features

- There is increased, homogenous density, which is bilaterally symmetrical throughout the skeleton. The trabeculae of the medullary cavity are not visible, as the internal radiopacity reduces the contrast between the outer cortical border and the cancellous portion of the bone. The entire bone may be mildly enlarged.
- The base of the skull is grossly thickened with increased radiodensity. A uniformly dense and radiopaque skull vault. There is loss of normal skull markings; the diploe is effaced and the head of the patient resembles a bladder of lard. There is narrowing of the foramina.
- There may be occasional involvement of the jaws, which is always bilateral and includes thickening of the lamina dura around the teeth in the early stages (an almost pathognomic finding in adults) and gradual thickening of the trabeculae and a reduction in the size of the marrow spaces producing an overall increase in bone density.
- The increased radiopacity of the jaws is so severe that the radiographs may not reveal the internal structures. The roots of the teeth may also not be apparent.
- The lamina dura and cortical border appear thicker than normal.
- The teeth are usually normal, but they may be deformed.

Differential Diagnosis

- *Polyostotic fibrous dysplasia*: This usually involves part of a bone rather than the complete bone.
- *Paget's disease*: It usually involves the skull, pelvis, vertebrae, femur, maxilla and mandible. There is marked elevation of the serum alkaline phosphatase levels.
- *Sclerotic cemental mass*: It have a predilection for black women over 30 years of age. Only the jaws are affected, with the radiographs showing radiopaque masses surrounded by radiolucent borders.
- *Infantile cortical hyperostosis*: Skeletal changes are subperiosteal and not endosteal. The mandible is more commonly involved.
- *Other bone dysplasias that produce a general sclerotic appearance*: They are sclerosteosis, pyknodysostosis, craniometa-physeal dysplasia, diaphyseal dysplasia, melorheostosis, osteopathia striata, osteosclerosis from fluoride poisoning, and secondary hyperthyroidism from renal disease.
- *Melorheostosis*: This is a rare unilateral abnormality of the bones with radiographic appearance of increased density and a deformity in shape that suggests the appearance of candle grease which has run down and collected at the side of the candle, the surface is very nodular. The jaws are rarely involved, but when affected the involvement is usually unilateral.

- *Idiopathic hypercalcemia*: This is seen more often in infants with mental retardation, skeletal underdevelopment, muscular weakness and anorexia. The child has an elfin appearance. The skull tends to be small with increased bone density especially in the frontal and basal regions. There are convolution markings on the skull. The jaws present with increased density, the lamina dura is indistinct, but the follicular walls enclosing the developing teeth is intact. In patients who survive there is a tendency for the bone to assume a more normal structure.

Management

Bone marrow transplants: Avoid major bone surgeries and any risk of infection.

Osteogenesis Imperfecta (Brittle Bone, Lobstein Disease)

Refer Chapter 19—Dental Anomalies and Developmental Disturbances of the Jaws (Page 254).

Leontiasis Ossea

Definition

The word 'Leontiasis' has been used to describe the leonine appearance of some patients with facial leprosy. The word 'ossea' is added to describe leonine appearance in bilateral bone disease. This is believed to result due to fibrous dysplasia, Paget's disease, metaphyseal dysplasia, diaphyseal dysplasia, periostitis of the jaw bones or osteitis fibrosa. *In recent literature the term 'Leontiasis Ossea' is not used as it requires a lot of imagination to see the lion in it.*

Clinical Features

- There is bilateral enlargement of the facial bones.
- A classical case is one where there is enlargement of the maxillae, mandible, malar bones, and in some cases changes in the frontal as well as the ethmoid, sphenoid and temporal bones.
- The orbital cavity is reduced in size and the eyes protruded. Blindness may follow due to compression of the optic nerve and there may be difficulty in breathing as a result of narrowing of the nasal passage.
- Clinically, there are three types of leontiasis ossea:
  - First type starts early in life and quickly extends until skeletal growth ends. The lesion then ceases to grow but it does not regress.
  - Second type starts in the early years and it may progress slowly or quickly, and it does not cease with the end of somatic growth but continues to grow and produces gross deformities.
  - Third type starts in early adulthood or even near the middle life and progresses slowly and inexorably.

Radiographic Features

- The affected bones may vary in size and density, and there may be a symmetrical thickening of the bones. The trabeculae may be thickened and dense with narrowing of the marrow spaces.
- The base of the skull appears homogeneously dense or granular.
- There is gross deformity of the face, with bone projecting from the mandible on one side and the paranasal region from the opposite side.
- The nasal bone is often thickened, and the nasal septum may or may not be involved.
- The mandible has a characteristic appearance; the inferior margins of the bone deep to the bicuspid and molar region project markedly downwards as compared to the either unchanged or slightly deeper incisor area. The effect of the altered configuration of the mandible results in a rough W-shaped caricature. The surface of the bony projection from the inferior aspect of the mandible may present an irregular appearance resembling a cumulus cloud.

Progressive Systemic Sclerosis (Scleroderma)

Definition

This is a generalized connective tissue disease that causes hardening of the skin and other tissues. The involvement of the gastrointestinal tract, heart, lungs and kidneys usually result in more serious complications. The cause of the disease is unknown.

Clinical Features

- This is a disease of the middle age, with women more affected than men.
- The skin is thickened and leathery, not mobile over the underlying soft tissues and involvement of the facial region may inhibit normal mandibular opening.
- Patients have xerostomia, increased number of filled, missing or decayed teeth, they have deeper periodontal pockets and higher gingivitis score.

Radiographic Features

- An unusual pattern of mandibular erosions at regions of muscle attachment such as the angles, coronoid process, digastric region or condyles. These lesions are usually bilateral and symmetrical. The erosive borders are smooth and sharply defined. This resorption is progressive with the disease.
- There is an increase (nearly double) in the width of the periodontal ligament spaces around the teeth, it is more pronounced around the posterior teeth (despite this the involved teeth are not mobile and their gingival attachments are intact).
- The lamina dura remains normal.

Differential Diagnosis

- *Tooth mobility*: Causes widening of the periodontal ligament space due to:
  - Orthodontic tooth movement.
  - Intermaxillary fixation with arch bars.
- *Invasion of the periodontal ligament by malignant neoplasms*: Here there is destruction of the lamina dura and irregular widening.
- *Sarcoma*: Here the thickening is not around the major portion of the root surface, and there is associated interdental bone destruction.

Management

The progressive loss of bone in the region of the mandibular angle, may lead to fracture, periodic radiographs are advised to help monitor the amount of bone involvement.

Pierre Robin Syndrome (Robin Anomalad)

Definition

This is a result of arrested development.

Clinical Features

- It consists of a triad of cleft palate, micrognathia and glossoptosis.
- The patient has a typical bird face, due to arrested development and ensuing hypoplasia of the mandible, giving a retrognathic appearance.
- The tongue is thus pushed between the palatal shelves resulting in a cleft palate.
- There is micrognathia, and the tongue tends to fall backwards, partially obstructing the epiglottis causing difficulty in respiration.
- There may be associated congenital heart defects, other skeletal abnormalities, ocular lesions and mental retardation.

Management

Surgical closure and orthognathic surgery.

Marfan's Syndrome (Marfan-Achard Syndrome, Arachnodactyly)

Definition

This is a hereditary disease transmitted as an autosomal dominant trait. It is basically a disease of connective tissue related to defective organization of collagen which is abnormally soluble.

Clinical Features

- The shape of the skull and face is characteristically long and narrow.
- There is excessive length of the tubular bones resulting in disproportionately long thin extremities. The fingers and toes are long, thin and tapering and are called spider fingers.
- There is hyperextensibility of the joints with habitual dislocations, kyphosis or scoliosis and flat foot.
- The patient might have bilateral ectopia lentis that is weakening or rupture of the suspensory ligaments.
- The patients may have cardiovascular complications like aortic aneurysm, aortic regurgitation, valvular defects and enlargement of the heart.
- There is usually a high arched palate, bifid uvula, malocclusion, multiple odontogenic cysts of the maxilla and mandible. There may be temporomandibular joint dysarthrosis.

Management

No specific treatment.

Down Syndrome

Definition

This is also called Trisomy 21 syndrome and mongolism. This is associated with a subnormal mentality in which an extremely wide variety of anomalities and functional disorders may occur. It results from excessive chromosomal material involving all or portion of chromosome 21. It is commonly believed to occur in children who are born at an advanced maternal age, or in case of uterine or placental abnormalities.

They are of three types:
1. *Typical type*: Trisomy 21 with 47 chromosomes (95% cases)
2. *Translocation type*: 46 chromosomes
3. Chromosomal mosaicism.

Clinical Features

- The skull is brachycephalic with frontal prominence and occipital flattening. The face is flat with large anterior fontanelle and open sutures.
- The palpebral fissures are almond shaped with superio-lateral or Mongolian obliquity.
- The eyes are small, slanting with epicanthal folds and ocular hypertelorism.
- There is flattening of the nasal bridge.

- There is sexual underdevelopment, cardiac abnormalities and hypermobility of the joints.
- The patient has prognathism, high arched palate. Hypoplasia or aplasia of the maxillary sinus.
- There is macroglossia with protrusion of the tongue, which may appear pebbly due to enlargement of the papilla.
- There is malocclusion due to small maxillary arch relative to the mandibular arch.
- The teeth are malformed, with enamel hypoplasia and microdontia.
- There may be severe destructive periodontal disease with no apparent local cause.

Achondroplasia (Chondrodystrophia Fetalis)

Definition

This is a disturbance of endochondral bone formation, which results in a characteristic form of dwarfism. It is a hereditary condition, which is transmitted as an autosomal dominant trait.

Clinical Features

- The patient is usually short (less than 14 meters), with thickened muscular extremities, brachycephalic skull and bowed legs. The patient has lumbar lordosis with prominent buttocks and a protruding abdomen. The joints exhibit limited motion. The arms do not hang freely at the sides, elbows cannot be straightened and the hands are small with stubby fingers.
- The base of the skull is small and constricted as a result of retarded growth of the cartilaginous portions. The calvarium is large and bulges frontally and laterally. There is depression of the bridge of the nose.
- The maxilla is retruded (due to restricted growth of the base of the skull), with a relative appearance of mandibular prognathism.
- There may be disturbances and variations in the shape of the teeth, congenitally missing teeth are often found.

Radiographic Features

- The long bones are shorter with thickening or clubbing at the ends. The epiphysis may either close early or late.
- The bone of the base of the skull fuse prematurely, producing a shortening as well as a narrow foramen magnum.

Management

No specific treatment.

Skeletal Fluorosis (Fluoride Toxicity)

Definition

These are of two types:
1. Acute.
2. Chronic.

Clinical Features

Acute

Nausea, vomiting and epigastric distress, excessive salivation and mucus discharge, headache and sweating. There may be a barely detectable pulse, hypotension, cardiac arrhythmias and disturbance in the electrolyte balance. The patient might develop complications like respiratory and metabolic acidosis and go into coma.

Chronic

- It may be a birth anomaly, or a mutation and/or genetic disorder.
- Stiffness of gait and limitation of movements occurs. Pain in the joints of the hands, feet and spine.
- In severe cases, there is crippling of the movement and extreme pain as the spine joints' become rigid and virtual immobilization of the individual occurs.

Radiographic Features

In the chronic cases there will be increased bone density. Here there is increased osteophytic activity which results in thickening of the bones of the extremities. There may be calcification of the tendons and ligaments.

Management

In the acute cases, detoxification with support to the vital signs is indicated.

Generalized Cortical Hyperostosis (von Buchem Disease)

Definition

Here there is excessive deposition of endosteal bone throughout the skeleton in a pattern that is suggestive of a hereditary condition, with an autosomal recessive characteristic.

Clinical Features

- There may be loss of visual activity and facial sensation. Facial paralysis and deafness may occur due to closure of the foramina, from where the cranial nerve emerges.

- The face appears swollen with widening of the angles of the mandible and at the bridge of the nose.
- Intraorally there may be over growth of the alveolar processes.

Radiographic Features

- There is increased density of bones of the entire skeleton
- The skull exhibits a diffuse sclerosis, which may also be seen in the jaws.

Management

There is no specific treatment, and the patient may lead abnormal life.

Massive Osteolysis (Vanishing Bone, Disappearing Bone, Phantom Bone, Progressive Osteolysis, Gorham Syndrome)

Definition

This is characterized by spontaneous, progressive resorption of the bone with ultimate total disappearance of the bone.

Clinical Features

- It affects both the sexes equally and is more common in older children and young and middle aged adults.
- The disease is not painful, it begins suddenly. Progresses rapidly until the involved bone is replaced by a thin layer of fibrous tissue surrounding a cavity.
- The most commonly affected bones are the clavicle, scapula, humerus, ribs, ileum, ischium and sacrum.
- In the oral cavity there may be complete destruction of the mandible, the maxilla is less commonly involved.

- The patients may present with pain and/or facial asymmetry, followed by pathological fracture of bone following even minor trauma.

Management

No specific treatment, although surgical resection may cease the progress of the disease.

BIBLIOGRAPHY

1. Garg P, Karjodkar FR, Garg S, Imaging findings in craniofacial polyostotic fibrous dysplasia. J Oral Sign. 2011;(13)2.
2. Goaz PW, White SC. Principles and Interpretation, In: Oral Radiology, 3rd edition. St. Louis: Mosby Year Book; 1994.
3. Miles DA, Van Dis MJ, Jensen CW, et al. Interpretation normal versus abnormal and common radiographic presentations of lesions. In: Radiographic and Imaging for Dental Auxillaries, 3rd edition. Philadelphia: WD Saunders; 1999.pp.231-80.
4. Oral and maxillofacial surgery. CNA. 1997;9(4).
5. Shafer WG, et al. A Text Book of Oral Pathology, Philadelphia: WB Saunders; 1983.
6. Sontakke SA, Karjodkar FR, Hemant R. Umarji Computed Tomographic features of Fibrous Dysplasia of Maxillfacial Region. J Imag Sci Dentis. 2011;41:23-8.
7. Van der Waal I. Diseases of the jaws diagnosis and treatment. Munksgaard: Copenhagen; 1991.
8. Wood NK, Goaz PW. Differential diagnosis of oral lesions. 4th edition. CV Mosby: St. Louis; 1991.
9. Wood RE. Handbook of signs in dental and maxillofacial radiology. Warthog Publications, Toronto; 1988.
10. Worth HM. Principles and practice of oral radiographic interpretation. Year Book Medical Publishers, Chicago; 1963.

Temporomandibular Joint Disorders 25

INTRODUCTION

The temporomandibular joint is a unique complex joint which executes both hinge and sliding movements. It is also called as the ginglymoarthroidal type of joint. It is formed by the mandibular fossa (glenoid fossa), the inferior surface of the temporal bone and the condylar process of the mandible. A disc composed of fibrocartilage is interposed between the condyle and the mandibular fossa. A fibrous capsule lined with synovial membrane surrounds and encloses the joint **(Fig. 25.1)**. Ligaments and muscles restrict or allow movement of the condyle. It is a synovial type of joint and is distinguished from most of the other joints by the following points:

- *Fibrocartilage*: The articulating surface of the bone is covered by avascular, fibrous connective tissue, which may contain variable number of cartilage cells
- *Point of closure*: The two articulating surface complex of bone carry teeth, whose shape and position influence the movement of the joint. It is the only joint with a rigid end point of closure.
- *Articulation*: It has a bilateral articulation with the cranium, so both the joints must function together as a single unit.

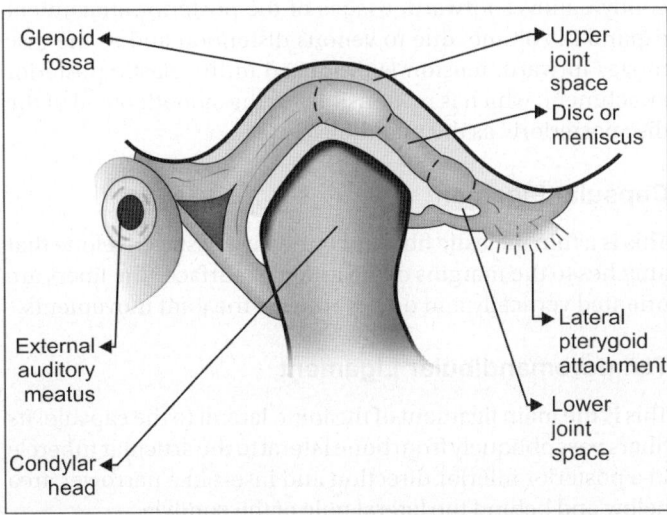

Figure 25.1 A sagittal section through the right TMJ showing the various components

The glenoid (mandibular) fossa is located at the inferior aspect of the squamous part of the temporal bone. The temporal component of TMJ is formed by the squamous portion of temporal bone. This portion of the temporal bone is made of a concave mandibular (glenoid) fossa. The articular eminence forms the anterior limit of the glenoid fossa and is convex in shape. Its most inferior aspect is called the summit or apex of the eminence. Normally, the roof of the fossa, the posterior slope of the articular eminence, and the eminence itself form an S shape when viewed in the sagittal plane. The most lateral aspect of the eminence consists of a protruberance called the articulate tubercule, which is a ligamentous attachment. The squamotympanic fissure and its medial extension, the petrotympanic fissure, form the posterior limit of the fossa. The middle portion of the roof of the fossa forms a small portion of the floor of the middle cranial fossa and only a thin layer of cortical bone separates the joint cavity from the intracranial subdural space. The spine of the sphenoid forms the medial limit of the fossa. The fossa depth varies, and the development of the articular eminence depends on the functional stimulus from the condyle. The fossa and the eminence develop during the first 3 years and mature by the age of 4, thus young infants lack a definite fossa and articular eminence.

All the aspects of the temporal components may be pneumatized with small air cells derived from the mastoid air cell complex.

The head or the condyle of the mandible forms the other osseous component of the joint. It forms the lower part of the bony joint. It is an ellipsoidal bar of bone connected to the mandibular ramus by a narrow neck. The condyle is approximately 20 mm long mediolaterally and 8–10 mm thick anteroposteriorly. The shape of the condyle varies; the superior aspect may be flattened, rounded or markedly convex, whereas the mediolateral contour is usually slightly convex. The extreme aspects of the condyle are called the medial pole and lateral poles. The long axis of the condyle is slightly rotated on the condylar neck such that the medial pole is angled posteriorly forming an angle of 15–33 degrees with the sagittal plane. The two condylar axis typically intersect near the anterior border of the foramen magnum in the submentovertex projection.

Most condyles have a pronounced ridge oriented mediolaterally on the anterior surface, marking the anteroinferior limit of the articulating area. This ridge is the upper limit of the pterygoid fovea, a small depression on the anterior surface at the junction of the condyle and the neck. This is the attachment site of the inferior head of the lateral pterygoid muscle this may be mistaken for an osteophyte (spur).

Radiographs of condyles of children may show little or no evidence of a cortical border as the mandibular and temporal components of the TMJ calcify by 6 months to 20 years of age.

The articular surfaces of the condyle and the fossa, including the eminence are covered with a white fibrocartilage. This is not visible radiographically.

The interarticular disc **(Figs 25.2A to C)** (meniscus) lies between the articular surfaces, and provides an interface for the condyle as it glides across the temporal bone. It is oval in shape and is made up of fibrous tissue. It divides the joint spaces into two synovial compartments, called the inferior (lower) and superior (upper) joint spaces. The disc is of varying thickness (concavo-convex structure biconcave shape), being the thinnest centrally and thicker at the margins. The disc is also thicker medially than laterally. The medial and lateral margins of the disc blend with the joint capsule. The thin central portion serves as an articulating cushion between the condyle and the articular eminence. The superior head of the lateral pterygoid muscle is inserted into the disc anteriorly, but there is no muscle attachment at

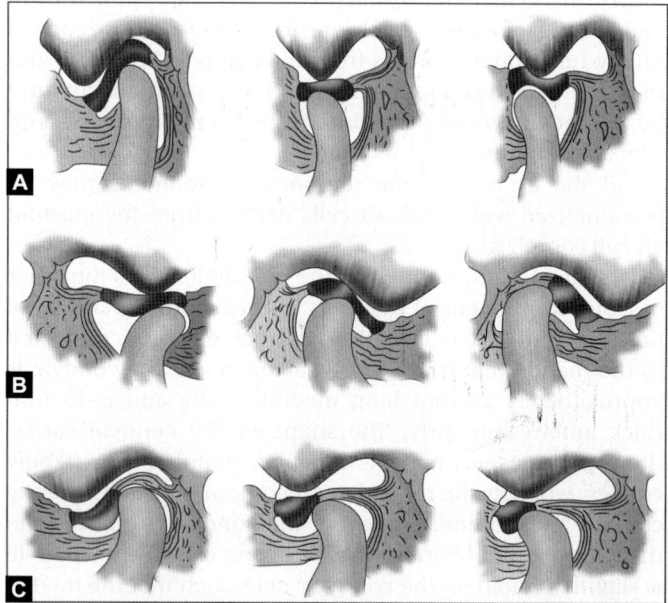

Figures 25.2A to C (A) Normal disc position in closed and open TMJ position; (B) Partially displaced disc; (C) Fully displaced disc

the posterior aspect of the disc. The posterior band attaches to the posterior retrodiscal tissues (posterior attachment). The junction between the posterior band and the posterior attachment usually lies within 10 degrees of vertical above the condylar head. The disc and posterior attachment are called the soft tissue component of the TMJ.

In the closed position of the jaws—apposition called centric, the disc occupies a position above the condyles, but when the mouth is opened, the condyles move downward and forward, and the disc moves forward and rotates so that the greater part of it is above and posterior to the condyle. Its thin central portion remains between the articulating convexities of the condylar head and the articular eminence. Laterally and medially the disc attaches to the condylar poles, and ensures passive movement of the disc with the condyle. There is no loss of contact between the condyle and the disc in any normal joint, irrespective to the degree of movement of the condyle. As the mandible opens, the condyle also rotates against the lower surface of the disc in the inferior joint space.

The disc is entirely made up of soft tissue and along with the cartilaginous coverings on the bone surface; it appears radiolucent on the radiograph and is known as the joint space, though it could be more accurate to call it cartilage space, as no actual empty space exists.

Posterior attachment (retrodiscal tissues), this consists of a bilaminar zone of vascularized and innervated loose fibroelastic tissue, which occupies the space behind the disc and the condyle. The superior lamina which is rich in elastin inserts into the posterior wall of the mandibular fossa. The superior lamina stretches and allows the disc to move forward with condylar translation. The inferior lamina attaches to the posterior surface of the condyle. The posterior attachment is covered with a synovial membrane that secretes synovial fluid, which lubricates the joint. As the condyle moves forward, tissues of the posterior attachment expand in volume, due to venous distention and as the disc moves forward, tension is produced in the elastic posterior attachment, which is responsible for the smooth recoil of the disc posteriorly as the mandible closes.

Capsular Ligament

This is a thin inelastic fibrous connective tissue envelope that attaches to the margins of the articular surface. The fibers are oriented vertically and do not restrain the joint movements.

Temporomandibular Ligament

This is the main ligament of the joint, lateral to the capsule. Its fibers pass obliquely from bone lateral to the articular tubercle in a posterior inferior direction and insert in a narrower area below and behind the lateral pole of the condyle.

Muscles of Mastication

The muscles of mastication are the paired masseter, medial and lateral pterygoid and the temporalis muscles. Mandibular movements towards the tooth contact position are performed by contraction of the masseter, temporalis and medial pterygoid muscles. Masseter contraction also contributes to moving the condylar head towards the anterior slope of the mandibular fossa. The posterior part of the temporalis contributes to mandibular retrusion, and unilateral contraction of the medial pterygoid contributes to a contralateral movement of the mandible. The masseter and the medial pterygoid muscles have their insertions at the inferior border of the mandibular angle. They join together to form a sling that cradles the mandible and produces the powerful forces required for chewing. The masseter is divided into a deep portion and a superficial portion.

The temporalis muscle is broadly attached to the lateral skull and has been divided into anterior, middle and posterior parts. The muscle fibers converge into a tendon that inserts on the coronoid process and anterior aspect of the mandibular ramus. The anterior and middle fibers are generally oriented in a straight line from their origin on the skull to their insertion on the mandible. The posterior part traverses anteriorly then curves around the anterior root of the zygomatic process before insertion.

The lateral pterygoid is the main protrusive and opening muscle of the mandible. It is arranged in parallel-fibered units whereas the other muscles are multipennated. This arrangement allows greater displacement and velocity in the lateral pterygoid and greater force generation in the jaw closing muscles. The lateral pterygoid is divided into two parts. The inferior part arises from the outer surface of the lateral pterygoid plate of the sphenoid and the pyramidal process of the palatine bone. The superior part originates from the greater wing of the sphenoid and the pterygoid ridge. The fibers of the upper and lower heads course posteriorly and laterally, fusing in front of the condyle. They insert into the anteromedial aspect of the condylar neck. Some of these fibers insert into the most anteromedial portion of the disc. The superior head of the lateral pterygoid is thought to be active during closing movements, and the inferior head is thought to be active during opening and protrusive movements. Translation of the condylar head onto the articular eminence is produced by contraction of the lateral pterygoid.

Accessory Masticatory Muscles

The diagastric muscle is a paired muscle with two bellies. The anterior belly attaches to the lingual aspect of the mandible at the parasymphysis and courses backward to insert into the round tendon attached to the hyoid bone. Contraction produces a depression and retropositioning of the mandible. The mylohyoid and geniohyoid muscles contribute to depressing the mandible when the infrahyoid muscles stabilize the hyoid bone during mandibular movement. These muscles may also contribute to retrusion of the mandible. The buccinator attaches inferiorly along the facial surface of the mandible, just behind the mental foramen and superiorly high on the alveolar surface behind the zygomatic process. The fibers are arranged horizontally. Anteriorly, fibers insert into mucosa, skin and lip. The buccinator helps position the cheek during chewing movements of the mandible.

Vascular Supply of Temporomandibular Structures

The external carotid artery is the main blood supply. The artery leaves the neck and crosses superiorly and posteriorly, embedded in the substance of the parotid gland. At the level of the condylar neck, the external carotid bifurcates into the superficial temporal artery and the internal maxillary artery. These two arteries supply the muscles of mastication and the TMJ. Arteries within the temporal bone or mandible may also send branches to the capsule.

Nerve Supply of Temporomandibular Structures

The masticatory structures are innervated primarily by the trigeminal nerve, but cranial nerves VII, IX, X and XI and cervical nerves 2 and 3 also contribute. The peripheral nerves synapse with nuclei in the brainstem that are associated with touch, proprioception and motor function. The large spinal trigeminal nucleus occupies a major part of the brainstem and extends to the spinal cord. The spinal trigeminal nucleus is thought to be the main site for the reception of impulses from the periphery involved in pain sensation. The mandibular division of the trigeminal supplies motor innervations to the muscles of mastication and the anterior belly of the digastric muscle. Branches of the auriculotemporal nerve supply the sensory innervation of the TMJ; this nerve arises from the mandibular division in the infratemporal fossa and sends branches to the capsule of the joint. The deep temporal and massetric nerves supply the anterior portion of the joint. These nerves are primarily motor nerves, but they contain sensory fibers distributed to the anterior part of the TMJ capsule. The autonomic nerve supply is carried to the joint by the auriculotemporal nerve and by nerves travelling along the superficial temporal artery.

Jaw jerk reflex: This reflex is thought to relate to the fine control of the jaw movements to take into account different consistencies of food.

Jaw opening reflex: This reflex results in an inhibition of the activity of the jaw closing muscles. It helps prevent injury when biting or chewing objects that may cause damage.

Condylar Movement (Fig. 25.3)

The movements of the joints are complicated and differ in the two compartments which are separated by the disc. When the joint is moved from occlusion position to the position of rest, the rotation of the condyle is purely a hinge movement, localized to the lower compartment only. On opening of the mouth from rest position, the disc slides forward on the eminence at the same time there is further hinge movement in the lower compartment. Thus, the sliding movement takes place in the upper compartment and the hinge movement takes place in the lower one. On closing the mouth, these movements are reversed, but the sliding and hinge movements are confined to the upper and lower compartments respectively. There are also slight rotatory movements as the jaw is moved to one or the other side.

The axis of rotation of the mandible is in line with the mandibular foramen, which gives ingress to the vessels and nerves, so that these structures are not subject to any tension during the various movements of the jaws.

The extent of normal condylar translation varies:
- Usually at maximal opening, the condyle moves down and forward to the summit of the articular eminence or slightly anterior to it. (The range is 2–5 mm posterior and 5–8 mm anterior to the crest of the eminence).
- Reduced condylar translation, where the condyle has little or no downward and forward movement and does not leave the mandibular fossa is seen in patients with reduced degree of mouth opening.
- Hypermobility of the joint may be suspected when the condyle translates more than 5 mm anterior to the eminence. This may permit anterior locking or dislocation of the condyle if a superior movement also occurs above and anterior to the summit of the articular eminence.

The diagnostic significance of:
- Mild or moderate condylar eccentricity is not clear.
- Markedly eccentric condylar positioning usually represents an abnormality. Inferior condylar positioning (widened joint space) is indicative of fluid or blood in the joint space.

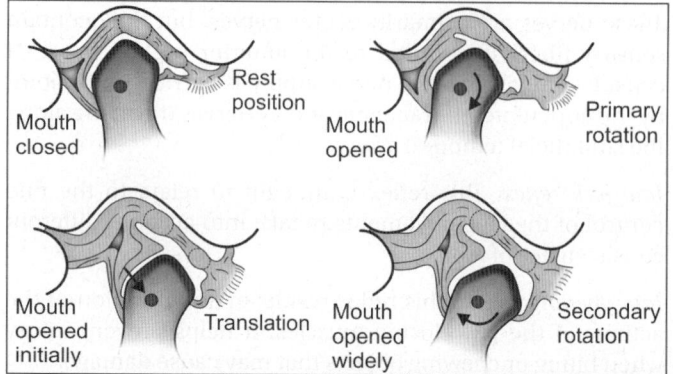

Figure 25.3 The rotary and translatory movements of the condyle during normal mouth opening

- Superior condylar positioning (decreased or no joint space, with osseous contact of joint components) may indicate loss, displacement or perforation of intracapsular soft tissue components.
- Posterior condylar positioning is seen in case of disc displacement.
- Anterior condylar positioning is seen in juvenile rheumatoid arthritis.

Normal Radiographic Appearance of the Temporomandibular Joint

On the lateral radiograph:
- The articular fossa appears as a concave recess with the eminentia articularis or zygomatic eminence at its anterior end.
- Posteriorly the tympanic plate of the temporal bone extends downwards, giving greater depth to the fossa.
- Behind the tympanic plate is an oval or rounded area of radiolucency, representing the external-auditory meatus and canal.
- The condyles occupy the anterior part of the concavity. The space between the condyles and the tympanic plate is wider than between the condyle and the eminence and between the condyle and the base of the fossa.
- The articular surface of the condyle is usually sharply convex. There is a flat beveled surface on the anterior aspect of the condyle, which corresponds to the site of approximation of the condyle to the posterior surface of the eminence.
- There are variations in the neck of the condyle. It may be straight and directed upwards and backwards in the same line as the posterior border of the ascending ramus of the mandible, or there may be a concavity in the neck of the condyle and the articular surface is directed upwards and slightly forwards. The length of the condylar process is variable and is sometimes accentuated by a deep concave sigmoid or mandibular notch in the posterior surface of the ramus.
- In the anteroposterior projection there is sometimes a concavity on the deep (medial) aspect of the neck of the condyle.

Radiographic examination of the temporomandibular joint is often difficult and despite the finest technical results, many a times no abnormality may be detected on a routine conventional radiograph.

DIAGNOSTIC IMAGING (TABLE 25.1)

When clinical presentation suggests a progressive pathologic condition of the TMJ, imaging should be a part of the assessment. Imaging is indicated for recent injury, sensory and motor abnormality, severe restriction in mandibular motion and acute alterations of the occlusion, degenerative changes of bone and disc displacement.

Table 25.1 Diagnostic terms and clinical criteria for temporomandibular disorders (adapted from McNeill C)

Diagnostic terms	Clinical criteria
Deviation in form (painless mechanical dysfunction or altered function due to irregularities or aberrations in form of the intracapsular soft and hard articular tissues)	Complaint of faulty or compromised joint mechanics Reproducible joint noise, usually at the same position during opening and closing Radiographic evidence of structural bony abnormality or loss of normal shape
Disc displacement with reduction (abrupt alteration or interference of the disc-condyle structural relation during mandibular translation with mouth opening and closing; from a closed mouth position, the "temporary" misaligned disc reduces or improves its structural relation with the condyle when mandibular translation occurs with mouth opening, which produces joint noise described as clicking or popping)	Pain (when present) is precipitated by joint movement Reproducible joint noise, usually at variable positions during opening and closing mandibular movements Soft-tissue imaging reveals displaced disc that improves its position during jaw opening. Clinical findings that may support the diagnosis: pain (when present) precipitated by joint movement; deviation during movement coinciding with a click, no restriction in mandibular movement (episodic and momentary catching of smooth jaw movements during mouth opening [< 35 mm] that self-reduces with voluntary mandibular repositioning)
Disc displacement without reduction (altered or misaligned disc-condyle structural relation that is maintained during mandibular translation)	Pain precipitated by function Marked limited mandibular opening Straight-line deviation to the affected side on opening Marked limited laterotrusion to the contralateral side Soft-tissue imaging reveals displaced disc without reduction. Clinical findings that may support the diagnosis: pain precipitated by forced mouth opening; history of clicking that ceases with the locking; pain with palpation of the affected joint; ipsilateral hyperocclusion
Synovitis or capsulitis (inflammation of the synovial lining or capsular lining)	Localized pain at rest exacerbated by function, especially with superior and posterior joint loading Limited range of motion secondary to pain T2-weighted MRI may show joint fluid
Osteoarthrosis (degenerative noninflammatory condition of the joint, characterized by structural changes of joint surfaces secondary to excessive straining of the remodeling mechanism)	Crepitus Limited range of motion causes deviation to the affected side on opening Radiographic evidence of structural bony change (subchondral sclerosis, osteophyte formation) and joint-space narrowing
Osteoarthritis (degenerative condition accompanied by secondary inflammation (synovitis) of the TMJ)	Same as for osteoarthritis, plus crepitus or multiple joint noises, pain with function due to inflammation, and point tenderness on palpation
Myofascial pain (regional dull aching pain and presence of localized tender spots [trigger points] in muscle, tendon, or fascia that reproduce pain when palpated and may produce a characteristic pattern of regional referred pain and/or autonomic symptoms on provocation)	Regional pain, usually dull Localized tenderness in firm bands of muscle and/or fascia Reduction in pain with local muscle anesthetic injection or vapocoolant spray and stretch of muscle trigger points
Myositis, delayed onset (painful condition due to intermittent overuse that results in interstitial inflammation)	Increased pain with mandibular movement Onset following prolonged or unaccustomed use (up to 48 hours afterward)
Myositis, generalized (constant, acutely painful, and generalized inflammation and swelling, usually of the entire muscle)	Pain usually acute in localized area Localized tenderness over entire region of the muscle Increased pain with mandibular movement Moderately to severely limited range of motion, due to pain and swelling Onset following injury or infection
Protective muscle splinting (restricted or guarded mandibular movement due to cocontraction of muscles as a means of avoiding pain caused by movement of the parts)	Severe pain with function but not at rest Marked limited range of motion without significant increase on passive stretch
Contracture (chronic resistance of a muscle to passive stretch, as a result of fibrosis of the supporting tendon, ligaments, or muscle fibers themselves)	Limited range of motion Unyielding firmness on passive stretch History of trauma or infection

MRI = magnetic resonance imaging; TMJ = temporomandibular joint.

Temporomandibular joints can be examined by using plain-film radiography, CBCT, tomography, arthrography, computerized tomography (CT), magnetic resonance imaging (MRI), single photon emission computed tomography, and radioisotope scanning.

As already mentioned, for majority of the cases diagnostic imaging has not proven to be a valuable test for directing treatment or for predicting outcome and long-term course.

- No differences were found in joint space narrowing in centric occlusion in symptomatic and asymptomatic patients by transcranial plain film radiography and tomography. A large variation exists in condylar position in plain film radiographic and tomographic studies making the condyle-fossa relationship and assessing disc position of little value in the diagnosis or treatment of TMD.
- In arthrography of the TMJ, radiopaque material is injected into the lower (sometimes upper) joint space under fluoroscopic guidance. Once the dye is in place, fluoroscopic recordings of the joint in motion may be made in order to assess the shape, location and function of the articular disc.
- Osteodegenerative joint disease may be studied by tomography.
- Computed tomography provides details for bony abnormalities and is an appropriate study when considering ankylosis, fractures, tumors of the bone and osteodegenerative disease.
- Magnetic resonance imaging has become the imaging method of choice to assess alterations in disc position in the open and closed positions. T2-weighted images may show a relationship between joint pain and joint effusion.

The typical MRI examination of the TMJ consists of both open and closed mouth views in an oblique sagittal plane, with the section oriented perpendicular to the long axis of the condyle. Images may also be obtained in the coronal plane which makes easier identification of the lateral or medial disc displacement.

The sagittal images are used to evaluate disc position with respect to the head of the condyle. The disc is considered in the normal position when the posterior band is superior to the condyle (twelve o'clock position) when the mouth is closed. In the open mouth views, the disc may be seen to be interposed between the condyle and the articular eminence (normal or reducing) or to remain anterior to the condyle (nonreducing).

Bone marrow abnormalities may also be detected by MRI. Abnormal signals on T2-weighted image from the condyle marrow, that is an increased signal indicated marrow edema, a reduced signal indicates marrow sclerosis or fibrosis. A combination of marrow edema and sclerosis signal in the condyle is most reliable for histological diagnosis of osteoradionecrosis.

Joint inflammation (e.g. pigmented villonodular synovitis) shows characteristic (almost pathognomonic) low signal because of hemorrhagic by products, on T1-weighted and T2-weighted MRI images.

Radioisotope scanning has been used to detect condylar hyperplasia and increase in metabolic activities, and shows a positive result in a joint that is undergoing physiological remodeling.

CBCT is also an important diagnostic aid for studying the bony components of the temporomandibular joint.

Arthrography

Arthrography of the TM joint is basically a method that will supply information on soft tissue state of the TM joint, especially the integrity and position of the disc and its posterior attachment. It also provides evidence of internal disc derangement or disc perforation.

This examination is most helpful in diagnosis of those cases in which little or no bony damage is evident on prearthrographic tomograms and in which clinical evidence (e.g. joint clicking or popping, painful limitation of opening or joint locking) suggests derangement of the disc.

It also helps in differentiating disc derangement from other nonbony problems such as capsulitis, myofascitis and myofacial pain dysfunction syndrome.

Temporomandibular joint arthrography is performed by catheterizing the upper and lower joint spaces and injecting 0.5–1 mL of radiographic contrast media first into the lower space and then into the upper space. The most commonly used contrast media are iodine compounds.

A series of radiographs are taken following joint space opacification with the jaws closed and in graded stages of opening.

The disc appears as a radiolucent void between two opaque areas of contrast media because there is no known normal situation where a communication exists between the superior and inferior joint spaces.

Opacification of both the joint spaces following injection of only one denotes a pathological condition:

Indications

- Long standing TMJ pain dysfunction unresponsive to simple treatments
- Persistent history of locking
- Limited opening of unknown etiology.

Diagnostic Information Provided

- Dynamic information on the position of the joint components and disc as they move in relation to one another.
- Static images of the joint components with the mouth closed and with the mouth open. Any anterior or anteromedial displacement of the disc can be observed.
- The integrity of the disc, i.e. presence of any perforations.

Limitations and Disadvantages

- Very painful
- Not indicated when the patient is hypersensitive to iodine or the contrast medium
- Iodine may bring about fibrosis
- Very strict asepsis has to be maintained
- Capsule may rupture if too much contrast media is injected
- Contraindicated in acute joint infection.

Arthroscopy

Arthroscopy of the TM joint is a procedure where direct visualization of the internal joint structure can be done.

This aids in doing surgical procedures and biopsy procedures, which may be performed under visual control.

Advantages

- Safe procedure
- Direct visualization yields information not achievable by other techniques
- Minimal postoperative complications
- Color change in inflammed tissues is clearly seen
- Biopsy and surgical procedures can be easily visualized
- It allows certain interventional procedures to be performed
  - Washing out the joint with saline
  - Introduction of steroids directly into the joint
  - Division of adhesions
  - Removal of loose bodies from within the joint

Arthroscopy is usually considered as the last line of investigation before full surgical exploration of the joint is carried out.

Disorders of the temporomandibular joint are abnormalities that interfere with the normal form or function of the joint. These disorders include dysfunction of the articular disc and associated ligament and muscles, joint arthritis and inflammatory lesions, neoplasms, and growth or developmental abnormalities (Tables 25.2 to 25.5).

DEVELOPMENT DISORDERS OF THE TEMPOROMANDIBULAR JOINT

These may be broadly categorized as anomalies in the form and size of joint components. The most striking changes are usually seen in the condyle and although the temporal component is also deformed, it often remodels to accommodate the abnormal condyle.

Table 25.2 First classification of TM joint disorders by C Weldon Bell

- Masticatory muscle disorders
  - Protective muscle splinting
  - Masticatory muscle spasm (MPD)
  - Masticatory muscle inflammation (myositis)
- Derangement of TMJ
  - Incoordination
  - Anterior disc displacement with reduction (clicking)
  - Anterior disc displacement without reduction (mechanical restriction, closed lock)
- Extrinsic trauma
  - Traumatic arthritis
  - Dislocation
  - Fracture
  - Internal disc derangement
  - Myositis
  - Myospasm
  - Tendonitis
- Degenerative joint disease
  - Noninflammatory phase (arthrosis)
  - Inflammatory phase (osteoarthritis)
- Inflammatory joint disease
  - Rheumatoid arthritis
  - Infective arthritis
  - Metabolic arthritis
- Chronic mandibular hypomobility
  - Ankylosis (fibrous and osseous)
  - Fibrosis of articular capsule
  - Contracture of elevator muscles
    - Myostatic contracture
    - Myofibrotic contracture
  - Internal disc derangement (closed lock)
- Growth disorders of the joint
  - Developmental disorders
  - Acquired disorders
  - Neoplastic disorders

Condylar Hyperplasia (Figs 25.4 to 25.6)

Definition

This results in the enlargement and/or deformity of the condylar head. It may be due to overactive cartilage or persistent cartilaginous rests, increasing the thickness of the entire cartilaginous and precartilaginous layers.

Clinical Features

- More common in males before the age of 20 years.
- The condition is usually unilateral and may be accompanied with some degree of hyperplasia of the ipsilateral mandible.
- The condition is self-limiting and is usually arrested with the termination of skeletal growth.

Table 25.3 Second classification of TM joint disorders

Intracapsular
- Degenerative joint changes
  - Osteoarthritis
    - Primary
    - Secondary
- Inflammatory (diffuse collagen diseases)
  - Juvenile rheumatoid arthritis (Still's disease)
  - Psoriatic arthritis
  - Systemic lupus erythematosus
  - Sjögren's syndrome
  - Systemic sclerosis
  - Polymyalgia rheumatica
  - Necrotizing vasculitis
  - Ankylosing spondylitis
  - Sinovitis
- Infection
  - Pyogenic or septic arthritis (spread from contiguous sites; skin, teeth, parotid, ear or hematogenous)
    - Staphylococci
    - Streptococci
    - Pneumococci
    - Gonococci
  - Gonorrhea
  - Syphilis
  - Tuberculosis
  - Actinomycosis
  - Rheumatic arthritis (rheumatic fever)
  - Osteomyelitis
  - Arthritis associated with secondary bowel disease
  - Secondary to hepatitis B infection
- Development
  - Condylar hyperplasia
  - Condylar hypoplasia
  - Agenesis of the condyle
  - Exostosis of the condyle
  - Double condyle
  - Juvenile arthrosis
  - Coronoid hyperplasia
- Traumatic
  - Effusion
  - Trauma to the disc
  - Trauma to the developing condyle or growth center
  - Trauma to the ligaments
  - Trauma to the condyle with
    - Subluxation
    - Dislocation
    - Dislocation with displacements
  - Ankylosis of the joint
    - Pseudo
    - Fibrous
    - Bony
  - Foreign body in joint space
    - Synovial chondromatosis
    - Chondrocalcinosis
- Trauma to the muscles
  - Internal derangement
    - Derangement of condyle—disc complex
  - Disc displacement

Contd...

Contd...
- Disc dislocation with reduction
- Disc dislocation without reduction
- Structural incompatibility of the articular surfaces
- Adhesions
- Alterations in the form of articulating surfaces
- Disc displacement with perforation
  - Fracture
- Metabolic
  - Crystal induced
    - Gout
    - Calcium pyrophosphate dihydrate chondrocalcinosis (pseudogout)
    - Oxalate (oxalosis)
  - Biochemical abnormalities
    - Amyloidosis
    - Scurvy
    - Specific enzyme deficiency (Falry's and Faber's syndrome)
    - Hyperlipoproteinemias
    - Mucopolysaccharidoses
    - Wilson's disease (hepatolenticular degeneration)
    - Gaucher's disease and other histiocytosis disorders
    - Hyperparathyroidism
    - Immunodeficiency diseases
    - Osteoporosis (localized/generalized)
    - Paget's disease
- Neoplasia
  - Benign
    - Osteoma
    - Chondroma
    - Osteochondroma
    - Osteochondromatosis
    - Fibromyxoma
    - Giant cell tumor
    - Synovioma
  - Malignant
    - Osteosarcoma
    - Chondrosarcoma
    - Synoviosarcoma
    - Carcinoma
    - Metastatic lesions
    - Lymphomas
- Neuropathic disorders
  - Charcot's joints
  - Reflex sympathetic dystrophy
- Drug Induced
  - Steroid

Extracapsular
- Psychophysiologic (MPDS)
- Costen's syndrome
- Myofacial pain
- Myofascial pain
- Myositis
- Myositis ossificans
- Iatrogenic
- Traumatic
- Those referred from local dental origin
- Infection
- Otologic
- Neoplastic

Table 25.4 Third classification of TM joint disorders (adapted from McNeill)

Diagnostic category	Diagnosis
Cranial bones (including the mandible)	Congenital and developmental disorders—aplasia, hypoplasia, hyperplasia, dysplasia (e.g. 1st and 2nd branchial arch anomalies, hemifacial microsomia, Pierre Robin syndrome, Treacher Collins syndrome, condylar hyperplasia, prognathism, fibrous dysplasia)
Temporomandibular joint disorders	Deviation in form
	Disc displacement (with reduction; without reduction) Dislocation Inflammatory conditions (synovitis, capsulitis) Arthritides (osteoarthrosis polyarthritides) Ankylosis (fibrous, bony) Neoplasia
Masticatory muscle disorders	Myofascial pain
	Myositis Spasm Protective splinting Contracture

Table 25.5 Fourth classification of TMJ disorders (adapted from Clark GT et al)

Diagnostic category	Diagnosis
Muscle and facial forceful jaw closure	Myalgia, muscle contracture, disorders splinting, hypertrophy, spasm, dyskinesia, habit, myositis (bruxism)
TMJ disorders	Disc condyle incoordination, osteoarthritis, disc condyle restriction, inflammatory polyarthritis, open dislocation, traumatic articular disease, arthralgia
Disorders of mandibular mobility	Ankylosis, adhesions (intracapsular), fibrosis of muscle tissue, coronoid elongation-hypermobility of TMJ
Disorders of maxillomandibular growth	Masticatory muscle hypertrophy/atrophy, neoplasia (muscle, maxillomandibular or condylar), maxillomandibular or condylar hypoplasia/hyperplasia

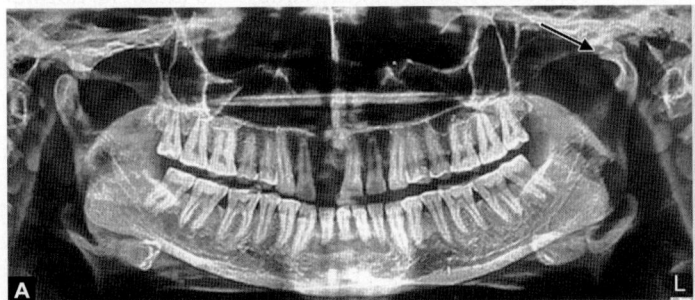
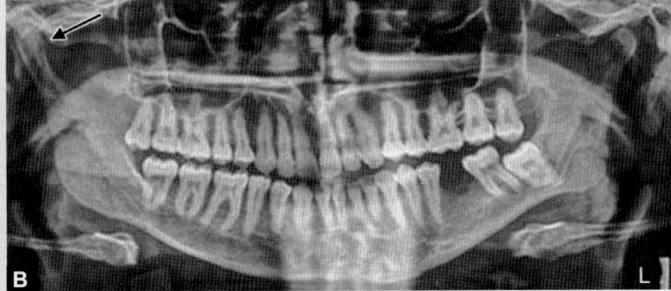
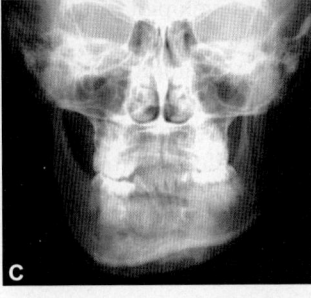

Figures 25.4A to C Condylar hyperplasia: (A) Hypertrophic left condyle is elongated and altered in shape as compared to right side. Constriction at the neck of the condyle. No growth, resorption, sclerosis seen; (B) Right condylar hyperplasia with elongation of the right condylar neck and condylar head compared with left condyle. Shift of the mandibular midline towards left side. Deepening of the antegonial notch of left side compared to right; (C) PA mandible showing abnormal, growth of mandibular condyle

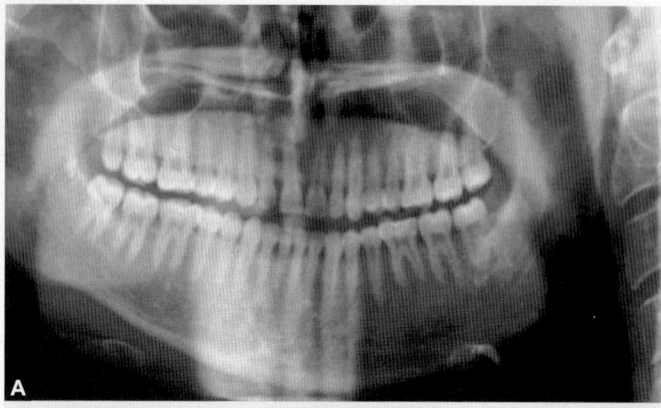

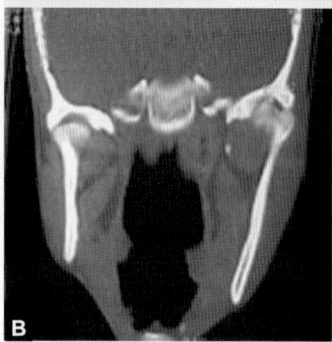
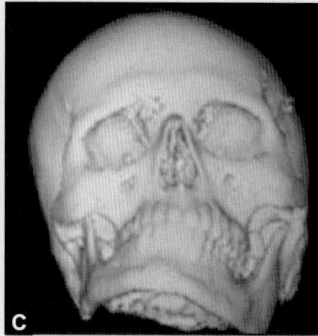

Figures 25.5A to C Left condylar hyperplasia: (A) Panoramic radiograph shows increased length of the condylar neck on the left side, hyperplasia of left condyle. Deep sigmoid notch on the left side. CT scan: (B) Coronal section; (C) 3D view shows—asymmetry of the mandible with increased length of the condylar neck on the left side and hyperplasia of left condyle

- The condition may progress slowly or rapidly, producing mandibular asymmetry. The chin may be deviated to the unaffected side and/or there may be an increase in the vertical dimension of the ramus, mandibular body or the alveolar process of the affected side.
- The patient may have a posterior open bite on the affected side.
- The patient may complain of limited and/or deviated mandibular opening, caused by the restricted opening due to the enlarged condyle.
- A bilateral hyperplasia of the condyle would produce an anterior crossbite, with an obtuse mandibular angle.

Radiographic Features

- The condyle may appear relatively normal but symmetrically enlarged.
- Sometimes it may have an altered shape—conical, spherical, elongated, lobulated or irregular in outline.
- There may be an elongation of the condylar head and neck with a compensating forward bend, forming an inverted L.

- In the anteroposterior plane the condylar neck may appear elongated, thick and laterally bent.
- The cortical thickness and trabecular pattern of the enlarged condyle is normal (this distinguishes it from condylar neoplasm).
- The glenoid fossa may be enlarged, usually at the expense of the posterior slope of the articular eminence.
- The ramus and mandibular body of the affected side may also be enlarged, resulting in a depression of the inferior border at the midline, where the enlarged side joins the contralateral normal mandible.
- The affected ramus may have an increased vertical height and may be thicker in the anteroposterior dimension. This prevents the occlusion of the posterior teeth.
- The angle of the jaw is right angled or more obtuse than in the normal cases.

Differential Diagnosis

- Condylar tumor (osteochondroma)—It is more irregular in shape. Surface irregularities and continued growth even after cessation of skeletal growth tends the diagnosis more in favor of a tumor.
- Condylar osteoma or large osteophyte that occurs in chronic degenerative joint disease may simulate condylar hyperplasia.

Management

Orthodontics with orthognathic surgery is the best line of treatment.

Condylar Hypoplasia (Fig. 25.7)

Definition

This occurs due to failure of the condyle to attain its normal size because of developmental and congenital abnormalities or acquired disease that affect growth. The condyle may be small but its morphology remains normal. The condition may be inherited or may appear spontaneously. Sometimes the cause may be birth injury or an intra-articular inflammatory lesion. It may be unilateral or bilateral.

Clinical Features

- This is a component of mandibular growth deficiency and is often associated with an under developed ramus and (occasionally) mandibular body.
- Congenital abnormalities may be unilateral or bilateral and are usually manifestations of a more general condition (e.g. micrognathia, Treacher Collins syndrome). They may also be associated with congenital defects of the ear and zygomatic arch.
- Developmental abnormalities that manifest during birth are usually unilateral.

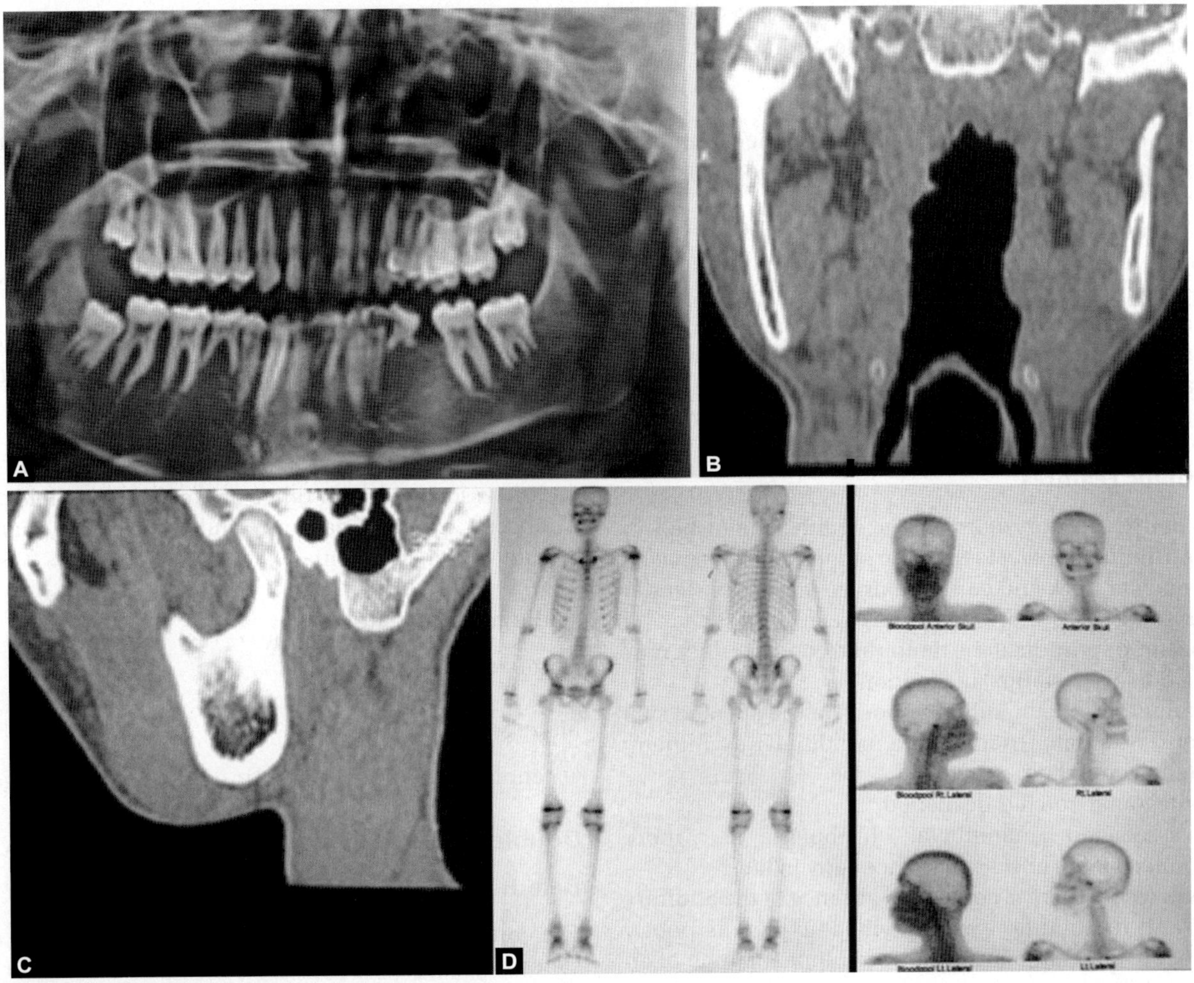

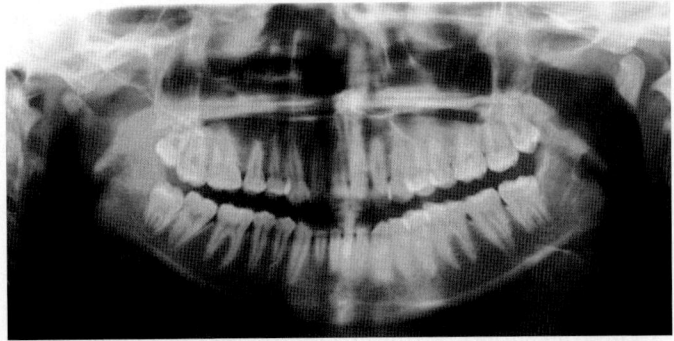

Figures 25.6A to D Condylar hyperplasia: (A) Panoramic radiograph shows increase in the height of right ramus. Elongation of right condyle. Reduction of the antegonial notch on right side. CT scan: (B) Coronal; (C) Sagittal shows a symmetry of the mandible. The right hemimandible is larger than the left side. The right and left coronoid and condylar processes are normal in morphology; (D) Bone scan with 99 MTc- MDP shows increased radiotracer uptake in the region of the right maxilla and infraorbital region

Figure 25.7 Condylar hypoplasia of left condyle which appears smaller than the right and out of the glenoid fossa, with shortening of the neck

- There is an elongation of the body of the mandible on the unaffected side and a flat appearance of the face.
- The body is short, with unerupted and impacted molars, leading to malocclusion.
- There may be deficiency of some parts of the adjacent auditory apparatus. The external ear may be small, deformed, partially or completely absent.
- Acquired abnormalities are the result of damage during growth period from sources such as therapeutic radiation or infection that diminish or prevent further condylar growth and development.
- Patients will have mandibular asymmetry and symptoms of temporomandibular joint dysfunction.

- The chin is deviated to the affected side and the mandible deviates to the affected side during mandibular movements.
- In case of bilateral hypoplasia:
  - There is a symmetrical lack of growth of the mandible.
  - Micrognathia with the chin retruded to the level of the hyoid bone.
  - The posterior growth of the ramus is affected, the length of the mandibular body is diminished and the ramus does not increase in height to open the space between the upper and the lower jaws, thus leading to disturbances of eruption and malocclusion.
- Degenerative joint disease is a long-term sequelae.

Radiographic Features

- The condyle appears normal but slightly diminished in size and the mandibular fossa is also proportionately smaller.
- The condylar neck and coronoid process are very slender and in some cases shortened or elongated.
- The posterior portion of the ramus and condylar neck may have a dorsal (posterior) inclination.
- The ramus and the mandibular body on the affected side may also be small, resulting in a mandibular asymmetry and dental crowding.
- The antegonial notch is deepened.
- The associated mandibular hypoplasia is more pronounced if the effect takes place early in life.
- In cases where there is congenital absence of the auditory canal and the middle ear, the tympanic plate is poorly developed, so that the articular fossa appears to be of an increased size.
- In cases of bilateral hypoplasia, all the above features are seen bilaterally.

Differential Diagnosis

- Condylar destruction from juvenile rheumatoid arthritis may appear similar. A survey of the other joints or testing for rheumatoid factor will help in the diagnosis.
- Changes in the condylar morphology in severe degenerative joint disease or other arthritic conditions have a similar appearance, but arthritic disease will not cause mandibular hypoplasia of the affected side unless it occurs during the period of growth and other signs of arthritis are usually visible in the affected joint.
- Changes in the condylar morphology in tuberculosis (**Figs 25.8A to E**).

Management

Orthognathic surgery, bone grafts and orthodontic therapy when required.

Agenesis of the Condyle (Fig. 25.9)

Definition

It may be caused due to various factors and is associated with hemifacial microsomia, Goldenhar syndrome and Hallermann-Streiff syndrome.

Clinical Features

- It is a rare condition and may occur unilaterally or bilaterally.
- There are free movements (eccentric movements) of the joint, with an anterior open bite, asymmetry of the face, altered occlusion and inability to masticate.
- In case of unilateral involvement, the mandible shifts to the affected side.
- It is associated with other anomalies like; defective and absent external ear, an underdeveloped mandibular ramus or microstomia.

Radiographic Features

Absence of the condyle.

Management

Osteoplasty may be advocated in case of severe derangements.

Double Condyle (Bifid Condyle) (Figs 25.10A to D)

Definition

The condyle may have a vertical depression, notch or deep cleft in the center of the head seen in the frontal or sagittal plane, or there may be an actual duplication of the condyle resulting in the appearance of a double or bifid condylar head. It may result due to an obstructed blood supply or other embryopathy, or due to trauma where it may be a result of a longitudinal linear fracture of the condyle.

Clinical Features

- The condition may be unilateral or bilateral.
- It is usually asymptomatic and discovered as an incidental finding in panoramic views or anteroposterior projections.
- Some patients may give signs and symptoms of temporomandibular dysfunction, like limitation of opening of mouth, a mild deviation with limited lateral movements, joint noises and pain.

Radiographic Features

- A depression or a notch may be present on the superior condylar surface, giving an anteroposterior silhouette of a heart shape.

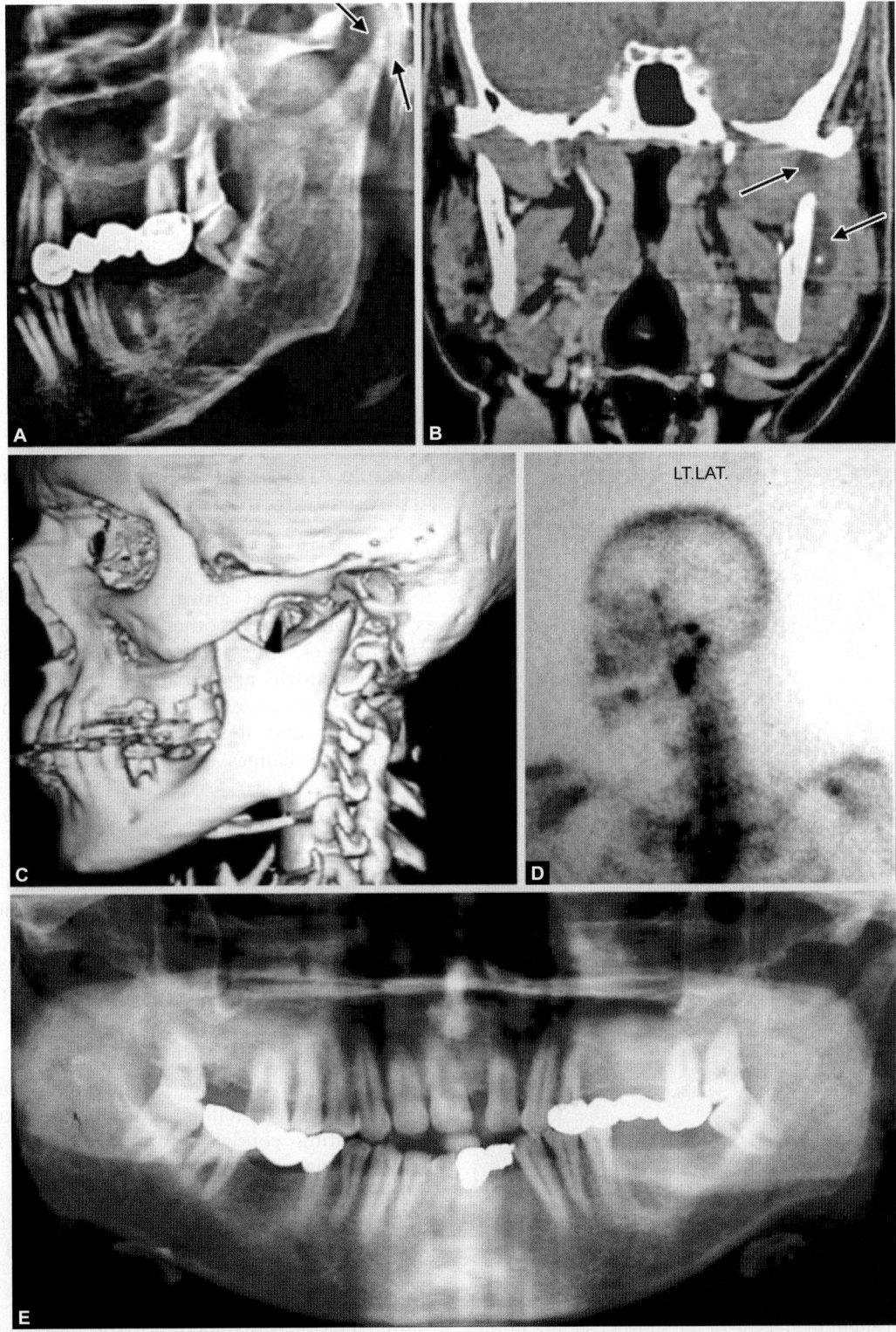

Figures 25.8A to E (A) Part of the panoramic radiograph showing resorption of the condylar head. The patient gave positive history of tuberculosis; (B) Coronal CT of the same patient, showing abscess formation (tuberculous) in the left TMJ with infectious destruction of the joint; (C) 3D CT of the same patient, showing the resorbed condyle due to tuberculous infection; (D) Bone scan shows increase uptake in the left ramus and condylar region; (E) The patient was started on Anti-Koch's therapy. The patient after 6 months showed remission of the swelling, clicking and trismus. Panoramic view revealed bone apposition seen on the left condyle

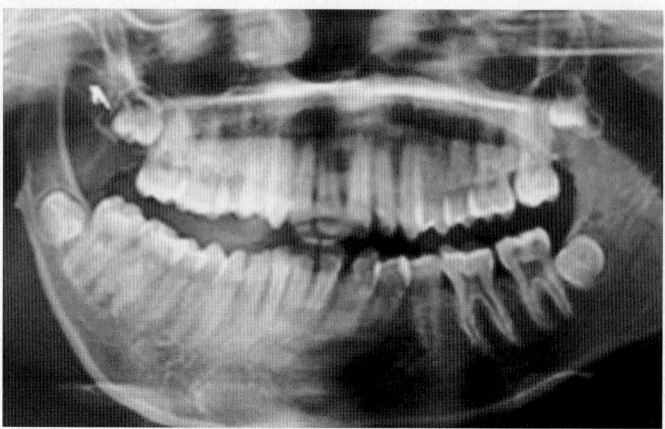

Figure 25.9 Agenesis of the condyle, panoramic radiograph showing absence of the condyle, ramus on the right side

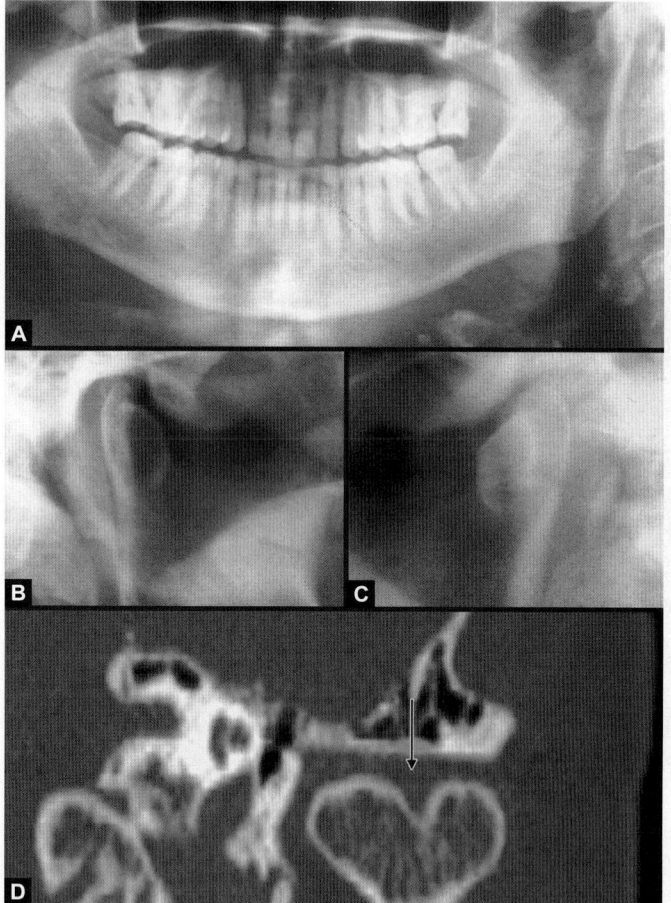

Figures 25.10A to D Bifid condyle: (A) Panoramic; (B and C) Cropped view showing well-defined linear vertical radiopaque line is seen running downwards from the middle of the superior surface of the condylar head bilaterally giving the appearance of double condyles. There is depression on the superior part of the head of both right and left condyles giving the appearance of double condyles; (D) CT Scan showing bifid condyle

- In severe cases a duplicate condylar head may be present in the mediolateral plane.
- The mandibular fossa may remodel to accommodate the altered condylar morphology.

Differential Diagnosis

- A slight medial depression on the superior condylar surface may be considered a normal variant (the point at which the depth of the depression signifies a bifid condyle is unclear).
- Vertical fracture through the condylar head.

Management

Treatment is not indicated unless pain and/or functional impairment is present.

Juvenile Arthrosis (Boeing's Arthrosis, Arthrosis Deformans Juvenilis)

Definition

This is a condylar growth disturbance which manifests as hypoplasia and other characteristic morphological abnormalities. This differs from hypoplasia in that the affected condyle at one time was normal and became abnormal during growth. Juvenile arthrosis may be unilateral or bilateral and it predisposes the TMJ to secondary degenerative changes.

Clinical Features

- It affects children and adolescents during the period of mandibular growth, and is more common in females.
- Usually the patient has no symptoms and it may be an incidental finding on the panoramic projection.
- The patient may present with mandibular asymmetry and signs and symptoms of TMJ dysfunction or both.

Radiographic Features

- The condylar head has a typical toadstool appearance, with marked flattening and apparent elongation of the articulating condylar surface and dorsal (posterior) inclination of the condyle and neck.
- The condylar neck may be shortened or even absent, with the condyle resting on the upper margin of the ramus.
- The articulating surface of the temporal component is often flattened.
- There is progressive shortening of the ramus on the affected side with depening of the antegonial notch, which indicates mandibular hypoplasia.
- In long standing cases, superimposed degenerative changes may be present.

Differential Diagnosis

- Developmental hypoplasia of the condyle.
- Destruction of the anterior portion of the condylar head from rheumatoid arthritis and severe degenerative joint disease.
- Severe condylar degeneration after orthognathic surgery or joint surgery may simulate juvenile arthrosis.

Management

Orthognathic surgery and orthodontic therapy may be required to correct the mandibular asymmetry.

Coronoid Hyperplasia (Figs 25.11A to E)

Definition

This is an elongation of the coronoid process which may be:
- Developmental
  - Unilateral
  - Bilateral
- Acquired (may be a response to restricted condylar movement caused by abnormalities such as ankylosis)
  - Unilateral
  - Bilateral.

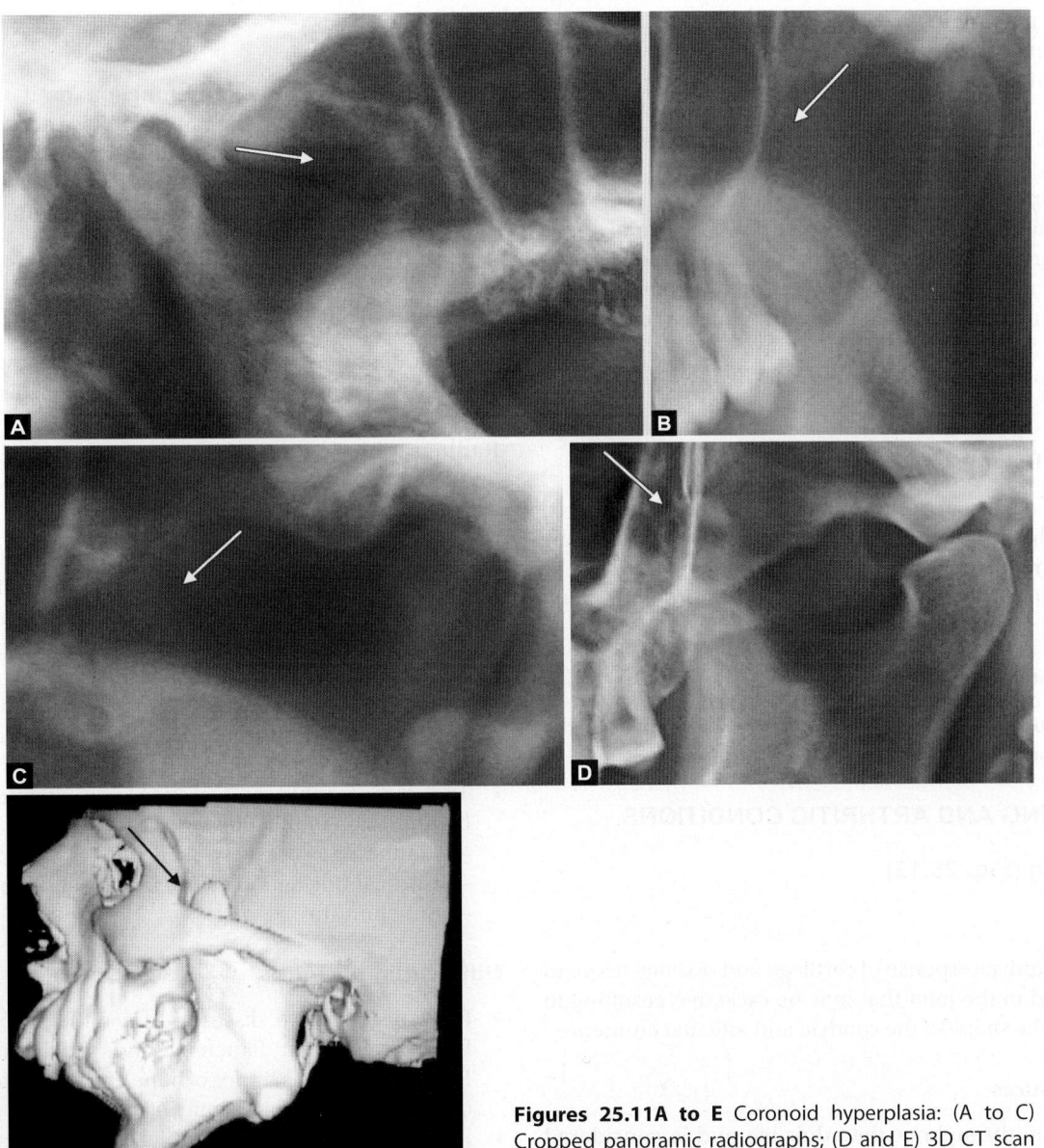

Figures 25.11A to E Coronoid hyperplasia: (A to C) Cropped panoramic radiographs; (D and E) 3D CT scan showing coronoid hyperplasia

Clinical Features

- Bilateral developmental coronoid hyperplasia is more common in males, commencing at the onset of puberty. A case of a 3-year-old has also been reported.
- Patients complain of progressive inability to open the mouth and may have an apparent closed lock.
- The condition is painless.

Radiographic Features

- This is best seen on the panoramic, waters and lateral tomographic views and CT scan.
- It is very important to include the image of the coronoid in all images taken for TMJ (especially in cases where there is inability to open the mouth). An axial CT image with the patient in a wide-open position is useful in establishing coronoid interference to opening.
- The coronoid appears elongated and the tip extends at least 1 cm above the inferior rim of the zygomatic arch (this may impinge on the medial surface of the zygomatic arch during opening, restricting condylar translation).
- The coronoid process may have a large but normal shape or may curve anteriorly and may appear very radiopaque.
- The posterior surface of the zygomatic process of the maxilla may be remodeled to accommodate the enlarged coronoid process during function.
- The radiographic appearance of the TMJ is usually normal.

Differential Diagnosis

- Osteoma or osteochondroma should be differentiated from unilateral coronoid hyperplasia. Tumors usually have an irregular shape.
- Other causes of trismus; soft tissue abnormalities and ankylosis.

Management

Treatment consists of osteotomy or surgical removal of the coronoid process and postoperative physiotherapy.

REMODELING AND ARTHRITIC CONDITIONS

Remodeling (Fig. 25.12)

Definition

This is an adaptive response of cartilage and osseous tissue to forces applied to the joint that may be excessive, resulting in alteration of the shape of the condyle and articular eminence.

Clinical Features

- This occurs throughout the adult life and is considered abnormal only if accompanied by clinical signs and

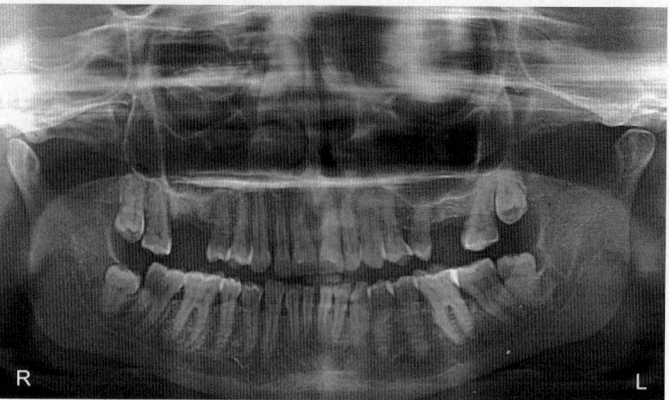

Figure 25.12 Flat condyle as seen on the panoramic radiograph

symptoms of pain or dysfunction or if the degree of remodeling seen on the radiograph is very severe.
- The clinical signs are usually related to the soft tissue components, associated muscles or ligaments. The accompanying internal derangement of the disc may be a factor.
- The adaptive response may result in the flattening of the curved joint surfaces, which effectively distributes the forces over a greater surface area.
- Remodeling may be unilateral and does not necessarily serve as a precursor to degenerative joint disease.

Radiographic Features

- These are seen affecting the condyle, temporomandibular component or both.
- The radiographic changes first occur on the anterosuperior surface of the condyle and posterior slope of the articular eminence. The lateral aspect of the joint is affected in the early stages and the central and medial aspects become involved as the remodeling progresses.
- The number of trabeculae also increases, increasing the density of subchondral cancellous bone (sclerosis), this is to better resist the applied forces.
- The radiographic appearance may include one or a combination of the following:
  - Flattening
  - Cortical thickening of articulating surfaces
  - Subchondral sclerosis.

Differential Diagnosis

- Early degenerative disease—It is difficult to differentiate from severe joint flattening and subchondral sclerosis. Radiographic appearance of bone erosions, osteophytes, loss of joint space are signs signifying degenerative joint disease.
- It is known that microscopic changes of degeneration occur before they can be detected radiographically.

Management

No treatment is indicated unless there are clinical signs and symptoms. Treatment is directed to relieve stress on the joint, by finding out the cause and/or such splint therapy.

DEGENERATIVE JOINT DISEASE (DJD)

Osteoarthritis (Figs 25.13 to 25.16)

Definition

This is a noninflammatory disorder of the joints characterized by:

- Joint deterioration, loss of articular cartilage and bone erosion. More common in acute disease.
- *Proliferation*: This is characterized by new bone formation at the articular surface and in the subchondral region. More common in chronic disease.

Usually a variable combination of the above-mentioned two changes occurs, sometimes one aspect may predominate.

Degenerative joint diseases (DJD) occurs when the ability of the joint to adapt to excessive forces (remodel) is exceeded. Though the etiology is unknown a number of factors play an important role, including:

- Acute trauma
- Hypermobility
- Loading of the joint (parafunction)
- Internal derangement (this factor is controversial)

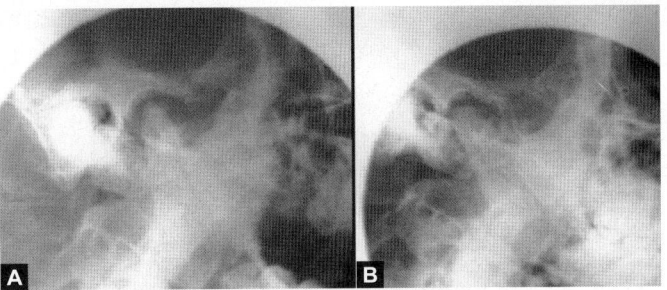

Figures 25.13A and B Transcranial view left TM joint in: (A) Open; (B) Close mouth positions show irregular bone loss and loss of cortical lining over the condylar head on right side with reactive bone formation over the glenoid fossa. Minimal movement of the right condylar head during mouth opening

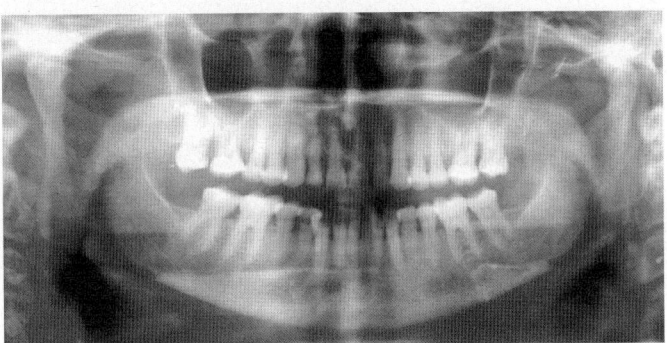

Figure 25.14 Panoramic radiograph showing mild flattening of both condyles in the anterosuperior aspect, indicative of early arthritic changes

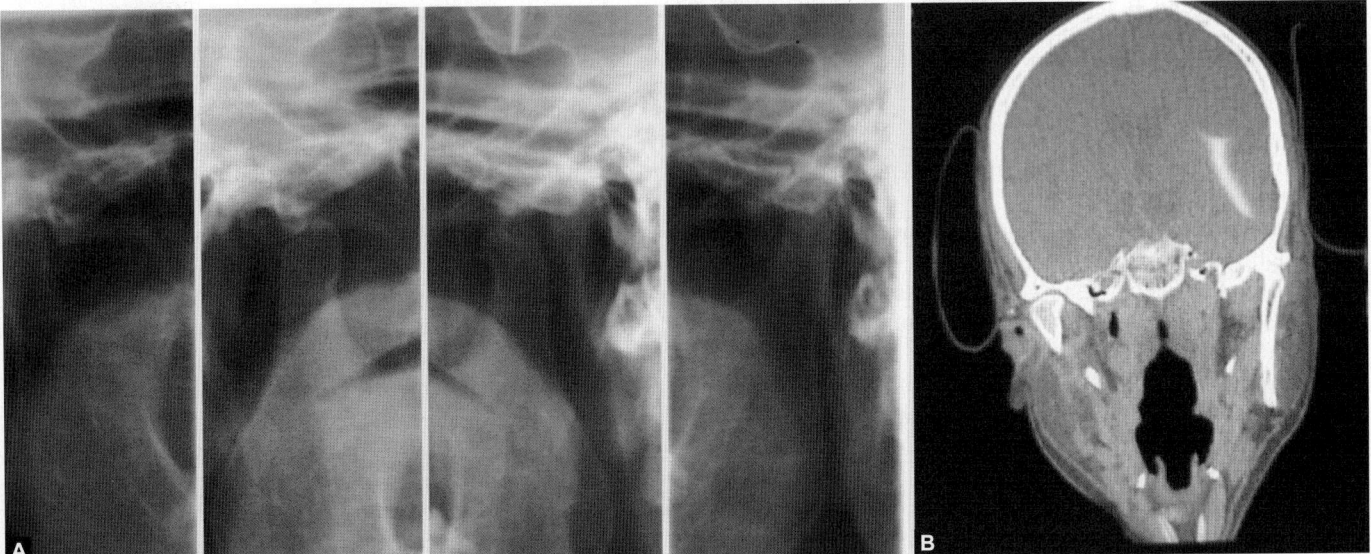

Figures 25.15A and B Osteoarthritis: (A) Panoramic TMJ showing widening of the posterior joint space on the left side. Erosion on the posterior aspect of the condyle. Osteophyte formation on the anterior aspect of the condyle. Normal forward translation while opening; (B) Coronal CT scan shows decreased left joint space, flattening, sclerosis and osteophyte formation on the articular surface of left condyle. Normal right TM joint. Features suggestive of osteoarthritis

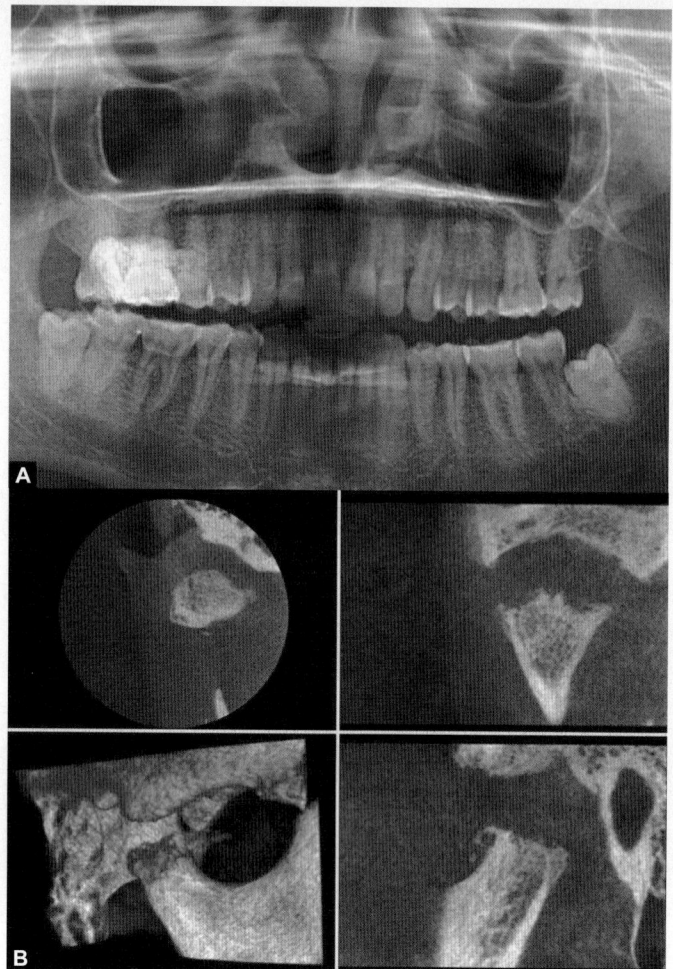

Figures 25.16A and B Temporomandibular (TMJ) osteoarthritis: (A) Panoramic radiograph; (B) CBCT sections showing extensive resorption of the condylar head

DJD may be categorized into different types:
- According to depth:
  - *Shallow*: The lesion of the joint surface is velvet like to slightly scalloped in nature.
  - *Deep*: The lesion results due to loss of substance in the soft tissues or in the region of the underlying hard structures.
- *According to etiology*:
  - *Primary*: This is generally described as a condition due to wear and tear and is more common with increasing age (more than 50 years of age).
  - *Secondary*: Here the joint changes occur in response to recognizable local or systemic factors (Developmental Perthes' disease; *Metabolic*: Wilson's disease, chondrocalcinosis, hemachromatosis, alkaptonuria, traumatic; *Endocrinal*: Acromegaly, gout; *Others*: Hemophilia, sickle cell anemia, etc.). This is more common in the younger patients.

Clinical Features

- This may occur at any age, and is more often found in the female population.
- The disease may be asymptomatic or the patient may complain of signs and symptoms of TMJ dysfunction which include, pain on palpation and movement, joint noises (crepitus), limited range of motion and muscle spasm.
- The onset of symptoms may be sudden or gradual and they even disappear spontaneously, only to return in recurring cycles.
- It has been reported in some studies that the disease may burn out or markedly decrease in severity over a long period of time.
- Presence of Ely cysts, which are not true cysts, but areas of degeneration that contain fibrous tissue, granulation tissue and osteoid.

Radiographic Features

- Signs of previous remodeling, such as flattening and subchondral sclerosis may be evident or they may be obscured by the degenerative changes.
- Degenerative joint disease (DJD) may have a spectrum of appearance ranging from substantial subchondral sclerosis and osteophyte formation (proliferative component) to extensive erosions (degenerative component).
- In maximal intercuspation position, the joint space may appear narrow or absent, which correlates with internal derangement. Perforation of the disc or posterior attachment, resulting in bone to bone contact of the joint components is common.
- There may be loss of cortex or erosions of the articulating surfaces of the condyle and/or the temporal component.
- Sometimes small, round, radiolucent areas with irregular margins surrounded by a varying area of increased density are visible deep to the articulating surfaces, these are called Ely cysts.
- The patient may have an anterior open bite in severe cases of DJD.
- As the disease progresses, there is bony proliferation at the periphery of the articulating surface, increasing the surface area. This new bone is called an osteophyte, which typically appears on the anterosuperior surface of the condyle and/or lateral aspect of the temporal component. Osteophytes may also form on the lateral, medial and posterosuperior aspect of the condyle.
- In severe cases, the osteophyte originating in the glenoid fossa may extend from the articular eminence to almost encase the condylar head.
- The osteophytes may break off and lie free within the joint space (joint mice).
- In severe DJD, the glenoid fossa may appear grossly enlarged because of the erosion of the posterior slope of

the articular eminence, and the condyle may be markedly diminished in size and altered in shape due to destruction and erosion of the condylar head.

- The enlargement of the fossa and reduced size of the condylar head allow the latter to move forward and superiorly into an abnormal anterior position that may result in an anterior open bite.

Differential Diagnosis

- A more erosive appearance may simulate inflammatory arthritis (rheumatoid arthritis)
- A more proliferative appearance with extensive osteophyte formation may simulate a benign tumor (osteoma, osteochondroma).

Management

Treatment is directed towards joint stress (splint therapy), reduction of secondary inflammation (nonsteroidal anti-inflammatory) increasing joint mobility and function (physiotherapy).

INFLAMMATORY JOINT DISORDERS

Rheumatoid Arthritis (Figs 25.17 to 25.19)

Definition

Rheumatoid arthritis (RA) is a heterogeneous group of systemic disorders that manifests mainly as synovial membrane inflammation in several joints. The TMJ is involved in 50% of the cases. The characteristic radiographic findings are because of villous synovitis, which leads to formation of granulomatous tissue (pannus) that grows into fibrocartilage and bone, releasing enzymes that destroy the articular surface of the underlying bone.

Clinical Features

- It is more common in females and the incidence increases with increasing age. There is also a juvenile variant of RA.
- The small joints of the hands, wrists, knee and feet are affected in a bilateral symmetrical fashion. The TMJ involvement varies, and is usually bilateral and symmetrical.
- When the TMJ is affected the patient may complain of pain, swelling, tenderness, stiffness on opening, limited range of movement and crepitus.
- The chin appears receded and an anterior open bite is a common finding, because of bilateral destruction and anterosuperior positioning of the condyles.
- Joint destruction leads to secondary DJD.
- Rose-Waller's test is positive in 70% of the cases. Antinuclear antibodies are detected by indirect immunofluorescense, in 30% cases.

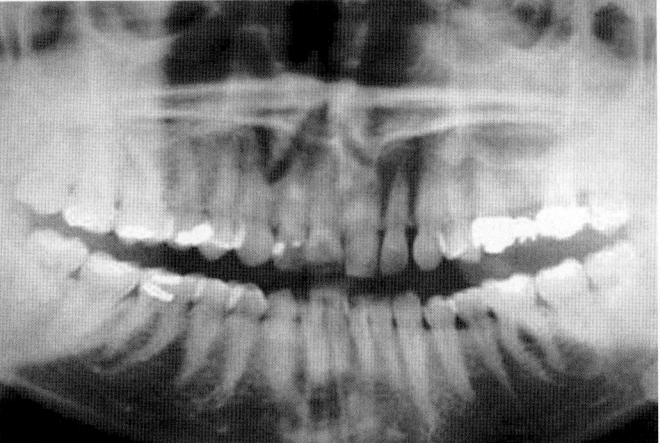

Figure 25.17 Panoramic view showing flattening of the condyles and exophytes, this was a case of rheumatoid arthritis

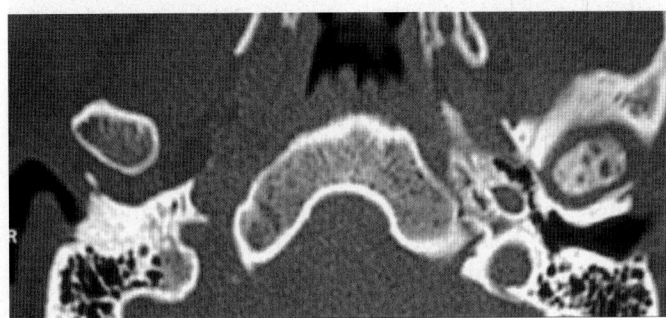

Figure 25.18 CT showing arthritis changes and sclerosis of the outer surface of the condyle. The CT showed very extensive degenerative joint disease on both right and left joints, superimposed on the patient's rheumatoid arthritis. There was extensive sclerosis of the outer surfaces of the condyles and the temporal component of the left joint. There was narrowing of the articular space of both joints (particularly on the right joint) and there were some impressive erosions on the condylar head of both joints. The small radiolucent areas of cystic appearance are degeneration areas that do not contain any fluid but fibrous tissue and poorly formed osteoid. They are always continuous with the articular surfaces though it is not always readily visible on radiographs

Radiographic Features

- The initial changes are seen as generalized osteopenia (decreased density) of the condyle and the temporal component.
- There may be diminished joint space due to destruction of the disc by the pannus.
- The pannus also causes bone erosions of the articular eminence and the anterior aspect of the condylar head, which permits anterosuperior positioning of the condyle when the teeth are in maximal intercuspation, this results in an anterior open bite.

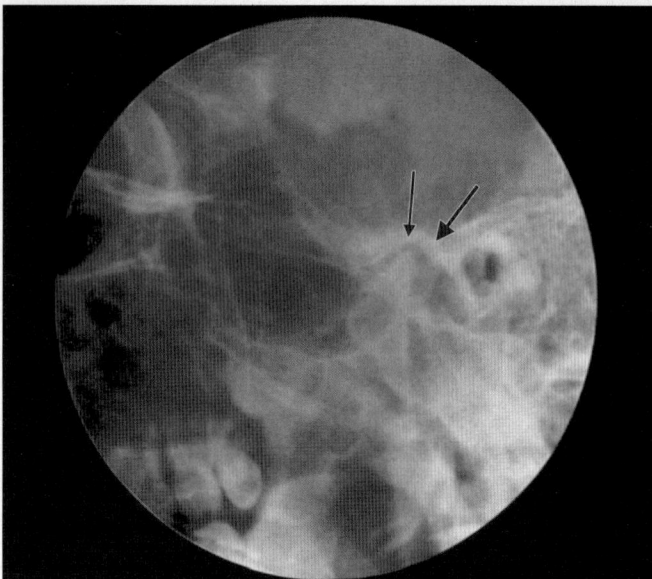

Figure 25.19 Lateral view showing arthritic changes in the right condyle, note the sharpened pencil appearance

- There may be sharpened pencil appearance of the condylar head due to erosion of the anterior and posterior condylar surfaces at the attachment of the synovial lining.
- Erosive changes may be so severe that the entire condylar head is destroyed, with only the neck remaining as the articulating surface.
- The articular eminence may also be destroyed to the extent that a concavity replaces the normally convex eminence.
- Secondary DJD changes are seen as—subchondral sclerosis, flattening of articular surfaces, subchondral cyst, osteophyte formation.
- Fibrous ankylosis or in rare cases osseous ankylosis may occur.
- The radiographic progression in rheumatoid arthritis may be staged as:
  – Stage I   : Periarticular stage
  – Stage II : Loss of articular cartilage
  – Stage III : Erosion
  – Stage IV : Subluxation and ankylosis

Differential Diagnosis

- *Degenerative joint disease (DJD)*: Osteopenia and severe erosions particularly of the articular eminence are more characteristic of RA.
- *Psoriatic arthritis*: Osteopenia and severe erosions particularly of the articular eminence are more characteristic of RA. Psoriatic arthritis may be ruled out by patient's history.

Management

Treatment is directed towards pain relief (analgesics), reduction of inflammation (nonsteroidal anti-inflammatory drugs, gold salts, corticosteroids) and prevention of muscle and joint dysfunction (physiotherapy). Joint replacement surgery may be necessary in some cases.

Juvenile Chronic Arthritis (JCA) (Still's Disease, Juvenile Rheumatoid Arthritis)

Definition

This is a chronic inflammatory disease that appears before the age of 16 years. It is characterized by chronic, intermittent synovial inflammation that results in synovial hypertrophy, joint effusion and swollen painful joints. As the disease progresses the cartilage and the bone are destroyed. Rheumatoid factor may be absent, thus this disease is now called JCA instead of juvenile rheumatoid arthritis.

Clinical Features

- There may be initial bilateral polyarthritis of both small and large joints including the cervical spine.
- There may be associated splenomegaly, lymphadenopathy, leukocytosis, pyrexia and rash.
- Temporomandibular joint (TMJ) involvement occurs in 40% of the cases.
- The involvement may be unilateral or bilateral. Unilateral onset is common, but involvement of the other joint is usual as the disease progresses.
- The patient complains of pain and tenderness in the affected joint or joints, and restricted opening of the mouth.
- Severe TMJ involvement results in inhibition of the mandibular growth causing micrognathia and posteroinferior chin rotation, resulting in a bird face appearance, which may be accompanied with an anterior open bite.
- When one joint is more severely affected the patient may have a mandibular asymmetry with the chin deviated to the affected side.
- The degree of micrognathia is proportional to the severity of the joint involvement and the early onset of the disease.

Radiographic Features

- Osteopenia (decreased density) is seen only in the initial radiographs.
- Impaired mandibular growth.
- Erosions may extend to the mandibular fossa and the articular eminence may be destroyed.
- Erosion of the anterior or superior aspect of the condyle may occur and in more severe cases only a pencil shaped small condyle remains, the condyle may be completely destroyed.

- As the inflammation is intermittent, during the quiescent periods the cortex of the joint surface may reappear, and the surfaces may appear flattened.
- Due to bone destruction, the condylar head is positioned anterosuperiorly in the mandibular fossa.
- Hypomobility at maximal opening is common and fibrous ankylosis may occur in some cases.
- Secondary degenerative changes, like sclerosis and osteophyte formation may be superimposed on the rheumatoid changes, and ankylosis may occur.
- Inhibited mandibular growth is manifested as, the deepening of the antegonial notch, diminished height of the ramus, dorsal bending of the ramus and condylar neck, and also unilaterally or bilaterally resulting in an obtuse angle between the mandibular body and ascending ramus.
- On MRI active disease is seen as enhancement of the synovial membrane and pannus after intravenous contrast injections.

Differential Diagnosis

Rheumatoid arthritis (RA): JCA has an earlier onset and the systemic involvement is more severe.

Management

The principles of management in JCA do not differ from those in RA.

Psoriatic Arthritis

Definition

This is a seronegative, systemic arthritides that may affect the TMJs. It is a chronic disease of unknown origin where the patient suffers from psoriasis of the skin with inflammatory joint disease occurring in 7% of the cases.

Clinical Features

- Skin lesions are found on the trunk, arm, face and scalp. They appear as broad irregular papules or plaques, which are dull red to brownish in color and are usually covered with a layer of fine silvery scales. Exacerbation may occur when exposed to ultraviolet light.
- When scraped they leave behind small bleeding points called Auspitz's sign.
- Arthritis may occur in the third decade with no sex predilection.
- Involvement of the TMJ causes unilateral preauricular pain and difficulty in opening the mouth.
- The TMJ is tender, with crepitus, deviation to the affected side and in a few cases deformities may also be seen.

Radiographic Features

- Generalized osteopenia.
- Irregularity of the condylar articular surface.
- Proliferative changes with diminution of the joint space.
- Temporomandibular joint (TMJ) radiographic changes are indistinguishable from those caused by RA, but profound sclerosis may be seen in psoriatic arthritis.

Differential Diagnosis

Rheumatoid arthritis (RA).

Management

Treatment includes: short wave diathermy, physiotherapy, drugs like salicylates, and steroidal applications for the skin lesions.

Septic Arthritis (Infective Arthritis)

Definition

This is an infection and inflammation of the joint that may result in joint destruction. It may be caused due to the direct spread of organisms from an adjacent cellulitis or from parotid, otic or mastoid infections. It may also be due to direct extension of osteomyelitis of the mandibular body and ramus or spread from a middle ear infection, hematogenous spread from a distant nidus. It may be acute or chronic.

Clinical Features

- It is rare in the TMJ when compared to the incidence of DJD and RA.
- There is no age or sex predilection.
- It usually occurs unilaterally.
- The patient may complain of:
  - Redness and swelling over the joint
  - Trismus
  - Severe pain on opening
  - Inability to occlude the teeth
  - Large tender lymph nodes
  - Fever and malaise
  - Pus formation in the joint space.
  - The mandible may be deviated to the affected side.
- Chronic cases are rare in the TMJ, ankylosis of the joint and facial asymmetry may occur if the growth centers are involved.

Radiographic Features

- There are no radiographic signs in the early stages, except for widening of the space between the condyle and the roof of the mandibular fossa, due to inflammatory exudates into the joint spaces.

- Osteopenic (radiolucent) changes of the joint component and mandibular ramus are seen.
- Obvious bony changes are seen about 7–10 days after the onset of the clinical symptoms.
- The osteolytic effect of inflammation causes the condylar articular surface to appear slightly radiolucent and discontinuity or subtle irregularities of the anterior cortical surface are evident.
- As the disease progresses, the condyle, articular eminence, including the disc may be destroyed.
- Osseous ankylosis occurs after the infection subsides.
- If the disease occurs during the period of mandibular growth, radiographic manifestations of inhibited mandibular growth may be evident.

Differential Diagnosis

- *Severe DJD*: Septic arthritis usually occurs unilaterally and the patient often has symptoms of infection.
- *Severe RA*: Septic arthritis usually occurs unilaterally and the patient often has symptoms of infection.

Additional Imaging

- CT images—show the inflammatory changes that may accompany septic arthritis, such as involvement of the mastoid air cells, osteomyelitis of the mandible and inflammation of the surrounding soft tissue.
- MRI using T2-weighted images may be helpful in diagnosing.
- Scintigraphy—using technetium bone scans followed by gallium scans are useful diagnostic aids.

Management

Treatment includes antimicrobial therapy, drainage of the effusion, and rest to the joint, followed by physiotherapy.

Ankylosing Spondylitis (Marie-Strumpell Disease, Rheumatoid Spondylitis)

Definition

This is a seronegative, systemic arthritides that may affect the TMJs. It is a chronic inflammatory connective tissue disease that affects the axial skeleton and central joints including the TMJ.

Clinical Features

- This occurs predominantly in males.
- This progresses to spinal fusion.
- Joint stiffness results from immobility (during sleep) and is typically relieved by heat and exercise.

Radiographic Features

- Temporomandibular joint (TMJ) radiographic changes are indistinguishable from those caused by RA.
- Flattening of the articular surface, osteophyte formation and erosions of the condylar head are commonly seen.

Differential Diagnosis

Rheumatoid arthritis (RA).

Management

Treatment includes NSAIDs, sulphasalazine and local corticosteroid injections.

Articular Loose Bodies

These are radiopacities of varying origin located in the synovium, within the capsule in the joint space or outside the capsule in soft tissue. They appear radiographically as soft tissue calcifications positioned around the condylar head. They might represent bone that has separated from the joint components, as in DJD (joint mice), hyaline cartilage metaplasia (calcifications) that occurs in synovial chondromatosis, crystals deposited in the joint space in crystal-associated arthropathy (pseudogout) or tumoral calcinosis associated with renal disease.

Synovial Chondromatosis (Synovial Chondrometaplasia, Synovial Osteochondromatosis)

Definition

This is an uncommon disorder characterized by metaplastic formation of multiple cartilaginous and osteocartilaginous nodules within connective tissue of the synovial membrane joints. Some of these nodules may detach and form loose bodies in the joint space, where they may increase in size (nourished by the synovial fluid). This condition is not as common in the TMJ as in the axial skeleton.

Clinical Features

- The patient may be asymptomatic or present with pain and swelling in the preauricular region, with limitation of movement and deviation to the affected side.
- It usually occurs unilaterally.
- There may be crepitus and other joint noises.

Radiographic Features

- It may appear radiographically normal or may exhibit osseous changes similar to those seen in DJD.

- The joint space may be widened.
- A radiopaque mass or several radiopaque masses may be seen surrounding the condylar head, in case of ossification of the cartilaginous nodules.
- CT images help:
  - To localize the exact location of the calcifications
  - To detect any erosion through the glenoid fossa into the middle cranial fossa.

Differential Diagnosis

- Chondrocalcinosis
- Degenerative joint disease (DJD) with joint mice
- Chondrosarcoma—there is severe bone destruction.

Management

Removal of the loose bodies and resection of the abnormal synovial tissue in the joint.

Chondrocalcinosis (Pseudogout, Calcium Pyrophosphate Dihydrate Deposition Disease)

Definition

This is characterized by acute or chronic synovitis and precipitation of calcium pyrophosphate dihydrate crystals in the joint space. It differs from gout in which urate crystals are precipitated.

Clinical Features

- The condition occurs unilaterally and is more common in males.
- The joints commonly affected are the knee, wrist, hip, shoulder and elbow. The TMJ involvement is rare.
- Patients may be asymptomatic or may complain of pain and joint swelling.

Radiographic Features

- The radiographic appearance simulates synovial chondromatosis.
- The radiopacities within the joint space are finer and have a more even distribution than in osteochondromatosis.
- There may be bone erosions and an increase in the condylar bone density.
- CT images help to detect erosions of the glenoid fossa, if present.

Differential Diagnosis

- Synovial chondromatosis
- Degenerative joint disease (DJD) with joint mice
- Chondrosarcoma, there is severe bone destruction.

Management

Treatment consists of surgical removal of crystalline deposits. Pain killers and anti-inflammatory drugs may be given to provide relief. Colchicine may be used to reduce acute symptoms and for prophylaxis.

METABOLIC DISORDERS

Gout

Definition

This is a chronic metabolic disorder characterized by acute exacerbation of joint pain and swelling associated with an elevated blood uric acid level and deposition of crystals of monosodium urate. The most likely predisposing factors are intake of drugs like thiazide diurectics, operations, trauma, alcohol and rapid weight loss.

Gout is of two types:
1. Acute gouty arthritis.
2. Chronic tophaceous gout.

Acute Gouty Arthritis

- Metacarpophalangeal joints are the first to be involved followed by joints of the foot, ankle, hand, wrist and elbow.
- The patient complains of excruciating pain, which increases at night and may be associated with anorexia, fever and general malaise.
- The joint returns to normal after a few days with desquamation of the overlying skin.

Chronic Tophaceous Gout

- As the disease becomes chronic, pain and stiffness persist with swelling.
- Tophi are found in the cartilage of the ear, nose or eyelids. In more than 50% of the cases the patient develops white streaks along the creases of the palms.

Clinical Features

- Involvement of the TMJ is seen in the middle age, and equally distributed among the sexes. It may have a hereditary tendency.
- The patient may complain of sudden excruciating pain in the TMJ, followed by a rapidly developing swelling.
- There is limitation of movement of the involved joint and deviation to the affected side while opening the jaws.

Radiographic Features

- Punched out radiolucency may be seen on the condylar cartilage.
- Sometime severe destruction of the cartilage may occur.
- The carpal bone of the hands also show punched out areas.

Management

Treatment consists of control of diet, especially excess intake of purive and alcohol which causes high uric acid and fat accumulation. Administration of uricosuric agents like colchicine and allopurinol to increase elimination of uric acid also helps.

TRAUMATIC DISORDER OF THE TEMPOROMANDIBULAR JOINT

Effusion (Figs 25.20A to C)

Definition

It is an influx of fluid into the joint, usually as a result of trauma (hemorrhage) or inflammation (exudates).

Clinical Features

- Patient may have a swelling over the affected joint with limited range of movement
- Pain in the TMJ, preauricular region or ear
- Patient may complain of sensation of fluid in the ear, tinnitus and hearing difficulties
- Patient may have difficulty in occluding the posterior teeth
- Joint effusion is more commonly seen in conjunction with internal derangements, though it has been described in normal joints.

Radiographic Features

- The joint space is widened
- T2-weighted MRI studies show a bright signal (white), indicating fluid adjacent to the disc.

Differential Diagnosis

- Septic Arthritis
  This is accompanied with signs and symptoms of infection.

Management

Treatment may include anti-inflammatory drugs; surgical drainage may sometimes be necessary.

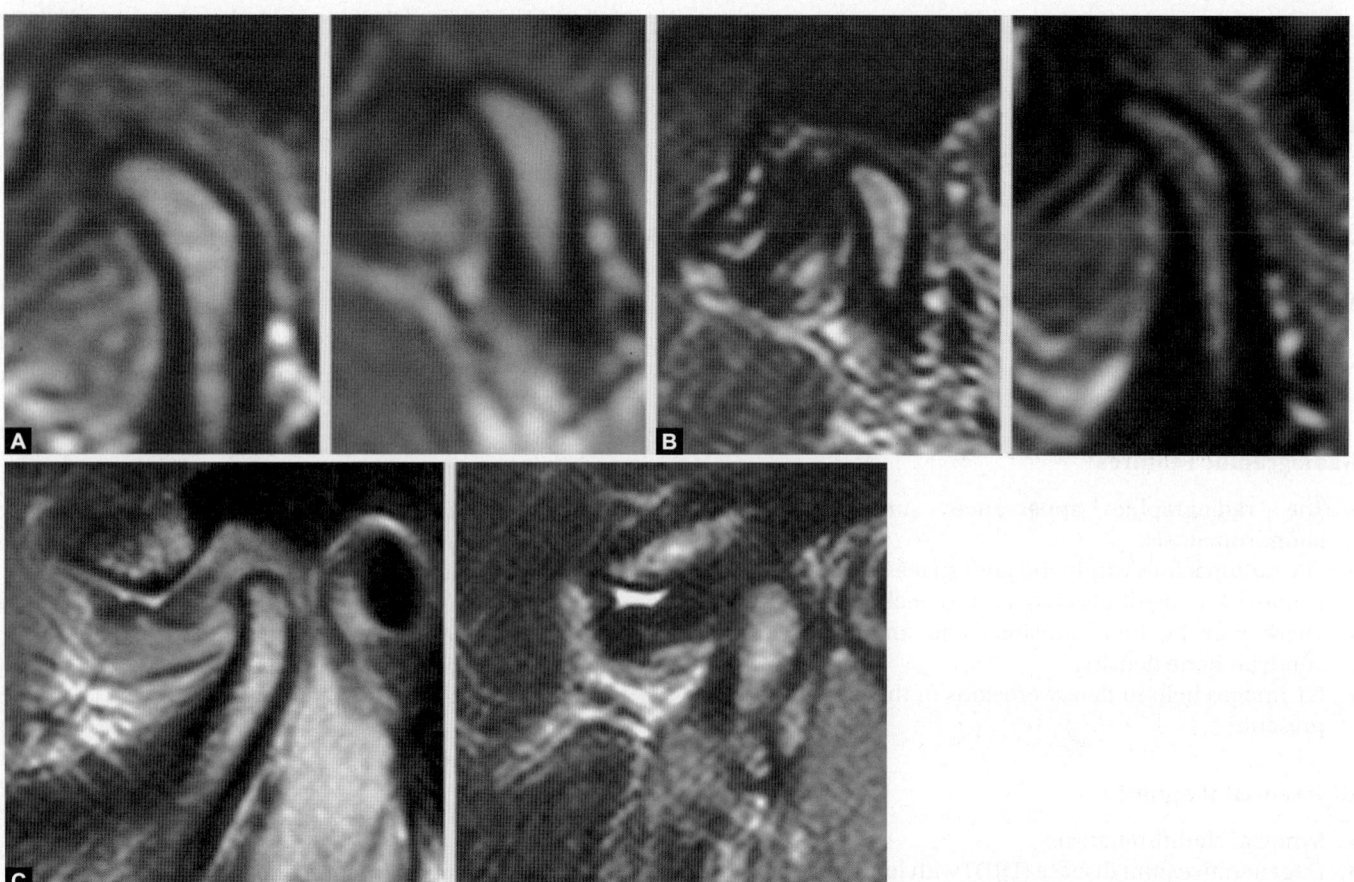

Figures 25.20A to C MRI images showing anterior disc displacement with effusion

Dislocation (Figs 25.21A to C)

Definition

This is abnormal positioning of the condyle out of the mandibular fossa but within the joint capsule. It usually occurs bilaterally and is most common in the anterior direction. It may be caused by a failure of muscular coordination, subluxation or external trauma and may be associated with a condylar fracture.

It may be classified as:

A. • Acute dislocation
   • Chronic dislocation
   • Recurrent dislocation.
B. • *Anterior dislocation*: This is the most common type of dislocation
   • *Posterior dislocation*: This is a rare type of dislocation and results due to severe injuries which are sustained on the end point of the chin or at the inferior border of the mandible.
   • *Central dislocation*: Occurence and cause similar to posterior dislocation.
   • *Medial or lateral dislocation*: This occurs as a result of injury to the neck of the condyle with a fracture. This type of dislocation is very rare.

Clinical Features

• Patients are unable to close the mandible to maximal intercuspation. In acute dislocation there may be history of injury, gagging of molar teeth and anterior open bite.
• Some patients cannot reduce the dislocation, and this is accompanied with:
  – Pain and muscle spasm.
  – There will be a depression where the condylar head is normally situated.
  – The mandible is postured forward and movement is extremely limited.
  – The condyle becomes locked anterior to the articular eminence and is prevented from sliding back by muscular spasm.
  – The patient has great difficulty in swallowing and saliva drools over the chin.
  – When unilateral dislocation occurs, the teeth will be gagged posteriorly on the side of the dislocation and the chin will be deviated towards the normal side.
• Whereas other may be able to reduce the mandible by manipulation.

Radiographic Features

In case of bilateral dislocation both the condyles are located anterior and superior to the summits of the articular eminentia.

Differential Diagnosis

• Normal range of motion may also extend anterior to the summit of the articular eminence. Clinical information is important.
• Fracture dislocations may be difficult to visualize on the radiograph, especially if the dislocation is very slight.

Management

Treatment consists of manual manipulation of the mandible to reduce the dislocation. Surgical intervention may sometimes be necessary, if mandibular function is not adequate.

Subluxation (Hypermobility)

Definition

This is unilateral or bilateral positioning of the condyle anterior to the eminence, with repositioning to normal accomplished by physiological activity. It is a self-reducing incomplete dislocation, which generally follows stretching of the capsule and ligaments.

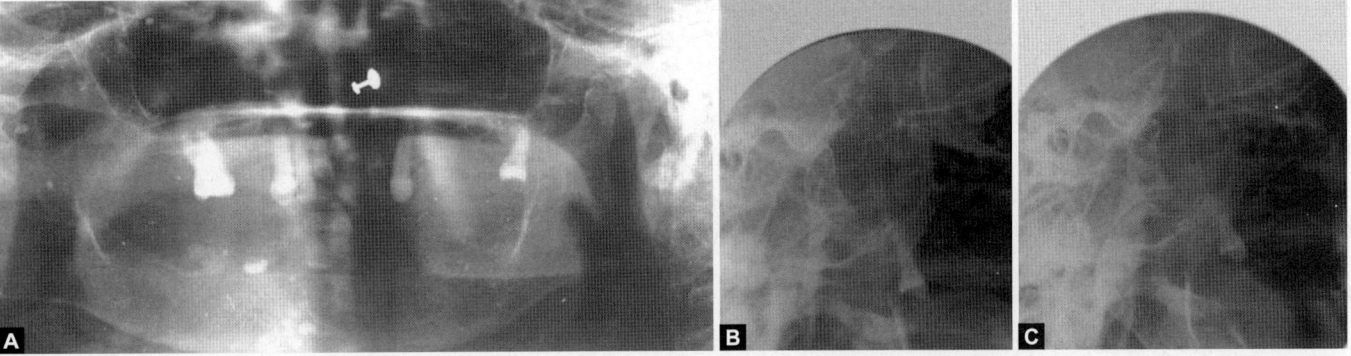

Figures 25.21A to C (A) Panoramic radiograph shows head of the condyle of left TMJ placed anterior to articular eminence. Right side head of condyle in its normal position; (B and C) Transcranial closed and open position showing dislocation of left TM joint

Clinical Features

- It may be unilateral or bilateral.
- The condyle may get locked when the mouth is opened wide and upon closing it will return with a jumping motion, accompanied by a sound caused due to the movement of the condyle over the articular eminence.
- On palpation a click on opening and sliding of the condyle over the articular eminence is common.
- Patient may describe weakness of the joint while yawning.
- Pain may be associated with the last few millimeters of mouth opening.

Radiographic Features

The radiographs will show excessive translation of the condyle from rest position to the position when the jaw is wide open.

Differential Diagnosis

Normal range of motion of condyle.

Management

Treatment may consist of injecting a sclerosing agent or surgical treatment or shortening of the temporalis tendon.

FRACTURE

Refer to Chapter 28—Trauma to Teeth and Facial Structures. (Page 536).

Trauma to the Developing Condyle

If the condylar fracture occurs during the period of mandibular growth, the growth may be inhibited due to damage to the condylar growth center. The degree of hypoplasia is related to the stage of mandibular development at the time of injury.

Injury to the joint may result in hemorrhage or effusion into the joint space that eventually may form bone during the healing process, which results in severe hypoplasia and limited joint function.

Neonatal Fractures

Definition

The use of forceps during delivery may result in the fracture and displacement of the rudimentary condyle.

Clinical Features

The result of the injury is later manifested as mandibular hypoplasia and lack of development of the glenoid fossa and articular eminence.

Radiographic Features

On the panoramic radiograph it has the appearance of a partly opened pair of scissors in place of the normal condyle. This is due to the overlapping images of the medially displaced 'carrot shaped' condyle and remnants of the condylar neck.

Differential Diagnosis

- The condition is not diagnosed until later in life, at which time the diagnosis of fracture may be made without a history that the fracture occurred at the time of birth.
- Developmental hypoplasia of the mandible—this condition is unrelated to birth injuries.

Management

The fracture is usually not treated but the mandibular asymmetry may be corrected with a combination of orthodontic and orthognathic surgery.

Ankylosis (Figs 25.22 to 25.25)

Definition

Ankylosis in Greek means 'stiff joint'. This is a condition in which the condylar movement is limited due to an abnormal consolidation of the joint. This may be:

- *True ankylosis (intra-articular)*: Movement is limited due to mechanical problem in the joint, which may be due to fibrous or bony adhesion between the articular surfaces of the TMJ. This may be:
- *Bony ankylosis*: The condyle or ramus is attached to the temporal bone by an osseous bridge. This may be:
  - *Partial ankylosis*: There is incomplete union between the articulating surfaces.
  - *Complete ankylosis*: There is complete union between the articulating surfaces.
  - *Fibrous ankylosis*: There is a soft tissue (fibrous) union of the joint components. The bony components appears normal.
- *False ankylosis (extra-articular)*: The movement is limited by a mechanical cause not related to the joint components. The condition may result due to pathological conditions outside the joint, such as, muscle spasm, myositis ossificans or coronoid process hyperplasia.

Clinical Features

- The patients may have oral problems depending on the duration. There may be poor oral hygiene, carious teeth, periodontal problems and malocclusion.
- Most unilateral cases are caused due of mandibular trauma or infection.
  - The patient may be able to produce a few millimeters of interincisal opening.

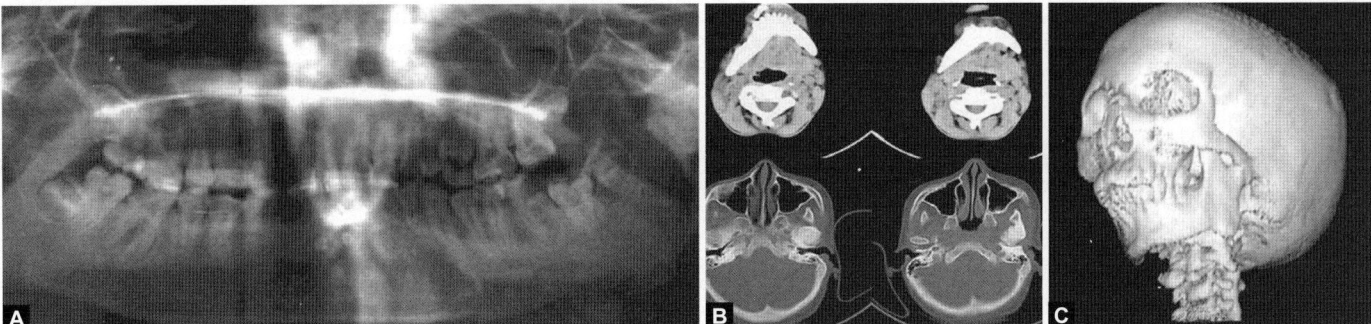

Figures 25.22A to C (A) Ankylosis as seen on a panoramic view, with a well-defined radiopaque area in relation to the left condyle. The outline of the left condyle cannot be determined. A prominent antegonial notch is observed on the left side; (B) CT scan axial views showed that condylar process and the condylar fossa of the left TMJ appeared expanded and sclerosed with irregularity of the articular surfaces and effacement of the joint space. Bony ankylosis was also seen. Right TMJ appears normal. Mandible appears hypoplastic and deformed, with the symphysis menti shifted to the left; (C) 3D CT showing the same case—ankylosis

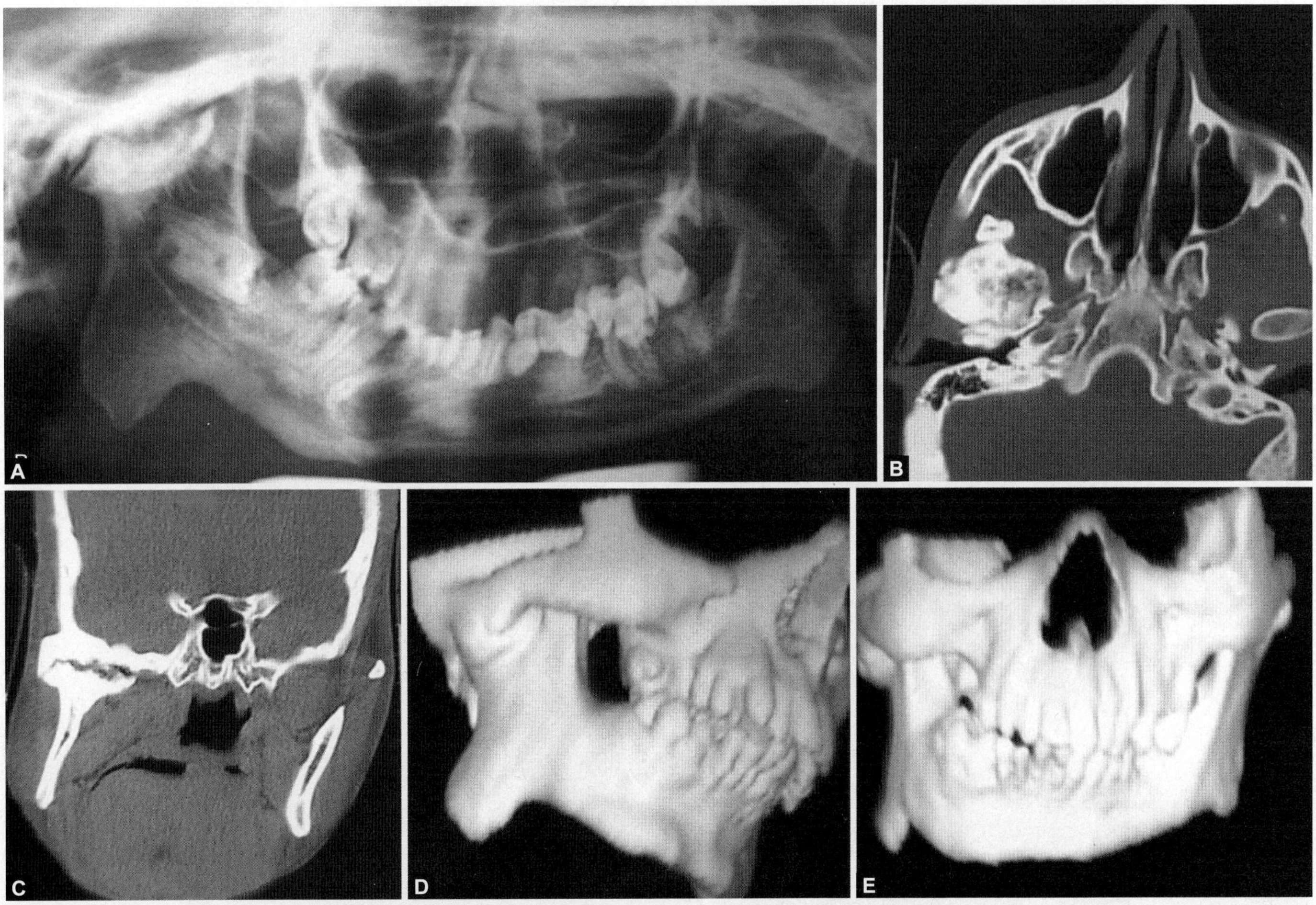

Figures 25.23A to E Ankylosis of right TMJ: (A) Panoramic radiograph showed prominent right antegonial notch. Both condyle and sigmoid notch could not be traced. Bony fusion of the condylar head, sigmoid notch and articular surface on right side. Elongated coronoid process. Inverted tooth mandibular molar impacted in the ramus. CT scan: (B) Axial; (C) Coronal; (D and E) 3D views show right glenoid fossa and condylar articular surface are sclerotic, irregular with no visible joint space. Right hemimandible is hypoplastic with malalignment of teeth. Left TMJ is normal

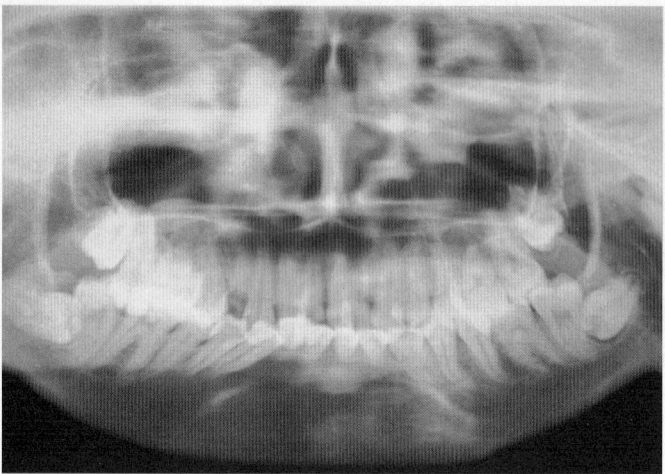

Figure 25.24 Panoramic radiograph showing complete obliteration of the joint space. Deepened antegonial notches

- There will be asymmetry of the face with fullness on and deviation towards the affected side and relative flattening of the unaffected side.
- Cross bite may be present.
- Bilateral TMJ ankylosis is usually due to rheumatoid arthritis, or in rare cases may be due to fractures.
  - The face is symmetrical with micrognathia, the patient has a bird face appearance.
  - The patient is neither able to do protrusive nor lateral movements.
  - In case of bony ankylosis there is no pain, but in case of fibrous ankylosis the patient may have pain.
  - Due to long standing ankylosis, atrophy or fibrosis of the muscles of mastication may result.
  - The patient will develop a class II malocclusion, protrusive incisors and an anterior open bite (This is developed due to the patients attempt at forcing food through the anterior teeth over the years).

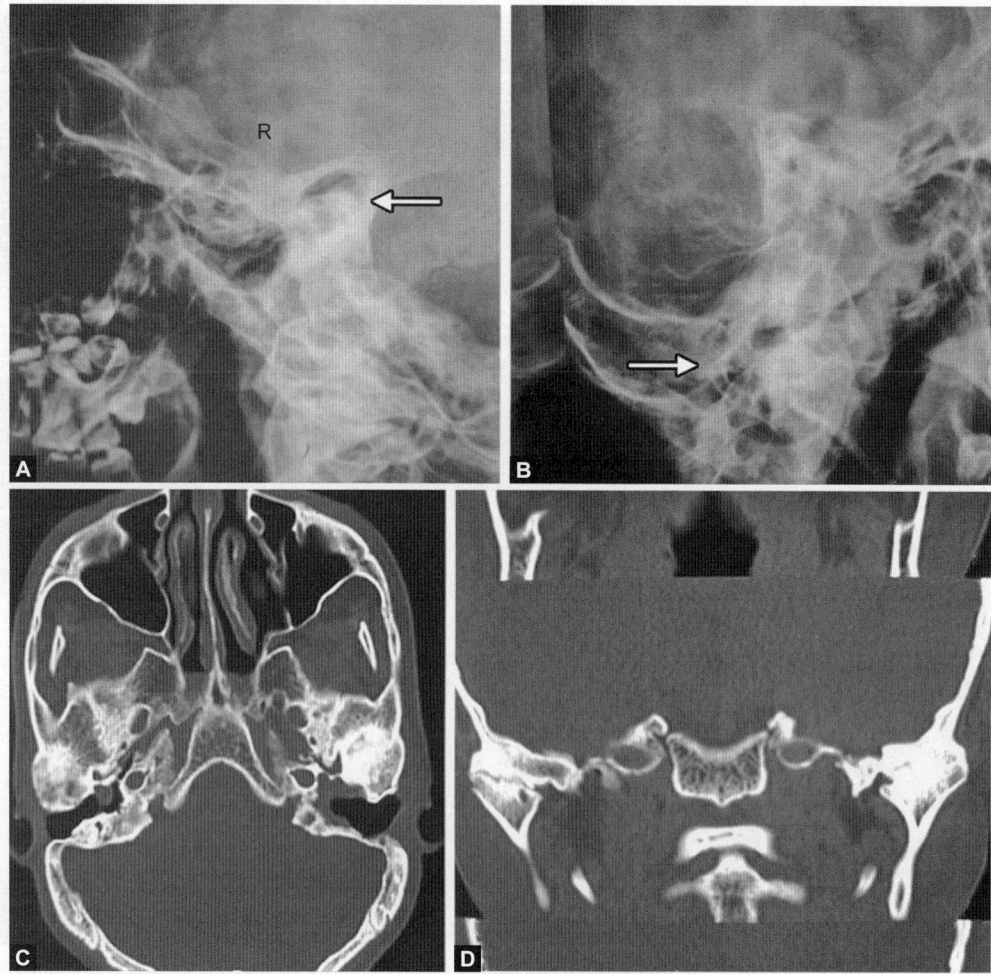

Figures 25.25A to D Bilateral TMJ ankylosis: Lateral skull views: (A) Right; (B) Left showed bilateral bony ankylosis of TMJ with reduced joint spaces. Some amount of arthritic changes were also suspected. CT scan: (C) Axial; (D) Coronal revealed bilateral fibrous ankylosis of the TM joints. There was reduced joint space, loss of articular cartilage, multiple erosions and irregularities within the joint spaces

- Most of the cases of TMJ ankylosis in infancy occur secondary to birth injuries.

Radiographic Features

- *Fibrous ankylosis*:
  - The articulating surfaces are usually irregular because of erosions.
  - The joint space is usually very narrow and the two irregular surfaces may appear to fit into one another like a jigsaw puzzle.
  - Little or no condylar movement is seen.
  - There may be radiographic signs of remodeling which may be seen as the joint components adapt to repeated attempts at mandibular opening.
- *Bony ankylosis*:
  - The joint space may be partly or completely obliterated by the osseous bridge, which may vary from a slender segment of bone (difficult to locate) to a large bony mass. This extensive new bone may fuse the condyle to the cranial base.
  - Secondary degenerative changes of the joint components are common.
  - Morphological changes such as:
    - Compensatory progressive elongation of the coronoid processes.
    - Deepening of the antegonial notch in the mandibular ramus on the affected side as a result of muscle function during attempted mandibular opening.
  - If ankylosis occurs before mandibular growth is complete, growth of the affected side of the mandible is inhibited.
- *Additional imaging*:
  - Ankylosed joint space is better seen on CT than MRI.
  - Coronal CT images are best diagnostic imaging method to evaluate ankylosis.
- *Differential diagnosis*:
  - *Condylar tumor*—There will be no history of trauma, infection or joint disease.
  - Fibrous ankylosis is difficult to detect on the radiograph and therefore difficult to differentiate from false ankylosis.

Management

Mobility is improved by surgical removal of the osseous bridge or creation of pseudarthrosis.

Internal Derangements (Figs 25.26 to 25.32)

Definition

This is an abnormality in the position and sometimes the morphology of the articular disc that may interfere with the normal function. The disc most often is displaced in an anterior direction, but it may be displaced anteromedially, medially

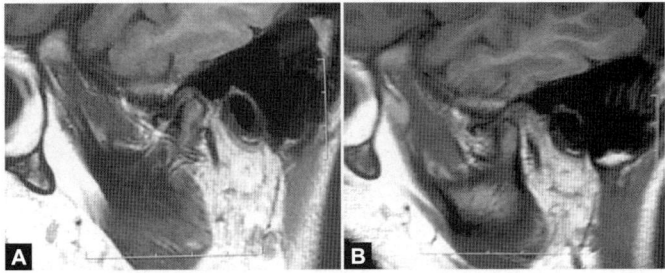

Figures 25.26A and B MRI showing: (A) Anterior disc displacement (closed mouth); (B) There is no reduction of the disc on opening the mouth. Deformation of the disc is noted

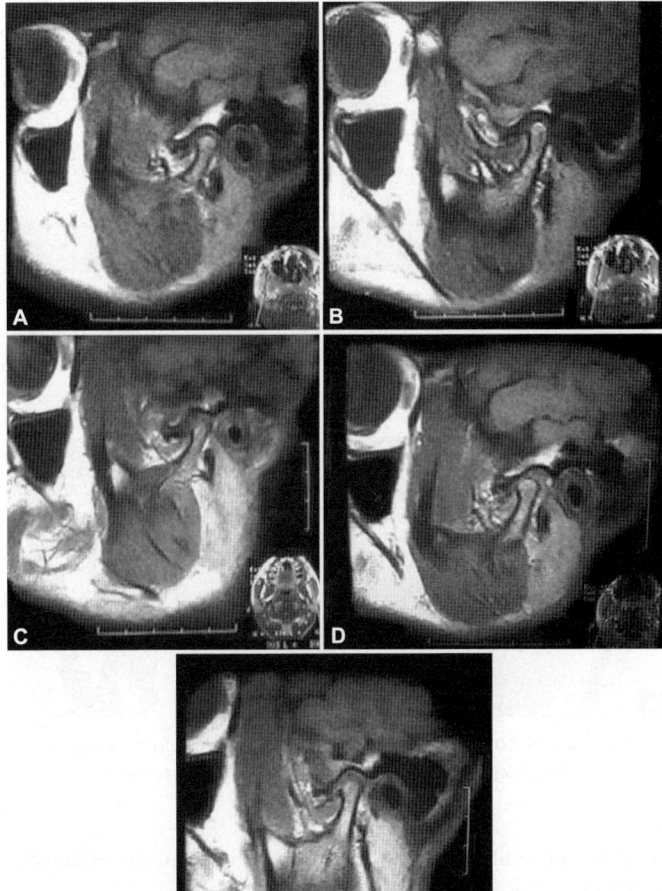

Figures 25.27A to E Disc displacement in a patient with complain of restricted mouth opening since two months: (A to C) MRI was suggestive of anteriorly displaced disc in closed mouth position, without obvious deformity. It's posterior aspect is seen at the level of the articular eminence. (D and E) MRI in open mouth position, shows limited forward translation of condylar head and deformity of the disc in the open position, and the anterior translation of the left condyle is slightly reduced

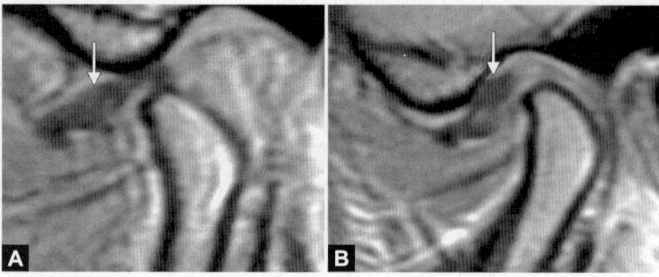

Figures 25.28A and B Magnetic resonance imaging medial section showing: (A) Open; (B) Closed position with complete anterior disc displacement

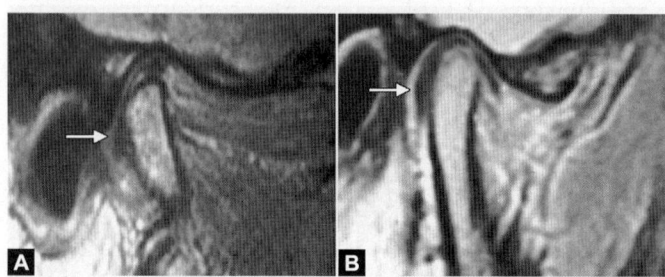

Figures 25.29A and B Magnetic resonance imaging medial section showing: (A) Open; (B) Closed position with posterior disc displacement

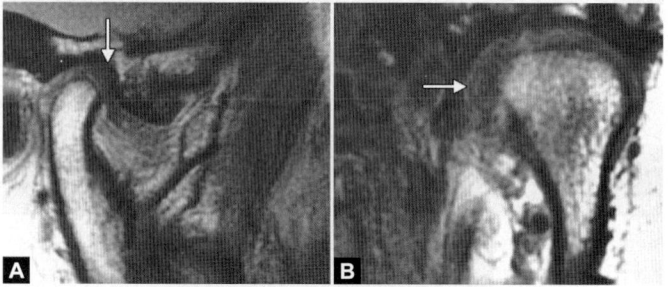

Figures 25.30A and B MRI medial section showing: (A) Open; (B) Closed position with medial disc displacement

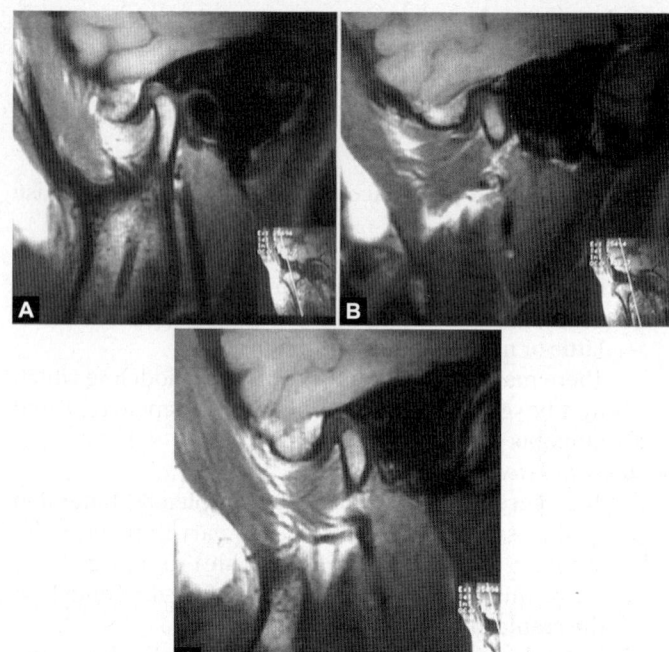

Figures 25.31A to C MRI medial section showing open and closed position with complete anterior disc displacement without reduction

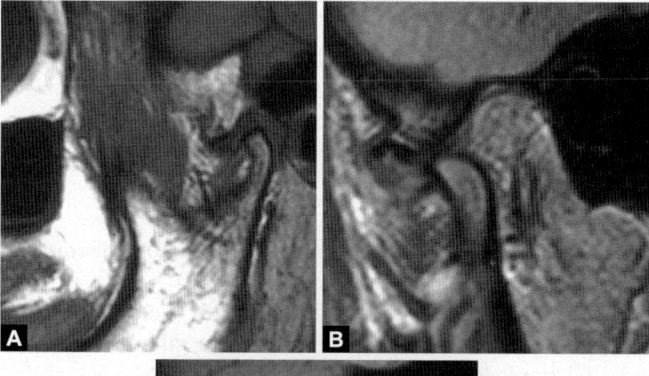

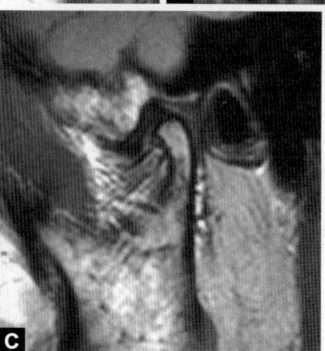

Figures 25.32A to C MRI medial section showing open and closed position with complete anterior disc displacement without reduction and crumpled disc

or anterolaterally. Lateral and posterior displacements are extremely rare.

The cause of internal derangements is unknown, although parafunction, jaw injuries, whiplash injuries and forces opening beyond the normal range have been implicated.

Reduction of the disc–here the disc resumes a normal position with respect to the condyle during mandibular opening.

Nonreduction of the disc—here the disc remains displaced throughout the entire range of mandibular movement.

A chronically displaced disc may become deformed, losing its normal biconcave shape, and it may become thickened and fibrotic, leading to complications such as DJD, perforation of the disc or posterior attachment.

Disc interferences may be classified as:

A. • Derangement of the condyle-disc complex—this occurs due to abnormal biomechanical function between the condyle and the disc
  – Disc displacement
  – Disc dislocation with reduction
  – Disc dislocation without reduction
  • Structural incompatibility of the articular surface
  – Adhesions and adherences
  – Alterations in the form of articulation surfaces

B. • Anterior displacement with reduction—here as the condyle moves forward, it snaps under the posterior edge of the disc producing an audible click and on closing the condyle may again snap under the posterior edge of the disc producing another click.
  • Anterior displacement without reduction—here there is no reduction of the disc in the mandibular fossa in the open position.
  • Disc displacement with intermittent locking
  • Disc displacement with perforation.

Clinical Features

• Disc displacement has been found both in symptomatic patients and healthy volunteers, thus indicating that it could be a normal variant and not a predisposing factor for TMJ dysfunction. The posterior border of the disc becomes thin and the retrodiscal lamina and collateral ligament become elongated, the disc may then slip anteriorly through the discal space, known as disc displacement. Hence, there is loss of contact between the articular surfaces of the condyle and the disc.
• Internal derangements may be unilateral or bilateral.
• Unilateral derangements show mandibular deviation to the affected side on opening.
• Joint noises are common and may manifest as a click as the disc reduces to a normal position during mandibular opening and occasionally as a softer click as the disc becomes displaced again during mandibular closing.
• Noises may be absent in chronically displaced, nonreducing discs, or crepitus may be heard.
• If there is an associated perforation crepitus and grinding noises may be heard.
• Symptomatic patients may have a decreased range of mandibular motion.
• Patients may complain of pain in the preauricular region or headaches.
• They may have episode of closed or open locking of the joint.
• Patients may have to manipulate the mandible to open it fully past an apparent closed lock by applying medially directed pressure to the affected joint or mandible with the hand.
• Adhesions may occur in either superior or inferior joint space due to changes in the articular surfaces and synovial fluid, leading to increased friction with resultant sticking or adhesion of the articulating surfaces.
• Fibrous adhesions are masses of fibrous tissue or scar tissue that form in the joint space, particularly after TMJ surgery.
• Alteration in the shape of the articulating surfaces occurs, leading to impairment of the smooth sliding movement of the joint.

Radiographic Features

• Internal derangements are best diagnosed using either arthrography or MRI, as the disc cannot be visualized with conventional radiography or tomography.
• A retruded condylar position has been associated with disc displacement, condylar position in maximal opening is not a reliable indicator of disc displacement.
• Diminished range of motion at maximal opening is not a reliable indication of a nonreducing disc.

Disc Displacement

• *Anterior displacement*: When the mandible is in maximal intercuspation, partial or full anterior disc displacement is indicated by anterior location of the posterior band of disc from the normal position, which is directly superior to the condylar head. The normal articulating surface of the disc (thin intermediate zone) is somewhat anteriorly positioned, and as a result the osseous structures of the joint articulate with the posterior band of the disc or the retrodiscal tissue.
• *Anteromedial displacement*: This is indicated in the sagittal image slices when the disc is in the normal position in the medial images of the joint but anteriorly positioned in the lateral images of the same joint.
• *Medial displacement*: This is indicated in the MRI coronal images when the body of the disc is positioned at the medial aspect of the condyle.

Disc Reduction and Nonreduction

• Videofluoroscopy of mandibular movements during arthrography may show a sudden movement of the disc from an anterior displacement to a normal position during normal opening and back to the abnormal anterior (displaced) position during mandibular closing (often, coinciding opening and closing (reciprocal) clicks are heard).
• If the disc remains anteriorly displaced (nonreduction) on opening, it may bend or deform as the condyle pushes against it. The nonreduced disc is clearly seen on MRI scans, though fibrotic changes of the bilaminar zone may alter the signal to approximate the signal of the disc and thus make identification of the disc itself difficult, and an erroneous diagnosis of the disc occupying abnormal position at maximal opening may be made.

Disc Perforations

- Disc perforations are not reliably detected with MRI.
- Arthrography may reveal a tear in the joint capsule or a perforation in the disc or posterior attachment by demonstrating the flow of contrast agent from the inferior to the superior joint space during the injection phase.

Adhesions

- These are best identified with arthrography by resistance to injection of contrast agent. The pressure of the injected contrast agent may tear some of these adhesions, resulting in increased joint mobility after the procedure.
- It may be detected in MRI studies as tissue with low signal intensity.

Disc Deformities

Both MRI and arthrography may indicate alterations in the normal biconcave outline of the disc, which may vary from enlargement of the posterior band to a bilinear or biconvex disc outline.

Effusion

Magnetic resonance imaging (MRI) may detect accumulation of fluid in joint spaces, which appears as a high signal in the joint spaces in T2-weighted images.

NEOPLASTIC CONDITIONS

Benign Tumors (Figs 25.33 to 25.35)

Definition

The most common benign intrinsic tumors affecting the TMJ are osteomas, osteochondromas, Langerhans histiocytosis and osteoblastomas. Other benign tumor which are less common involving the TMJ are chondroblastomas, fibromyxomas, benign giant cell lesions and aneurysmal bone cysts.

Benign cysts and tumors of the mandible (ameloblastoma, odontogenic keratocyst, simple bone cyst) may involve the entire ramus and in some cases the condyle.

Clinical Features

- Condylar tumors grow slowly and need to attain considerable size before they become clinically noticeable.
- Patients may complain of TMJ swelling, with pain and decreased range of motion.
- There may be facial asymmetry, malocclusion and deviation of the mandible to the unaffected side.
- There may be symptoms of TMJ dysfunction.

- Tumors of the coronoid are painless, but the patient may complain of progressive limitation of movement.

Radiographic Features

- Condylar enlargement with an irregular outline. They may appear as a bulbous or globular expansion of the condyle, or commonly a pedunculated growth.
- The trabecular pattern may be altered. Regions of destruction seen as radiolucencies or increased density due to new abnormal bone formation with abnormal trabeculae.
- An osteoma or osteochondroma may appear as an abnormal pedunculated mass attached to the condyle.
- Osteochondroma extends from the anterior or superior of the condyle.
- Osteochondroma is the most common benign tumor affecting the condyle and the coronoid process; it interferes with joint function and erodes adjacent osseous structures.

Differential Diagnosis

- *False ankylosis*: The TMJ may appear radiographically normal. Hyperplasia or tumor of the coronoid process must be ruled out.
- Unilateral condylar hyperplasia, osteomas and osteochondromas give an irregular appearance, the characteristic condylar shape and proportions are better preserved in condylar hyperplasia.
- Coronoid tumors must be differentiated from coronoid hyperplasia.
- *Coronoid tumours*: The coronoid remains regular in shape, which is not the case with condylar tumors.

Management

This consists of surgical excision of the tumor or sometimes excision of the condylar head or the coronoid process.

Malignant Tumors

Definition

The malignant tumors of the jaws are more often metastatic. Primary intrinsic malignant tumors of the condyle are rare. These include chondrosarcoma, osteogenic sarcoma, synovial sarcoma and fibrosarcoma of the joint capsule.

Extrinsic malignant tumors may represent direct extension of adjacent parotid salivary gland malignancies, rhabdomyosarcoma (especially in children), other regional carcinomas from the skin, ear and nasopharynx.

The most common metastatic lesions include neoplasms originating in the breast, kidney, lung, colon, prostrate and thyroid gland.

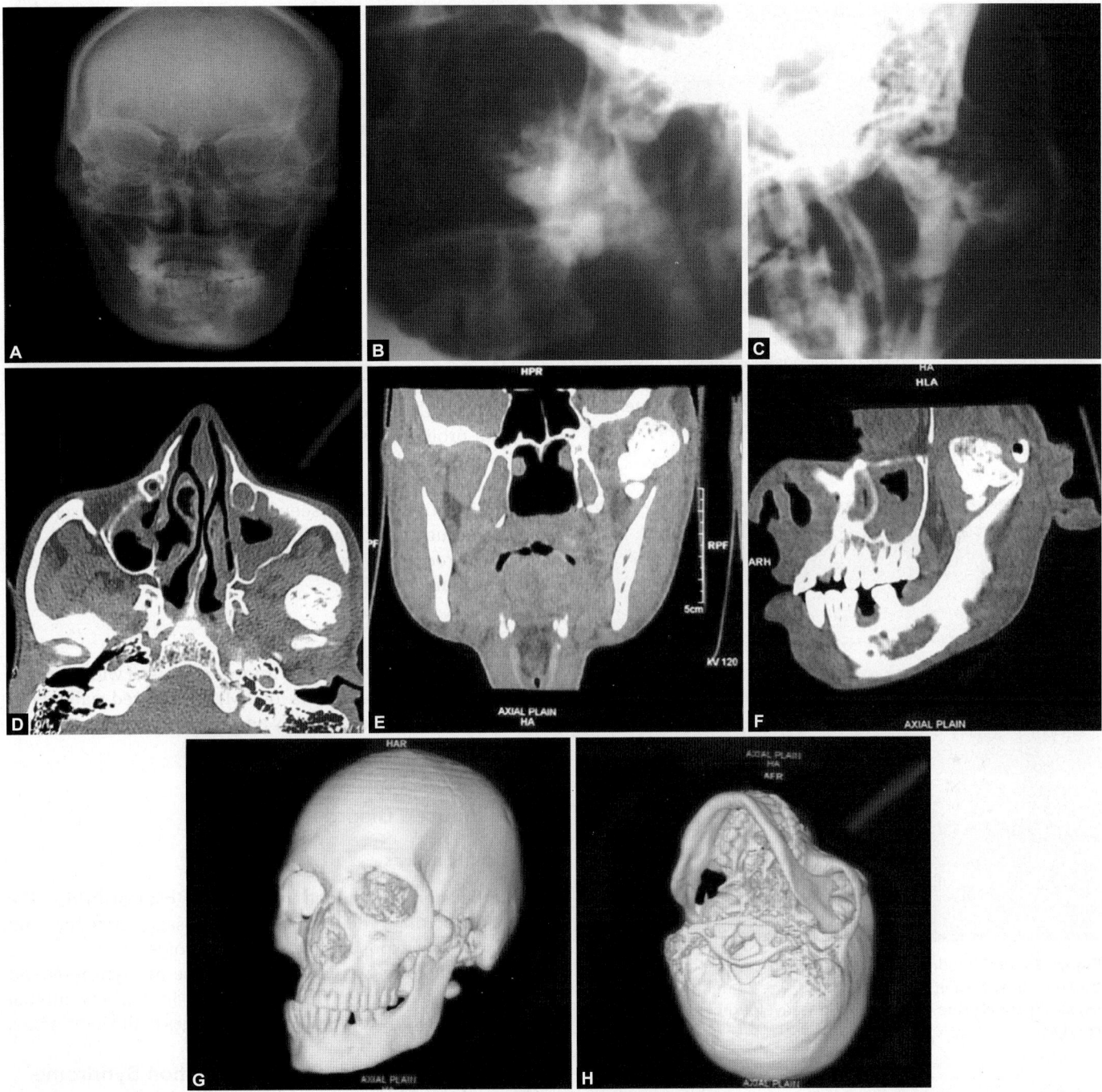

Figures 25.33A to H Osteochondroma: (A) PA mandible showed a faint radiopacity arising from left TMJ with deviation of the mandible to the right side. Right posterior cross-bite was noted; (B) Transcranial; (C) Transorbital view showed well-defined bony outgrowth of heterogeneous density arising from the anterior aspect of the left mandibular condyle. The lesion was pedunculated with anteromedial, inferior and superior extensions. CT scan: (D) Axial; (E) Coronal; (F) Sagittal views showed a well-defined cauliflower-shaped, pedunculated bony lesion predominately radiopaque (3.8 × 3.1 × 1.8 cm in size) originating from the anteromedial surface of the left condylar head and projecting anteromedially the infratemporal fossa and inferiorly till lingula of mandible. The lesion displayed superior indentation of the left greater wing of the sphenoid, which exhibited thinning. Anteromedially, the tumor indented into the posterolateral wall of the left maxillary sinus; laterally, the tumor contacted the left zygomatic arch. The cortex of the tumor was continuous with that of the normal condylar bone. Anterior subluxation of the left temporomandibular joint was noted. Evidence of ipsilateral pterygoid muscle atrophy and contralateral masseter muscle hypertrophy was observed mucosal thickening in bilateral maxillary sinus. CT scan: (G and H) 2D shows enlargement of the condyle

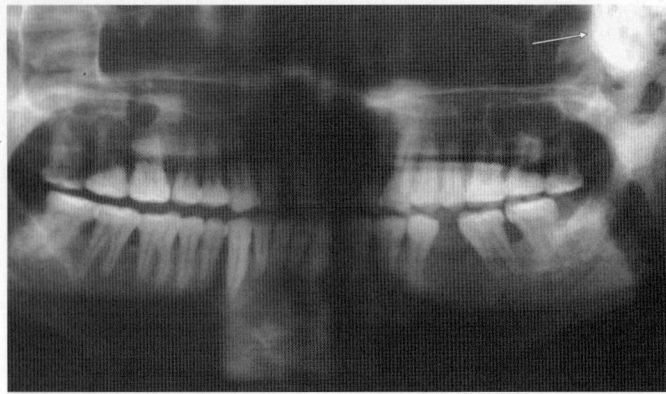

Figure 25.34 Osteochondroma: Panoramic radiograph demonstrated a well-defined bony outgrowth of heterogeneous density arising from the anterior aspect of the left mandibular condyle. The lesion was pedunculated with anteromedial, inferior and superior extensions. Anteromedially, the lesion caused indentation of the posterolateral wall of the left maxillary sinus

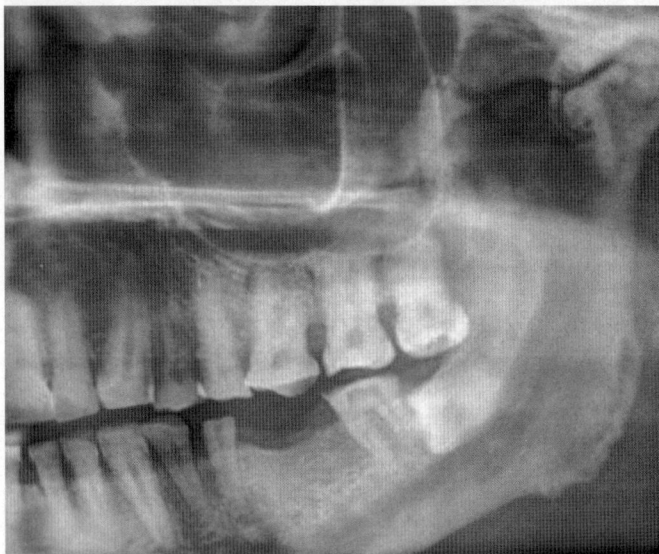

Figure 25.35 Chondroma, panoramic radiograph shows radiopaque bulbous growth seen over left condyle. Size of right side condyle is smaller then left side of condyle suggestive of growth of left side of condyle

Clinical Features

- The primary or metastatic malignant tumors may be asymptomatic or
- The patient may complain of TMJ dysfunction such as pain, limited mandibular opening, mandibular deviation, and swelling.
- Many a times the patient is only treated for TMJ dysfunction without recognizing that the underlying condition is malignancy.

Radiographic Features

- There will be varying degree of bone destruction with ill-defined irregular margins.
- Most lesions lack tumor bone formation except in the case of osteogenic sarcoma.
- Chondrosarcoma may appear as an indistinct, radiolucent destructive lesion of the condyle with surrounding discrete soft tissue calcifications that may simulate the appearance of articular loose bodies.
- In case of metastatic tumors the radiographic appearance is nonspecific condylar destruction (with exception of metastatic tumor of the prostrate) and does not indicate the site of origin.

Differential Diagnosis

- *Severe DJD*: This causes more peripheral bone destruction, with proliferative changes such as osteophyte formation, but no soft tissue mass of swelling is evident. Malignant tumors cause more central bone destruction, no proliferative changes seen and there may be presence of soft tissue mass or swelling.
- *Chondrocalcinosis or pseudo gout*: The bone destruction in malignancy is more.

Management

Treatment in case of primary tumor consists of wide surgical excision. Metastatic tumors of TMJ are treated palliatively and may include radiotherapy and chemotherapy.

NEUROPATHIC DISORDERS

Drug Induced Disorders (Steroids)

Clinical Features

- Corticosteroids induce mandibular osteoarthritis. The manifestations depend on the dosage, potency and duration of exposure to excessive steroids.
- Triamcinolone was found to enhance the synthesis and secretion of parathyroid hormone in various animal studies, leading to degenerative changes in the joint tissue.

Temporomandibular Pain Dysfunction Syndrome (Flow chart 25.1)

Myofascial pain dysfunction syndrome is a pain disorder, in which unilateral pain is referred from the trigger points of the myofacial structures to the muscles of the head and neck. The pain is constant, dull aching type which is in contrast to the sudden sharp, shooting, intermittent pain of neuralgias (chronic pain). But the pain may range from mild to intolerable. Clinically, it has typical features such as a zone of reference, trigger points in muscles, occasional associated symptoms and presence of contributing factors.

Flow chart 25.1 The first three choices of treatment for a patient with confirmed TMJ disorder

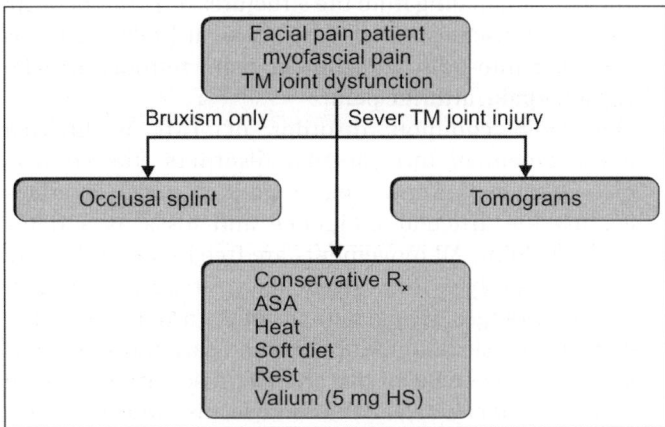

It is believed to arise from multifactorial origins, which may be put in the following groups: Psychologic or central etiology, occlusal or peripheral etiology and the third group which is recently considered as due to intrinsic joint disorder etiology.

Etiology

- *Occlusal status*: Occlusal interferences cause altered proprioceptive feedback causing muscle spasm.
- *Periodontal view point*: Self-protective system modifies the path of closure and prevents painful contacts. The corrective movements elicit muscle strain eliciting abnormal pressure on temporomandibular joint.
- *Prosthetic view point*: Faulty complete or partial dentures over a period of time result in temporomandibular joint pain. This causes changes in myotatic stretch reflex resulting in pain.
- *Orthodontic view point*: Malocclusion leads to temporomandibular joint dysfunction. Discrepancies in occlusion or maxillomandibular relationship can lead to pain.
- *Emotional status*: Pattern of overall behaviors relating to care of teeth, food habits or attitude towards the dentist. Oral habits that cause structural damage, or persistent pain. Dysfunction of autonomic nervous system, resulting from anxiety, and eventually producing structural change in the end organs.
- *Psychophysiological theory*: The masticatory muscle spasm is responsible for the pain. Spasm is initiated by muscular over-extension due to dental restoration, muscular over contraction, muscle fatigue due to oral habits such as clenching or grinding of teeth, dental irritation like maloccluding restorations or overhanging margin.
- Persistent myospasm.

Classification

- *Spasms of lateral pterygoid muscles*: It occurs when teeth are brought into maximum intercuspation and extended translatory movement. Pain reduces on biting against a separator (as it prevents the intercuspation required to stretch the spastic muscles). It is accompanied with very acute malocclusion expressed as anterior displacement of the mandible.
- *Spasms of elevator muscles*: It occurs when biting and chewing efforts are made while opening the mouth. Pain is not decreased on biting on a separator and is accompanied by trismus with little or no restriction of excursive movements.
- *Spasms of lateral pterygoid and elevator muscles*: In it, pain occurs while biting, chewing, opening, maximum intercuspation and extended translatory movement. Pain is not affected by biting against a separator, except for some decrease in pain with maximum intercuspation and accompanied by acute malocclusion, trismus but with little or no restriction of excursive movements.

Clinical Features

- Laskin's four cardinal signs:
  1. *Unilateral pain*: It is generally a dull ache felt in the ear or the preauricular area or at the angle of the mandible. The pain is more often moderate on rising in the morning or relatively mild, but gradually becomes worse as the day progresses.
  2. *Muscles tenderness*: The most frequent areas are the neck of the mandible and the region distal and superior to the maxillary tuberosity.
  3. Clicking or popping noise in the TMJ.
  4. Limitation of jaw function or deviation of the mandible on opening.
- Laskin emphasized that the patient must also have these negative characteristics:
  - Absence of clinical, radiographic or biochemical evidence in the TMJ.
  - Lack of tenderness in TMJ area, on palpation via the external auditory meatus.
- Other signs:
  - Restrictions of opening and protrusion may be accompanied by deflection of the mandibular incisal path.
  - Soreness of muscles, when palpated. Myofascial trigger zones are stimulated by pressure and produce referred pain.
- Symptoms:
  - Masticatory pain may be due to myalgia, arthralgia or from both.
  - There is difficulty in chewing and restriction of mandibular excursion.

- Interference with mandibular movement with a noise on rubbing, clicking and with popping snapping sounds.
- Other features:
  - Oral or parafunctional habits, such as bruxism, present as indentation on lateral borders of the tongue, ridging of the buccal mucosa and extensive attrition of teeth.
  - Occurs in episodes of several times a day, at times, with extended symptom-free intervals. Usually episodes are seen during increased emotional tension, resulting in increased intra-articular pressure in the joint.
  - Acute malocclusion with abnormal relationship of teeth, due to mandibular displacement.

Treatment

The first important task is counseling of the patient and giving the assurance regarding prognosis and planning for symptomatic pain relief. Nature of the myofacial pain resulting from parafunctional habits secondary to stress and anxiety should be explained to the patient and the patient should be encouraged for behavior modification. Modification of diet, home exercise should be prescribed along with medication.

- *Medication*:
  - Nonsteroidal anti-inflammatory drugs—to reduce inflammation and to provide pain relief, both in muscles as well in the joints. For 14–21 days.
  - Muscle relaxants—are recommended only for short duration, as they produce sedation and addiction. Chlorzoxazone, diazepam 2–5 mg or cyclobenzaprine 10 mg at bedtime can be given for 10 days or meprobamete 400 mg/3 times a day for 7 days.
  - Ethyl chloride spray—or vasodilators like intramuscular local anesthetic injection like lidocaine are injected in the affected muscles can also give relief.
  - Antidepressants are used to inhibit neurotransmitters in the CNS and promote release of endomorphins and enkephalins. The patients are asked to follow the stretch exercise after that. Two percent lignocaine or 0.05% bupivacaine can be used.
- Intra-articular injections
- Hydrocortisone intra-articular injections can be used to treat the inflammation within the joint. 0.5 cc of 2% lignocaine can be mixed with hydrocortisone for relieving pain. These injections should not be used routinely, but may be given once a month with supportive and corrective treatment.
- Physiotherapeutic modalities
- Stress management
- Occlusal splints
- Temporomandibular joint arthrocentesis.

Temporomandibular Joint Pain

- The pain emanating from the structures of TMJ is of deep, somatic musculoskeletal type. This arthralgic pain is classified into—disc attachment pain, retrodiscal pain, capsular pain, arthritic pain.
- The most common disorder of TMJ is internal derangement or intracapsular disorders. The condyle disc complex is a movable hinge joint which operates against the articular eminence and fossa as a freely movable joint. All movements are free between the disc and the condyle. Its movements are restricted only in the outer ranges. Displacements of the articulating parts constitute dislocation. Subluxation (partial dislocation) is the displacement of the anterior disc without loss of surface contact between the condyle, disc and eminence. Luxation or complete dislocation is displacement of the articular disc with loss of surface contacts between the condyle, disc and eminence with resulting collapse of the articular space. Sensation of interference and abnormal disc sounds relate chiefly to movements of roughened or irregular articular surfaces, which may result from trauma, abusive use or derangement. Disc interference pain relates chiefly to strain and inflammation of the discal ligaments which resist abusive movements that tend to displace the disc from the condyle. Advanced radiological imaging techniques like computerized tomography, arthrography, magnetic resonance imaging, etc. help in accurate judgment of the disc space and to study internal derangements present. Pain depends chiefly on the extent of displacement and the condition of neural structures that innervate the discal ligaments. Pain occurs intermittently in conjunction with occlusal disharmony, when teeth are in maximum intercuspation. Sometimes restricted mandibular movement is displayed.
- Arthritic pain may be due to trauma or rheumatoid arthritis or osteoarthritis. Pain is of dull aching or burning sensation associated with capsulitis and synovitis and occlusal pressure increases the discomfort. In acute arthritis condition joint function is decreased due to pain, inflammatory exudates or secondary muscle effects. If osseous resorption decreases the vertical height of the ramus, some occlusal disharmony will be present. In severe cases, anterior open bite may result.
- Radiographic evidence of inflammatory arthritis is variable. There may be diffuse articular surface resorption of bone. Fibrous ankylosis may be present with restriction of jaw movements.
- Degenerative jaw disease may appear as decrease in the width of interarticular space with change in the contour

Table 25.6 Classification of different causes of trismus

- Traumatic
  - Intra-articular
    - Trauma to the growth center
    - Monoarticular arthritis like spasm or subluxation due to chronic malocclusion
    - Trauma to the articular disc
    - Trauma to the capsular or temporomandibular ligament
    - Fracture with or without dislocation of the condylar head
    - Ankylosis
    - Foreign bodies in the joint area
- Extra-articular
  - Trauma to the muscle
  - Trauma during extraction
  - Faulty mandibular block
  - Fracture of the coronoid process
  - Fracture of the zygomatic arch
  - Fracture of the styloid process
  - Misplaced fixative or augmentative device
  - Scar tissue formation
- Inflammatory
  - Intra-articular
    - Pyogenic infection
    - Rheumatic fever
    - Rheumatoid arthritis
    - Gout
    - Tuberculosis
    - Syphilis
    - Actinomycosis
    - Osteomyelitis
    - Synovitis
  - Extra-articular
    - Pericoronitis
    - Acute and chronic osteomyelitis
    - Acute and chronic dentoalveolar abscess
    - Infections of the mandible (tuberculosis, syphilis, actinomycosis)
    - Cancrum oris (noma)
    - Abscess in various spaces like: infratemporal, lateral pharyngeal, submasseteric and pterygomandibular spaces.
    - Phosphorous necrosis
    - Quinsy (peritonsillar abscess)
    - Infection of the ear (otitis media)
    - Mumps
    - Acute generalized stomatitis
    - Angular cheilitis
    - Pharyngitis
    - Parotitis
- Neoplastic
  - Intra-articular
    - Benign
    - Osteoma
    - Chondroma
    - Osteochondroma
    - Myxoma
    - Benign giant cell tumor
    - Trotter's syndrome

Contd...

Contd...

  - *Malignant*
    - Osteosarcoma
    - Chondrosarcoma
    - Fibrosarcoma
    - Metastatic carcinoma
  - Extra-articular
    - Benign and malignant tumors of the mandible and maxilla especially in the premolar and molar region
    - Malignant tumors of the nasopharynx
    - Malignant tumors of the maxillary sinus
    - Benign and malignant tumors of the parotid gland
- Cystic
  - Extra-articular
    All large cystic lesions affecting the mandible, ramus and posterior aspect of the maxilla.
- Systemic
  - Tetanus
  - Tetany
  - Fibrous dysplasia
  - Paget's disease
  - Acromegaly
  - Epilepsy and hysteria
  - Hydrophobia
  - Sudden shock (physical, chemical, electrical)
  - Hemorrhage
  - Brain tumors
  - Scleroderma
  - Strychnine poisoning
  - Myelofibrosis
  - Amyotrophic lateral sclerosis
  - Hypocalcemia
- Congenital or developmental
  - Unilateral or bilateral condylar hyperplasia
  - Unilateral or bilateral exostosis of coronoid
  - Hyperplasia of coronoid process and /or zygomatic arch
  - Fusion of coronoid process with zygomatic arch
  - Absence of coronoid process
  - Arthrogryposis multiplex congenita of TMJ—(multiple contraction of muscles, rigidity of joints, atrophy of muscle groups involved, fusiform extremities, muscle ligament contractures)
  - Fusion of maxillary and mandibular process
  - Unilateral hyperplasia of the jaw
- Miscellaneous
  - Oral submucous fibrosis
  - Osteoradionecrosis
  - Myositis ossificans
  - Disuse atrophy
  - Myofascial pain dysfunction syndrome (MPDS)
  - Extensive burns of the face with keloid and scar formation
  - Dystrophic epidermolysis bullosa
  - Catalepsy—accompanied with mental distress
  - Trichinosis (from ingestion of infected pork)
  - Drugs (like metoclopramide, phenothiazine may cause extra-pyramidal reactions)

of the condyle with flattened surface, anterior lipping and loss of definition, suggestive of osseous resorption. Traumatic arthritis may show evidence of trauma or malocclusion due to fracture. Periarticular inflammation may occur as a result of trauma or otitis media. Rarely neoplastic disorders involve the TMJ. The characteristic features are slow progressive immobilization of the joint without any pain. Early signs and symptoms are similar to fibrous ankylosis.

- *Retrodiscal pain*: Is due to the inflammation of tissues that comprises the retrodizal pad, this is basically caused when the condyle is displaced posteriorly due to posterior overclosure from missing teeth or from trauma, the resultant inflammatory swelling displaces the condyle anteriorly causing acute malocclusion with contralateral premature contact of the anterior teeth and disocclusion of the posteriors ipsilaterally.
- *Capsular pain*: Also called capsulitis, which is the inflammation of the fibrous and synovial capsule, and results in pain every time the capsule is stretched by the translatory movement of the condyle.

Trismus (Mandibular Hypomobility, Lock Jaw) (Table 25.6)

This is defined as a motor disturbance of the trigeminal nerve, producing spasms of the muscles with difficulty in opening of the mouth.

This limited opening of the mouth is a challenging problem that may result from several different causes and which not only impairs the patients chewing, swallowing and patient's oral hygiene but also limits the access to the mouth, creating problems for the dentist in carrying various treatment procedures.

BIBLIOGRAPHY

1. Aggressive Condylar Resorption Journal of Cranoiofacial Surgery. 2013;115:1.
2. Brooks SL, et al. Imaging of the TMJ. Position Paper of the American Academy of Oral and Maxillofacial Radiology; Oral Surg Oral Med Oral Pathol Oral Radiol Endod. 1997;83:609.
3. Dworkin S, LeResche L. Research Diagnostic Criteria for TMJ Disorders: review, criteria, examinations and specifications, critique. J Craniomandib Disord. 1992;6:301-35.
4. Goaz PW, White SC. Principles and Interpretation. In: Oral Radiology, 3rd edition. St Louis: Mosby Year Book, 1994.
5. Heffez LB, Mafee MF, Rosenberg H. Imaging atlas of the temporomandibular joint. Williams and Wilkins Baltimore; 1995.
6. Helms CA, Kalpan P. Diagnostic imaging of the TMJ: recommendations of various techniques. Am J Roentgenol. 1990;154:319.
7. Miles DA, Van Dis MJ, Jensen CW, et al. Interpretation normal versus abnormal and common radiographic presentations of lesions. In: Radiographic and Imaging for Dental Auxillaries, 3rd edition. Philadelphia: WB Saunders; 1999.pp.231-80.
8. Norman J de B, Bramley P. A Textbook and Colour Atlas of the Temporomandibular Joint. Wolfe Medical Publications; 1990.
9. Rees A. The structure and function of the mandibular joint. Br Dent J. 1954;96:125-33.
10. Shafer WG, et al. A Textbook of Oral Pathology. Philadelphia: WB Saunders; 1983.
11. Wood NK, Goaz PW. Differential diagnosis of oral lesions, 4th edition. CV Mosby: St Louis; 1991.
12. Wood RE. Handbook of signs in dental and maxillofacial radiology.Warthog Publications, Toronto: 1988.
13. Worth HM. Principles and practice of oral radiographic interpretation. Year Book Medical Publishers, Chicago; 1963.

Disorders of the Maxillary Sinus | 26

The paranasal sinuses are air filled cavities of the craniofacial complex, comprising the maxillary, frontal, and sphenoidal sinuses and the ethmoidal air cells. The maxillary sinuses because of their close proximity to the dental structures are of importance to the dental surgeon. The diseases of the sinuses may mimic odontogenic disease, and also, odontogenic disease may spread to the sinuses or mimic sinus disease.

FUNCTIONS

- Air conditioning (heating and humidification)
- Acting as an air reservoir
- Ventilation
- Aiding in olfaction
- Reduction in weight of the cranium
- Addition of resonance to the voice
- Protection
- Insulation of the cerebrum and orbits
- Participation in formation of the cranium.

The mucosal lining of the paranasal sinuses is similar to that found in the nasal cavity, but with slightly fewer mucous glands. In the absence of disease, the epithelial cilia move mucous toward their respective communications with the nasal fossae.

ANATOMY OF THE MAXILLARY SINUS (ANTRUM OF HIGHMORE) (FIGS 26.1A AND B)

These are paired structures located in the body of the maxilla and are a mirror image of each other. It contains air and is lined by mucoperiosteum which has a pseudostratified ciliated columnar epithelium. The average size is approximately 3.5 cm in height, 2.5 cm in width and 3.2 cm anteroposteriorly. It opens into the middle meatus of the nose in the lower part of the hiatus semilunaris.

They are pyramidal in shape with the base directed medially towards the lateral aspect of the nose and the apex directed laterally in the zygomatic process of the maxilla.

The roof of the sinus is formed by the floor of the orbit, which is transversed by the infraorbital nerve. The roof is flat and slopes slightly anterior and laterally. The most medial part of the roof forms the sloping wall of the ethmoidal sinuses (from where disease may spread to the maxillary sinus). Antral infection may involve infraorbital vessels and nerves and malignant tumors growing in the sinus may involve the orbit.

The floor of the sinus is curved and formed by the alveolar process of the maxilla and lies about 1 cm below the level of the floor of the nose. The roots of the upper molars and

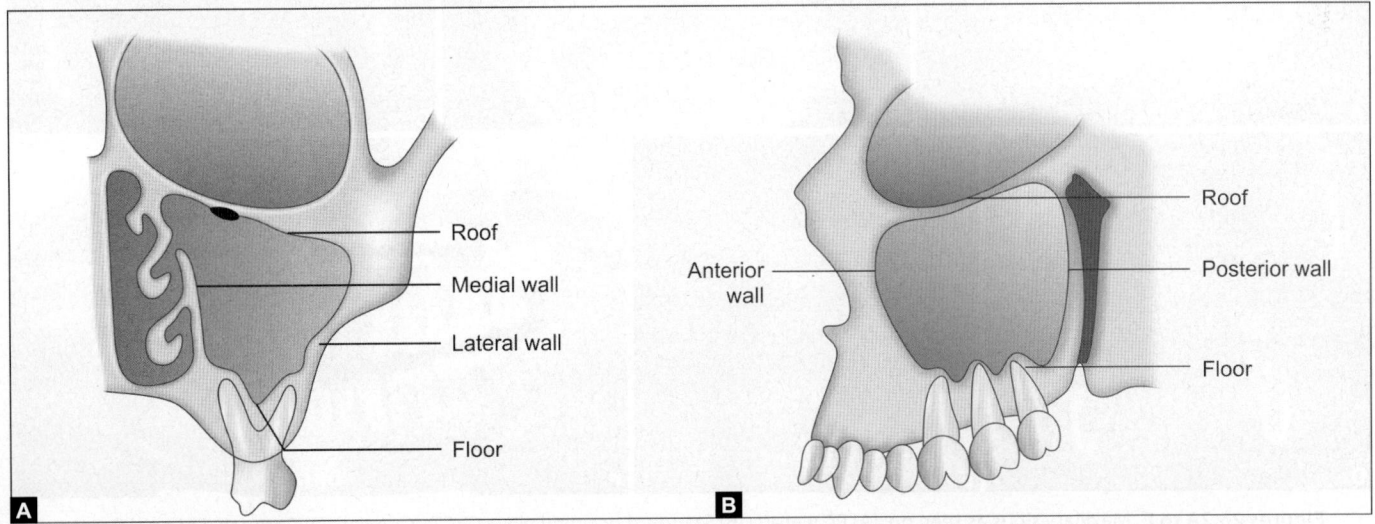

Figures 26.1A and B Diagram of a left antrum showing the basic shape and various walls and margins: (A) From the front; (B) From the side

premolars may ridge the floor or project into it. The floor may be subdivided by the incomplete bony septa lying between the roots of the teeth, especially in the posterior part of the sinus.

The medial wall is bounded by the nasal cavity and is slightly convex towards the sinus.

The posterior wall is related to the pterygopalatine fossa and bulges posterior towards the infratemporal fossa.

The lateral wall is in relation with the zygoma.

The anterior wall is depressed by the canine fossa on the anterior surface of the maxilla and is convex towards the interior of the sinus.

Blood supply is by the facial, infraorbital and greater palatine arteries, which drains into the facial and pterygoid plexus of veins.

The lymphatics drain into the submandibular lymph nodes.

The maxillary sinuses are innervated by the infraorbital and the posterior superior alveolar nerves.

Radiographic Anatomy (Figs 26.2A to F)

The antrum appears as a radiolucent cavity in the maxilla, with well-defined, dense, corticated radiopaque margins or walls. The internal bony septa and blood vessels canals in the walls produce their own shadows.

Diseases associated with the maxillary sinuses include both intrinsic (primarily originating from within the sinus) and extrinsic diseases (those that originate from outside the sinus, and either impinge or infiltrate into the sinus) (**Table 26.1**).

General Clinical Features

- Feeling of pressure
- Altered voice characteristics
- Pain on movement of head
- Percussion sensitivity of teeth or cheek region
- Regional paresthesia or anesthesia
- Swelling of the facial structures adjacent to the maxilla.

Applied Diagnostic Imaging

- Intraoral periapical radiograph will show the floor, the base of the antral cavity and relationship with upper posterior teeth.
- Maxillary lateral occlusal radiograph gives a more extensive view of the sinus.

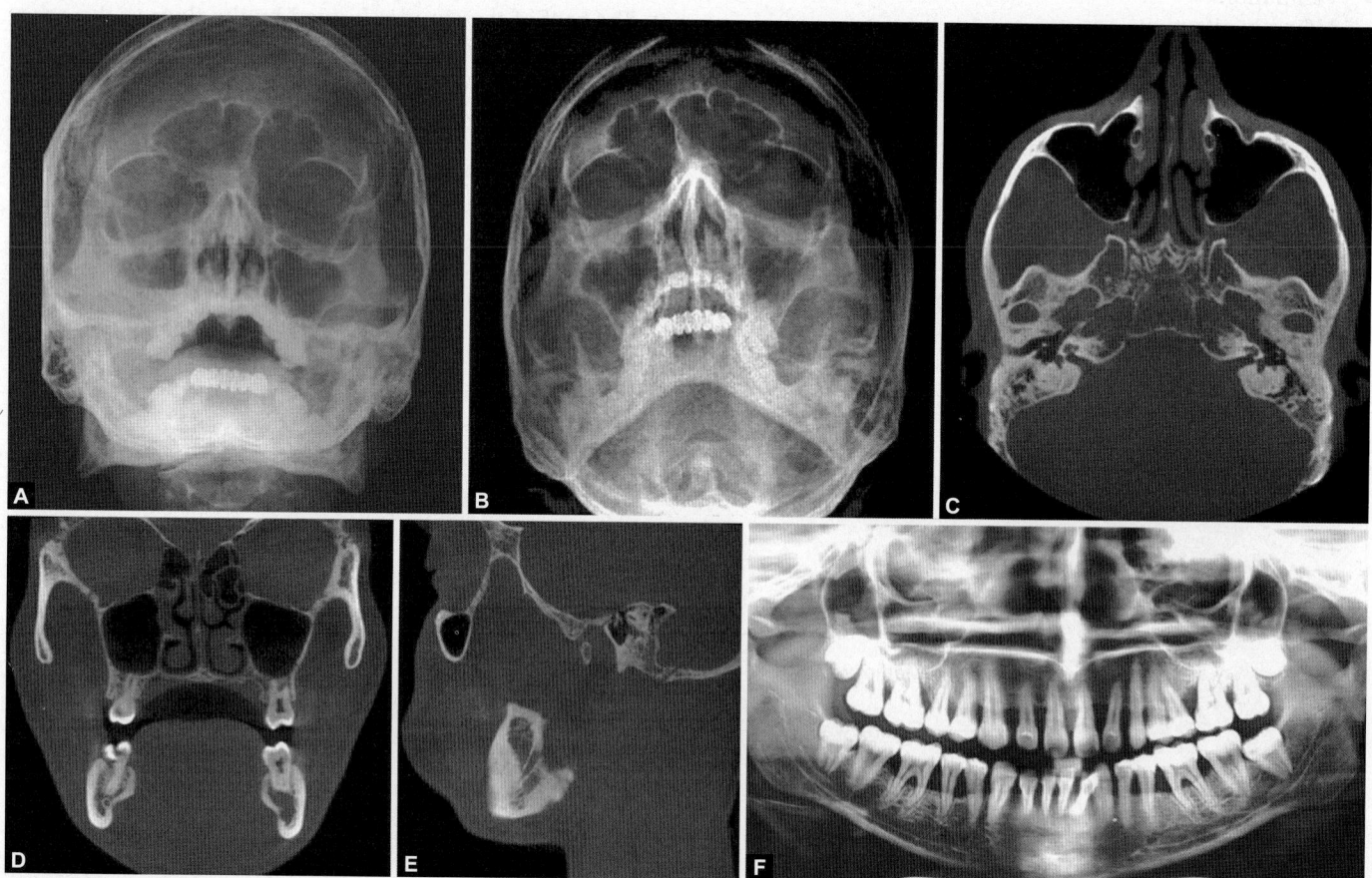

Figures 26.2A to F Maxillary sinus as seen on: (A) PA waters; (B) Standard occipital view, CBCT: (C) Axial; (D) Coronal; (E) Sagittal view; (F) Panoramic radiograph showing right and left sinus note the variation of the sinus wall of both sides

Table 26.1 Classification of disorders of the maxillary sinus

- Traumatic
  - Fracture of maxilla, tuberosity, nasal bone, zygoma and orbital floor
    - Blow out fracture
    - Isolated injury
    - Complex fracture
  - Hematoma due to traumatic injury
  - Foreign bodies displaced into the sinus; fractured root/ tooth, bullets, anthroliths
  - Oral antral fistula; during extraction of, or from pulpoperiapical infections of the maxillary teeth
  - Sinus contusion
- Infection/inflammatory
  Nonspecific
  - Mucositis
  - Acute sinusitis
  - Chronic sinusitis
  - Empyema
  - Local hyperplasia from odontogenic infections/periosteitis
  - Antral polyps
  - Osteomyelitis
  - Osteoradionecrosis
  Specific (these infections involve the sinus secondarily)
  - Actinomycosis
  - Aspergillosis
  - Blastomycosis
  - Coccidioidomycosis
  - Histoplasmosis
  - Leprosy
  - Mucormycosis
  - Sarcoidosis
  - Syphilis
  - Rhinosporidiosis
  - Tuberculosis
  - Wegner's granulomatosis
  - Pseudotumor (diseases of fungal origin)
- Cysts
  Intrinsic
  - Mucous retention cyst
  - Serouscyst
  - Psuedocyst
  - Benign mucosal cyst of the maxillary sinus
  - Surgical ciliated cyst
  - Mucocele
  - Dermoid cyst
  Extrinsic (these secondarily encroach upon the sinus)
  Odontogenic
  - Radicular
  - Dentigerous
  - Primordial
  - Keratocyst
  Nonodontogenic
  - Globulomaxillary
  - Traumatic cyst
  - Aneurysmal bone cyst

Contd...

Contd...

- Neoplasms
  Benign
  Odontogenic
  - Ameloblastoma and its variants
  - Adenoameloblastoma
  - Compound and complex composite odontomes
  - Calcifying odontogenic epithelial tumor
  - Cementifying fibroma
  - Cementoma
  Nonodontogenic
  - Antral polyp
  - Antral papilloma
  - Exostosis
  - Enostosis
  - Tumors of the salivary glands
  - Myxomas
  - Fibromas–juvenile cementofibroma
  - Giant cell granuloma
  - Osteoma
  - Chondroma
  - Central hemangioma
  - Pseudo cholesteatoma
  - Plasmacytoma
  - Neurogenic tumors
  Malignant
  - Squamous cell carcinoma
  - Invasion of the maxillary sinus by local malignant disease
  - Metastatic carcinoma of the maxillary sinus
  - Multiple myeloma
  - Midline lethal granuloma
- Metabolic and endocrinal
  - Hyperparathyroidism
  - Fibrous dysplasia
  - Cherubism
  - Paget's disease
  - Langerhan's cell histiocytosis
  - Leontiasis ossea
  - Caffey's disease
  - Osteopetrosis
  - Cooley's anemia
- Calcifications
  - Anthroliths
- Syndromes (Developmental)
  - Crouzon's syndrome
  - Treacher Collins syndrome
  - Binder's syndrome

- The panoramic radiograph depicts both maxillary sinuses, revealing greater internal structure and parts of the inferior, posterior and anteromedial walls. It may be difficult to compare the internal radiopacities of the right and left sinus due to the variations that result from the overlapping phantom images of other structures that appear on the panoramic radiograph.
- Caldwell's posteroanterior view gives a good visualization of the frontal sinus, ethmoidal air cells, nasal cavity and superior portion of the maxillary antrum.

- Water's view, is optimal for visualization of the maxillary sinuses, especially to compare internal radiopacities, as well as the frontal sinuses and ethmoidal air cells, when the mouth is open the sphenoidal sinus is also seen. This view shows the roof, medial walls and allows the comparison of both the maxillary sinuses.
- Lateral skull helps to view the sphenoidal and maxillary sinuses the anterior and superior walls. It allows examination of all four pairs of paranasal sinuses, but each member of a pair is superimposed on the other.
- Submentovertex is useful in evaluating the lateral and posterior borders of the maxillary sinus as well as the ethmoid air cells.
- Tomography is useful for viewing solid masses such as antroliths, in the anterior wall, posterior wall, lateral wall, or roof of the sinus.
- *Computed tomography provides multiple sections through the sinuses in different planes*: High-resolution axial and coronal CT provide the most revealing, noninvasive technique for visualizing the paranasal sinuses and adjacent structures and areas. CT helps to determine the extent of the disease in patients who have chronic or recurrent sinusitis. Coronal CT provides superior visualization of the osteomeatal complex (the region of the ostium of the maxillary sinus and the ethmoid ostium) and nasal cavities, as well as for demonstrating any reaction in the surrounding bone to sinus disease.
- Scintigraphy, the radioactive isotopes can be used diagnostically to demonstrate physiological changes. In case of extension of the antral carcinoma to involve bone, the osteoblastic response produced is clearly evident in the delayed phase of a radionuclide bone scan.
- Ultrasound is effective in distinguishing normal sinuses, chronically inflamed sinus lining and if the sinus is filled with fluid, tumor or scar.
- Magnetic resonance imaging also provides multiple sections through the sinuses in different planes, high-resolution axial and coronal MRI provide the most revealing, noninvasive technique for the paranasal sinuses and adjacent structures and areas. It is extremely sensitive in demonstrating maxillary antrum pathology due to the high signal intensity of T2-weighted image of almost all the soft tissue abnormalities, contrasted by the absence of signal from both air within the sinus and the surrounding cortical bone. It helps to delineate soft tissues in the sinus, and gives a very clear comparative view of the two sinuses. It helps to differentiate retained fluid secretions from soft tissue masses in the sinuses.
- Cone beam computed tomography is the breakthrough in dental imagining of the maxillary sinus and gives

adequate information of this anatomical region which much reduced exposure to the patient.

INTRINSIC DISEASES INVOLVING THE MAXILLARY SINUS

Developmental Condition

Crouzon's Syndrome

Early synostosis of the sutures produces hypoplasia of the maxilla and therefore the maxillary sinus, together with a high arched palate.

Treacher Collin's Syndrome

Mandibulofacial dysostosis is associated with a grossly and symmetrically underdeveloped maxillary sinuses and malar bones.

Binder's Syndrome

Maxillonasal dysplasia, involves hypoplasia of the middle third of the face. There is maxillary retrognathism, smaller maxillary length and maxillary sinus hypoplasia.

INFLAMMATORY DISEASE

Mucositis (Thickened Mucous Membrane) (Figs 26.3 and 26.4)

Definition

The normal mucosal lining of the paranasal sinus is composed of respiratory epithelium and is approximately 1 mm thick, and is not visualized on the radiograph. When the mucosa becomes inflamed from either an infectious or allergic process, it may increase in thickness 10–15 times and is then seen on the radiograph. This thickening is called mucositis; any thickening greater than 3 mm is most likely to be pathological.

Clinical Features

It is usually asymptomatic and is discovered on a routine radiograph.

Radiographic Features

- It is seen as a non-corticated band noticeably more radiopaque than the air filled sinus, paralleling the bony wall of the sinus.
- Mucosal thickening seen distinctly on Denta Scan Images.

Management

Removal of the cause.

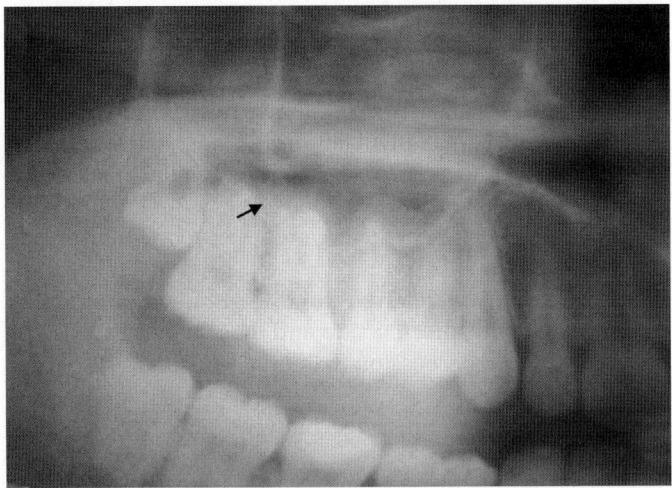

Figure 26.3 Panoramic radiograph shows increased width of sinus epithelium in right maxillary sinus

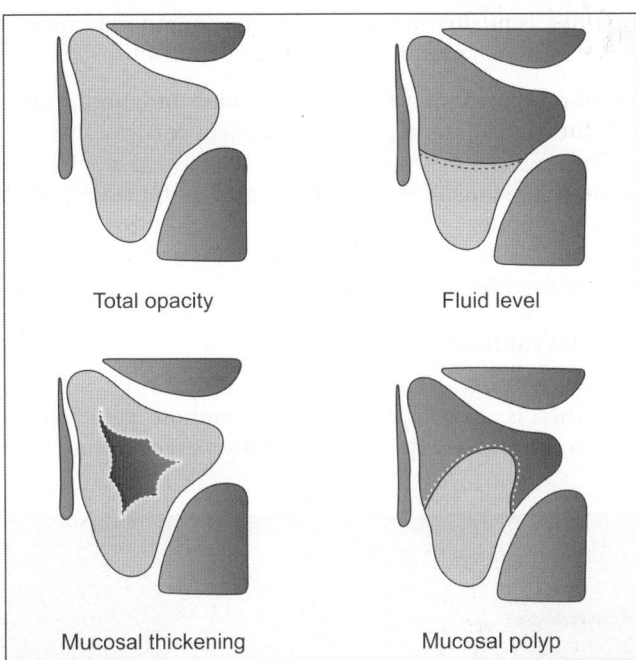

Total opacity   Fluid level

Mucosal thickening   Mucosal polyp

Figure 26.5 Simplified line diagrams of a left antrum (as depicted on a 0° OM) illustrating the various radiographic changes in the antrum caused by acute and chronic sinusitis

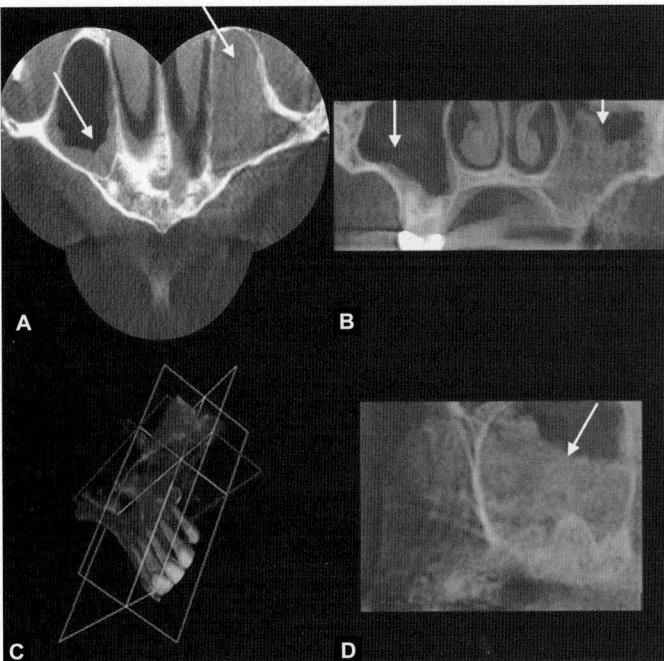

Figures 26.4A to D Cone beam computed tomography showing sinus pathology; Crown on the maxillary left first molar causing a periapical lesion and endo antral syndrome. This patient also has sinusitis. Note white arrows showing sinus thickening: (A) Axial; (B) Coronal; (C) 3D; (D) Sagittal section

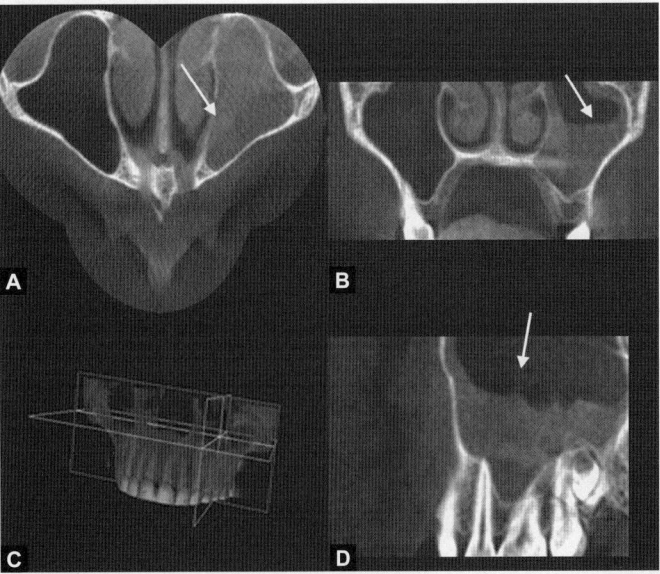

Figures 26.6A to D Cone beam computed tomography image of maxillary sinus of the left side: (A) Axial; (B) Coronal; (C) 3D; (D) Sagittal section shows the level of the inflammatory exudate commonly referred to as the waters level in PA Water's view indicative of sinusitis

Maxillary Sinusitis (Figs 26.5 to 26.8)

Definition

There is generalized inflammation of the paranasal mucosa; the etiologic agent may be an allergen, bacterial or viral. It may be caused due the blockage of drainage from the ostiomeatal complex. Inflammatory changes may lead to ciliary dysfunction and retention of sinus secretions. About 10% of the inflammatory conditions of the maxillary sinus are extensions of dental infections. The term pansinusitis describes sinusitis affecting all the paranasal sinuses. Pansinusitis in children is suggestive of cystic fibrosis.

Maxillary sinusitis may be broadly divided into three types:
1. Acute sinusitis is a condition present for less than two weeks.
2. Subacute sinusitis is a condition present for two weeks to three months.
3. Chronic sinusitis is a condition present for more than three months.

Clinical Features

- *Acute sinusitis*:
  - This is a complication of common cold and is accompanied by a clear nasal discharge or pharyngeal

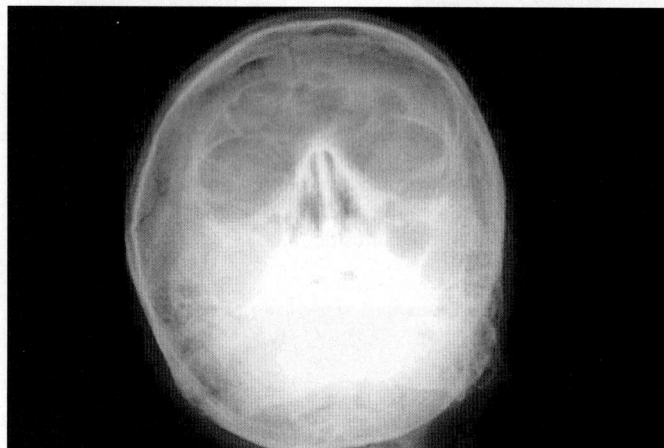

Figure 26.7 PA view showing bilateral maxillary sinusitis. Radiopacity seen over the floor of the right maxillary sinus extending up to the roof of the sinus having a concave superior surface suggestive of air fluid level

drainage, which may eventually become green or greenish- yellow colored.
  - After a few days the stuffiness increases and the patient complains of pain and tenderness to pressure or swelling over the involved sinus.
  - There will be signs of sepsis; fever, chills, malaise and an elevated leukocyte count.
  - Pain may be felt in the areas of the eyeballs, cheek and frontal region.
  - Pain may be referred to the premolar and molar teeth on the affected side and these teeth may also be sensitive to percussion (bacterial sinusitis).
- *Subacute sinusitis*:
  - This is an interim stage between acute and chronic sinusitis.
  - It is devoid of symptoms associated with the acute condition, such as pain and toxemia.
  - The nasal discharge is purulent with an associated nasal voice and stuffiness.
  - There may be a sore throat.
  - Patient may be unable to sleep due to a persistent irritating cough.
- *Chronic sinusitis*:
  - This is sequela of the former two, which has failed to resolve by 3 months.
  - There are no external signs, except in case of an acute exacerbation when increased pain and discomfort is apparent.
  - This type is usually associated with anatomical derangements that inhibit the outflow of mucous, like deviation of the nasal septum and presence of a concha bullosa (pneumatization of the middle concha).
  - It is also associated with allergic rhinitis, asthma, cystic fibrosis and dental infections.

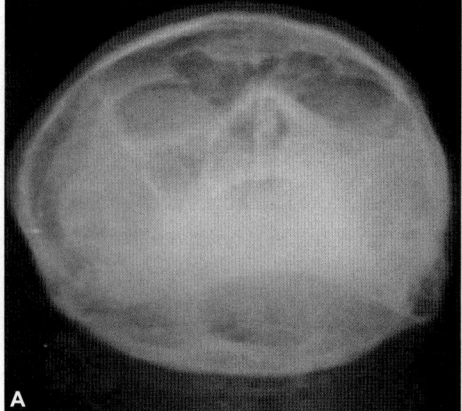
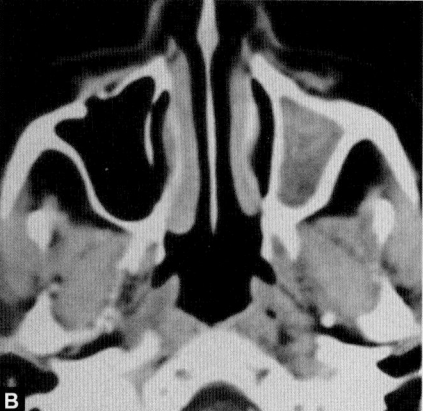
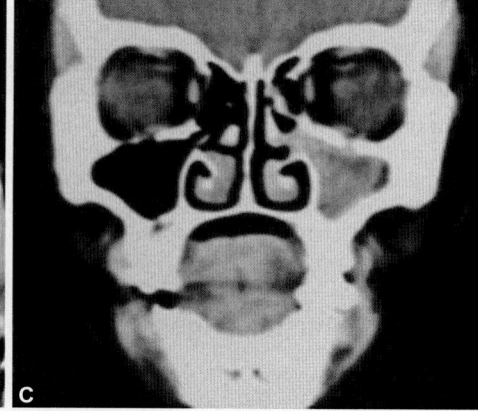

Figures 26.8A to C Chronic sinusitis: (A) Water's view radiograph: It shows haziness of the left maxillary sinus region. CT scan; (B) Axial; (C) Coronal view shows mucosal thickening and presence of secretions in the left maxillary sinus. Mucosal thickening also noted in the left anterior ethmoidal sinuses and the left half of the frontal sinus. Left OMU is blocked. Final diagnosis—left maxillary, ethmoidal and frontal sinusitis

Radiographic Features

- Thickening of the sinus mucosa and the accumulation of secretions that accompany sinusitis reduce the air content of the sinus and cause it to become increasingly radiopaque
- The most common radiopaque patterns as seen on the Water's view are:
  - Localized mucosal thickening along the sinus floor.
  - Generalized thickening of the mucosal lining around the entire wall of the sinus.
  - Complete filling of the sinus except in the region of the ostium on the medial wall.
  - Complete opacification of the sinus.
- The frontal and the sphenoidal sinuses may be similarly affected
- The image of the thickened sinus mucosa on the radiograph may vary from:
  - Being uniform or polypoidal.
  - In case of an allergic reaction the mucosa tends to become lobulated.
  - In case of infection, the thickened mucosal outline tends to be smoother, with its contour following the sinus floor.

Air fluid level resulting from the accumulation of secretions may be present:
- Radiopacities of transudates, exudates, blood and pathologically altered mucosa are similar; the differentiation depends on their shape and distribution.
- Fluid appears radiopaque and occupies the inferior aspect of the sinus. The border between the radiopaque fluid and the relatively radiolucent antrum is horizontal and straight with a meniscus.
- Air-fluid interface may be confirmed by tilting the patient's head and making another radiograph. To demonstrate an air-fluid level, the central ray of the X-ray beam must be horizontal and at the level of the air-fluid interface. Sufficient time should be allowed after the change in position, between the two radiographs for the fluid level to change.
- Chronic sinusitis may result in persistent radiopacification of the sinus with sclerosis and/or thickening of the sinus wall. Resorption of the bony border is unusual
- The resolution of acute sinusitis becomes apparent on the radiograph as a gradual increase in the radiolucency, beginning from the interior of the sinus; the thickened mucosa gradually shrinks, till the sinus appears normal.

Additional Imaging

- *CT images*: may reveal the presence of thickened mucosal tissue, which may cause blockage of the ostium.
- Chronic sinusitis has a varying mucosal swelling which may be smooth or irregular due to edema or secretions. The sinus walls may be thickened, sclerotic or fibrotic.

There may be dystrophic calcifications present. These change may be seen on T1-weighted MRI images as low to intermediate signals, T2-weighted MRI usually shows high signal of the inflamed mucosa, low signal of sclerosis and fibrosis. Inspissated mucus may be dark on all sequences resulting in false negative MR diagnosis of chronic sinusitis. T1-weighted post Gd RI shows intense enhancement of inflamed mucosa, with no enhancement of the fluid.

Management

The goals of the treatment are to control the infection, promote drainage and relieve pain.

Empyema

Definition

This is a cavity filled with pus. It may result as a possible sequela of a sinus ostium blocked by a thickened, inflamed mucous membrane or some other pathologic process, especially in the maxillary sinus. Empyema is probably a variant of a mucocele or pyocele.

Radiographic Features

- The sinus appears completely radiopaque
- Decalcification of the surrounding bony walls and haziness of trabecular bone next to the sinus wall is seen
- It may extend into the adjacent bone with the development of osteomyelitis.

CYST (FIG. 26.9)

(Retention Pseudocysts, Antral Pseudocyst, Benign Mucous Cyst, Mucous Retention Cyst, Mesothelial Cyst, Pseudocyst, Interstitial Cyst, Lymphangiectatic Cyst, False Cyst, Retention Cyst of the Maxillary Sinus, Benign Cyst of the Antrum, Benign Mucosal Cyst of the Sinus, Serous Nonsecretory Retention Pseudocyst, Mucosal Antral Cyst, Intramural Cyst)

Definition

The term retention pseudocyst is used to describe several related conditions, the pathogenesis is controversial, but as their clinical and radiographic features are similar, no attempt is made here to differentiate them. It is suggested that it results due to blockage of the secretory ducts of seromucous glands in the sinus mucosa leading to accumulation of secretions and swelling of the tissue, or it may be a result of cystic degeneration within an inflamed, thickened sinus lining. Both are not lined by epithelium and are called pseudocysts.

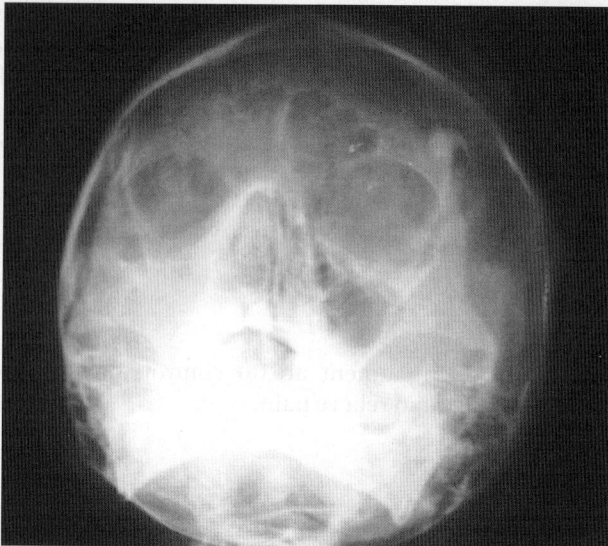

Figure 26.9 Pseudocyst/benign cyst of antrum. PA waters shows haziness of right maxillary sinus. Medial, posteroinferior and floor of right maxillary sinus are not traceable. A well defined cortication is noted along the borders of the right maxillary sinus which is unilocular and irregular in shape. Discontinuation noted in the right floor of orbit. Erosion of lateral nasal wall also noted. Frontal and ethmoidal sinuses seems clear. Differential diagnosis: Benign cystic lesion, mucocele

Clinical Features

- It may be found in any of the sinuses, more in the months of April and November (related to changes in seasons) and more often in males
- They are the most common in the maxillary sinus and are not related to extractions nor associated with periapical disease. These cysts may also be found in the frontal or sphenoidal sinuses
- It is usually asymptomatic and may be an incidental finding on a routine radiograph.
- When the pseudocyst completely fills the maxillary sinus, there may be localized pain and feeling of fullness or numbness. It may prolapse (extrude) through the ostium and cause nasal obstruction and postnasal discharge
- The pseudocyst may rupture as a result of abrupt pressure changes caused due to sneezing or blowing the nose, or it may herniate into the nasal cavity and subsequently rupture
- There may be copious discharge of yellow fluid from the nostrils.

Radiographic Features

- Pseudocysts may occur bilaterally, or there may be more than one cyst in the sinus. They project from the floor of the sinus or from the lateral walls
- The size may vary from that of a finger tip to a size large enough to completely fill the sinus and make it radiopaque

- Both varieties are noncorticated, smooth dome-shaped radiopaque masses. As they originate within the sinus no osseous border surrounds it. The base may be narrow or broad
- It appears homogeneous and radiopaque in comparison with the surrounding air sinus, due to the accumulation of fluid
- The sinus floor is intact, with a persistent thin radiopaque line of the antral cortex

Additional Imaging

- Partial images may be seen on the posterior periapical radiographs
- They are best demonstrated on the panoramic radiographs
- The smooth spherical soft tissue masses are seen on T1-weighted MRI images as low to intermediate signal but may show high signal if the cyst has high protein content. T2-weighted MRI images show a high signal

Differential Diagnosis

- Inflammatory lesions of the sinus where the patient may complain of persistent pain.
- Odontogenic cyst have a characteristic corticated border. These are more rounded or tear drop shaped and not as homogenous. The floor of the antrum is missing or displaced. Apical radicular cyst, dentigerous cyst, odontogenic keratocysts and cyst of the globulomaxillary area are the most common.
- Antral polyps of infectious or allergic origin are more opaque, more heterogeneous and multiple and are commonly associated with thickened mucosa.
- *Benign neoplasms*: If originating outside the sinus, is separated from the cavity by a radiopaque border. It is less likely to be dome-shaped.
- *Malignant neoplasms*: It may be destroy the osseous border of the sinus, whether it arises from within the sinus or from the alveolar process.

Management

These require no treatment.

Mucocele (Pyocele, Mucopyocele)

Definition

This is an expanding, destructive lesion that results from a blocked sinus ostium, due to intra-antral or intranasal inflammation, polyp or neoplasm. As the mucous is accumulated and the sinus cavity filled, the increase in intra-antral pressure results in the thinning, displacement and in some cases destruction of the sinus walls. If the mucocele becomes infected, it is called pyocele or a mucopyocele.

Clinical Features

- Ninty percent of the mucoceles occur in the ethmoidal and frontal sinuses and are rare in the maxillary and sphenoidal sinuses
- In the maxillary sinus it may exert pressure on the superior alveolar nerves causing radiating pain, with a swelling and fullness of the cheek. The swelling may be first observed over the anteroinferior aspect of the antrum, where the wall may be thinned or destroyed
- If the lesion expands inferiorly, it may cause loosening of the posterior teeth
- If the medial wall of the sinus is expanded, the lateral wall of the nasal cavity will deform and the nasal airway may be obstructed
- If it expands into the orbit, it may cause diplopia (double vision) or proptosis (protrusion of the globe of the eye).

Radiographic Features

- The normal shape of the maxillary sinus is changed into a more circular shape as the mucocele enlarges
  - Septa and bony walls may be thinned or destroyed.
  - Teeth may be displaced and/or roots resorbed.
  - The supramedial border of the orbit is displaced or destroyed.
- The scalloped border of the frontal sinus is usually smoothed by expansion, and the intersinus septum may be displaced
- In the ethmoidal air cells, displacement of the lamina papyracea may occur, displacing the contents of the orbit
- In the sphenoid sinus the expansion may be in the superior direction, suggesting a pituitary neoplasm
- The sinus cavities appear uniformly radiopaque.

Additional Imaging

- *Computed tomography*: It helps to differentiate and observe any remnants of the internal aspect of the antrum between the wall of a cyst and the wall of the antrum, and to help differentiate between a large odontogenic cyst and a mucocele
- The T1 and T2 weighted MRI images show variable signals depending on the protein content, state of dehydration and viscosity of the contents. The most frequently observed patterns are moderate to marked high signal on T1 and T2 weighted images, moderate to marked low, and/or usually low to intermediate signal on T1 and T2 images. On T1 weighted post Gd MRI images there is no enhancement except in the area of the thin peripheral rim.

Differential Diagnosis

- Cyst
- Benign tumor
- Malignancy

- Any suggestion of a lesion associated with occluded ostium should be a mucocele. A large odontogenic cyst displacing the maxillary antral floor may mimic a mucocele.

Management

Surgical removal by the Caldwell-Luc operation.

Surgical Ciliated Cyst of the Maxilla (Postoperative Maxillary Cyst)

Definition

It is a delayed complication arising years after surgery involving the maxilla.

Clinical Features

- It usually occurs in the 4th–5th decade of life, more in males
- The patient may complain of pain, discomfort or swelling of the face or intra oral swelling of the palate or alveolus, with pus discharge.

Radiographic Features

- It is seen as a well-defined radiolucency closely related to the maxillary sinus
- There is sclerosis of the surrounding bone
- As the cyst enlarges it produces pressure effects, with thinning of the sinus walls which may eventually perforate (resembles a malignant neoplasm)
- There may be resorption of the maxillary alveolar process
- There is no communication between the cyst and the maxillary sinus which may be demonstrated by injecting the sinus with radiopaque material.

Management

Enucleation.

CALCIFICATIONS

Antroliths

Refer to Chapter 27 Soft Tissue Calcifications and Ossifications (Page 510).

BENIGN NEOPLASMS

Benign neoplasms of the paranasal sinuses other than inflammatory polyps are rare. The radiographic images of such benign neoplasms are nonspecific. Usually the involved portion of the sinus appears radiopaque because of the presence of mass, and they may cause displacement of the adjacent sinus borders.

Polyps (Antral Polyp) (Figs 26.10 to 26.12)

Definition

The thickened mucous membrane of a chronically inflamed sinus frequently forms into irregular folds called polyps. Polyposis of the sinus mucosa may develop in an isolated area or in a number of areas throughout the sinus.

Clinical Features

- It usually occurs in young persons
- It may arise from any part of the sinus wall and occasionally pass through the opening to appear in the nose as antrochoanal polyp

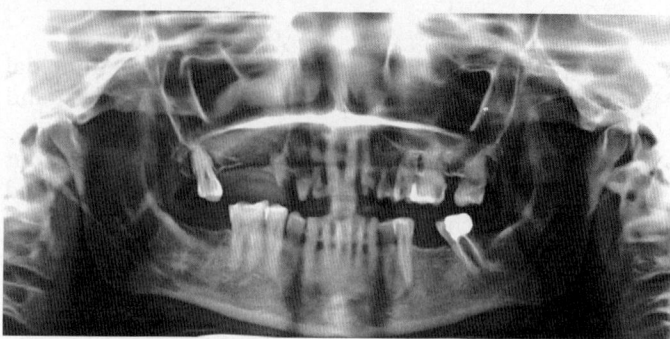

Figure 26.10   Panoramic radiograph showing right antral polyp with radiopacity in the right maxillary sinus

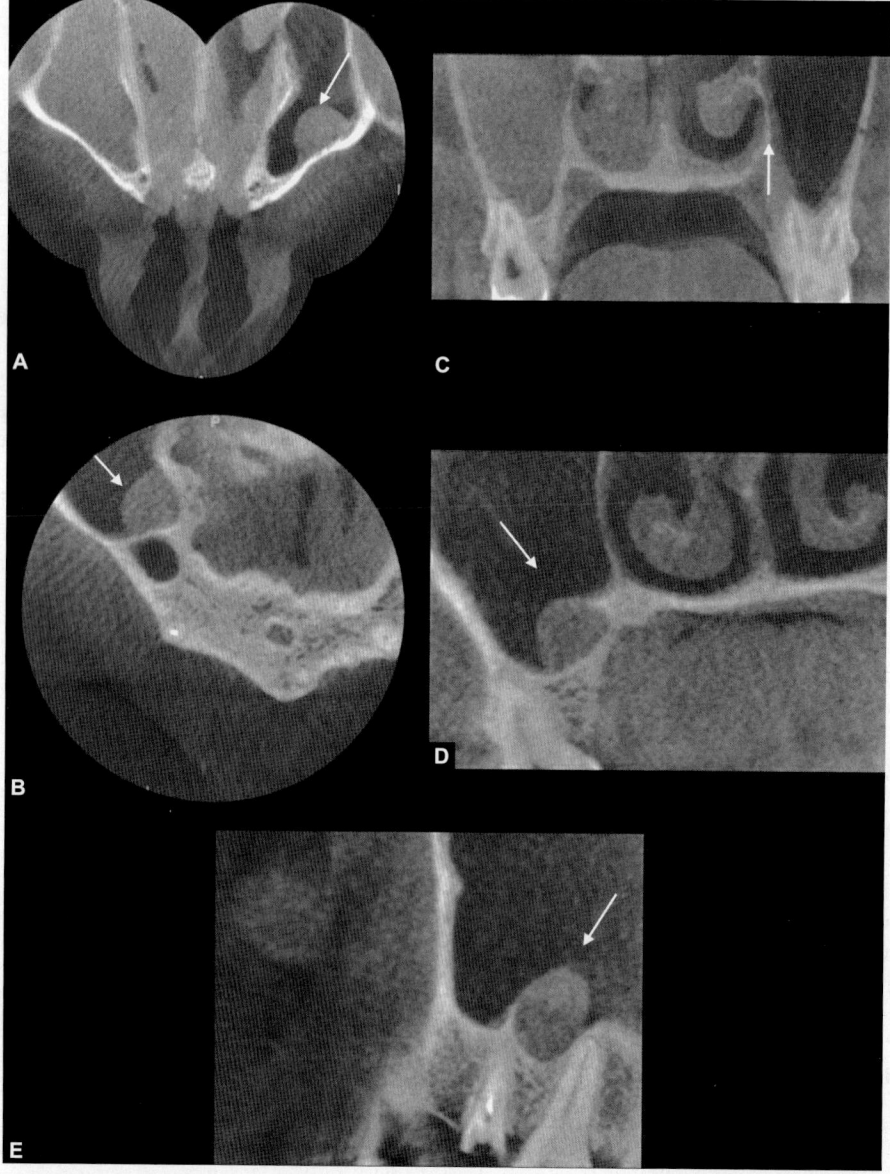

Figures 26.11A to E   Cone beam computed tomography images showing antaral polyps: (A and B) Axial; (C and D) Coronal; (E) Sagittal views

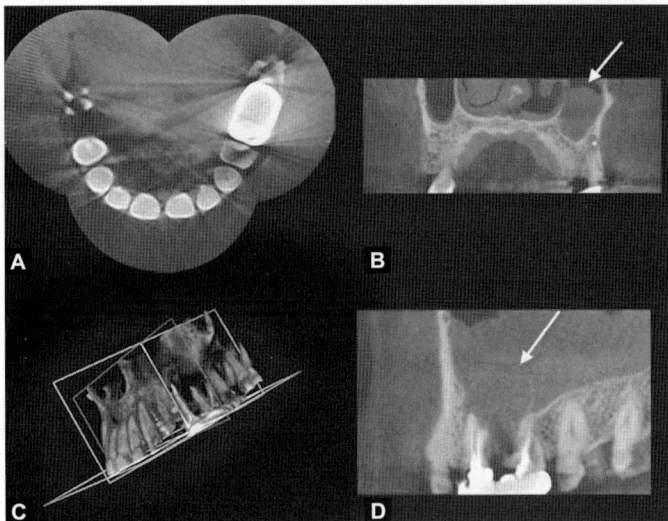

Figures 26.12A to D CBCT: (A) Axial; (B) Coronal; (C) 3D; (D) Sagittal section shows. Mucosal polyp; chronic inflammation of the lining of the maxillary sinus

- It may cause bony displacement or destruction of bone
- In the ethmoidal air cells it may cause destruction of the medial wall of the orbit (lamina papyracea of the ethmoid bone), and a unilateral proptosis may develop.

Radiographic Features

- It appears as an isolated homogeneous radiopaque mass of soft tissue density in the nose or sinus
- Bone destruction may occur due to pressure destruction
- This smooth spherical soft tissue mass, which may be multiple and causing complete opacification of the nasal cavity and the sinus, is seen on T1-weighted MRI as low to intermediate signal and T2-weighted MRI as a high signal. A heterogeneous MRI signal is characteristic in chronic polyps, which may also enhance.

Differential Diagnosis

- *Retention pseudocyst*: Polyp usually occurs with a thickened mucous membrane lining, whereas in case of the pseudocyst the adjacent mucous membrane is not usually apparent. If multiple lesions are seen in the sinus it is more likely to be sinus polyposis.
- *Benign tumor, malignancy*: The bone displacement and destruction associated with polyps may mimic a benign or a malignant lesion, and many sinus neoplasms are asymptomatic. Bone destruction with radiopacification is an indication for biopsy.

Epithelial Papilloma (Antral Papilloma)

Definition

It is a rare neoplasm of respiratory epithelium that occurs in the nasal cavity and paranasal sinuses.

Clinical Features

- It predominantly occurs in men, more common in the ethmoidal and maxillary sinus. It may also appear as an isolated polyp in the nose
- It causes unilateral nasal obstruction, nasal discharge, pain and epistaxis
- They patient may have a history of recurring sinusitis and a subsequent nasal obstruction of the same side
- Ten percent of these papillomas are associated with carcinoma.

Radiographic Features

- It appears as a homogeneous radiopaque mass of soft tissue density
- Bone destruction may be caused due to pressure erosion
- The radiographic features are not specific and diagnosis is based only on histological examination.

Osteoma (Fig. 26.13)

Definition

It is the most common of the mesenchymal neoplasms in the paranasal sinuses.

Clinical Features

- It is more common in males, in the second, third and fourth decades
- It is slow growing, asymptomatic and thus may be detected as an incidental finding
- It is more common in the frontal and ethmoidal sinus. The incidence in the maxillary sinus varies between 3.9 and 28.5% of the incidence in all paranasal sinuses
- Symptoms occur due to obstruction of the sinus ostium or infundibulum or are secondary to erosion or deformity, orbital involvement or intracranial extension
- Those growing in the maxillary sinus may:
  - Extend into the nose causing nasal obstruction
  - They may expand the sinus producing swelling of the cheek or hard palate
  - Extending to the orbit causing proptosis
  - It may produce an external fistula
- It may occur in the maxillary sinus after a Caldwell-Luc operation.

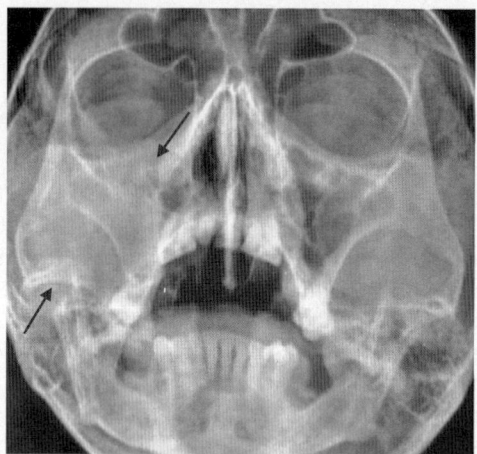

Figure 26.13 Osteoma of right maxillary sinus; PA Water's view shows radiopaque mass involving right side maxillary sinus involving its roof, mesial wall and floor. There is loss of normal pneumatization of right maxillary sinus. The radiopaque mass is also involving zygomatic malar complex and definite portion of left maxilla. Differential diagnosis: Osteochondroma, fibro-osseous lesion

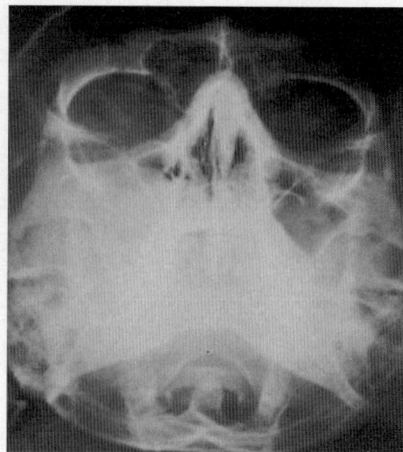

Figure 26.14 Squamous cell carcinoma involving the maxilla. PA waters showed haziness in the right and destruction of walls of the right sinus

Radiographic Features

The osteoma is usually lobulated or rounded, homogeneous radiopacity with sharply defined margins.

Differential Diagnosis

- Anthroliths
- Mycoliths
- Teeth
- Odontogenic neoplasms (odontomas).

MALIGNANT NEOPLASMS

The most common primary malignant neoplasms of the paranasal sinus are the squamous cell carcinomas and to a lesser extent, malignant salivary gland neoplasms. Other primary neoplasms include adenocarcinomas, soft and hard tissue sarcomas, melanoma and malignant lymphomas. Of the carcinomas of the paranasal sinuses 74% originate in the maxillary sinus, but involvement of the frontal and sphenoid sinuses is also comparatively common. Although opacification is a feature of both the inflammatory conditions and neoplasms, bone destruction is more common in malignant neoplasms, before symptoms become apparent. Therefore any unexplained radiopacity of the maxillary sinus of an individual older than 40 years should be investigated thoroughly.

Squamous Cell Carcinoma (Figs 26.14 and 26.15)

Definition

This originates from metaplastic epithelium of the sinus mucosal lining.

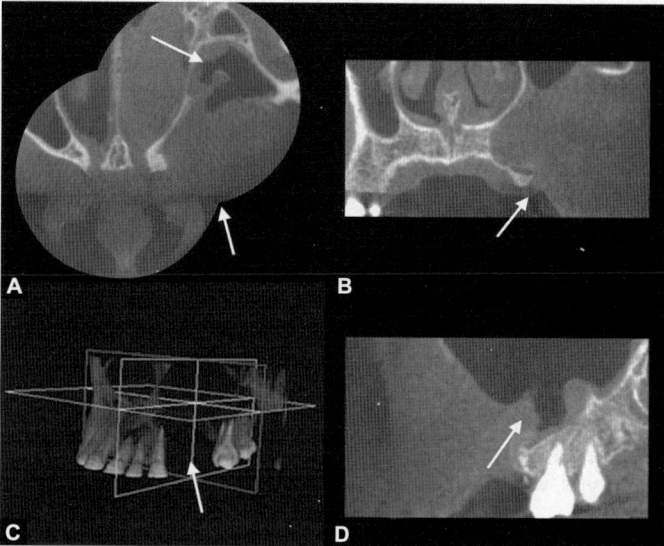

Figures 26.15A to D Cone beam computed tomography showing squamous cell carcinoma of the upper left alveolus: (A) Axial; (B) Coronal image shows destruction of the inferior and lateral border of the maxillary sinus; (C) 3D; (D) Sagittal image shows loss of inferior border as well

Clinical Features

- The males are more commonly affected and the mean age is approximately 60 years (range from 25–89 years)
- The most common symptom is facial pain or swelling, nasal obstruction and a lesion in the oral cavity. Lymph nodes are involved in 10% of the cases

In the maxillary sinus the symptoms produced depend on which wall is involved:

- Erosion of the medial wall causes nasal obstruction, nasal discharge, bleeding and pain
- Lesions that arise on the floor of the sinus produce dental signs and symptoms like, expansion of the alveolar process, unexplained pain and numbness of the teeth, loose teeth, swelling of the palate or alveolar ridge and ill-fitting dentures. The neoplasm may erode the floor and penetrate into the oral cavity
- When the lesion involves or penetrates the lateral wall, facial and vestibular swelling becomes apparent, patient may complain of pain and hyperesthesia of the maxillary teeth
- Involvement of the sinus roof and floor of the orbit causes symptoms related to the eye, diplopia, proptosis, pain and hyperesthesia or anesthesia and pain over the cheek and upper teeth
- Invasion and penetration of the posterior wall leads to invasion of the muscles of mastication, causing painful trismus, obstruction of the Eustachian tube causing a stuffy ear and referred pain and hyperesthesia over the distribution of the second and third division of the trigeminal nerve
- If the neoplasm invades the cranium it may cause paresthesia of the mandibular nerve.

Radiographic Features

- In the early stages the radiographic features are non-specific, and it is thus difficult to differentiate from the radiopacity due to sinusitis and polyp formation
- As the lesion enlarges it may destroy the sinus walls and in general, cause irregular radiolucent areas in the surrounding bone
- Adjacent alveolar process may show bone destruction around the teeth or irregular widening of the periodontal ligament space
- The medial wall of the sinus may be thinned or destroyed and it may also extend into the nasal cavity
- Destruction of the floor and anterior and posterior walls may be detected.

Additional Imaging

- The medial wall of the sinus is best seen on the Caldwell and Water's projections
- Destruction of the floor and anterior and posterior walls may be detected on the panoramic film
- CT shows the invasion into the soft tissue planes beyond the sinus walls. It is helpful in revealing the extent of the paranasal sinus neoplasms, especially when extension into the orbit, infratemporal fossa, or cranial cavity has occurred.

- *Magnetic Resonance Imaging*: It is excellent for revealing the extent of the soft tissue penetration into adjacent structures and in differentiating mucous accumulation from the soft tissue mass of neoplasm.

Differential Diagnosis

- Sinusitis
- Large retention psuedocysts
- Odontogenic cysts.

Neoplasm should be suspected in any older patient in whom chronic sinusitis develops for the first time without obvious cause.

Management

Treatment generally is a combination of surgery and radiation therapy.

Pseudotumor (Invasive Fungal Sinusitis, Inflammatory Pseudotumor, Fibroinflammatory Pseudotumor, Plasma Cell Granuloma, Sinonasal Fungal Disease, Mucormycosis, Aspergillosis, Zygomycosis of the Paranasal Sinuses, Rhizopus Sinusitis) (Figs 26.16A to D)

Definition

This is a descriptive name for a group of apparently related diseases of fungal origin that occur in the paranasal sinuses, as well as other parts of the head and neck.

Clinical Features

- This occurs after a series of recurrent infections, with symptoms that may not be very specific
- There may be complain of recurring pain with the presence of a mass simulating a neoplasm, which may cause erosion of the walls of the involved sinus and proptosis if the orbit is involved
- Altered nerve function resulting from involvement of the nerve or occlusion of blood vessels by the mass, may be seen
- Many a times the patient may be immunocompromised or have systemic diseases like diabetes mellitus, von Willebrand disease or myelodysplasia.

Radiographic Features

The radiographic features simulate that of malignant neoplasms that cause erosion of the bony walls of the involved sinuses.

Differential Diagnosis

Benign and malignamt neoplasms.

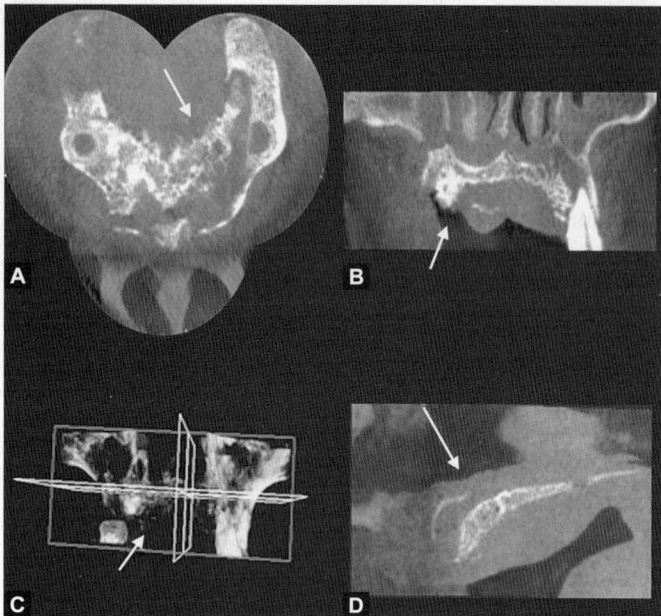

Figures 26.16A to D Cone beam computed tomography showing mucormycosis involving the maxillary sinus, irregular bone loss with thickening of the mucosal lining is noted. The diagnosis was confirmed by laboratory testing: (A) Axial; (B) Coronal; (C) 3D; (D) Sagittal section

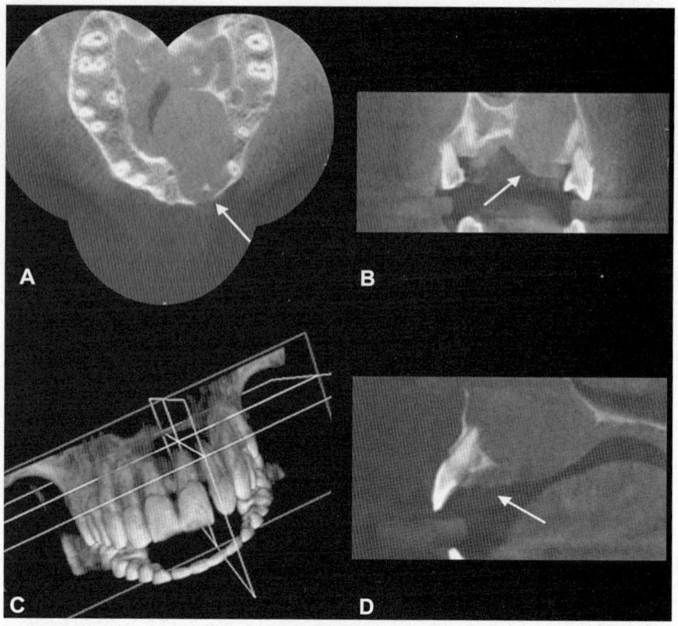

Figures 26.17A to D Cone beam computed tomography showing periapical lesion associated with the upper anterior region. Complete loss of the palatal cortical plate on the sagittal image coronal image shows extension of the lesion in the nasal fossa: (A) Axial; (B) Coronal; (C) 3D; (D) Sagittal section

Management

Treatment includes debridement of the sinuses and administration of antifungal medication (amphotericin B and rifampin), a Caldwell-Luc approach and therapy.

EXTRINSIC DISEASES INVOLVING THE MAXILLARY SINUS

Inflammatory Disease (Figs 26.17A to D)

Dental inflammatory lesions such as periodontal or periapical disease may cause a localized mucositis in the adjacent floor of the maxillary antrum, due to the diffusion of inflammatory exudates (mediators) beyond the cortical floor of the antrum and into the periosteum and the mucosal lining of the sinus. The localized type of mucositis related to dental inflammatory disease usually resolves in days or weeks after successful treatment of the underlying cause.

On the radiograph the mucosa presents as a homogeneous radiopaque ribbon shaped shadow that follows the contour of the floor of the maxillary sinus, and is centered directly above the inflammatory lesion.

Periostitis

Definition

The exudates from the dental inflammatory lesions can diffuse through the cortical boundary of the antral floor, this

strips and elevates the periosteal lining of the cortical bone of the floor of the maxillary antrum, stimulating the periosteum to produce a thin elevated layer of new bone adjacent to the root of the involved tooth, which appears as a halo-like layer (which indicates inflammation of the periosteum).

Radiographic Features

The periosteal new bone formation, is always centered directly above the inflammatory lesion and may appear as a single thin radiopaque line, a very thick radiopaque line, or has a laminated (onion skin) appearance.

BENIGN ODONTOGENIC CYSTS AND TUMORS

Odontogenic Cysts (Figs 26.18 to 26.21)

These are common group of extrinsic lesions that encroaches the maxillary sinus. The most common are radicular cysts, dentigerous cysts and odontogenic cysts. These cysts originate outside the maxillary sinuses and encroach on the space of the sinuses by displacing the sinus borders. The cyst cortex and the sinus wall may be indistinguishable from one another and thus as the cyst enlarges the sinus decreases in size. There is a radiopaque line dividing the cyst and the sinus, which in not present in the case of a retention pseudocyst, which is in the sinus and thus will not have a cortex around its periphery.

- *Apical radicular cyst*: There is presence of a nonvital tooth, (usually first molar and lateral incisor). Lamina dura is not intact. They cause elevation of the floor of the sinus resulting in a halo appearance. Large-cysts may obliterate the sinus and make differentiation from sinusitis difficult.
- *Dentigerous cyst*: Most commonly related to the third molar; when they expand into the sinus, the radiograph shows radiolucency elevating the floor of the sinus. If it is small it appears as a dome- shaped opacity in the base of the antrum, with well-defined radiopaque corticated margins. Sometimes there may be displacement of the associated tooth. If the cyst is large it may cause total obliteration of the antral region due to complete compression of the antral cavity. There may be loss of the antral outline. Large cysts can displace third molars as far as the floor of the orbit.
- *Cyst in the globulomaxillary area*: These may expand so as to obliterate or alter the typical pattern or border of nasal fossa and anterior recess of the maxillary sinus.

Radiographic Features

- The invading cyst has a curved or oval shape defined by a corticated border
- It appears homogeneous and radiopaque relative to the sinus
- It may displace the floor of the sinus, and sometimes encroaches the entire sinus, so that the residual sinus space appears as a thin saddle over the cyst.

Differential Diagnosis

- *Retention pseudocyst*: Has no cortex at the periphery. Only in case of infected odontogenic cyst is the periphery lost and it becomes difficult to differentiate it from pseudoretention cyst. Odontogenic cysts will show some relation to the neighboring teeth.
- *Maxillary sinusitis*: The walls of a cyst completely filling the sinus are much thicker and more regular than that of the sinus, and the normal vasculature markings on the walls of the sinus wall are not present on the walls of the cyst.

  A cyst that occupies the entire sinus usually causes expansion of the medial wall (middle meatus) of the sinus and will alter the sigmoid contour of the posterolateral wall of the sinus (this may be seen in an axial CT image).
- *Antral loculation*: These may occasionally have a round shape and sometimes appear to be corticated, but since the loculations contain air, they are more radiolucent than the fluid filled cysts, and also more radiolucent than the surrounding antrum.

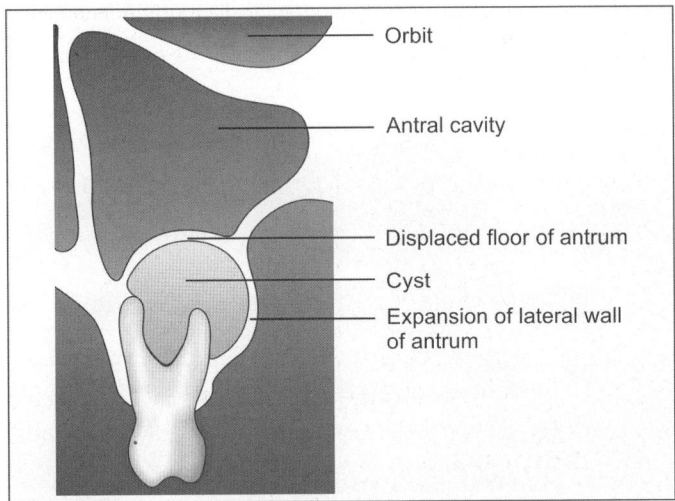

Figure 26.18 Simplified line diagram illustrating the essential radiographic features of a small odontogenic cyst and its effects on the antrum (as depicted on an 0° OM)

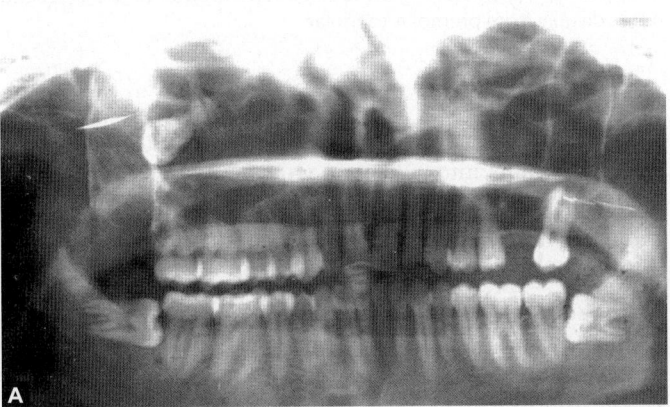
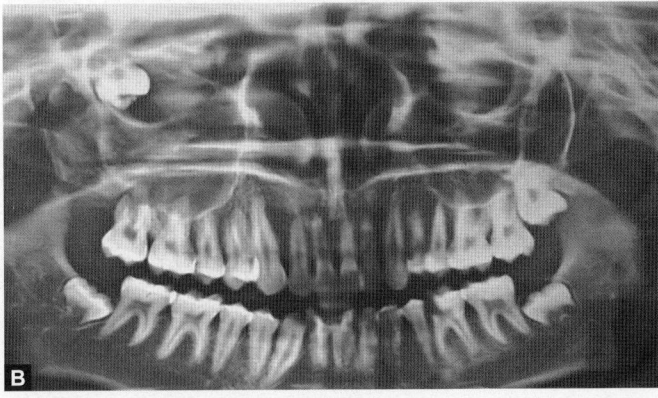

Figures 26.19A and B (A) Panoramic radiograph showing cystic expansile lesion was seen arising from alveolar margin of right maxilla and extending into the maxillary sinus with an unerupted tooth (18) within it. Bony defect seen in its inferior wall allowing cyst to communicate with roof of oral cavity. Dentigerous cyst; (B) Panoramic radiograph showing dentigerous cyst associated with impacted 18 within the maxillary sinus. Radiolucent well defined lesion within the maxillary sinus attached to 18 with displacement of floor of maxillary sinus

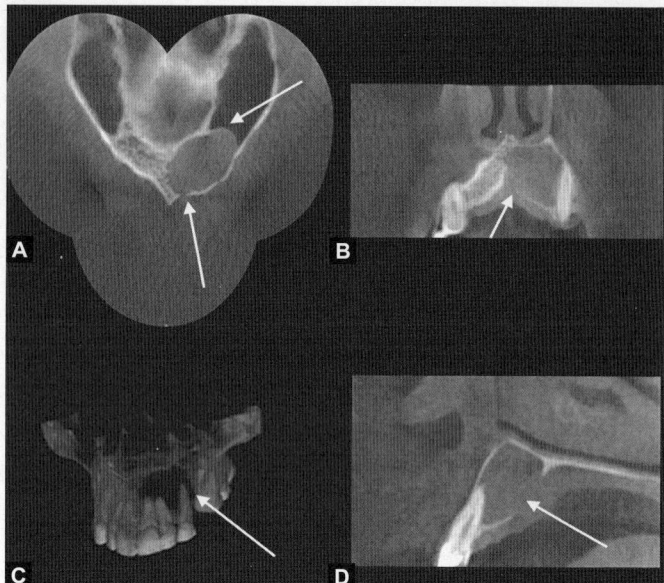

Figures 26.20A to D Cone beam computed tomography showing radicular cyst associated with the upper anterior region encroaching in to the maxillary sinus of the left side: (A) Axial image; (B) Coronal; (C) 3D section; (D) Sagittal image shows perforation of the palatal cortex

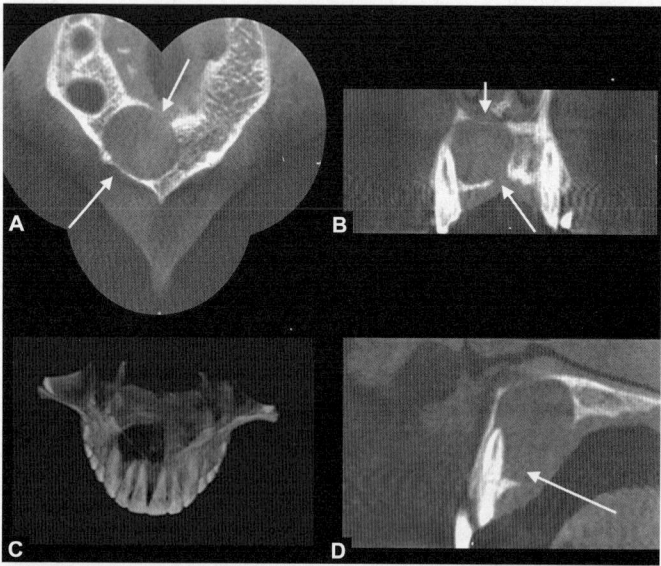

Figures 26.21A to D Cone beam computed tomography showing radicular cyst associated with right central and lateral incisor: (A) Axial; (B) Coronal image shows perforation of the palatal cortex and the nasal floor; (C) 3D; (D) Sagittal section

Odontogenic Tumors (Figs 26.22 to 26.24)

These usually cause facial deformity, nasal obstruction, and displacement or loosening of teeth. The nature of bony barriers in this region of the face, and the relatively good blood supply are responsible for the efficient local spread. The aggressive

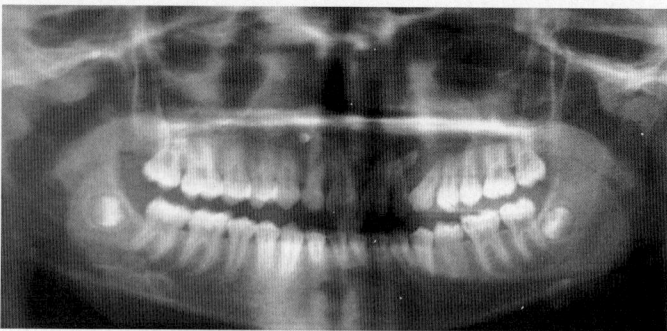

Figure 26.22 Panoramic radiograph view shows well defined, unilocular, corticated, and irregular in shape radiolucency in upper left side in relation to upper left in anteriors. Superiorly it is extended till middle of nasal septum displacing the floor of left maxillary sinus inferiorly till crestal bone of the anterior teeth. Haziness of left maxillary sinus was also noted. Radiographic diagnosis: Adenomatoid odontogenic tumor

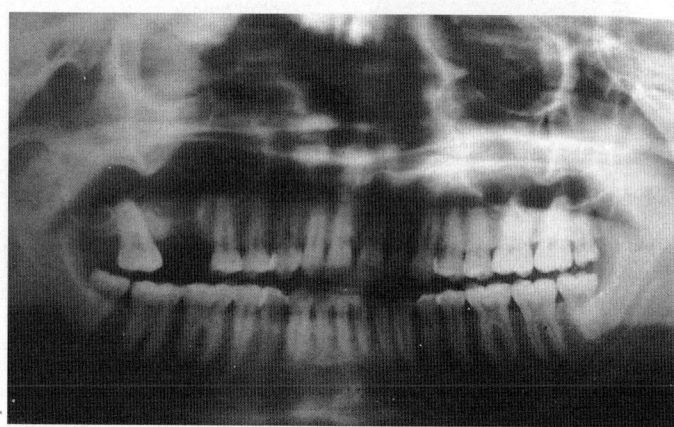

Figure 26.23 Pleomorphic adenoma of the palate seen on the panoramic radiograph as a solitary unilocular well defined radiolucency in the right maxilla extending from the alveolar margin of upper right premolar region to the inferior border of the sinus and mesiodistally from premolar to molar

growth pattern of some tumors (e.g. ameloblastoma) may directly invade into adjacent vital anatomical structures, including the skull base and compromise patients.

Radiographic Features

- The tumor may have a curved, oval or multilocular shape that is usually defined by a thin cortical border. The border may be absent in case of aggressive tumors
- The tumors usually have coarse or fine septae, or regions of dystrophic calcification depending on the histopathologic nature of the tumor
- It may displace the floor of the antrum and cause thinning of the peripheral cortex

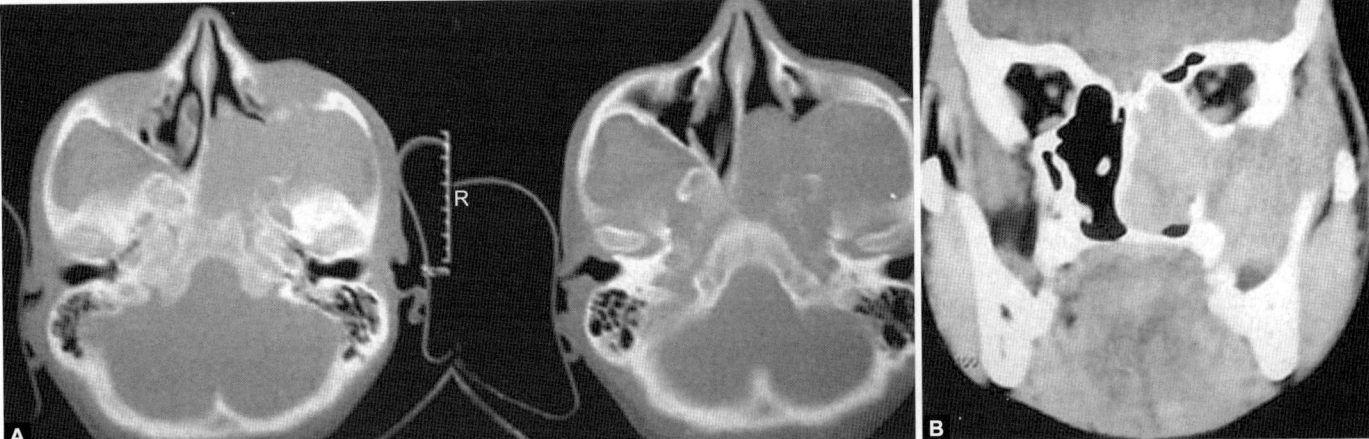

Figures 26.24A and B (A and B) Nasopharyngeal angiofibroma—Patient came with a complain of a diffuse swelling on the left cheek since the last 2 years. Panoramic view showed no finding. USG indicated presence of a subcutaneous mass. (A and B) CT scan revealed a massive expansile mass involving the nasal cavity, sinus, orbit, middle cranial fossa and the oral cavity. Anterior bowing of the posterior wall of the maxillary sinus can be noted

- The tumor may completely fill the sinus, and as in the case of odontogenic cysts, the residual sinus space may appear as a thin saddle over the tumor
- The bony walls of the sinus may be thinned or eroded and adjacent structures displaced.
- A tooth or part of a tooth may be embedded in the neoplasm

Malignant Tumors (Figs 26.25A to D)

Invasion of the maxillary sinus by local malignant disease.

Malignant tumors of the upper jaw spread easily into the sinus. Pleomorphic adenoma which arises from the palatal minor salivary gland may bulge into the floor of the sinus and adenocystic carcinoma may invade it.

Metastatic Carcinoma of the Maxillary Sinus

The most common site of the primary disease is the kidney, breasts and testicles. Maxillary sinus is a rare site for metastasis.

OTHER DISEASES

Craniofacial Fibrous Dysplasia

Definition

This may arise in the maxillary, sphenoid, frontal, ethmoid and temporal bones, causing displacement of the sinus borders and resulting in a smaller sinus on the affected side.

Clinical Features

- It is more common in children and young adults and tends to stop growing when skeletal growth ceases. It may

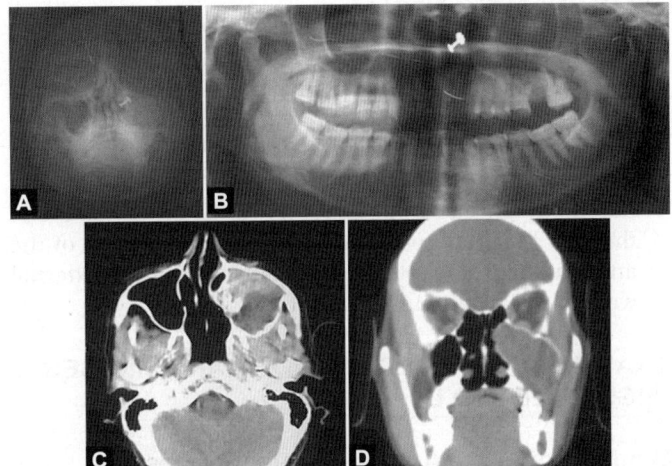

Figures 26.25A to D Mucoepidermoid carcinoma involving the sinus: (A) PA Water's; (B) Panoramic radiograph showed a diffuse mixed radiolucent-radiopaque shadow involving left maxilla extending from inferior wall of orbit to palate, mediolaterally from nasal septum to posterior wall of right maxilla. Walls of left maxillary sinus were not traceable. CT scan: (C) Axial; (D) Coronal view showing a lytic expansile destructive lesion measuring 5 × 3 × 3 cm with adjacent heterogeneously enhancing soft tissue was noted involving the medial, lateral and anterior walls of left maxillary sinus, hard palate, alveolus, left middle and inferior turbinates, ethmoidal septae and inferomedial wall of left orbit. Lesion extended anteriorly into buccal space, inferiorly into mucobuccal sulcus, superomedially into the nasal cavity. Few densely calcified flecks were seen in medial aspect of lesion

occasionally, be found in adults. The posterior maxilla is the most common location for fibrous dysplasia
- It results in facial asymmetry, nasal obstruction, proptosis, pituitary gland compression, impingement on the cranial nerves or sinus obliteration

- The sinus obliteration results due to the expansion and encroachment of the dysplastic bone lesion
- The lesion may displace the roots of the teeth and cause the teeth to separate or migrate. It does not cause root resorption.

Radiographic Features

- The lesion is not well-defined, and tends to blend with the surrounding bone. The external cortex of the bone is maintained intact, although in may be displaced
- The normal radiolucency of the maxillary sinus is partially or totally replaced by the increased radiopacity of the lesion. The degree of radiopacity depends on the stage of development and the relative amount of bone present. The radiopaque areas have a characteristic ground glass appearance on extraoral radiographs or an orange peel appearance on the intraoral views.

Differential Diagnosis

- *Paget's disease*: This does not obliterate the sinus. The person is usually older.
- *Complex odontoma*: It is usually associated with one or more unerupted teeth and is surrounded by a radiolucent line (soft tissue capsule), in turn surrounded by a radiopaque line.
- *Ossifying fibroma*: It may have a similar radiopaque appearance, but has a definite border. But in some cases differentiating ossifying fibroma involving the antrum and fibrous dysplasia can be extremely difficult. The shape of the new bone encroaching on the internal aspect of the antrum often parallels the original shape of the external walls of the antrum in fibrous dysplasia.

TRAUMATIC INJURIES TO MAXILLARY SINUSES (FIGS. 26.26A TO D)

Sinus Root in the Antrum/Foreign Bodies (Figs 26.27 to 26.29)

Definition

Tooth roots may be fractured as a result of various forms of trauma, including iatrogenic reasons. Fractured roots may be forced into the sinus during extraction or subsequent attempts to retrieve them.

Excess root canal filling material may be forced through the apex of an upper posterior tooth during endodontic therapy. Foreign material may be pushed into the antrum via an existing oroantral fistula. Metallic objects such as pellets, bullets and fragments of shells or bombs may be found if the patient has been exposed to the same.

Clinical Features

- No visible signs and symptoms if the root is displaced recently

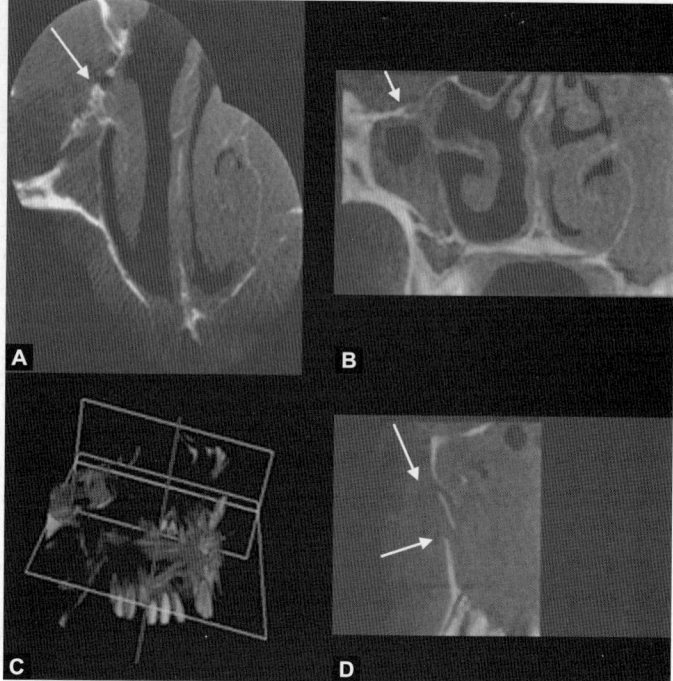

Figures 26.26A to D Cone beam computed tomography showing fracture of lateral wall of sinus: (A) Axial; (B) Coronal; (C) 3D; (D) Sagittal views

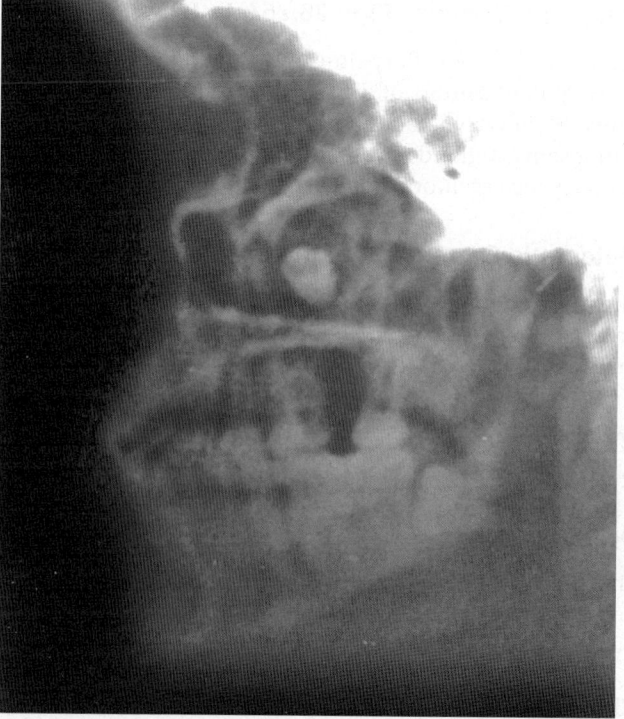

Figure 26.27 Lateral cephalogram shows upper right third molar present within the maxillary sinus

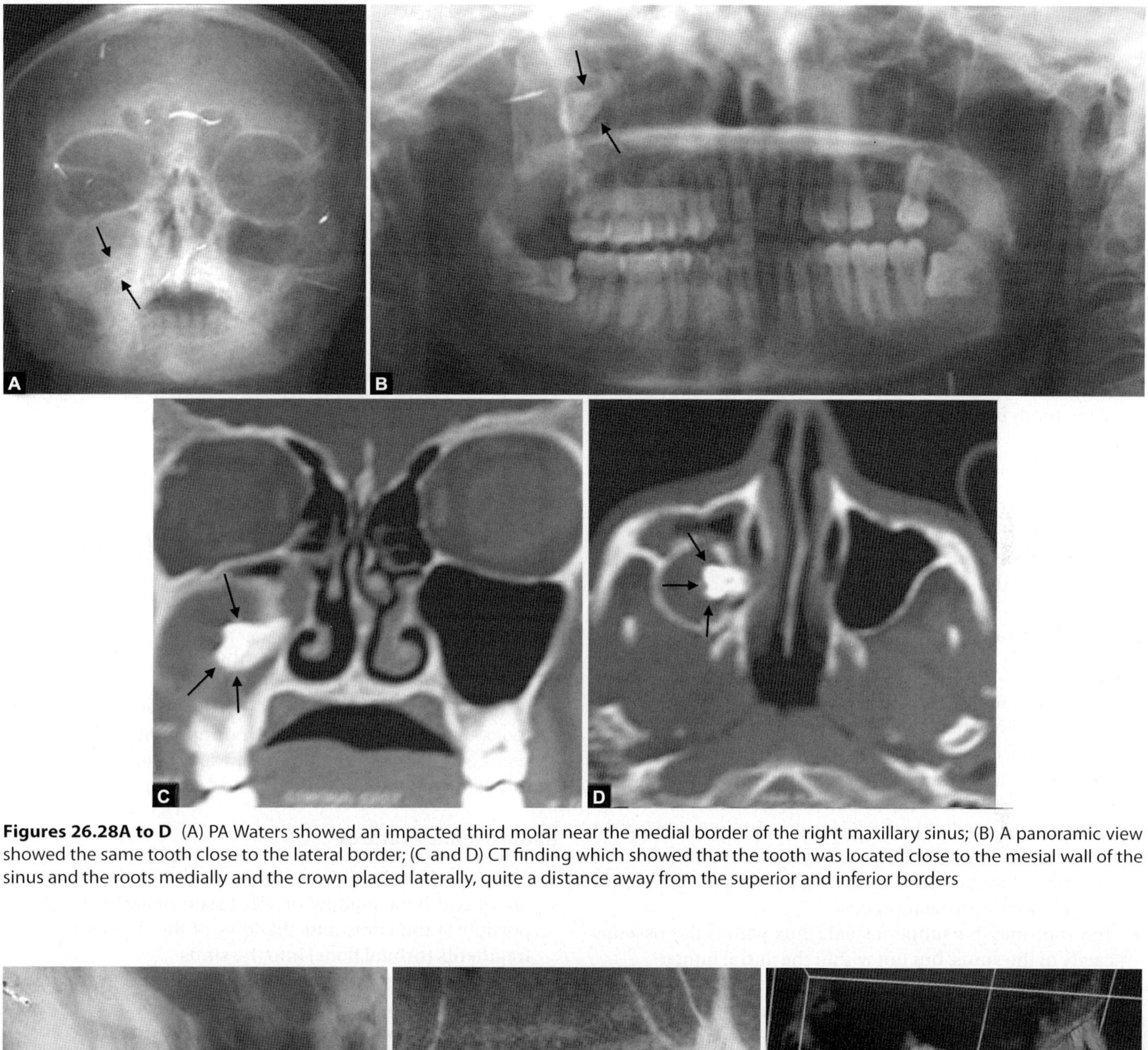

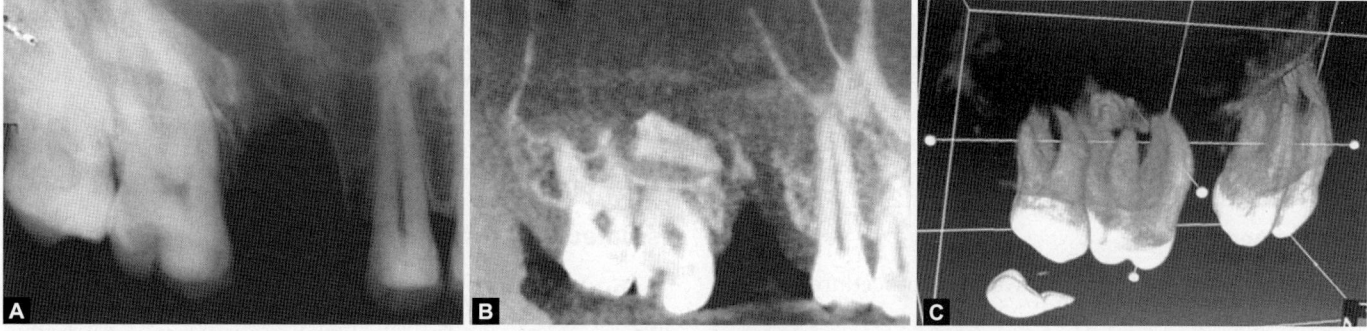

Figures 26.28A to D (A) PA Waters showed an impacted third molar near the medial border of the right maxillary sinus; (B) A panoramic view showed the same tooth close to the lateral border; (C and D) CT finding which showed that the tooth was located close to the mesial wall of the sinus and the roots medially and the crown placed laterally, quite a distance away from the superior and inferior borders

Figures 26.29A to C Tooth luxated into sinus during extraction as seen on the: (A) Intraoral periapical radiograph and CBCT; (B) Reformatted panoramic; (C) CBCT 3D view

- Ask the patient to hold his/her nose while attempting to breathe out through, similar to a Valsalva maneuver, it will cause bubbles to appear within the blood contained within the fresh extraction
- If the patient has had the root or tooth in the sinus for a number of days, he may present with sinusitis
- The associated roots are usually of molars and premolars as the sinus is in close proximity to these teeth.

Radiographic Features

- The dislodged fragments are usually found near the floor of the sinus because of gravity. Sometimes the displaced structure may be mucosal, between the osseous wall of the sinus and the periosteum
- The floor of the sinus may break due to the displacement of the tooth fragment into the sinus.

Additional Imaging

- *Lateral maxillary occlusal views*: They are useful for examining root tips in the maxillary sinus.
- *Water's projection*: Alongwith the occlusal view, may help in the three dimensional localization.

Differential Diagnosis

- Exostoses of the sinus wall or floor and septa within the sinus, may mimic dental root fragments or even whole teeth.
- *Antroliths*: The shape of the radiopacity or the presence of a pulp canal or a layer of enamel may help to differentiate. The tooth fragment may be made to move by tilting the head of the patient abruptly between views.
- If the root tip remains in the socket it may be superimposed radiographically over the maxillary sinus, but the presence of lamina dura and periodontal ligament space indicate a position in the alveolar process
- The root may be subperiosteal, thus within the osseous cavity of the sinus, but not within the antral lumen
- Sometimes the root may be forced out of the socket into the surrounding bone or even through the bone to lie between the soft tissue of the oral mucosa and the bone of the alveolar process
- The root may be forced into surrounding structures, such as the infratemporal fossa.

Management

Surgical removal using the Caldwell-Luc procedure.

Sinus Contusion

Definition

This occurs due to a blow to the face that damages the lining of the paranasal sinuses without fracturing the facial bone. There may be a green stick fracture of the sinus with a resultant tearing injury to the mucosal lining.

Clinical Features

- There is a bloody nasal discharge, extreme tenderness of the involved sinus on pressure
- There is rapid resolution of the soft tissue changes.

Radiographic Features

- Haziness of the sinus due to edema
- An opaque sinus or fluid level resulting from hemorrhage from the mucosal tear.

Differential Diagnosis

Sinusitis.

Blow-out Fracture

Definition

This results from sudden increase in the intraorbital pressure, due to may be a direct blow to the eye.

Clinical Features

- The pressure of the blow forces the inferior orbital content (fat and muscle) through the fracture
- It results in diplopia (double vision) when the victim looks upwards (caused by the entrapment of the inferior rectus) and enophthalmus (backwardly depressed eyelid) following reduction of edema and fat atrophy.

Radiographic Features

- Opacification of the sinus with or without a fluid level.
- There will be a shadow of soft tissue mass in the upper portion of the sinus and shadows of the depressed bone fragments (orbital floor) into the sinus
- A tear drop shaped radiopacity is produced in the upper part of the sinus, due to the herniation of the orbital content downwards into the sinus following the collapse of the antral roof
- The depression fracture of the orbit may be accompanied by the fracture of the antrum wall of the maxillary sinus.

Isolated Fracture (see Fig. 26.27)

Definition

This involves a single wall which may appear as a bright line on the radiograph.

The most common sites are the anterolateral wall of the antrum and the floor of the antrum, during extraction of the upper posterior teeth whose roots are in close proximity to the antral floor.

Zygomatic Complex Fracture

Refer Chapter 28—Trauma to Teeth and Facial Structures (Page 533).

Definition

This fracture occurs at the line of weakness and passes through the orbital floor, usually medial to the zygomaticomaxillary suture.

Clinical Features

- The fractured zygoma is forced into the sinus
- There may be tearing of the lining membrane with subsequent bleeding into the antrum.

Radiographic Features

The antrum appears cloudy or will show a fluid level.

Fractured Tuberosity

Definition

This occurs most frequently while extracting a lone standing upper third molar.

Oroantral Fistula (Figs 26.30 and 26.31)

Definition

This is a pathological pathway connecting the oral cavity and the maxillary sinus. It may be caused due to extraction of teeth having chronic periapical infections, extraction of a solitary tooth. Extraction of teeth having apices very close to the antral floor, blind instrumentation, surgical removal of large lesions in the upper jaws, malignant tumors, osteomyelitis, syphilis, malignant granulomatous lesions, facial trauma and inadequate blood clot formation.

Clinical Features

- *Immediate*:
  - History of recent traumatic extraction or disappearance of the roots during extraction
  - Passage of fluid into the nose from the oral cavity
  - Inability to blow the cheek or smoke
  - Unilateral epitaxis, due to blood in the antrum escaping through the nasal ostium
  - Alteration in vocal resonance.
- Delayed (the defect may have been occluded by a blood clot and only after it is dislodged or degenerates due to infection that the signs and symptoms become apparent).
  - A simple dimple on the alveolar ridge may be the only sign
  - There may be invasion of an antral polyp through the fistula into the oral cavity
  - Foul, sweetish or salty taste
  - Facial pain and headache, with unilateral nasal discharge
  - Aspiration of the air into the mouth through the tooth socket
  - Sinusitis and tenderness over the maxillary sinus
  - Postnasal drip
  - Painless lump at the site of extraction.

To confirm the diagnosis the patient should be asked to blow air into the pinched nose with the mouth open. This forces the air into the sinus through the ostium. If an oroantral opening is present, bubbles appear in the extraction socket.

Radiographic Features

- There will be a break in the continuity of the floor of the maxillary sinus, which may be seen as a disalignment of a small portion of the cortical layer of bone
- Radiographic features of acute or chronic sinusitis are present
- There may be evidence of the displaced root or tooth, and a second view of the sinus with the head in a different position may be required to ascertain the exact location of the displaced object.

Additional Imaging

- Confirmation of the presence of the fistula may be done by the introduction of a silver probe or a gutta-percha point into the orifice, followed by the radiograph
- CT with denta scan imaging gives exact location of OAF.

Management

Treatment consists of repair and surgical closure under antibiotic therapy.

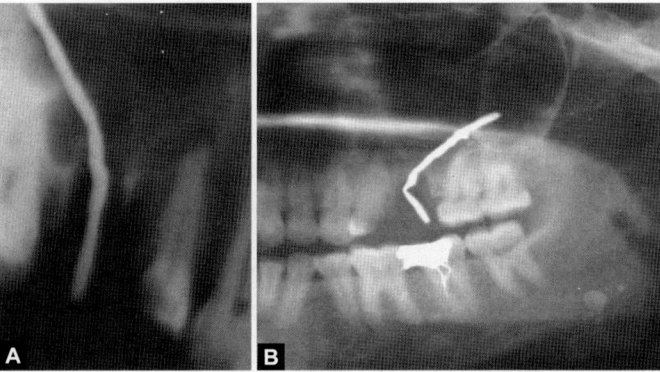

Figures 26.30A and B Oroantral fistula with respect to maxillary right molar: (A) Intraoral radiograph; (B) Panoramic view shows a discontinuity in the floor of the sinus, as demonstrated

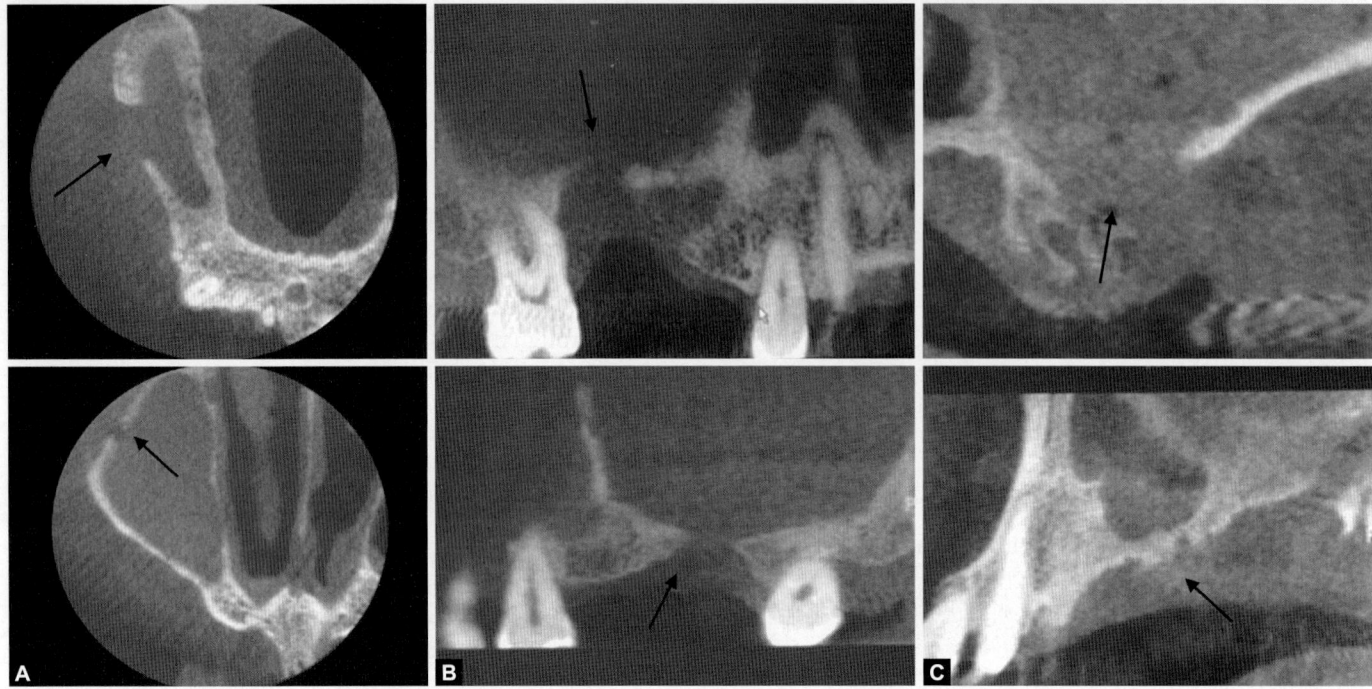

Figures 26.31A to C Oroantral fistual as seen on CBCT. Different sections of axial, coronal and sagittal views

BIBLIOGRAPHY

1. Goaz PW, White SC. Principles and Interpretation. In: Oral Radiology, 3rd edition. St. Louis: Mosby Year Book; 1994.
2. McGowan DA, Baxter PW, James J. The maxillary sinus and its dental implications. Butterworth-Heineman, Oxford;1993.
3. Miles DA, Van Dis MJ, Jensen CW, et al. Interpretation normal versus abnormal and common radiographic presentations of lesions. In: Radiographic and Imaging for Dental Auxillaries, 3rd edition. Philadelphia: WD Saunders; 1999.pp.231-80.
4. Shafer WG, et al. A textbook of oral pathology. Philadelphia: WB Saunders; 1983.
5. Som PM. The paranasal sinuses. In: Som PM, Curtin HD (Eds), Head and Neck Imaging, 4th edition, St Louis: Mosby; 2003.
6. Wood NK, Goaz PW. Differential diagnosis of oral lesions, 4th edition. CV Mosby: St Louis; 1991.
7. Wood RE. Handbook of signs in dental and maxillofacial radiology. Warthog Publications, Toronto; 1988.
8. Worth HM. Principles and practice of oral radiographic interpretation. Year Book Medical Publishers, Chicago; 1963.

Soft Tissue Calcifications and Ossifications | 27

The deposition of calcium salts, primarily calcium phosphate usually occurs in the skeleton. Pathologic calcifications or heterotrophic ossification is said to occur when calcium is deposited in soft tissue in an unorganized manner. This pathologic mineralization of soft tissue may occur in many unrelated disorders and degenerative processes. The term heterotropic indicates that the bone has formed in an abnormal (extraskeletal) location. This bone may be compact bone or it may show trabeculae and fatty marrow. The deposits may range from 1 mm to several centimeters in diameter and one or more may be present. The causes range from post-traumatic ossification, bone produced by tumors, and ossification caused by diseases such as progressive myositis ossificans and ankylosing spondylitis (**Table 27.1**).

GENERAL CLINICAL FEATURES

Sites of heterotopic calcifications may not cause significant signs or symptoms. They are most often detected as an incidental finding during radiographic examination.

Table 27.1 Classification of soft tissue calcification in head and neck region

- Dystrophic calcifications
  - General dystrophic calcification of the oral regions
  - Calcified lymph nodes
  - Dystrophic calcification in the tonsils
  - Cysticercosis
  - Arterial calcification
    - Monckerberg's medial calcinosis (Arteriosclerosis)
    - Calcified atherosclerotic plaque
- Idiopathic calcifications
  - Sialoliths
  - Phleboliths
  - Laryngeal cartilage calcifications
  - Rhinolith/Antrolith
- Metastatic calcifications
  - Ossification of the styloid ligament
  - Osteoma cutis
  - Myositis ossificans

GENERAL RADIOGRAPHIC FEATURES

- Soft tissue opacities are seen in 4% of panoramic radiographs.
- If the calcification is adjacent to bone, it may be difficult to determine whether it is within bone or soft tissue, another radiographic view at right angles is thus useful.
- Knowledge of the soft tissue anatomy, such as the position of lymph nodes, stylohyoid ligaments, blood vessels, laryngeal cartilages, the major ducts of the salivary glands is important to interpret the anatomical location, number, distribution and shape of the calcification.

DYSTROPHIC CALCIFICATIONS

Dystrophic calcification refers to calcification that forms in degenerating, diseased and dead tissue despite normal serum calcium and phosphate levels. The soft tissue may be damaged by blunt trauma, inflammation, injections, the presence of parasites, soft tissue changes arising from disease, and many other causes. This type of calcification is usually localized to the site of injury.

General Dystrophic Calcification of the Oral Regions

Definition

This is the precipitation of calcium salts into primary sites of chronic inflammation or dead and dying tissue. The process is usually associated with a high local concentration of phosphatase, as in normal bone calcification, an increase in local alkalinity, and anoxic conditions within the inactive or devitalized tissue. A long standing, chronically inflamed cyst is a common location of dystrophic calcification.

Clinical Features

- It is commonly found in tissues affected by tuberculosis, necrosis, blood vessels in arteriosclerosis, scars and areas of fatty degeneration.
- The common soft tissue sites in the oral cavity are gingiva, tongue, lymph nodes and cheek.

- It usually does not produce any signs or symptoms.
- Occasionally there may be enlargement and ulceration of the overlying soft tissues.
- A solid mass of calcium salts may be palpated.

Radiographic Features

The most common sites are that of long standing, chronically inflamed cysts.

The appearance varies from being barely perceptible, fine grains of radiopacities to larger irregular radiopaque particles that rarely exceed 0.5 cm in diameter.

One or more of the radiopacities may be seen, they may be homogenous or may contain punctate areas.

The outline is usually irregular or indistinct.

Calcified Lymph Nodes (Figs 27.1 and 27.2)

Definition

This occurs in lymph nodes that have been chronically inflamed because of various diseases (usually granulomatous disorders).

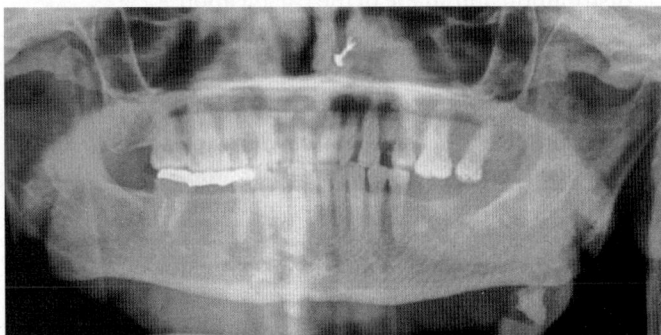

Figure 27.1 Lymph node calcification, large, cauliflower shaped heterogeneous radiopaque mass just inferior to the lower border of the mandible in the antegonial notch region on the left side. The mass shows radiolucent serration in between the radiopacity

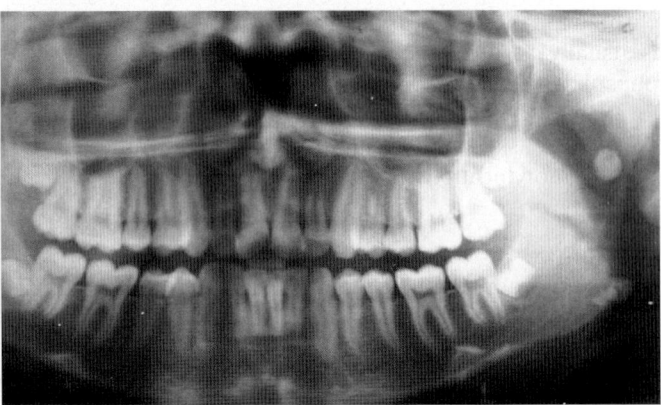

Figure 27.2 Lymph node calcification, heterogenous radiopaque mass seen in the condylar region

The lymphoid tissue is replaced by hydroxyapatite, like calcium salts nearly effacing all of the nodal architecture. The common disease that cause calcified lymph nodes are— tuberculosis (scrofula or cervical tuberculous adenitis), BCG vaccination, sarcoidosis, cat-scratch disease, lymphoma treated with radiation therapy, fungal infections, and metastases from distant calcifying neoplasms.

Clinical Features

- The most commonly involved nodes are submandibular and cervical nodes (superficial and deep) and less commonly the preauricular and submental nodes.
- There are no significant signs or symptoms. They are most often detected as an incidental finding during panoramic radiographic examination.
- On palpation these nodes, which may be single or multiple or sometimes chain of nodes, which are found to be mobile, hard, round or oblong masses, whose outline is well contoured and well defined.

Radiographic Features

- The most common site is the submandibular region, either at or below the inferior border of the mandible near the angle, or between the posterior border of the ramus and cervical spine.
- The image of the calcified node may sometimes overlap the inferior aspect of the ramus.
- The node calcification may be single, or a series of nodes called *lymph node chaining.*
- The periphery may be well-defined, irregular and sometimes may even have a lobulated appearance (*cauliflower like*). The irregular outline helps to differentiate lymph node calcification from other potential soft tissue calcification in the area.
- It may have a varying degree of radiopacity, giving an impression of a collection of spherical or irregular masses, which may look like *mass of coral.*
- Occasionally the lesion may have a laminated appearance.

Differential Diagnosis

- *Sialoliths*: This is painful and has a smooth outline. The patient may have symptoms related to the submandibular salivary gland. Sialography will aid in the differentiation.
- *Phleboliths*: These are smaller and have concentric radiopaque and radiolucent rings, and its shape may mimic a portion of a blood vessel.

Management

Usually require no treatment, but the underlying cause should be determined in case treatment is required; as in the case of lymphoma.

Dystrophic Calcification in the Tonsils (Tonsillar Calculi, Tonsil Concretions, Tonsilloliths)

Definition

Tonsillar calculi are formed when repeated bouts of inflammation enlarge the tonsillar crypts. Incomplete resolution of dead bacteria and pus serve as the nidus for dystrophic calcification.

Clinical Features

- These occur between the 20 and 68 years of age, more in the older age group.
- Tonsilloliths are usually hard, round, white or yellow objects projecting from the tonsillar crypts.
- The small calculi may not produce any signs or symptoms.
- In case of larger calcifications, pain, swelling, fetor oris dysphagia and a foreign body feeling on swallowing has been reported.
- In rare cases there may be giant tonsilloliths, which stretch the lymphoid tissue, resulting in ulcerations and extrusion.

Radiographic Features

- On the panoramic film, tonsilloliths appear as single or multiple radiopacities that overlap the mid-portion of the mandibular ramus in the region where the image of the dorsal surface of the tongue crosses the ramus in the palatoglossal air spaces.
- It appears as clusters of multiple small ill-defined radiopacities. This may vary from 0.5–14.5 cm in diameter.
- The radiopacity is of the same density as that of cortical bone, and a little more radiopaque than cancellous bone.

Differential Diagnosis

- *Calcified granulomatous disease*
- *Syphilis*
- *Mycosis*
- *Lymphoma*
- Radiopaque lesion within the mandibular ramus, such as a dense bone island. A right angled view to the panoramic field such as a posterior skull view or an open Towne's view may help to differentiate whether the calcification lies to the medial aspect of the ramus.

Management

Larger calcifications with associated symptoms should be removed surgically.

Cysticercosis

Definition

When eggs or gravid proglottids from *Taenia solium* (pork tapeworm) are ingested by human, their covering is digested in the stomach and the larval form cysticercus cellulosae of the parasite is hatched. These larvae penetrate the mucosa, enter the blood vessels and lymphatics and are distributed in the tissues all over the body, but preferentially locate to the brain, muscle, skin and heart. They are also found in the oral and perioral tissues, especially the muscles of mastication. After the larva die, they are treated as foreign bodies causing granuloma formation, scarring and calcification, this takes approximately 3 months. These areas in the tissues are called cysticerci.

Clinical Features

- Multiple small nodules may be felt in the region of the masseter and suprahyoid muscles and in the buccal mucosa and lip.
- Examination of the head and neck region may disclose palpable, well circumscribed soft fluctuant swellings, which resemble a mucocele.
- Mild cases are completely asymptomatic.
- Moderate cases have symptoms that range from mild to severe gastrointestinal upset with epigastric pain and severe nausea and vomiting.
- Invasion of the brain may result in seizures, headaches, visual disturbances, acute obstructive hydrocephalus, irritability and loss of consciousness.

Radiographic Features

- When alive the larva is not visible radiographically.
- They are usually found in the muscles of mastication and facial expression, the suprahyoid muscle, and the postcervical musculature.
- They appear as multiple, well-defined, elliptical, homogeneous, radiopacities, which resemble *grains of rice*.

Differential Diagnosis

Sialolith: These are not as small in size and multiple with wide spread dissemination, especially in the brain and muscles as the calcified nodules of cysticerci.

Management

Medical management by using an anthelmintic, in the initial stage. After the larvae have settled and calcified in the oral tissues, they are harmless.

Arterial Calcification

There are two different patterns of arterial calcifications which can be identified both radiographically and histologically—Monckerberg's Medial Calcinosis and Calcified Atherosclerotic Plaque.

Monckerberg's Medial Calcinosis (Arteriosclerosis)

Definition

This is characterized by the fragmentation, degeneration and eventual loss of elastic fibers followed by the deposition of calcium within the medial coat of the vessel.

Clinical Features

- Initially most patients are asymptomatic.
- Eventually they may develop cutaneous gangrene, peripheral vascular disease and myositis due to vascular insufficiency.
- Patients with Sturge-Weber syndrome also develop intracranial arterial calcifications.

Radiographic Features

- Those involving the facial or the carotid artery may be seen on the panoramic radiographs.
- The calcific deposits in the walls of the artery outline an image of the artery.
- From the side, it may appear as a parallel pair of thin, radiopaque lines, that may have a straight or tortuous path (pipe stem or tram track appearance).
- In cross-section the involved vessels display a circular ring like pattern.

Differential Diagnosis

Other calcific deposits: The linear nature of arteriosclerosis is distinctive and pathognomic of the condition.

Management

Evaluation of the patient for occlusive arterial disease, and in some cases hyperparathyroidism should be considered as medial calcinosis frequently develops as a metastatic calcification in these patients.

Calcified Atherosclerotic Plaque

Definition

This is found in the extracranial carotid vasculature and is a major contributing source of cerebrovascular embolic and occlusive disease. Dystrophic calcifications can occur in the evolution of plaque within the intima of the involved vessel.

Radiographic Features

- This first develops at the arterial bifurcation as a result of increased endothelial damage at these sites.
- When calcification occurs, these lesions may be visible on the panoramic radiograph in the soft tissues of the neck adjacent to the greater cornu of the hyoid bone and the cervical vertebrae C3, C4 or the intervertebral space between them.
- The soft tissue calcifications are usually seen as heterogeneous radiopacities, which are multiple and irregular in shape, sharply defined from the surrounding soft tissues and have a vertical linear distribution.

Differential Diagnosis

Calcified Triticeous cartilage: The uniform size, shape and location of calcified triticeous cartilage in the laryngeal cartilage generally aids in the identification of this condition.

Management

The patient should be referred to the physician for cerebrovascular and cardiovascular workup.

Idiopathic Calcification (Or Calcinosis)

This results from deposition of calcium in normal tissue despite normal serum calcium phosphate levels. (e.g. chondrocalcinosis, phleboliths).

Sialoliths (Salivary Gland Stone, Salivary Gland Calculus) (Figs 27.3 and 27.4)

Definition

Sialolithiasis is the formation of calcified obstruction within the salivary duct, resulting in chronic retrograde infection

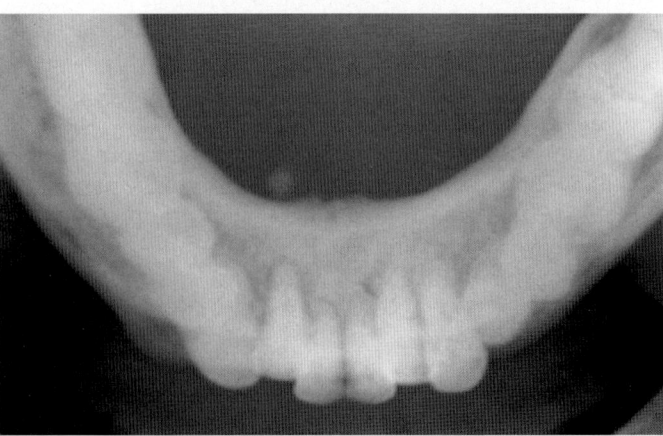

Figure 27.3 Sialolith: Occlusal view—this view revealed a well-delineated, solitary radiopaque shadow, about 5 mm diameter in right premolar-canine region

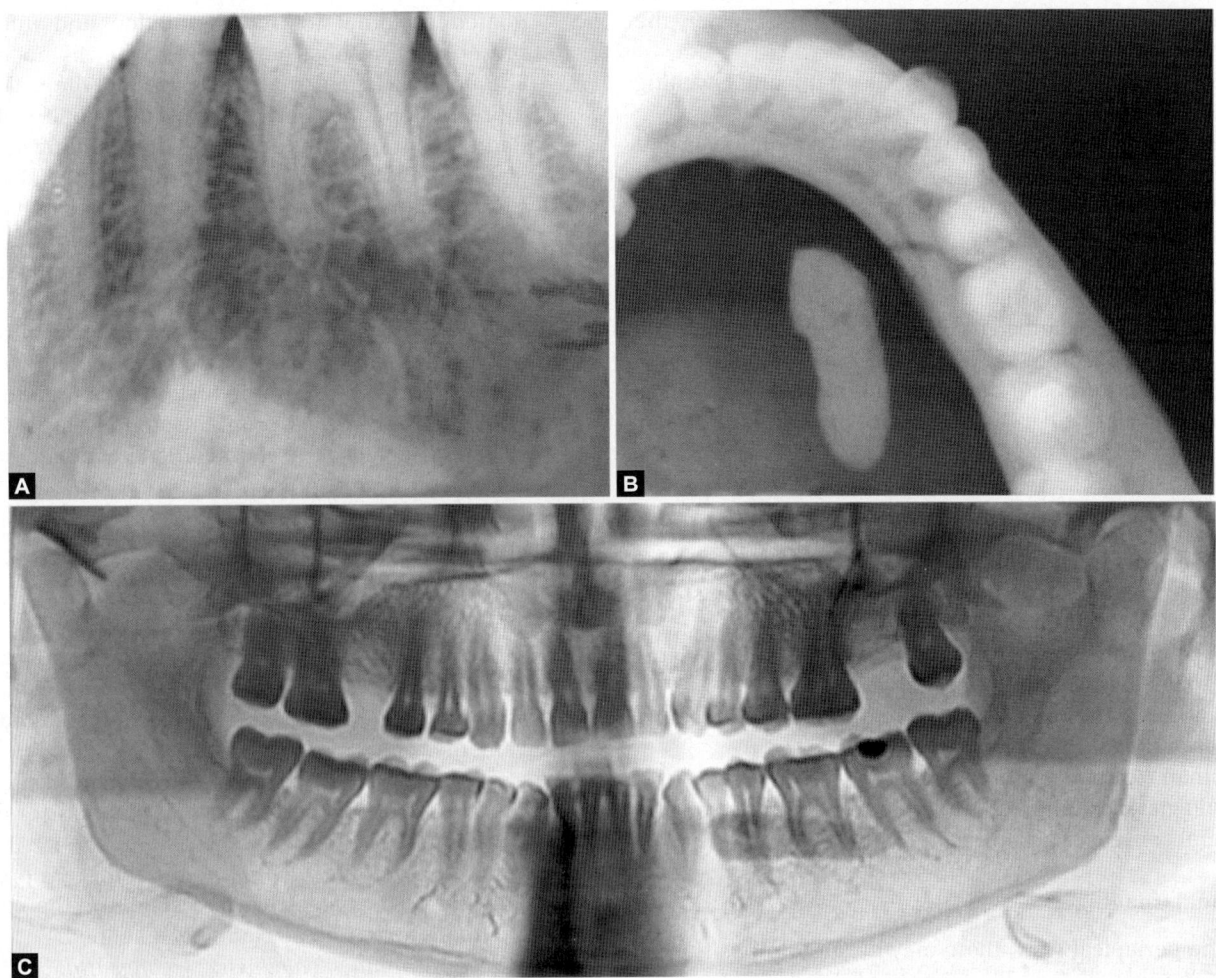

Figures 27.4A to C Sialolith of the left submandibular duct: (A) Intraoral periapical radiograph showing long cylindrical homogenous radiopaque mass in the periapical region of the left mandibular premolar and molar region; (B) Mandibular occlusal view showing long cylindrical homogenous radiopaque mass in the left side of the floor of the mouth; (C) Panoramic radiograph showing a long cylindrical homogenous radiopaque mass in the inter-radicular area of the lower left premolar and molars

because of a decreased salivary flow. Sialoliths may also form in any of the major or minor salivary glands (glandular sialolith) or their ducts (ductal sialolith), usually only one gland is involved.

Mechanical conditions contributing to the slow flow rate and physiochemical characteristics of the gland secretions both contribute to the formation of a nidus and subsequent precipitation of calcium and phosphate salts.

Accordingly, the submandibular gland and ductal system lie in a dependent position. The Wharton's duct is long and has an irregular tortuous course, an uphill flow in the proximal portion and the orifice is much smaller than the lumen. The salivary secretion of the submandibular gland is more viscous and has higher mineral content.

The sialolith is made up of laminated layers of organic material covered with concentric shells of calcified material, which is crystalline in structure (Hydroxyapatite crystals with octacalcium and phosphate). The chemical composition is principally of calcium phosphate and carbon with traces of magnesium, potassium, chloride and ammonium.

Clinical Features

- These are common in the middle age with a slight predilection for men.
- The submandibular gland and the Wharton's duct are by far the most frequently involved (83% of the cases), followed by the parotid (10%) and sublingual (7%) glands. About half of the submandibular stones lie in the distal portion of the Wharton's duct, 20% in the proximal portion, and 30% in the gland.
- The patient may be asymptomatic, or they may history of pain and swelling in the floor of the mouth and in the involved gland. Intraglandular stones cause less severe symptoms than the extra-glandular or the intraductal types.

- The discomfort may intensify at meal times, when the salivary flow is stimulated.
- If the blockage is partial, then the pain and swelling gradually subsides.
- Nine percent of patients have recurrent sialolithiasis and 10% have nephrolithiasis.
- Pus may exude from the duct orifice, the surrounding soft tissue may be inflamed, and tender, and the overlying mucosa may ulcerate.
- Stones in the more peripheral portion of the duct may be palpated, if it is of sufficient size.
- Sialolithiasis of minor salivary gland is a rare occurrence, the most common site being buccal mucosa either near the commissure or in the proximity to the mandibular mucobuccal fold.

Radiographic Features

- The sialoliths located in the duct of the submandibular glands are usually cylindrical. But they may vary in shape from long cigar shapes to oval or round shapes.
- Stones that form in the hilus of the submandibular gland tend to be larger and more irregularly shaped.
- The stones are homogeneously radiopaque, and show evidence of multiple layers.
- Less than 20% of the submandibular gland and 40% of the parotid gland sialoliths are radiolucent because of the low mineral content of parotid secretions.

Additional Imaging

- On the periapical view, there may be superimposition of the stone over the mandibular premolar and molar apices.
- A standard mandibular occlusal view, using half the usual exposure time, displays the floor of the mouth without overlap of the mandible and is the best view for visualizing stones in the distal portion of the Wharton's duct.
- A lateral oblique view or a panoramic view, helps to visualize stones in a more posterior location.
- A periapical film, placed in the buccal vestibule, with reduced exposure and time and the central ray directed through the cheek, helps to demonstrate stones in the parotid gland duct.
- An anteroposterior skull view, of the patient with 'blow-out' cheek, or an open-mouth lateral skull projection, helps to demonstrate stones in the parotid duct.
  - When producing radiographs to detect sialoliths, the exposure time should be reduced to about half of normal, this helps to detect stones that are highly calcified.
  - If noncalcified stone are suspected, then sialography; is helpful in locating obstructions that are undetectable with plain radiography. The contrast agent usually flows around the sialolith, filling the duct proximal to the obstruction. The ductal system is frequently

dilated proximal to the obstruction and infers the presence of an obstruction even when is not visible. The contrast agent that flows around the sialolith is more radiopaque and may obscure small sialoliths. Radiolucent sialoliths appear as ductal filling defects.
  - Sialography should not be performed if the radiopaque stone is shown by plain radiography to be in the distal portion of the duct, because the procedure may displace it proximally into the ductal system, complicating its subsequent removal.
- *Computed tomography*: It also helps to detect minimally calcified sialoliths which are not visible on plain films.
- *USG*: It is of limited use in the diagnosis of inflammatory and obstructive diseases, but if the stone is large (2 mm), it will be detected as a characteristic acoustic shadow showing echo-dense spots.

Differential Diagnosis

- *Gas bubble*: These are more easily removed and are more circular than sialoliths.
- *Hyoid bone*: These are seen bilaterally on the panoramic film.
- *Myositis ossificans*: There will be restriction of mandibular movements.
- *Phleboliths*: There will be no sialadenitis, and these are more or less rounded and contain laminations or central dark (radiolucent) areas.
- *Calcific submandibular lymph nodes*: If there is presence of pain then it is suggestive of a sialolith. The calcified lymph nodes appear to be cauliflower shaped.
- *Chondrodystrophia calcificans congenita*: This is associated with calcifications in the neck which resemble the submaxillary calculi in the radiographs.
- *Palatine tonsillitis*: On the panoramic image it has a similar location to parotid sialoliths, superimposed over the ramus, but can be differentiated in that they are typically multiple and punctate.

Other Causes of Obstructions

- *Mucous plugs*: These are incompletely mineralized sialoliths.
- *Strictures and stenosis*: This may be papillary or ductal obstruction due to chronic irritation, acute trauma or presence of intra ductal growth or tumor.
- *Foreign bodies*: Food particles, toothbrush bristles, tooth picks.
- *Extraductal causes*: Like muscle pressure, tumors, lymph nodes and denture flanges.
- Parotid fistula; this may open into the oral cavity or on to the exterior of the face. It may be due to trauma, rupture of parotid abscess or complication of superficial parotidectomy.

Management

It is best to encourage spontaneous discharge through the use of sialogogues or piezoelectric extracorporeal shock wave lithotripsy or surgical removal is indicated.

Phleboliths (Figs 27.5 to 27.7)

Definition

Intravascular thrombi, which arise secondary to venous stagnation, may get organized or mineralized. The mineralization begins at the core of the thrombus and consists of crystals of apatite with calcium phosphate and calcium carbonate. Phleboliths are calcified thrombi found in veins, venulae, or the sinusoidal vessels of hemangiomas (especially the cavernous type).

Clinical Features

- In the head and neck region, phleboliths always indicate the presence of a hemangioma.
- In an adult it may be the sole residual of a childhood hemangioma, which has long since regressed.
- The involved soft tissue may be swollen, throbbing or discolored by the presence of veins or a soft tissue hemangioma, which often fluctuate in size, associated with changes in body position or during a Valsalva maneuver. The vascular nature may be confirmed by the presence of blanching or change in color on applying pressure. Auscultation may reveal bruit in case of cavernous hemangioma but not in the capillary type.

Radiographic Features

- These are commonly found in hemangiomas.
- In cross-section the shape is round or oval, up to 6 mm in diameter with a smooth periphery. If the involved blood vessel is viewed from the side, the phlebolith may resemble a *straight* or a *slightly curved sausage.*
- It may be homogeneously radiopaque but more commonly has the appearance of laminations, giving phleboliths a bull's eye or target appearance. A radiolucent center may be seen, which may represent the remaining patent portion of the vessel.

Differential Diagnosis

Sialolith: These usually occur singly, if multiple sialoliths are present, they are usually oriented in a single line, whereas phleboliths are usually multiple and have a more random, clustered distribution, and is usually associated with a vascular lesion.

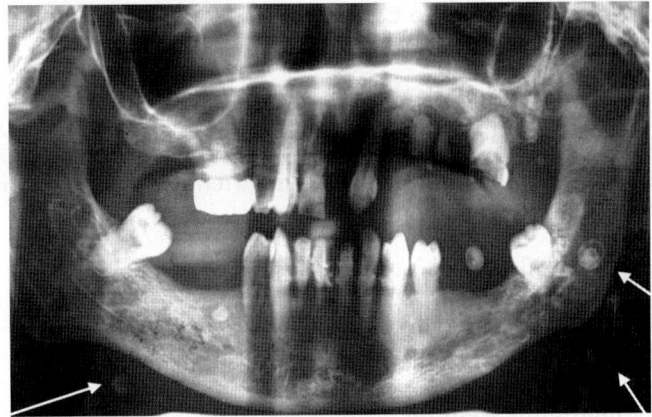

Figure 27.5 Panoramic radiograph showing calcification foci seen on the left side over body and angle of mandible and one on the right side in submandibular region

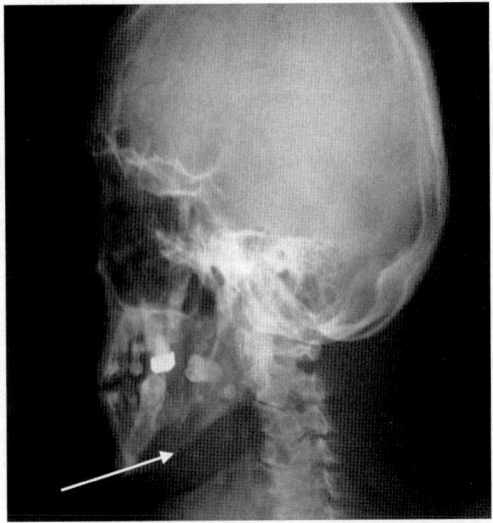

Figure 27.6 Lateral skull view showing calcification foci in pharynx and neck region

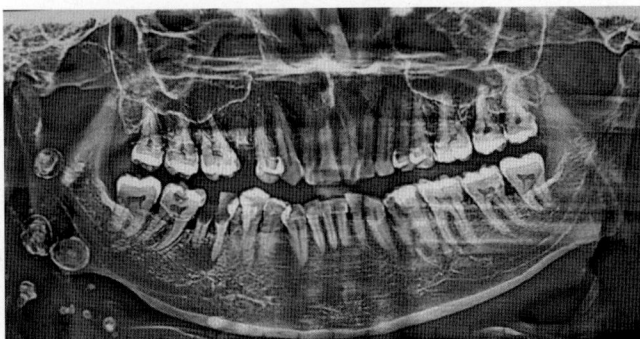

Figure 27.7 Calcifications in AV malformations

Laryngeal Cartilage Calcifications

Definition

Both the thyroid and the triticeous (means grain of wheat) cartilages (found within the lateral thyrohyoid ligaments) consist of hyaline cartilage, which has a tendency to calcify or ossify with advancing age.

Clinical Features

It has no clinical features and usually is an incidental radiographic finding.

Radiographic Features

- The calcified cartilage is located on a lateral view within the pharyngeal air space inferior to the greater cornu of the hyoid bone and adjacent to the superior border of C4. The superior cornu of a calcified thyroid cartilage appears medial to C4 and is superimposed on the prevertebral soft tissue.
- The triticeous cartilage measures 7–9 mm in length and 2–4 mm in width. The periphery is well-defined and smooth, and only the top 2–3 mm of the calcified thyroid cartilage is visible at the lower edge of a panoramic radiograph.
- The calcified tracheal cartilages usually present a homogeneous radiopacity, with an occasional outer cortex.

Differential Diagnosis

Calcified atheromatous plaque in the carotid bifurcation, the calcified triticeous cartilage has a solitary nature and an extremely uniform shape and size.

Management

No treatment required.

Rhinolith/Antrolith (Fig. 27.8)

Definition

Hard calcified bodies or stones that occur in the nose (rhinoliths) or the antrum (antroliths) arise from the deposition of mineral salts such as calcium phosphate, calcium carbonate, and magnesium around a nidus. In case of a rhinolith the nidus is usually an exogenous foreign body (coin, beads, etc) whereas the nidus for an antrolith is usually endogenous (root tip, bone fragment, masses of stagnated mucus, etc.).

Clinical Features

- The patient may be asymptomatic initially.
- With the increase in size of the expanding mass, it may impinge on the mucosa, producing pain, congestion and ulceration.
- The patient may develop a unilateral purulent rhinorrhea, sinusitis, headache, epistaxis, nasal obstruction, anosmia, fetor, fever and facial pain.

Radiographic Features

- These stones have a variety of shapes and sizes. They have well-defined smooth or irregular borders.
- They may be homogeneous or heterogeneous radiopacities, depending on the nature of the nidus and sometimes have laminations. Occasionally the density may exceed the surrounding bone.
- Antroliths occur within the maxillary sinus above the floor of the antrum and may be seen on the periapical, occlusal and panoramic radiographs.
- Rhinoliths are seen in the nasal fossae. A posteroanterior skull view will help to identify the location of a rhinolith.

Differential Diagnosis

- *Osteoma*
- *Healing odontogenic cyst*
- *Mycolith*
- *Root fragments*: It should be differentiated from antroliths by the presence of the root anatomy and presence of a root canal. A displaced fragment in the sinus will move when the radiography is performed with the head in different positions, unless it is lodged between the bone and the sinus lining.

Management

Patients should be referred to an otorhinolaryngologist for the removal of the stone.

METASTATIC CALCIFICATION

Metastatic calcification results when minerals precipitate into normal tissue as a result of higher than normal serum

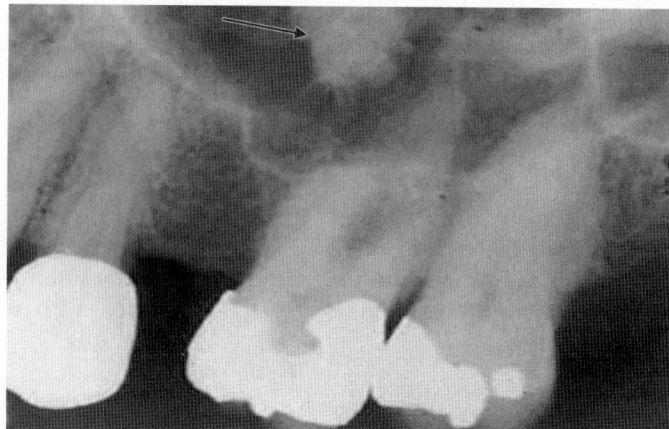

Figure 27.8 Anthrolith in the sinus

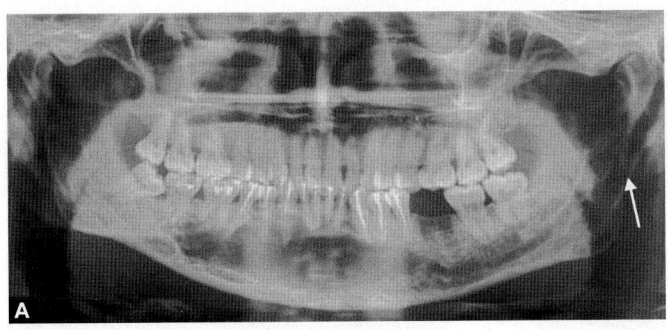
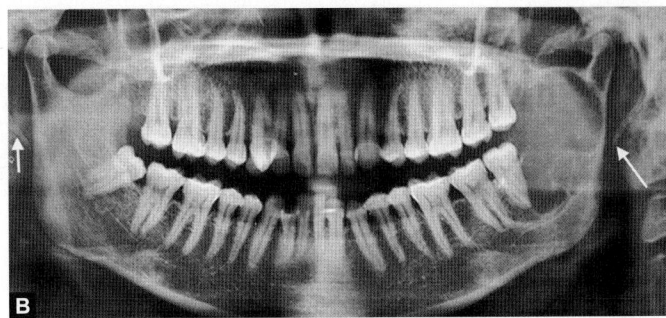

Figures 27.9A and B Panoramic radiographs: (A and B) Showing ossification of the styloid process

calcium (e.g. hyperparathyroidism, hypercalcemia of malignancy) or phosphate (e.g. chronic renal failure). Metastatic calcifications usually occur bilaterally and symmetrically. The deposits of calcium occur in the kidney, lung, gastric mucosa and media of blood vessels.

Ossification of the Styloid Ligament (Figs 27.9 to 27.11)

Definition

Ossification of the styloid ligament usually extends downwards from the base of the skull and commonly occurs bilaterally. In rare cases the ossification begins at the lesser horn of the hyoid or in the central area of the ligament. The associated conditions are Eagle's syndrome, Styloid syndrome and Styloid chain ossification.

Clinical Features

- Patients are more than 40 years of age and are usually clinically symptom less.
- It may be detected by palpation over the tonsil as a hard pointed structure.
- The patient may present with a complaint of a vague nagging to intense pain in the pharynx on swallowing, turning the head or opening the mouth, especially on yawning.
- If the patient gives an associated history of neck trauma (e.g. tonsillectomy), the condition is called Eagle's syndrome. The elongated styloid process and local scar tissue probable cause symptoms by impinging on the glossopharyngeal nerve.
- Similar clinical findings without a history of neck trauma constitute stylohyoid (carotid artery) syndrome.
  - The patient may also describe attacks of otalgia, tinnitus, temporal headache and vertigo or transient syncope.
  - The pain may be produced by mechanical irritation of sympathetic nerve tissue in the arterial wall, producing regional carotidynia.
  - This condition is more prevalent than Eagle's syndrome.

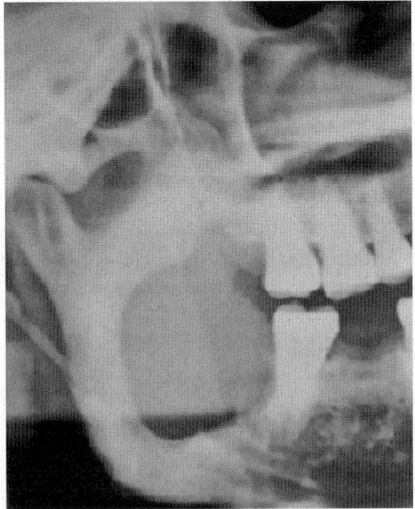

Figure 27.10 Cropped panoramic radiograph showing calcified styloid process with radiolucency in the ramus region which has well-defined borders indicative of a cystic lesion

Radiographic Features

- The styloid ligament ossification is quite common in individuals of any age and may be detected as an incidental feature on any panoramic radiograph.
- In the panoramic image it is seen as a linear, long, tapering, thin, radiopaque process that is thicker at its base, extending forward from the region of the mastoid process and crosses the posteroinferior aspect of the ramus towards the hyoid bone. The hyoid bone is positioned approximately parallel to or superimposed on the posterior aspect of the inferior cortex of the mandible.
- It varies in length from 0.5–2.5 cm.
- The ossified ligament has a more or less straight outline, but it may sometimes show irregularity in the outer surface. The further the radiopaque ossified ligament extends towards the hyoid bone, the more likely it is that it will be interrupted by radiolucent, joint like junctions (pseudoarticulations).

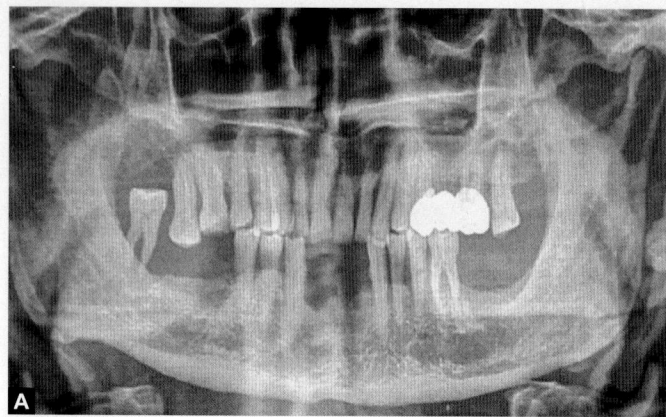
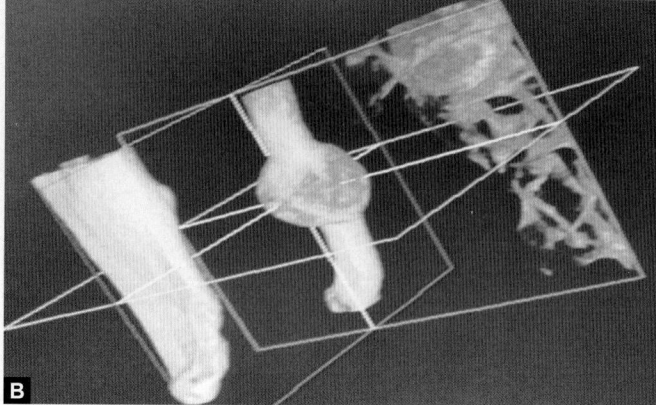

Figures 27.11A and B (A) Panoramic radiograph showing elongated styloid processes left and right. The left styloid process has a dilated shape, which may indicate; pseudoarthrosis in styloid or if the styloid process is disturbed or fractured during tonsilectomy in childhood, it reforms in the form of bulb, normal variation of styloid or focal fibrous dysplasia; (B) CBCT 3D image of the same styloid process

- Small ossifications of the styloid ligament appear homogeneously radiopaque. As the ossification increases in length and girth, the outer cortex of this bone appears as a radiopaque band at the periphery.

Differential Diagnosis

Temporomandibular joint dysfunction: There is no radiographic evidence of ligament ossification.

Management

Amputation of the stylohyoid process.

Osteoma Cutis

Definition

These are sites of normal bone formation in abnormal locations. It is a rare soft tissue calcification in the skin. It may develop secondary to acne of long duration, in a scar or chronic inflammatory dermatosis. Histologically these are seen as areas of dense viable bone in the dermis or subcutaneous tissue. They are occasionally found in diffuse scleroderma, replacing the altered collagen in the dermis and subcutaneous septa.

Clinical Features

- It may occur on the face (extraoral) in the cheek and lip region, and tongue (intraoral) where it may be called osteoma mucosae or osseous choristoma.
- It does not cause any visible change in the overlying skin, except in some cases where the color may change to yellowish white.

- It varies in size from 0.1 mm to 5 cm in diameter, if the lesion is large. The individual osteoma may be palpated. A needle inserted into one of the papules usually meets with stone like resistance.
- Osteoma may be single or multiple.
- Some patients develop numerous lesions (dozens to hundreds), usually on the face in females and on the scalp or chest in males. This is known as multiple miliary osteoma cutis.

Radiographic Features

- An intraoral film placed between the cheek and the alveolar bone gives accurate localization.
- A posteroanterior skull view with the cheek blown outward using a soft tissue technique of 60 kVp helps localize osteomas of the skin.
- If present in the cheek or lip region the shadow may be superimposed over a tooth root or alveolar process, giving the appearance of dense bone.
- The osteoma cutis appears as smoothly outlined, radiopaque, washer-shaped images.
- These single or multiple radiopacities may be of various sizes.
- It appears as a homogeneous radiopacity with a radiolucent center that represents normal fatty marrow, giving the lesion a dough-nut appearance radiographically.
- Trabeculae usually develop in the marrow cavity of the larger osteomas.
- Lesions of calcified cystic acne resemble a snow-flake radiopacity which corresponds to the clinical location of the scar.

Differential Diagnosis

- *Myositis ossificans*: It is of greater proportions, in some cases causing noticeable deformity of the facial contour.
- *Calcinosis cutis*.
- *Osteoma mucosae*: If the blown out cheek technique is used, the lesions of osteoma cutis appear much more superficial than mucosal lesions.

Management

They may be removed for cosmetic reasons. The methods used are excision, resurfacing of the skin with Er:YAG laser using tretinoin cream (especially in cases of multiple miliary osteoma cutis).

Myositis Ossificans

In this case, there is the fibrous tissue and heterotopic bone that form within the interstitial tissue of the muscle and associated tendons and ligaments. There is secondary destruction and atrophy of the muscle as the fibrous tissue and bone interdigitate and separate the muscle fibers.

It is of two types:
1. Localized myositis ossificans.
2. Progressive myositis ossificans.

Localized Myositis Ossificans (Post-traumatic Myositis, Myositis Ossificans, Solitary Myositis)

Definition

This results due to acute or chronic trauma, heavy muscular strain, muscle injury which may lead to considerable hemorrhage into the muscle or associated tendons or fascia. The hemorrhage organizes and undergoes progressive scarring. During the healing process, heterotopic bone and in some cases cartilage is formed. There is no inflammation (the term myositis is thus misleading). The fibrous tissue and bone form within the interstitial tissue of the muscle, there is no actual ossification of the muscle fibers.

Clinical Features

- It may develop at any age, in either gender, but is more common in young men who engage in vigorous activities. The commonly involved oral sites are, the masseter, sterno-cleidomastoid and lateral pterygoid muscle.
- The site of the precipitating trauma remains swollen, tender and painful for a long time. The overlying skin may be red and inflamed.
- If the lesion involves a muscle of mastication, opening the jaw may be difficult.

- After a period of 2–3 weeks the area of ossification may become apparent, as a firm, intramuscular palpable mass, which enlarges slowly, but eventually stops growing. The lesion may appear fixed or may be freely movable on palpation.

Radiographic Features

- A radiolucent band may be seen between the areas of ossification and adjacent bone, and the heterotopic bone may lie along the long axis of the muscle.
- The periphery is more radiopaque than the internal structure. The shape may vary from irregular, oval to linear streaks (pseudotrabeculae) running in the same direction as the normal muscle fibers.
- The internal structure varies with time:
  - In the third or fourth week after injury, the appearance is faintly homogeneous radiopacity.
  - By the second month, it is organized and appears as delicate lacy or feathery radiopaque internal structure, which indicate the formation of bone. This bone does not have a normal appearing trabecular pattern.
  - Gradually the image becomes denser and better defined, maturing fully in about 5–6 months.
  - After this the lesion may shrink.

Differential Diagnosis

- Ossification of the stylohyoid ligament, dystrophic calcifications in areas of necrosis, pathological calcifications, phleboliths. The form and location of myositis ossifications and the presence of pseudotrabeculae are enough to differentiate it from them.
- *Bone forming tumors*: Although tumors like osteogenic sarcoma can form a linear bone pattern, the tumor is contiguous with the adjacent bone and signs of bone destruction are present.

Management

Sufficient rest to the injured part, and if necessary excision.

Progressive Myositis Ossificans

Definition

This is a rare disease of unknown cause that usually affects children before 6 years of age, and occasionally as early as infancy. Progressive formation of heterotopic bone occurs within the interstitial tissue of muscles, tendons, ligaments and fascia, and the involved muscle atrophies. This condition may be inherited or may be a spontaneous mutation affecting the mesenchyma.

Clinical Features

- It usually affects children before 6 years of age, and occasionally as early as infancy, males are more affected. It may affect the striated muscles including the heart and diaphragm.
- It starts in the muscles of the neck and upper back and moves to the extremities.
- It begins as a soft tissue swelling that is tender and painful and may show redness and heat, indicating the presence of inflammation.
- As the acute symptoms subside, a firm mass remains in the tissue.
- Sometimes the spread of ossification is limited, in other cases it may be very extensive; affecting, almost all the muscles of the body, resulting in stiffness and limitation of motion of the neck, chest, back and extremities (especially the shoulders), which gradually increases.
- Advanced stages of the disease result in the 'petrified man' like appearance.
- During the third decade the process may spontaneously arrest, however most of the patients die young during the 3rd or 4th decade, due to respiratory embarrassment or from inanition through the involvement of the muscles of mastication.

Radiographic Features

- The radiographic appearance is similar to that of localized myositis ossificans.
- The heterotopic bone more commonly is oriented along the long axis of the involved muscle, with coarser linear striae of increased density which represent new bone formation, and there is evidence of dense osseous replacement of the greater part or whole of the muscle.
- The bone that is laid down does not show normal bone structure, and appears as a rather structure less mass of variable density.
- Osseous malformations of the regions of muscle attachment, such as the mandibular condyles, may also be seen.
- Skeleton becomes osteoporotic because of lack of function as muscles atrophy and joints become ankylosed.

Differential Diagnosis

- *Rheumatoid arthritis*: In the initial stage it may be difficult but as the disease progresses specific anomalies confirm the diagnosis.

- *Calcinosis*: The deposists of amorphous calcium salts frequently resorb, but in progressive myositis ossificans that bone never disappears.

Management

There is no effective treatment. The treatment is symptomatic and supportive as per the requirement of each case. Nodules that are traumatized and then ulcerate should be excised.

ABBERENT CALCIFICATIONS IN THE OROFACIAL REGION (FIGS 27.12 TO 27.14)

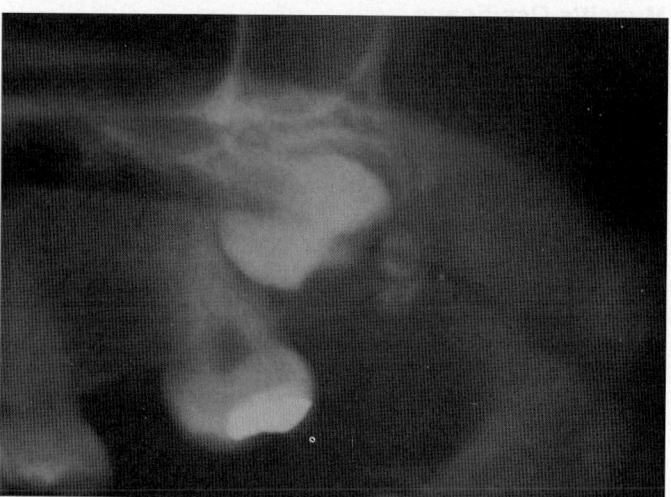

Figure 27.12 Calcifications in follicular space

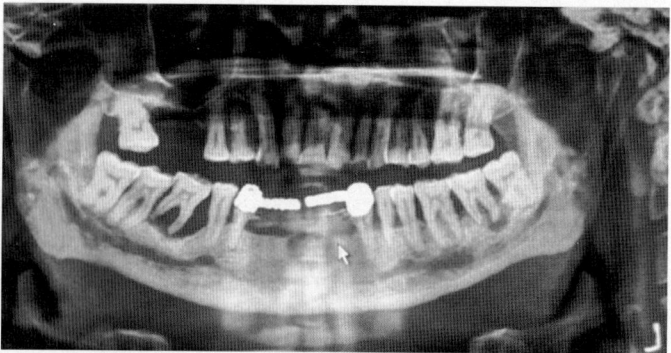

Figure 27.13 Calcification in the thyroid region

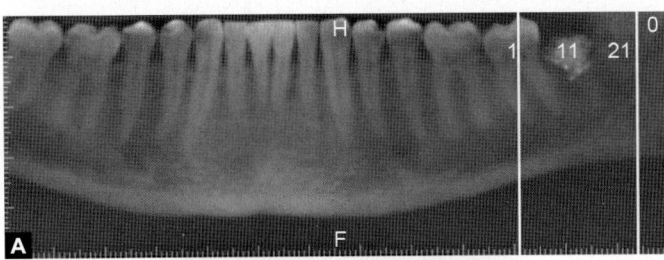

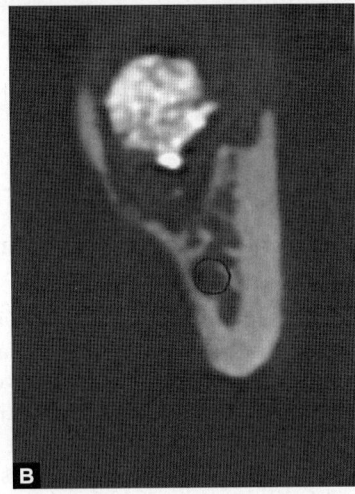

Figures 27.14A and B Cone beam computed tomography image: (A) Panoramic; (B) Cross-sectional showing radiopacity in the region of 3rd molar, zinc oxide pack placed in socket for treatment of dry socket

BIBLIOGRAPHY

1. Almog DM, Horev T, Illig KA, et al. Correlating carotid artery stenosis detected by panoramic radiography with clinically relevant carotid artery stenosis determined by duplex ultrasound. Oral Surg Oral Med Oral Pathol Oral Radiol Endod. 2002;94(6):768-73.

2. Friedlander AH, Altman L. Carotid artery atheromas in postmenopausal women. Their prevalence on panoramic radiographs and their relationship to atherogenic risk factors. JADA. 2001;132(8):1130-6.

3. Friedlander AH, Freymiller EG. Detection of radiation-accelerated atherosclerosis of the carotid artery by panoramic radiography: a new opportunity for dentists. JADA. 2003;134(10):1361-5.

4. Goaz PW, White SC. Principles and Interpretation. In: Oral Radiology, 3rd edition. St Louis, Mosby Year Book, 1994.

5. Miles DA, Van Dis MJ, Jensen CW, et al. Interpretation normal versus abnormal and common radiographic presentations of lesions. In: Radiographic and Imaging for Dental Auxiliaries, 3rd edition. Philadelphia, WB Saunders. 1999.pp.231-80.

6. Monsour PA, et al. Soft tissue calcifications in the differential diagnosis of opacities superimposed over the mandible by dental panoramic radiography. Aust Dent J. 1991;36:94.

7. Ohba T, Takata Y, Ansai T, et al. Evaluation of calcified carotid artery atheromas detected by panoramic radiograph among 80-year-olds. Oral Surg Oral Med Oral Pathol Oral Radiol Endod. 2003;96(5):647-50.

8. Ravon NA, Hollender LG, McDonald V, et al. Signs of carotid calcification from dental panoramic radiographs are in agreement with Doppler sonography results. J Clin Periodontol. 2003;30(12):1084-90.

9. Shafer WG, et al. A textbook of oral pathology. Philadelphia, WB Saunders, 1983

10. Wood NK, Goaz PW. Differential diagnosis of oral lesions. 4th edition. CV Mosby, St Louis; 1991.

11. Wood RE. Handbook of signs in dental and maxillofacial radiology. Warthog Publications, Toronto; 1988.

12. Worth HM. Principles and practice of oral radiographic interpretation. Year Book Medical Publishers, Chicago; 1963.

Trauma to Teeth and Facial Structures | 28

Injuries to the teeth and facial skeleton are, unfortunately, common. The type and severity of injuries can vary considerably, from minor damage to the teeth to grossly comminuted fractures of the skull. Whatever the suspected injury, radiography is an essential requirement both in the initial assessment and in the follow-up appraisal. However, the radiographic examination may be restricted and limited by the general state of the patient and the type and severity of other injuries. For example, severe facial injuries are often associated with intracranial damage and/or cervical spine injuries, the importance of which far outweighs any damage to the teeth and their supporting structures. The radiographic investigation must therefore be tailored to each patient's needs.

Though radiography plays an important role in the diagnosis, location and determination of the extent of injury in cases of traumatic injuries to the jaws, there are however serious limitations to radiology in the study of teeth and bones when searching for evidence of fracture. There is often good clinical evidence of fracture while the radiographs appear normal. The reverse is also true, where radiographs have revealed hair-line fractures with undisplaced fragments in the absence of clinical signs and symptoms. This being the case, no examination of suspected injury is complete that does not include careful clinical examination as well as radiographic investigation. With the advent of newer imaging modalities like CT, MRI and CBCT detection of minuest fractures and extent of deformities is now much easily detected.

CLASSIFICATION OF TRAUMA TO THE TEETH AND FACIAL STRUCTURES

- Traumatic injury to the soft tissue
- Traumatic injury to the teeth
- Traumatic injury to the maxilla
- Traumatic injury to the mandible.

TRAUMATIC INJURY TO THE SOFT TISSUE

Mechanical trauma may produce:
- Keratotic lesion, necrotic white lesion, reddish erythematous macule
- Purplish macule (subepithelial hematoma) within tissue space, bleb (pooling of fluid into tissue)

- Erosion, ulcer and exophytic lesion (inflammatory hyperplasia)
- Electric burns
- Cervicofacial emphysema.

General Radiographic Features Indicating Fracture of Bone

- Demonstration of the line of cleavage, which depends on the passage of the rays through the space that exists between the fragments and is best shown when the axis of the X-rays and the plane of the fracture are in the same direction. The presence of a radiolucent line (usually sharply defined) between the fragments (within the anatomical boundaries of the structures). If the line extends beyond the boundaries of the mandible, for instance, it is more likely to represent overlapping structure.

  In cases where the fracture is very oblique the X-rays cannot pass through it and the fracture may not be seen.

  Many fractures pass slightly obliquely across the bone and the line of cleavage of the inner and outer cortices are not superimposed on the radiograph and may appear as two dark lines of fracture with a bone fragment between them. On carefully studying the radiograph the two lines will be found to be continuous at the lower border.
- A fracture that has become impacted does not have any space between the fragments and the line of cleavage is obscured by the superimposition of the bony trabeculae, a slight increase in density may be seen due to the double number of trabeculae which interdigitate. In short, an increase in the density of bone which may be caused by the overlapping of two fragments of bone.
- *Displacement*: Instead of the normal continuity of the surface of the bone. There is a disalignment of the two fragments. A defect in the outer cortical boundary, which may appear as a deviation in the smooth outline, a gap in the outer cortical bone, or a step like defect.
- *Deformity*: A change in the normal anatomical outline or shape of the structure. For example, an alteration in the outline shape of the root and discontinuity of the periodontal ligament shadow, or a mandible that is noticeably asymmetrical between the left and the right sides may indicate a fracture. A fracture of the mandible often shows a sharp change in the occlusal plane at the

location of the fracture. An abrupt angulation of the bone where bone is normally present is seen in cases associated with green stick fractures.

Limitations of Radiographic Interpretation of Fractured Bone and Tooth

Unfortunately, as a result of the inherent limitations of a two-dimensional image, radiographic interpretation is not always as straight forward, the radiographic appearances can be influenced by:

- The position and severity of the fracture
- The degree of displacement or separation of the fragments
- The position of the film and X-ray tube-head in relation to the fracture line(s). A fracture may be missed if the plane of the fracture is not in the same direction as the X-ray beam.

  It is for these reasons that a minimum of two views, from two different angles, is essential.

Radiographic Investigation (Fig. 28.1)

Although the type of injury may be evident clinically, radiographic investigation of all traumatized teeth is needed initially, to assess fully the degree of underlying damage. Radiographs are also required later to assess healing and/or the development of post-trauma complications.

The ideal radiographic requirements include:

- Two views of the injured tooth from different angles, ideally at right angles to one another, but more usually

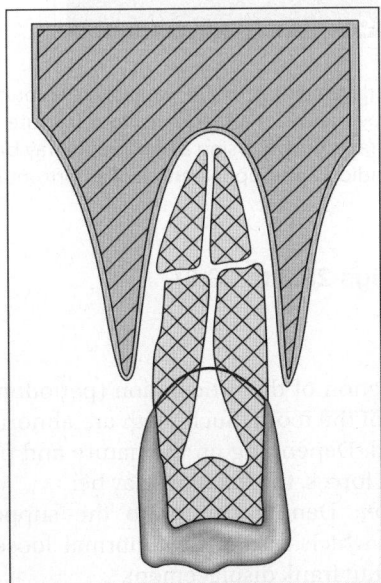

Figure 28.1 Diagram illustrating the radiographic appearance of a theoretical root fracture showing a radiolucent line between the fragments, alteration in the outline shape of the root and discontinuity of the periodontal ligament shadow

with the X-ray tube head in two different positions in the vertical plane. For example, in the anterior region (**Figs 28.2A to D**):
  - A periapical (paralleling technique)
  - An upper standard occlusal
- Reproducible views to provide a base-line assessment and to allow subsequent follow-up evaluation
- Views of the chest and/or abdomen if a tooth or foreign body is thought to have been inhaled or swallowed, including:
  - Soft tissue lateral and AP of the larynx and pharynx.

The diagnostic information provided by these radiographs may include:

- The type of injury to the teeth
- The site(s) of fractures
- The degree of displacement of the tooth fragments
- The stage of root development
- The condition of the apical tissues
- The presence, site and displacement of alveolar bone fractures
- The condition of adjacent or underlying teeth
- Evidence of healing
- Post-trauma complications, including:
  - Resorption
  - Infection
  - Cessation of tooth development
- The location of the tooth if swallowed or inhaled.

TRAUMATIC INJURY TO THE TEETH (TABLE 28.1)

Concussion

Definition

This indicates a crushing injury to the vascular structures at the tooth apex and to the periodontal ligament, resulting in inflammatory edema. Only minimal loosening or displacement of the tooth occurs. There may be elevation of the tooth out of the socket so that its occlusal surface makes premature contact on mandibular closing.

Clinical Features

- Patient may complain of pain and tenderness.
- Traumatized tooth is sensitive to percussion (horizontal and vertical)
- Complain of pain and inability to bite, patient may modify their occlusion to reduce the pressure on the tooth or teeth.

Radiographic Features

- Widening of the periodontal ligament space, more so in the apical region (due to the elevation of the tooth from the socket).

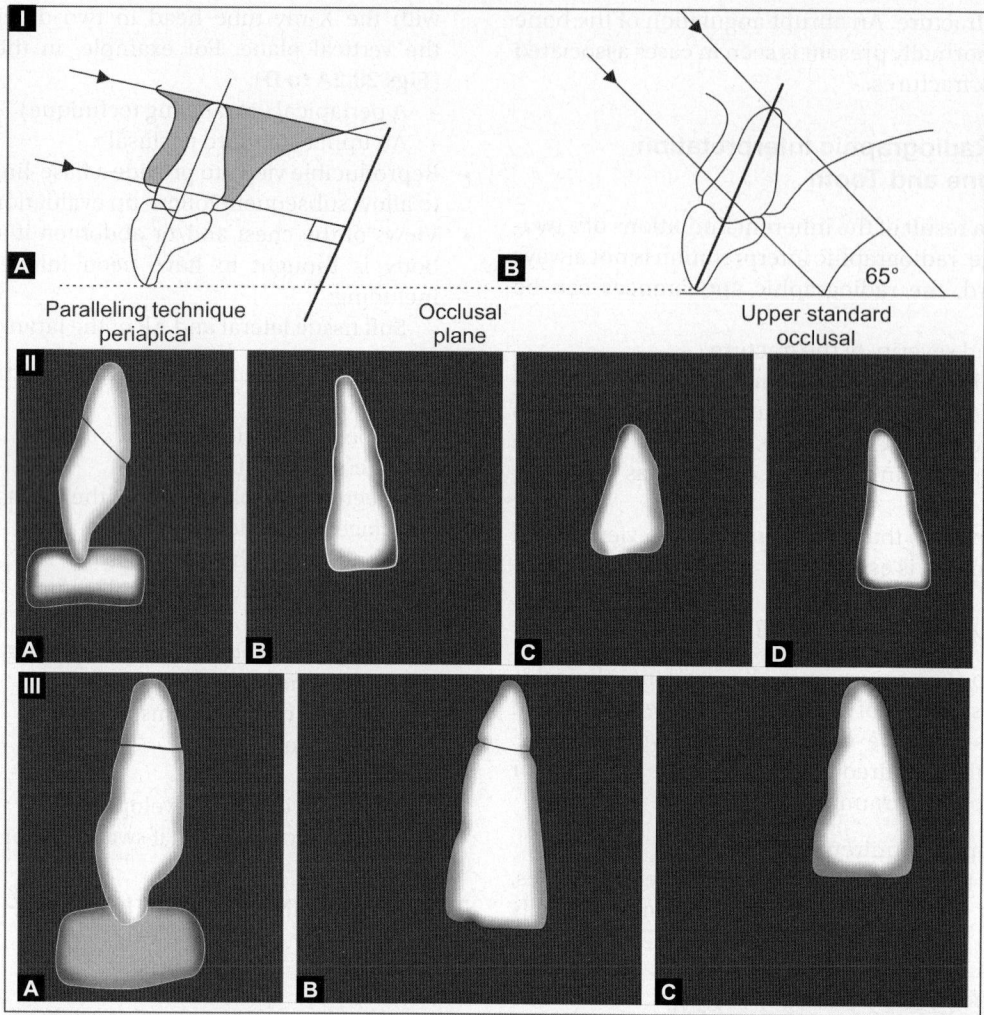

Figures 28.2 (I) Diagram showing the difference in vertical angulation of the X-ray tubehead: A. For a paralleling technique periapical; B. An upper standard occlusal of the maxillary incisors; (II) The different radiographic appearances of a tangential root fracture using different projections: A. From the side showing the direction of the fracture and separation of the fragments; B. Using a horizontal X-ray beam; C. Using a steeply angled (75°) X-ray beam; D. Using an angled (65°) X-ray beam; (III) The different radiographic appearances of a horizontal root fracture: A. From the side; B. Using a horizontal X-ray beam; C. Using an angled (65°) X-ray beam

- Reduction in the size of the pulp chamber and pulp canals may develop in months and years after the traumatic injury.
- There may be a slow developing pulp necrosis which may result in a comparative increase in width of the pulp chamber and canals due to the death of the odontoblasts, which lay down secondary dentine.
- Pulpal necrosis may cause a periapical lesion.
- In rare cases internal resorption may be seen.

Management

Conservative treatment with slight adjustment of the apposing teeth, repeated vitality tests and radiographic examination during the period and after the injury.

Luxation (Figs 28.3 to 28.5)

Definition

This is dislocation of the articulation (periodontal ligament attachment) of the tooth. Such teeth are abnormally mobile and displaced. Depending on the nature and orientation of the traumatic forces, the luxation may be:

- *Subluxation*: Denotes injury to the supporting tooth structures which results in abnormal loosening of the tooth without frank displacement.
- *Intrusive luxation*: Denotes the displacement of the tooth into the alveolar bone. This is accompanied by comminution (crushing) or fracture of the supporting alveolar bone.

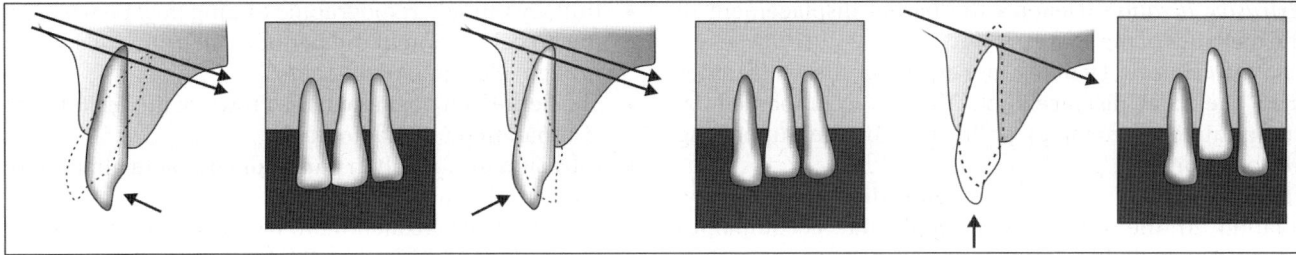

Figure 28.3 Diagram of radiographic signs of subluxation

Table 28.1 Classification of traumatic injury to the teeth

- Injuries to the hard dental tissue and pulp
  - Crown infarction; incomplete fracture of the enamel without loss of tooth substance.
    - Pulp may be devitalized
    - Internal resorption may develop
    - External resorption may develop
  - Uncomplicated crown fracture; fracture may be restricted to the enamel and /or dentin, but does not expose the pulp.
  - Complicated crown fracture; fracture involving enamel, dentin and exposing the pulp.
  - Complicated crown root fracture; fracture of the enamel, dentin and cementum and exposing pulp or coronal fracture extending subgingivally.
  - Root fracture; fracture involving dentin, cementum and pulp, with or without loss of crown structure
    - Horizontal fracture
    - Vertical fracture (chisel fracture)
- Injuries to the periodontal tissue
  - Concussion
  - Luxation
  - Avulsion
- Injuries to the supporting bone
  - Comminution of alveolar socket; crushing and compression of the alveolar socket, usually found in intrusive and lateral luxation.
  - Fracture of the alveolar socket; fracture contained to the facial or lingual socket walls.
  - Fracture of the alveolar process; fracture of the alveolar process, which may or may not involve the alveolar socket.
  - Fracture of the mandible and maxilla; fracture of the base of the mandible or maxilla and/or the alveolar process which may or may not involve the alveolar socket.
- Injuries to the gingiva and oral mucosa
  - Laceration of the gingiva or oral mucosa; a shallow or deep wound in the mucosa resulting from a tear, usually produced by a sharp object.
  - Contusion of the gingiva and oral mucosa; a bruise produced by impact from a blunt object, not accompanied by a break of the sub-mucosal tissues.
  - Abrasion of gingiva or oral mucosa; superficial wound produced by rubbing or scrapping of the mucosa leaving a raw bleeding surface.

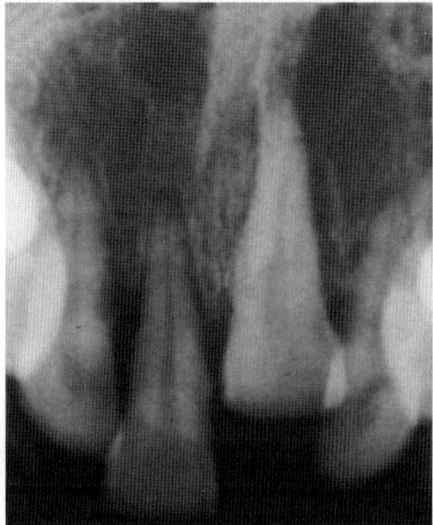

Figure 28.4 Intrusion of maxillary central incisor

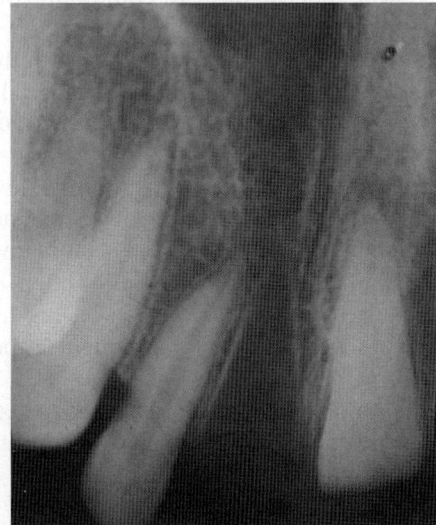

Figure 28.5 Intrusion and avulsion. Maxillary left central incisor shows displacement of the tooth in the alveolar process suggestive of intrusion with normal enamel, dentin and pulp chamber. The region of maxillary right central incisor shows empty socket suggestive of avulsion

- *Extrusive luxation*: Denotes the partial displacement of the teeth out of the socket.
- *Lateral luxation*: Denotes movement of the teeth other than the axial displacement. This is accompanied by comminution (crushing) or fracture of the supporting alveolar bone.

The movement of the apex and disruption of the circulation to the traumatized tooth that accompanies luxation usually induce temporary or permanent pulpal changes, which may result in complete or partial pulpal necrosis. If the pulp survives, the rate of hard tissue formation by the pulp accelerates and continues until it obliterates the pulp chamber and canal. This can affect both deciduous and permanent teeth.

Clinical Features

- *Subluxated teeth are usually*:
  - In their normal location, but are abnormally mobile
  - There may be some blood flowing from the gingival crevice (indicating periodontal ligament damage)
  - These are extremely sensitive to percussion and masticatory forces.
- *Intruded teeth have*:
  - Clinical crowns which appear to be shortened.
  - Maxillary incisors may be driven so deeply into the alveolar ridge that they may appear to be avulsed.
  - The displaced tooth may cause some damage to the adjacent teeth, including any developing or succedaneous teeth.
  - Depending on the orientation and magnitude of the force and the shape of the root, the root may be pushed through the buccal or less commonly the lingual alveolar plate.
- On repeated vitality testing, the sensitivity of the luxated tooth may be temporarily decreased, especially shortly after the accident. Vitality may return after several weeks or even several months.
- The teeth most often subjected to luxation are the maxillary central incisors in both deciduous and permanent dentitions. The mandibular teeth are seldom involved.
- Intrusions and extrusions are more often found in decidous teeth.
- Intrusive type of luxation is less frequent in permanent teeth.
- In either dentition when teeth are luxated, usually two or more are involved, seldom is a single tooth luxated.

Radiographic Features

- A radiograph made at the time of injury serves as a valuable reference point for comparison with subsequent radiographs

- Initially the sole radiographic finding may be widening of the apical portion of the periodontal ligament space, due to slight elevation of the tooth
- The depressed position of the crown of the intruded tooth is apparent on the radiograph
- Intrusion may result in partial or complete obliteration of the periodontal ligament space
- An extrusively luxated tooth results in increased width of the periodontal ligament space, especially in the apical region
- A severely extruded tooth will show all the periodontal space increased
- A laterally luxated tooth may show a widened periodontal ligament space, with greater width on the side of impact. Often these teeth are somewhat extruded.

Additional Imaging

Multiple radiographic projections, including occlusal views, may show the direction of displacement and its relationship to the outer cortical bone and developing teeth.

Management

A subluxated tooth may be restored back to its position by digital pressure. Stabilization by splinting may be necessary.

Avulsion (Fig. 28.5)

Definition

Exarticulation or avulsion is the term used to describe the complete displacement of the tooth from the alveolar process. This may occur due to direct or indirect trauma, fights are responsible for the avulsion of most permanent teeth and accidental falls account for the traumatic loss of deciduous teeth.

Clinical Features

- Maxillary central incisors from both dentitions are more commonly involved.
- Usually occurs in young adults when the permanent incisors are erupting and the periodontal ligament is immature.
- Usually a single tooth is lost with fracture of the alveolar wall and lip injuries.

Radiographic Features

- In a case of recent avulsion the lamina dura is apparent and persists for several months
- As the new bone forms the socket width is reduced
- Ultimately only a thin vertical radiolucent shadow remains which may have an appearance similar to a pulp canal

- In some cases the new bone replacing the socket is very dense and may appear similar to a retained root.
- Sometimes the missing tooth may be in the adjacent soft tissue and its image may project on the radiograph, giving a false impression that it is lying within the bone.
- If the avulsed tooth is not found a chest radiograph should be considered to rule out aspiration.

Differential Diagnosis

To differentiate between an intruded tooth and an avulsed tooth lying within the soft tissues, a radiograph of the lacerated lip or tongue should be produced.

Management

Reimplantation of avulsed permanent teeth often restores the function. Sometimes endodontic treatment may be necessary.

Dental Crown Fracture (Figs 28.6A and B)

Definition

This usually involves the anterior teeth of both the dentitions, caused by a fall, automobile accidents or blows from foreign objects striking the teeth.

The different types are:
- *Infraction of the crown or crack*: The fracture involves only the enamel without the loss of enamel substance.
- *Uncomplicated fracture*: Fracture that involves enamel or enamel and dentin with loss of tooth substance but without pulpal involvement.

- *Complicated fracture*: Fractures that pass through enamel, dentine and pulp with loss of tooth substance.

Clinical Features

Infarction of the crown or crack: These are not readily detected. Illuminating crowns with indirect light (directing the beam in the long-axis of the tooth) causes cracks to appear distinctly in the enamel.

Uncomplicated Fracture

- Uncomplicated fractures that involve both the enamel and dentine of permanent teeth are more common than complicated fractures
- Incidence of complicated and uncomplicated fractures is about equal in the deciduous teeth
- Those which do not involve the dentine usually occur at the mesial or distal corner of the tooth
- Loss of the central portion of the incisal edge is also common
- Fractures that involve the dentine can be recognized by the contrast in color between dentine and the peripheral layer of enamel. The exposed dentine is usually sensitive to chemical, thermal and mechanical stimulation
- In deep fractures the pink image of the pulp may shine through the remaining thin dentinal wall.

Complicated Fracture

- There will be bleeding from the exposed pulp.
- The pulp is visible and may extrude from the open pulp chamber if the fracture is old.
- The exposed pulp is sensitive to most forms of stimulation.

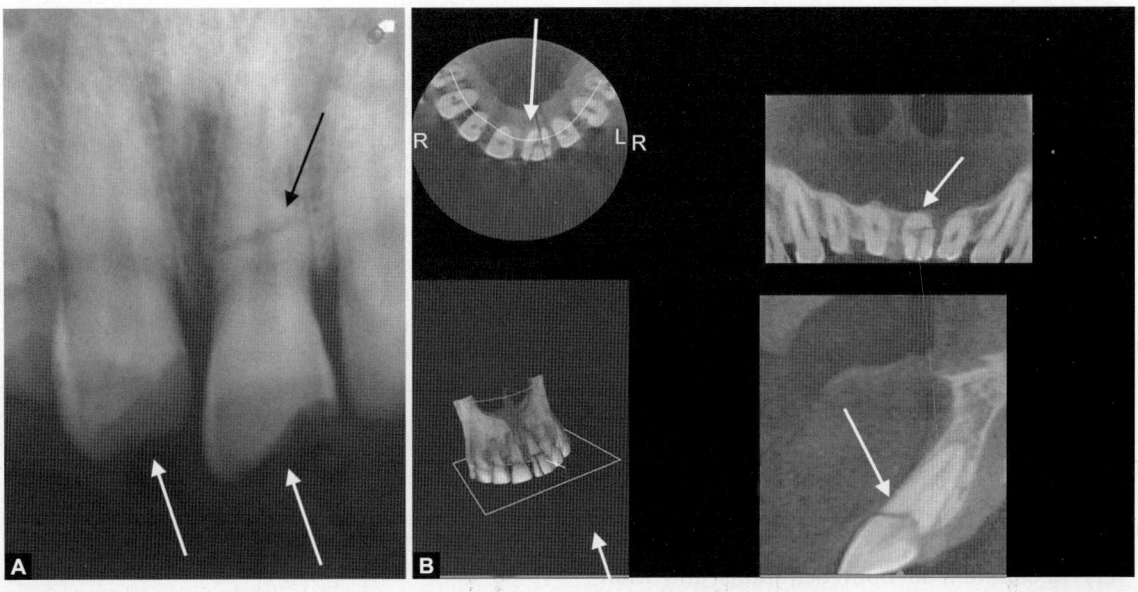

Figures 28.6A and B (A) Crown and horizontal root fracture (white arrows) of maxillary centrals with pulp exposure and horizontal root fracture (black arrow) of the right central; (B) Oblique crown fracture. As seen on CBCT axial, reformatted panoramic, 3D and sagittal views

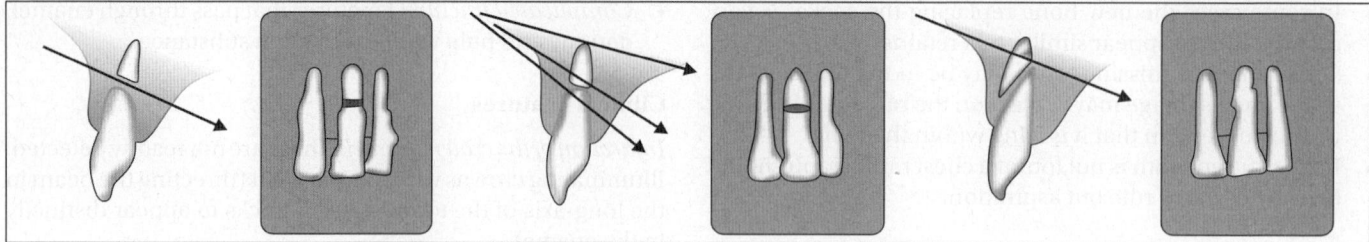

Figure 28.7 Diagram of radiographic signs of root fracture

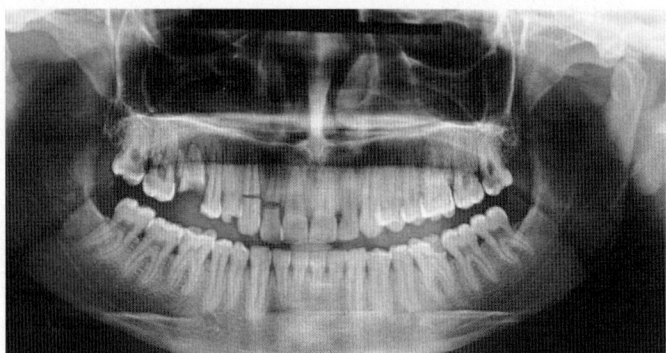

Figure 28.8 Horizontal fracture of central incisior and lateral incisior at cervical 1/3rd of roots

Radiographic Features

- The radiograph provides information regarding the location and extent of the fracture, the relationship to the pulp chamber and the stage of the root development of the involved tooth.
- The initial radiograph also provides a means of comparison for follow-up studies of the involved teeth.

Management

Crown infractions do not require any treatment except for rounding off of the sharp edges.

Uncomplicated oblique fractures have a worse prognosis than horizontal fractures, with higher degree of pulpal necrosis.

Complicated fractures of permanent teeth may be treated by pulp capping, pulpotomy or pulpectomy depending on the stage of root formation. In cases of coronal fracture of deciduous teeth involving the pulp the best treatment is to extract the tooth.

Dental Root Fracture (Figs 28.6A, 28.7 to 28.11)

Definition

These are very uncommon in both dentitions and more uncommon in deciduous teeth, may be for the fact that they are less firmly anchored in the alveolus.

Clinical Features

- Most involve the maxillary central incisors.
- Fractures of the dental root may occur at any level and involve one or all the roots of a multirooted tooth. Most of the fractures confined to the root occur in the middle third of the root.
- The coronal fragments are usually displaced lingually and slightly extruded.
- The degree of mobility of the crown relates to the level of the fracture. Closer the fracture to the apex, the more stable is the tooth. (This can be tested by placing a finger over the alveolar bone of the traumatized tooth and then gently test the mobility. If the movement of only the crown is detected, root fracture is likely).
- Fractures of the root may occur with fractures of the alveolar bone. This is more common in the case of anterior teeth of the mandible.
- Root fractures are usually associated with temporary loss of sensitivity, which usually returns to normal within about 6 months.

Radiographic Features

- The ability of the film to reveal the presence of the root fracture depends on the degree of distraction of the fragments and whether the X-ray beam is in alignment with the plane of the fracture.
- When visible:
  – The fracture appears as a sharply defined radiolucent line, confined to the anatomic limits of the root.
  – If the orientation of the beam is not directly through the plane of the fracture, the image appears as a more poorly defined gray shadow.
- Most nondisplaced fractures are difficult to demonstrate on the radiograph, and several views at different angles may be necessary.
- Sometimes the only evidence of a fracture may be a localized increase in the periodontal ligament space adjacent to the fracture site.
- Transverse and oblique fracture produce a shadow of the fracture line at the buccal and lingual surfaces which may suggest the presence of more than one (comminuted) fracture.

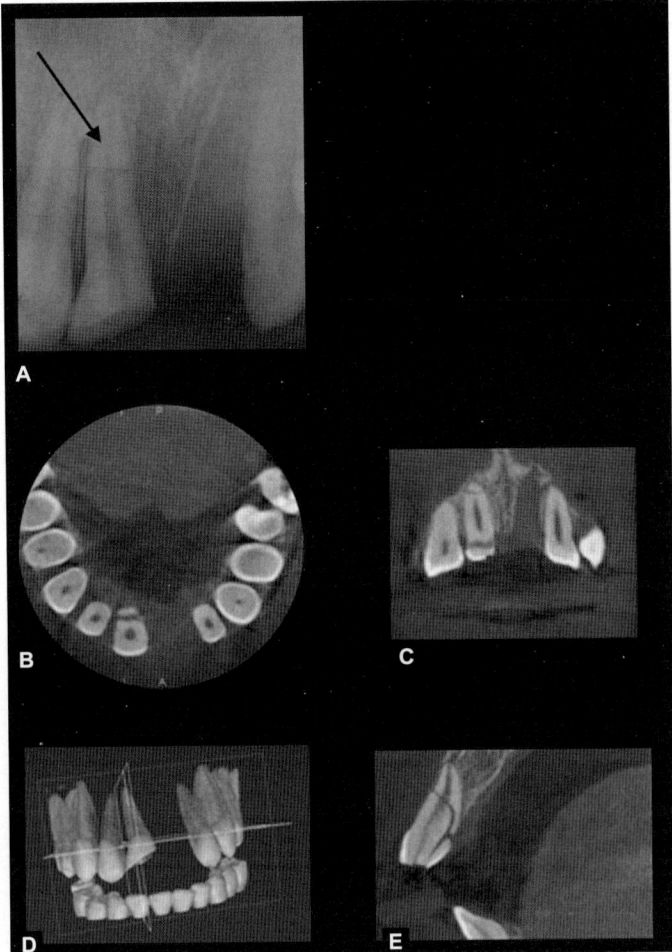

Figures 28.9A to D Horizontal fracture of the root as viewed on: (A) Periapical radiograph and CBCT; (B) Axial; (C) Coronal; (D) 3D; (E) Sagittal view show a much clearer picture of the extent of the fracture and the fracture on the lingual aspect of the tooth is also clearly appreciated

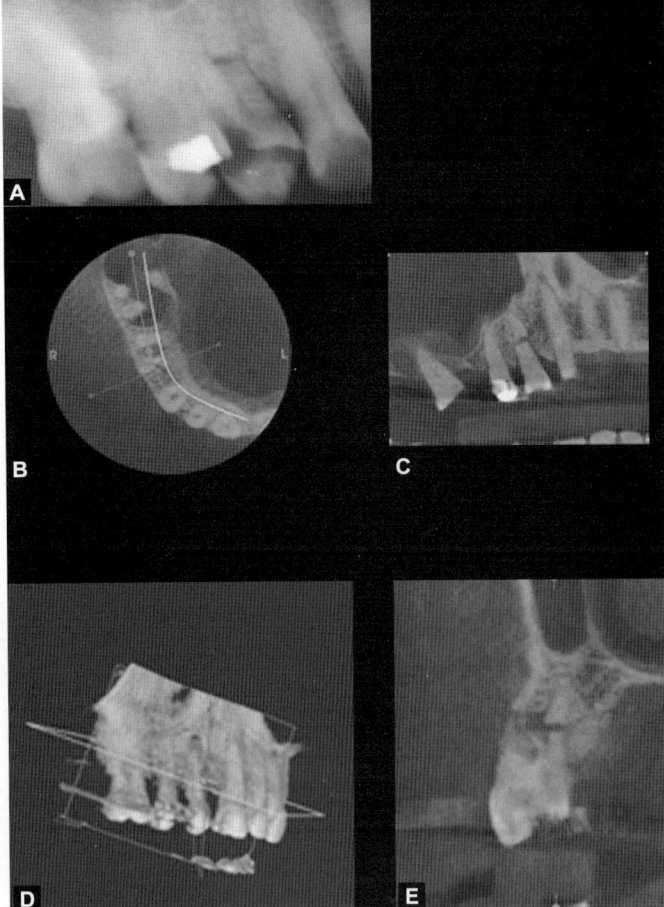

Figures 28.10A to D Root fracture of premolar as observed on: (A) Periapical radiograph and CBCT; (B) Axial; (C) Coronal; (D) 3D; (E) Sagittal views

- Longitudinal fractures are uncommon and more likely in teeth which have posts.
- The width of the fractures tends to increase with time (resorption of the fractured surfaces), and subsequently there is calcification and obliteration of the pulp chamber and the canal.

Differential Diagnosis

Superimposition of soft tissue structures such as the lip, ala of the nose and the nasolabial fold over the image of the root may suggest a root fracture. It should be noted that the soft tissue image of the lip line usually extends beyond the tooth margins.

Fractures of the alveolar process may also overlap the root and suggest a root fracture.

Management

Treatment consists of reduction with immobilization of fractures of the middle or apical third, with endodontic treatment in case of pulp necrosis. Fractures of the coronal third have a poor prognosis and usually the tooth needs to be extracted.

Vertical Root Fractures

Definition

These run lengthwise from the crown toward the apex of the tooth. The crack is usually oriented in the facial-lingual plane in both anterior and posterior teeth. The cause is usually iatrogenic, following insertion of retention screws or pins into vital or nonvital teeth. Uncrowned endodontically treated posterior teeth are more at risk, especially from large occlusal forces.

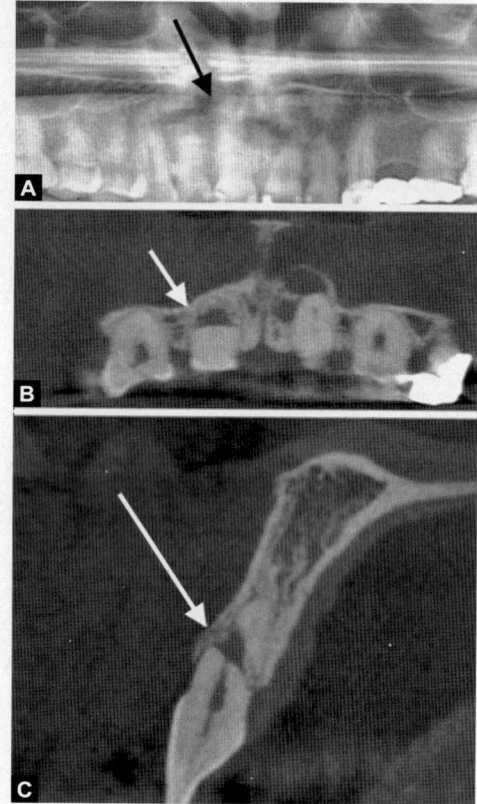

Figures 28.11A to C Horizontal fracture of the root as viewed on: (A) Panoramic view the fracture line is not seen clearly in relation the maxillary right central incisor; CBCT; (B) Coronal; (C) Sagittal section clearly shows horizontal fracture line passing through the root of the central incisor

Clinical Features

These fractures are more common in posterior teeth, especially in the mandibular molars.

Patient will complain of persistent dull pain (cracked tooth syndrome), often of long duration, which may be elicited by applying pressure to the involved tooth. Sometimes the pain may be nonexisting or very mild.

The patient may have a periodontal lesion (chronic abscess) or give history of repeated failed endodontic treatment.

Many a times a definitive diagnosis may only be made by inspection after surgical exposure.

Radiographic Features

- If the central beam lies in the plane of the fracture, the fracture may be visible as a radiolucent line.
- Usually this is not detected on the radiograph in the early stages and later after the development of an inflammatory lesion, with evidence of bone loss the fracture may be diagnosed.

- The widening of the periodontal ligament space and bone loss may not be centered at the apex but often positioned coronally towards the alveolar crest.
- Lesions may extend apically from the alveolar crest, may resemble periodontal lesions.
- Vertical fractures are best seen on denta scan images.

Management

Single rooted teeth with these fractures need to be extracted. Multirooted teeth may be hemisected and the intact remaining half restored with endodontic therapy and a crown.

Crown and Root Fractures (Fig. 28.6A)

Definition

These fractures usually involve the pulp, and about twice as many affect the permanent as the deciduous teeth. Crown-root fractures of anterior teeth are a result of direct trauma and those of the posterior teeth are due to presence of extensive caries or large restorations.

Clinical Features

- In the anterior teeth, the fracture has a labial margin in the gingival third of the crown and courses obliquely to exit below the gingival attachment on the lingual surface.
- Displacement of the fragments is usually minimal
- There may be bleeding from the pulp.
- The patient may complain of pain during mastication.
- The teeth are sensitive to occlusal forces, which may cause separation of the fragments.

Radiographic Features

- These are usually not visible on the radiographs as the X-ray beam is rarely aligned with the plane of the fracture. Distraction of the fragments is also usually not present
- Those fractures of the crown and root that are tangential to the direction of the X-ray beam (very rare) are readily apparent on the radiograph.

Management

Treatment includes removal of the coronal fragment, with conservative restorations, endodontic treatment, along with crown lengthening procedures. If the crown root fracture is vertical the prognosis is poor.

TRAUMATIC INJURY TO THE MAXILLA (FIG. 28.12 AND TABLE 28.2)

Interpretation of Middle Third Fractures

In view of the numerous possible fracture sites, an ordered sequence to viewing is essential. One suggested approach can be summarized as follows:

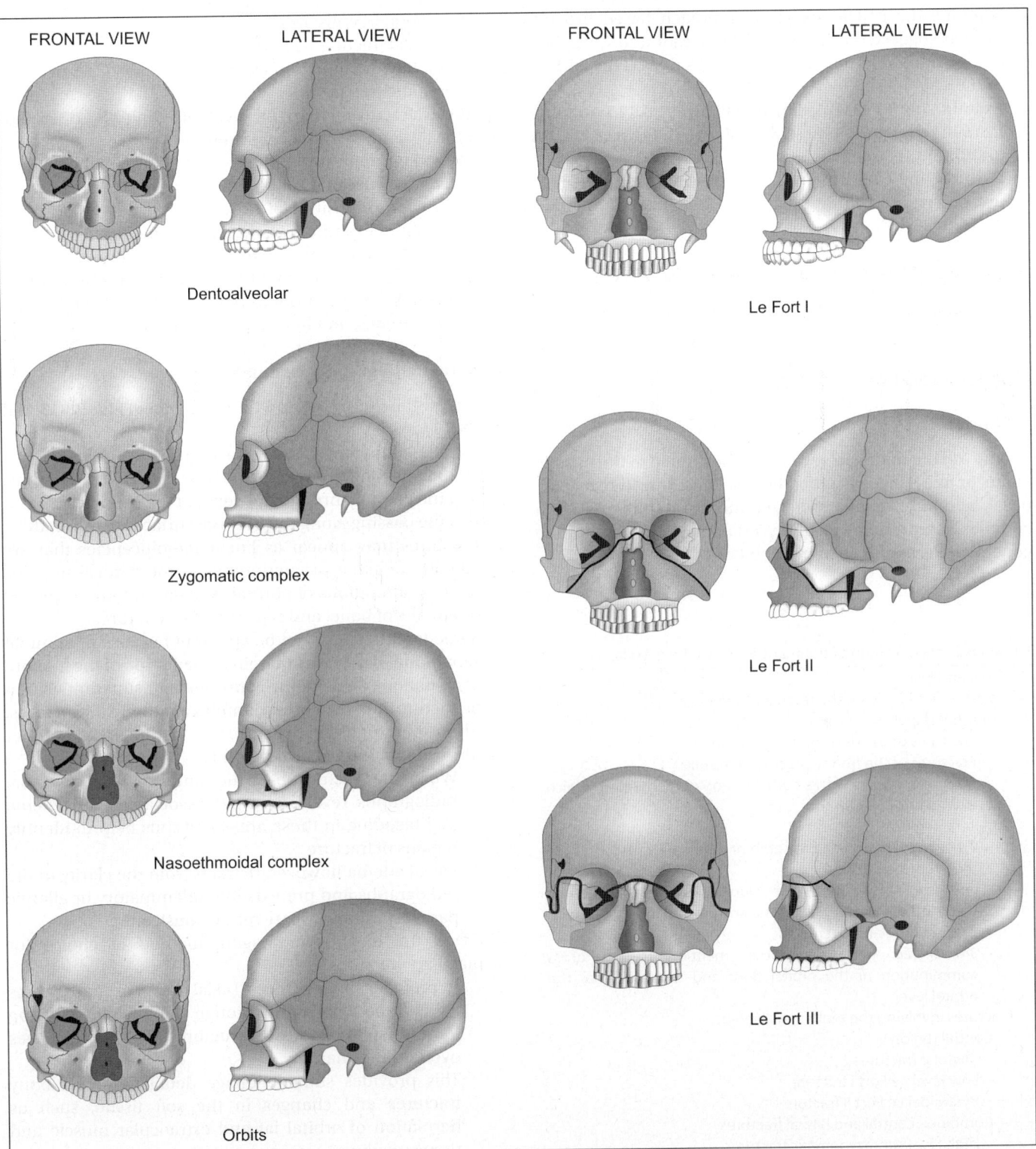

FRONTAL VIEW   LATERAL VIEW   FRONTAL VIEW   LATERAL VIEW

Dentoalveolar

Le Fort I

Zygomatic complex

Le Fort II

Nasoethmoidal complex

Le Fort III

Orbits

Figure 28.12 Diagram of the skull from the front and side illustrating the main sites of middle third fractures

- Examine the 0° OM using an approach based broadly on that suggested originally by McGregor and Campbell (1950), often referred to as Campbell's lines (**Figs 28.13A and B**).
- Examine the 30° OM as shown in **Figures 28.14A and B.**
- Examine the true lateral skull as shown in **Figures 28.15A and B.**
- With CT and CBCT many of the conventional views may not be required to detect fractures in this region (**Figs 28.16 to 28.18**).

Fractures of the Alveolar Process (Fig. 28.19)

Refer traumatic injury to the mandible–fractures of the alveolar process.

Midface Fractures (see Fig. 28.12)

Definition

Fracture of the midfacial region may be limited to the maxilla alone or may involve other bones, including the frontal, nasal, lacrimal, zygoma, vomer, ethmoid and sphenoid. Such complex fractures may be quite variable but often follow the general patterns classified by Léon Le Fort.

Table 28.2 Classification of traumatic injury to the maxilla

By Rave and Killey
• Fractures not involving the teeth and alveolus
– Central region
- Fractures of the nasal bone or septum
- Fractures of the frontal process of maxilla
- Fractures involving the both the above mentioned, which extend into the ethmoid
– Lateral region
- *1st degree*: Fractures of the arch or minimal displacement of the zygomatic bone
- *2nd degree*: Fracture of the zygomatic bone and/or arch involving the lateral walls of the antrum and interfering with the mandibular movements
- *3rd degree*: Both the above mentioned with gross comminution of the orbital floor and depression of the orbital level
• Fractures involving the teeth and alveolus
– Central region
- Alveolar fractures
- Low level Le Fort I fracture
- Pyramidal Le Fort II fracture
– Combined central and lateral fractures
- High level suprazygomatic fractures
- Same as the above mentioned along with a midline split separating the maxillae into two
- Same as both the above mentioned, but associated with fracture of the roof of the orbit or frontal bone

- Horizontal fracture Le Fort I
- Pyramidal fracture Le Fort II
- Craniofacial disjunction Le Fort III
- Zygomatic fracture.

These fractures may be evident clinically or radiographically and are rare in children.

The radiographic interpretation of fractures of the midface is difficult because of the complex anatomy of the region and multiple superimposition of structures.

A plain film examination should include Posteroanterior, Water's, Reverse Towne's, Lateral skull and submentovertex projections. Each film should be systematically scrutinized for fractures in the frontal bone, nasion, orbital walls, zygomatic arches, and maxillary antrum.

General Radiographic Features

- Follow the McGregor and Campbell lines (**Figs 28.13 and 28.14**):
  1. Line joining the frontomalar sutures.
  2. Line passing through the inferior margins of the orbits.
  3. Line passing through the necks of the condyles.
  4. Line passing along the occlusal surfaces of the teeth.
- Fractures may appear as linear radiolucencies that are usually widest at discontinuities in the cortical margins of bone, alterations of normal skeletal contour, displaced fragments of bone, and separated bony sutures.
- Some fractures may not be apparent because of minimal separation of the bony margins, orientation of the fracture at an oblique angle to the X-ray beam or superimposition of fracture lines over other complex anatomical structures.
- Abnormal soft tissue densities may both help and hinder the examination of facial trauma.
  - When the fracture tears the antral or nasal mucosa, radiographs reveal densities associated with edema and bleeding in those areas and thus help to identify regions of fracture.
  - Facial edema however, detracts from the clarity of the radiographs and pre-existing inflammatory or allergic paranasal sinus disease may be misleading.
- CT is the diagnostic imaging method of choice for maxillary fractures:
  - It provides image slices (axial and coronal images using bone algorithm) through the maxilla, allowing for the display of osseous structures without the images overlapping anatomy.
  - This provides suitable image detail to detect bony fractures and changes in the soft tissue, such as herniation of orbital fat and extraocular muscle and tissue swelling.
  - It is an aid in determining the spatial orientation of fractures or bone fragments.
  - CT images may be reformatted in three-dimensional images.

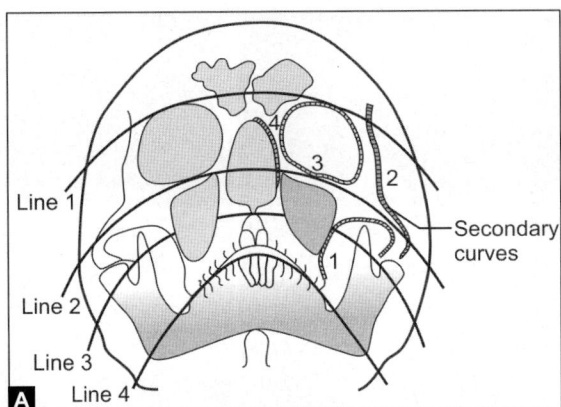
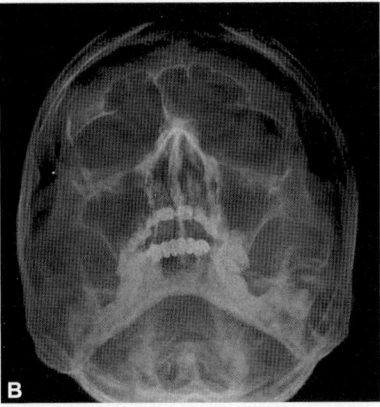

Figures 28.13A and B Suggested systematic approach to interpretation of the 0° OM: (A) Diagram of a O° OM showing Campbell's curvilinear lines and the secondary curves; (B) An example of a 0° occipitomental

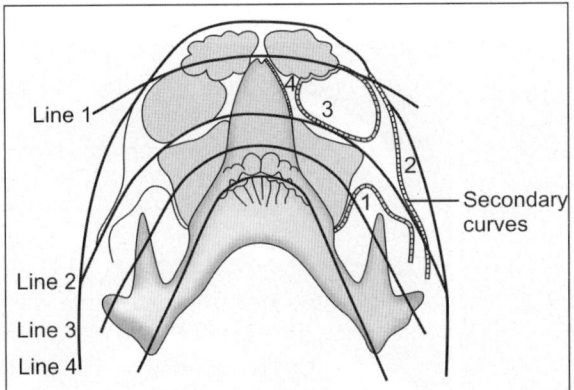
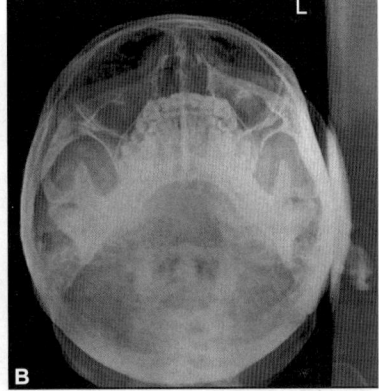

Figures 28.14A and B Suggested systematic approach to interpretation of the 30° OM: (A) Diagram of a 30° OM showing Campbell's curvilinear lines and the secondary curves; (B) An example of a 30° occipitomental

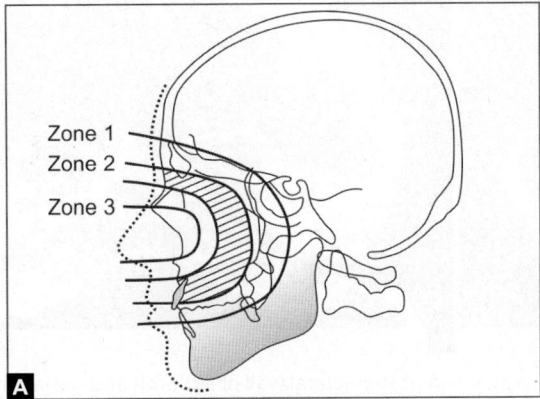
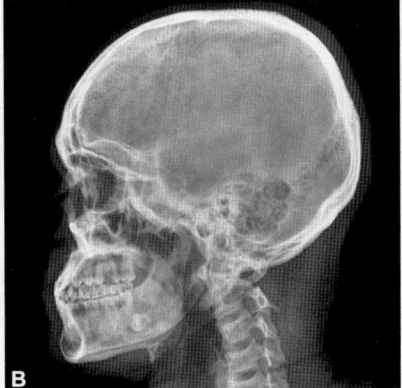

Figures 28.15A and B Suggested systematic approach to interpretation of the true lateral skull: (A) Diagram of a lateral skull showing the three curved zones; (B) An example of a true lateral skull

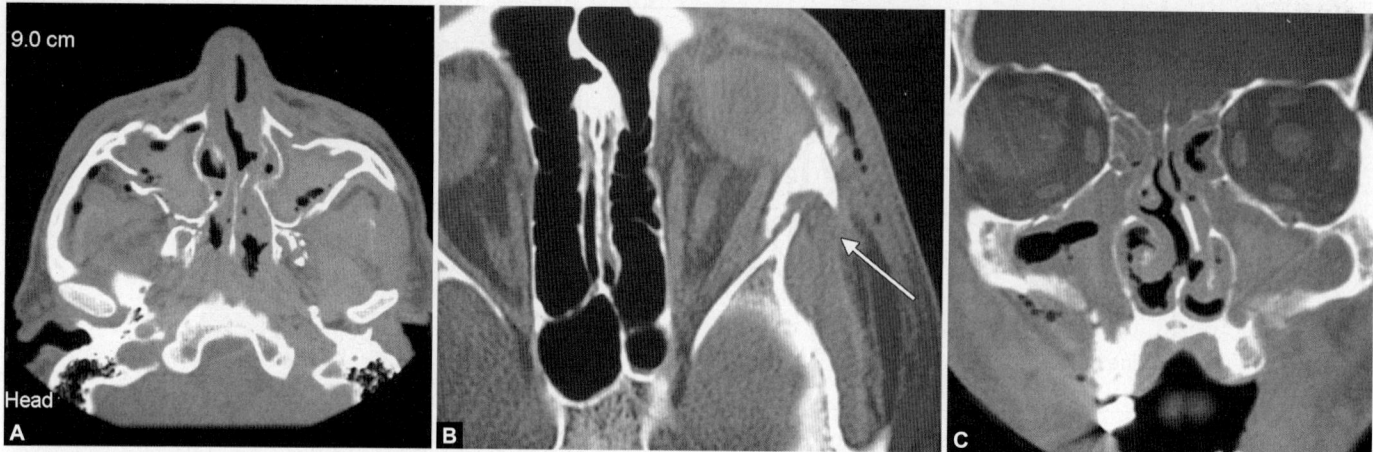

Figures 28.16A to C CT scan axial: (A) Showing fracture of the walls of the sinus; (B) Showing orbital wall fracture; (C) Coronal section showing involvement of the sinus and orbits

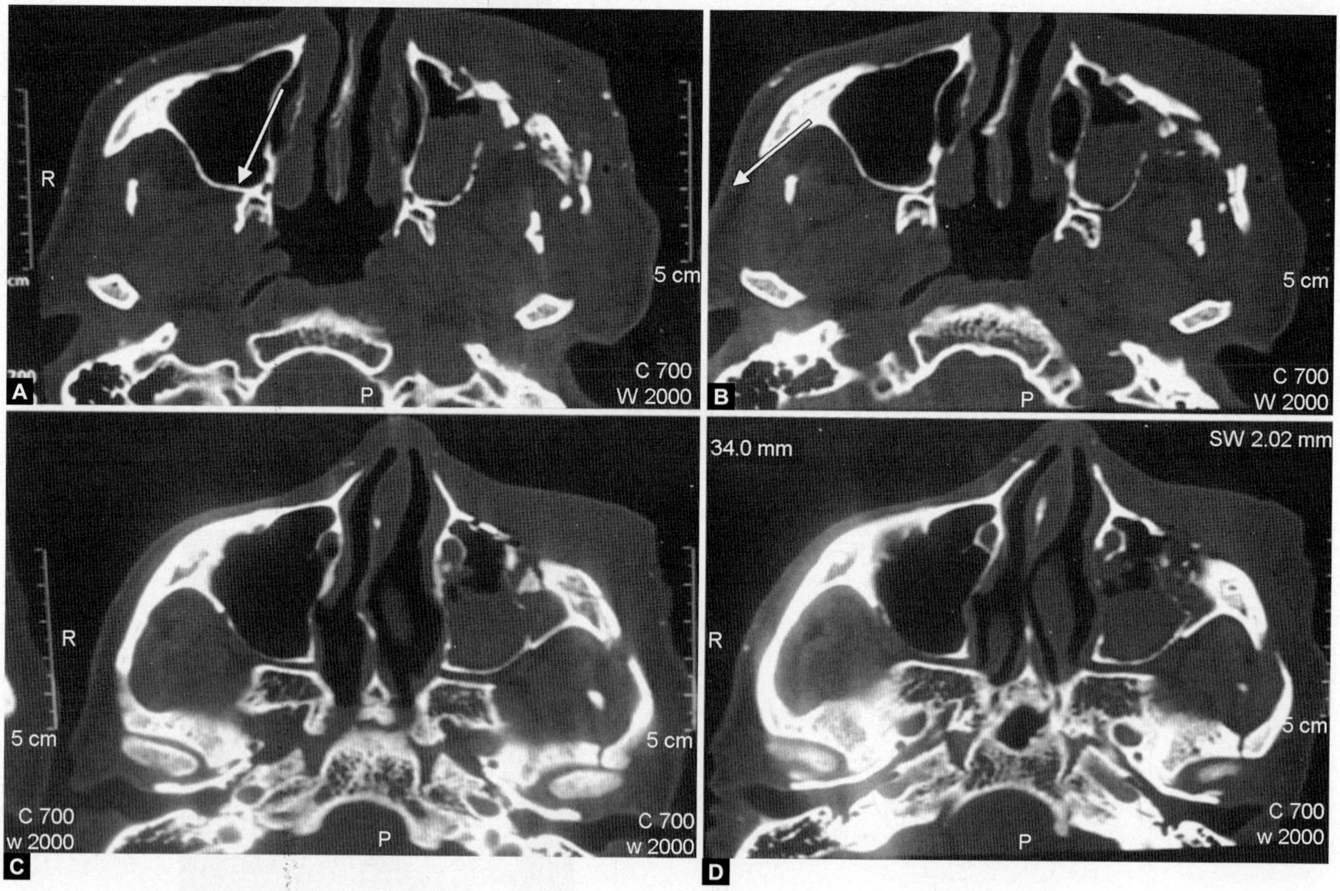

Figures 28.17A to D CT scan showing fracture of anterolateral, medial and posterolateral wall of left orbit and deviation of nasal septum

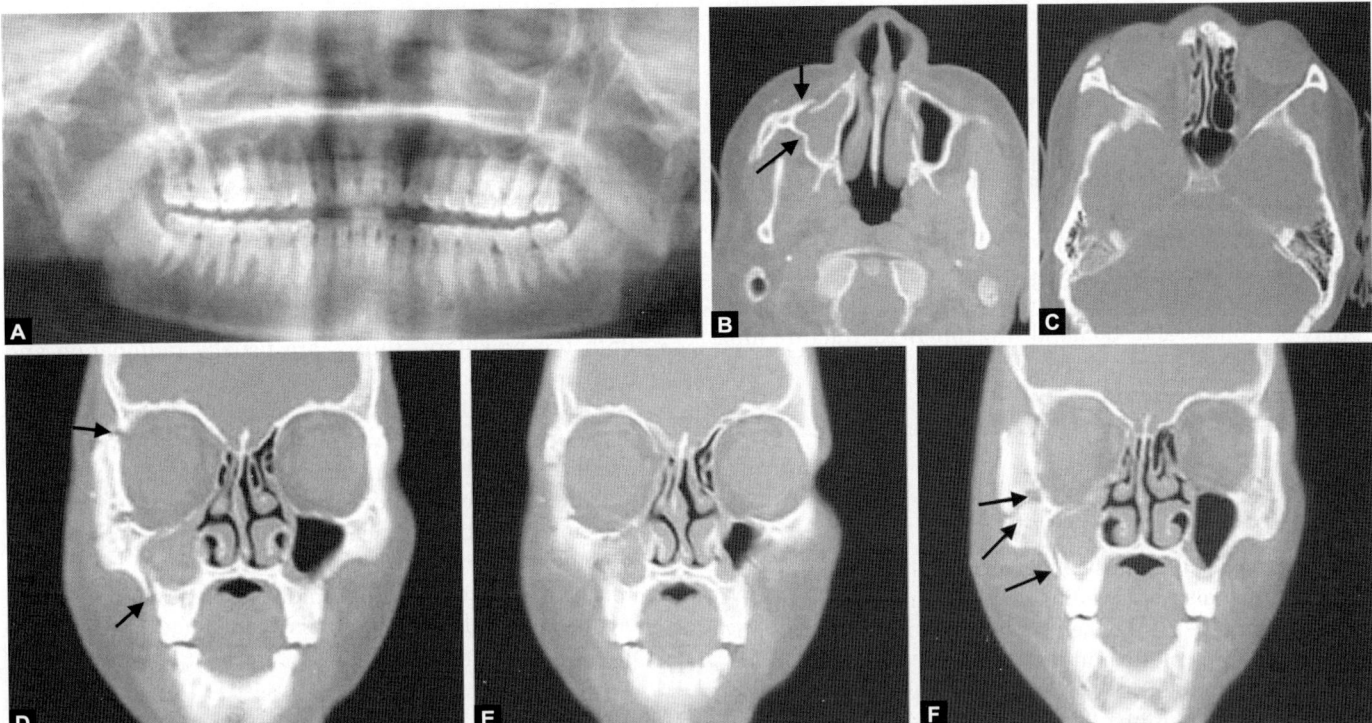

Figures 28.18A to F Multiple fractures after trauma: (A) Panoramic showed fracture right lateral wall of the orbit; (B) CT scan axial section showed fracture of the anterior wall, posterolateral and medial wall of the right maxillary sinus, with soft tissue shadow in the right sinus; (C) CT axial section shows fracture of the right greater wing of sphenoid Coronal sections show; (D) Fracture of the lateral wall of the orbit and posterolateral wall of the sinus; (E) Fracture of the floor of the frontal sinus and bilateral lacrimal plates, deviation of the nasal septum; (F) Communited fracture seen involving right zygoma and lateral wall of the orbit

Differential Diagnosis

- Shadow of the infraorbital canal is thrown over the inferior orbital margin, and this dark line may be mistaken for a fracture.
- In the PA view, there is often a dark line on the outer wall of the antrum, vertical in direction and situated where the inferior margin of the malar bone joins the facial bone, this represents a suture and may be mistaken for a fracture. But this is usually present bilaterally, and a white line is seen on either side of the dark line representing the cortex of the suture which will not be seen in case of a fracture.
- On the intraoral periapical radiograph of posterior teeth dark lines are often seen in the antral shadow which represent normal vascular canals and should not be mistaken for fracture lines. They will show radiopaque corticated borders.
- In the upper cuspid region a fracture may be misdiagnosed from the appearance of the lip line.
- The intermaxillary suture is seen as a dark line in the center of the palate. It is also corticated and should not be mistaken for a fracture line.

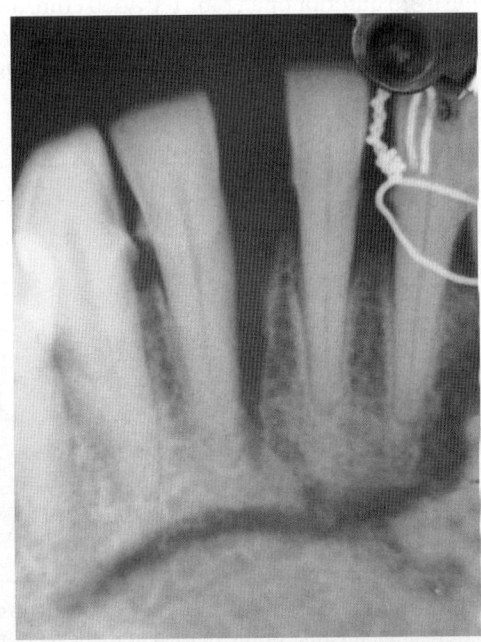

Figure 28.19 Periapical radiograph showing dentoalveolar fracture of the anterior mandible

Horizontal Fracture Le Fort I (Figs 28.12 and 28.20)

Definition

This is a relatively horizontal fracture in the body of the maxilla that results in the detachment of the alveolar process of the maxilla from the middle face. It is a result of a traumatic force directed to the lower maxillary region.

The fracture line passes above the teeth, below the zygomatic process, and through the maxillary sinuses and tuberosities to the inferior portion of the pterygoid process. It may be unilateral or bilateral. The unilateral fracture must be distinguished from a fracture within the alveolar process which does not extend to the midline. Fractures of the mandible (54%) and the zygoma (23%) may also be found in these patients.

Clinical Features

- There may be a slight swelling around the upper lips
- There may also be swelling and bruising about both the eyes, pain over the nose and face, deformity of the nose and flattening of the middle face
- Epistaxis, double vision and varying degree of paresthesia over the distribution of the infra-orbital nerve
- If the fragment is not distally impacted, it can be manipulated holding on to the teeth
- Manipulation may reveal a mobile maxilla and crepitations
- If the fracture line is at a high level, the fragment may include the pterygoid muscle attachment, which will pull the fragment posteriorly and inferiorly. Due to this the posterior maxillary teeth contact the mandibular teeth first, resulting in an anterior open bite, retruded chin, and a long face, an appearance characteristic of this type of fracture
- If the fracture is at a low level, no displacement may occur

- If it is an impacted type of fracture, there may be damage to the cusps of the involved teeth caused by the impaction of the mandibular teeth against them
- The complete Le Fort I fracture is often associated with a split in the palate.

Radiographic Features

- The fractures may be difficult to detect radiographically. The recommended views are: posteroanterior, lateral skull, Water's projection and CT scans.
- Both the maxillary sinuses are usually radiopaque and may show fluid levels.
- The lateral view may disclose a slight posterior displacement of the fragment (inferior portion of the maxilla below the fracture line) and if present, the fracture line through the pterygoid bones.
- The intervertebral spaces of the cervical spine may simulate fracture lines in the PA Skull view.
- This type of fracture unites rapidly, thus a fracture may not be detected, if the radiograph is taken a few days after the injury.

Management

- *Low level*: Intermaxillary fixation
- *High level*: Intermaxillary and craniomaxillary fixation.

Pyramidal Fracture Le Fort II (Figs 28.12 and 28.21)

Definition

This fracture has a pyramidal appearance on the PA skull radiograph. The fracture results from a violent force applied to the central region of the middle third of the facial skeleton.

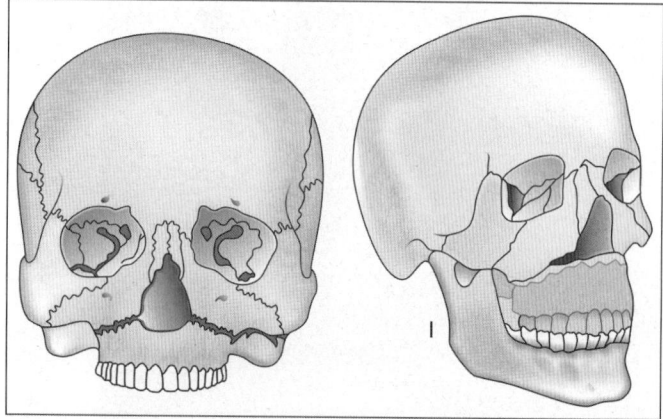

Figure 28.20 Le Fort I Maxillary fractures Le Fort I/Guerin's may be defined as horizontal fracture of the maxilla at the level of the nasal fossa which allows motion of the maxilla while the nasal bridge remains stable

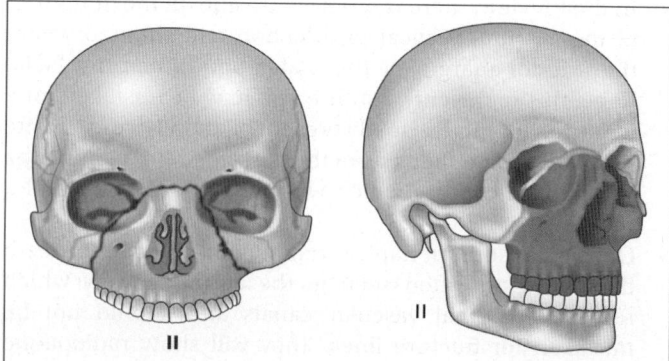

Figure 28.21 Le Fort II—Maxillary fractures Le Fort II/high central midface are defined as pyramidal fractures which involve the: maxilla; nasal bones; medial aspect of the orbits; plain facial films will reveal the presence of facial fractures, but are less helpful in determining the type or extent. Head and facial CT, including three dimensional recreations, offer much more useful information

This force separates the maxilla from the base of the skull by causing fractures of the nasal bones and frontal processes of the maxilla. The fractures extend laterally through the lacrimal bones and floors of the orbit and inferiorly through the zygomaticomaxillary sutures. Frequently, on one side the fracture passes through the suture or through the zygomatic complex, and on the other side it passes around and beneath the base of the zygomatic process of the maxilla. From here, the fracture then passes posteriorly along the lateral wall of the maxilla, across the pterygomaxillary fossa, and through the pterygoid plates. It usually extends through the maxillary sinuses. The frontal and the ethmoidal sinuses are involved in about 10% of cases, especially in comminuted fractures.

Clinical Features

- There is massive edema and marked swelling of the middle third of the face.
- There is ecchymosis around the eyes that develops within minutes of the injury. The edema around the eyes is so severe that it is difficult to see the eyes without prying the eyes open. The conjunctivas over the inner quadrants of the eyes are blood shot. And if the zygomatic bones are involved the ecchymosis extends to the outer quadrant.
- The broken nose is displaced and because the face has fallen the nose and face are lengthened.
- An anterior open bite occurs (premature contact of the molars)
- Epistaxis with cerebrospinal fluid rhinorrhea is common.
- Palpation reveals discontinuity of the lower borders of the orbits.
- If pressure is applied to the bridge of the nose and the palate, the pyramid bone can be moved.
- Other symptoms include, double vision, variable degree of paresthesia over the distribution of the infraorbital nerve.

Radiographic Features

- CT examination is required to supplement plain views of the skull because of multiple superimpositions of the structures.
- The radiographic examination reveals fractures of the nasal bones, both frontal processes of the maxilla (ethmoid and frontal sinuses, if involved), and the infraorbital rims on both sides (floor of both the orbits). Fractures of the zygoma or zygomatic process of the maxilla, separation of the zygomaticomaxillary sutures on both sides deformity and discontinuity of the lateral walls of the maxillary sinuses, and fractures through both pterygoid plates.
- Thickening of the lining mucosa or increased radiopacity of the maxillary sinus and sometimes the frontal and ethmoidal sinuses.

Differential Diagnosis

On the water's projection it may be difficult to examine the floor of the orbit because two different radiopaque lines often represent the lower limit of the orbit. One is the actual floor of the orbit, which is often thin and difficult to discern. The other is the inferior rim of the orbit, which is usually thicker bone and appears above the floor of the orbit. The presence of a less distinct orbital floor may suggest a blow-out fracture of the orbital floor. The presence of herniated orbital contents through the floor and into the maxillary sinus is a useful sign for blow-out fracture but orbital floor fractures are not always associated with soft tissue herniation.

Management

- Reduction followed by intermaxillary fixation
- Open reduction and interosseous wiring of infraorbital rims.

Craniofacial Disjunction Le Fort III (Figs 28.12 and 28.22)

Definition

This results when the traumatic force is of sufficient magnitude to completely separate the middle third of the facial skeleton from the cranium. The fracture line usually extends through the nasal bones and the frontal processes of the maxilla or nasofrontal and maxillofrontal sutures, across the floors of the orbits and through the ethmoid and sphenoid sinuses and the zygomaticofrontal sutures. It passes across both the pterygomaxillary fissures and separates the pterygoid plates where they arise from the sphenoid bone (at their roots). If the maxilla is displaced and freely movable, a fracture must also have occurred in the area of the zygomaticotemporal suture. As the zygoma or zygomatic arch is involved, these injuries are as a rule associated with multiple other maxillary fractures. Mandibular fractures may also be observed in more than 50% of the cases.

Clinical Features

- The clinical appearance is similar to that of pyramidal fractures however the injury is considerably more extensive
- The soft tissue injuries are severe with massive edema.
- The nose may be blocked with a blood clot or blood, serum or cerebrospinal fluid rhinorrhea may be present.
- Bleeding may occur in the periorbital tissues and all quadrants of the conjunctiva—a number of eye signs of neurological importance are likely to be present. There is lowering of the ocular level due to the fracture line passing above the Whitnall's tubercle, removing the support

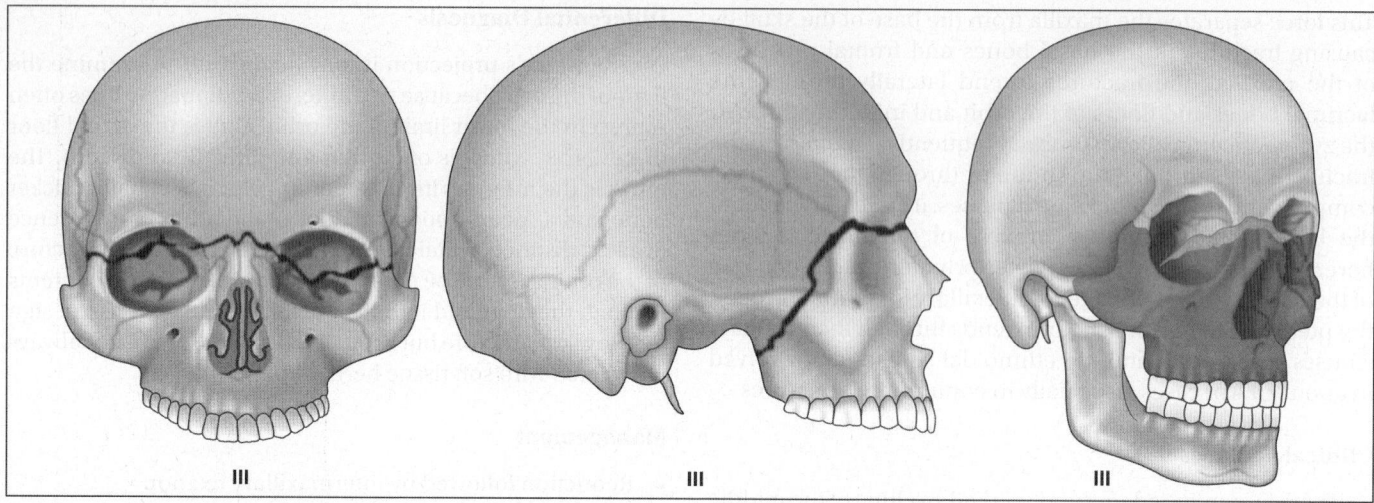

Figure 28.22 Le Fort III—LeFort III/centrolateral midface/craniofacial disjunction involves fractures through the maxilla, zygoma, nasal bones, ethmoid bones and the bones of the base of the skull

given to the eye by Lockwood's suspensory ligament. As one or both eye-drops, the upper eyelid follows the globe down, producing unilateral or bilateral hooding of the eyes.

- A dish face deformity is characteristic of these fractures.
- An anterior open bite (because of the retro position of the maxillary incisors) with the posterior teeth in occlusion. Although the mandible is wide open, the patient is unable to separate the molars.
- Intraoral and extraoral palpation reveals irregular contours and step deformities, and crepitations are also apparent when fragments are moved.

Radiographic Features

- The radiographic projections are hazy due to extensive soft tissue swelling.
- It is extremely difficult to document these multiple fractures with plain films alone; therefore CT images along with the clinical information are very important.
- The main radiographic findings are separated naso-frontal, maxillofrontal, zygomaticofrontal and zygomaticotemporal sutures.
- The nasal bones, frontal processes of the maxilla, both orbital floors and pterygoid plates may show radiolucent lines and discontinuity in some areas (**Fig. 28.23**).
- The ethmoid and sphenoid sinuses are radiopaque, indicating presence of fractures. The frontal sinus may also be frequently involved.
- There may be associated fractures of the walls of the maxillary sinus, which gives a radiopaque appearance.

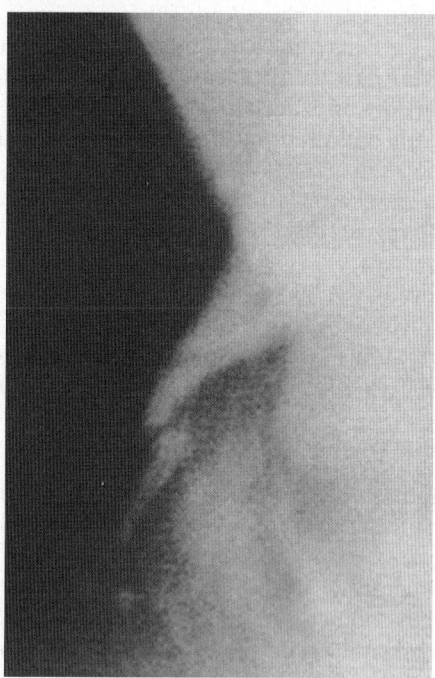

Figure 28.23 Lateral view of the nose showing fracture of the nasal bones

Management

Control hemorrhage and maintain airway. Surgery is delayed till the edema subsides. External immobilization.

Zygomatic Fracture (Figs 28.12, 28.24 to 28.26)

Definition

These are of two types:

1. *Zygomatic arch fractures*: In which just the arch is fractured.
2. *Zygomatic complex fractures*: In which the zygomatic bone is separated from its frontal, maxillary and temporal connections.

Bilateral zygomatic fractures occur in association with Le Fort II and III fractures. Injuries to the zygomatic arch usually result from a forceful blow to the side of the face. Although the blow may displace the fragment medially, the arch is so well supported superiorly by the temporalis muscle and inferiorly by the masseter muscle that it is rarely displaced upward or downward.

The arch may fracture at the center, resulting in a V-shaped medial displacement, or near its articulation with the zygomatic process of the maxilla, resulting in medial displacement of the anterior end of the zygomatic bone.

Figure 28.24 Submentovertex (reduced exposure) showing a depressed fracture of the right zygomatic arch (arrow)

Clinical Features

- There will be flattening of the upper cheek with tenderness and dimpling of the skin over the arch and zygomaticofrontal suture and a fullness of the lower cheek may occur after the zygomatic complex fracture
- Step defects may be palpated in the zygomaticofrontal area and along the orbital rim
- The clinical characteristics and signs of trauma are masked by edema within an hour after the injury, and the edema may persist for nearly a week
- There may be circumorbital ecchymosis and hemorrhage into the sclera (near the outer canthus)
- There may be unilateral epistaxis (for a short time after the accident), anesthesia or paresthesia of the cheek, and an altered level of the eye. There may be diplopia which may suggest a significant injury to the floor of the orbit
- The zygomatic arch may fracture at its weakest point, about 1 cm posterior to the zygomaticotemporal suture
- Separation of fracture of the frontozygomatico suture may occur
- Fractures do not usually occur through the zygomaticomaxillary suture, but medially within the thin bone comprising the lateral wall of the antrum
- Mandibular movements may be limited if the displaced zygomatic bone impinges on the coronoid process.

Radiographic Features

- The radiographic examination may be the only determining factor for the presence and extend of injury, due to the edema obscuring the clinical features
- The occipitomental (Water's) radiograph provides an image of the whole zygoma and maxillary sinus
- The submentovertex projection provides a good view of the zygomatic arch
- CT images provide valuable three-dimensional information

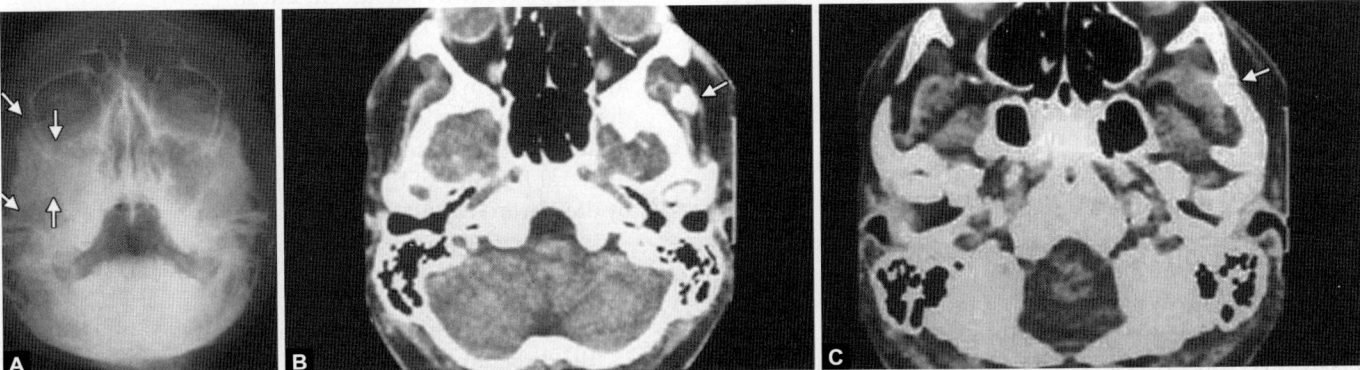

Figures 28.25A to C (A) Fracture of the right zygomatic bone and zygomatic arch, clinically the patient gave history of difficulty in opening the mouth; (B) Same case CT scan-13 shows the zygomatic bone fracture (arrow) and the limitation of movement of the coronoid process by the fragments of the zygomatic arch (arrow); (C) Same case CT scan-22 shows the medial position of the zygomatic arch fragments (arrow)

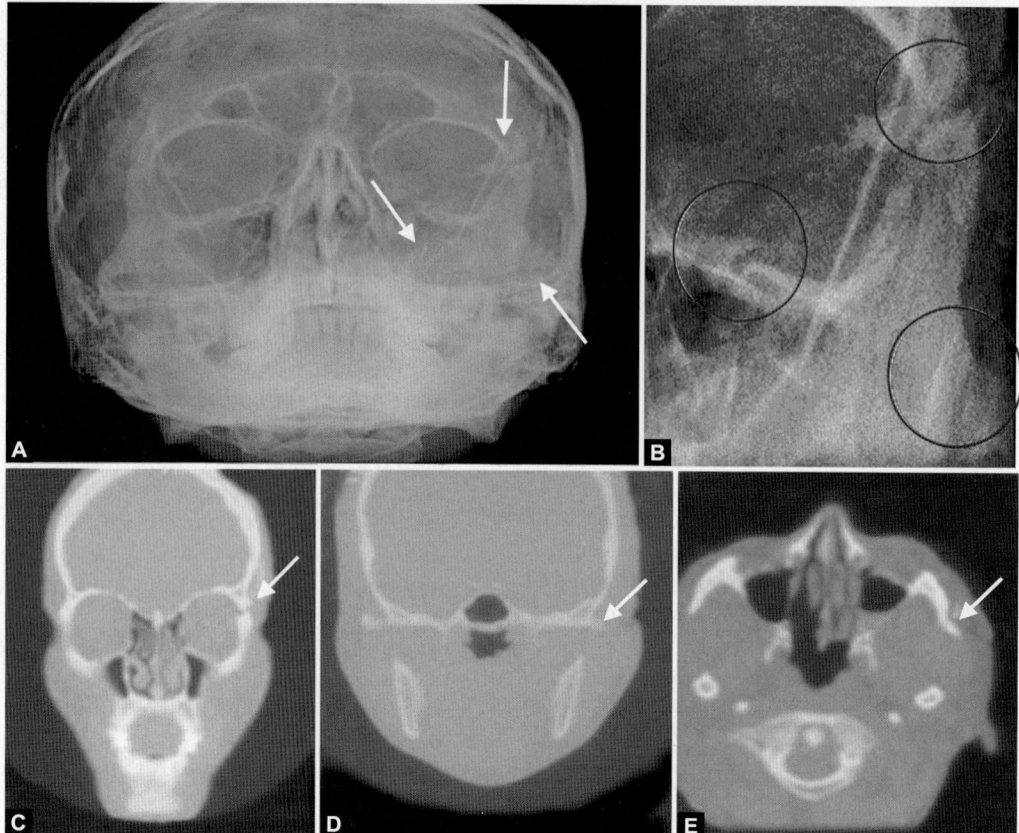

Figures 28.26A to E Tripod fracture: (A and B) PA waters and magnified image which shows—left zyomatic arch fracture, left zygomatic bone fracture and lateral wall of left orbit seen. CT scan; (C) Coronal view showing fracture Lateral wall of orbit; (D) Coronal view showing fracture of left zygomatic bone; (E) Axial view showing fracture of zygomatic arch

- Fracture of the lateral wall of the antrum may cause the maxillary sinus to appear radiopaque and may also demonstrate a fluid level resulting from bleeding into the sinus.

Differential Diagnosis

Panoramic views of the zygomatic arch often reveal the zygomaticotemporal suture as a radiolucent line, which may even have the appearance of a discontinuity in the inferior border. This is a variation of the normal and should not be misinterpreted as a fracture.

Management

Minimal displacement of the zygomatic arch and no cosmetic deformity or impairment of the eye movement, requires no treatment, otherwise reduction is indicated.

TRAUMATIC INJURY TO THE MANDIBLE (TABLE 28.3)

The typical radiographic features of mandibular fractures include (**Figs 28.27 to 28.29**):

- The most common sites are the condyle, body and angle, followed less frequently by the parasymphyseal region, ramus, coronoid process, and alveolus.
- There are sharp well-defined radiolucent line(s) between the bone fragments if they are separated.
- Fractures through the buccal and lingual cortical plates may produce two radiolucent lines.
- A radiopaque line is apparent, if the fragments overlie one another.
- An alteration in the outline of the bone if the fragments are displaced, producing a step deformity of the lower border or the occlusal plane.
- Bilateral fracture of the mandible is sometimes followed by downward angulation of the anterior fragment.

Important Points to Note

- The extent/severity of any displacement depends on:
  - The direction and strength of the fracturing force
  - The direction of the resultant fracture line
  - The relevant muscles attached to each fragment and their direction of pull.

Table 28.3 Classification of traumatic injury to the mandible

- Kruger's general classification
  - *Civilian type fractures*: Fractures with no gross comminution of the bone, and no loss of hard and soft tissue
  - *Simple*: This includes closed linear fractures of the condyle, coronoid, ramus and edentulous body of the mandible.
  - *Compound*: Fracture of the tooth bearing area of the mandible which communicate into the mouth via the periodontal membrane and sometimes externally on the face
  - *Complicated or complex*: Fractures associated with damage to the important vital structures complicating the treatment as well as prognosis
  - *Comminuted*: Occurs due to direct violence to the mandible from a relatively sharp penetrating object and missiles which strike the bone. They are usually of the Compound Type, further complicated by bone and soft tissue loss
  - *Pathological*: May occur on minimum trauma to the mandible which is already weakened by existing disease (e.g. osteomyelitis, neoplasm)
- *Green stick*: This is a rare variant of a simple fracture, usually seen in children
  - *Gunshot fractures*: Fractures with gross comminution of the bone and where there is extensive destruction of both hard and soft tissue
  - *Excessive muscular contracture*: Occasionally fractures of the coronoid process occur because of the sudden reflex contracture of the temporalis muscle
- According to the site of fractures
  - *Unilateral*: Caused by direct violence
    - Dentoalveolar
    - Condyle
    - Coronoid
    - Ramus
    - Angle
    - Body (molar and premolar region)
    - Parasymphysis
    - Symphysis
  - *Bilateral*: Caused by direct and indirect violence
  - *Multiple*: Also associated with direct or indirect violence causing more than two fractures
  - *Comminuted*: Seen in war missile injury

- If the fracture line runs in such a manner that the associated muscles tend to hold the fragments together, the fracture is described as favorable.
- If the associated muscles tend to pull the fragments apart, the fracture is described as unfavorable.

Fractures of the Alveolar Process (see Figs 28.19)

Definition

Simple fractures of the alveolar process may involve the buccal or lingual cortical plates of the alveolar process of the maxilla or mandible. These are commonly associated with traumatic injuries to the teeth that are luxated with or without dislocation. Several teeth are usually affected and the fracture line is mostly horizontal. The labial plate of the alveolar process is more prone to fracture than the palatal plate.

Some fractures extend through the entire alveolar process (in contrast to simple fractures that involve only one cortical plate) and may be apical to the teeth or involve the tooth socket. They are usually associated with dental injuries and extrusive luxations with or without root fractures.

Clinical Features

- There may be injury to the lips with laceration on the inner aspect. Foreign bodies may get lodged in the soft tissue of the lip.
- There may be laceration of the gingiva due to deformity of the alveolus.
- There may be associated trauma to the teeth.
- The alveolar fractures are more common in the maxilla than the mandible, and simple alveolar fractures are more common in the anterior region. Fractures of the entire alveolar process may occur in the anterior and premolar regions and in the older age group.
- These fractures are characteristically marked by malocclusion with displacement and mobility of the fragment. The teeth in the fragment will have atypical dull sound when percussed.
- An impacted alveolar fracture may be virtually immobile. Sometimes crepitation may be detected on palpation and a cracked pot noise is detected when the teeth within the alveolar fracture are percussed.
- The detached bone may include the floor of the maxillary sinus which may be accompanied with epistaxis, and ecchymosis of the buccal vestibule.
- A complete alveolar fragment may be displaced into the soft tissue of the floor of the mouth.

Radiographic Features

- Intraoral radiographs do not reveal fractures of a single cortical wall of the alveolar process.
- Fracture of the anterior labial cortical plate may be apparent on a lateral extraoral radiograph if some bone displacement occurs and if the direction of the X-ray beam profiles the fracture site.
- Closer the fracture to the alveolar crest more likely that a root fracture has occurred. It may be difficult to differentiate a root fracture from an overlapping fracture line of the alveolar bone.
- Posterior palatal fracture is best demonstrated on the occlusal radiograph.
- By taking several radiographs with different projection angles, it may help to diagnose whether the fracture line

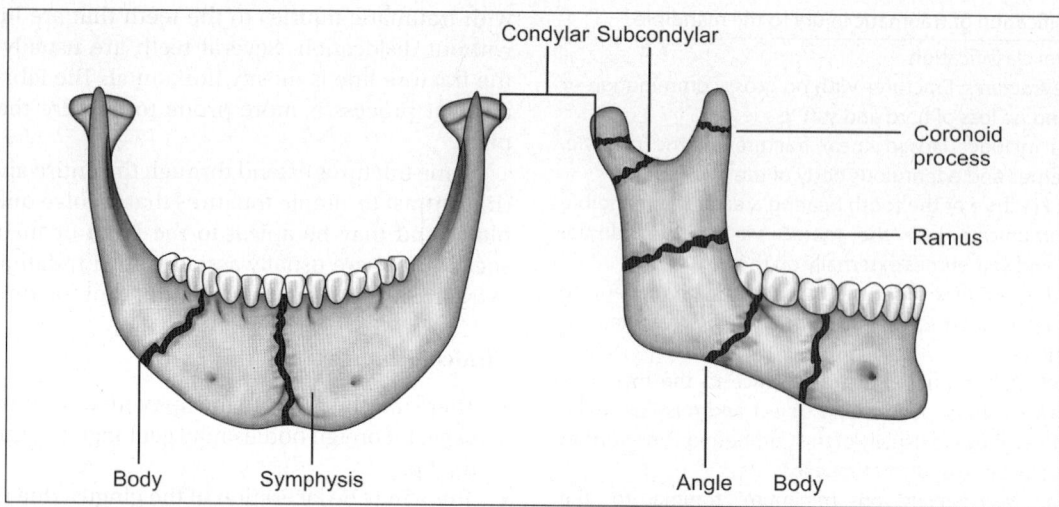

Figure 28.27 Diagram showing the main fracture sites of the mandible. Although only one side of the jaw is illustrated, mandibular fractures are often bilateral

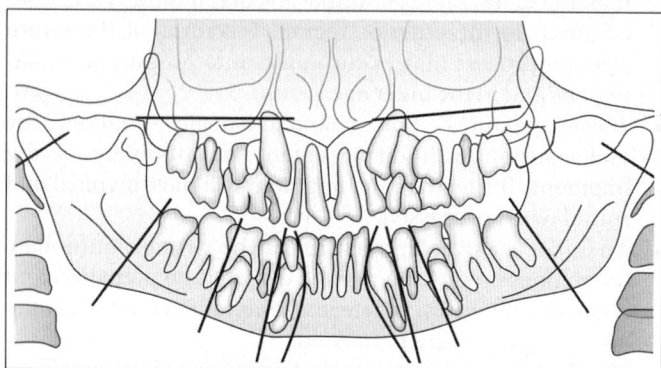

Figure 28.28 Diagram of common fracture locations in the mandible during mixed dentition

is truly associated with the tooth (the line will not move relative to the tooth structure) or not.
- Fractures of the posterior alveolar process may involve the floor of the maxillary sinus and result in abnormal thickening of the sinus mucosa.

Management

Manual reduction and fixation of fractured segments using arch bars or splints.

Mandibular Condyle Fractures (Figs 28.30 to 28.32 and 28.40)

Definition

Condylar fractures may be classified as:
- Intracapsular fractures
  - Fractures involving the articular surface

- High condylar fractures—fractures above or through the anatomical neck.
  - Fractures associated with injury to the capsule, ligament and meniscus.
- Extracapsular fractures
  - The fracture runs from the lowest point of the curvature of the sigmoid notch, obliquely downwards below the surgical neck of the condyle, to the posterior aspect of the upper part of the ramus.
  - Low or subcondylar fracture; the fracture is influenced in its site and direction by the insertion of part of the masseter muscle and the temporomandibular joint ligament. The fracture takes the line of least resistance.
  - The condylar head may be split in the anteroposterior or sagittal plane, the split extends through the neck and produces a combined intra and extracapsular fracture.

They may also be broadly divided into condylar neck fractures and condylar head fractures. The condylar neck fractures are more common. When the condylar neck fracture occurs, the head is usually displaced medially, inferiorly, and anteriorly (as a result of the pull of the lateral pterygoid muscle). Severe trauma may displace the head into the skull or sinuses. Fractures of the condylar head are fissure like, with a vertical cleft dividing the head; this may result in multiple fragments in a compression-like fracture. More than half the patients with condylar fractures also have fractures of the mandibular body. In rare cases the fractures may involve the temporal component.

Clinical Features

- Unilateral fractures are more common than bilateral fractures and may be accompanied by a parasymphyseal or mandibular body fracture on the contralateral side

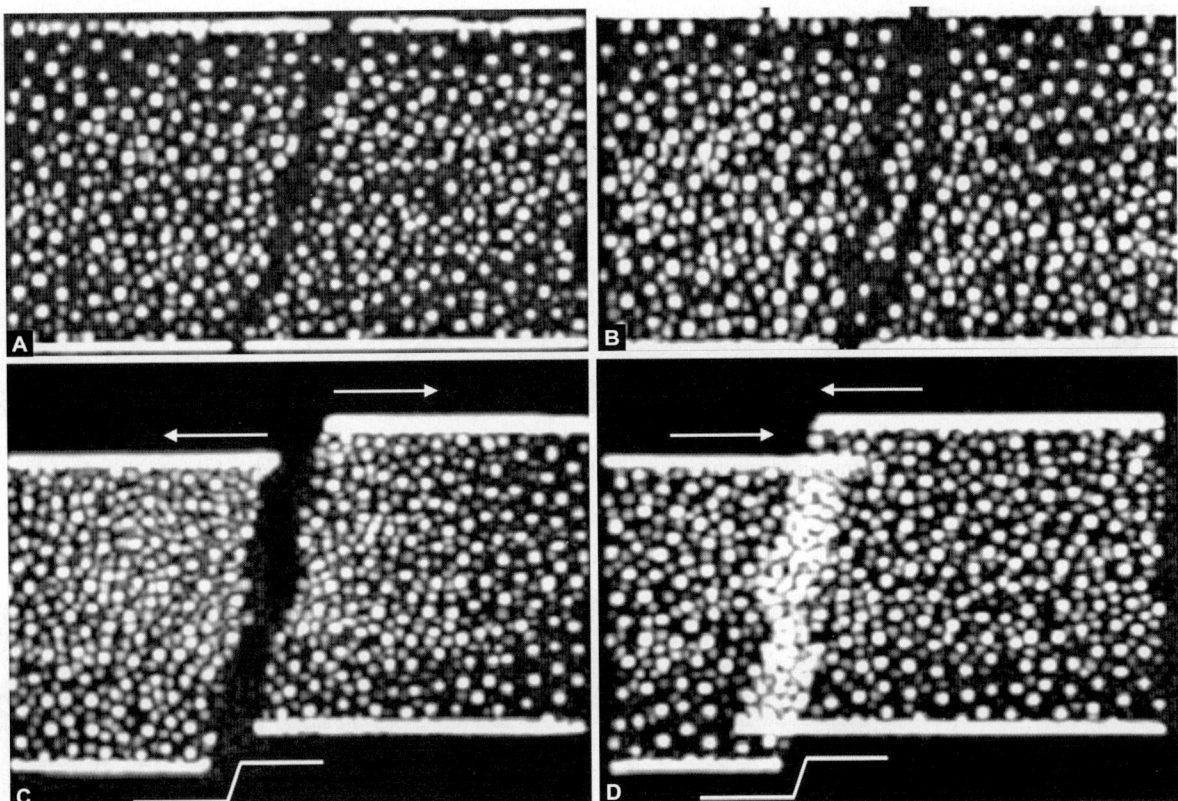

Figures 28.29A to D Diagrams showing the different radiographic appearances of fractures depending on the bony displacement, separation or overlap; (A) One rediolucent fracture line with no displacement of the fragments; (B) Two radiolucent fracture line with no displacement of the fragments; (C) Wide radiolucent fracture line and step deformity due to separation and displacement of the fragments; (D) Radiopaque line due to overlap of the fragments step deformity also evident

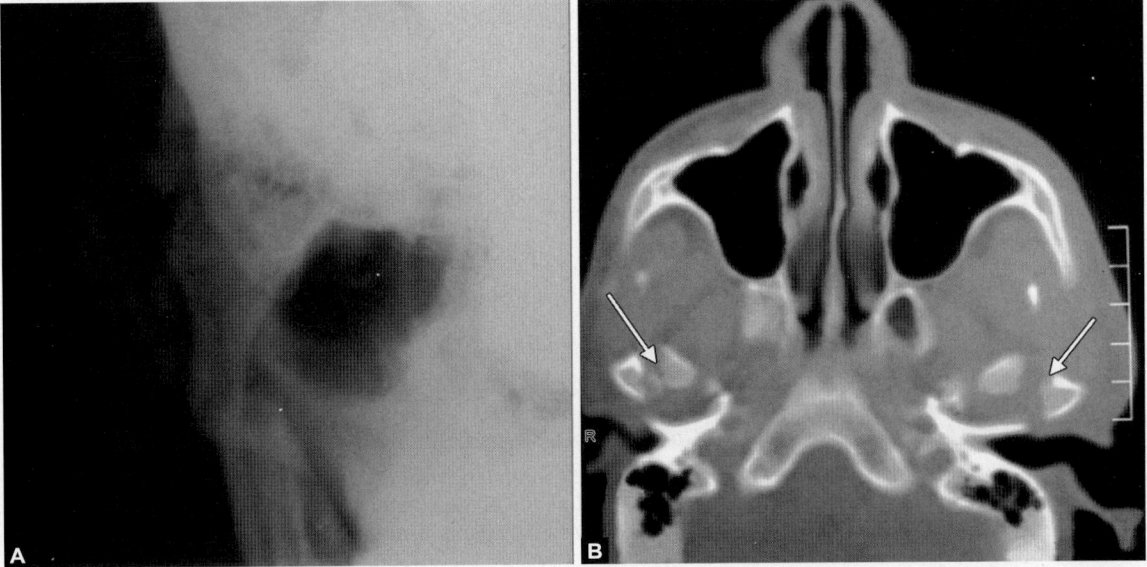

Figures 28.30A and B (A) Subcondylar fracture viewed on transorbital radiograph; (B) CT axial section showing bilateral condylar fracture

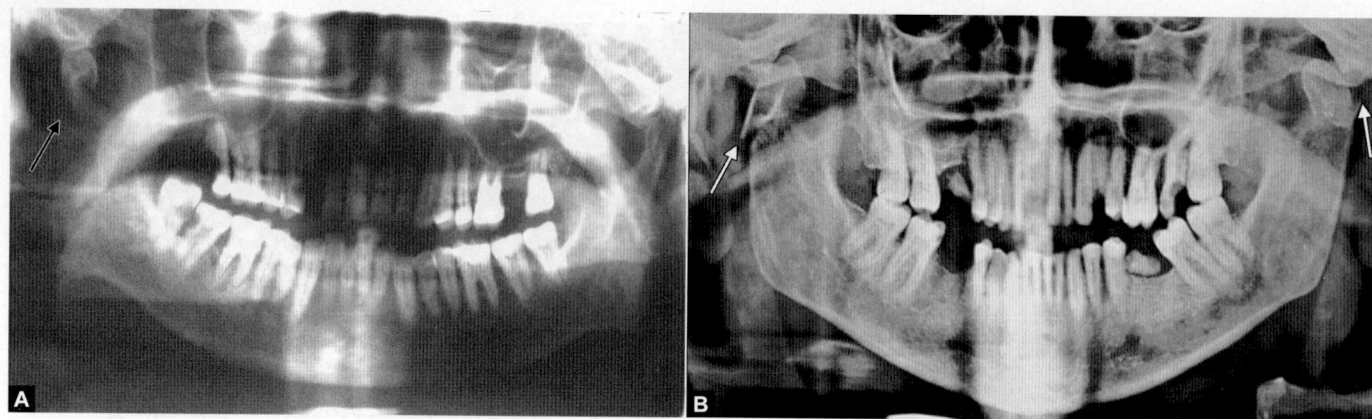

Figures 28.31A and B Panoramic radiograph showing: (A) Left condylar neck fracture; (B) Discontinuity in the posterior border of ramus and the condyles bilaterally. The fractured condylar fragments seen overlapping each other and displaced anteriorly

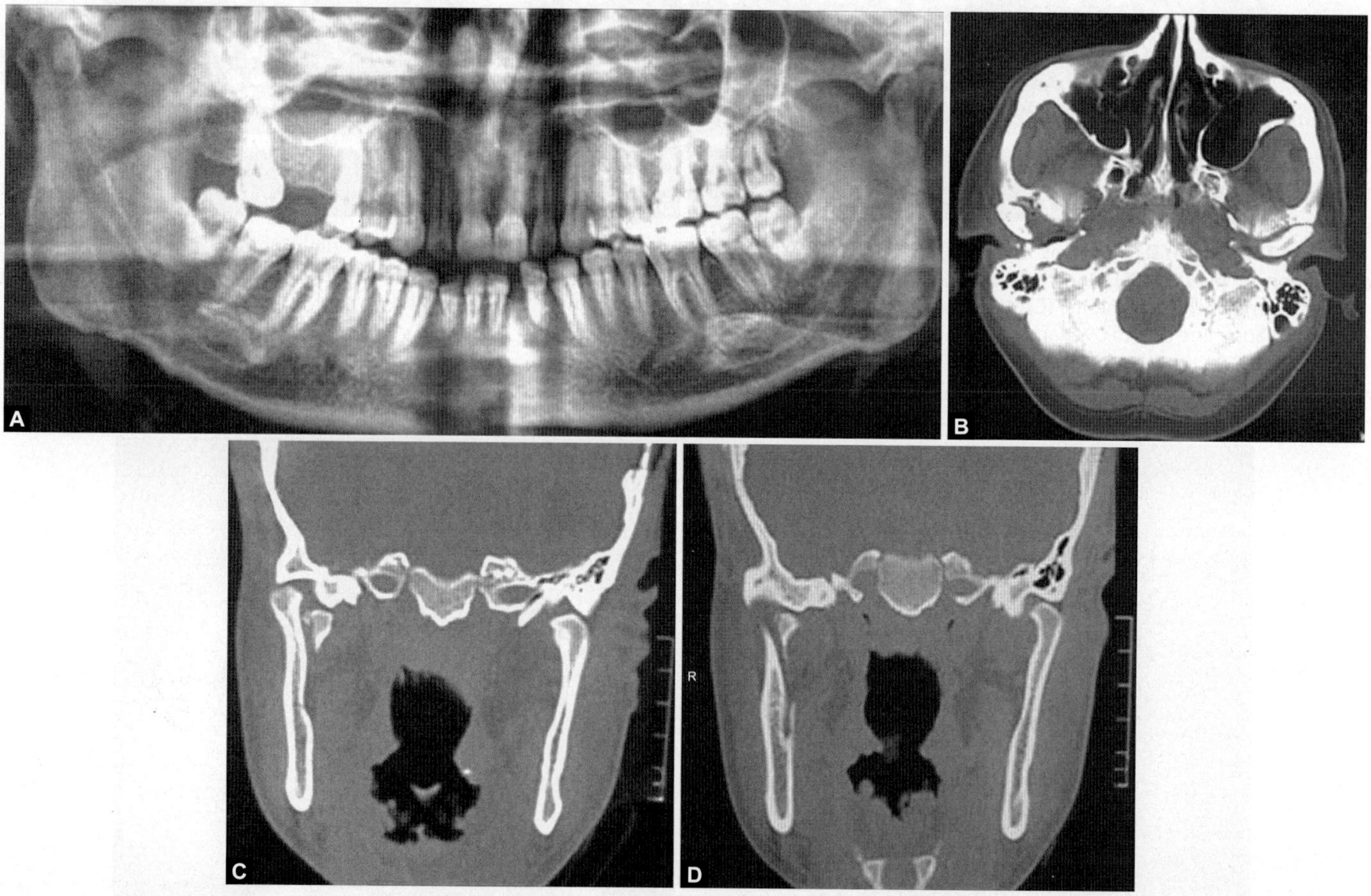

Figures 28.32A to D A 32-year-old patient having history of trauma 3 months back came with restricted opening and deranged occlusion: (A) Panoramic view showed no fracture detected; (B) Axial CT showing fracture of the greater wing of the right sphenoid, with displacement of the TMJ of that side; (C and D) Coronal CT showing fracture of the condyle with inferior displacement

- The periauricular region should be carefully examined and palpated as there may not be any clinical symptoms. A condylar fracture must be suspected if the condyle cannot be palpated in the external ear canal when the jaw is closed
- Movement of the jaw may cause crepitus
- The patient may have pain on opening and closing the mouth, or there may be swelling and trismus which inhibits the patient from moving the jaw
- There may be an anterior open bite with the last molars in contact
- The mandible may be displaced forward, or in the case of a unilateral fracture, it may be deviated towards the side of fracture (especially on opening)
- The patient will be unable to bring the jaw forward because the external pterygoid muscle is attached to the condyle.

Radiographic Features

- Some TMJ fractures are relatively asymptomatic and may not be discovered at the time of trauma; instead they come to light as an incidental finding at a later time when radiographs are taken for other reasons.
- Nondisplaced fractures of the condylar process may be difficult to detect on lateral views and are best demonstrated on anteroposterior views.
- Careful tracing of the outer cortical plate of the posterior border of the ramus, the condylar head, and the condylar notch on the lateral and posteroanterior projections may reveal the presence of fractures.
- If there is contraction of the lateral pterygoid muscle, it rotates the transverse axis of the condylar head, so that the medial end moves anteriorly, thus increasing the apparent width of the fractured condyle.
- In complete fracture dislocation the condylar head may be inclined medially at an approximate 45° angle to the vertical axis of the ramus.
- In case of an anterior displacement of the condyle which has been turned at 90° to the vertical axis of the ramus, when viewed on from the lateral aspect, only the articular surface of the condylar head will be seen, which will appear as a narrow radiopaque bar situated in the infratemporal fossa.
- The condylar head may split with little or no displacement of the fragments, or some portion may be separated from the head of the bone. Rarely, the whole of the articular portion is crushed and flattened.
- The fracture line:
  - Is often transverse but usually oblique, starting from the base of the mandibular notch and passing slightly or even markedly downwards. In the absence of any displacement it is difficult to visualize such fractures.
  - In the lateral projection there is often no evidence of any fracture line; but when the posterior margin of the ramus is followed, a sudden step may be seen.

- In some cases there is displacement of the adjacent margins of the fragments, so that the inferior borders of the condylar fragment are superimposed over the adjacent ramus.
  - The outercortical boundary may have an irregular outline or a step defect.
- The articular surface of the condyle is usually rotated inwards with fracture dislocation.
- In cases of remodeling of the fractured condyle it has been observed that:
  - Young persons have greater remodeling potential than adults.
  - The extent of remodeling is greater with fractures of the condylar head than with fractures of the condylar neck with displacement of the the condylar head.
  - The most common deformities are the medial inclination of the condyle, abnormal shape of the condyle, shortening of the neck, erosion and flattening, with loss of vertical height on the affected side.
  - The condyle may eventually show degenerative changes, osteophytes and ankylosis. These changes are more severe if the condyle is displaced.
  - Early condylar fractures commonly result in hypoplasia of the ipsilateral side of the mandible.
- Radiographic examination of the condyle should always include:
  - Lateral and anteroposterior views of each condyle. Lateral projections include panoramic, parma and lateral oblique views of the ramus and condylar regions.
  - Frontal views include reverse—Towne's and transorbital projections, are useful when there is minimal or medial displacement of the condylar head.
  - Computed tomography is an excellent imaging modality for detecting condylar fractures.

Differential Diagnosis

Old fractures that have remodeled are difficult to differentiate from developmental abnormalities.

Management

Treatment may not be indicated if mandibular mobility is adequate otherwise, the fracture is reduced surgically.

Coronoid Fractures

Definition

These fractures are rare but may result from reflex contracture of the powerful anterior fibers of temporalis muscle or during the surgical removal of large cysts of the ramus.

Clinical Features

There may be tenderness over the anterior part of the ramus with the presence of a hematoma.

The patient may complain of pain and trismus, especially on protrusive movements.

Radiographic Features

The tip of the coronoid process may be ditched, and the fragment pulled upwards towards the infratemporal fossa by the temporalis muscle.

Mandibular Ramus Fractures (Figs 28.33 and 28.34)

The fracture may be:

- *Single*: Low condylar fracture with both the coronoid and condylar process on the upper fragment.

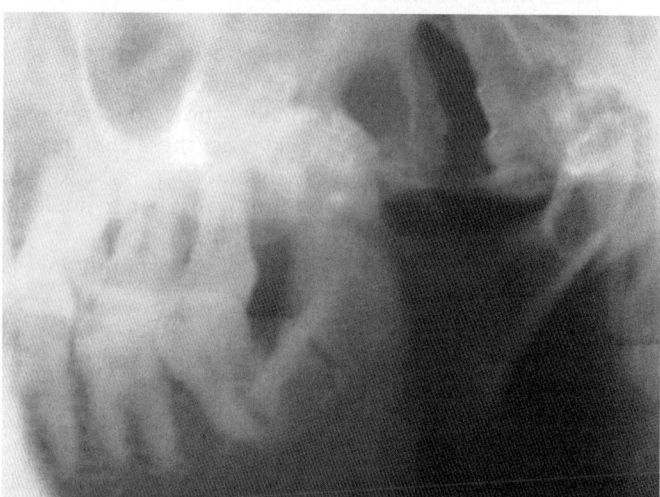

Figure 28.33 Lateral oblique view showing right side fracture of the mandibular ramus

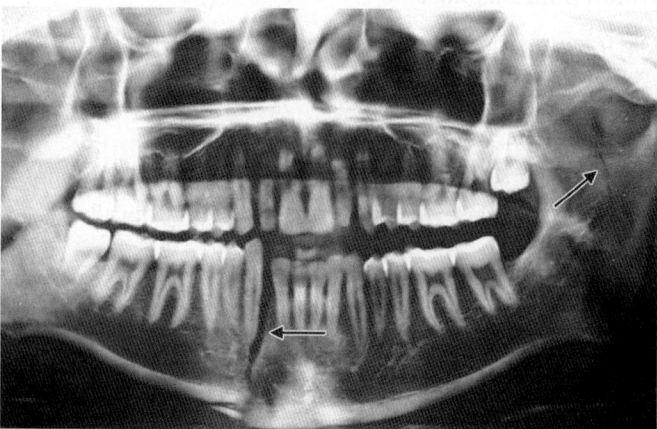

Figure 28.34 Panoramic view revealed fracture right side parasymphysis with minimal displacement extending from mesial of mandibular right canine to inferior border of mandible. Another fracture line extending from left side sigmoid notch not involving the posterior border of body of mandible

- *Comminuted*: This results from direct violence to the side of the face. The fragment tends to be splinted between the masseter and medial pterygoid muscle with little or no displacement, unless the violence is very severe.

Clinical Features

- Intraoral and extraoral swelling and ecchymosis is usually present.
- Tenderness over the ramus.
- Severe trismus or very restricted painful movements.

Management

Open reduction can be done for stabilization of fracture segments.

Mandibular Angle Fractures (Figs 28.35, 28.36, 28.38 and 28.41)

Clinical Features

- There may a swelling and tenderness at the angle externally over an obvious deformity
- There may be anesthesia or paresthesia of the lower lip on the side of the fracture
- Intraorally there may be a step-deformity seen behind the last molar
- Occlusion is deranged
- If the ramus is steadied between the finger and the thumb and the body of the mandible is moved gently with the other hand, movement and crepitus at the fracture site, may be felt
- There will be trismus and pain on even slight movement.

Radiographic Features

- Displacement of the fragments results in a cortical discontinuity or step like deformity.
- Irregularity of the occlusal plane is apparent at the fracture site.

Management

Open reduction using intraosseous wiring or bone plating should be done.

Mandibular Body Fractures (Figs 28.37A and B)

Definition

The mandible is the most common fractured facial bone. Mandibular fractures may be broadly classified, depending on their orientation as:

- Favorable—in these fractures the muscle action tends to reduce the fracture.
- Unfavorable—in these fractures, the actions of the muscles attached to the mandible are likely to displace the

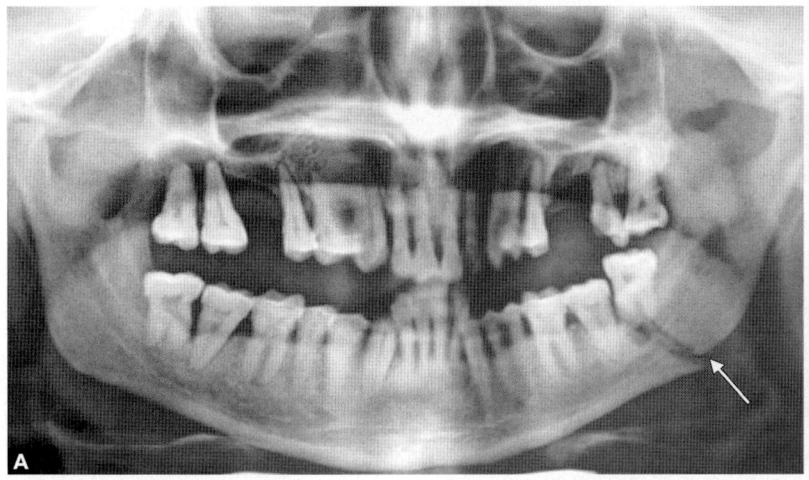
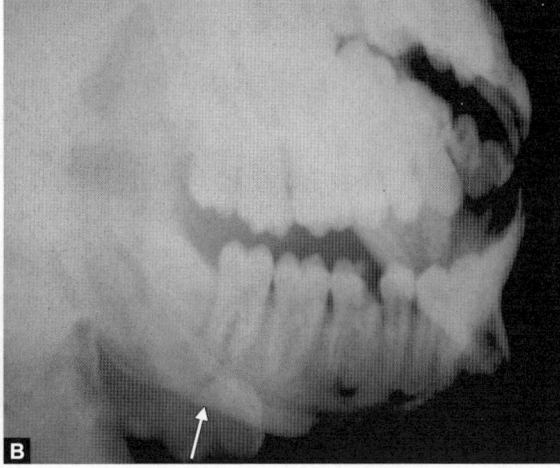

Figures 28.35A and B (A) Panoramic view showing a fracture of the mandible through the left angle; (B) Left lateral oblique shows—fracture line extending for apical end of 38 up to inferior border of mandible. Fractured segments appear to be undisplaced

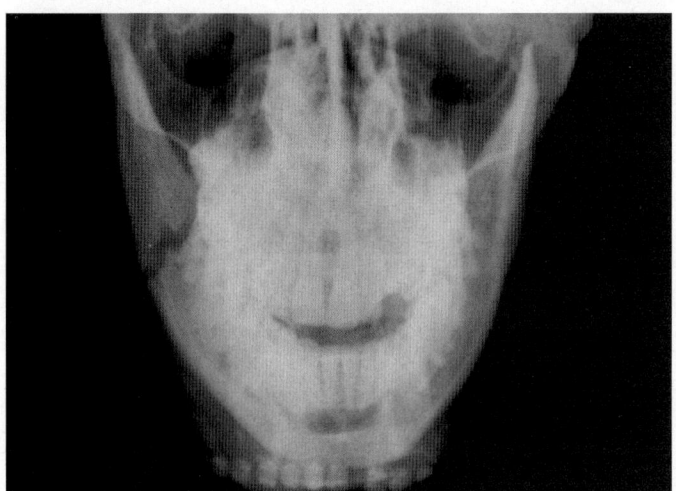

Figure 28.36 PA mandible showing fracture of the angle of the mandible

fracture margins. (e.g. if a fracture site in the body of the mandible slants posteriorly and inferiorly such that the masseter and internal pterygoid muscles pull the ramus segment away from the body of the mandible, the fracture is unfavorable).

Clinical Features

- History of injury and evidence of trauma that caused the fracture such as contusions or wounds in the skin.
- The swelling and deformity is accentuated when the patient opens the mouth.
- There may be a discrepancy in the occlusal plane.
- Manipulation of the fragment will produce crepitus or abnormal mobility.

- Intraoral examination may reveal ecchymosis in the floor of the mouth. If the inferior dental artery is damaged their may be severe hemorrhage.
- A fracture of the mandibular body on one side is frequently accompanied by a fracture of the condylar process on the opposite side.
- Trauma to the anterior mandible may result in a unilateral or bilateral fracture of the condylar processes.
- When a heavy force strikes a small area laterally, fracture of the angle, ramus or even the coronoid may result.
- In children fracture of the mandible usually occurs in the anterior region.
- In case of bilateral fracture to the mandible, the diagastric and mylohyoid muscles may pull the mandible against the pharynx and compromise the airway. Since the tongue is also attached to the anterior fragment it may fall back and obstruct the glottis.

Radiographic Features

- The margins of the fractures usually appear as sharply defined radiolucent (dark) lines of separation that are confined to the structure of the mandible. These are best visualized when the X-ray beam is oriented in the plane of the fracture.
- Displacement of the fragments results in a cortical discontinuity or step like deformity.
- Irregularity of the occlusal plane is apparent at the fracture site.
- Sometimes the margins of the fracture overlap each other, resulting in an area of increased radiopacity at the fractured site.
- Nondisplaced fractures may involve both, buccal and lingual cortical plates or only one cortical plate.

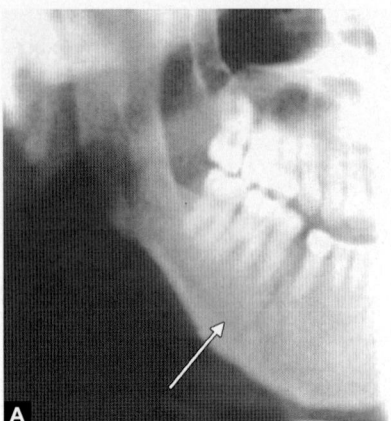 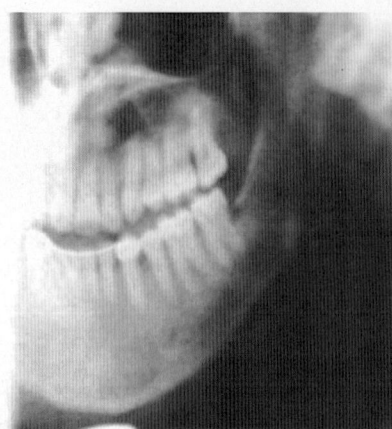 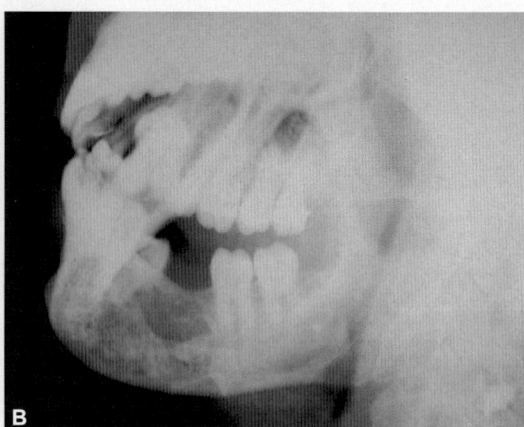

Figures 28.37A and B (A) Panoramic view showing fracture of the body of the ramus; (B) Lateral oblique showing fractured buccal cortical plate with region of missing 46

- An incomplete fracture involving only one cortical plate, called green stick fracture, is usually seen in children.
- An oblique fracture that involves both the cortical plate may cause some diagnostic difficulty if the fracture lines in the buccal and lingual plates are not superimposed; in this case two distinct fractures may be apparent when in reality only one exists. Another right-angled view may help, and also the fact that the two fracture lines join at the same point on the inferior border of the mandible may guide to reach the right diagnosis.
- The radiographic examination of the suspected fracture should include a panoramic view but it is important to supplement this film with right-angled views such as occlusal and extraoral views such as posteroanterior and submentovertex skull views. These supplementary views may disclose fractures which may have not been evident on panoramic projections. Intraoral periapical films have a greater resolution.

Management

Open or closed reduction may be needed.

Fracture of Symphysis and Parasymphysis (Figs 28.34, 28.38 to 28.42)

Clinical Features

- As the fracture is usually a result of direct violence there is frequently associated soft tissue injury to the chin and lower lip.
- There will be presence of bony tenderness and a small lingual hematoma.
- In some cases there may be detachment of the genioglossus muscle which may contribute to the loss of tongue control and obstruction of the airway.

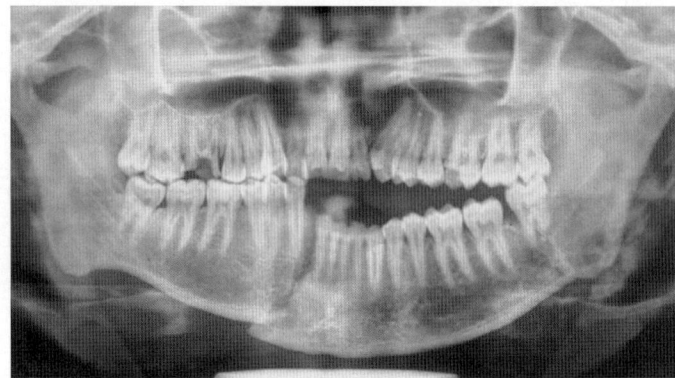

Figure 28.38 Right parasymphyseal and left angle fracture of mandible. Panoramic view showing a radiolucent line passing from distal of lower right lateral downwards obliquely to the right premolar region. A step at the inferior border of the mandible in region of premolars with upward displacement of distal fragment. Another radiolucent line extending from mesial of left third molar downward backward to inferior border of mandible at angle with displacement of fractured fragment

Radiographic Features

These fractures are usually associated with the fracture of one or both condyles.

Radiographic Differential Diagnosis of Fractures of Mandible

- The superimposition of soft tissue shadows on the image of the mandible may simulate fractures:
  - A narrow air space between the dorsal surface of the tongue and the soft palate are superimposed across the angle of the mandible in a panoramic image may appear as a fracture.

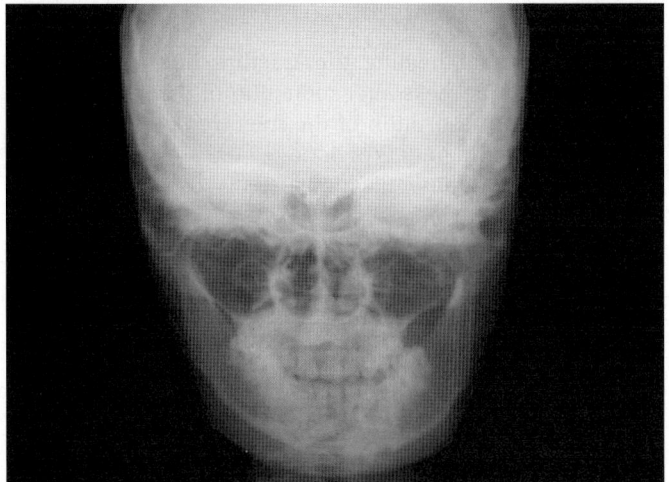

Figure 28.39 Mandibular symphyseal fracture. This is an postero-anterior view of mandible showing discontinuity at the inferior border of mandible in the symphysis region. An oblique radiolucent line passing from distal of left mandibular central to the right side downwards up to inferior border of mandible

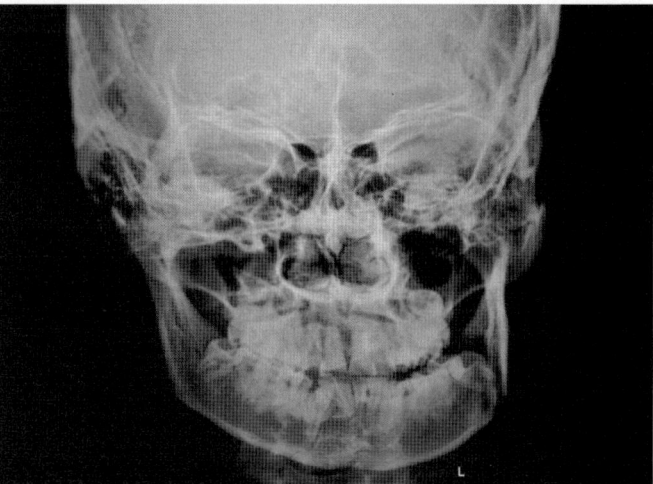

Figure 28.41 Mandibular symphyseal and left angle fracture. This is an posteroanterior view of mandible showing discontinuity at the inferior border of mandible in the symphysis region. Oblique radiolucent line passing from distal of lower left central incisor to the right side downwards up to inferior border of mandible. Linear radiolucency extending from distal of lower left third molar downwards posteriorly to the inferior border of mandible at the angle. Radiographic diagnosis: Mandibular symphyseal fracture and left mandibular angle fracture

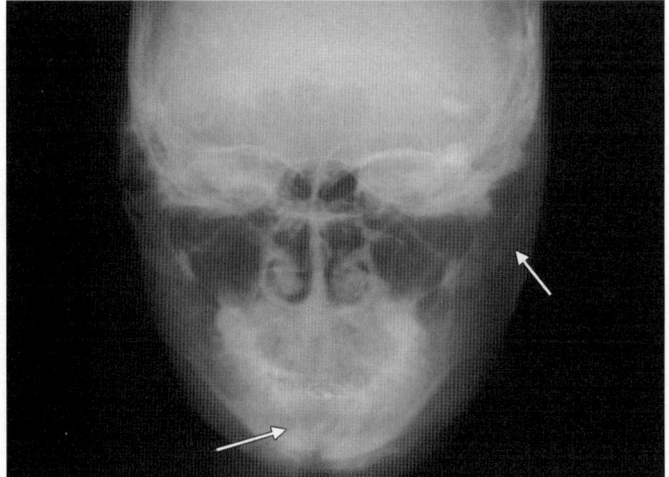

Figure 28.40 This is an posteroanterior view of mandible showing discontinuity at the inferior border of mandible in the symphysis region. Oblique radiolucent line passing from distal of lower left central incisor to the right side down words up to inferior border of mandible. Linear radiolucency seen at the medial side of the ramus in the subcondylar region Radiographic diagnosis: Mandibular symphyseal fracture and left subcondylar fracture with interdental wiring of the lower central incisor

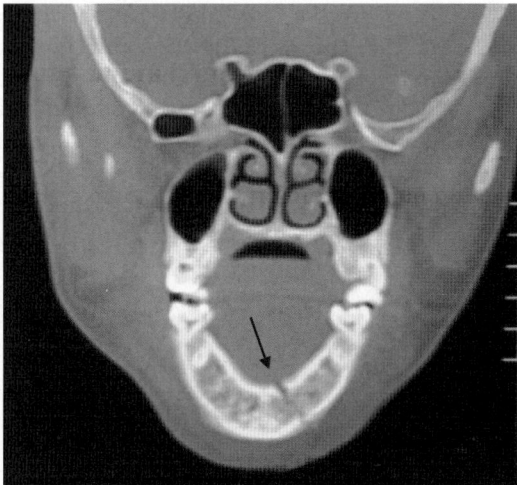

Figure 28.42 Computed tomography coronal section showing fracture of right parasymphysis region

– Similar appearances may occur in the region of the soft palate superimposition on the ramus.

In all the above cases careful study will show that the dark line or the shadow is continuing on the bone and no fracture can produce such an effect.

- The shadow of the hyoid bone may be mistaken for a fracture line
- On lateral radiographs.

– The air space between the dorsal surface of the tongue and the posterior pharyngeal wall may appear similar to a fracture on lateral views of the mandible.

The shadow of the neck intervenes over some part of the bone and where it ends anteriorly, there is a difference in the radiographic density. The line of demarcation between the two densities may be mistaken for a fracture line, or a thin dark line which in fact represents the subcutaneous fat and the anterior aspect of the neck may be mistaken for a fracture line, or a thin dark line which in fact represents the subcutaneous fat and the anterior aspect of the neck may be mistaken for a fracture line.

In all the above cases careful study will show that the dark line or the shadow is continuing on the bone and no fracture can produce such an effect.

- On the PA view, the shadow of the cervical vertebrae (especially the joint space between the lateral articular process) are superimposed over the anterior portion of the mandible, which presents as a dark shadow which may be mistaken for a fracture line. In this case an occlusal view of the same region gives an excellent diagnostic radiograph.
- In young jaws unerupted teeth and teeth follicles may obscure bone structure and make it difficult to diagnose a fracture.
- Nutrient canals may be mistaken for fracture line.

Orbital Blow-out Fracture

Following a direct blow to the globe of the eye, the orbital rim remains intact but the force of the blow is transmitted either downwards or medially. The very thin bones of the orbital floor can break and allow the contents of the globe to herniate downwards into the antrum. Superimposition on conventional radiographs makes this type of fracture difficult to detect, hence the need for CT (if available) or tomography to determine the site and severity of the injury.

Other Fractures and Injuries

Facial fractures are often associated with some other injury involving the head and neck. These can be divided broadly into:
- Fractures of the skull vault
- Fractures of the cranial base
- Fractures of the cervical spine
- Intracranial injuries.

Radiographic Monitoring of Healing in Fractures

Radiographic examination of the facial bones after trauma is usually necessary to measure the degree of reduction from treatment and to monitor the continued immobilization of the fracture site during repair. The monitoring should include:
- Examination of the alignment of the cortical plates of the involved bone.
- Remodeling and remineralization of the fractured site.

Radiographic Features

- During normal healing the fracture line increases in width about 2 weeks after reduction of the fracture. This is due to the resorption of the fractured ends and small sequestrated fragments of bone
- Evidence of remineralization usually occurs 5–6 weeks after treatment.
- Unlike long bones of the skeleton, callus formation is rare in healing jaw fractures.
- The complete remodeling of the fractured site with obliteration of the fracture line may take several months.
- Sometimes the fracture lines may persist for years, even when the patient has made a complete clinical recovery.
- Complications of healing include:
  - Malalignment of fractured segments.
  - Inflammatory lesions related to nonvital teeth near or in the line of the fracture.
  - Nonunion of the fractured segments seen as increased width of the fracture line.
  - Cortication of the fractured surfaces and rounding of the sharp edges of the segments.
  - The development of osteomyelitis of the fractured site, which will appear as an increased sclerosis of the surrounding bone, inflammatory periosteal new bone and development of sequestra.

BIBLIOGRAPHY

1. Andreasen JO, Andreasen FM. Textbook and colour atlas of traumatic injuries to the teeth, 3rd edition. Munksgard, Copenhagen; 1994.
2. Gerlock AJ Jr, Sinn DP, McBride KL. Clinical and radiographic interpretation of facial fractures. Boston, Little Brown; 1981.
3. Goaz PW, White SC. Principles and interpretation. In: Oral Radiology, 3rd edition. St Louis, Mosby Year Book, 1994.
4. Miles DA, Van Dis MJ, Jensen CW, Ferretti A. Interpretation normal versus abnormal and common radiographic presentations of lesions, in radiographic and imaging for dental auxillaries, 3rd edition. Philadelphia, WD Saunders; 1999.pp.231-80.
5. Newman J. Medical imaging of facial and mandibular fractures. Radiol Technol. 1998;69 (5):417.
6. Rowe NL, Williams JL. Maxillofacial injuries. Churchill Livingstone, Edinburgh, 1985;(1).
7. Wood NK, Goaz PW. Differential diagnosis of oral lesions, 4th edition. CV Mosby, St Louis; 1991.
8. Wood RE. Handbook of signs in dental and maxillofacial radiology. Warthog Publications, Toronto; 1988.
9. Worth HM. Principles and practice of oral radiographic interpretation. Year Book Medical Publishers, Chicago; 1963.

Salivary Gland Disorders | 29

The salivary glands are exocrine glands whose secretions flow into the oral cavity. Patients with salivary gland disease most frequently present with complaints of oral dryness, swelling or a mass in the gland. A familiarity with salivary gland disorders and applicable current imaging techniques is an essential armamentarium of a dental diagnostician who is responsible for detecting the disorders of salivary glands.

The salivary glands may be classified into:
- *Major salivary glands*: These are paired glands located at some distance from the oral mucosa with which they connect by extraglandular ducts.
  These include:
  - Parotid glands
  - Submandibular glands
  - Sublingual glands.
- *Minor salivary glands*: These are located in the mucosa and submucosa opening directly through the mucosa or indirectly via short ducts. The function is not only to secrete saliva for digestion but also to keep the oral mucosa moist.
  These include:
  - Anterior glands of the tongue
  - Labial glands
  - Numerous small lingual glands
    - von-Ebner's gland
    - Glands of Blandin and Nuhn
    - Posterior lingual glands
  - Buccal glands
  - Palatine glands
  - Glossopalatine glands
  - Incisive glands.

PAROTID GLAND

Parotid gland is the largest salivary gland, it has a shape of an inverted flattened pyramid. It lies between the mastoid process and the ramus of the mandible. The bulk of the parotid is situated in the retromandibular fossa. The broad base of the gland lies subcutaneously and the apex lies deep between the parotid fascia. A part of it forms an irregular lobulated yellowish mass lying below the external acoustic meatus, between the mandible and the sternocleidomastoid. A smaller part of it lies between the zygomatic arch superiorly and the parotid duct inferiorly. It is divided into superficial and deep lobes by the facial nerve and its branches.

The parotid duct or Stenson's duct is about 5 cm long and has thick walls. It emerges from the substance of the gland to course anteriorly till it reaches the anterior border of the masseter muscle. As it crosses the masseter muscle it is joined by the duct of the accessory lobe. At the border of the masseter muscle the duct turns sharply medially and is often embedded in the furrow of the protruding buccal fat pad. In its medial course the duct reaches the outer surface of the buccinator muscle, which it perforates in an oblique direction anteriorly and medially, runs a short distance obliquely forward between the buccinator and the mucous membrane of the oral cavity and opens on the oral surface of the cheek opposite the upper second molar.

The gland is supplied by the external carotid artery and its branches. The lymphatic drainage first drains into the parotid nodes and then goes to the deep cervical nodes. The nerve supply is via the auriculotemporal nerve, plexus around the external carotid artery and greater auricular nerve.

SUBMANDIBULAR GLAND

Submandibular gland is a round biconvex salivary gland which is situated in the anterior part of the digastric triangle, about the size of a walnut. It is enclosed by two layers of deep cervical fascia. The inner surface of the gland is in contact with the styloid, digastric and styloglossus muscle, posteriorly with the hyoglossus and posterior border of the mylohyoid muscle anteriorly.

The submandibular gland duct is called the Wharton's duct which is also about 5 cm long but its wall is much thinner than that of the parotid duct. It emerges from the middle of the deep surface of the superficial part of the gland, runs forward beneath the deep part of the gland, between the mylohyoid and hyoglossus muscle, it runs further forward between the medial surface of the sublingual gland and the genioglossus muscle and finally ends by opening into the summit of the sublingual papilla, situated in the floor of the mouth, on the side of the frenum.

It is supplied by the lingual and facial branches of the carotid artery, and drains into the facial and lingual vein. The lymphatic drainage is into the submandibular lymph nodes.

The nerve supply is via the branches from the submandibular ganglion through which it receives fibers from chorda tympani.

SUBLINGUAL GLAND

Sublingual gland lies above the mylohyoid and below the mucosa of the floor of the mouth. It is medial to the sublingual fossa of the mandible on either side of the symphysis menti and lateral to the genioglossus muscle. It has approximately 15 ducts that open directly into the floor of the mouth.

There are 8–20 small ducts of the sublingual gland which open into the sublingual fold (caruncula sublingualis), in the floor of the mouth on either side of the frenum, some open into the submandibular duct and others unite to form the principle sublingual duct (Bartholin's duct) which opens in the floor.

It is supplied by the sublingual and submental arteries and the lymphatic drainage is to the submandibular lymph nodes. The nerve supply is by the lingual and chorda tympani nerve.

DIFFERENTIAL DIAGNOSIS OF SALIVARY GLAND ENLARGEMENTS (TABLE 29.1)

Enlargement of the Parotid Area

Unilateral enlargements of the parotid area are categorized by the presence of a discrete, palpable mass or a diffuse swelling.

If no mass is apparent:
- Sialadenitis should be considered. Sialadenitis may be primary or secondary to ductal obstruction (retrograde).
- Sialodochitis.

A mass intrinsic to the gland suggests:
- A neoplasm (benign or malignant)
- Cyst
- Intraglandular lymph node
- Hamartoma.

Rapid growth, facial nerve paralysis, rock hard texture, and an older age occurrence are clinically suggestive of:
- Malignant neoplasm.

Asymptomatic bilateral enlargements of the parotid area include:
- Benign lymphoepithelial lesion
- Sjögren's syndrome
- Alcoholism
- Medication (iodine and certain heavy metals)
- Warthin tumor.

Painful bilateral enlargement of the parotid glands:
- Secondary to radiation treatment
- Secondary to bacterial or viral sialadenitis (including mumps) (there will be presence of other systemic symptoms).

Table 29.1 Summary of the main salivary gland complaints and their causes

Salivary gland complaint	Causes
Acute intermittent generalized swelling	Obstructive disorders including: Sialolithiasis—salivary stones Stricture or stenosis of the duct, usually secondary to surgery, stones or infection Recurrent parotitis of childhood
Acute generalized swelling	Infection, either Viral, e.g. mumps Bacterial, e.g. ascending sialadenitis
Chronic generalized	Sjögren's syndrome, either primary or secondary Sialosis Cystic fibrosis Sarcoidosis
Discrete swelling	Intrinsic tumor, benign or malignant Extrinsic tumor Cyst Overlying lymph nodes
Dry mouth	Sjögren's syndrome Postradiation damage Mouth breathing Dehydration Functional disorders, including: Drugs such as tricyclic antidepressants, used to treat Neurosis, particularly chronic anxiety states
Excess salivation	Psychological (false ptyalism) Reflex, e.g. due to local stimulation Heavy metal poisoning

Diffuse facial swelling in the parotid region not related to abnormalities of the gland:
- Hypertrophy of the Masseter muscle (unilateral or bilateral)
- Accessory parotid gland
- Lesions related to temporomandibular joint and other osseous structures
- Osteomyelitis of the ramus of the mandible
- HIV-associated multicentric cysts (bilateral)

A palpable mass superficial to the gland:
- Lymphadenitis
- An infected preauricular or sebaceous cyst
- Benign lymphoid hyperplasia
- Extraparotid tumor.

Enlargement of the Submandibular Area

Unilateral enlargement of the submandibular area associated with tender lymph nodes:

Sialadenitis, which may be primary or secondary to ductal obstruction or decreased salivary flow (retrograde).

Unilateral enlargement of the submandibular area associated without tender lymph nodes:

- Neoplasm
- Cyst
- Lymphoepithelial lesion
- Fibrosis.

An intraglandular mass is suggestive of:

- Neoplasm
- Cyst.

Rapid growth, pain, rock hard texture, and an older age occurrence are clinically suggestive of:

Malignancy (neoplasms of the submandibular gland have a greater chance of being malignant than those of parotid gland and neoplasms of the sublingual gland have an even greater chance of being malignant than those of submandibular gland).

Masses superficial or adjacent to the submandibular gland are assumed to be:

- Lymph nodes
- Extraglandular neoplasms.

Bilateral enlargement of the submandibular gland:

- Bacterial sialadenitis
- Viral sialadenitis (mumps is primarily an infection of the parotid gland, it may also occur in the submandibular gland)
- Sialodochitis.

Other causes of swelling in the submandibular region:

- Sjögren's syndrome
- Enlarged lymph nodes
- Submandibular space infection
- Brachial cleft cyst.

APPLIED DIAGNOSTIC IMAGING OF THE SALIVARY GLANDS

A number of imaging techniques are useful in evaluation of the salivary glands. Depending on the technique used, imaging can provide information on salivary function, anatomical alterations, and space occupying lesions within the glands.

Plain Film Radiology (Figs 29.1A to C)

Since the salivary glands are located relatively superficially, radiographic images may be obtained with standard dental radiographic techniques.

Symptoms suggestive of salivary gland obstruction (swelling of the gland with pain), warrant plain film radiography of the major salivary glands in order to visualize possible radiopaque sialoliths (stones).

Panoramic or lateral oblique and anteroposterior (AP) projections are used to visualize the parotid glands. Panoramic views overlap anatomic structures that can mask the presence of a salivary stone.

A standard occlusal film/intraoral periapical film may be placed intraorally adjacent to parotid duct to visualize a stone close to the gland orifice. However, this technique will not capture the entire parotid gland.

Sialoliths obstructing the submandibular gland may be visualized by panoramic, occlusal or lateral oblique views.

Smaller stones or poorly calcified sialoliths may not be visualized radiographically. If a stone is not evident with plain film radiography but clinical evaluation and history are suggestive of salivary gland obstruction, then additional images are necessary.

Sialography

Sialography is the radiographic visualization of the salivary gland following retrograde instillation of soluble contrast material into the ducts. It is the imaging technique of choice for delineating ductal anatomy and for identifying and localizing sialoliths. It is useful in evaluating intrinsic and acquired abnormalities of the ductal system as it provides the clearest visualization of the branching ducts and acinar end-pieces. It is also a precious tool in presurgical planning prior to removal of salivary masses.

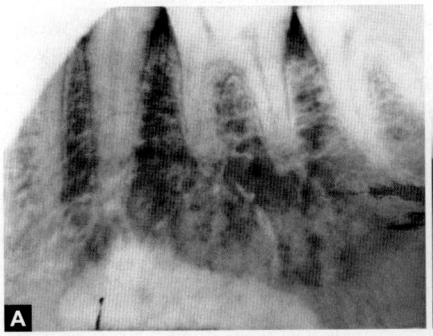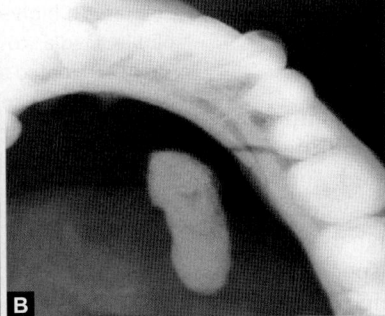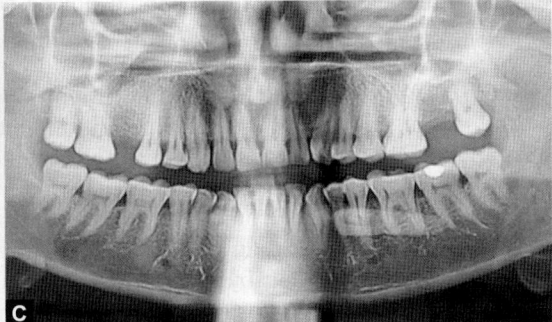

Figures 29.1A to C Plain films showing sialolith: (A) Intraoral periapical radiograph showing long cylindrical homogeneous radiopaque mass in the periapical region of the manibular left premolar molar region; (B) Mandibular occlusal view shows long cylindrical hemogeneous radiopaque mass in the left side of the floor of the mouth; (C) Panoramic radiograph shows a long cylindrical hemogeneous radiopaque mass in the interradicular area of the mandibular left premolar molar region. *Final diagnosis*: Sialolith of the left submandibular duct

The glands are cannulated and filled with a radiopaque contrast agent to make them visible on the radiographs. The procedure reveals the location and integrity of the salivary glands, and indicates the presence of diseases that change the internal architecture.

Indications

- Detection of calculus or calculi or foreign bodies, whether these are radiopaque or radiolucent.
- Determination of the extent of destruction of the gland secondary to obstructing calculi or foreign bodies. This will aid in deciding whether a total excision of the gland or a simple lithotomy should be performed.
- Detection and portrayal of fistulae, diverticula or strictures.
- Determination and diagnosis of recurrent swellings and inflammatory processes.
- Demonstration of a tumor and the determination of its location, size and origin, whether the radiograph suggests a benign or a malignant lesion.
- Selection of a site for biopsy.
- Outline of the plane of the facial nerve as a guide in planning a biopsy or dissection.
- Detection of residual stone or stones, residual tumor, fistula or stenosis; or retention cysts following simple lithotomy or other surgical procedures.
- Sialography has also been recognized as a therapeutic procedure because:
  - The dilatation of the ductal system produced during the study may aid in the drainage of the ductal debris.
  - The therapeutic effect produced by the iodinated contrast media when injected into the ductal system has also been seen.

Contraindications

- Patient with a known sensitivity to iodine compounds and patients who have experienced severe asthmatic attacks or anaphylaxis following use of iodine compounds in a prior radiologic examination, should not be considered subjects for this technique. A history of nausea and vomiting following the intravenous injection of contrast media is not considered a contraindication.
- The use of sialography during a period of acute inflammation of the salivary system is contraindicated. During this period the ductal epithelium may be disrupted, and escape of the contrast medium from the ductal system into the parenchyma can produce severe foreign body reaction, accompanied by severe pain. This is specially true when the oily contrast medium is used. Foreign body reaction following the use of water soluble media has not been reported.

- The administration and retention of the iodinated contrast material may interfere with subsequent thyroid function tests, such function studies if required, should be done prior the sialography procedure.

Contrast Media (Table 29.2)

An ideal sialographic contrast media should have the following characteristics:
- Physiological properties similar to that of saliva
- Miscibility with saliva
- Absence of local or systemic toxicity
- Pharmacological inertness
- Satisfactory opacification
- Low surface tension and low viscosity to allow filling of fine components of the ductal system
- Easy elimination, but should be durable for sufficient time so as to permit time for satisfactory radiographs
- Residual contrast media should be absorbed by the salivary gland and detoxified by the liver or excreted by the kidney.

Table 29.2 Types of contrast media

- Water soluble media
  - These are principally iodinated benzene or pyridone derivatives.
  - These compounds have a low viscosity, less surface tension and are more miscible with the salivary secretions.
  - These physical characteristics permit filling of the finer ductal system under lower pressure and facilitate prompt drainage.
  - Causes less pain or discomfort, with no granulomatous reaction, in the glands.
  - Opacification of the water based media is not as good as that of oil media.
  - The excretion of the contrast media is very rapid.
  - Hydropaque and Renografin are the available water soluble contrast media.
- Fat soluble media (Oil based)
  - There are two types of fat soluble contrast media: 1. Iodized oil, 2. Water insoluble organic iodine compounds.
  - These compounds are more viscous have more surface tension and are less miscible with the salivary secretions.
  - It requires a higher injection pressure than that of the water soluble media, to visualize finer ducts. Oil based media is poorly eliminated and causes ductal obstruction.
  - Usually accompanied with pain and a lot of discomfort. Extravasation of the fat soluble media can produce severe foreign body reaction with focal necrosis of the parenchyma and stroma.
  - The fat soluble contrast media on the whole produces a satisfactory degree of opacification. This is an excellent media if the ductal systems under examination are intact.
  - The excretion of the contrast media is slow and gives adequate time to carry out the various radiographic procedures. Ethidol is the available fat soluble contrast media.

Procedure

Before starting with the procedure, collect all data sheets containing pertinent and clinical data including patient's name, age and hospital identifying data, the chief complaint, the physical findings and clinical impression, previous history of allergy, prior radiologic study and reports, and the volume and type of contrast media previously used.

Before the initiation of the examination and injection of the contrast media, the patient is instructed to raise his right hand if he experiences any discomfort during the procedure. The amount of contrast media to be injected should be governed by the production of pain.

This is divided into three main steps:
1. The preliminary plain film evaluation
2. The injection or filling phase
   Equipment required:
   - Polyethylene tubing with a special blunt end metallic tip with
     - Side hole for parotid gland.
     - End terminal hole for submandibular gland.
   - 5 or 10 cc syringe
   - Lacrimal dilators
   - Contrast media
   - Sialagogue, like 5 lemon slices or lemon extract or chewing gum.
     - The parotid orifice is located at the base of the papilla in the buccal mucosa adjacent to the first or second molar. The area over the mucosa where the duct orifice is expected to be located should be dried with a small sponge. If the gland has some degree of function, a drop of saliva can be expressed by applying gentle pressure to the skin over the main parotid areas, thus identifying the location of the orifice.
     - The submandibular excretory duct orifice is situated on the summit of the small papilla at the side of the lingual frenum, but care should be taken to differentiate it from the sublingual gland orifices in the same region.
     - After the appropriate orifice has been identified, the duct can be explored with the lacrimal probe.
     - In case of the submandibular gland, the probe should pass through the length of the floor of the mouth to the level of the posterior border of the mylohyoid muscle, a penetration of about 5 cm.
     - Because of the tortuous course of the parotid duct, the cheek has to be turned outward before the probe is inserted into the duct. The eversion of the cheek will help reduce the possibility of penetrating the duct at one of the sharp angles in its course.
     - In both the parotid and submandibular ducts, the probe should slide easily back and forth and also rotate freely without dragging.

   - When the duct orifice has been adequately sized and enlarged, the sialographic cannula is inserted into the duct so that the tissue stop presses firmly into the orifice to prevent dye reflux. The cannula may be held in place by taping the tubing to the face or by having the patient bite on the tubing wrapped in sponge.
   - After insertion of the cannula, the radiographic dye is slowly introduced into the duct. The amount of dye to be placed in the gland for adequate filling varies from patient to patient and depends on the condition of the gland.
   - The amount used is best determined by fluoroscopic observation; the patient should be instructed to inform the operator when the gland area feels tight or full.
   - Appropriate volumes of dye required vary from 0.76–1.00 mL, for the parotid glands, and 0.0–0.75 mL for submandibular glands. The cardinal rule is that the injection should be stopped when the gland is full, if the dye is extravasated, or when the patient experiences mild discomfort.
   - *Radiographic projections*: The filming procedure is carried out with the patient in the supine position. All dentures should be removed. Often several films are obtained during the injection in order to monitor the filling phase and degree of filling. Because geometrical artifacts are introduced by all techniques, it is important to use the same procedure consistently.
   - The lateral oblique projection and/or mandibular occlusal view is used to delineate the submandibular gland. In the lateral oblique the duct pattern is not distorted and a sialolith is seen well on the occlusal view.
   - The AP view of both glands demonstrates the medial and lateral gland structures. In case of the parotid gland the patient should be asked to keep the mouth open.
   - The panoramic projection may also be taken. This is helpful in studying erosion of bone or destruction of the mandible, in case of salivary tumors.
3. The evacuation (fat soluble medium) or the parenchymal phase (water soluble medium).
   - After the final sialographic views have been made, the cannula should be removed from the duct orifice. The patient is instructed to chew gum or the lemon slice and then asked to rinse. This is done to stimulate the gland and cause excretion of the dye.
   - Lateral jaw, lateral oblique or AP radiographs should be made 5 minutes after removal of the cannula. They provide the information about the excretory function of the gland.
   - Normal salivary gland will excrete 100% of the contrast dye within 5 minutes after removal of the cannula.

Additional views which may be taken to study special features are:

- Reverse basilar view to demonstrate the deep portion of the parotid.
- A film made with the cheek in the blow-out position in the anteroposterior view to demonstrate the superficial portion of the course of the Stenson's duct of the parotid gland.
- Occlusal view for demonstration of the distal submandibular gland's Whartons duct.
- Filming of the filling phase with the mouth open will reduce superimposition of the mandible on the parotid gland.
- Stereoscopic studies are invaluable for the study of the spatial relationships of the gland and the duct.
- Subtraction views are of great value in the delineation of the finer ducts and of the sublingual ductal system.
- Plesioradiography is a technique in which a small X-ray tube is placed in contact with the facial soft tissues contralateral to the gland being examined in an attempt to eliminate the obscuring overlying bony structures.

Sialography may be performed both on the submandibular and parotid glands.

The normal ductal architecture has a leafless tree appearance. As the ductal structure branches through the major glands, the submandibular gland demonstrates a more abrupt transition in ductal diameter whereas the parotid gland demonstrates a gradual decrease in ductal diameter. Ductal stricture, obstruction, dilatation, ductal ruptures and stones are better visualized by sialography.

Nonopaque sialoliths appear as voids: Sialectasis is the appearance of focal collections of contrast medium within the gland, seen in cases of sialadenitis and Sjögren's syndrome. The progression of severity is classified as punctate, globular and cavitary.

Following the procedure the patient should be encouraged to massage the gland and/or to suck on lemon drops to promote the flow of saliva and contrast media out of the gland. Postprocedure radiography is done approximately one hour later. If a substantial amount of contrast material remains in the salivary gland at that time, follow-up visits should be scheduled until the contrast material empties or is fully resorbed.

Incomplete clearing can be due to obstruction of salivary outflow, extraductal or extravasated contrast, collection of contrast material in abscess cavities or impaired secretory function.

Sialography should not be performed if a radiopaque stone has been shown by plain radiography to be in the distal portion of the duct, because the procedure may displace it proximally into the ductal system, complicating subsequent removal.

Normal Sialographic Appearances

Parotid Gland

These include:

- The main duct is of even diameter (1–2 mm wide) and should be filled completely and uniformly.
- The duct structure within the gland branches regularly and tapers gradually towards the periphery of the gland, the so-called tree in winter appearance (**Fig. 29.2**).

Submandibular Gland

These include:

- The main duct is of even diameter (3–4 mm wide) and should be filled completely and uniformly.
- This gland is smaller than the parotid, but the overall appearance is similar with the branching duct structure tapering gradually towards the periphery—the so-called bush in winter appearance.

Pathological Appearances

Based on the suggested systematic approach to sialographic assessment, the main pathological changes can be divided into:

- Ductal changes associated with:
  - Calculi
  - Sialodochitis (ductal inflammation/infection)
- Glandular changes associated with:
  - Sialadenitis (glandular inflammation/infection)
  - Sjögren's syndrome
  - Intrinsic tumors.

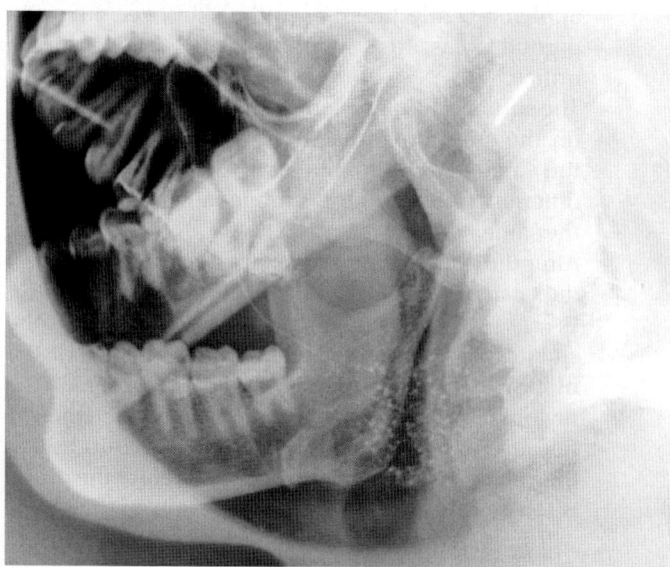

Figure 29.2 Sialogram showing a normal left parotid gland, the tree in winter appearance

Sialographic Appearances of Calculi

Sialographic appearances of calculi include:
- Filling defect(s) in the main duct
- Ductal dilatation proximal to the calculus
- The emptying film usually shows contrast medium retained behind the stone.

Sialographic Appearances of Sialodochitis

Sialographic appearances of sialodochitis include:
- Segmented sacculation or dilatation and stricture of the main duct, the so-called sausage link appearance.
- Associated calculi or ductal stenosis.

Sialographic Appearances of Sialadenitis

Sialographic appearances of sialadenitis include:
- Dots or blobs of contrast medium within the gland, an appearance known as sialectasis (**Figs 29.3A and B**) caused by the inflammation of the glandular tissue producing saccular dilatation of the acini.
- The main duct is usually normal.

Sialographic Appearances in Sjögren's Syndrome

Sialographic appearances in sjögren's syndrome include:
- Widespread dots or blobs of contrast medium within the gland, an appearance known as punctate sialectasis or snowstorm. This is caused by a weakening of the epithelium lining the intercalated ducts, allowing the escape of the contrast medium out of the ducts
- Considerable retention of the contrast medium during the emptying phase
- The main duct is usually normal.

An understanding of the underlying disease processes explains why the sialographic appearances of sialadenitis and Sjögren's syndrome (two totally different conditions) are so similar. This is shown diagrammatically in (**Figs 29.4A to C**).

Sialographic Appearances of Intrinsic Tumors include

Sialographic appearances of intrinsic tumors include:
- An area of underfilling within the gland, owing to ductal compression by the tumor.
- Ductal displacement—the ducts adjacent to the tumor are usually stretched around it, an appearance known as ball in hand.
- Retention of contrast medium in the displaced ducts during the emptying phase.

Interventional Sialography

Conventional sialographic techniques can be supplemented and expanded into minimally invasive interventional procedures by using balloon catheters and small Dormia baskets under fluoroscopic guidance. The balloon catheter, as the name implies, can be inflated once positioned within a duct to produce dilatation of ductal strictures. The Dormia basket may be used to retrieve mobile ductal salivary stones (**Figs 29.5A to D**). Both these procedures are now being used successfully to relieve salivary gland obstruction without the need for surgery.

Ultrasonography (Figs 29.6 and 29.7)

Ultrasonography is a noninvasive and cost-effective imaging modality that can be used in the evaluation of masses, in the salivary glands. Due to their superficial location,

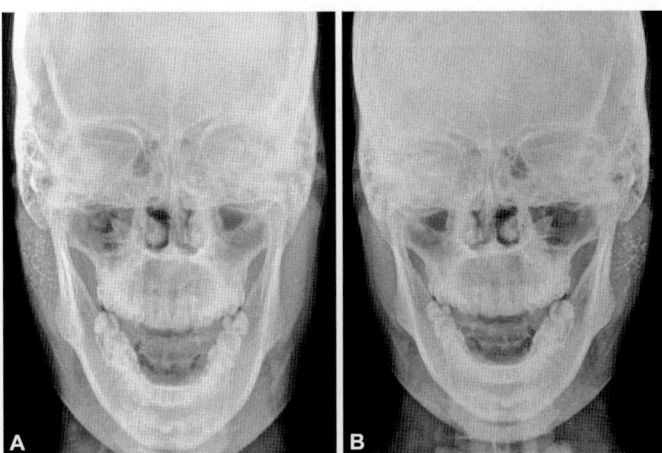

Figures 29.3A and B Sialogram of a right and left parotid gland showing the dots or blobs of contrast medium within the gland—the appearance known as sialectasis, caused by sialadenitis. Note the main duct is normal

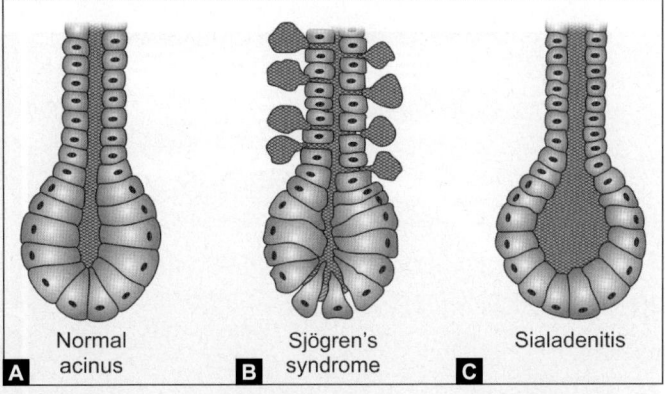

Figures 29.4A to C Diagrams showing an intercalated ductule and acinus: (A) In a normal gland; (B) In Sjögren's syndrome, the epithelium lining the intercalated ductule becomes weakened allowing escape of the contrast medium out of the duct producing the dots or blobs; (C) In sialadenitis, the acinus becomes dilated allowing the collection of contrast into a dot or blob

parotid and submandibular glands are easily visualized by ultrasonography although the deep portion of the parotid gland is difficult to visualize because the mandibular ramus lies over the deep lobe. Ultrasonography is best at differentiating between the intra and extra-glandular masses as well as between cystic and solid lesions.

In general, solid benign lesions present as well circumscribed hypoechoic intraglandular masses.

Ultrasonography can demonstrate the presence of an abscess in an acutely inflamed gland, as well as the presence of sialoliths which appear as echogenic densities that exhibit acoustic shadowing.

Indications

- Discrete and generalized swellings both intrinsic and extrinsic to the salivary glands.
- Salivary obstruction.

Advantages

- Ionizing radiation is not used
- Provides good imaging of superficial masses
- Useful for differentiating between solid and cystic masses and for identifying nature and location of the margins of a lesion

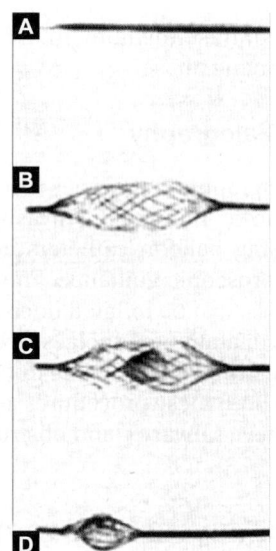

Figures 29.5A to D The meditech (Boston scientific) Dormia basket: (A) Closed for insertion down the main duct and beyond the stone; (B) Open ready to draw back over the stone; (C) Open with the stone inside; (D) Closed around the stone ready for withdrawal back along the duct

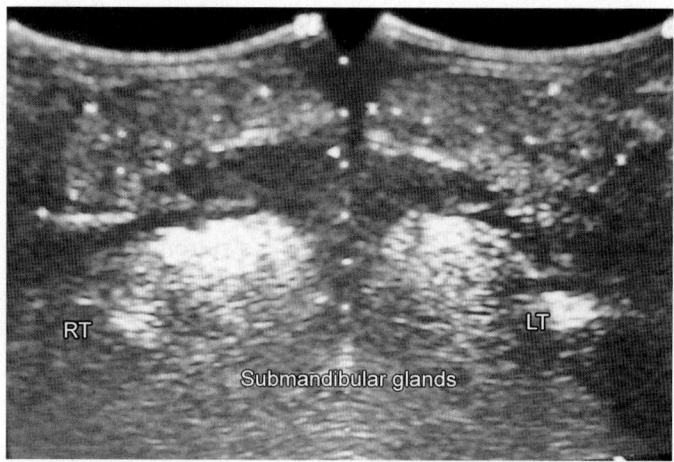

Figure 29.6 An ultrasound scan showing a horse shoe shaped hypoechoic area in the submental region measuring 3.9 × 5 × 1.5 cm extending on either side towards the submandibular glands

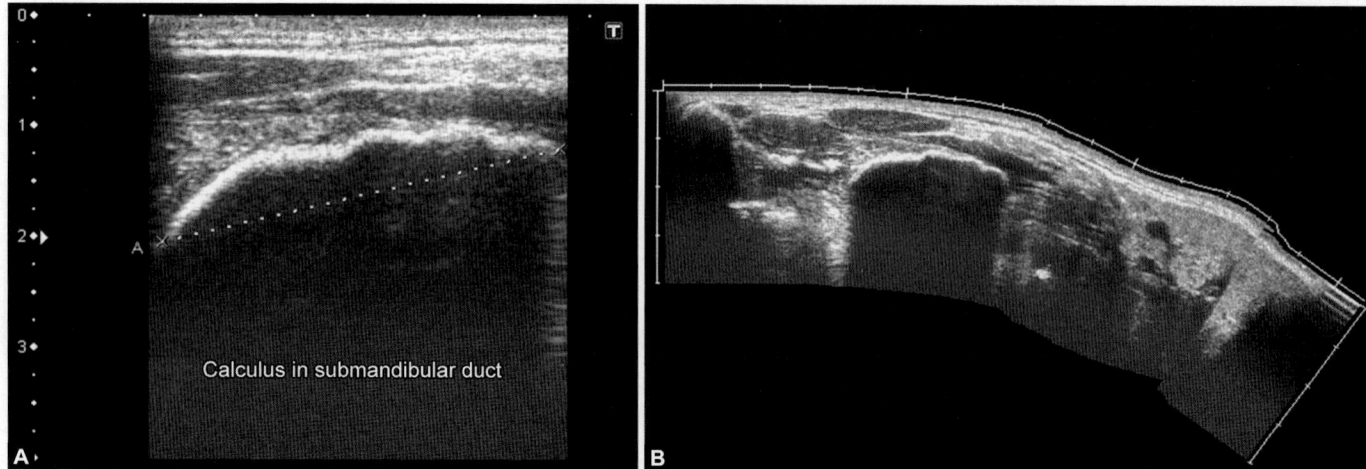

Figures 29.7A and B Ultrasonography of right submandibular gland showing: (A) Length of the sialolith; (B) Calculus in submandibular duct and with normal submandibular gland

- Different echo signals are obtained from different tumors
- Identification of radiolucent stones
- Lithotripsy of salivary stones
- Ultrasound-guided fine-needle aspiration (FNA) biopsy possible
- Intraoral ultrasound possible with small probes.

Disadvantages

- The sound waves used are blocked by bone, so limiting the areas available for investigation.
- Provides no information on fine ductal architecture.

Radionuclide Salivary Imaging

Scintigraphy with technetium Tc 99m pertechnetate is a dynamic and minimally invasive diagnostic test to assess salivary gland function and to determine abnormalities in gland uptake and excretion. This is the only salivary imaging technique that provides information on the functional capabilities of the glands. Technetium is a pure gamma ray emitting radionuclide that is taken up by the salivary glands (following intravenous injection), transported through the glands, and then secreted into the oral cavity. Uptake and secretion phases can be recognized on the scans.

Uptake of Tc 99m by a salivary gland indicates that there is functional epithelial tissue present. The Tc 99m scan can be used as a measure of secretory function as it has been shown to correlate well with salivary output.

Tc 99m is capable of substituting for chloride (Cl⁻) in the sodium-potassium $(Na^+/K^+)/2Cl^-$ salivary transport pump and serves as a measurement of fluid movement in the salivary acinar glands. Duct cells can also accumulate Tc 99m.

Scintigraphy is indicated for evaluation of patients when sialography is contraindicated or cannot be performed (such as in cases of acute gland infection or iodine allergy) or when the major duct cannot be cannulated successfully.

It has also been used to aid in the diagnosis of ductal obstruction, sialolithiasis, gland aplasia, Bell's palsy, and Sjögren's syndrome.

Salivary gland imaging is performed following the injection of 10–20 mCi of Tc 99m pertechnetate. The uptake, concentration and excretion of the pertechnetate anion by the major salivary glands and other organs is imaged with a gamma detector that records both the number and the location of gamma particles released in a given field during a period of time. This information can be stored in a computer for later analysis or recorded directly on film from the gamma detector, to give static images.

Several rating scales exist for the evaluation of salivary scintiscans, however, no standard rating method presently exists. Current approaches to functional assessments include visual interpretation, time activity curve analysis, and numeric indices. A semiquantitative method exists in which Tc 99m uptake and secretion is calculated by the computer analysis of a user-defined region of interest (ROI). Time activity ROI studies are time consuming and are commonly used for research.

Radionuclide imaging can provide information regarding salivary gland function by generating a time activity curve. A normal time activity curve has three phases: flow, concentration and washout.

The flow phase is about 15–20 seconds in duration and represents the phase immediately following injection when the isotope is equilibrating in the blood and accumulating in the salivary gland at a submaximal rate.

The concentration phase represents the accumulation of Tc 99m pertechnetate in the gland through active transport. This phase starts about one minute after administration of the tracer and increases over the next ten minutes. With normal salivary function, tracer activity should be apparent in the oral cavity without stimulation after 10–15 minutes. Approximately 15 minutes after administration, tracer begins to increase in the oral cavity and decrease in the salivary glands. A normal image should demonstrate uptake of Tc 99m by both parotid and submandibular glands and the uptake should be symmetrical.

The last phase is the excretory or washout phase. During this phase, the patient is given a lemon drop, or citric acid is applied to the tongue to stimulate secretion. Normal clearing of Tc 99m should be prompt, uniform and symmetrical. Activity remaining in the salivary gland after stimulation is suggestive of obstruction, certain tumors and inflammation.

With few exceptions, neoplasms arising within the salivary gland do not concentrate Tc 99m. However, Warthin's tumor and oncocytomas, which arise from the ductal tissue, are capable of concentrating the tracer. They retain Tc 99m because they do not communicate with the ductal system, and they appear as areas of increased activity on static images. The difference is accentuated during the washout phase, when normal tissue activity decreases with stimulation and activity is retained in the tumors. Other salivary gland tumors may appear as areas of decreased activity on scintiscans.

Radioisotope Imaging

Indications

- Dry mouth as a result of salivary gland diseases such as Sjögren's syndrome
- To assess salivary gland function
- Positron emission tomography (PET) for salivary gland tumors.

Advantages

- Provides an indication of salivary gland function
- Allows bilateral comparison and images of all four major salivary glands at the same time
- Computer analysis of results is possible

- Can be performed in cases of acute infection
- Co-localization of PET with CT or MRI scans.

Disadvantages

- Provides no indication of salivary gland anatomy or ductal architecture
- Relatively high radiation dose to the whole body
- The final images are not disease-specific.

Flow-Rate Studies

These are used to investigate salivary gland function. Comparative flow rates of saliva from the major salivary glands are measured over a time period.

Indications

- Dry mouth
- Poor salivary flow
- Excess salivation.

Advantages

- Ionizing radiation is not used
- Simple to perform
- Provides information on salivary gland function.

Disadvantages

- Provides only limited information— no indication of the nature of underlying disease
- Time consuming.

Computed Tomography (Fig. 29.8)

Potential neoplasms are better visualized by cross-sectional imaging techniques such as CT or MRI. Computed tomography images are produced by radiographic beams that penetrate the tissues. Computerized analysis of the variance of absorption produces a reconstructed image of the area. Coronal and axial images are usually obtained.

Computed tomography (CT) is useful for evaluating salivary gland pathology, adjacent structures and the proximity of salivary lesions to the facial nerve.

The retromandibular vein, carotid artery and deep lymph nodes can also be noted on CT. Osseous erosions and sclerosis are better visualized by CT than by MRI.

Since calcified structures are better visualized by CT, this modality is especially useful for the evaluation of inflammatory conditions that are associated with sialoliths. Abscesses have a characteristic hyper-vascular wall that is evident in CT imaging.

CT also provides definition of cystic walls, making it possible to distinguish fluid filled masses (i.e. cysts) from abscess.

CT images of salivary glands should be obtained by using continuous cuts through the involved gland. Axial-plane cuts should include the superior aspect of the salivary glands, continuing to the hyoid bone and visualizing potentially enlarged lymph nodes in the supra hyoid neck region.

Dental restorations may interfere with CT imaging and may require repositioning the patient to a semiaxial position.

Nonenhanced and enhanced CT images are routinely obtained. The initial nonenhanced scans are reviewed for the presence of sialoliths, masses, glandular enlargements and/or asymmetrical, nodal involvement, and loss of tissue planes. Glandular damage from chronic diseases often alters the density of salivary glands and makes the identification of the masses more difficult. Contrast enhanced images are more defined and accentuate pathology. Tumors, abscesses and inflamed lymph nodes have abnormal enhancement compared to that of normal structures.

Ultra fast CT and three-dimensional CT sialography have been reported to be an effective method of visualizing masses that are poorly defined on the MRI. Ultra fast CT is also useful for patients who are unable to lie still long enough for MRI (pediatrics, geriatric, claustrophobic and mentally or physically challenged patients) and for patients for whom MRI is contraindicated.

Indication

Discrete swellings both intrinsic and extrinsic to the salivary glands.

Advantages

- Provides accurate localization of masses, especially in the deep lobe of the parotid
- The nature of the lesion can often be determined
- Images can be enhanced by using contrast media, either in the ductal system or more commonly intravenously
- Co-localization possible with PET scans
- CT sialography may be performed.

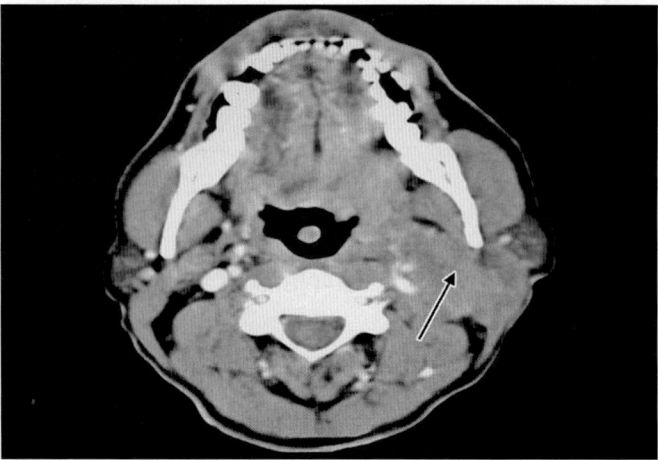

Figure 29.8 Computed tomography axial view showing metastasis to the left parotid space

Disadvantages

- Provides no indication of salivary gland function
- Risks associated with intravenous contrast media if used for enhancement
- Fine duct detail is not well imaged
- Radiation exposure
- Potential scatter from dental restorations.

Magnetic Resonance Imaging (Figs 29.9A to C)

Magnetic resonance imaging (MRI) is also useful for evaluating salivary gland pathology, adjacent structures and the proximity of salivary lesions to the facial nerve. It has become the imaging modality of choice for preoperative evaluation of salivary gland tumors because of its excellent ability to differentiate soft tissues and its ability to provide multiplanar images.

The varying water content of the tissue allows for magnetic resonance imaging to distinguish tissue types. Tissues absorb and then re-emit electromagnetic energy when exposed to a strong electromagnetic field. Analysis of the net magnetization by radiofrequency is reconstructed to provide an image. Images are described as T1 or T2-weighted images, according to the rate constant with which magnetic polarization or relaxation occurs.

In T1-weighted images, the normal parotid gland has greater intensity than muscle and lower intensity than fat or subcutaneous tissue.

In T2-weighted images, the parotid has greater intensity than adjacent muscle and lower intensity than fat.

Structures and conditions that are dark on both T1 and T2-weighted images include calcifications, rapid blood flow, and fibrous tissue.

The use of intravenous MRI contrast can improve imaging and aid in defining neoplastic processes, in specific cases.

Indication

Discrete and generalized swellings both intrinsic and extrinsic to the salivary glands.

Contraindications

- Patients with pacemakers or metallic implants such as aneurysmal bone clips
- Patients who have difficulty in maintaining a still position
- Patients who are claustrophobic and may have difficulty tolerating the MRI procedure, which may result in poor image quality.

Advantages

- Ionizing radiation is not used
- Provides excellent soft tissue detail, readily enables differentiation between normal and abnormal
- No intravenous contrast media is required routinely
- Provides accurate localization of masses
- The facial nerve may be identifiable
- Images in all planes are available
- Co-localization possible with PET scans
- MR sialography may be performed
- There are minimal artifacts from dental restorations.

Disadvantages

- Provides no information on salivary gland function
- Limited information on surrounding hard tissues
- May not distinguish benign lesions with high water content from cysts.

SALIVARY GLAND DISORDERS (TABLE 29.3)

Sialolithiasis (Calculus, Salivary Stone) (Figs 29.10A to E)

Definition

It is the formation of calcific concretions within the parenchyma or ductal system of major or minor salivary glands.

The submandibular (83%) calculi are more common than the parotid (10%) or sublingual (7%), due to the following factors:

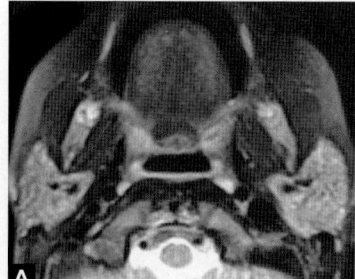 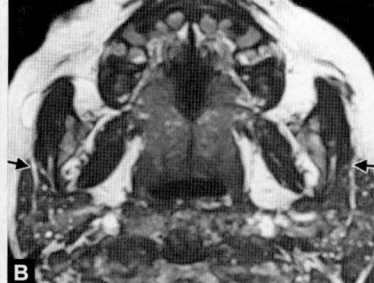 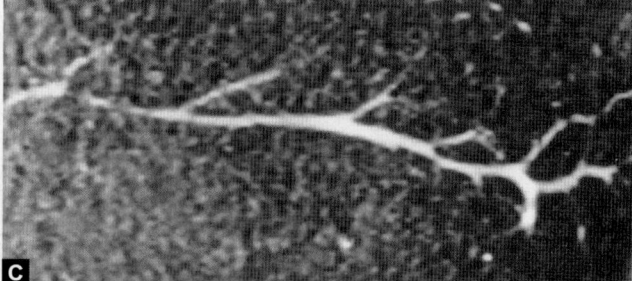

Figures 29.9A to C MRI showing: (A) Axial T2-W (a) Images show enlarged bilateral parotid glands that are of hyperintense signal on T2-W; (B) Hypointense signal shows, multiple intraglandular hyperintense foci. The main parotid duct is normal (Arrow); (C) MR sialogram of the normal parotid gland duct in a healthy volunteer. Main duct and intraglandular ducts are well seen

Table 29.3 Classification of salivary gland disorders

- Developmental disorders
  - Aberrant or ectopic gland
  - Aplasia (Agenesis)
  - Hypoplasia
  - Hyperplasia
  - Atresia (congenital occlusion or absence of one salivary duct)
  - Accessory duct
  - Diverticuli
  - Congenital fistula
- Functional disorders
  - Sialorrhea
  - Xerostomia
- Obstructive disorders
  - Sialolithiasis
  - Mucous plug
  - Stricture and stenosis
  - Foreign bodies
  - Extraductal causes
- Cysts
  - Mucocele
  - Ranula
  - Lymphoepithelial cyst
  - Brachial cyst
- Asymptomatic enlargements
  - Sialosis
  - Allergic
  - Associated with malnutrition and alcoholism
- Infections
  - Viral infection
  - Bacterial infection
  - Mycotic infection
- Autoimmune disorders
  - Sjögren's syndrome
  - Mikulicz's disease
  - Uveoparotid fever
  - Recurrent nonspecific parotitis
- Neoplasms
  Benign but seldom recurrent
  - Warthin's tumor
  - Oncocytoma
  - Monomorphic salivary adenomas
  Benign but often recurrent
  - Pleomorphic adenoma
  - Mucoepidermoid tumor (low grade)
  - Acinic cell tumor
  Malignant
  - Carcinoma in pleomorphic adenoma
  - Adenoid cystic carcinoma (cylindroma)
  - Mucoepidermoid tumor (high grade)
  - Acinic cell tumor
  - Squamous carcinoma
  - Adenocarcinoma
  - Undifferentiated carcinoma

Contd...

Contd...

  Others
  - Lymphomas (Hodgkins and non-Hodgkins)
  - Metastatic tumors
  Others
  - Frey's syndrome (due to injury to auriculo temporal nerve)
  - Melkersson Rosenthal syndrome (sarcoidosis)
  - Postl-irradiation complications
  - Stomatitis nicotina
  - Salivary fistula

Anatomical Factors

- The length and irregular course of the Wharton's duct
- The submandibular gland and the ductal system lies in a dependent position
- The position of the orifice
- The orifice is much smaller than the duct lumen.

Physiological Factors

- High mucin content in saliva
- Great degree of alkalinity with high percentage of organic matter
- Greater concentration of calcium and phosphate salts
- Low content of carbon dioxide
- Richness in phosphatase enzyme.

Clinical Features

- Sialoliths obstruct the secretory ducts, resulting in chronic retrograde infection, due to decreased salivary flow
- There may be intermittent swelling and pain when eating
- *Signs of infection*: Inflammation, tenderness and sometimes pus exudates
- Sometimes there may be no signs or symptoms and may be discovered on a routine radiographic examination.

Radiographic Features

- Depending on the degree of calcification the sialolith may appear radiopaque or radiolucent. When visible they usually have a homogeneous radiopaque internal structure.
- Sialolith vary in shape from long cigar shapes to oval or round shape, with smooth borders.
- It may vary in size from a little more than a pin head to a length of an inch or more, with a girth of about 5 mm.
- It may be solitary or multiple.
- Sialography is useful in detecting obstructions that are not visible on plain radiographs. The contrast agent usually flows around the sialolith, filling the duct proximal to the obstruction.

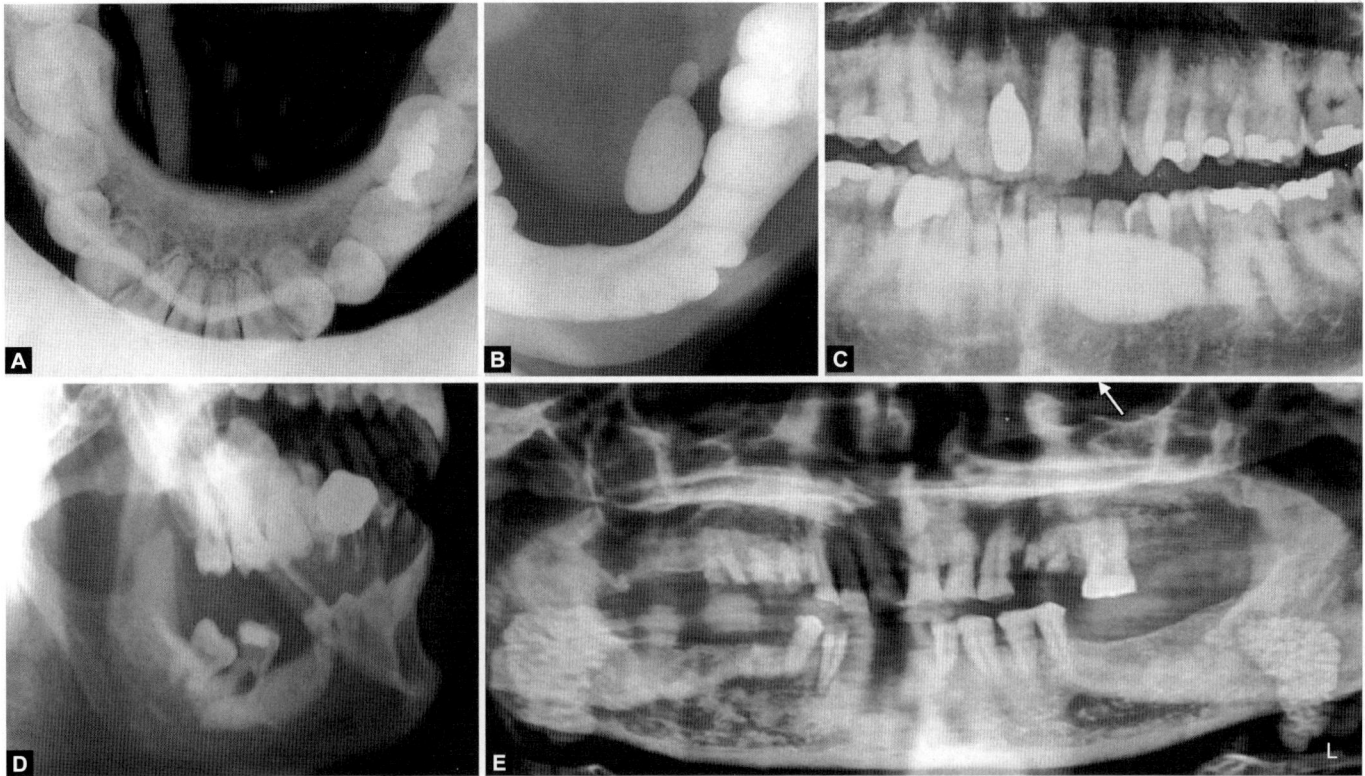

Figures 29.10A to E Sialoliths: (A) Mandibular occlusal radiograph showing a well-defined cylindrical radiopacity seen extending from first premolar posteriorly upto the distal of first molar; (B) Mandibular occlusal showing well-defined radiopacity near lower left premolars and molars; (C) Panoramic radiograph shows superimposition of the shadow on the lower left premolars and molars; (D) Lateral oblique showing a large sialolith; (E) Panoramic radiograph showing Sialothiasis of left submandibular gland; two large cauliflower like radiopacities in mandibular angle region bilaterally, consisting of smaller clusters of multiple ill-defined radiopacities. The right one is the ghost image of the left one

- The ductal system is usually dilated proximal to the obstruction and infers the presence of an obstruction even when it is not visible.
- Sometimes the contrast agent may be more radiopaque and may obscure the small sialolith.
- Radiolucent sialoliths appear as ductal filling defects.
- Computed tomography (CT) may help to detect minimally calcified sialoliths not detected on plain films.
- Ultrasonography (USG) though having a limited value in diagnosing inflammatory and obstructive cases, has recently shown to be fairly reliable in demonstrating sialoliths. The larger stones are detected as echo-dense spots with characteristic acoustic shadows.

Differential Diagnosis

- *Gas bubbles*: Which may be introduced during sialography are more easily removed and are more circular in shape.
- *Hyoid bone*: This is seen bilaterally on the panoramic film.
- *Myositis ossificans*: Here there is restriction of the mandibular movements.

- *Phleboliths*: There will be no sialadenitis. These are more or less rounded and contain laminations or central dark (radiolucent) area.
- *Calcific submandibular lymph nodes*: If painful swelling accompanies the calcified mass it is usually a sialolith. The calcified lymph nodes are usually cauliflower shaped.
- *Palatine tonsillolith*: On a panoramic image these have a similar location as parotid sialoliths, superimposed over the ramus, but can be differentiated in that they are typically multiple and punctate.
- *Chondrodystrophia calcificans congenita*: This is sometimes associated with calcification in the neck which may resemble the submaxillary calculi in radiographs.

Management

Treatment of sialolithiasis may be encouraged with spontaneous discharge through use of sialogogues to stimulate secretions. Sialography (oil-based contrast) may also stimulate discharge. Sometimes surgical removal may be indicated.

Bacterial Sialadenitis (Parotitis) (Figs 29.11 and 29.12)

Definition

This is an acute or chronic bacterial infection of the terminal acini or parenchyma of the salivary glands.

Clinical Features

Acute bacterial infections:
- These most commonly affect the parotid gland
- Most cases are unilateral

- It may occur at any age, but those commonly affected are:
  - Older adults
  - Postoperative patients
  - Debilitated patients who have poor oral hygiene as a result of reduced salivary secretion and retrograde infection by the oral flora (usually *Staphylococcus aureus* and *S. viridans*).
  - Reduced salivary secretion may also be drug related or secondary to occlusion of a major duct.
- The patient will present with swelling, redness, tenderness and malaise

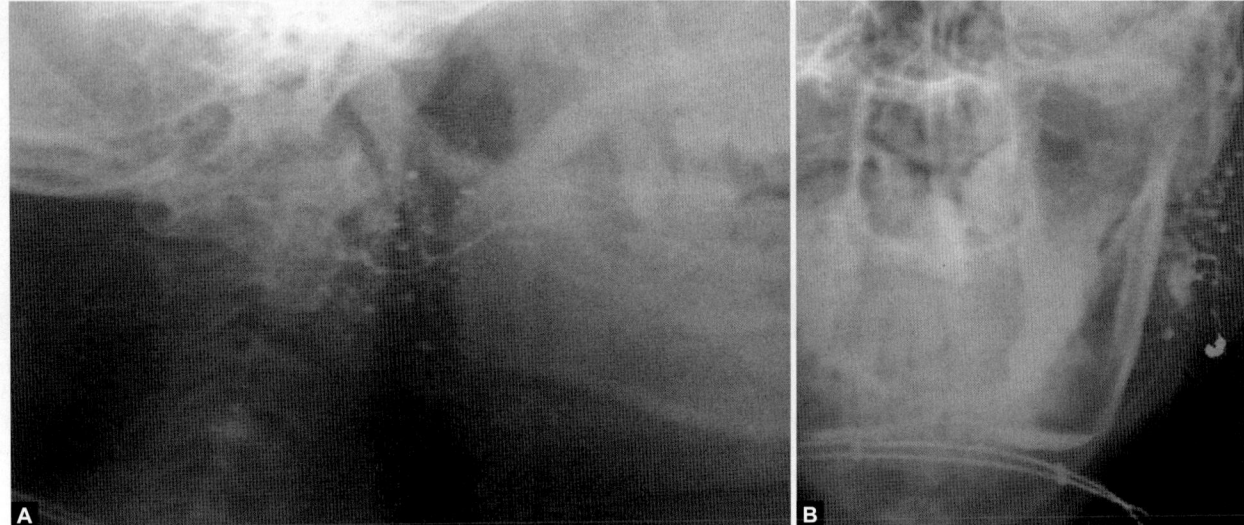

Figures 29.11A and B Chronic sialadenitis: Sialography of right parotid gland showed a cherry blossom appearance of the acini in lateral and cheek blow out PA view of mandible

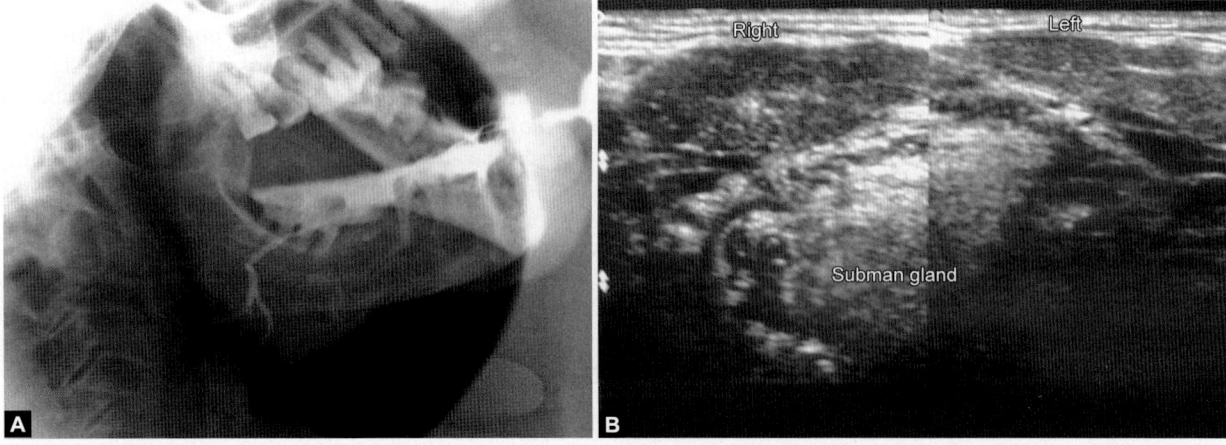

Figures 29.12A and B Sialadenitis: (A) Sialography-showed normal ductal pattern; (B) USG-Rt submandibuar gland is bulky, however normal in position and axis. It shows altered echo texture and decreased echogenecity. There is mild increased vascularity. Few internal echoes are seen in the right submandibuar gland. Rt submandibular gland measures 3.3 × 1.8 × 1.2 cm. Evidence of few lymph nodes are seen in the Rt submandibuar gland

• Enlarged regional lymph nodes and suppuration may be present
• Untreated acute suppurative infections may form abscesses.

Chronic Bacterial Infections

• This may affect any of the major salivary glands, causing extensive swelling and culminating in fibrosis. The parotid is most often involved
• It may be due to an untreated acute sialadenitis or associated with some type of obstruction resulting from sialolithiasis, noncalcified organic debris, or strictures (scar or fibrosis) formation in the excretory ducts.
• The obstruction may be due to congenital or secondary to trauma, infection or neoplasia.
• During periods of painful swelling, pus may be expressed from the ductal orifice and salivary stimulation may cause pain.
• Pain and swelling may be typically associated with eating.
• Advanced sialadenitis may be present in combination with sialolithiasis, sialodochitis, abscess formation and fistula.

Radiographic Features

• Sialography is contraindicated in acute cases but may be carried out in suspected chronic infections.
• Sialectasia (epithelial flattening leading to mildly dilated terminal ducts and sac like acini) are demonstrated with sialography.
• If connected to the ductal system, abscess cavities:
  – May fill with contrast media during sialography.
  – On the CT they appear as walled off areas of lower attenuation within an enlarged gland.
  – Ultrasonography (USG) may also demonstrate abscess cavities.
• Ultrasonography (USG) may help distinguish between diffuse inflammation (echo-free light image) and suppuration (less echo-free darker image).
• Contrast-enhanced CT may demonstrate glandular enlargements.
• Magnetic resonance imaging (MRI) shows inflamed glands (localized abscess) at a lower tissue signal on T1-weighted images, and higher signal on T2-weighted images than that of the surrounding muscle, diffuse or localized abscess may also show low signal depending on whether edema or cellular infiltration dominates. T1-weighted post GdMRI shows moderate diffuse contrast enhancement or only enhanced peripheral rim (abscess).

Management

Treatment begins with attention to oral hygiene, increased fluid intake, use of oral sialogogues (sour citrus fruit wedges or salivary stimulants), and an appropriate antibiotic regimen.

Sialodochitis (Ductal Sialadenitis)

Definition

This is an inflammation of the ductal system of the salivary glands.

Clinical Features

This is common in both parotid and submandibular gland.

Radiographic Features

• Dilatation of the ductal system is a prominent sialographic presentation.
• If interstitial fibrosis develops, it is apparent in sialograms as sausage-string appearance of the main duct and its major branches produced by alternative strictures and dilatations.
• Similar changes can be detected on a thin section MRI.
• MRI sialography can be done with heavily T2 weighted images without injection of contrast medium. This visualizes the main parotid duct and submandibular duct with secondary ducts but not finer ducts as seen with conventional sialography. However MR sialography may be useful in cases in which cannulation of the duct cannot be performed.

Management

The treatment is the same as that for sialadenitis.

Autoimmune Sialadenitis (Myoepithelial Sialadenitis, Sjögren's Syndrome, Benign Lymphoepithelial Lesion, Mikulicz Disease, Sicca Syndrome, Autoimmune Sialosis) (Figs 29.13A to C)

Definition

These are a group of disorders that affect the salivary glands and share an autosensitivity. The range of clinical and histopathologic manifestations suggests that these disorders represent different developmental stages of the same immunologic mechanisms, differing only in the extent and intensity of tissue reaction.

Clinical Features

• The disease is more common in adults, occurring primarily in the 40–60 age group, with a more female prevalence.
• A presumptive diagnosis may be made on the basis of any two of the three features: dry mouth, dry eyes and rheumatoid disease.
• In this disorder there is gradual cavitation and fibrosis as a result of recurrent inflammation.
• There may be recurrent painless swelling of the salivary glands (more commonly the parotid) which may also cause enlargement of the lacrimal glands.

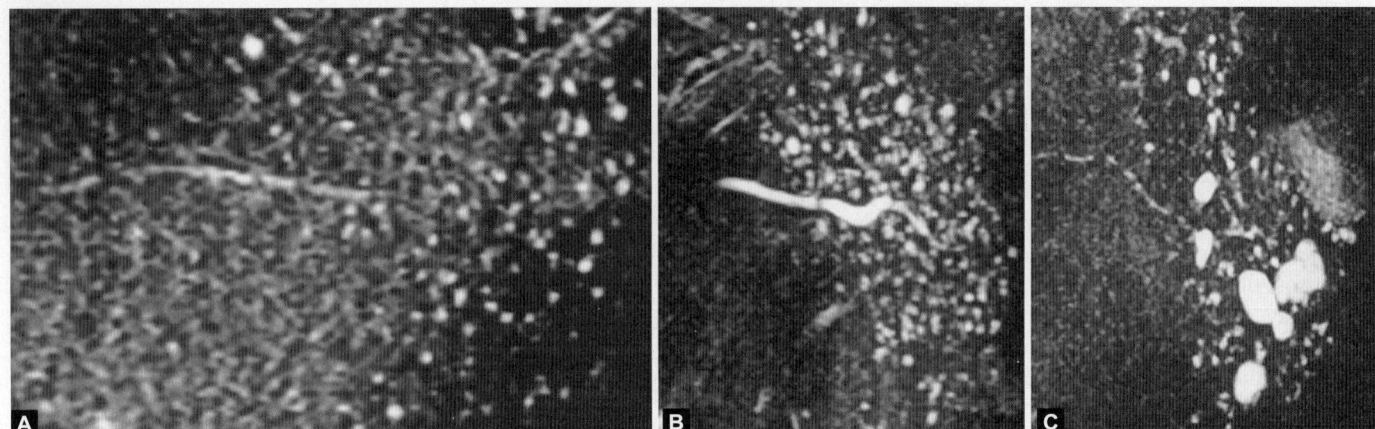

Figures 29.13A to C MRI showing ductal pattern in Sjögren syndrome: (A) Diffuse areas of punctate high signal intensity 1 mm or less in diameter are distributed throughout the duct (stage 1, punctate appearance); (B and C) Areas of spherical high signal intensity 1–2 mm in diameter are evident (stage 2, globular appearance)

- Glandular swelling may be accompanied by xerostomia and xerophthalmia (primary Sjögren's syndrome).
- This may progress to produce a connective tissue disease like arthritis, progressive systemic sclerosis, systemic lupus erythematosus, or polymyositis (secondary Sjögren's syndrome).
- The process may progress to benign lymphoepithelial lesions that may assume the proportions of a tumor.

Radiographic Features

- Sialography is helpful in the diagnosis and staging of autoimmune disorders.
- Sialectases are seen in the early stages as punctate (less than 1 mm) and globular (1–2 mm) spherical collections of contrast agent evenly distributed throughout the glands. The main duct may appear to be normal but intraglandular ducts may be narrowed or not evident. Sialectasia remains after administration of a sialogogue, which is indication that the contrast agent is pooled extraductally.
- *Cavitary sialectases*: As the disease progresses the collections of contrast increase in size (greater than 2 mm in diameter) and are irregular in shape. These larger sialectases are fewer in number and less uniformly distributed throughout the gland.
- Progressively larger cavities of the contrast agent and dilatation of the main ductal system may also be present.
- At the end point of the disorder, there is complete destruction of the gland.
- CT and MRI images are normal in early stage of the disease.
- T1-weighted MRI images show multiple punctate changes of low density uniformly distributed in the gland as the earliest sign, diagnostic for Sjögrens syndrome.
- T2-weighted MRI shows multiple punctate changes with high signal reflecting watery saliva. The punctate

changes will progress to globules, cavitary and destructive abnormalities. At the end stage a honey comb appearance may develop with multiple cystic lesions and abnormally dense parenchyma.
- MR sialography has been found to correlate with conventional sialography and with labial biopsy findings.

Differential Diagnosis

- Chronic bacterial or granulomatous infections
- Multiple parotid cysts associated with HIV infection; diffuse cervical lymphadenopathy is common in HIV disease, which is uncommon in Sjögren's syndrome.

Management

Treatment is directed towards relief of symptoms.

Sialadenosis (Sialosis)

Definition

This is a non-neoplastic, noninflammatory enlargement of primarily the parotid salivary gland. It is usually related to metabolic and secretory disorders of the parenchyma associated with diseases of nearly all the endocrinal glands (hormonal sialadenosis), protein deficiencies, malnutrition in alcoholics (dystrophic metabolic sialadenoses), vitamin deficiencies and neurologic disorders (neurogenic sialadenoses).

Clinical Feature

Affected glands are typically enlarged.

Radiographic Features

- Sialography may demonstrate enlargement of the affected gland or a normal appearance

- In enlarged glands the ducts will be splayed
- CT and MRI provide a more straight forward depiction of the glands, but are nonspecific and require correlation with the clinical findings and history.

Management

Treatment depends on identifying the etiology and correcting the deficiency.

Cystic Lesions (Fig. 29.14)

Definition

Cysts of the salivary glands most commonly occur unilaterally in the parotid gland. They may be congenital (brachial), lymphoepithelial, dermoid, or acquired, including mucous retention cysts (obstructions with any etiology).

Clinical Features

- Cystic salivary lesions may be intraglandular or extra-glandular in nature.
- Mucous-extravasation pseudocysts lack an epithelial lining and result from ductal rupture.
- Ranulas are retention cysts which usually occur secondary to obstruction of sublingual duct.
- Benign lymphoepithelial cysts are believed to be sequelae of cystic degeneration of salivary inclusions within lymph nodes.
- Multicentric parotid cysts are often associated with HIV, are usually in the superficial portion of the gland. These

are accompanied by bilateral lymphadenopathy, and secondary parotitis may develop.

Radiographic Features

- Cystic masses are indirectly visualized by displacement of the ducts arching around them.
- These lesions appear as well-circumscribed, nonenhancing (with contrast), low density areas when examined on CT.
- T1-weighted images show low signal.
- They appear as well-circumscribed, high-signal areas (cyst) on T2-weighted MRI, but do not enhance after gadolinium contrast (as do benign mixed tumors).
- T1-weighted post Gd MRI shows rim enhancement of cysts and heterogenous or homogeneous enhancement of the solid masses.
- On the USG they appear as sharply marginated and echo free (dark) areas.

Differential Diagnosis

- The cystic lesions may progress to such proportions that are clinically palpable and must be distinguished from neoplasia.
- Vascular lesion—may be differentiated from superficial nonkeratin cyst by aspiration.
- Early mucoepidermoid tumor and adenocarcinoma—induration is present.
- Sublingual dermoid—is more often in the midline and not translucent and may be differentiated from ranula which is translucent.
- Submandibular lymph nodes—are hard and firm in consistency.

Management

Treatment is surgical removal of the cyst or total excision of the gland.

Benign Tumors (Table 29.4)

Definition

Neoplasms arise both in major and minor salivary glands.

Clinical Features

- Salivary gland tumors are relatively uncommon
- The parotid is the most common involved gland
- Most of the tumors occur in the superficial portion of the gland
- Most of lesions are benign or low grade malignancies.

Radiographic Features

- Most of the benign or low grade malignancies have a well-defined margin which is observed well on CT or MRI examinations.

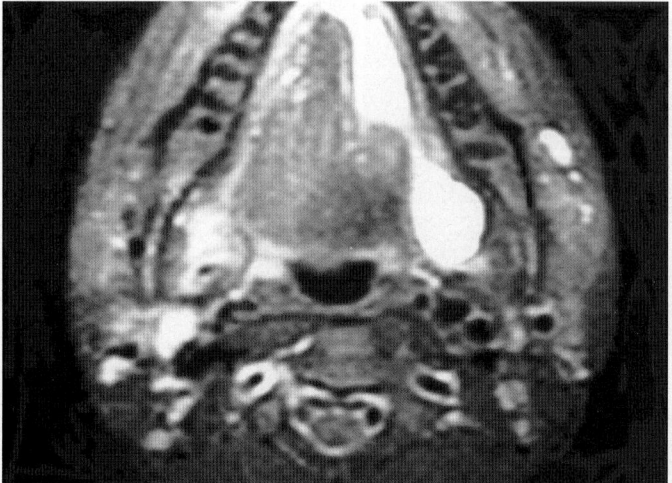

Figure 29.14 T2 weighted MRI image—contrast material in the submandibular gland and extending into the Wharton's duct MRI showing cystic lesion of about 6.3 x 2 cm in the region of the right submandibular duct involving the duct. It extends from the gland to the opening of the duct. No focal obstructive lesion is seen in the duct. The submandibular gland appears normal. Final diagnosis; Ranula or mucous retention cyst of the submandibular duct

Table 29.4 WHO classification of salivary gland tumors

- Epithelial tumors
  - Adenoma
    - Pleomorphic adenoma
    - Monomorphic adenoma
    - Adenolymphoma
    - Oxyphilic adenomas
    - Other types
  - Mucoepidermoid tumor
  - Acinic cell tumor
  - Carcinoma
    - Adenoid cystic carcinoma
    - Adenocarcinoma
    - Epidermoid carcinoma
    - Undifferentiated carcinoma
    - Carcinoma in pleomorphic adenoma
- Nonepithelial tumors
- Unclassified tumors
- Allied conditions
  - Benign lymphoepithelial lesion
  - Sialosis
  - Oncocytosis

- In case of the submandibular gland which has higher or equal density as that of the neoplasm, and may thus obscure the tumor an intravenous contrast enhancement is required during the CT examination, which makes the tumor more radiopaque as the vascularity of the tumor is greater than the adjacent salivary gland tissue.
- In the USG examination the benign masses are typically sharply defined, less echogenic than parenchyma, and essentially of homogenous echo strength and density.
- Benign tumors may present as low intensity (dark) and high intensity (light) tissue signals on MRI. The relative intensity of the signal may indicate the presence of lipid, vascular or fibrous tissues.
- Sialography may suggest a space occupying lesion when the ducts are compressed or smoothly displaced around the lesion (the ball-in-hand appearance).

Differential Diagnosis

- The following tumors are firm on palpation
  - Pleomorphic adenoma
  - Adenoid cystic carcinoma

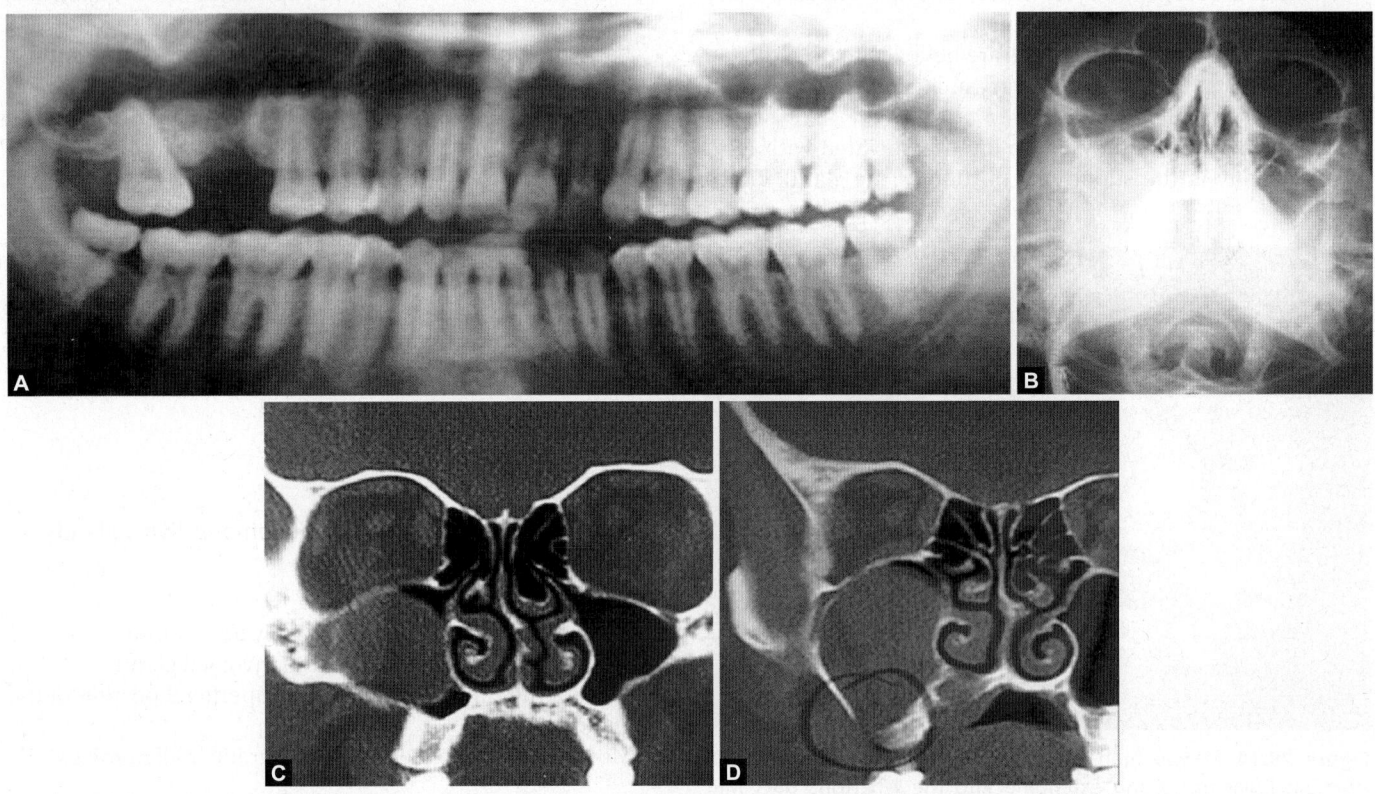

Figures 29.15A to D Pleomorphic adenoma of the palate: (A) Panoramic view revealed a solitary unilocular well-defined radiolucency in the right maxilla extending from the alveolar margin of first premolar region to the inferior border of the sinus and mesiodistally from first premolar to second molar; (B) PA Water's view showed haziness in the right maxillary sinus indicative of a large soft swelling with a convex superior border; (C and D) CT scan revealed a focal cystic lesion measuring 4.2 × 2.5 cm in coronal dimensions projecting into the right maxillary sinus. Discontinuity is seen in the right maxillary alveolar bone and the inferior wall of the maxillary sinus

– Carcinoma in pleomorphic adenoma
– Acinic cell carcinoma
– Oncocytoma
• The following tumors are soft on palpation
– Well-differentiated mucoepidermoid tumor
– Papillary cyst adenoma
– Mucous producing adenocarcinoma
– Warthin's tumor.

Management

Treatment is usually surgical.

Benign Mixed Tumor (Pleomorphic Adenoma) (Figs 29.15 to 29.20)

Definition

The benign mixed tumor is a neoplasm arising from the ductal epithelium of major and minor salivary glands exhibiting epithelial and mesenchymal components.

Clinical Features

• These account for 75% of all salivary gland tumors
• 80% of which are found in the parotid gland
• They usually occur in the fifth decade of life as a slow growing, unilateral, encapsulated, asymptomatic mass
• There is a slight female predilection
• Recurrence rate is nearly 50% of cases after excision.

Radiographic Features

• CT presents a sharply circumscribed, infrequently lobulated, round homogeneous lesion that has a higher density than the adjacent glandular tissue.
• Calcifications in the tumors are well-depicted on the CT.
• On the MRI the tumor shows various signals depending on the technique:
– Relatively low (dark) in T1-weighted images
– Intermediate on proton density weighted images

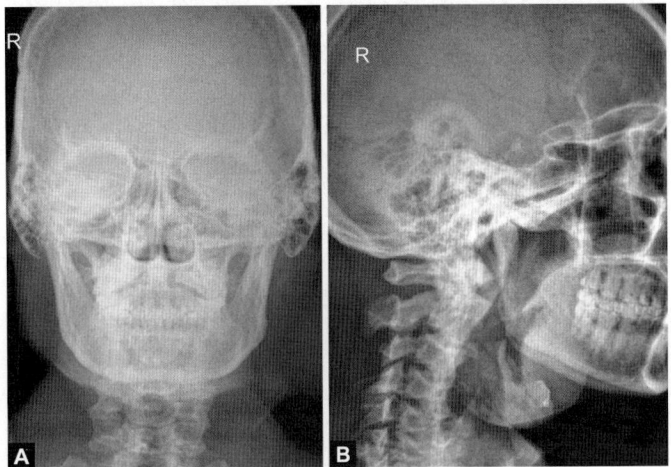

Figures 29.16A and B Pleomorphic adenoma: (A) PA skull; (B) Lateral cephalogram showing soft tissue swelling

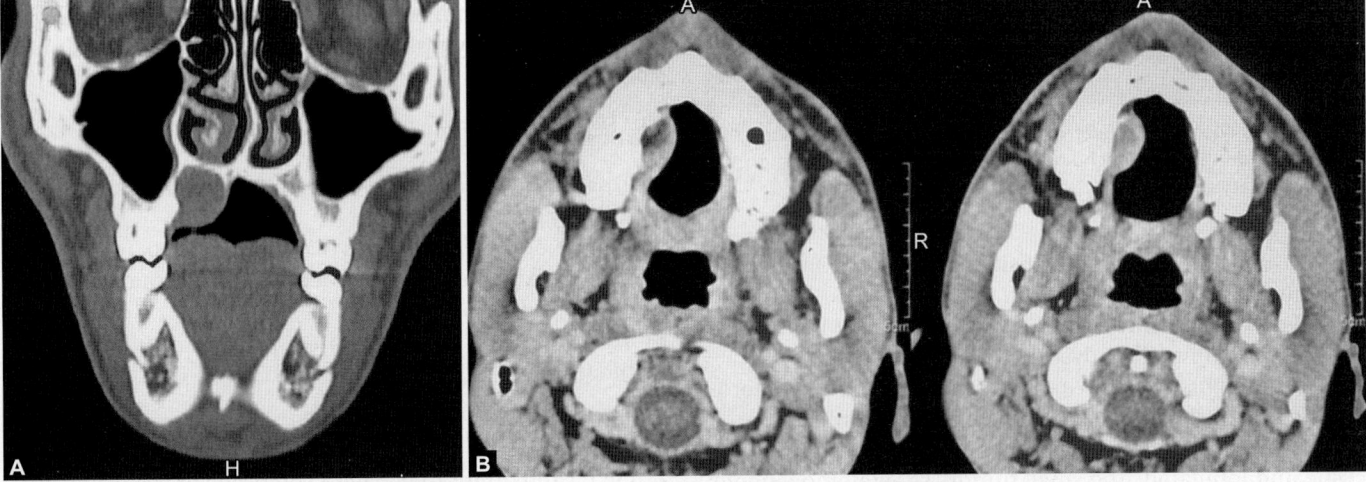

Figures 29.17A and B Pleomorphic adenoma CT reveals a 2.1 × 2 cm well-defined enhancing soft tissue lesion in relation to right half of the soft palate. It is causing attenuation, scalloping of adjacent portion of the hard palate. Anteriorly and laterally it is reaching up to right maxillary alveolus ridge. Posteriorly reaching up to the soft palate, and medially just short of the midline. Diagnosis; salivary gland neoplasm, proved to be pleomorphic adenoma on biopsy

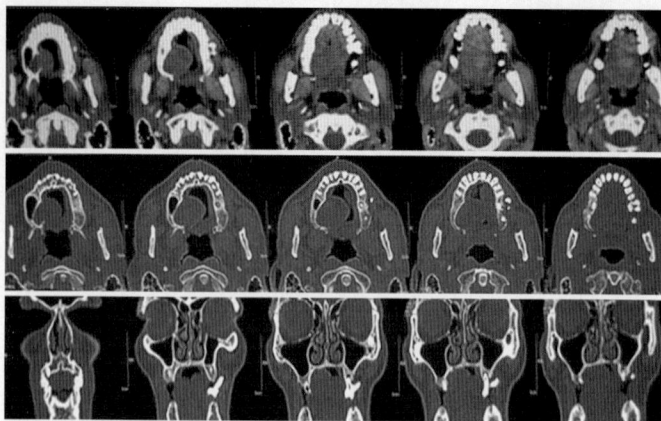

Figure 29.18 Pleomorphic adenoma: CT scan shows a fairy well circumscribed lobulated enhancing mass 4 × 3 cm is seen overlying the hard palate and protruding in to the oral cavity. Scalloping of hard palate and superior alveolus seen

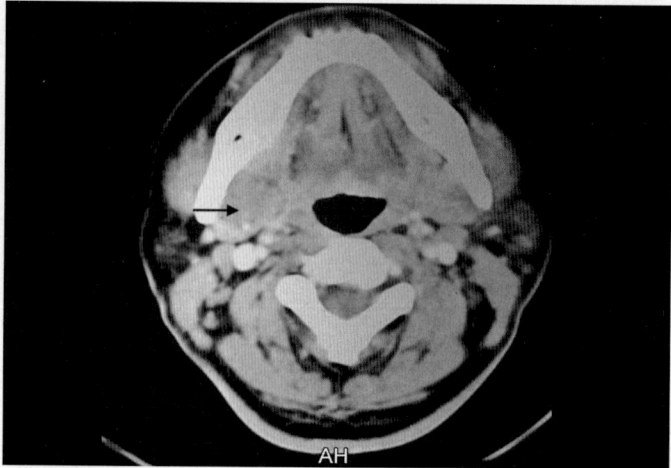

Figure 29.20 Pleomorphic adenoma: CT scan—enlarged right submandibular gland with mild heterogeneous enhancement

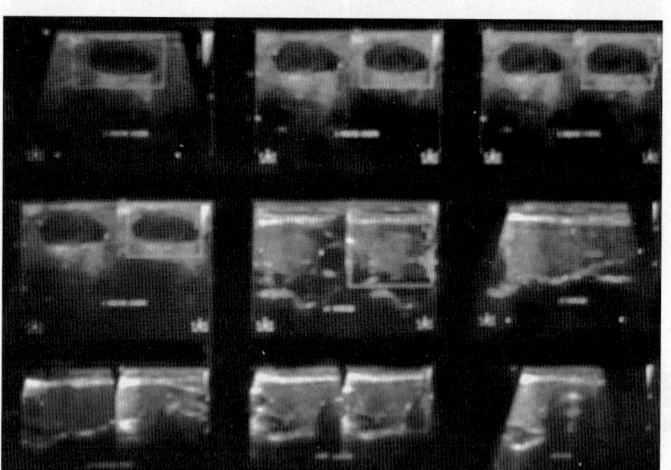

Figure 29.19 Pleomorphic adenoma of parotid gland. Ultrasonography shows well-defined hypoechoic area in the left parotid region s/o benign salivary gland tumor

- Homogeneous high intensity (bright) on T2 weighted images
- Foci of low intensity (dark area) usually represents areas of fibrosis or dystrophic calcifications
- T1-weighted post Gd MRI shows variable heterogeneously mild to moderate enhancement.

It is seen as a well-defined mass of highly variable size, cystic and lobulated. The small tumors show homogeneous enhancement, large lobulated tumors show heterogeneous enhancement. Some calcifications may also be seen.

On scintigraphy examination, as the tumor does not concentrate 99mTc-pertechnetate, it appears as a cold spot. Solid tumors larger than 5 mm are well visualized.

Differential Diagnosis

Other parotid masses—If on the MRI a calcification is present (signal void) the diagnosis favors a mixed benign tumor, otherwise it is difficult to differentiate this tumor from other parotid masses.

Warthin Tumor (Papillary Cystadenoma Lymphomatosum) (Figs 29.21A to C)

Definition

This is a benign tumor arising from proliferating salivary ducts trapped in lymph nodes during embryogenesis of the salivary glands.

Clinical Features

- This is the second most common benign lesion of the salivary glands.
- It more often affects males over the age of 40.
- Two to six percent of these occur in the parotid, usually in the inferior lobe.
- This tumor is slow growing, painless and frequently bilateral.

Radiographic Features

- On CT the tumor may have a soft tissue or cystic density.
- On the MRI it is heterogeneous and may demonstrate hemorrhagic foci.
- On 99m Tc-pertechnetate scans it appears intensely hot.
- The USG shows a solid mass (hypoechoic), unless the tumor happens to be cystic in nature.

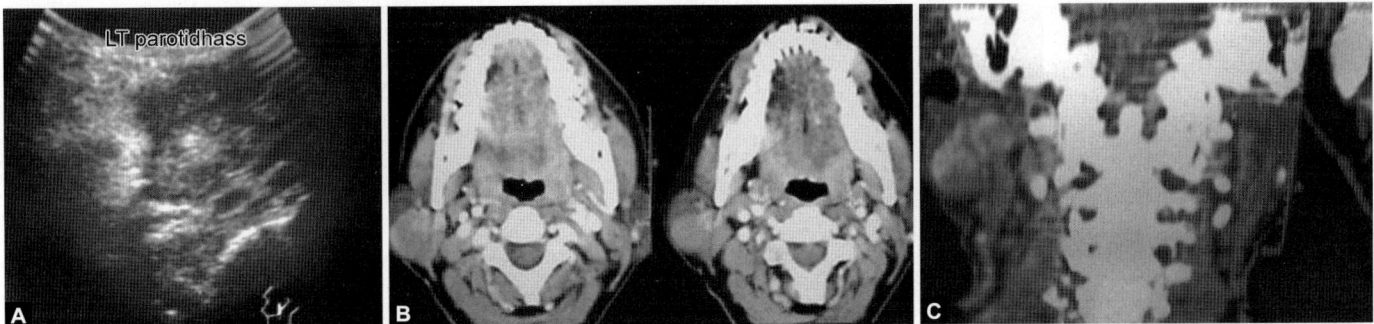

Figures 29.21A to C Warthin's tumor: (A) Ultrasonography reported a 3.6 × 2.7 sized lobulated hypoechoic lesion with internal echoes, noted behind the angle of mandible on the right side in the parotid gland. CT scan: (B) Axial; (C) Coronal view reported a well-defined is to hyperdense mass in superficial and deep part of right parotid gland with bilateral level I and level II lymphadenopathy

Differential Diagnosis

Oncocytoma (oxyphilic adenoma)—may also accumulate the 99m Tc-pertechnetate but are uncommon and less likely to be bilateral, and in the over 70 years age group.

Hemangioma (Vascular Nevus)

Definition

This is a benign neoplasm of proliferating endothelial cells (congenital hemangioma) and vascular malformations, including lesions resulting from abnormal vessel morphologies.

Clinical Features

- It is one of the most frequently occuring nonepithelial neoplasm in over 50% of the cases
- Eighty five percent arise in the parotid gland
- It is more common in infancy and childhood. And has a female predilection
- They usually occur unilaterally and are asymptomatic
- Phleboliths are common in this tumor.

Radiographic Features

- On sialography, displaced ducts curving around the mass are apparent.
- The CT shows the hemangioma as a soft tissue mass that is well-distinguished from the surrounding tissue, especially when intravenous contrast is used.
- The soft tissue mass, is frequently lobulated, isodense to muscle, contrast enhancing. It may be unilateral or bilateral, single or multiple. On MRI, the tumor has a similar signal as adjacent muscle on T1-weighted images and a very high signal on T2-weighted images. T1 post Gd MRI shows intense contrast enhancement.
- Ultrasonography (USG) demonstrates well-defined margins in hemangiomas. A strongly hypoechoic he-

mangioma may have a complex USG appearance, resulting from multiple interfaces of the lesion.
- Phleboliths image as multiple hyperechoic areas within the body of the parotid on the USG. They are best identified on plain films and CT where they appear as calculi with a radiolucent center.

Management

Treatment is local excision for those that do not undergo spontaneous remission.

Malignant Tumors (Figs 29.22A to H)

Definition

Sublingual tumors (90%) are more prone to malignant changes, followed by minor salivary glands (60–75%), submandibular (50–60%) and parotid (20%).

Clinical staging of salivary gland tumors:
- *By spiro*
    - T1—0 to 3 cm, solitary and freely mobile, CRVII intact.
    - T2—3.1 to 6 cm, solitary and freely mobile or skin fixed, CRVII intact.
    - T3—6 cm, or multiple nodes or ulceration or deep fixation or CRVII dysfunction.
    - Patients with T1 and T2 lesion are placed in Stage I and II respectively.
    - Any patient with clinical evidence of metastases to lymph nodes or with T3 lesion is considered Stage III.
- By American Joint Committee
    Primary tumor (T)
    - Tx—Tumor that cannot be assessed by the rules.
    - T0—No evidence of primary tumor.
    - T1—Tumor 2 cm or less in diameter without significant local extension.
    - T2—Tumor 2-4 cm in diameter without significant local extension.

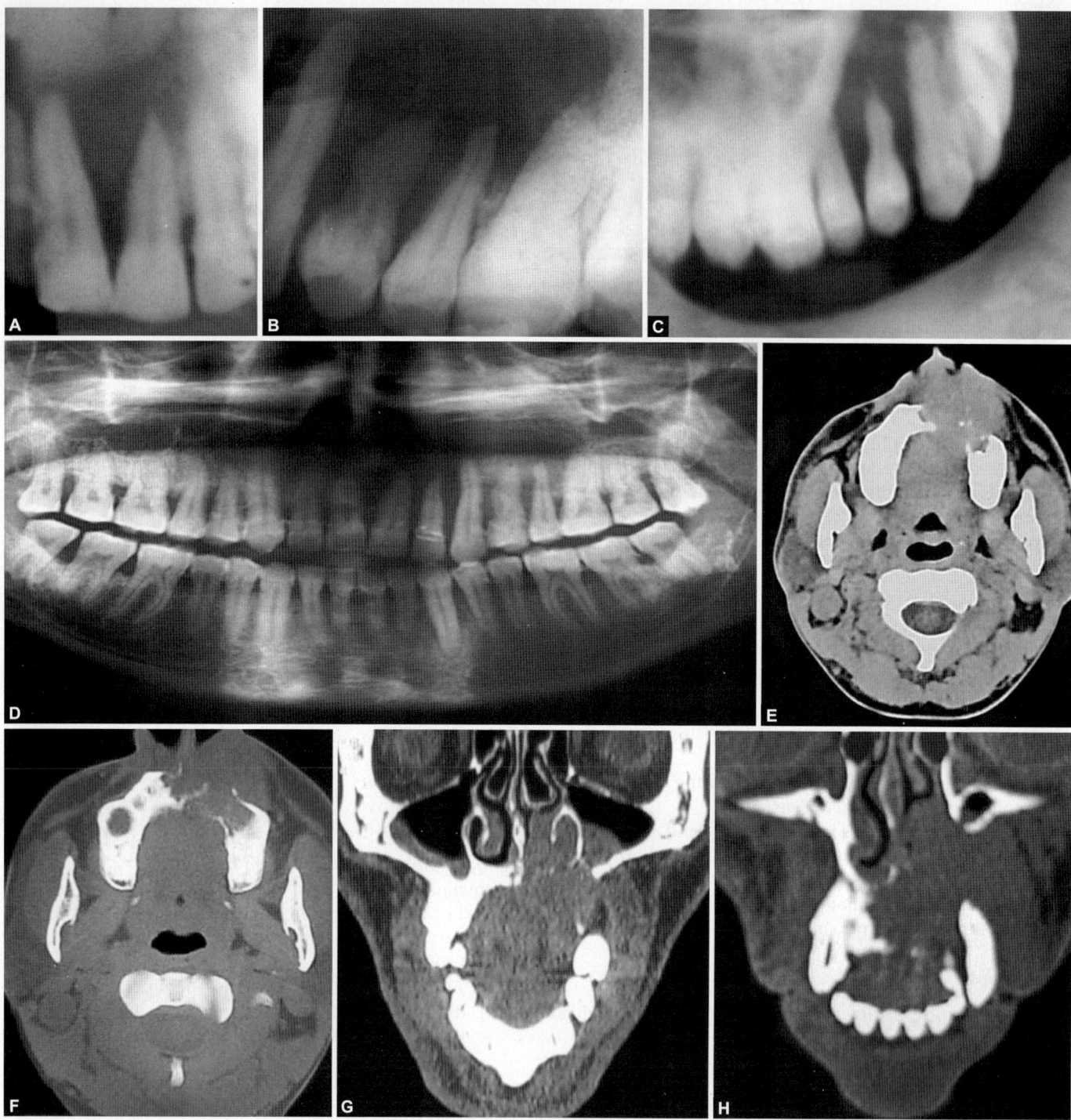

Figures 29.22A to H Salivary duct carcinoma: (A and B) Periapical radiographs; (C) Occlusal radiograph showed ill-defined osteolytic lesion extending till maxillary left second premolar region with spiked root resorption of the first premolar; (D) Panoramic radiograph showed ill-defined osteolytic defect extending from periapical region of right premolar region to anterior teeth with floating tooth appearance. Anterior wall and floor of the maxillary sinus are not traceable. Shadow of the hard palate is discontinuous in the center. Lateral root resorption of the upper left premolars present giving a spiked appearance to the roots. CT scan: (E and F) Axial view soft and bone window; (G and H) Coronal soft tissue and bone window showed an 3.7 × 3.5 cm expansile lytic lesion with adjacent soft tissue component extending from incisors to premolar region. Destruction of both the buccal and lingual cortices, anterior left half of the hard palate, floor and lateral wall of left nasal cavity and floor of the left maxillary sinus. Soft tissue extension present in the nasal vestibule and the maxillary sinus. Loosening of left incisors, canine and premolars seen. Bilateral level 5 lymph nodes were visualized

- T3—Tumor more than 4 cm but not more than 6 cm in diameter without significant local extension.
- T4a—Tumor over 6 cm in diameter without significant local extension.
- T4b—Tumor of any size with significant local extension.

Nodal Involvement (N)

- Nx—Regional lymph node cannot be assessed
- No—No regional lymph node metastasis
- N1—Clinical or histologically positive regional lymph node.

Distant Metastasis (M)

- Mx—Distant metastasis cannot be assessed
- Mo—No distant metastasis
- M1—Distant metastasis.

Stage grouping is performed as follows:
- Stage I — T1 NO MO or T2 NO MO
- Stage II — T3 NO MO
- Stage III — T1 or T2 N1 MO or T4a or T4b NO MO
- Stage IV — T4 N1 MO , T4a or T4b N1 MO, any T any N M1.

Radiographic Features

- The radiographic presentation is variable depending on the grade, aggressiveness, location and type of tumor.
- They, however, have some of the general features like ill-defined margins, invasion of adjacent soft tissues (fat spaces), and destruction of adjacent osseous structures.

Management

Treatment is usually surgical with combination of therapeutic radiation and chemotherapy. High grade tumors may require radical neck dissection.

Mucoepidermoid Carcinoma

Definition

This is a malignant tumor of epidermoid intermediate, and mucous cells of the salivary glands.

Clinical Features

- This is the most common tumor of the salivary glands. And most commonly involving the parotid.
- It is more common in the fifth decade of life, with a slight predilection for females.
- The aggressiveness of the lesion varies with its histological grade.
- The low grade variety rarely metastasizes. The tumor clinically is movable, slowly growing, painless nodule,

approximately 1–4 cm in diameter and has a good prognosis.
- The high grade tumors cause facial pain and paralysis, have ill-defined margins, and are relatively immobile. Metastasis by blood and lymph are common with a poor prognosis and 50% recurrence after excision.

Radiographic Features

Low grade mucoepidermoid carcinoma:
- No changes seen on plain films unless destructive changes to adjacent osseous structures have occurred
- Sialographic, CT, MRI, USG and scintigraphic presentations are similar to that of benign tumors
- On CT it may show:
  - A lobulated or irregularly sharply circumscribed appearance
  - Cystic areas may be present
  - Calcifications may be seen.

High Grade Mucoepidermoid Carcinoma

- CT section shows an irregular homogeneous mass, not much more dense than the parenchyma.
- CT with intravenous contrast enhancement shows the tumor as a sharply defined homogeneous mass that is considerably more opaque than on the CT images without contrast.
- CT also helps to detect any bony invasion.
- MRI also shows:
  - The appearance of irregular margins and ill-defined form.
  - Low signal intensity on T1-weighted images, suggestive of high grade malignancy. The images have a lower intensity (darker) than the surrounding structures and are relatively homogeneous.
  - T2-weighted images are more heterogeneous and intense (brighter) than the T1-weighted images and are just slightly darker than the surrounding tissues.
- Sialography may show cavitary sialectasia and ductal displacement.

Malignant Mixed Tumor (Carcinoma Ex Mixed Tumor, Carcinoma Ex Pleomorphic Adenoma, Malignant Pleomorphic Adenoma)

Definition

There are three distinct types of malignant mixed tumors:
1. *Carcinoma Ex-mixed tumor*: Arises from the epithelial components of a pre-existing benign mixed tumor.
2. *True malignant mixed tumor*: Arises from both epithelial and mesenchymal components of a mixed tumor.
3. *Metastasizing mixed tumor*: This appears histologically benign but behaves like a malignant lesion.

Clinical Features

- These begin as slow growing masses that suddenly undergo rapid proliferation, often accompanied with pain and facial paralysis
- Metastasis is early and prognosis is poor.

Radiographic Features

- The presentation is similar to high grade mucoepidermoid carcinoma
- Magnetic resonance imaging (MRI) gives a superior definition as compared to the CT image.

Other Malignant and MetastaticTumors

Definition

Incidence of other malignant tumors of the major salivary glands is low. Adenocystic carcinomas account for 23% of all salivary gland malignancies (usually involve the minor salivary glands) followed by adenocarcinomas (6.4%). Acinic cell carcinoma, primary lymphoma, and squamous cell carcinoma occur with less frequency.

Clinical Features

- Patient with high grade tumors, may complain of pain, paresthesia and paralysis. Pain of acinic cell carcinoma is not considered to be as grave a sign as in other malignant salivary tumors.
- Tumor spread may be direct invasion or metastasis. Adenoid cystic carcinoma spreads along nerve sheaths and is best demonstrated on post contrast MRI, where nerve enhancement and enlargement is present.
- Metastatic lesions in the parotid are more common than in any other salivary gland tumor because of extensive lymphatic and circulatory components of the parotid gland. Most of the metastatic tumor are via the lymphatic system which include squamous cell carcinoma, lymphoma and melanoma.
- Hematogeneous dissemination is lesser with metastasis from the lung, breast, kidney and gastrointestinal tract.

Radiographic Features

- The presentation is similar to that of high grade mucoepidermoid carcinoma.
- Ultrasonography (USG) may demonstrate echo free cystic areas in adenoid cystic carcinomas.
- Adenoid cystic carcinoma spreads along nerve sheaths and is best demonstrated on postcontrast MRI, where nerve enhancement and enlargement is present.

Causes of salivary gland hypofunction (xerostomia)

- Pharmaceuticals
  - Anticholinergic
  - Antidepressants
  - Sympathomimetics
  - Opium derivatives
  - Barbiturates
  - Antihistaminics
  - Antipsychotics
  - Diuretics
  - Sedatives, hypnotics and tranquilizers
  - Digitalis
  - Chemotherapeutics
  - Steroids
- Radiation therapy
  - External beam radiation
  - Internal radionuclide therapy
- Oncologic chemotherapy
- Systemic diseases
  - Sjögren's syndrome (primary and secondary)
  - Granulomatous diseases (sarcoidosis, tuberculosis)
  - Graft versus host reactions
  - Cystic fibrosis
  - Bell's palsy
  - Diabetes
  - Amyloidosis
  - Human immunodeficiency virus infection
  - Thyroid disease (Hyper and Hypo-function)
  - Congestive cardiac failure
  - Ascites
  - Liver cirrhosis
  - Encephalitis
  - Brain tumors
  - Nutritional and vitamin deficiency (Iron deficiency anemia, pernicious anemia)
- Psychological factors (affective disorder)
  - Emotional disturbances (stress and strain)
  - Depression
  - Hysteria
  - Neurosis
- Alteration in fluid or electrolytic balance
  - Malnutrition
  - Anorexia
  - Bulimia
  - Dehydration
  - Diarrhea
  - Vomiting
- Disorders of salivary gland
  - Developmental—aplasia
  - Inflammation and infections
  - Tumors
  - Atrophy
  - Obstruction
  - Excision or irradiation of the gland

Contd...

Contd...

- Miscellaneous
  - Menopause
  - Toxemia
  - Mouth breathing habit
  - Poisoning
  - Chronic alcoholism
  - Habits like smoking, local snuff application, betel nut chewing, etc.
  - Neurological operations

Causes of sialorrhea (ptyalism)

- Acute inflammation of the oral mucosa
  - Stomatitis
  - Glossitis
  - Pharyngitis
  - Tonsillitis
- During eruption of teeth in infants
- Mental retardation
  - Neurosis
  - Psychosis
- Parkinsonism
  - Schizophrenia
  - Epilepsy
- Poisoning
  - Acrodynia (Mercury poisoning)
- Epilepsy
- Rabies
- Familial dysautonomia (Riley-Dey syndrome—excess salivation and sweating)
- Local oral diseases
  - Herpetic stomatitis
  - Anug
  - Apthous ulcer
  - Carcinoma of the oral cavity
- Fracture of the jaw bones

BIBLIOGRAPHY

1. Bryan N, Miller R, Roque I, et al. Computed tomography of the major salivary glands. AJR. 1982;139:547-54.
2. Goaz PW, White SC. Principles and Interpretation. In: Oral Radiology, 3rd edn. St Louis, Mosby Year Book, 1994.
3. Keith, Thornton, Gordon. CT of salivary glands. Radiologic clinics of North America. 22(1):145-59.
4. Manashil GB. Clinical Sialography. Charles C Thomas, Illinois; 1978.
5. Miles DA, Van Dis MJ, Jensen CW, et al. Interpretation normal versus abnormal and common radiographic presentations of lesions. In: Radiographic and Imaging for Dental Auxillaries, 3rd edn. Philadelphia, WB Saunders; 1999.pp.231-80.
6. Rabinov K, Weber AL: Radiology of the salivary glands, Boston. GK Hall Medical Publishers; 1985.
7. Shafer WG, et al. A Textbook of Oral Pathology. Philadelphia, WB Saunders; 1983.
8. Van den Akker HP: Diagnostic imaging in salivary gland disease. Oral Surg. 1988;66:625.
9. Wood NK, Goaz PW. Differential diagnosis of oral lesions. 4th edn. CV Mosby, St Louis; 1991.
10. Wood RE. Handbook of signs in dental and maxillofacial radiology. Warthog Publications, Toronto; 1988.
11. Worth HM. Principles and practice of oral radiographic interpretation. Year Book Medical Publishers, Chicago; 1963.

Section VII

Role of Radiology in Specialized Dental Fields

Implant Radiology | 30

Dental implants are metal posts that are surgically implanted in the jaw to support a fixed dental prosthesis. In the early development of implants, dentist attempted to imitate the natural anchorage system of the teeth, which are attached to the bony socket by the periodontal ligament. In addition to supporting the teeth, this ligament permits slight degree of tooth motion within the socket. The initial efforts to reproduce this ligament promoted growth of soft tissue between the oral implants and the bone. These implants were often referred to as pseudoligaments or fibrous osseointegrated implants. However, the long-term results of these soft tissue anchored implants were poor.

Dental implantology has experienced explosive growth during last few years. It has expanded from a technique practiced on the fringe of acceptability to one embraced by mainstream dentistry. As the biology and mechanics of any procedure are better understood, refinements in technique are made. One aspect of implantology that requires further emphasis and refinement is that of treatment planning. An insufficiently planned case can bring poor results and dissatisfaction on the part of surgeon, dentist and the patient. Dental implants are a widely used modality in the restoration of complete or partial edentulous arch. Regardless of the type of intraosseous implant system used, the radiographic examination is an essential part.

Diagnostic imaging and techniques help to develop and implement a cohesive and comprehensive treatment plan for the implant team and the patient.

Various radiographic techniques were introduced for preoperative implant site assessment. However, it was not possible to determine the exact position for optimal implant placement, using those techniques. Before the development of CBCT/CT with third party software, attempts were made to obtain this information with intraoral, panoramic and cephalometric films. But, accurate measurements were impossible. Also, the width of the alveolar bone could not be determined by any of these techniques. Therefore, the surgeon had to rely primarily on clinical assessment to determine the quantity of bone available.

It is important to note that; implant imaging objectives would depend on the stage when the image is taken.

PREPROSTHETIC IMPLANT IMAGING

The objectives of this phase of imaging include all necessary surgical and prosthetic information to determine the quantity, quality and angulation of bone; the relationship of critical structures to the prospective implant sites; and the presence or absence of disease at the proposed implant sites.

This phase of implant imaging is intended to evaluate the current status of the patient's teeth and jaws and to develop and refine the patient's treatment plan. Before planning an implant, a screening radiograph should be taken which give the clinician an indication of:
- The overall status of teeth and supporting bone.
- Those sites where it is possible to place implant using a straight forward protocol.
- Those sites where it is unlikely that implants can be placed without using complex procedures such as grafting.
- Anatomic anomalies or pathological lesions.

The use of imaging stents helps to relate the radiographic image and its information to a precise anatomical location or potential surgical site.

Various interactive software packages have also been developed to allow presurgical simulation of implant orientation and placement on a computer screen.

CAD/CAM stereotactic surgical templates: It can be produced from CT examinations that have used interactive CT to develop a three-dimensional treatment plan for the position and orientation of dental implants. Anatomically accurate three-dimensional models of the patient's alveolar anatomy can be produced by a number of CAD/CAM and rapid protyping procedures.

Magnetic resonance imaging is used in implants as a secondary imaging technique when the primary imaging techniques such as complex tomography, CT or ICT fail. The latest imaging modality is CBCT.

The specific objectives of preprosthetic imaging are to:
- Identify disease
- Determine bone quantity
- Determine bone density
- Identify critical structures at the proposed implant regions
- Determine the optimum position of implant placement relative to occlusal loads.

SURGICAL AND INTERVENTIONAL IMPLANT IMAGING

It is focused upon assisting in the surgical and prosthetic intervention of the patient. The objectives of this phase are to evaluate the surgical sites during and immediately after surgery, assist in the optimal position and orientation of dental implants, evaluate the healing and orientation of dental implants, evaluate the healing and integration phase of implant surgery, and ensure that abutment position and prosthesis fabrication are correct.

The purpose of this phase includes:
- Evaluation of depth of implant placement
- To evaluate the surgery sites during and immediately after surgery
- Assist in the optimal position and orientation of implants/osteotomies
- To evaluate donor and graft sites
- To evaluate the healing and integration phase of implant surgery
- To evaluate any impairment in the proper seating of abutment and transfer copings due to antirotation devices of implant body
- To evaluate whether the metal framework or final restoration is seated completely
- To evaluate whether the margins are acceptable around the implant and teeth.

Because most implant surgeries are performed in doctor's office rather than in a hospital, the modalities are usually limited to periapical and panoramic radiography.

POSTPROSTHETIC IMPLANT IMAGING

This phase commences just after the prosthesis placement and continues as long as the implants remain in the jaws. The objectives of this phase are to evaluate the long-term maintenance of implant rigid fixation and function, including the crestal bone levels around each implant, and to evaluate the implant complex.

The successful healing of dental implants result in osseointegration, which is defined as contact between the implant and bone at the light microscopic level. Unfortunately, histological examination is not possible without compromising the implant. Therefore, radiographs are an alternative method to assess the fate of dental implant *in vivo*.

The purpose is to evaluate the status and prognosis of the dental implant. The bone adjacent to the dental implant should be evaluated regularly for changes in mineralization or bone volume. Changes in bone mineralization in the region of bone adjacent to the dental implant may indicate:
- Successful integration
- Fibrous tissue artifacts
- Inflammation, infection
- Loss of crestal bone volume adjacent to the dental implant

- Excessive functional loading
- Bone damage during implant placement
- Integration failure with an epithelial bone implant interface.

IMAGING MODALITIES (TABLE 30.1)

Analog Imaging Modalities

Analog imaging modalities are two-dimensional systems that use X-ray film as the image receptors. The image quality of these systems is characterized by resolution, modulation transfer function, contrast, H and D curve, noise, Wiener spectrum and sensitivity. This includes:
- Periapical radiography
- Occlusal radiography
- Cephalometric radiography
- Panoramic radiography.

Digital Two-Dimensional Imaging Modalities

A digital two-dimensional image is described by an image matrix that has individual picture elements called pixels. A digital image is described by its width and height and pixels. For larger digital images, the image is alternately described as a 1.5-M image, where M is mega pixels. Each picture element or pixel has a discrete digital value that describes the image intensity at that particular point. This include:
- Periapical radiography
- Panoramic radiography
- Cephalometric radiography.

Quasi Three-Dimensional Imaging Modalities

A digital three-dimensional image is described by an image matrix that has individual image/picture elements called voxels. A digital three-dimensional image is described not only by its width and height and pixels, but also by its depth/thickness. An imaging volume or three-dimensional characterization of the patient is produced by contiguous images, which produce a three-dimensional structure of volume elements.

These include:
- Computed tomography
- Magnetic resonance imaging
- Interactive computed tomography
- Cone beam computed tomography.

Periapical Radiography (Figs 30.1 and 30.2)

Advantages

- They are the highest resolution images produced by radiographic procedures
- It is a useful high yield modality for ruling out local bone or dental disease

Table 30.1 Valuation of implant imaging techniques for presurgical assessment of implant sites

| | 2D sources | | | | 3D sources | |
Imaging goal	Cephalometric	Tomographic	Panoramic	Periapical	CT	Cone beam CT
Bone height	*	* * *	* *	* * *	* * * *	* * * *
Bone width	–	* * *	–	–	* * * *	* * * *
Long axis or ridge	–	* * *	–	–	* * * *	* * * *
Identify internal anatomy	*	* * *	* *	* * *	* * * *	* * * *
Localize anatomy	*	* * *	*	*	* * * *	* * * *
Determine jaw boundaries	–	* * *	* *	–	* * * *	* * * *
Pathology detection	*	* *	* * *	* *	* * *	* * *
Bone quality	–	* *	* *	* *	* * * *	* * *
Communication	*	* *	* *	*	* * * *	* * * *
Anatomy overview	* *	*	* *	*	* * *	* * * *
Benefit/risk/cost ratio	*	* * *	* *	*	* * *	* * * *

Table 30. 1 shows a list of commonly used imaging techniques and associated goal. The relative application value for each imaging technique has been rated as follows: No value; * = Low value; * * = Moderate value; * * * = High Value; * * * * = Highest value
Source: David C Hatcher, Craig Dial, Comille Mayorga, CDA, Journal. 2003;31(11).

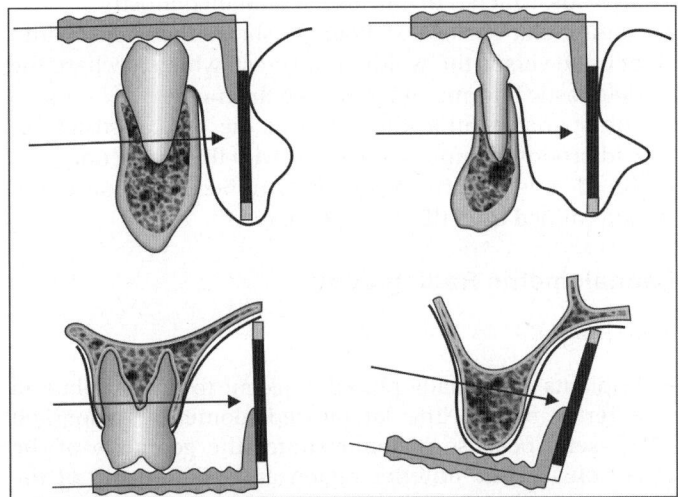

Figure 30.1 Paralleling technique used in intraoral radiographs

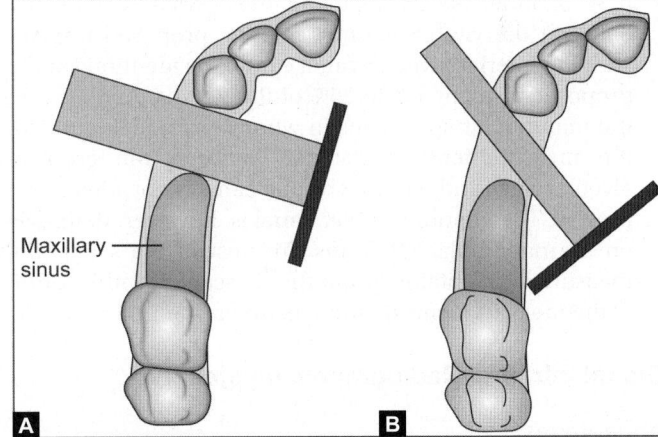

Maxillary sinus

Figures 30.2A and B (A) Correct horizontal angulation to obtain exact mesiodistal dimensions of edentulous area; (B) Incorrect horizontal angulation

- Valuable in identifying critical structures, but, of little use in depicting the spatial relationship between the structures and the proposed implant site
- Approximate vertical height of alveolar ridge can be determined
- Best image detail with minimal image distortion
- Some information about bone quality (density, trabecular pattern) and presence/absence of pathosis is revealed
- Films readily available to clinician and low cost to patient.

Disadvantages

- Periapical radiograph provides a lateral view of jaws and no cross-sectional information. Even with adjacent periapical radiographs, made with limited oblique orientations, two-dimensional information is of little use for the implant imaging.
- Periapical radiograph may suffer from distortion and magnification. The long cone paralleling technique eliminates distortion and limits magnification to less than 10%.
- Limited area viewed on a single film, no buccal-lingual or horizontal dimension of alveolar ridge, no bone volume information is revealed, no accurate assessment of vertical bone dimension or the 'precise' location of anatomic structures.
- Millimeter radiopaque grids, sometimes used in endodontics, may be superimposed over the film, before it is

exposed, but, are of little quantitative value and provide misleading information because they lie on the film and obfuscate the underlying anatomy and do not compensate for magnification.

- The opposing landmark of available bone in implant dentistry is beyond lingual muscle attachments in the mandible and beyond the palatal vault in the maxilla. As such, the image most often must be foreshortened to visualize the opposing cortical plate. Also, it is difficult to standardize focus-film distance. As a result, it becomes impossible to make precise measurements of the vertical height of the alveolar process.
- Burnout effects are common when standard kilovolt and milliampere settings are used, making crestal bone loss evaluation difficult. Digital intraoral systems are of benefit in these situations.
- It is of little value in determining bone density or mineralization (the lateral cortical plates prevent accurate interpretation and cannot differentiate subtle trabecular bone changes).
- It is of little use in depicting the spatial relationship between the vital structures and the proposed implant site. The inferior alveolar canal cannot be identified at the proposed implant site in 25% of the IOPA's. And even in the mandibular specimens in whom it can be identified, the measurement of distance between the crest of alveolar ridge and inferior alveolar canal is not adequately precise. The inferior alveolar canal is, however, definable on all mandibular CT scans. In most of the scans, the measurement obtained from the CT scans is within 1 mm of the measurements on the specimen.

Digital Intraoral Radiographic Images

Advantages

- Reduces patient exposure to radiation
- Increased patient comfort while the radiographic image is taken
- Instant results
- Elimination of inconvenience associated with developing
- Cost saving
- Images can be manipulated for the desired contrast, color enhancement, inversion or rotation of the image
- Distance measurement in 0.1 mm increments is possible, which is invaluable in implant procedure
- Pseudo three-dimensional views, oriented at 450 inclinations are available in both reverse and in color
- These images can be stored within an electronic chart and can also be sent via modem to other specialists and team members.

Limitations

The senors are very rigid and the area covered very limited.

Occlusal Radiography

Advantages

- Provides generalized information about bone density
- Indication of buccal-lingual dimension of mandible
- Determination of jaw size, jaw curve at proposed implant site
- Standard occlusal film provides width of the inferior border of mandible
- Laterally exposed film shows the width of the bone in the midline
- Readily accessible to clinician and low cost to the patient.

Disadvantages

- Although helpful, these views are two-dimensional, only reveals maximum buccal-lingual dimension, medial and lateral extent of cortical bone not seen
- Mandibular alveolus generally flares anteriorly and demonstrates a lingual inclination posteriorly, producing an oblique and distorted image of the mandibular alveolus, which is of little use in implant dentistry
- Mandibular occlusal radiograph shows the widest width of bone versus the width at the crest, which is where the diagnostic information is needed the most
- The spatial relationship between the critical structures and proposed implant site is lost with this projection
- The degree of mineralization of trabecular bone is not determined from this projection.

Cephalometric Radiography

Advantages

- Implants are usually placed adjacent to lingual plate in anterior region. The lateral cephalometric radiograph is useful because it demonstrates the geometry of the alveolus in the anterior region and relationship of the lingual plate to the patient's skeletal anatomy.
- The width of bone in the symphyseal region and the relationship between the buccal cortex and the roots of anterior teeth may also be determined before harvesting this bone for ridge augmentation (height/width information is revealed in the anterior mandible/maxilla).
- Images are cross-sectional
- Together with regional periapical radiograph, quantitative spatial information is available to demonstrate the geometry of the implant site and spatial relationship between the implant site and critical structures.
- Lateral cephalogram also can help to evaluate a loss of vertical dimension, skeletal arch inter-relationship, anterior crown/implant ratio, anterior tooth position in the prosthesis and resultant movement of forces.
- The soft tissue profile also is apparent on this film and can be used to evaluate profile alterations after prosthodontic rehabilitation.

- Image magnification is constant.
- Low radiation dose, low cost to patient.

Disadvantages

- Not useful for demonstrating bone quality
- Only demonstrates a cross-sectional image of the alveolus where the central rays of the X-ray device are tangent to the alveolus
- Limited use (anterior region only)
- Superimposition of structures
- Reveals only maximum buccal-lingual width and not depression in ridge.

Panoramic Radiography

Advantages

- Excellent 'screening' radiograph for presurgical implant planning. Gross anatomy of the jaws and other related pathologic findings could be evaluated.
- Indication of anatomical spatial relationship. Opposing landmarks are easily identified. Panoramic radiographs demonstrate anatomic vital structures adjacent to potential implant receptor sites. When implants are to be inserted between teeth, between a tooth and the mental foramen or between a tooth and the anterior border of the maxillary sinus, supplementary intraoral radiographs should always be obtained by paralleling technique.
- The vertical height of the bone initially can be assessed.
- The procedure is performed with convenience, ease and speed in most dental offices.
- Low cost to patient with minimal radiation dose.

Disadvantages

- Panoramic radiography is characterized by an image of the jaws that demonstrates vertical and horizontal magnification, along with a tomographic section thickness that varies according to the anatomic position. The X-ray source exposes the jaws from a negative angulation and produces a relatively constant vertical magnification of approximately 10%. The horizontal magnification is approximately 20% (0.70–2.2 mm) and variable depending upon the anatomic location, position of the patient, the focus-object distance and the relative location of the rotation center of the X-ray system. Structures of the jaws become magnified more as the object-film distance increases and the object-source distance decreases. Structures those are located obliquely in relation to the implant receptor produce aspects of the structures that are magnified more when they are farther from the image receptor and less when they are closer to the image receptor.
- Uniform magnification of the structures produces images with distortion that cannot be compensated for

in treatment planning. The posterior maxillary regions are generally the least distorted regions of a panoramic radiograph. The tomographic section thickness of panoramic radiography or trough of focus is thick, approximately 20 mm in posterior region and thin 6 mm in the anterior region. Consequently, in only 17% of cases, did measurements made from panoramic tomograms accurately represent the true osseous height on the dried specimen.

- Presence of artifacts may limit diagnostic accuracy.
- Image distortion (technique sensitive to patient positioning errors).
- Panoramic radiography is of some use in demonstrating critical structures but of little use in depicting the spatial relationship between the structural and dimensional quantitation of the implant site.

A technique for evaluating the panoramic radiograph for mandibular posterior implants and comparing this to the clinical evaluation during surgery was developed by identifying the mental foramen and the posterior extent of the inferior alveolar canal. Studies have demonstrated that the mandibular foramen cannot be identified 30% of the times on the X-ray films; and when visible may not be identified correctly.

- The maxillary anterior edentulous region is generally oblique to the film and is often the most difficult area of a panoramic radiograph to evaluate because of the curvature of the alveolus and the inclination of the bone. The dimensions of the inclined structures and linear measurements in panoramic radiography are not reliable.
- Little or no information about width or ridge inclination.
- The negative vertical angulation of the X-ray beam also may cause lingually positioned objects such as mandibular tori to be projected superiorly on the film, which may result in an over estimation of vertical bone height.
- Panoramic radiography does not demonstrate bone quality mineralization.
- Resolution and sharpness of the image is less.

Conventional Tomography

Advantages

- For dental implant patients, high quality complex motion tomography demonstrates the alveolus and taking magnification into consideration, enables quantification of the geometry of the alveolus. Conventional tomography was shown to be superior to panoramic radiography for bone height determination and for location of the mandibular canal.
- It produces cross-sectional images of specific proposed implant sites.
- It helps in assessment of bone height, width and inclination of ridge, bone quality, and determination of anatomic spatial relationship.

- As there is little or no superimposition, assessment of exact imaging and detailed view of specific implant site with selection of varying slice thickness and slice location is possible.
- Postimaging digitization of tomographic implant images enables use of digital ruler to aid in the determination of alveolar bone for implant placement.
- Image enhancement can aid in identifying critical structures such as inferior alveolar canal.
- Use of tomography increases the efficacy of periapical/panoramic images to predict the appropriate implant size. In a study by Schropp et al. 70% of cases, the dimensions of implant were changed after the surgeon had access to tomograms, when compared with conventional tomography in predicting the appropriate implant size as an adjunct to panoramic or periapical examination for treatment of single tooth implant. Length of the planned implant was changed on viewing tomograms in 64% cases in upper anterior region, 40% in upper premolar and 56% in mandible. With respect to the width of implant, the tomography resulted in a change in 32% of cases in upper anterior region, 13% of upper premolar sites and 44% in mandible. So, the use of conventional tomograms can increase the efficacy of periapical/panoramic images to predict appropriate implant size by a factor of 2.5. So, it is usually considered as a method of choice for single tooth implant.
- The cost of conventional tomography is much less than computed tomography.
- The deterioration of section due to scatter artifact on computed tomogram is not a problem with conventional tomography.
- The radiation exposure to the patient is reduced significantly as compared to computed tomography.

Disadvantages

- Conventional tomography is not particularly useful in determining bone quality or identifying dental or bone diseases.
- Image blurring and magnification error can affect the accuracy of measurements.
- The wider cortical bone mesial and distal to ridge resorption at the proposed implant site results in greater blurring of tomographic images. This may be significant if a ridge is narrow and could result in a dehiscence or fenestration if one attempts to engage the cortical plate. LT magnification ranges from 27.1% less to 27.9% greater than CT images.
- Accurate localization of critical structures is sometimes not possible.
- The angulation of the X-ray beam during LT may also result in the radiographic image of the mandible having a more vertical representation than the actual anatomic position. Misinterpretation of the actual angulation

may result in improper placement or angulation of the proposed implant.
- Multiple sites in a jaw necessitate additional calculations and changing of the angle of the patient's head, if the long axis of the proposed sites is not parallel to each other.
- Anatomic variation may result in images that are difficult to interpret.
- The equipment is costly and recommends availability of trained oral radiologist to perform imaging and calculate bone dimensions, which is time consuming when multiple sites are indicated.
- Transfer of radiographic information to clinical site may necessitate imaging stent.
- Variable definition of specific anatomic structures dependent of imaging system and availability.

Tuned Aperture Computed Tomography

In a study of peri-implant bone changes using axial tomosynthesis, tuned aperture computed tomography (TACT) was reported to provide a greater probability of correct identification of bone loss around titanium implants placed in edentulous dry mandibles than conventional images. A comparison of the diagnostic performance of film radiographs, digital radiographs and TACT images to locate the crestal defects around endosseous titanium implants found TACT, both with and without digital subtraction, to be significantly better at the same level of confidence for accuracy compared with the other X-ray modalities. So, TACT may provide an alternative to conventional tomography for dental implant imaging.

Computed Tomography

Advantages

- CT scanners produce very high-resolution images. There are two types of resolution—geometric and contrast.
  - Geometric resolution is defined as the ability to distinguish between closely spaced objects. It translates in nonspecific terms to sharpness, when edges and borders are distinct.
  - Contrast resolution means the ability to distinguish between objects that are similar anatomically and chemically, such as neural tissue and fat.
  - Conventional diagnostic radiographic technique provide images with fewer than 30 variations of gray, whereas CT scanning technology generates images with more than 200 shades of gray. The increased CT scan gray scale shows subtle variations in tissue density that is not discernable with conventional radiology.
- Evaluation of jaws with CT requires very precise patient positioning. Without specialized machines, it is necessary to reorient the patient for each series of images to keep image plane perpendicular to the alveolar ridge. The reformatted CT examination on the other hand, permits the

production of all possible cross sections from a single data acquisition without moving the patient or reconfiguring the X-ray machine. Each of these pictures produced in this manner can be localized in a three-dimensional space so that there is never a doubt as to which position of the alveolar ridge is included in the image.

- The dimensional accuracy of three-dimensional rendered images has been established. Linear measurements of anatomic structures are accurate to within 0.19 mm (0.28%) and angular measures are correct within 0.380 mm (1.39%). The linear measures of anthropologic dimensions of the skull using three-dimensional CT compared favorably with measurements made from original two-dimensional slice data and are generally accurate to within 1 mm. Hence, it gives accurate assessment of bone height, width, ridge inclination, bone quality, anatomic spatial relationship, without any superimposition.

- Special dental processing software programs, which are capable of greater enhancement of CT scan, shows three-dimensional image and one-to-one correspondence in contrast to conventional tomograms. These programs were introduced in 1987 and provide panoramic and cross-sectional views in addition to three-dimensional images of either the maxilla or mandible. Measures can be made directly from the CT films.

- The use of CT scan splint lined with barium sulfate and methyl methacrylate in the tooth portion of the template permits the implant team to evaluate proposed tooth position, abutment selection and implant placement before initiating therapy, especially in maxillary anterior region.

- Position of critical structures can be accurately assessed, with better contrast sensitivity than film tomography, and less time consuming for multiple sites.

- It is helpful in patient education and motivation.

Disadvantages

- Radiation dose factor for CT is much higher than the conventional cross-section tomograms. According to a recent study, the effective organ dose for CT is 100 times higher than the conventional cross-section tomography.

- Resolution of CT is also lower than that of conventional spiral tomograms.

- The CT scan must be recorded on a special optical disc that is send to a processing center for use on a personal computer using a proprietary software program. This all adds to the cost of treatment.

- The images obtained are very accurate, but only as accurate as the fit of the radiographic template. If the fit of the template is different during surgery than it was during CT scan, then, placement of implant will be in error by the same factor. This is especially true with complete upper and complete lower template, which is inherently unstable.

- Often CT scan does not add any useful information to the diagnostic process. If a proper examination, diagnostic wax up and two radiographic views of the proposed site are obtained; very often there is no need for any other further information.

- Expensive and time-consuming procedure very claustrophobic for the patient with higher radiation exposure.

- There may be degradation of image by metallic restorative materials (amalgam, crowns, post, pins) known as 'scatter'.

- Patient movement including swallowing results in distortion of image.

Cone Beam Computed Tomography

The cone beam computed tomography (CBCT) technology introduces an innovation in modes of image scanning and volumetric reconstruction of CT data. Due to rapid volumetric image acquisition (as low as 18 sec) from a single low radiation dose scan of the patient and the low mA, the effective dose with the CBCT technique is significantly smaller than that achieved with other CT imaging methods and is within the range of traditional dental imaging modalities (**Table 30.2**).

Cone beam computed tomography (CBCT) has been operational now for several years in areas such as implantology, surgery and oral diagnosis. It was found that although

Table 30.2 Comparative dosage to patients undergoing various radiographic exams for implant planning

Type of examination	Approximate effective dose in µSv
Digital/F speed, with rectangular collimation FMX	34.9
Digital/F speed, with round collimation FMX	170.7
Conventional single IOPA	<8.3
Panoramic	2.7–24.3
Lateral cephalometric	2.3–5.6
CT maxillomandibular	180–2100
CT maxilla	1400
Intraoral radiographs (FMX), panoramic, and lateral cephalometric radiographs	43.2–200.6
CBCT large FOV	260-136
CBCT medium FOV	166-84
CBCT small FOV	122-92

Cone beam computed tomography and radiographs in dentistry: Aspects related to radiation dose, Diego Coelho Lorenzoni, 1 AnaMaria Bolognese, Daniela Gamba Garib, Fabio Ribeiro Guedes, and Eduardo Franzotti Sant, Anna International Journal of Dentistry Volume 2012, Article ID 813768, 10 pages doi: 10.1155/2012/813768

CBCT underestimates the real distances between skull sites, differences are only significant for the skull base and therefore it is reliable for linear evaluation measurements of other structures more closely associated with dentomaxillofacial imaging.

When compared to panoramic and CT imaging for dental implants CBCT gives (**Figs 30.3 and 30.4**):

- An undistorted or accurate dimensional views of the jaws
- Provides cross-sectional (buccolingual), axial, coronal, sagittal, and panoramic views
- It is possible to separate out the various structures, for example, the left condyle from the right one
- Reproduces the whole anatomy of the area of interest
- Allows accurate dimensional measurements
- Allows accurate determination of relative bone density
- It virtually eliminates claustrophobia and greatly enhances patient comfort and acceptance. The upright position is also thought by many to provide a more realistic picture of condylar positions during a TMJ examination
- The lower cost of the machine may be passed on to the patient in the form of lower fees
- Both jaws can be imaged at the same time (depending on the specific cone beam machine). Easy acquisition with low scan time

- Smaller area can be scanned
- Radiation dose is considerably less than with a medical CT (**Table 30.2**).

Applications of CBCT in Implant Planning

- Determine bone height and width (bone dimensions)
  - Precise measurement of distance, area and volume
  - Used for sinus lift, augmentations
- Determine bone quality
  - Bone density proportional load bearing capacity of bone
  - Low bone density responsible for implant failure
- Determine long axis of alveolar bone
  - To help determine alignment of implant
- Identify and localize internal anatomy
- Determine jaw boundaries
- Pathology detection
- Determine post implant placement status.

Determine Bone Height and Width (Bone Dimensions)

- Bone height and width allow the clinician to determine how much bone is available in the proposed implant site. There are various classifications available (**Tables 30.3 to 30.5**). Most of the linear measures to be accurate have

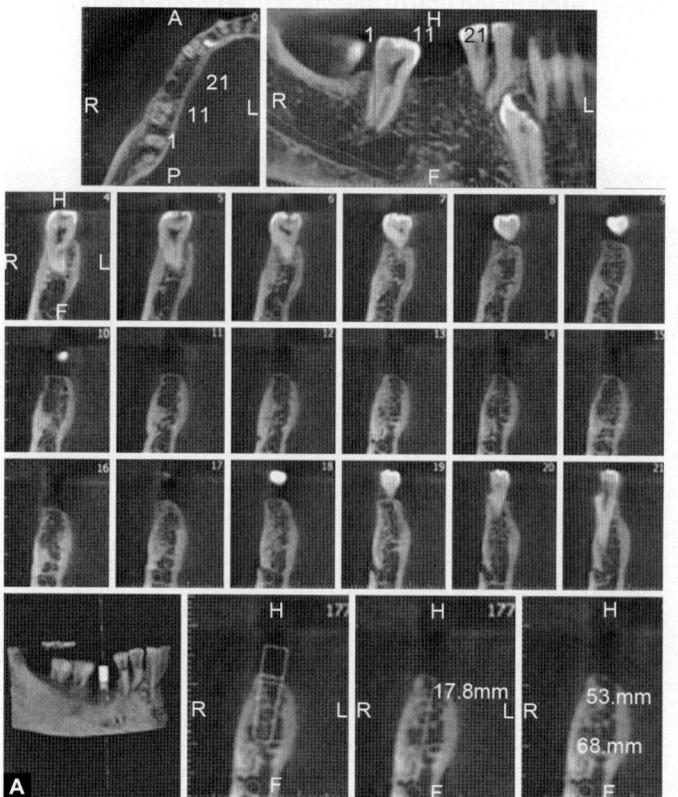
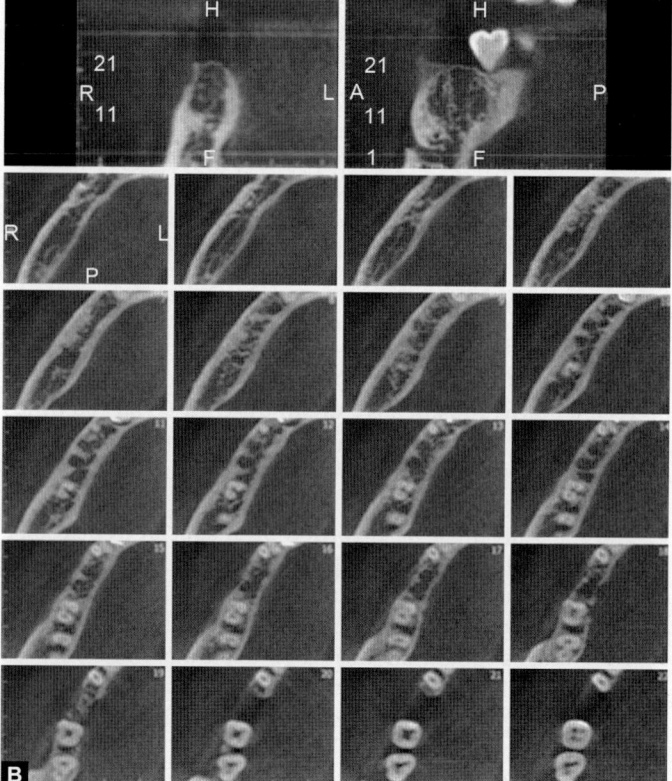

Figures 30.3A and B CBCT: (A) Axial view, panoramic view, sagittal cross-sections with available bone width and height measured, 3D view with virtual implant; (B) Sagittal view, and axial views showing the relation of the roots of the adjacent teeth to the area of implant placement

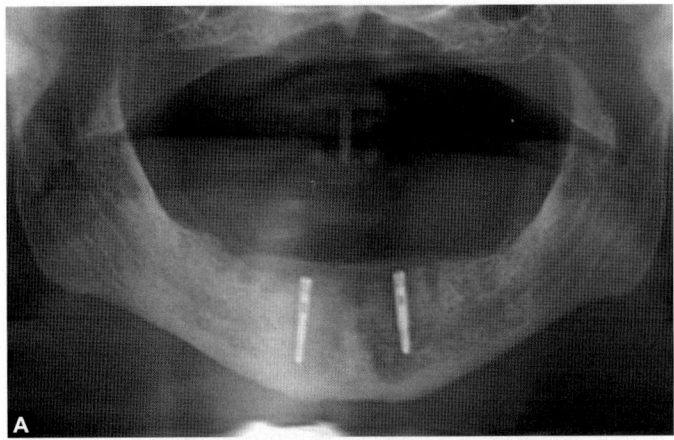

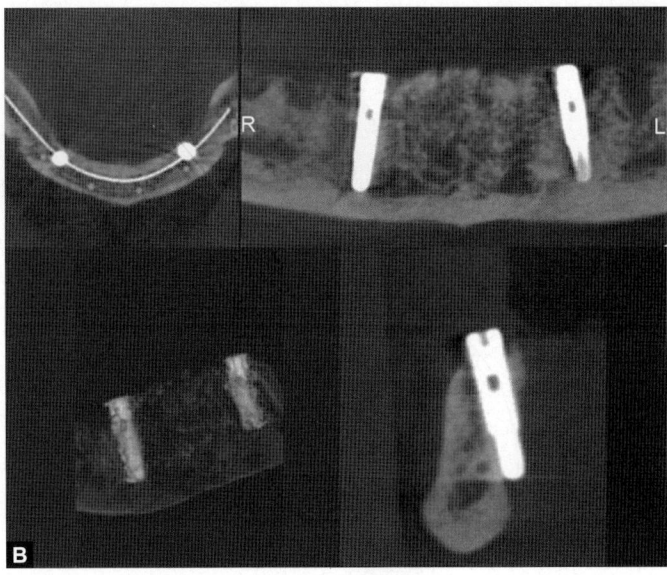

Figures 30.4A and B (A) Panoramic view showing implants adequately placed; (B) CBCT axial, panoramic, 3D and cross-sectional view, of the same patient reveals in the cross-sectional view that one of the implants have perforated the cortical plate

Table 30.3 Classification of bone dimensions for implant planning by Chanavaz*

Category	Dimension	Other features
A	Height: 9 mm	• Abundant bone in all dimensions
	Width: 5 mm	• Intact basal bone
B	Height: 9 mm	• Abundant bone except width
	Width: 3 mm	• Intact basal bone • Partially resorbed alveolar bone [5–9 years after extraction]
C	Inadequate bone	• Totally resorbed alveolar bone • Intact basal bone
D	Severe bone atrophy	• Totally resorbed alveolar bone • Partially resorbed basal bone except symphysis region and external oblique ridge

*Chanavaz M, Donazzan: Maxillomandibular bone reconstruction and implantology. Bone and biomaterials. French classification of available bone for implantology. The book of 30th Congress of Stomatology and Maxillofacial Surgery. Paris 1986.pp.189-204.

Table 30.4 Classification of bone dimensions as per height available for implant planning

Group	Height available at implant site (mm)
1	>12 mm
2	10–12 mm
3	5–10 mm
4	< 5 mm

Table 30.5 Classification of bone dimensions as per mesiodistal space of edentulous span for implant planning (N = Narrow. R = Regular. W = Wide. P = Platform)

Type of implant	Distance
NP	6 mm
RP	7 mm
WP	8 mm

to be done in the cross-sectional imaging which is easily available with CBCT (**Figs 30.5A to C**).

• Evaluation of alveolar bone for sharpness of the crest and ridge resorption:
  – Thin and flabby ridges are not favorable for implant placement and ride augmentation should be done before implant surgery. There are 3 types of shapes of alveolar crest normally encountered during implant procedure: knife edge, round, hour glass shaped (**Fig. 30.6**)
  – Vertical bone resorption evaluation helps to evaluate the discrepancy between the bone level at implant site and adjacent teeth. Implants should not be placed

deeper than 3 mm from the line connecting the CEJ of adjacent teeth as this may cause problems in alignment and represents risk to peri-implant tissue and esthetics.

– Bone volume has been classified as **Table 30.6** and correlated with CBCT cross-sectional images of maxilla and mandible showing corresponding bone volume (**Figs 30.7 and 30.8**).

– The ridge shape can also be determined from the cross-sectional views available on the CBCT (**Fig. 30.6**).

Determine Bone Quality

There is an assumption that bone density is directly proportional to load bearing capacity of the bone and that implant failure is associated with low bone density.

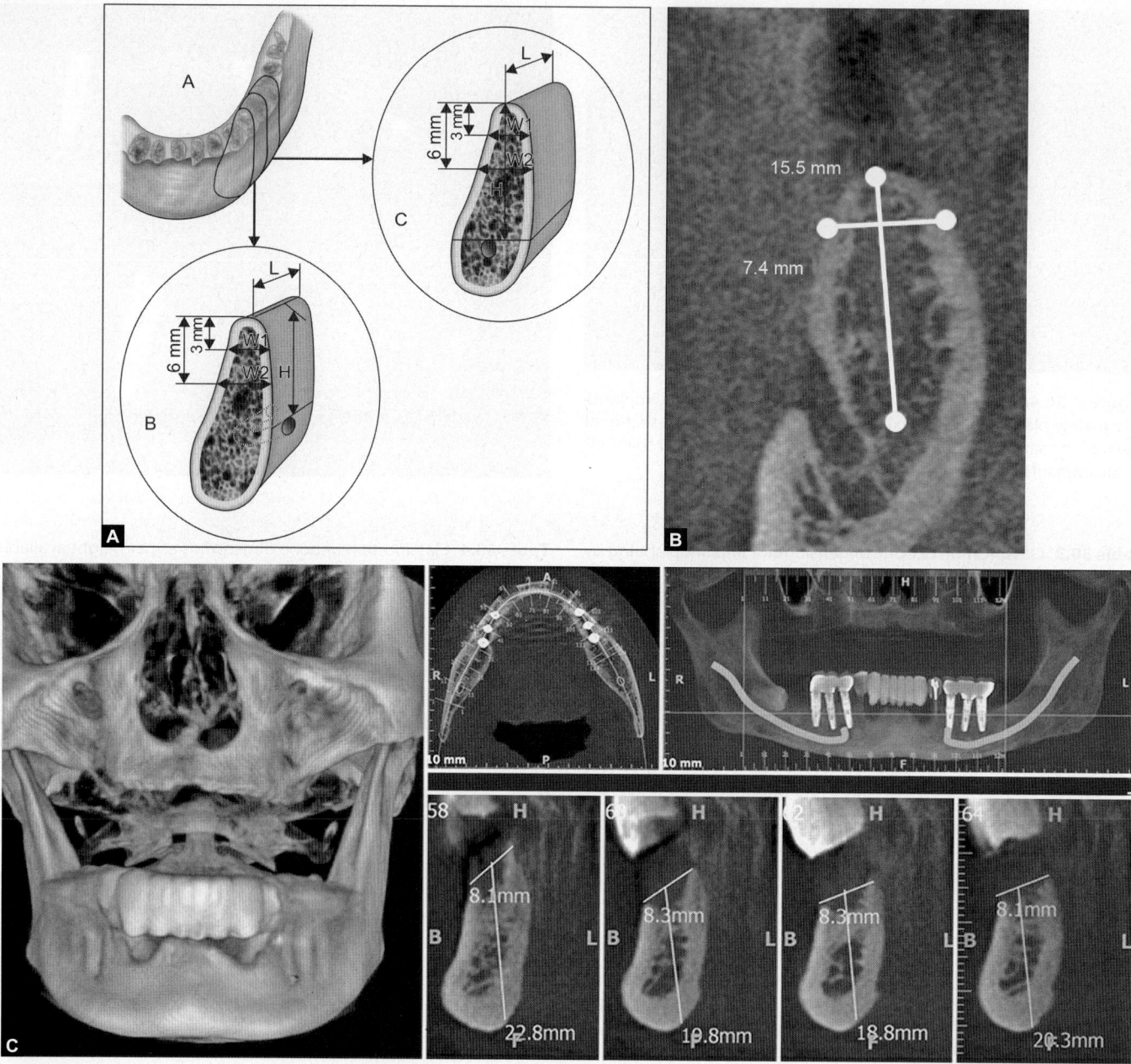

Figures 30.5A to C (A) Assessment of bone-width and height; (B) Precise measurements of height and width of available bone can be determined in the cross-sectional CBCT views-using the linear measurement tools available with the software. A = Mandible is divided into edentulous jaw segments that consists of alveolar and basal bone for planned implant bed. B = The vertical dimension (H) of the planned implant is determined by the distance between the alveolar ridge crest and mental foramen. C = The vertical dimension (H) of the planned implant is determined by the distance between the alveolar crestal ridge and mandibular canal. The horizontal EJS dimensions: length (L) in all cases is determined by the distance between neighboring teeth or implants and width (W) is determined by the alveolar process width measured at the level of 3 mm (W1) and 6 mm (W2) from the crest of alveolar ridge. EJC: Edentulous jaw segment.; (C) The stent can be used as a reference for radiographic planning and to transfer the simulation product to the mouth

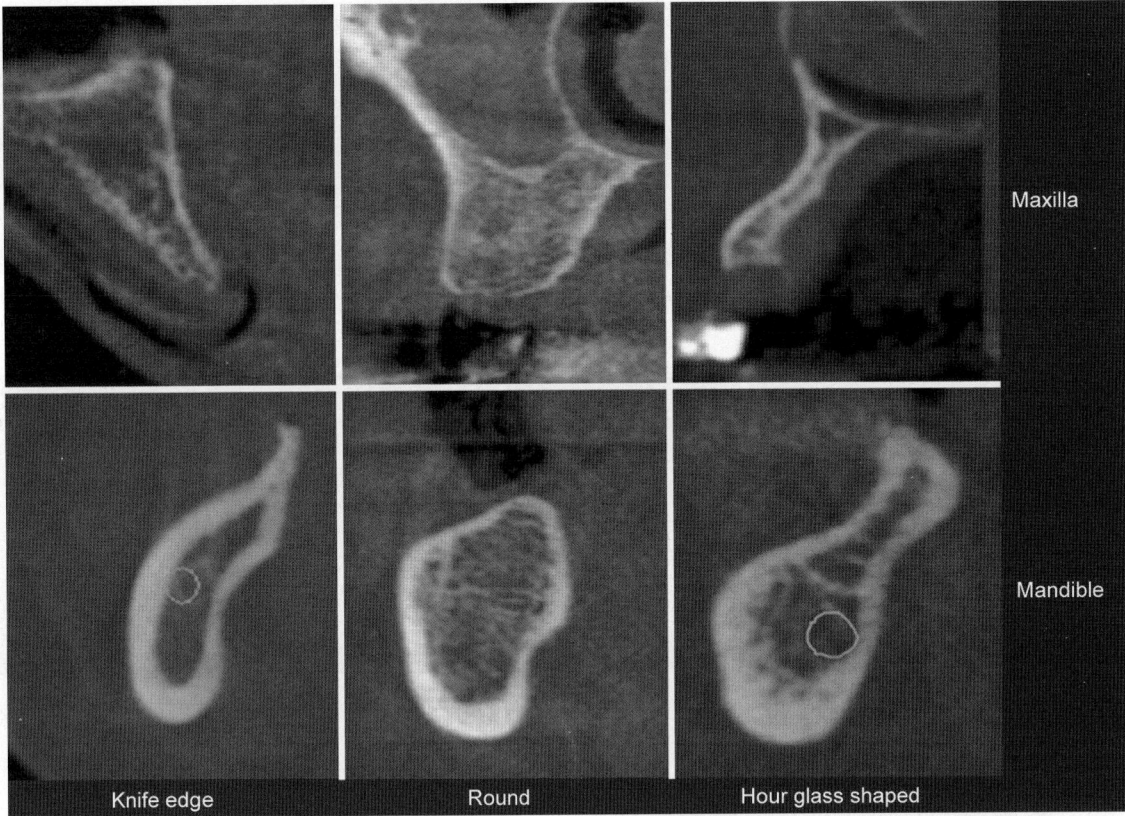

Figure 30.6 Alveolar ridge shapes seen in CBCT cross-sections

Table 30.6 Bone volume classifies as per availability of bone

	Bone volume
A	Abundant bone
B	Adequate bone height but reduced bone width
B-w	Reduced width
C-w	Advanced bone width loss
C-h	Further loss of bone height
D	Severe atrophy

Bone density helps to:
- To select the proper implant diameter.
- Decide about the optimal drilling sequence
  - *In soft bone*: Use final drill to half depth only
  - Minimal use of counter sink
    - Use smaller drill diameter than standard
- Determine the length of the healing period
- Evaluate the occlusal load capacity of different implants
- Determine implant number
- Implant design (angulation)
  - As bone density decreases—the angle of load on the implant body should be more axial.

Bone Density Measurement

It is likely that the amount of medullary bone at the implant site is important to the overall success rate of the surgical procedure. The most important factor for the successful integration of implant with the surrounding bone is the presence of sufficient amount of compact bone in which the implant can be anchored.

The two simplest assessments described in the literature and possibly the most appropriate for application in general practice, are the bone quality index (BQI) and mandibular cortical index (MCI).

Four types of bone quality are described in the BQI, based on subjective evaluation of the cortical thickness and trabecular pattern, proposed by Lekholm and Zarb. This is a four point index and was assessed using the following criteria (**Table 30.7**).
- *Clinical significance of bone quality and density*:
  - *Class 1 (Fig. 30.9)*: (D1) bone provides a poor blood supply, and surgical preparation is difficult. It is often found when alveolar bone has resorbed, and basal bone remains. There is an assumption that bone density is directly proportional to load bearing capacity of the bone and that implant failure is associated with low bone density.

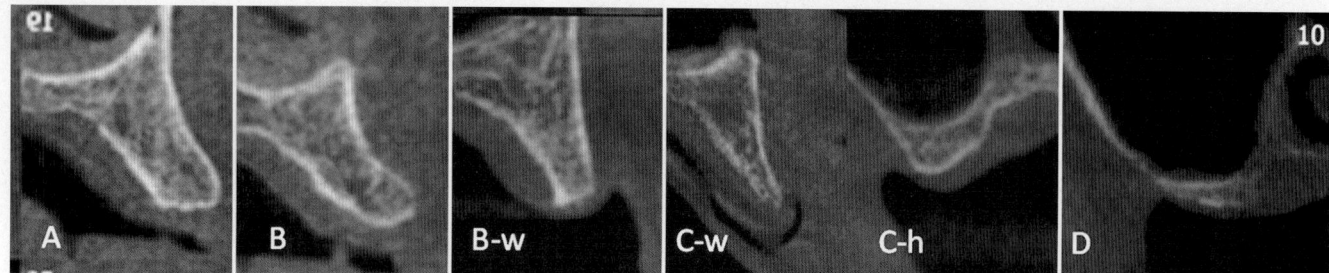

Figure 30.7 Cross-sectional view of maxilla of different patients showing availability of bone as per the Table 30.6 classification

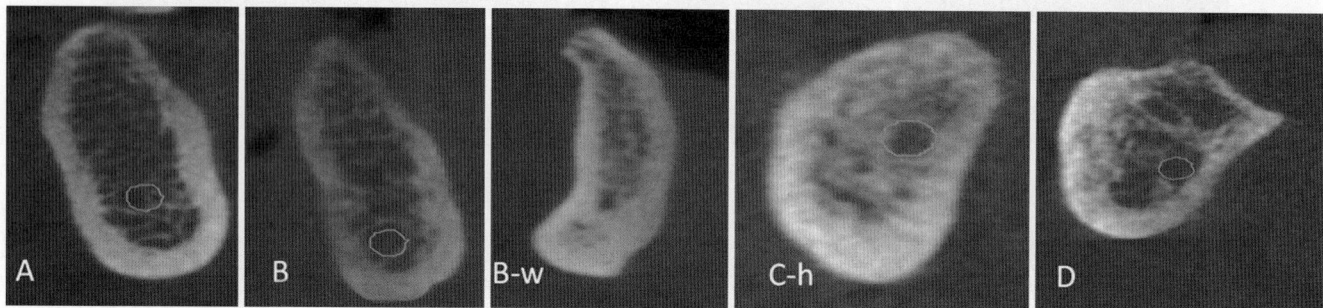

Figure 30.8 Cross-sectional view of mandible of different patients showing availability of bone as per the Table 30.6 classification

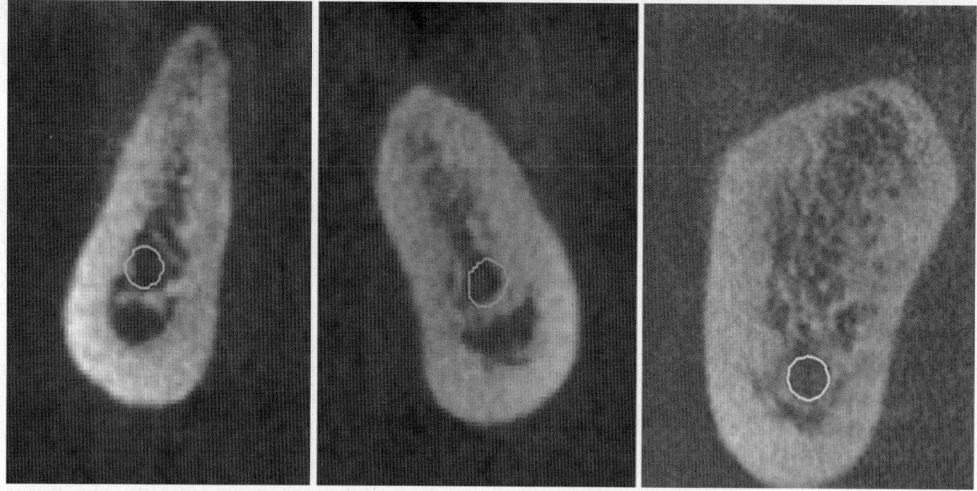

Figure 30.9 Class I type of bone seen in CBCT cross-sectional images

Table 30.7 Lekholm and Zarb classification of bone quality

	Bone quality	*HU*
Class 1	Compact cortical bone	> 1250
Class 2	Thick cortical bone surrounding highly trabecular bone	850–1250
Class 3	Thin cortical bone surrounding highly trabecular bone	350–850
Class 4	Thin cortical bone and spongy core	< 400

- *Class 2 (Fig. 30.10)*: It has slightly larger cancellation spaces with less uniformity of the osseous pattern. Satisfactory for implants. It has dense to thick porous cortical bone on the crest and within coarse trabecular bone. The architecture of the supporting bone is also a factor associated with the functional capacity of these tissues.
- *Class 3 (Fig. 30.11)*: Large marrow filled spaces exist between bony trabeculae. Results in loose fitting

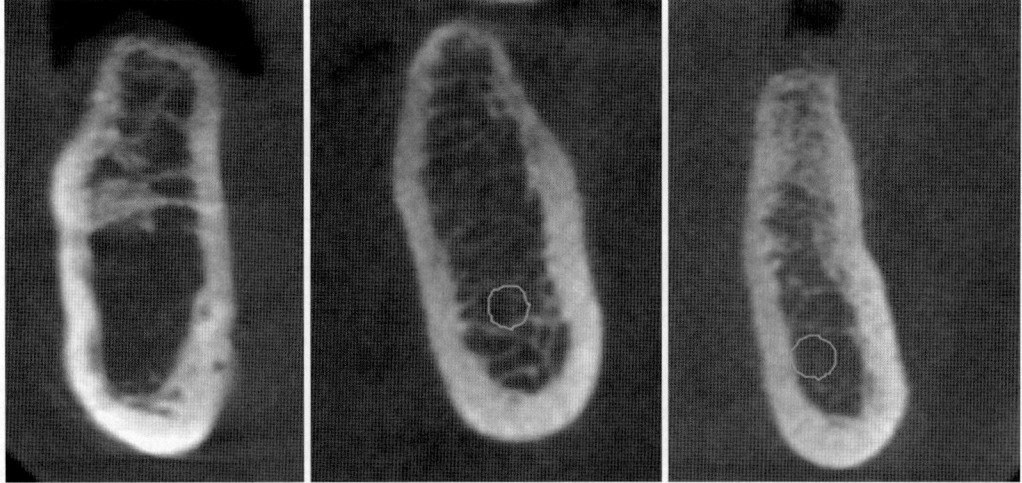

Figure 30.10 Class II type of bone seen in CBCT cross-sectional images

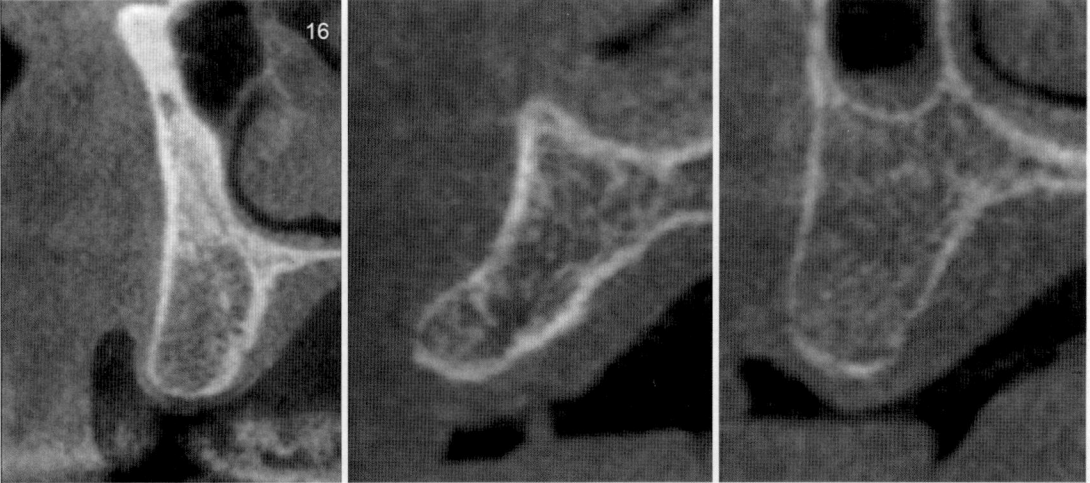

Figure 30.11 Class III type of bone seen in CBCT cross-sectional images

implant. It has thinner porous cortical crest and fine trabecular bone. Dynamic loads received by the implants may strain the supporting bone and induce changes in that bone.

– *Class 4 (Fig. 30.12)*: (D4) bone has been associated with higher implant failures. No crestal cortical bone. Bone requires a certain amount of strain for maintenance, but excessive strain may cause fatigue failure of the trabeculae.

Implant placement in denser, but not highly dense bone is to be preferred.

WP implants are not preferred in type 1 bone, as this may lead to marginal bone resorption during the healing period.

'Bone quality' is a term which is widely used but includes various factors, including cortical thickness and density and

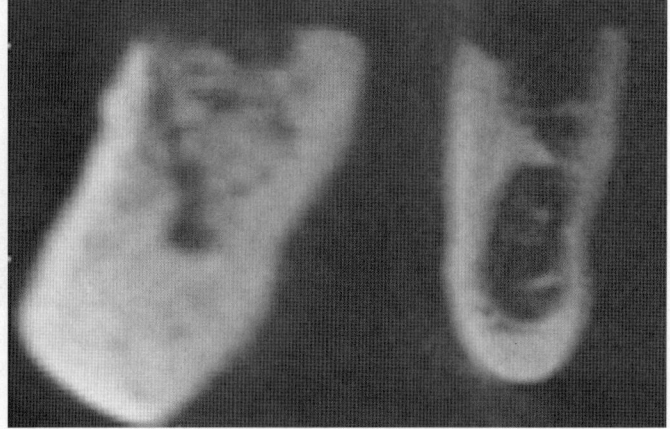

Figure 30.12 Class IV type of bone seen in CBCT cross-sectional images

importantly, BMD (Bone mineral density). A number of *in vivo* methods are available for the measurement of BMD, including:

- Single photon absorptiometry
- Dual photon absorptiometry
- QCT
- Single energy X-ray absorptiometry
- Dual energy X-ray absorptiometry.

The radiographic methods also allow topographic precise assessments of bone densities in region of interest. Currently, DXA (Dual energy X-ray absorptiometry) is widely accepted as the 'gold standard' method of clinical bone mineral measurement.

It showed significant correlation between bone density values in jaws and those of lumbar spine, femoral neck and forearm.

Many of the problems which arise during treatment or once the prosthesis is in function are most readily diagnosed using standard intraoral views. These include:

- Burning mouth syndrome
- Bone loss
- Component loosening
- Screw breakage
- Implant fracture
- Adjacent endodontic lesions
- Loss of integration.

However, some researchers argue that since the resolution level of an optimal radiographic technique is close to 0.1 mm, and the size of a fibroblast is at least 10 times smaller, it becomes evident that radiographs cannot be used to exclude the possibility of intervening soft tissue.

Determine Long Axis of Alveolar Bone (Fig. 30.13)

Axis orientation describes the angle formed by the vertical long axis of the alveolar-basal bone complex when viewed in cross-section. Information about the axis orientation is important for successful alignment of the implant within the boundaries of the jaws. Determining the long axis of the alveolar bone allows the clinician to optimize the trajectory of implant placement with the emergence profile and loading characteristics of the implant.

Identify and Localize Internal Anatomy

Adjacent teeth and identifying internal structures aid the clinician in determining the boundaries for implant placement. The important anatomical landmarks to be noted when doing implant placement are given in **Table 30.8**.

- *Maxillary sinus (Figs 30.14 to 30.16)*: The maxillary sinus is pyramidal in shape and of low-density (black or dark)

Table 30.8 Important anatomical landmarks for implant planning

Maxilla	*Mandible*
Maxillary sinus	Inferior alveolar canal
Posterior superior alveolar artery	Mental foramen with lingula
Nasal fossa	Mental foramen
Incisive/nasopalatine canal	Genial tubercles
Pterygoid plates	Groove for lingual artery
	Digastric fossa
	Submandibular fossa

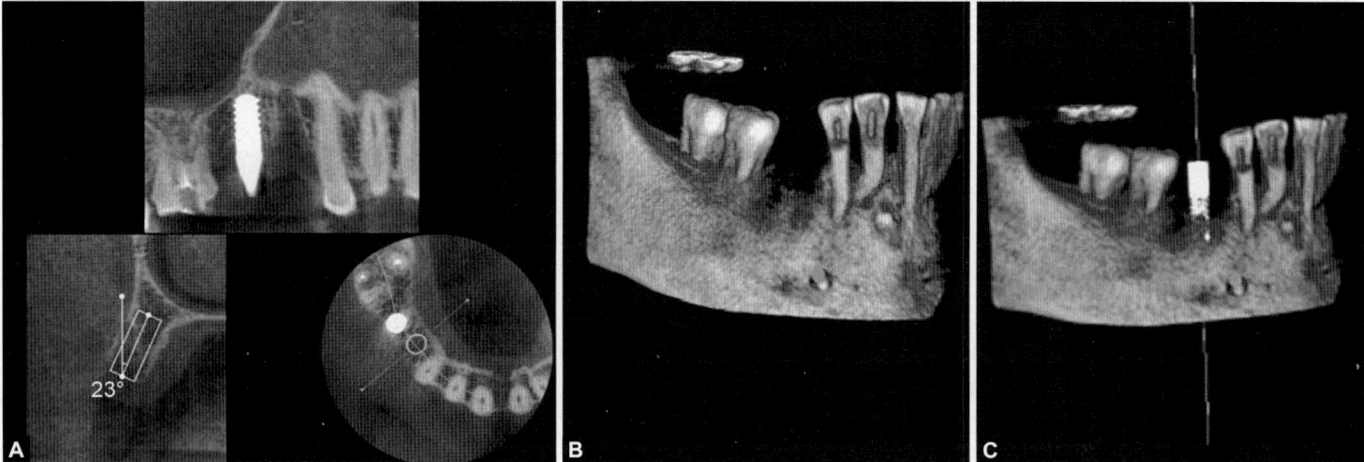

Figures 30.13A to C (A) Cone beam computed tomography scan showing virtual implant in panoramic, cross-sectional and axial view, the angulation of the implant can be simulated using the measurement tools; (B) 3D view of mandible; (C) Virtual implant inserted and angulation viewed in the 3D view

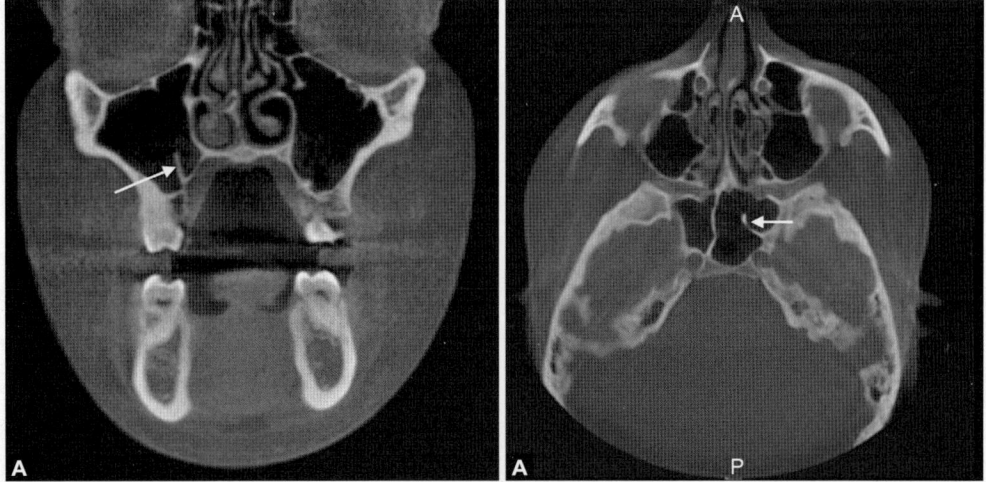

Figure 30.14 CBCT: (A) Coronal; (B) Axial images showing septa in the maxillary sinus

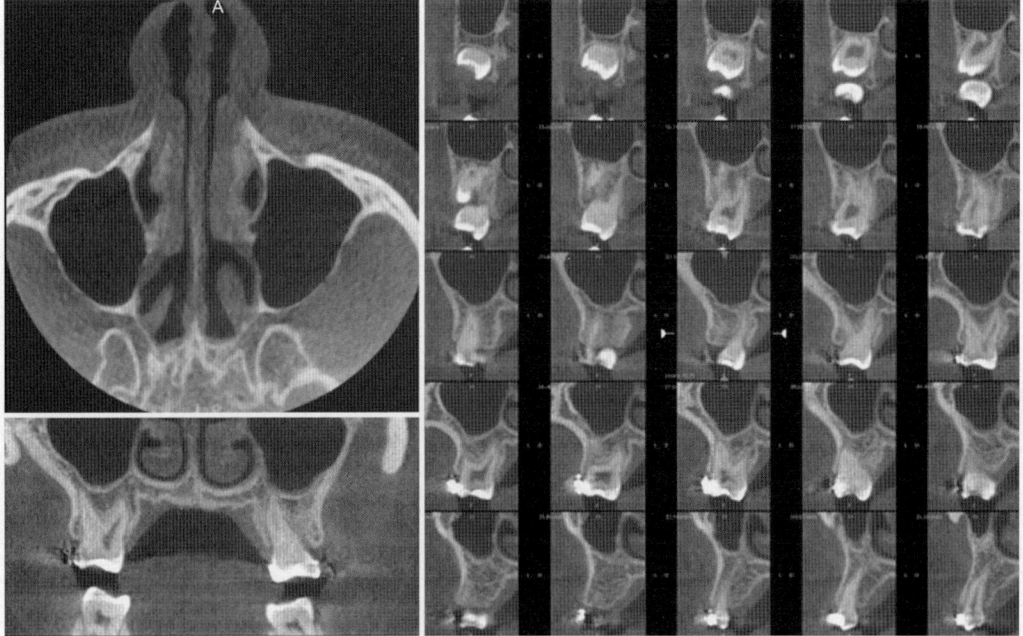

Figure 30.15 CBCT, axial, coronal and cross-sectional images giving an overview of the maxillary sinus region

structure. The appearance of healthy air cavities in the maxillary sinuses is dark (black) because of the fact that air attenuates x-rays minimally. The thin cortical outline of the buccal and medial sinus walls can be identified in these images. The medial wall of the maxillary sinus borders the sinus cavity from the nasal cavity. Standard implant placement in the posterior maxilla is often limited by the lack of vertical bone height due to the pneumatization of the sinus which may then require sinus lift procedures or graft placement before the implant procedure. Determination of septa and various

pathologies like poly etc. are important before implant placement in this region.

- *Posterior superior alveolar artery (**Figs 30.17A to C**)*: This is a vascular canal (or groove) in the wall of the maxillary sinus. Care should be taken during implant placement as encroachment may lead to profuse bleeding.
- *Nasal cavity and nasal septum (**Fig. 30.18**)*: The floor of the nasal cavity and position of the nasal septum are critical when placing implants in the anteriomaxillary region.
- *Nasoplalatine canal (**Figs 30.19 to 30.21**)*: Implant surgery in the anterior maxilla is often challenging because the

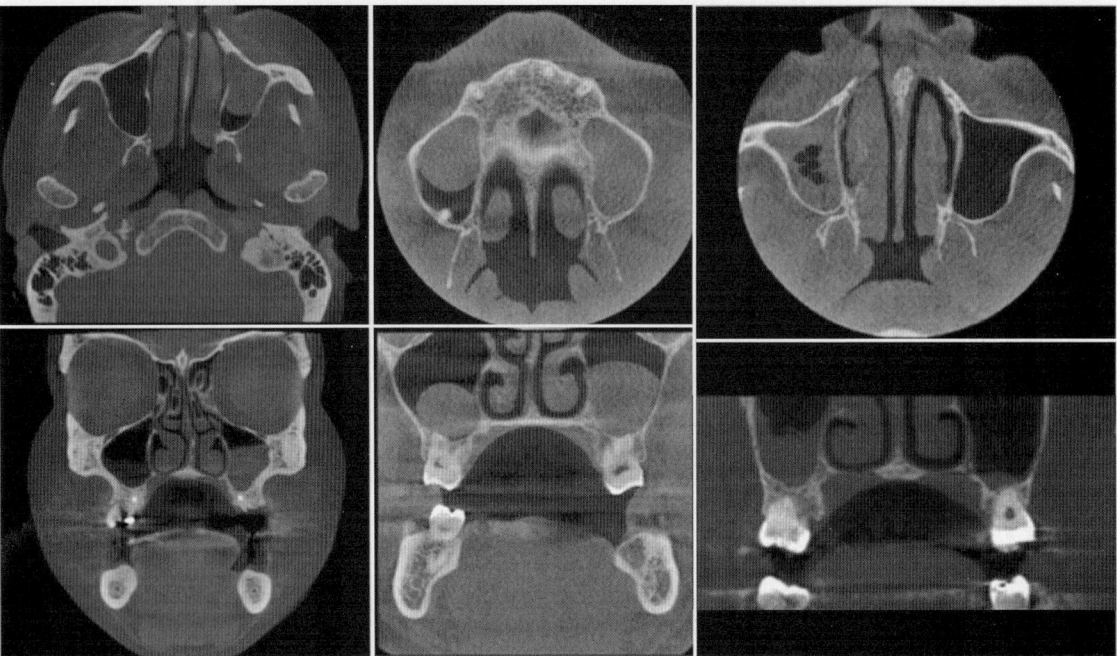

Figure 30.16 CBCT, axial and coronal images showing polyps and fluid levels in the maxillary sinus

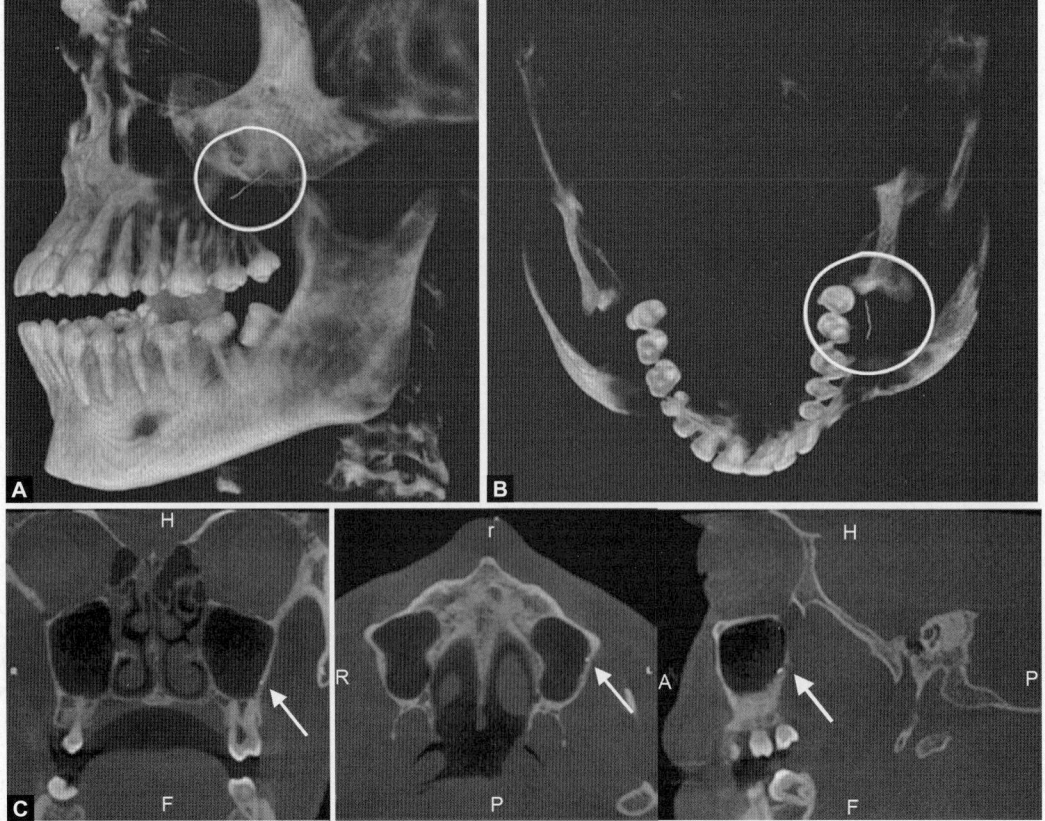

Figures 30.17A to C The posterior superior alveolar artery as seen on: (A) 3D CBCT lateral view; (B) 3D CBCT submento vertex view; (C) Coronal, axial and sagittal CBCT views

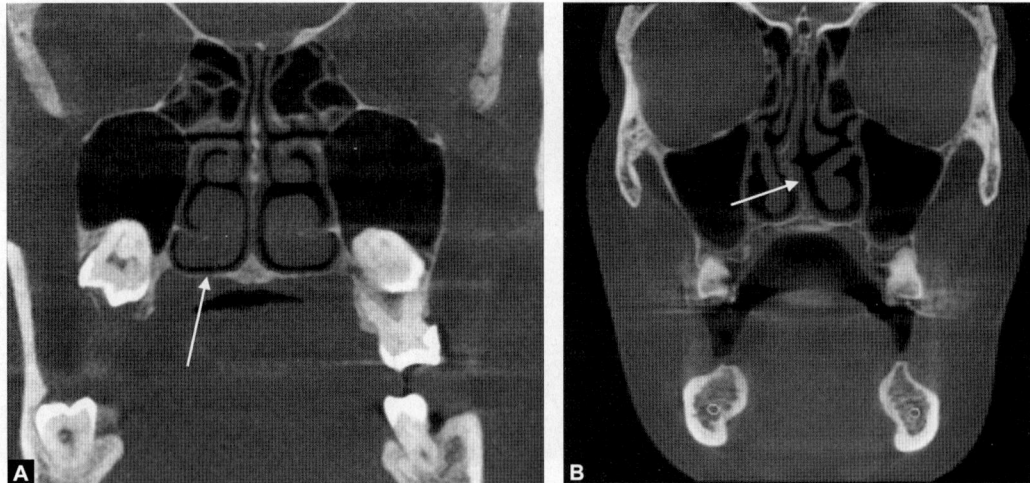

Figures 30.18A and B Cone beam computed tomography coronal images showing: (A) Floor of the nasal cavity; (B) Nasal septum

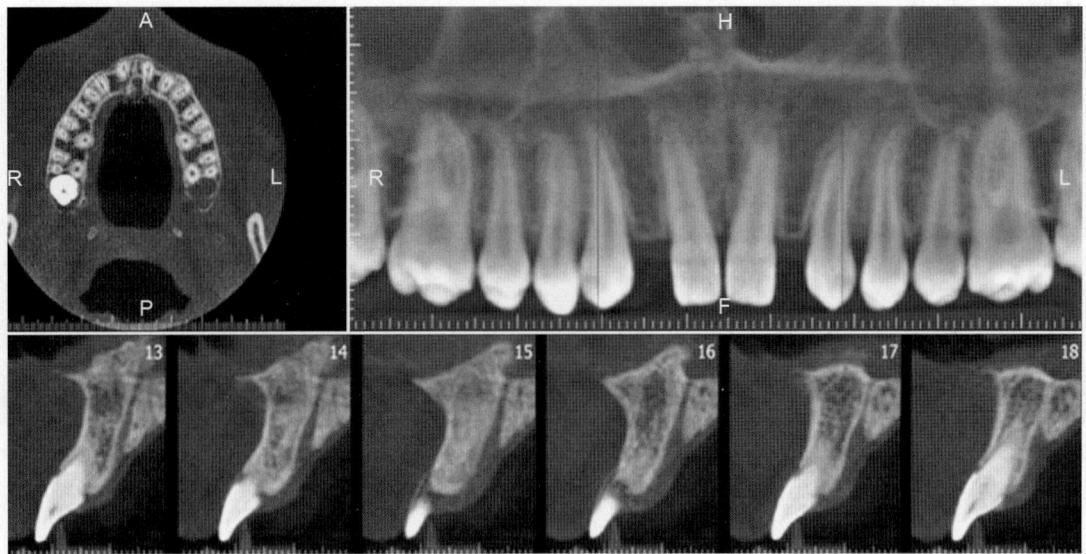

Figure 30.19 Cone beam computed tomography axial, panoramic and cross-sectional views of the nasopalatine canal

biomechanical, esthetic and phonetic demands need to find a perfect compromise with the anatomical limitations. In this perspective, it is important to consider the presence of the nasopalatine canal. Nasopalatine canal may vary in dimensions and may pose limitation in placing implant in this esthetic zone.

- *Pterygoid plates (Fig. 30.22)*: These bony landmarks should be determined when placing implants in the maxillary posterior region.
- *Mandibular foramen (Fig. 30.23)*: This landmark is only seen on a CBCT image. Inferior alveolar canal start from mandibular foramen and transverse within the body of

mandible to mental foramen. It traverses the mandible from the lingual to the buccal side. The nerve is midway between the buccal and lingual cortical plates in the first molar vicinity.

- *Mandibular canal (MC) (Fig. 30.24)*: The mandibular canal houses the inferior alveolar nerve, the inferior alveolar artery and inferior alveolar vein. The canal is seen bilaterally as it enters the mandible at the mandibular foramen on the lingual side of the ramus. The canal appears lucent with corticated borders and is usually seen inferior to the roots of the mandibular teeth.

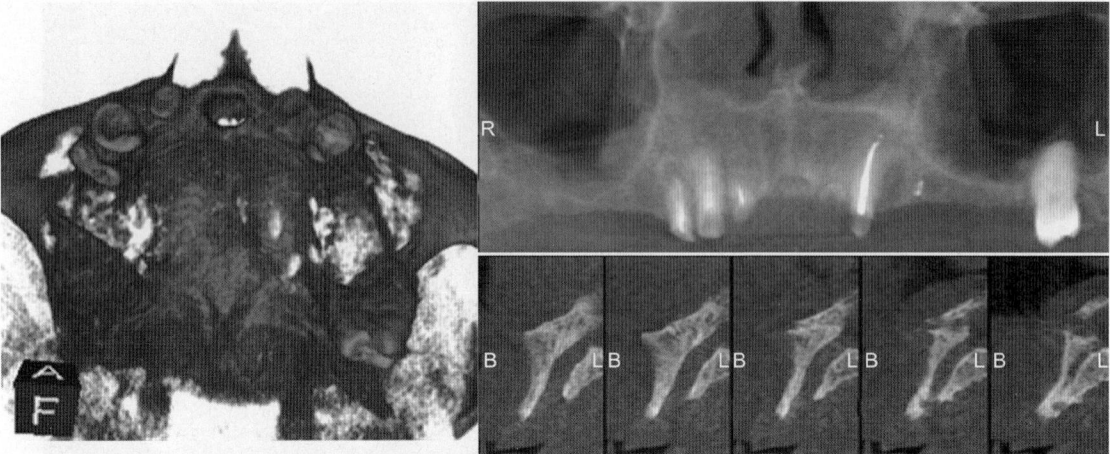

Figure 30.20 Cone beam computed tomography 3D, panoramic and cross-sectional views of the nasopalatine canal, showing a wide foramen which may lead to esthetic issues in anterior implant placement like diastema

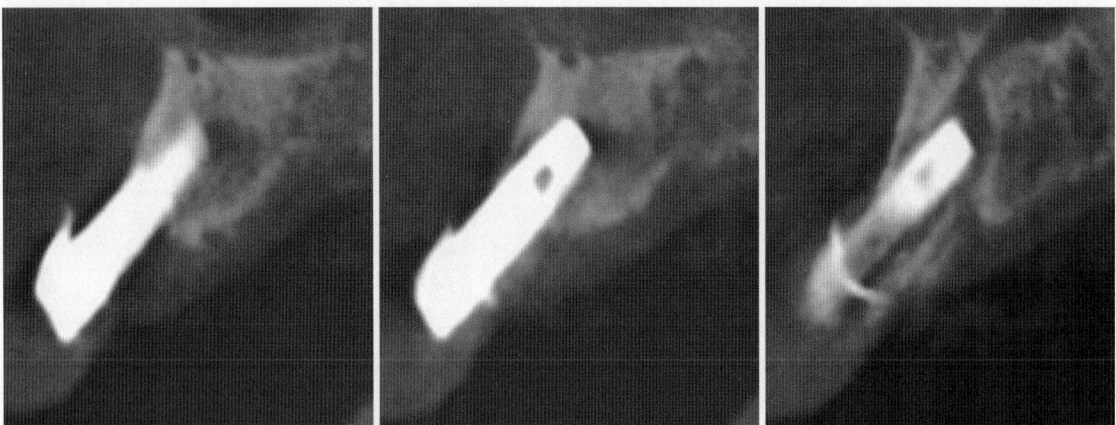

Figure 30.21 CBCT cross-sectional view shows implant placement complications due to encroachment into the naso palatine canal

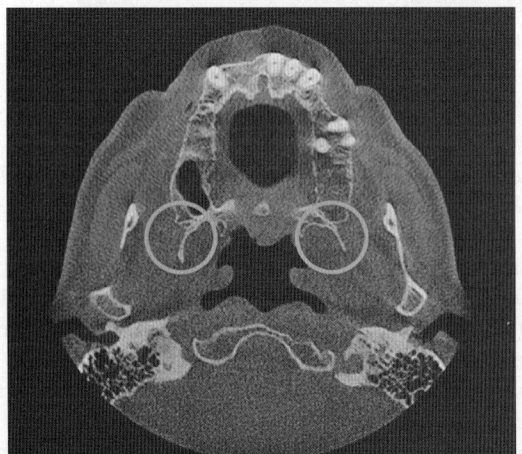

Figure 30.22 Cone beam computed tomography axial section showing left and right pterygoid plates

It is classified: According to its path (Classification by Anderson et al./ Classification by Nortje et al.).

- A = A steep ascent from anterior to posterior or a high MC (within 2 mm of the apices of the first and second molars).
- B = A gentle, progressive curve rising from anterior to posterior or an intermediate MC.
- C and D = A catenary-like canal/ or C = A low MC; D = Other variations.
- Classification of the topography of the inferior alveolar nerve.
  - I = The nerve has a course near the apices of the teeth
  - II = The main trunk is low down in the body
  - III = The main trunk is low down in the body of the mandible with several smaller trunks to the molar teeth (McManners 2000).

The mandibular canal has various shapes as can be noted in the cross sectional images, oval, circular or pyriform **(Fig 30.25)**.

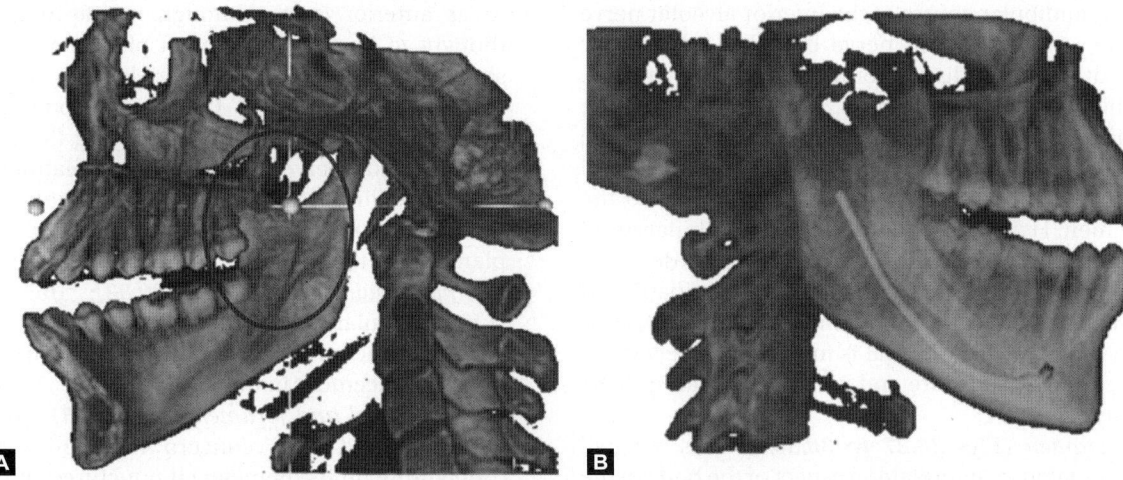

Figures 30.23A and B 3D Cone beam computed tomography: (A) Showing mandibular foramen on the lingual aspect of the mandible; (B) Path of the inferior alveolar nerve from the mandibular foramen to the mental foramen

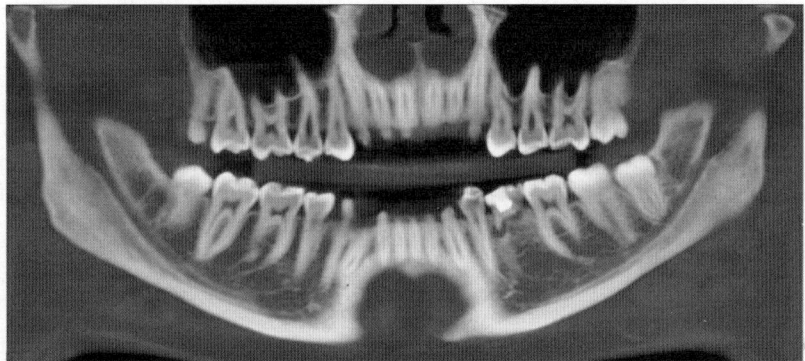

Figure 30.24 Cone beam computed tomography panoramic image in the thinnest slice will enable tracing of the mandibular canal, which is seen as a single channel, enclosed by bony tissue, forming an upward concave curve

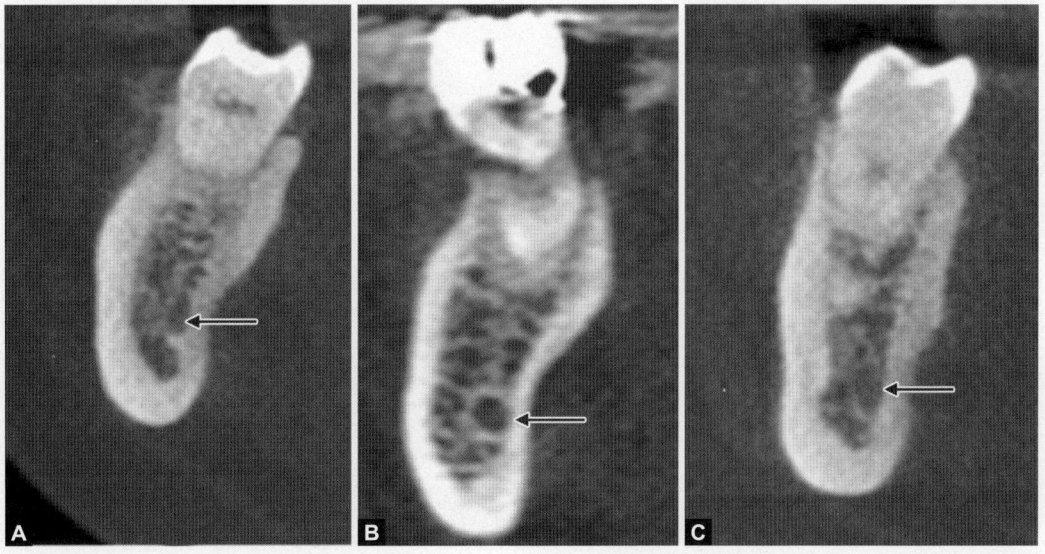

Figures 30.25A to C Different shape of the mandibular canal seen on cross-sectional images; oval, circular or pyriform

The intramandibular course of the inferior alveolar nerve has a number of vessels and nerve branches which may be spread out so that a distinct bone canal is not present. Neurovascular components may course through the mandible as a single entity or as a plexus, presenting a range of different-sized bundles, which do not necessarily travel within a bony canal from the mandibular foramen to the mental foramen. Hence many a times the mandibular canal cannot be identified or is visible, but has diffuse borders.

Variation in the anatomy of the MC is quite rampant with bifid canal being the most common finding (**Fig. 30.26**). This variation in inferior alveolar canal is important to recognize before any surgical procedure and its presence can only be confirmed by CBCT/CT.

- *Mental foramen (Figs 30.27 to 30.30A)*: It is a small foramen situated in anterolateral aspect of the body of the mandible. The mental nerve which enters the mandibular incisive canal, which continues anteriorly within the body of mandible. The size shape, location and direction of the opening of mental foramen have many variations. There is variation in its horizontal (**Table 30.9**) and vertical (**Table 30.10**) position which needs to be determined before implant procedures in its vicinity. Consequently, placement of immediate implants in the premolar area is associated with complications as in 25–38% of the cases the foramen is located coronal to the premolar apex.
- *Mandibular incisive canal and nerve (Fig. 30.30B)*: The mandibular nerve exits from the mental foramen into the incisive canal and proceed forward as the incisive nerve.
- *Anterior loop (Fig. 30.31)*: When the inferior alveolar nerve arises from the mental canal and runs outward, upward and backward to open at the mental foramen. It is referred to as anterior loop. Although interformina region are thought to be safe for implant placement consideration should be given to anterior loop when placement of implant is planned. Clinicians should not rely on panoramic radiographs for identifying the anterior loop of the mental nerve during implant treatment planning. A safe guideline of 4 mm, from the most anterior point of the mental foramen, is recommended for implant treatment planning on the basis of our anatomical findings.
- *Submandibular fossa (Fig. 30.32)*: This houses the submandibular gland and the undercut can be rather severe at times and may impose an anatomic limitation in implant placement in the region.
- *Lingual canal and foramen (Fig. 30.33)*: This canal has been reported as a concern for significant bleeding (depending on its diameter) if punctured during implant surgery. These foramina are identified fairly inferior, unless severe bone resorption is noted. Although not as frequently additional vascular channels may be present anterior to the premolar locations unilaterally or bilaterally. Depending on their diameter, they may pose a similar limitation to implant surgery as their midline counterparts.
- *Genial tubercle (Figs 30.34A to C)*: This landmarks have various muscle attachment and precaution should be taken while placing implants in the mandibular anterior region.

Determine Jaw Boundaries

Imaging can be used to identify the outer boundary of the jaws including impressions into the jaws, such as fossae.

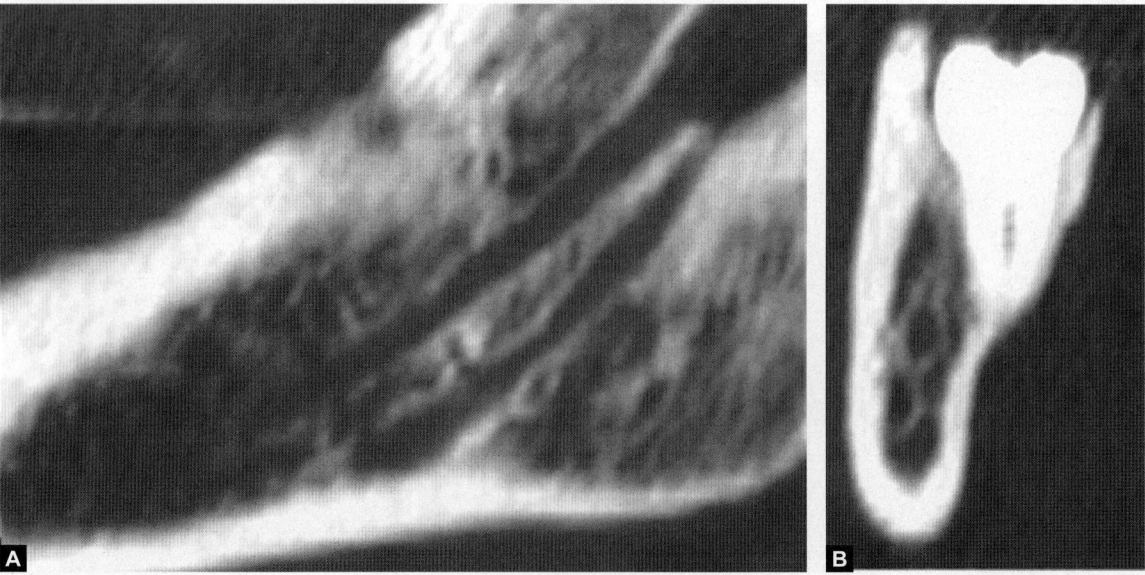

Figures 30.26A and B Bifid canal seen in cone beam computed tomography cropped reconstructed panoramic image and cross-section image

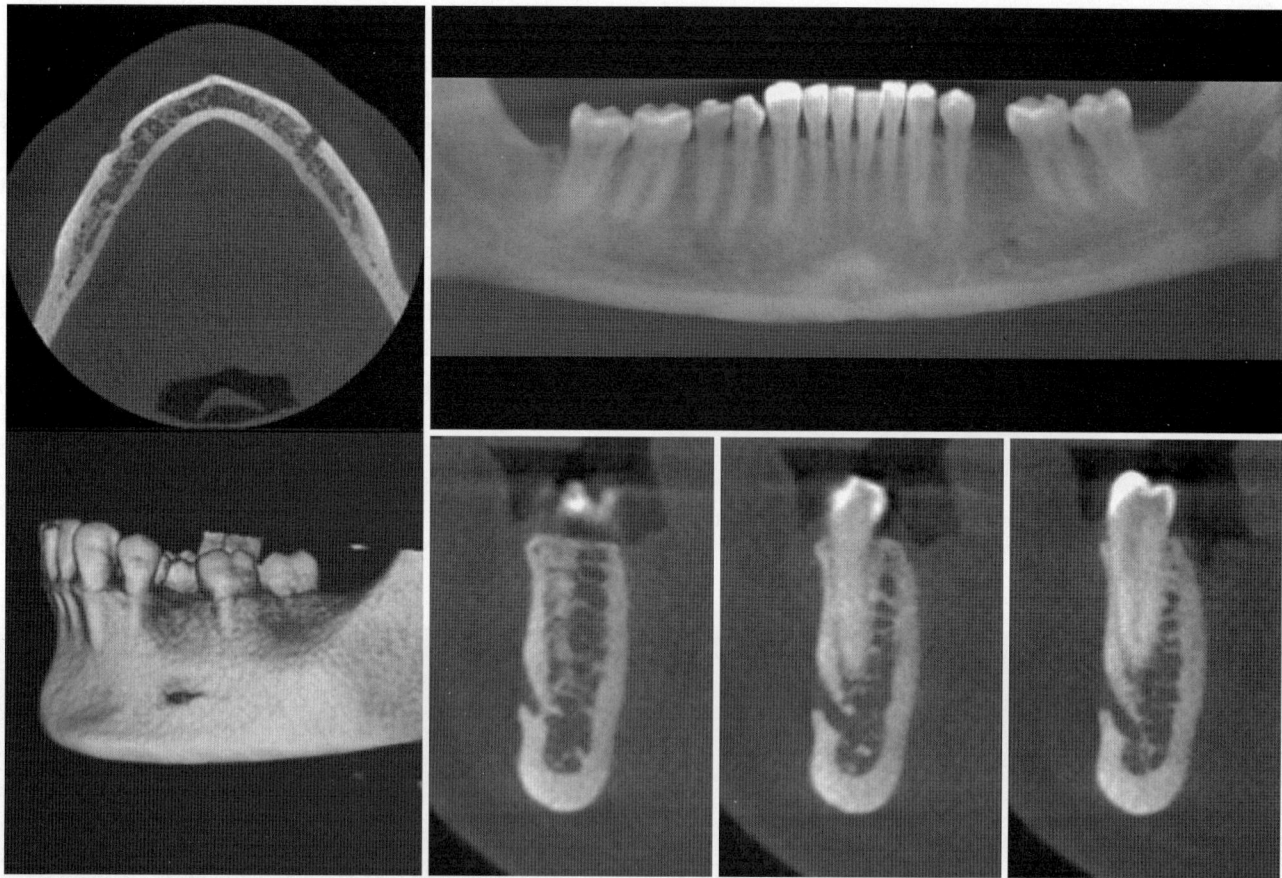

Figure 30.27 Mental foramen as seen on cone beam computed tomography; axial, panoramic, 3D and cross-sectional views

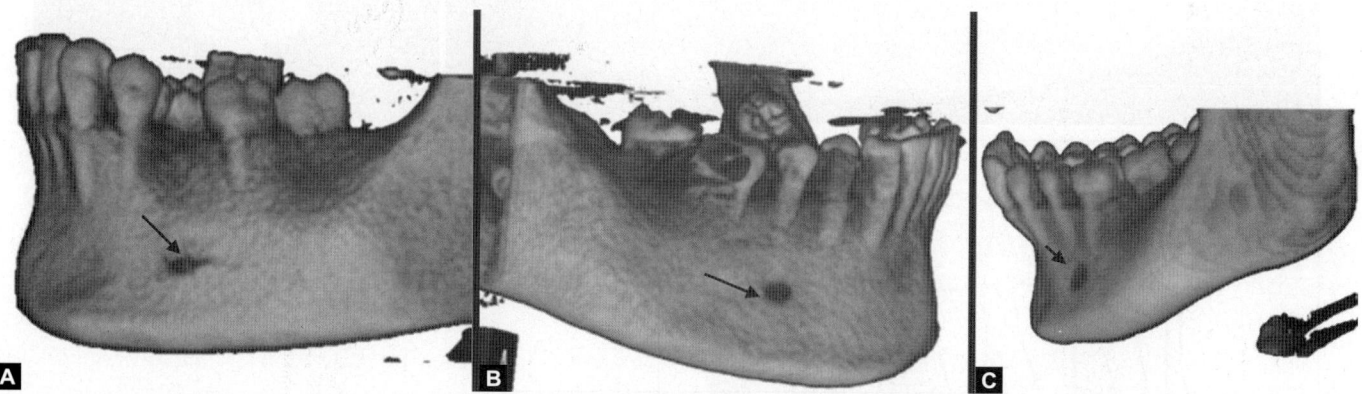

Figures 30.28A to C Different shapes of the mental foramen: (A) Oval horizontal; (B) Round; (C) Oval vertical

Pathology Detection

Abnormalities involving the alveolar ridge include retained root tips, inflammatory processes, cyst, and tumors. In addition, anomalies involving other maxilofacial structures such as maxillary sinuses and TMJs may complicate the successful implant process. For example, changes in stress (force/area) directed at poorly adapted TMJs may increase TMJ symptoms. Changes in TMJ stress levels may result from operative manipulations, changes in masticatory abilities and changes in vertical dimension or maxillomandibular spatial relationships.

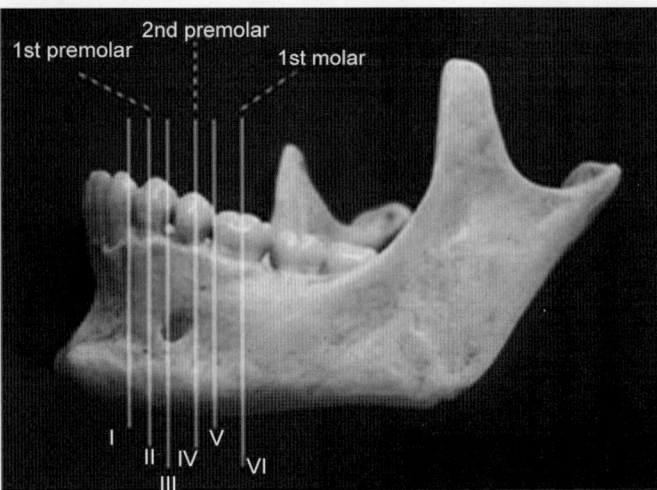

Figure 30.29 Relationship of mental foramen to the lower teeth as per classification in Table 30.9

Determine Post Implant Placement Status

Besides clinical evaluation, the interpretation of radiographic images is a frequently applied diagnostic procedure. Imaging plays an important part of treatment with tissue- integrated prostheses, both at the preoperative stage to obtain full assessment of the bony host and at the post-operative stage to assess the clinical result (**Table 30.11**). Intervention, at an early stage might save early-failing implants from complete loss of osseointegration. Hence, radiographic examination is an essential diagnostic evaluation prerequistite for evaluation of success and/ or failure of oral implants (**Figs 30.21, 30.35 to 30.41**).

Radiographic assessment is valuable measures of implant success when:

• Area due to constricted implant neck cannot be probed
• To assess future mobility without FPD removal
• To accurately determine amount of bone loss in absence of increased crevicular depth.

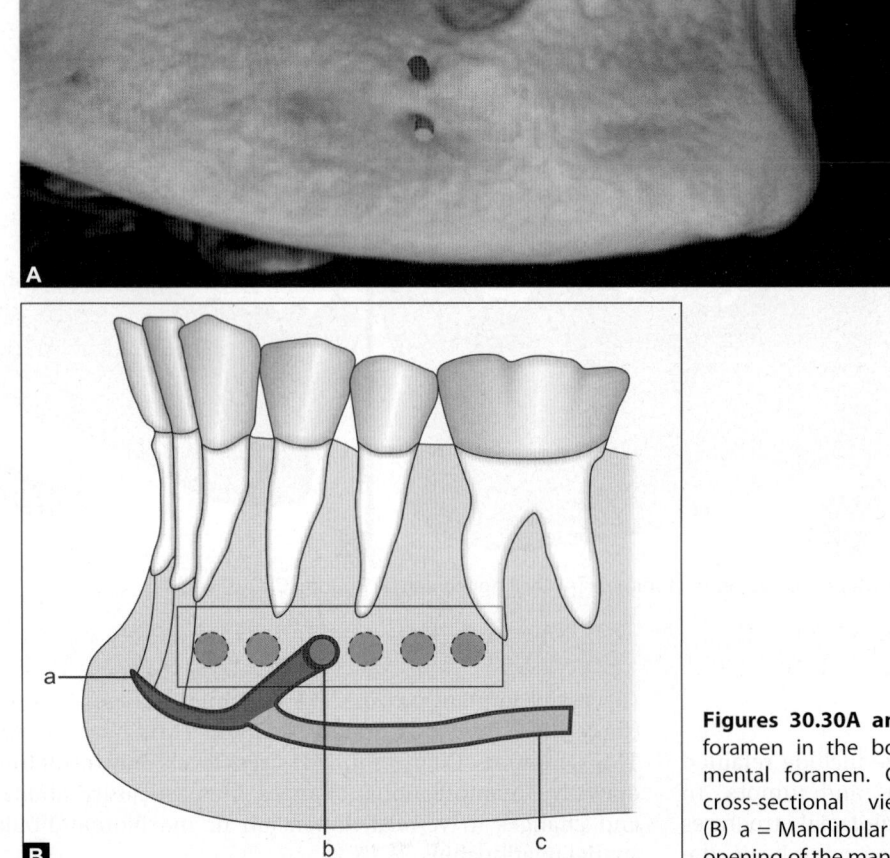

Figures 30.30A and B (A) Any foramen in addition to mental foramen in the body of the mandible is known as accessory mental foramen. Cone beam computed tomography 3D and cross-sectional views showing accessory mental foramen; (B) a = Mandibular incisive canal (MIC); b = Mental canal (Anterior opening of the mandibular canal); c = Mandibular canal

Table 30.9 Position of mental foramen described anterior posteriorly (Fig. 30.29)

Position 1 : MF situated anterior to the first premolar tooth
Position 2 : MF situated in the line with the long axis of first premolar tooth
Position 3 : MF situated between the apices of the first and second premolar teeth
Position 4 : MF situated in the line with the long axis of second premolar tooth
Position 5 : MF situated between the apices of the second premolar and first molar teeth
Position 6 : MF situated in the line with the long axis of mesial root of first molar tooth.

Table 30.10 Superio-inferior position of the mental foramen recorded in relation to the adjacent teeth

I : Above the level of apices of 1st and 2nd premolar
II : At the level of the apices of 1st and 2nd premolar
III : Below the apices of the 1st and 2nd premolar

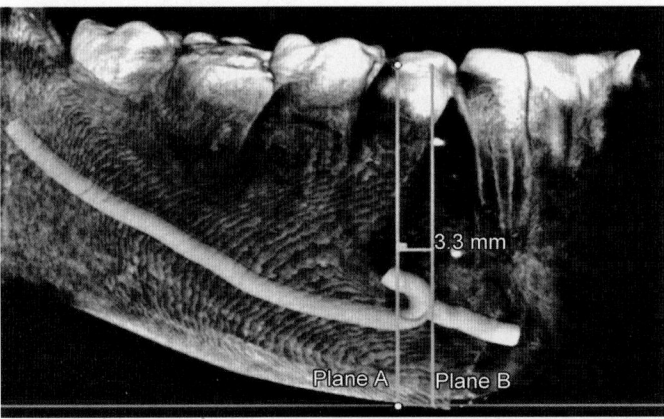

Figure 30.31 Anterior loop traced and determined on cone beam computed tomography

How to do radiographic postimplant assessment?
- Compare bony changes with stable landmarks—implant threads—(one-half thread = 0.3 mm)
- Expect 1.0 mm marginal bone loss during first year post insertion
- 0.1 mm per year anticipated thereafter
- Greater bone loss observed in maxilla.

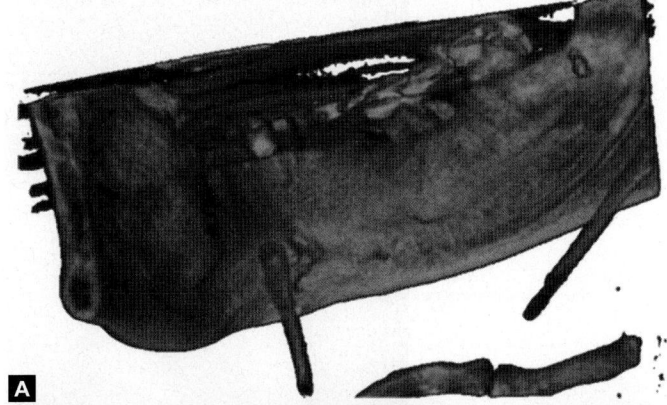

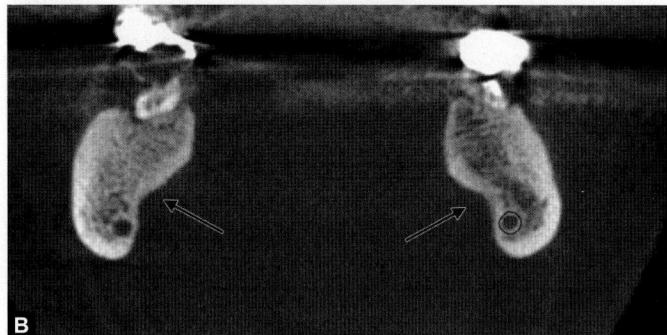

Figures 30.32A and B: Submandibular gland fossa seen on cone beam computed tomography: (A) 3D; (B) Coronal section

Evaluation of Osseointegrated Implants

In fibrointegrated implants, a faint line is visible surrounding the implant. This line may not be continuous, depending upon the intimacy of the contact between the bone and the implant. The osseointegrated implants forms a solid chemical bond to the host bone, which results in an intimate contact. The space between the implant fills in, except for the most superficial portion of the implant. A faint halo can be seen on the axial CT slices near the mucosal border. Determination of the presence of osseointegration should be made on the axial views, because they are the images with the highest resolution.

In patients with two or more adjacent implants, there will often be a very subtle black space between the implants on the axial views. This is a 'beam-hardening' artifact caused by passage of X-ray beam through two relatively dense objects in a single plane. A disproportionate amount of the X-ray beam is absorbed by the two implants and an error occurs in those picture elements between the two implants.

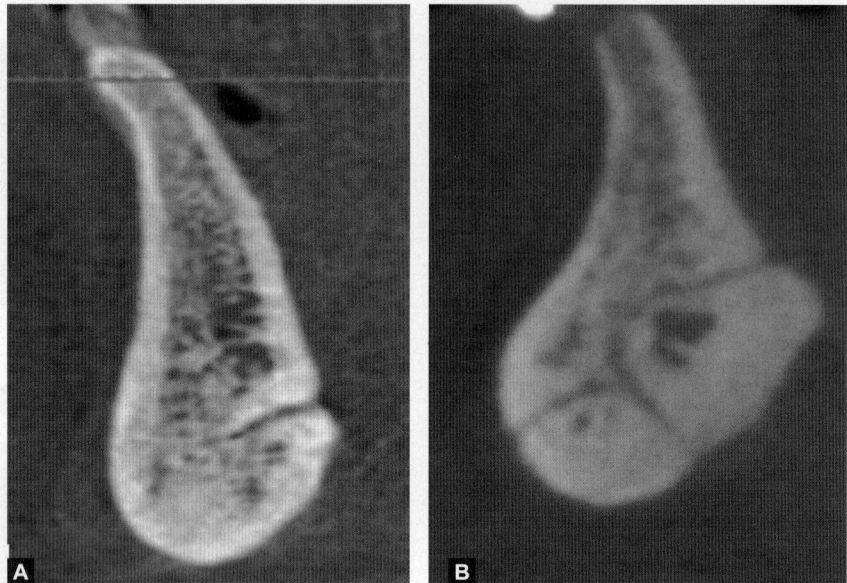

Figures 30.33A and B Cone beam computed tomography cross-sectional view showing: (A) Lingual foramen; (B) Accessory lingual foramina

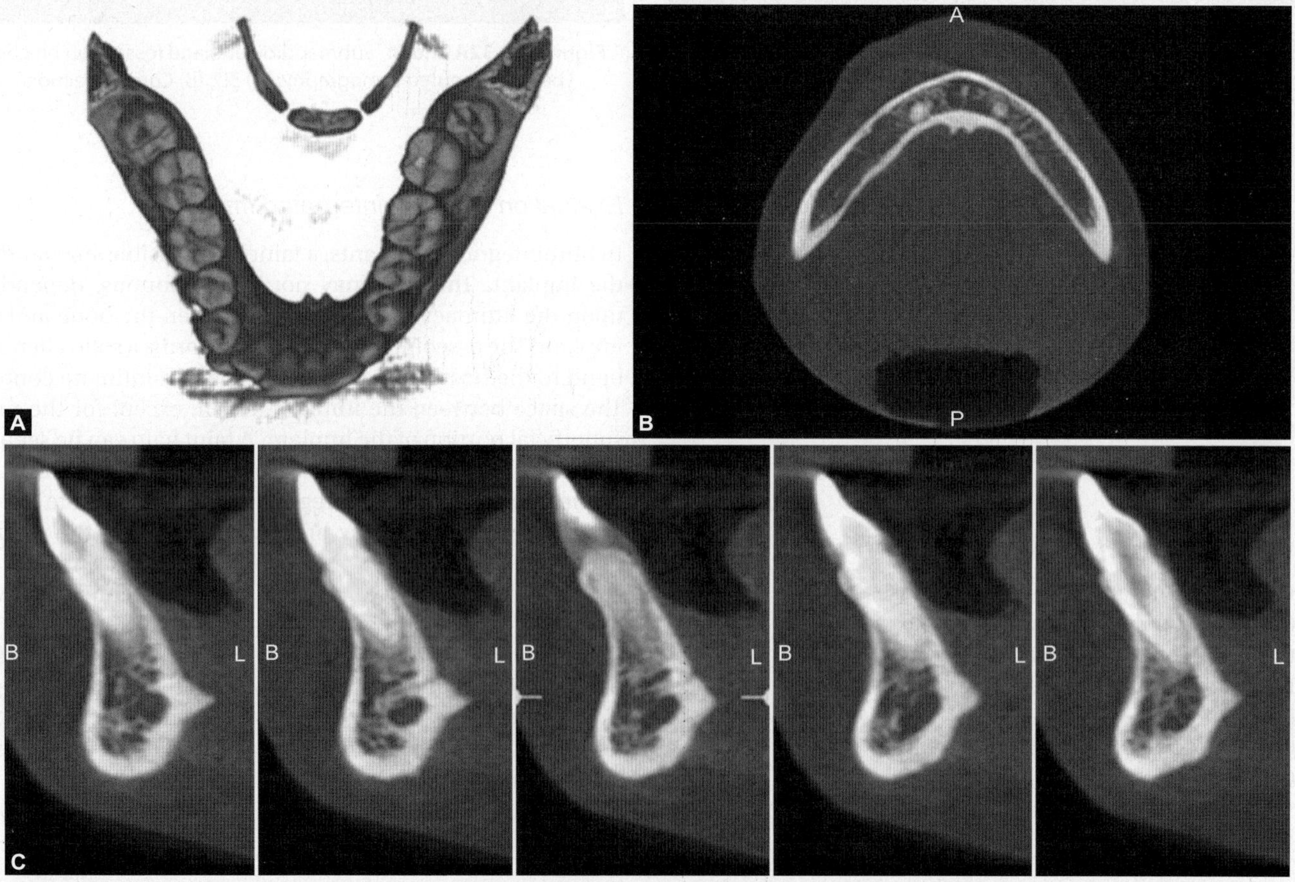

Figures 30.34A to C Genial tubercule seen on cone beam computed tomography: (A) 3D; (B) Axial section; (C) Cross-sections

Table 30.11 Radiographic signs associated with failing endosseous implants

Radiographic appearance	Clinical implications
Thin radiolucent area that closely follows the outline of the implant	Failure of the implant to integrate with the adjoining bone
Crestal bone loss around the coronal portion of the implant	Adverse loading or osteitis resulting from poor plaque control, or both
Apical migration of alveolar bone on one side of the implant	Nonaxial loading resulting from improper angulation of the implant
Widening of the periodontal ligament space of the nearest natural abutment	Poor stress distribution resulting from biomechanical inadequate prosthesis implant system
Fracture of the implant fixture	Unfavorable stress distribution during function
Rapid bone loss	Fractured fixture, initial osseous trauma at insertion, fixture over-tightening, occlusal trauma, poor adaptation of prosthesis to abutment, 'normal' physiologic response, plaque-associated infection (peri-implantitis)

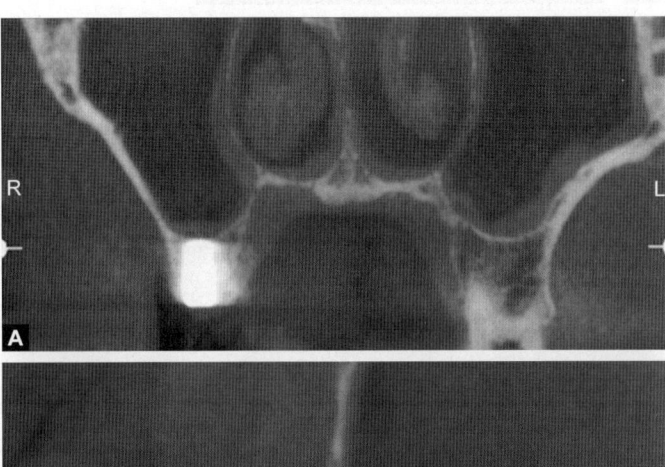

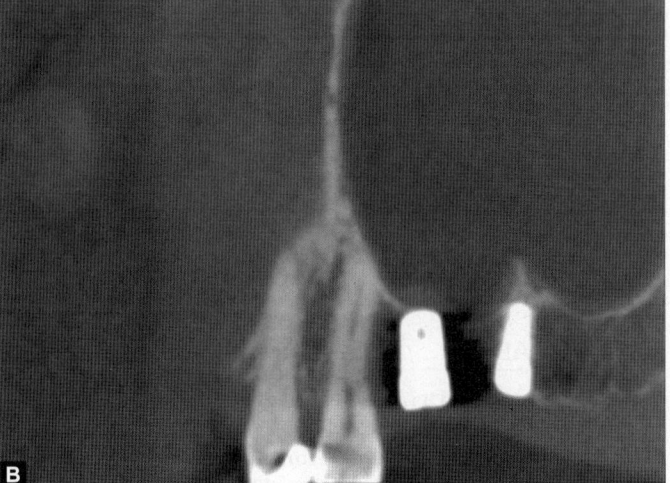

Figures 30.35A and B CBCT cross-sectional and sagittal view showing proximity of implant to the floor of the maxillary sinus

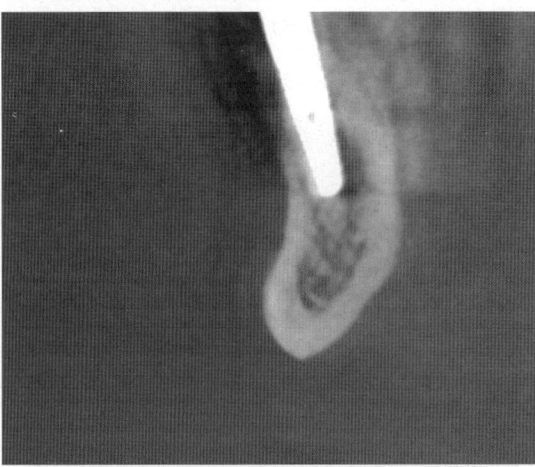

Figure 30.36 CBCT, cross-sectional view showing peri implantitis

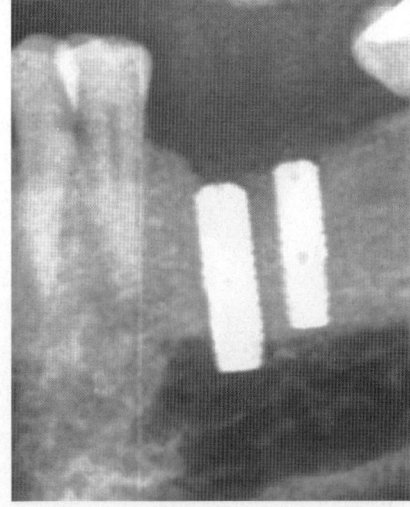

Figure 30.37 Close approximation between the surrounding bone and screw depicting a successful implant

The position and orientation of implants are easily determined from the cross-sectional oblique reformations. It is ideal that the implants parallel the plane of adjacent teeth. The screw access hole will then lie in the center of the prosthesis.

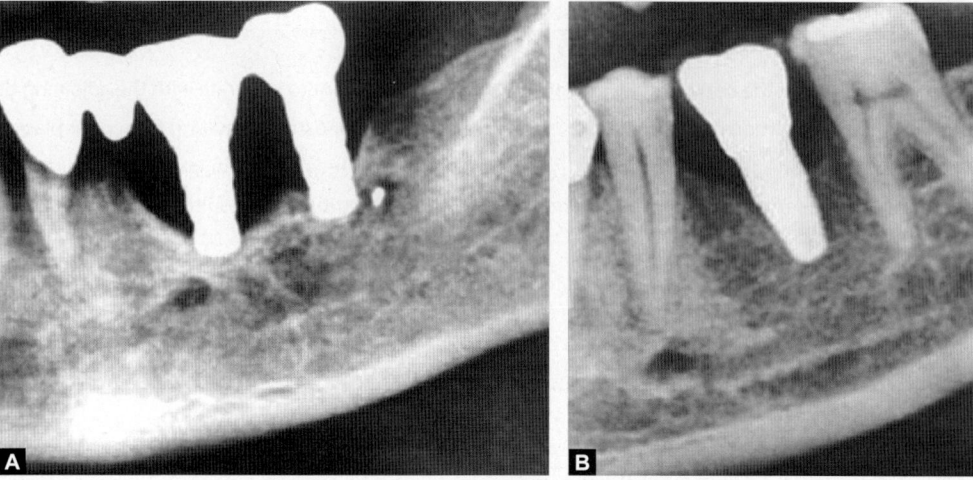

Figures 30.38A and B (A) Complete bone loss around implant; (B) Saucerization type of moderate bone loss in cervical region

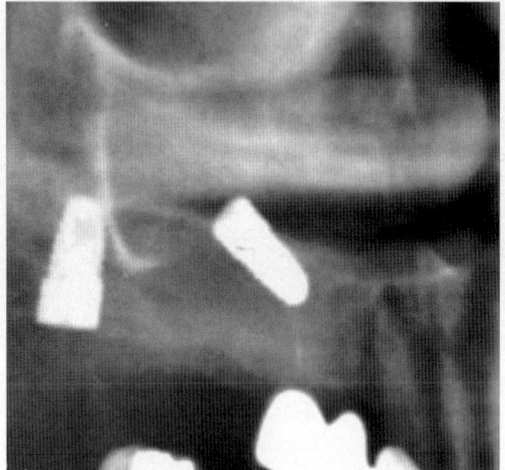

Figure 36.39 Failed implant in maxillary sinus

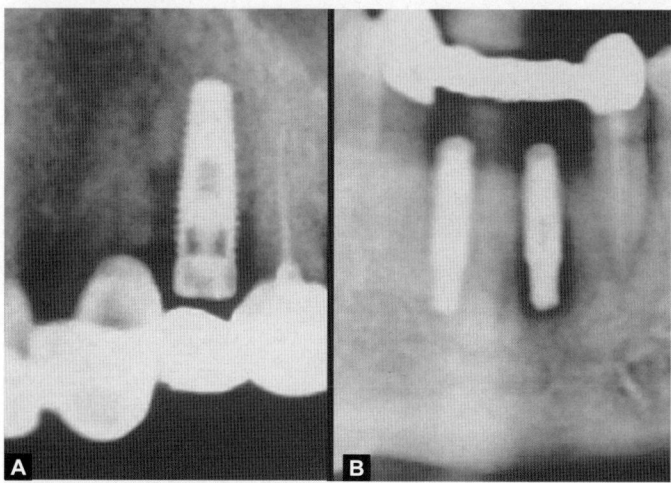

Figures 30.40A and B: (A) Vertical bone loss; (B) Peri-implantitis

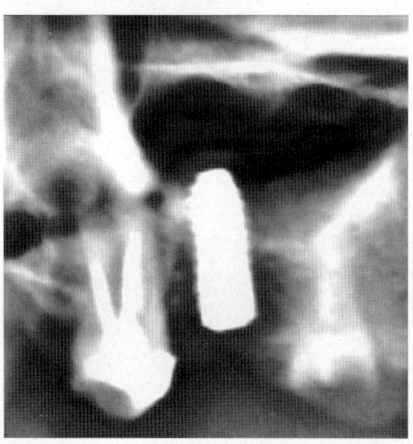

Figure 30.41 Conventional tomogram reveals the perforation of maxillary sinus floor

BIBLIOGRAPHY

1. Abrahams JJ. Dental CT imaging: a look at the jaw. Radiology. 2001;219(2):334-45.
2. Angelopoulos C, Aghaloo T. Imaging technology in implant diagnosis. Dent Clin North Am. 2011;55(1):141-58.
3. Clark DE, Danforth RA, Barnes RW, et al. Radiation absorbed from dental implant radiography: a comparison of linear tomography, CT scan and panoramic and intra-oral techniques. J Oral Implantol. 1990;16(3): 156-64.
4. Curry TS, Dowdey JE, Murry RC Jr. Christensen's physics of diagnostic radiology. 4th edn, Philadelphia: Lea & Febiger; 1990.pp.242-8.
5. DelBalso AM, Greiner FG, Licata M. Role of diagnostic imaging in the evaluation of the dental implant patient. Radiographics. 1994;14:699-719.

6. Ekestubbe A, Grondahl K, Grondahl HG. The use of tomography for dental implant planning. Dentomaxillofac Radiol. 1997;26(4):206-13.

7. Frederiksen NL, Benson BW, Sokolowski TW. Effective dose and risk assessment from computed tomography of the maxillofacial complex. Dentomaxillofac Radiol. 1995; 24(1):55-8.

8. Frederiksen NL. Diagnostic imaging in dental implantology. Oral Surg Oral Med Oral Pathol Oral Radiol Endod 1995; 80(5):540-54.

9. Frederiksen NL. X rays: what is the risk? Tex Dent J. 1995; 112(2):68-72.

10. Garg AK, Vicari A. Radiographic modalities for diagnosis and treatment planning in implant dentistry. Implant Soc. 1995;5(5):7-11.

11. Garg AK. Dental implant imaging: TeraRecon's Dental 3D Cone Beam Computed Tomography System. Dent Implantol Update. 2007;18(6):41-5.

12. Guerrero ME, Jacobs R, Loubele M, et al. State of the art on cone beam CT imaging for preoperative planning of implant placement. Clin Oral Investig. 2006;10(1):1-7.

13. Hatcher DC, Dial C, Mayorga C. Cone beam CT for presurgical assessment of implant sites. J Calif Dent Assoc. 2003;31:825-33.

14. Jeffcoat MK. Application of digital radiography to implantology. J Dent Symp. 1993;1:30-3.

15. Klein M, Abrams M. Computer-guided surgery utilizing a computer milled surgical template. Pract Proced Aesthet Dent. 2001;13(2):165-9.

16. Manz MC. Factors associated with radiographic vertical bone loss around implants placed in a clinical study. Ann Periodontol. 2000;5(1):137-51.

17. Miles DA, Van Dis ML. Implant radiology. Dent Clin North Am. 1993;37(4):645-8.

18. Misch CE. Density of bone: effect on treatment plans, surgical approach, healing and progressive bone loading. Int J Oral Implant. 1990;6(2):23-31.

19. Mupparapu M, Beideman R. Imaging for maxillofacial reconstruction and implantology. In: Fonseca RJ (Ed). Oral and maxillofacial surgery: reconstructive and implant surgery. Philadelphia: WB Saunders; 2000.pp.17-34.

20. Mupparapu M, Singer SR. Implant imaging for the dentist. J Can Dent Assoc. 2004;70(1):32.

21. Reisken AB. Implant imaging: status, controversies and new developments. Dent Clin North Am. 1998;42(1):47-56.

22. Rosenfeld AL, Mecall RA. The use of interactive computed tomography to predict the esthetic and functional demands of implant-supported prostheses. Compend Contin Educ Dent. 1996;17(12):1125-8,1130-20.

23. Rugani P, Kirnbauer B, Arnetzl GV, et al. Cone beam computerized tomography: basics for digital planning in oral surgery and implantology. Int J Comput Dent. 2009;12(2):131-45.

24. Sahiwal IG, Woody RD, Benson BW, Guillen GE. Radiographic identification of threaded endosseous dental implants. J Prosthet Dent. 2002;87(5):563-77.

25. Sahiwal IG, Woody RD, Benson BW, Guillen GE. Radiographic identification of nonthreaded endosseous dental implants. J Prosthet Dent. 2002;87(5):552-62.

26. Sansare KP, Singh D, Karjodkar FR, Changes in the fractal dimension on pre and post implant panoramic radiograph. Oral Radiology Nov 2011:DOI:10.1007/s11282-011-0075-8 .

27. Sawyer-Glover AM, Shellock FG. Pre-MRI procedure screening: recommendations and safety considerations for biomedical implants and devices. J Magn Reson Imaging. 2000;12(1):92-106.

28. Scaf G, et al. Dosimetry and cost of imaging osseointegrated implants with film-based and computed tomography. Oral Surg Oral Med Oral Pathol Oral Radiol and Endod. 1997;83:41.

29. Small BW. Surgical templates for function and esthetics in dental implants. Gen Dent. 2001;49(1):30-2.

30. Smith RA. New developments and advances in dental implantology. Curr Opin Dent. 1992;2:42-54.

31. Truhlar RS, Morris HR, Ochi S. A review of panoramic radiography and its potential use in implant dentistry. Implant Dent. 1993;2(2):122-30.

32. Tyndall DA, Brooks SL. Selection criteria for dental implant site imaging: a position paper of the American Academy of Oral and Maxillofacial Radiology. Oral Surg Oral Med Oral Pathol Oral Radiol Endod. 2000;89(5):630-7.

33. White SC, Heslop EW, Hollender LG, Mosier KM, Ruprecht A, Shrout MK. An official report of the American Academy of Oral and Maxillofacial Radiology. Oral Surg Oral Med Oral Pathol Oral Radiol Endod. 2001;91(5):498-511.

34. Wyatt CC, Pharoah MJ. Imaging techniques and image interpretation for dental implant treatment. Int J Prosthodont. 1998;11(5):442-52.

Role of Dental Radiology in Forensic Odontology | 31

INTRODUCTION

Forensic odontology has been with us since the beginning, when, according to the old testament, Adam was convinced by Eve to take a bite of the forbidden apple, and left behind a bite mark.

The word forensic is derived from the latin word 'Forensis' meaning public. Forensic science refers to areas of endeavor that can be used in a judicial setting and accepted by court and the general scientific community to separate truth from untruth.

The youngest and the corner stone of forensic sciences is forensic odontology; which is defined as the positive identification of the living or deceased persons using the unique traits and characteristics of teeth and jaws.

The teeth and bones of the craniofacial complex, represent a constellation of features, useful as identification tools. Forensic odontological examination is the primary means of identification in situations where exposure, time elapsed after death and destruction of body (fire, explosion, etc.) has made other means of identification impossible.

The main aspects of forensic odontology include:
- Dental identification
  - Identification of unknown
  - Confirmation of identification.
- Age estimation of an individual from teeth
- Sex determination
- Role in mass disasters
- Role in domestic violence, abuse and neglect
- Identification from bite marks
- Identification from lip prints
- Blood group determination
- Recent advances.
  - DNA typing
  - Computer assisted dental identification
  - Digital analysis of bite marks
  - Digital autopsy.

The oral structure findings that contribute to identification are:
- Age determination (gross, microscopic, radiologic and surface scanning)
- Sex determination (dental and skeletal comparison)
- Racial characteristics

- Blood group determination
- Other genetic findings
- Occupational markings
- Prosthetic markings
- Individual habits
- Tooth alignment (occlusion) and abnormalities
- Jaw deformities (developmental and functional)
- Dental pathology (developmental and post developmental)
- Dental therapy (fillings, crowns, bridges and dentures)
- Dental radiology
- Microscopic examination
- Holography (where individual tooth prints can be stored in a computer data files, later to be retrieved for identification purposes, as well as for other kinds of data treatment involving oral diagnosis).

METHODS OF IDENTIFICATION

Currently there are three types of personal identification that uses teeth, jaws and orofacial characteristics.

1. *Comparative dental identification*: This involves the comparison of antemortem and postmortem dental records to determine if the body is that of the person of interest.
   - Antemortem records are sought for the individual to enable comparison with the body and help to identify. For this all available dental records available for the patient are used. It is important for the dentist to release all the patient records, original records are more useful rather than photocopies or duplicated photographs. Poor quality dental records may result in inability to establish identification.
   - Intraoral and extraoral radiographs, clinical photographs, odontograms, study casts, orthodontic appliances, dental prostheses and sports mouth guards all have been used in forensic casework to identify human remains.

2. *Reconstructive postmortem dental profiling:* This is used in cases in which there is no suspicion as to who the decedent may be. The information can be gathered and provided to authorities by dentists about certain criteria, such as age, race and sex of the decedent, to reduce the scope of the search for antemortem records of potential victims.

- To determine who the deceased person may have been, it is often necessary to assess personal features such as:
- Age estimation
- Sex and race determination
- Other associated findings.

3. *DNA profiling*: This focuses on the application of modern forensic DNA profiling methods to oral tissues to establish identity. This method can be used when dental treatments or other traits of dental records are not available for comparison.

RADIOGRAPHY OF POSTMORTEM MATERIAL

Radiography can play an important role in forensic odontology, mainly to establish identification. This may take the precise form of comparison between antemortem and postmortem radiographs. Radiographs may also be taken to determine the age of a minor victim and even help in the assessment of the sex and ethnic group. Comparable radiographs are an essential factor to confirm the identification in a mass disaster, when there may be a passenger list and consequently antemortem radiographs are available from general practitioners. These are usually in the form of bitewing radiographs, but may also include other intraoral techniques such as periapical and occlusal views. Extraoral projections such as oblique views or panoramic views may also be available. The frontal sinus view taken for sinus complaints are very useful as it is an established fact that the frontal sinus is a unique feature of every individual. Consequently it is necessary for the forensic odontologist to be familiar with the relevant maxillofacial views as well as the radiographic techniques for the dental arches, both intraoral and extraoral. These views establish identification by the comparison of amalgam, crowns and other prosthesis, as well as endodontics procedures such as root canal treatment and apicotomies. Radiography may have to be carried out in the field or at the scene of autopsy. This may require certain modifications in the normal procedures followed, requiring the operator to adapt techniques to individual patients, and the ability to think laterally is an essential requirement of the forensic odontologist.

- *Density of the object:* This is of paramount importance as the variations in forensic field are extreme. The range is very low density specimens due to fire, or perhaps the remains of an early fetus, through specimen in varying stages of decalcification, to waterlogged skull at the other extreme. If in any doubt it is always recommended that at least two radiographs should be taken initially, with different exposure factors.
- *Exposure factors:* Many factors combine to produce radiographs and it is particularly important for the forensic odontologist to be aware of the many possible variations. This is of particular significance when identical reproduction of antemortem films is required. The

exposure factors need to be modified as per the need and situation (**Table 31.1**).

- *X-ray apparatus and the X-ray beam*: Most types of dental apparatus have a fixed output, in other words, the kilovoltage and milliamperage are constant. If the apparatus is old and has a low kilovoltage it may limit the work that can be carried out in surgery. If the kilovoltage is between 45–50 kVp it has little penetrating power. This is adequate for intraoral techniques and perhaps for lateral oblique techniques with appropriate auxillary equipment, but inadequate for maxillofacial projections. Ideally variable kVp apparatus is recommended.
  - *Kilovoltage*: Low kilovoltages will give high contrast but little detail. High kilovoltages will penetrate to greater densities, and will also give more detail as more differentials between different densities are demonstrated. Low kilovoltages are essential for specimens such as an early fetus and can be an advantage for dry dental specimens. Alternately, if an 'as found' fresh, complete skull is to be radiographed, kilovoltages of 65–75 kVp are to be preferred.
  - *Milliamperage*: Dental apparatus operates with a low milliamperage to allow for easy movement of the tube head. The density of the X-ray beam is measured in milliampere seconds (milliamperes × time). Time is

Table 31.1 Modified exposure time

Type of techniques and film used	kVp	mAs	Anode film distance (cm)	Time (s)
Bite wing and periapical technique using D-speed films	50	7.5	10	0.5
	60	10	20	0.6
	70	10	20	0.3
	80	15	40	1
Bite wing and periapical technique using E-speed films	50	7.5	10	0.25
	60	10	20	0.3
	70	10	20	0.15
	80	15	40	0.5
Occlusal technique	50	7.5	20	1.0
	60	10	30	1.0
	70	10	30	0.5
	80	15	40	0.75
Extra oral maxillofacial views				
PA view, Townes view	65	30		0.3
Whole skull	65	60		0.6
Lateral oblique	55	30		0.3
Lateral skull	55	60		0.6
Occipito mental view	65–75	30		0.3

not a problem in the forensic field as the object will not move and the exposure timer can simply be reactivated.

- *Distance*: The anode distance is of great importance when calculating exposure factors. If a large field of irradiation is required to cover a larger specimen, then the anode-object distance must be increased. A two meter anode object distance will give an effectively parallel beam of X-rays and so will produce an image of exact size. This factor is utilized in cephalometry and could have forensic applications.

- *Field of irradiation*: An X-ray apparatus with an adjustable diaphragm, should be used to limit the beam to the area to be reproduced, as this will reduce the scatter or secondary radiation, and help obtain a radiographic image with maximum contrast.

Radiography in forensic odontology is greatly assisted by some simple items of auxiliary equipment:

- Metal or other tape measure, to measure the anode-object distance.
- Radiopaque measure—to assess enlargement or exact size of specimen, e.g. a fetus.
- Rigid, clear plastic surface—to place specimen over cassette or film.
- Plastic foam pads of different shapes e.g. wedge and skull rest (**Fig. 31.1**) for general immobilization.
- Sandbags, dental wax and cotton rolls, for fine immobilization.
- Plastic bags and rubber gloves—to protect film, cassette and general area from specimen and operator's hands; also for esthetic reasons if specimen is to be taken to a hospital X-ray department.
- 'R' and 'L' lead letters.
- For emergency field work, a small manual processor.
- *Venues for radiography*: Radiographs may need to be taken at the scene of the accident or crime, at the mortuary, or in the hospital X-ray department or dental surgery. In practicality, for accurate assessment of age and other identification details, quite apart from exact reproduction

of antemortem radiographs, necessitates the separation of the skull from the spine so that the skull can be taken to a dental surgery or X-ray department.

- *Cadavers in the field*: A portable X-ray apparatus is used. The only radiographic projection possible is an anteroposterior view of the skull. In these circumstances the information required will be to establish injury or presence of a foreign body such as a missile. The X-ray cassette protected by a plastic bag is placed under the skull and the X-ray tube positioned as far as possible above the object (anode object distance usually about 80–120 cm). Another instance where radiography is required in the field is the investigation of a decomposed object too fragile to be moved. This is usually combined with soil and gravel, in which case it is very radiolucent and the exposure factors must be reduced, preferably with a low kilovoltage. Alternately the specimen could be set in concrete like a fossil; here a high kilovoltage giving greater differentials is recommended.

- *In the mortuary or scene of autopsy*: A mobile X-ray unit is required; if the cadaver is frozen the only views possible are the anteroposterior and lateral.

- *In the dental surgery or X-ray room*: Here the situation is entirely different, the specimen, whether it is a complete skull or a small portion of the mandible, maxilla or facial bones, down even to individual teeth, the main problem is to immobilize and control the position of the object. This combined with the ultra mobility of the dental X-ray apparatus, makes careful monitoring essential.

  - *Procedure*: Leave the specimen on a plastic or other radiolucent rigid surface. Immobilize the specimen in the required position with plastic foam pads or other radiolucent material. Cotton wool rolls make an excellent stabilizing medium for the finer differences in positioning.

    Place the film or cassette under the rigid surface. Position the X-ray tube as required. Document exposure factors including anode-object distance. Remove the film or cassette carefully without changing the position of the specimen or the X-ray tube.

  - *Process*: This can be done manually or by the automatic processor.

RADIOGRAPHIC VIEWS

- *Anteroposterior view* (**Figs 31.2A and B**): Place the cassette, protected by plastic under the skull and position the tube as far away as possible from the cadaver. The X-ray beam should be parallel to the orbitomeatal line (**Fig. 31.2B**), so in most cases the X-ray tube should be angled downwards from the vertex.

- *Lateral view* (**Figs 31.3A and B**): Place the cassette supported by sand bags parallel to the sagittal plane. Raise the skull above the table, insert a polystyrene foam pad or

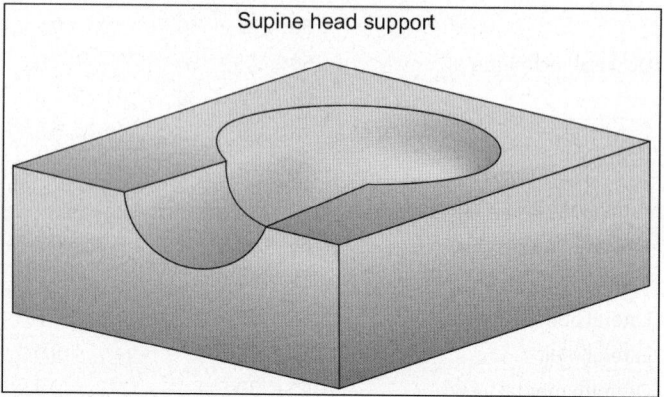

Supine head support

Figure 31.1 Skull foam pad

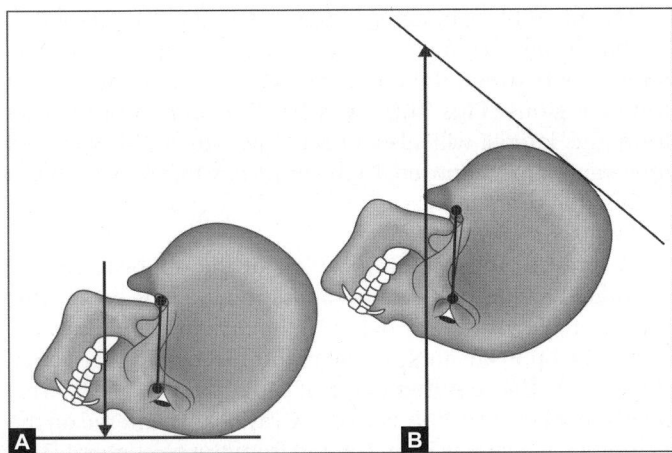

Figures 31.2A and B (A) Position for the head for a posteroanterior projection of the facial bones taken with the tube vertical and the film horizontal; (B) Compensated projection of this view taken anteroposterior when it is impossible to adjust the orbitomeatal line. Note how the X-ray beam has to be parallel to this line. The film should be below the occipital bone

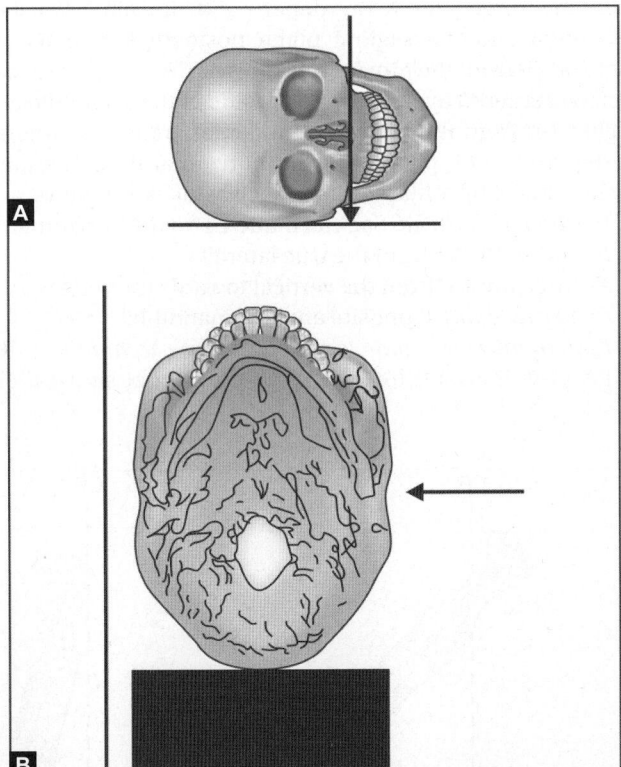

Figures 31.3A and B (A) Position of the head for a lateral view of the facial bones with the tube vertical and the film horizontal at 90 degrees to the infraorbital line; (B) Position of the film vertical and parallel to the sagittal plane when the body is supine. The tube is horizontal. Note that the head must be raised from the table with a radiolucent pad

wooded block underneath. Turn the X-ray tube head so the X-ray beam is parallel to the floor and centered over the skull towards the cassette **(Fig. 31.3B)**. If the cadaver is not frozen then other views are possible. The only possible intraoral view may be to insert an occlusal film if the mandible is released.

- *Occlusal techniques*: As the cadaver is supine new orientation is necessary.
  - *Maxilla*: Place the film in position in the occllusal plane. Position the X-ray tube head above the skull, angling the X-ray beam over the bridge of the nose downwards onto the film at 60° with an anode distance of 30 cm **(Fig. 31.4)**. If it is possible to shorten the anode distance, adjust the exposure factors accordingly.

    If posterior teeth are to be demonstrated, then the cadaver must again be rotated until the central beam is directed over the appropriate area. Remember that the X-ray tube head cannot be rotated in a lateral direction, as with dental X-ray equipment.
  - *Mandible*: Place the film in the occlusal plane. Position the X-ray tube below the mandible and angle upwards at 45° towards the occlusal plane in the midline **(Fig. 31.5)**.

If the area to be demonstrated is posterior, the cadaver must again be rotated. The difficulty with these views is that if *rigor mortis* has set in with the chin downwards it will be impossible to bring the tube head low enough; the body gets in the way.

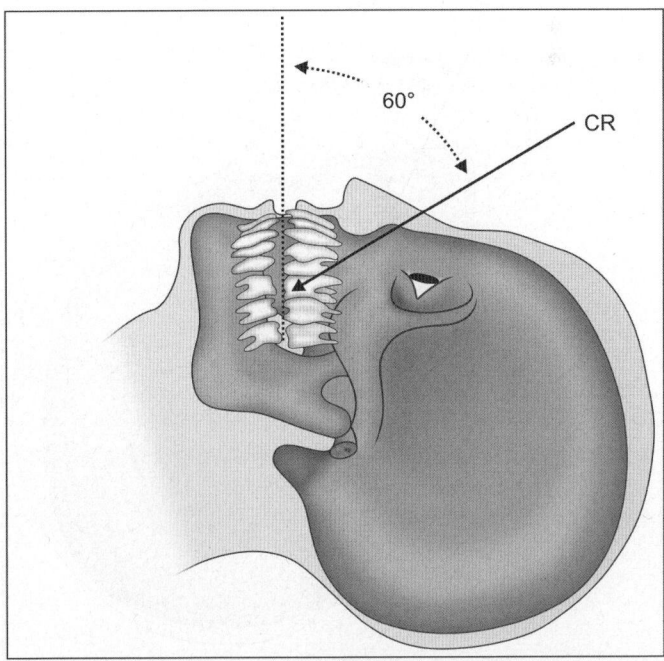

Figure 31.4 Upper midline oblique occlusal *Abbreviation*:
CR = central ray

- *Intraoral views*: Put the film into the dental cavity and immobilize in the appropriate position with the use of a film holder or Spencer Wells forceps. The relationship of the tooth and the film is of great importance if one is trying to reproduce antemortem radiographs.
- *Oblique lateral view*: This is one of the best view to demonstrate the dentition in general, as it prevents the superimposition of one side of the jaws over the other.

The cadaver is rotated so that the premolar or molar region is obliquely placed—enough to allow the tube head to be angled upward and forward from the lateral position. In the mortuary the cadaver must be raised with a radiolucent substance such as wood or plastic foam. Rotate the body so that the film can be placed parallel to the dental arches and vertically supported, this may be done with various auxiliary aids for immobilization such as foam pads, sand bags. The X-ray tube head must be horizontally positioned and the beam angled upwards towards the film.

Even with a complete specimen skull without the spine in the dental surgery, the problem of the superimposition of the opposite side of the dental arches to that being examined still occur. At the mortuary it may be even more difficult as the spine will also be present in addition the cadaver which is almost impossible to maneuver and the X-ray apparatus is also relatively immobile. The following problems must be considered.

The mandible is horse-shoe shaped, so it is important that the film is placed parallel to the area of interest. There will be difference between the molar region and the premolar and canine regions (**Figs 31.6A and B**). The amount of rotation from the lateral will also effect how much the spine, if present, is superimposed. In the mortuary this may prove an impossible problem, except for small areas of the mandible and maxilla.

To prevent the superimposition of the opposite side of the dental arches an angle of separation must be given. This means angling the X-ray beam so that it is directed upwards below the opposite angle of the mandible towards the vertex (**Fig. 31.7**). The required angle of separation is 20–30°. This may be achieved entirely with the X-ray beam centered on the mandible, which has been rotated from the true lateral. This positioning will produce an elongated image, which may not be important, but for comparison with previous radiographs the distortion may prevent positive identification. Ideally the sagittal plane should be tilted to make an angle with the film and so help to open out the mandible; the angle of separation can then be divided between the mandible of the specimen and the X-ray beam, and the image will be much more diagnostic.

In the surgery or X-ray department the film is placed horizontal and the sagittal plane positioned to make an angle of 10° from the film (vertex down). The X-ray beam can then be centered over the opposite side of the mandible and angled 10° from the vertical. The dental arches are rotated as required to be parallel to the horizontal film. The ideal positioning of the oblique lateral technique is as follows:

- *Position of the head*: Sagittal plane 10° to the horizontal.
- *Rotation*: 10–20° from the true lateral.
- *X-ray beam*: 10° from the vertical towards the vertex
- *Centering point*: Opposite angle of mandible
- *Posteroanterior and anteroposterior technique*: The PA view is useful for observing the frontal sinuses. For

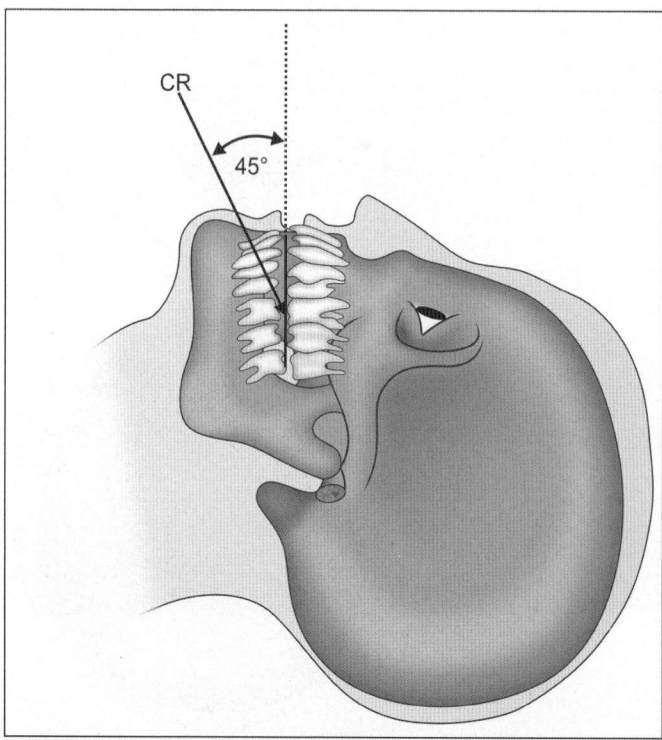

Figure 31.5 Anterior midline oblique lower occlusal technique
Abbreviation: CR = central ray

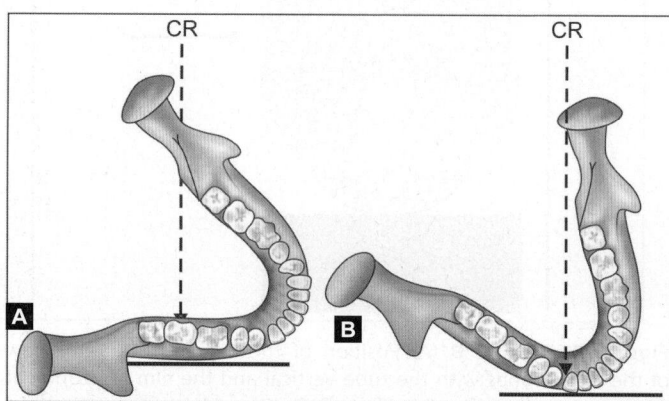

Figures 31.6A and B Diagram showing how the rotation of the mandible is necessary for oblique lateral radiograph of: (A) Molar; (B) Premolar and canine regions. *Abbreviation*: CR = central ray

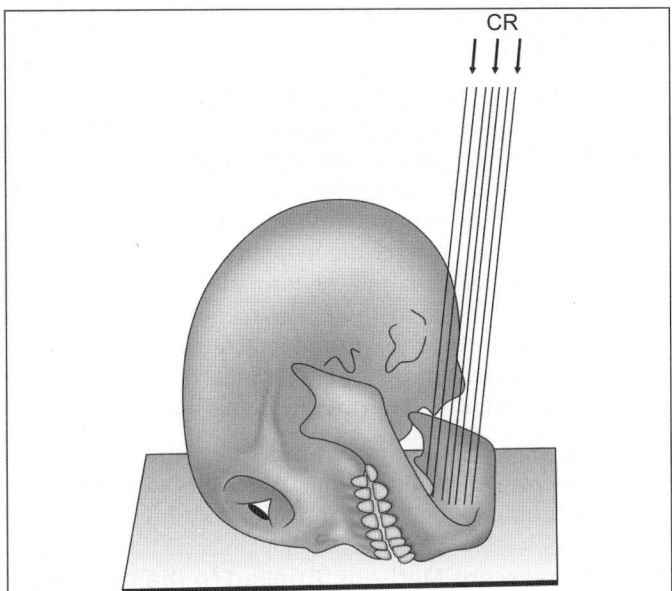

Figure 31.7 The position for an lateral oblique radiograph of the mandible. The side of the mandible to be radiographed is parallel to the film and the opposite side in angled away in an upward plane

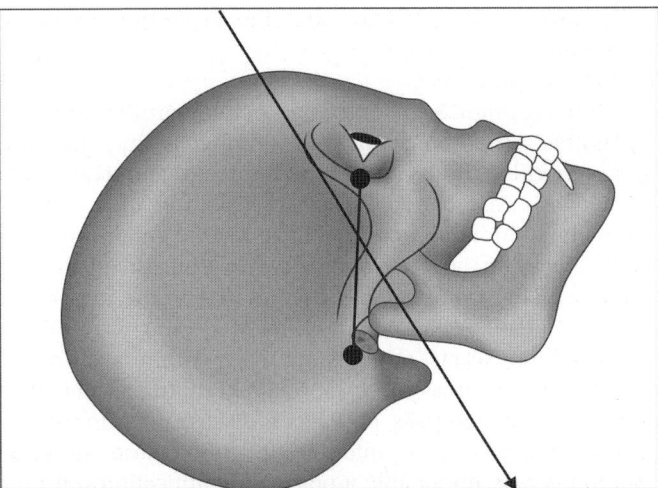

Figure 31.8 Position of the head for the 30° fronto-occipital (Townes) projection. This view is taken to demonstrate fracture of the neck of the condyle

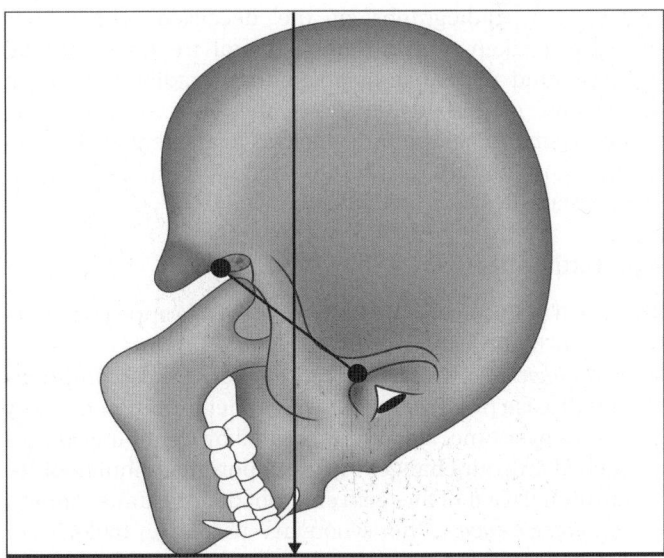

Figure 31.9 Position of the head for the occipitomental view routinely taken for the sinuses

comparison this must be simulated, but in the mortuary or in the field the AP view would be the only projection possible (**Fig. 31.2A**).

The skeletal measurements obtained from posteroanterior films are:

- Bigonal breadth
- Mastoid to apex height
- Bimaxillary breadth
- Bizygomatic breadth
- Maximum cranial breadth
- Sinus breadth
- Incisor height
- Total facial height.
  - *Position of the head*: Orbitomeatal line 90 degrees to the film.
  - *X-ray beam*: Parallel to the orbitomeal line.
  - *Centering point*: In the midline below the occipital protuberances at the level of the angle of the mandible (PA) or midline over the bridge of the nose (AP).
- *Thirty degree fronto-occipital (Townes) technique*: This view is taken for the neck of the condyles (**Fig. 31.8**). (It may be taken as a Reverse Townes view with the skull PA).
  - Position of the head: Back of the head to the film.
  - *Orbital-meatal line*: 90° to the film.
  - *X-ray beam*: 30° to the orbitalmeatal line.
  - *Centering point*: 5 cm above the nasion.
- *Occipitomental technique*: This is a routine view taken for the maxillary and frontal sinuses and is always in the PA position. To simulate this projection for the pattern of the

frontal sinuses the exact situation must be reproduced, so the skull must be positioned PA to the film. This is easier to achieve with the film horizontal (**Fig. 31.9**).

It was noted by Schuller that the frontal sinuses as observed radiographically; were useful in identifications. The frontal sinus in particular has been long established as a unique feature in every individual.

It has been found that the frontal sinuses of no two persons were alike. The frontal sinuses appear in the second year of life and increase in size until about the twentieth year of life. These are larger in males than females.

- *Position of head*: Orbitomeatal line 45° to the horizontal and film-sagittal plane
- *X-ray beam*: Vertical
- *Centering point*: 5 cm above the occipital protuberance.

Another importance of radiography is in detection of systemically produced defects in teeth and jaws such as ankylosis, ectodermal dysplasia resulting in partial or complete anodontia, increased incidence of supernumerary teeth occuring in cleidocranial dysostosis, disturbed eruption pattern of permanent teeth seen in the hyper and hypopituitarism, retarded eruption of deciduous teeth in cretinism and rickets, changes occurring within facial bones like radiolucent areas in eosinophilic granuloma, increased density in osteopetrosis or Paget's disease, or monostotic fibrous dysplasia. The information from these systemic conditions may not enable a positive identification but may lead to trace the hospital record thus may at least enable some suspects to be eliminated from inquiry.

COMPARISON RADIOGRAPHY

Antemortem radiographs of the deceased which may have been taken during routine dental treatment should be compared with that of postmortem radiograph taken at the time of investigations. For this, it is essential that, postmortem radiographs are obtained in an identical fashion to antemortem radiograph. The antemortem radiographs can be made available with the dentist.

Age Estimation

The use of dentition for the assessment of age appears to date from early in the last century.
- *Pathologic age*: This is related to the various conditions and disease processes that result in deterioration of many tissues over time. It can be estimated by examining factors such as arthritic changes in the temporomandibular joints, attritional wear of the teeth and root dentine transparency.
- *Physiologic age*: (The synonyms used are biologic or developmental age). This is determined by natural, expected changes that occur through growth and development. Maturation is scaled by occurrence of one or the sequence of multiple events that are reversible. An estimate of age can be determined from an examination of the development of roots (apical closure) and comparison with tables that record the amount of development versus age.
- *Chronologic age*: This is the time from birth to death. The age that investigators are most interested in is chronologic age.

Forensic dentists normally take into account estimates of a person's pathologic and physiologic age to arrive at an assessment of the most likely chronologic age at the time of death.

The dentition is one of the four systems used. The other three developmental indicators refer to bone development, secondary sexual characteristics and stature or weight which

is limited by the fact that they can be applied only after inception of puberty.

There are two main categories of dental age:
- *Calcification age*: The stage sequence of tooth development from the first appearance of cusps to root apical closure.
- *Eruption age*: The progressive emergence of the tooth from its alveolus into functional occlusion.

Dental age can be determined by the emergence of tooth or by radiographic analysis of formation of teeth. Tooth formation is superior to tooth emergence as the latter is influenced markedly by environmental factors. The measure of calcification (maturation) at different levels will provide a more precise index for determining dental age.

Dental age may be broadly classified into:
- Age determination during the first two decades of life.
- Age determination after the first two decades of life.

Age Assessment Methods Applied to the Dentition

- Tooth germs
- Earliest trace of mineralization
- Degree of completion of unerupted tooth
- Formation of enamel and neonatal line
- Emergence of tooth crown in the oral cavity
- Root completion of erupted teeth
- Root resorption
- Attrition
- Secondary dentine
- Cementum apposition
- Root translucency
- Gingival recession
- Tooth discoloration
- Chemical composition of teeth
- Disease or malnutrition.

Age Determination Methods Applied during the First Two Decades of Life

Histological characteristics of bone, tooth and salivary gland formation enable to estimate the age from seven weeks in the uterus to about 3 years of age.

During first six months of life no teeth are clinically visible in the baby's mouth therefore the methods used to study the changes occurring within the jaw of intact body or skeletal remains or even putrefied specimen are:
- Noninvasive radiographs should be taken and/or
- Sections should be taken for histopathologic examination.

Ageing of unknown body can be done by studying:
- The eruption status of teeth
- The degree of their development and the data may be compared with the standard chart of development. Such as those given by:
  - Kronfield (1933) (**Figs 31.10A and B**)

- Schour and Massler (1941), based on jaw sections (**Fig. 31.11**).
- Moorees, Fanning and Hunt (1963), based on radiographic survey (**Figs 31.12A to C**)
  - The eruption sequence of teeth in oral cavity (as given in the chart).
  - In mixed dentition—root resorption is considered.
  - The erupted teeth position whether attaining their functional position.

The method used, and tabulated data, make the survey of Morees et al. a useful development standard for the forensic dentist. Morees et al. defined 14 stages of mineralization for developing single and multirooted permanent teeth. The results are expressed as the mean of the age of attainment for each of the 14 stages for the developing tooth studied ± 2 standard deviations. Examination of their data indicates that the crown formation stages show less variation when compared with the root formation stages; this should be kept in mind when accuracy is of prime importance. The earliest age in the survey is 6 months, and the data include development of the third molar.

Other points of forensic interest to emerge from this study are:

- Differences in the crown formation between the sexes were minimal. Sexual difference in development became apparent during root formation, where females developed ahead of males.
- The teeth emerge clinically at the $R_{3/4}$ stage.
- The greatest sexual dimorphism is expressed in the mandibular canine, females being up to 11 months in advance of males with this particular tooth.

The radiograph can detect the earliest stages of calcification which affect each tooth germ in the dentition. Gleiser and Hunt (1953) studied the development of mandibular first molars using lateral oblique view radiograph and found tooth development occurs earlier in females.

Female age = 0.95 × Male age.

The development of roots of third molars is a more reliable guide to age rather than timing of eruption. Shirolkar RP (1984), reported 96% accuracy by using lateral oblique radiographs for third molars, for age determination in Indian subjects particularly of the age group of 16–20 years. He concluded in his extensive radiographic study entailing the degree of development of 3rd molars in Indian cases, that the roots of the 3rd molar fully develop (The apical foramina may not have closed) by the time a person in 18-years-old. At 19 even the apical foramina shows closure in the vast majority.

Nolla (1960) surveyed the development of the permanent dentition in the sample of American boys and girls using serial annual radiography.

Nolla's standards for determination of age of teeth are as follows (**Figs 31.13A and B**):

- Absence of crypt
- Presence of crypt
- Initial calcification
- 1/3rd crown completed
- 2/3rd crown completed
- Crown almost completed

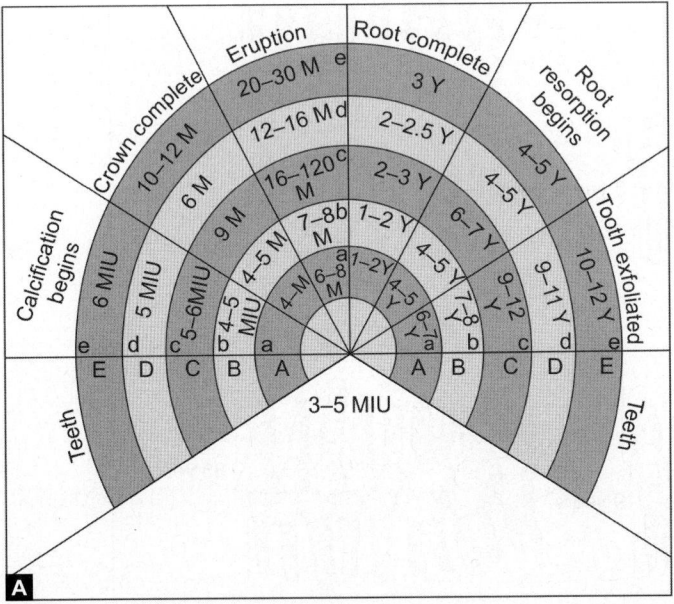

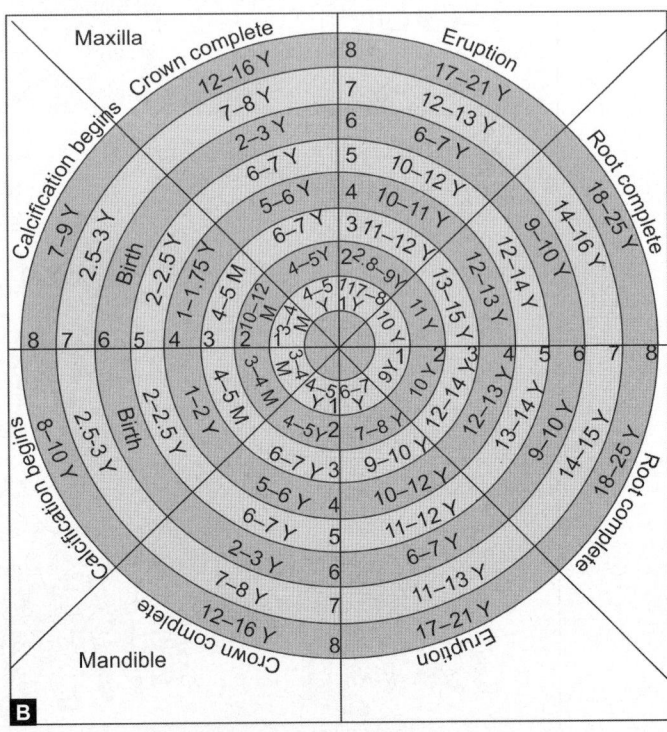

Figures 31.10A and B (A) Development of the deciduous teeth. Data from Kronfield (1935), Y = Age in years; M = Age in months; MIU = months intrauterine; A = deciduous central incisor; E = deciduous second molar; (B) Development of the maxillary and mandibular permanent teeth. Data from Kronfield (1935) 1 = First permanent incisor; 8 = Third permanent molar

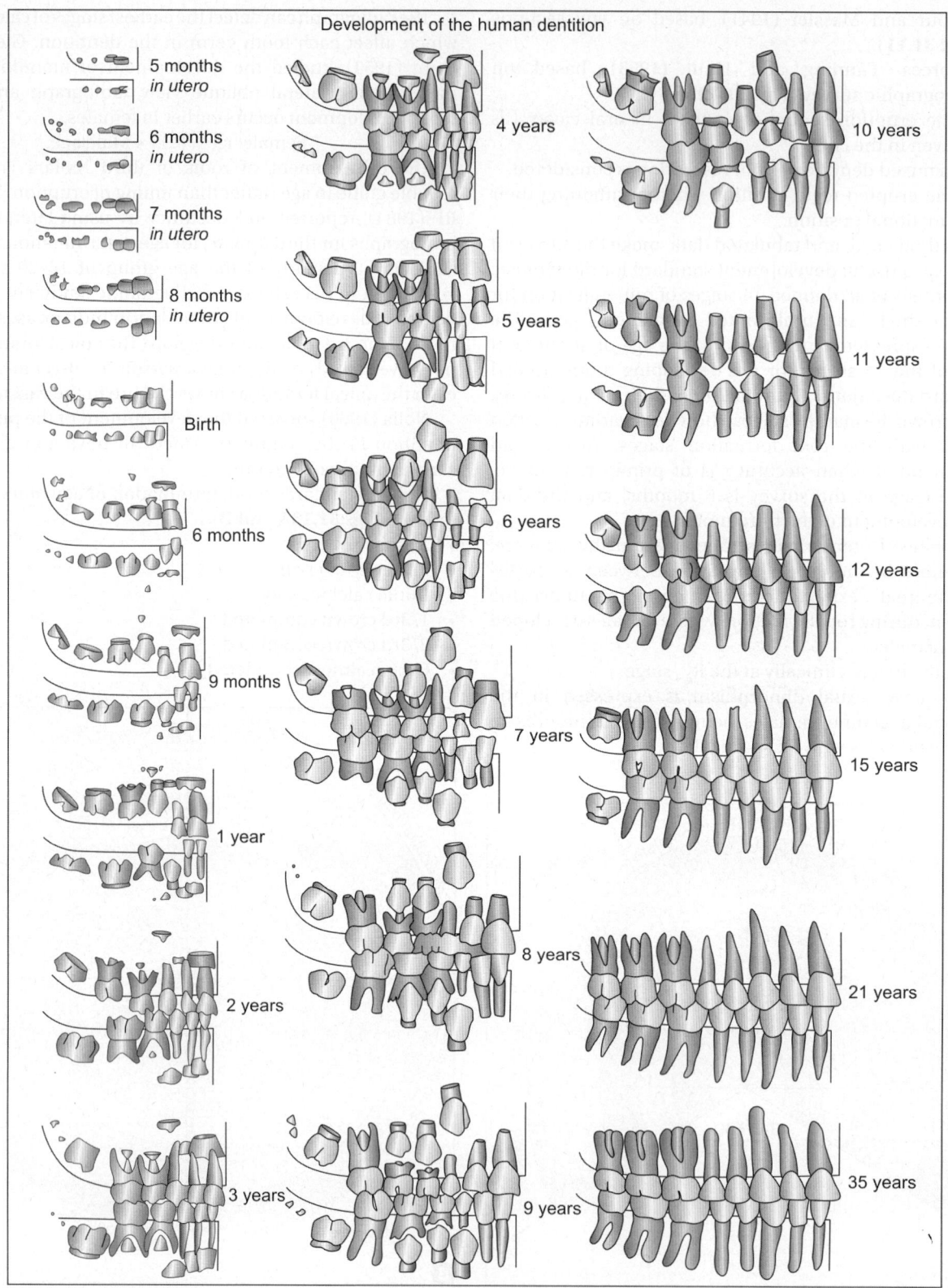

Figure 31.11 Schour and Massler, the sequence of formation of the human dentition. [Chart shown produced by ADA (1982)]

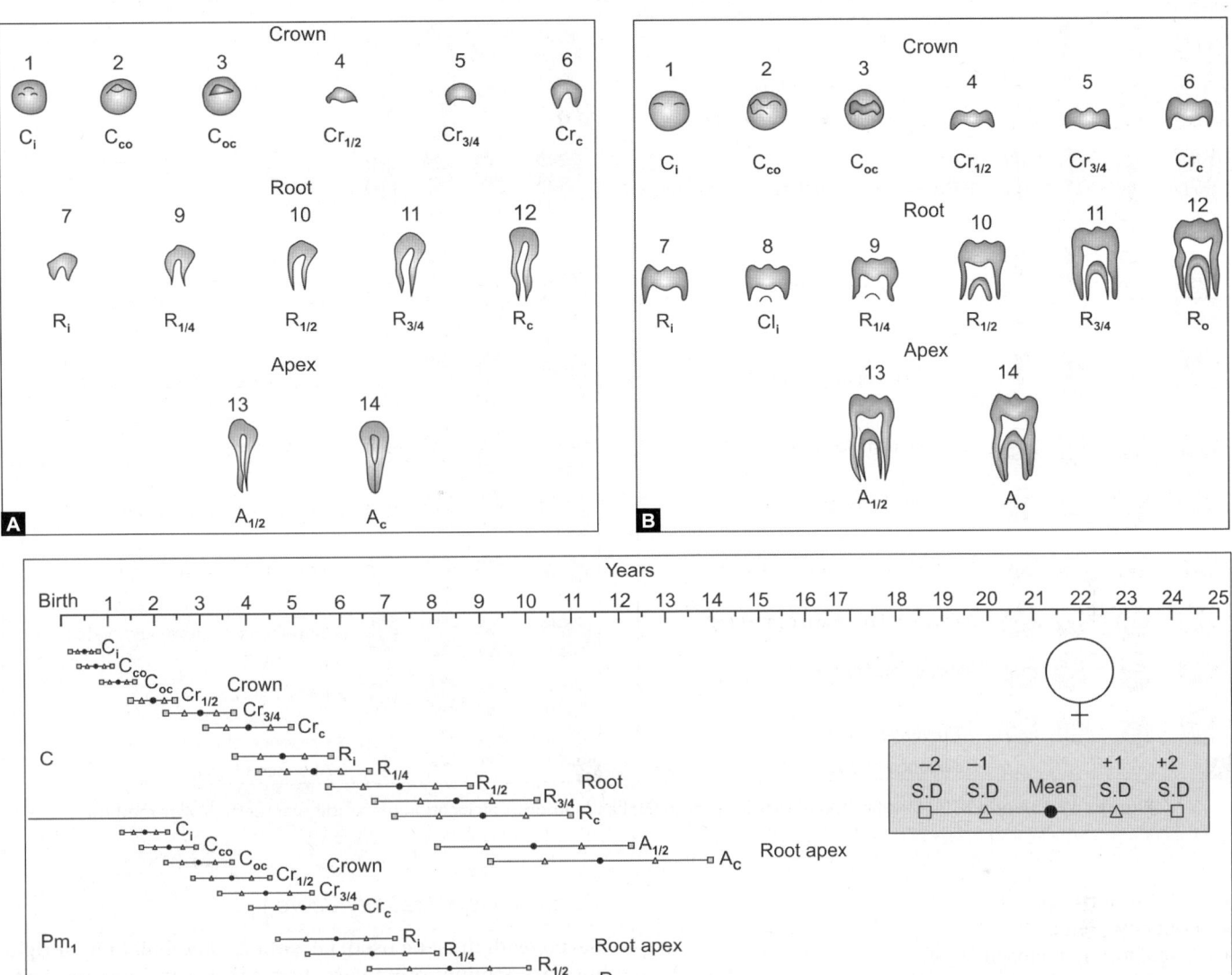

Figures 31.12A to C (A) Stages of tooth formation for assessing the development of single-rooted teeth (Moorees et al. 1963). The numbers above the diagram indicate the stage of development corresponding to the following coded symbols: C_i = initial cusp formation, C_{co} = coalescence of cusps, C_{oc} = cusp outline complete, $Cr_{1/2}$ = crown half complete, $Cr_{3/4}$ = crown three quarters complete, C_{rc} = crown complete, R_i = initial root formation, $R_{1/4}$ = root length one quarter, $R_{1/2}$ = root length one-half, $R_{3/4}$ = root length three quarter, R_c = complete, $A_{1/2}$ = apex half closed, Ac = apical closure complete; (B) Stages of tooth formation for assessing the development of multirooted teeth (from Moorees et al. 1953). Coded symbols as for Figure 37.12A, with the addition of Cl_i = initial cleft formation; (C) An example of data available for development of female permanent mandibular canines and premolars from Moorees et al. (1963). Mean age = + 2 standard deviations for attainment of 14 stages of calcification are given

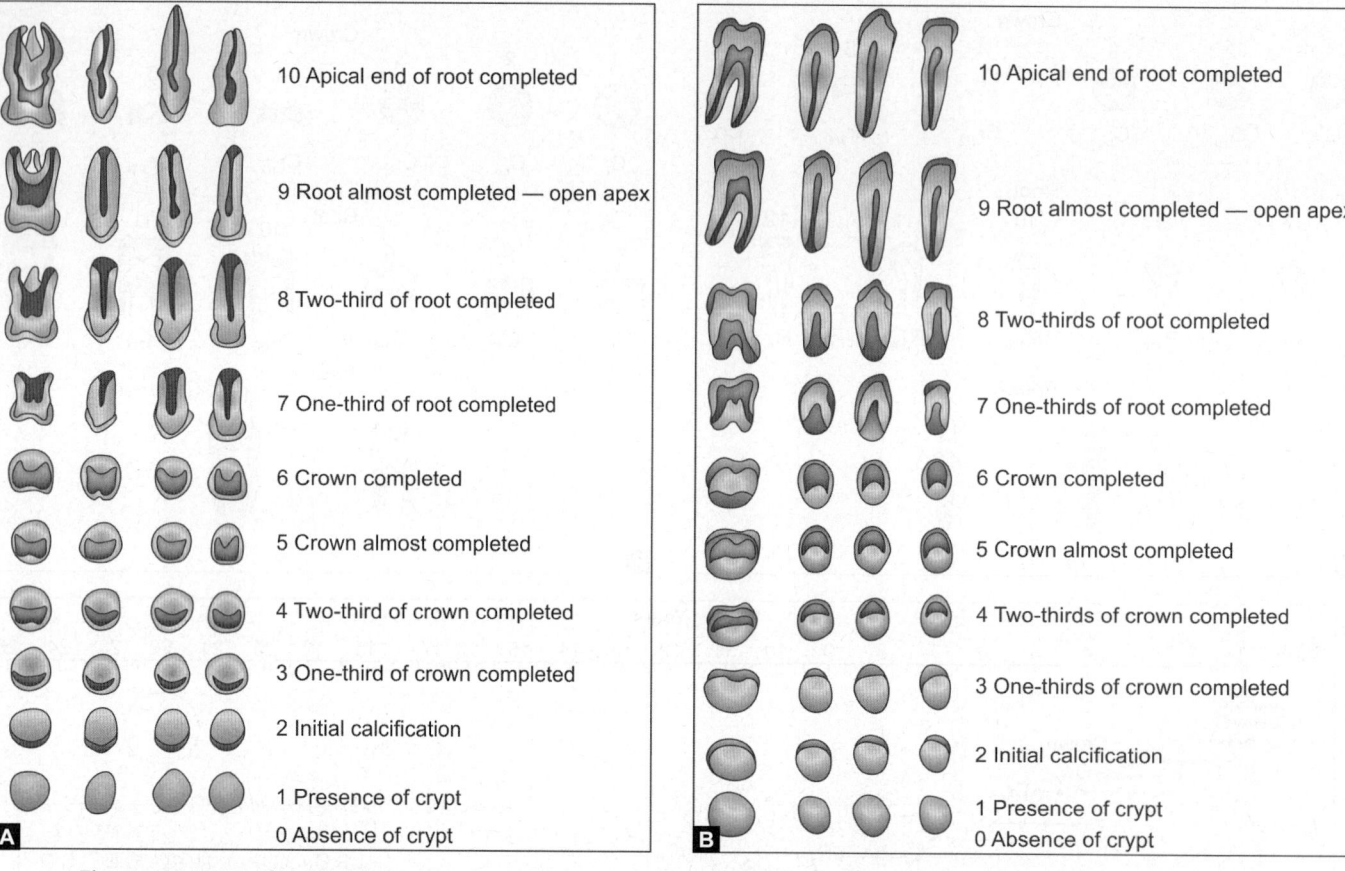

Figures 31.13A and B (A) Calcification of maxillary teeth (Nolla's method); Calcification of mandibular teeth (Nolla's method)

- 1/3rd root completed
- Root completed
- Apical foramen closed.

Demirjian, Goldstein and Tanner (1973), suggested a method, where in each stage of mineralization is given a score which provides an estimate of dental maturity on a scale of 0–100. This system is the most highly developed of all dental age surveys. There are two options when using this method, one involving the rating of seven mandibular teeth (Demirjian,1978) and the second using four mandibular teeth (Demirjian and Goldstein,1976). Missing teeth from one side can be substituted by those from the other side. Should the first molar be absent the central incisor can be substituted (Demirjian,1978). Griffin and Malan (1987) reviewed this system with emphasis on its possible forensic use, producing a pocket version of the system which can be used in the field.

Demirjian seven-tooth system for age determination:

Technique: Radiographs take two periapical radiographs of the left and right mandibular incisors, canines, premolars, first and second molars. Or right and left lateral oblique radiographs together with right and left lower anterior occlusal oblique films. Or rotational tomographs.

Calculations of Maturity Score

Seven teeth must be used, i.e. either mandibular left or right incisors, canine, premolars, first and second molars. Note the missing teeth from one side may be substituted with corresponding teeth from the opposite side.

Using the pictorial guide (**Fig. 31.14**) together with reference to written criteria (**Table 31.2**), determine the mineralization of each tooth, i.e., A, B, C, D, etc.

Mark X in the appropriate square of (**Fig. 31.15**) (or zero if mineralization is completely absent).

For each completed square of (**Fig. 31.15**), convert X to a number using (**Table 31.3**).

Add the numbers to find the total score, i.e. the maturity score.

Age Determination after the First Two Decades of Life

Once the development of crown and roots is completed and the teeth are in functional occlusion, age determination using dental findings becomes difficult. After the age of about 24 years dental estimate depends upon:

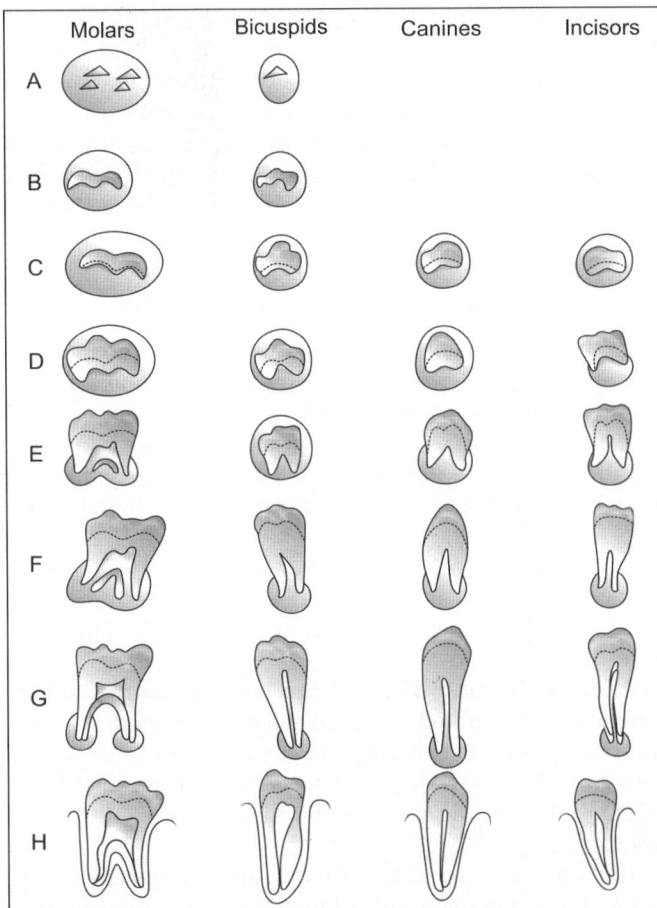

	Molars	Bicuspids	Canines	Incisors
A				
B				
C				
D				
E				
F				
G				
H				

Figure 31.14 Pictorial guide to mineralization assessment

Table 31.2 Mineralization assessment of developing teeth

- In both uniradicular and multiradicular teeth, a beginning calcification is seen at the superior level of the crypt, in the form of an inverted cone or cones. There is no fusion of these calcified points.
- Fusion of the calcified points forms one or several cusps, which unite to give a regularly outlined occlusal surface.
- Enamel formation is complete at the occlusal surface. Its extension and convergence toward the cervical region is seen.
    - The beginning of a dentinal deposit is seen
    - The outline of the pulp chamber has a curved shapes at the occlusal border.
- The crown formation is completed down to the cementoenamel junction
    - The superior border of the pulp chamber in uniradicular teeth has a definite curved form, being concave toward the cervical region. The projection of the pulp horns, if present, gives an outline like an umbrella top. In molars, the pulp chamber has a trapezoidal form
    - Beginning of root formation is seen in the form of a spicule.
- Uniradicular teeth
    - The walls of the pulp chamber now form straight lines, whose continuity is broken by the presence of the pulp horn, which is larger than in the previous stage
    - The root length is less than the crown height
    Molars:
    - Initial formation of the radicular bifurcation is seen in the form of either a calcified point or a semilunar shape
    - The root length is still less than the crown height.
- Uniradicular teeth
    - The walls of the pulp chamber now form a more or less isosceles triangle. The apex ends in a funnel shape
    - The root length is equal to or greater than the crown height.
    Molars:
    - The calcified region of the bifurcation has developed further down from its semilunar stage to give the roots a more definite and distinct outline, with funnel-shaped endings
    - The root length is equal to or greater than the crown height.
- The walls the root canals are now parallel (distal root in molars.
    - The apical ends of the root canals are still partially open (distal root in molars).
- The apical end of the root canal is completely closed (distal root in molars)
    - The periodontal membrane has a uniform width around the root and the apex.

- Changes in the teeth independent upon increasing age.
- The effects of wear and tear by:
    - Preparation of sections through teeth, or
    - Mandible or maxilla should be cut through alongside a standing permanent tooth.
    - Gustafson G (1950) developed a comprehensive compact chart of dental development for forensic use, using four stages of development described a method (**Figs 31.16A and B**).

$$= A + S + P + C + T + R$$

where,

A = Attrition
S = Secondary dentine
P = Periodontosis
C = Cementum apposition
T = Translucency (apical)
R = Root resorption

The total value of the points assigned for the teeth were plotted against the known age of teeth.

Standard error of estimation by Gustafson's method is ± 3.6 years.

- Modified Gustafson's method
    - Regressive changes as mentioned in Gustafson's method were observed under microscope using micrometer. Each index value of various parameters were calculated.

where,

A = Attrition index
D = Secondary dentine index
T = Translucency index
CE = Cementum apposition

Stages	Mandible						
	I_1	I_2	C	PM_1	PM_2	M_1	M_2
A							
B							
C							
D							
E							
F							
G							
H							

Figure 31.15 Chart for recording the mineralization stages determined from Figure 31.14 and Table 31.2

Table 31.3 Self-weighted scores for dental stages, seven teeth stage

Tooth	0	A	B	C	D	E	F	G	H
Boys									
M_2	0.0	1.7	3.1	5.4	8.6	11.4	12.4	12.8	13.6
M_1				0.0	5.3	7.5	10.3	13.9	16.8
PM_2	0.0	1.5	2.7	5.2	8.0	10.8	12.0	12.5	13.2
PM_1			0.0	4.0	6.3	9.4	13.2	14.9	15.5	16.1
C				0.0	4.0	7.8	10.1	11.4	12.0
I_2				0.0	2.8	5.4	7.7	10.5	13.2
I_1				0.0	4.3	6.3	8.2	11.2	15.1
Girls									
M_2	0.0	1.8	3.1	5.4	9.0	11.7	12.8	13.2	13.8
M_1				0.0	3.5	5.6	8.4	12.5	15.4
PM_2	0.0	1.7	2.9	5.4	8.6	11.1	12.3	12.8	13.3
PM_1			0.0	3.1	5.2	8.8	12.6	14.3	14.9	15.5
C				0.0	3.7	7.3	10.0	11.8	12.5
I_2				0.0	2.8	5.3	8.1	11.2	13.8
I_1				0.0	4.4	6.3	8.5	12.0	15.8

Changes in the mandible as seen in oral orthopantomogram, particularly on the right side, were determined to be of more value for age estimation than those on the left side.

The handedness of the person is related to the dominance of the cerebral hemisphere. Therefore, in a right-handed person, as is the case with majority of the population, use of the dominant hand, i.e. the right hand for brushing the teeth. A right-handed person will exert more pressure on the right side of the mandible while brushing the teeth than a left handed person, which will induce more age related changes on the right side than the left side.

Age Determination from Cementum Annulation

It has been observed that cementum appears to increase with age and the deposition of cementum in an apical area can compensate for loss of tooth substances from occlusal wear. It is also believed that cementum deposition is in layers and throughout life indicating incremental lines present in cementum. It is found that cementum increases by 0.030 mm every ten years.

In two studies in Nair Hospital, Department of Forensic Science and Department of Oral Radiology two formulae were devised for age estimation in male and female adult patients.

Using statistical analysis of the data, linear regressions graphs were prepared on a specially developed software program by plotting five significant variables (CSS, CBFS, MRD2, MRA and MLA) against the depended variable of age. MRD2, MRA and MLA were determined on the OPG of the patient.

The following equation for estimation of age (Male and Female) between the age of 25 to 45 years was derived from these graphs.

- Age (Male) = 8.442 (Constant) + 2.562 (CSS) + 3.514 (CBFS) + 8.687 (MRD2) + 0.436 (MRA) – 0.263 (MLA)
- Age (Female) = 22.673 (Constant) + 2.074 (CSS) + 0 (CBFS) + 9.550 (MRD2) + 0.273 (MRA) – 0.242 (MLA).

where,

CSS – Combined skin score
CBFS – Combined bone fusion score
MRA – Mandibular right angle
MLA – Mandibular left angle
MRD2 – Least perpendicular distance between the mandibular canal on the right side and a tangent drawn along the lower border of the body of the mandible.

From a statistical standpoint, the fitness of the formula (i.e. its accuracy) is very high (88%). Using this formula, the ages of the 32 subjects in the study group were predicted, and were found to tally almost exactly with the ages as claimed by 22 (69%) of them.

Cephalometry

It is mainly used for the study of growth and development of the craniofacial complex, but there is no known literature available for age estimation by cephalometric analysis.

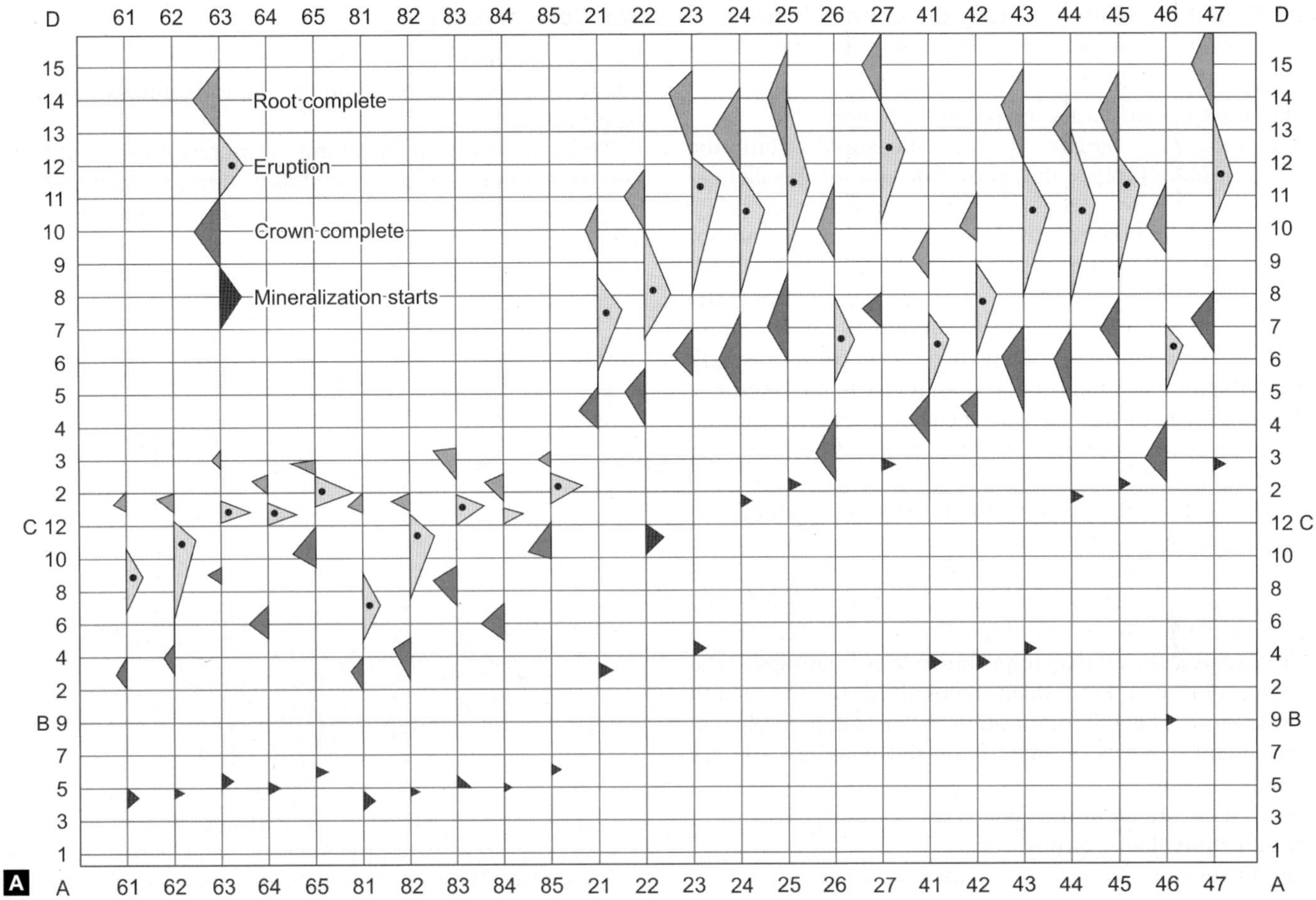

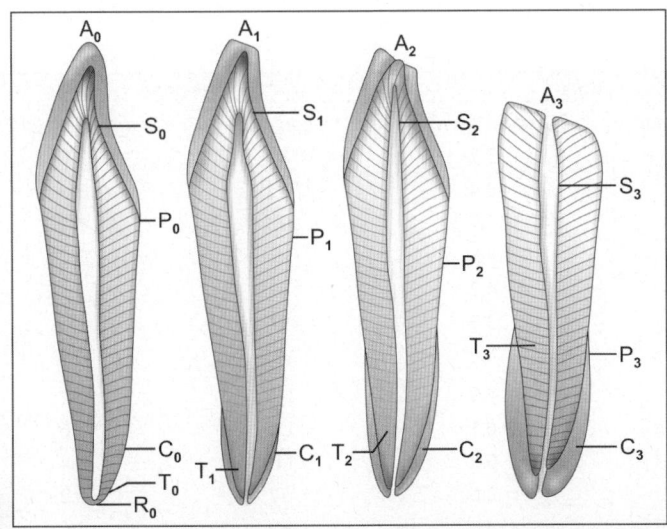

Figures 31.16A and B (A) Schematic representation of tooth formation and eruption. A–B = Intrauterine life, B–C = First year of life, and C–D = 2–16 years-of age. The base of the triangle represents range and the peak mean age (from Gustafson and Koch, '74) Gustafson's (1966) chart of formation and eruption of deciduous and permanent teeth (excluding the third molars). The peaks of the triangles represent the mean ages for attainment of the four stages, viz mineralization starts, crown complete, eruption and root complete. The bases of the triangles represent the variation. A–B = Intrauterine life, B–C = First year of life, and C–D = 2–16 years of age; (B) Age changes in teeth, Gustafson G (1958): A–Attrition; S–Secondary dentine deposition, P–Apical migration of periodontal ligament membrane, T–Root translucency, C–Cementum deposition, R–Root apical closure

Harvold used his analysis to study the severity of degree of jaw disharmony, using various linear measurement for a particular chronological age.

Cephalometric landmarks and planes used are:
- *The maxillary length*: It was measured from the temporomandibular joint, posterior wall of the glenoid fossa to the lower shadow of the anterior nasal spine, defined as the point on the lower shadow of the anterior nasal spine where the spine is 3 mm thick.
- *The mandibular length*: It was measured from the temporomandibular joint to the prognathion, the point on the bony chin contour giving the maximum length from the temporomandibular joint (close to pogonion).
- *Lower height of face*: It was measured from the upper anterior nasal spine (the point where it is 3 mm thick) to the menton.

   Harvold has formed a comparative table (**Table 31.4**) of the above mentioned measurements for a particular age. Hence, by taking a cephalogram, doing the analysis the obtained measurements may be compared with the given table to determine the age of the patient (**Fig. 31.17**).
- *Skeletal age*: The clinical importance of evaluating skeletal maturation has long been recognized by the health profession. Skeletal maturation is an integral part of individual patterns of growth and development and are studied as under:
- Hand wrist radiographs (**Fig. 31.18**)
- Ossification of long bones
- Ossification and bony fusion of the epiphysis.

Sex Determination

Sex determination is an important step for identification of human remains and for dentolegal investigations in forensic odontology.

   Teeth may prove to be an important factor for identifying the individual through cellular, immunological and enzymological examination of their pulp. Therefore, sexing of teeth could be of immense help in identification of human

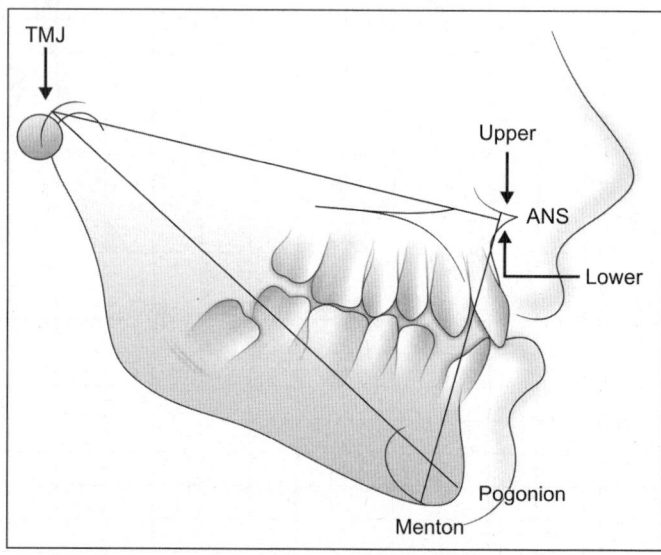

Figure 31.17 The linear measurements in the Harvold's analysis

Table 31.4 Harvold standard values (mm)

	Age	Male		Female	
		Mean value	*Standard deviation*	*Mean value*	*Standard deviation*
Maxillary length	6	82	3.2	80	3.0
	9	87	3.4	85	3.4
	12	92	3.7	90	4.1
	14	96	4.5	92	3.7
	16	100	4.2	93	3.5
Mandibular length	6	99	3.9	97	3.6
	9	107	4.4	105	3.9
	12	114	4.9	113	5.2
	14	121	6.1	117	3.6
	16	127	5.3	119	4.4
Lower face height	6	59	3.6	57	3.2
	9	62	4.3	60	3.6
	12	64	4.6	62	4.4
	14	68	5.2	64	4.4
	16	71	5.7	65	4.2

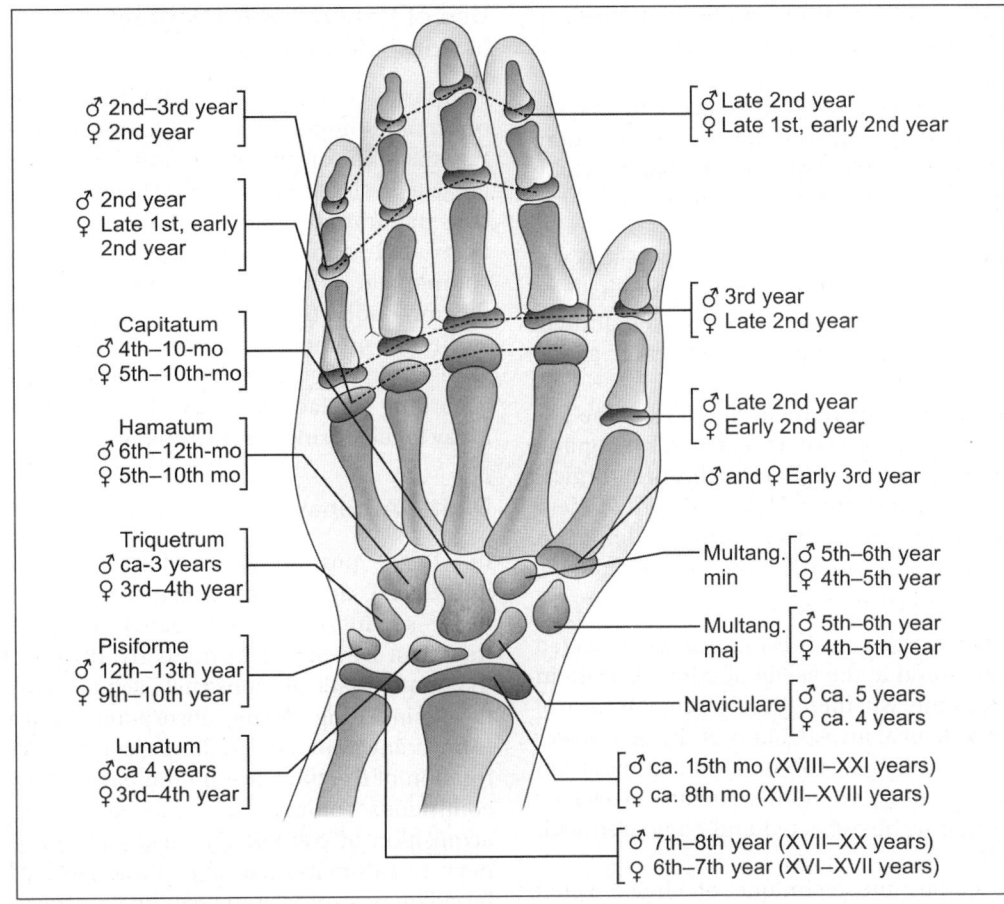

Figure 31.18 The time of appearance of carpal ossifications in boys and girls

remains investigation and solving crimes. During last five decades many workers have contributed for evolving different techniques of sex determination from human skeleton. These can be considered under following headings:

- Determination of sex by anatomical method which includes
  - Skull
  - Pelvis, sacrum, long bones and other bones of the skeleton
  - Tooth morphology.
- Determination of sex by radiological method
- Determination of sex by nuclear testing:
  - From blood stains
  - From hair
  - From saliva
  - From tooth pulp.
    - X-chromosomes
    - Y-chromosomes.

Some researchers believe that if the dental and bone ages correspond closely, the skeleton is probably male; if the bone age is advanced in comparison with the dental age, it is probably female.

Radiology in Race Determination

Radiology plays important but limited role in race determination.

- It has been suggested that the enamel of the molar teeth may extend down between the roots in Chinese race more commonly than in Europeans.
- The presence of enamel pearls on the roots of teeth may also be visible radiographically and this might indicate a person of Eskimo origin.
- Pulp cavity in molars of the Mongoloid race is said to be exceptionally deep and wide.

Reconstruction of Radiographs and Antemortem Photographs

There are very few cases in the forensic dental literature in which use has been made of 'superimposition technique' involving antemortem photographs and postmortem radiographs.

Surgical intervention may also be recorded radiographically and therefore may be useful in identification procedure. For example, extraction of teeth or roots may provide useful information for estimation of the time since extraction by careful observation of alveolar socket in relation to healing wound on a radiograph.

Occasionally sockets may remain unhealed and may be unchanged on the radiography up to 15 years after extraction, even lamina dura remains intact and sclerotic bone fills the socket giving the appearance of a retained root with a central root canal.

Infrequently a radiopaque steel bur may be left at the site of surgical removal of a tooth or radiopaque amalgam may get dislodged from tooth at the extraction site and get incorporated, and remains as a permanent marker in the bone.

Circumferential bone wiring done for fracture of the jaw and complex orthodontic treatment as seen in a radiograph will indicate that patient had undergone lengthy oral surgical procedure or orthodontic treatment. Usually record of these two treatment procedures are available with the dentist in the form of complete history, dental casts (study models), dental chart and X-rays even photographs.

Dental fragments: Small fragments become either impacted in soft tissues or are found at the scene of crime or even in food stuff. To determine whether these fragments are of dental origin, morphological investigation under low power microscope can be done. By using serological method, from fragments less than 1 mm^3 of tooth structure especially antigen from dentine can be extracted and compared with the known antibodies.

Radiography becomes the technique of choice when above technique cannot be applied or fragment is in soft tissue.

Postmortem intraoral radiography can reveal the status of the crowns of teeth when visual access is limited or impossible with antemortem means of achieving identification by comparison with antemortem clinical records.

Difficulties are often encountered in placing and retaining intraoral film in the mouth of deceased person whose musculature is been fixed in *rigor mortis*. Du Saucey MJ et al. (1991) used balloon catheter which can be inflated within the oral cavity and serve to support the film in place during radiographic exposure.

Smith BC (1992) presented a reversible technique in which root morphology of missing teeth in skeletonized human remain can be reconstructed and radiographs are made which will highlight the antemortem morphology of root and even may guide the discovery of antemortem dental evidence.

Cameron and Sims (1973) noted that the teeth may loosen when jaws dryout, and in such cases teeth should be pressed firmly back into the socket to avoid confusing variation in periodontal ligament thickness.

Seward (1972) noted that tissues immersed in fixing solution for a period of time tend to become some what opaque than fresh tissues.

Use of Panoramic Radiograph in Forensic Odontology

Happonen RP et al. (1991) recommended use of orthopantomography in identification which enables visualization of the structures of the jaws and related areas as a single radiograph. Haerting A et al. (1991) stated that panoramic dental radiography is the only regularly up dated and 'truly reliable identification card' for comparison radiography in forensic odontology. He further recommended that panoramic radiographs should be taken earlier for members concerned of the armed forces serving abroad as well as airline personnels. These radiographs according to Haerting A can be taken at the time of chest X-ray taken during medical check up.

Digital Autopsy

In 1989, postmortem radiographic examination was introduced. In recent decades, classic radiography has been used in the search for bullets, other foreign bodies and fractures. Developed in the early 1970s, CT is a technique that mathematically constructs digital cross-sectional images by assimilating tissue absorption information obtained from many transaxial radiographic projections during one rotation of the tube around the patient. Spiral CT allows for continuous volume data collection within one scan. This acquisition of volume data also makes it possible to create new two-dimensional and three-dimensional depictions based on post-processing sectional images, two-dimensional 'multiplanar' reformations, three-dimensional shaded surface display (SSD) and three-dimensional volume rendering.

The newest generation of CT scanners, multisliced computed tomography (MSCT) was introduced in 1998 and allows for scanning complete anatomic regions within a few seconds.

Alternatives to the classic autopsy for collecting forensically relevant data have been considered for many years. Some procedures have been discussed in the forensic literature for example, an 'endoscopic autopsy'.

When the modern method of multisliced computed tomography is used, the scan time for a full body examination of a fatality with a gunshot wound to the head is approximately 60 seconds.

The advantages of the forensic application of MSCT:
- This method is more rapid
- It is based on a nondestructive documentation process
- It is more precise than the standard forensic autopsy
- By the MSCT technique any new two-dimensional views can easily be reconstructed from the native data set and used for visualization
- Two-dimensional multiplanar reformation creates coronal, sagittal and any other oblique views from the axial data set
- Furthermore, it is possible to reconstruct three-dimensional views to visualize soft tissues and bone.

Table 31.5 Radiographic image of various dental implant fixtures

Implant type	Implant/Radiograph	Description
Osstem GS II implant fixture		*Straight body structure*: • Flat apical end • Finer radiopaque ring outlines in the upper one-third and well defined radiopaque serrations in the middle and apical third suggestive of dual combining micro and macro threads • A radiolucent area in the middle third • Reduced radiopacity along the borders of the fixture in the apical part due to blade of cutting edge
Dentsply XIVE implant		*Gradually tapering body*: • Rounded apical end • Uniform thread thickness • Radiolucency at the center corresponding to the internal cylindrical perforation • Apical vertical cuts causing reduced radiopacity along the borders in the apical one-third
Uniti equinox implant fixture		*Upper one-third is parallel body without prominent thread units*: • Well tapered lower two-thirds with prominent thread pattern • Rounded apical end • A rectangular radiolucency at the junction of middle and lower one-third • Reduced radiopacity in the apical third due to vertical cuts
Nobel biocare implant fixture		*Expanding tapered body*: • Flattened end apically • Radiopaque ring at the top • Implant in implant appearance • Rectangular radiolucent window in the upper half with a radiopaque bar passing through it • Crescent shaped radiolucency in the lower one-third area
Lifecare endopore implant fixture		*Truncated body*: • Shorter length • No radiopaque serrations due to lack of threaded units • Straight cut flat apical end • Rectangular radiolucency in the middle third • No reduced radiopacity at apical borders due to lack of vertical cuts

Oliver et al. made the first three-dimensional forensic visualization of a bullet path based on classic orthogonal radiographs using a treatment planning tool for radiation oncology.

Another advantage in comparison to the classic autopsy is that the documentation of the radiographic examination is produced nondestructively.

Limitations of the Forensic Application of Multisliced Computed Tomography

Because in bodies there is no circulation clinically established, use of intravenous contrast agents is not available, preventing the method from being used for questions like the assessment of vascular flow and detailed vascular morphology, tissue perfusion, bleeding sites or tissue differentiation. Radiographic documentation offers certain advantages in comparison with the standard forensic autopsy. It is rapid, objective, noninvasive and nondestructive.

The documentation and analytic process in the use of multisliced computed tomography may lead toward a minimally invasive virtual forensic autopsy in selected cases. Digital images are subject to modification and illegal tampering for which proper precautions need to be taken.

Identification of Dental Implants on Radiographs

The number of patients being treated with dental implants is increasing, thus the precise recognition of implants on radiographs is of increasing importance in victim identification. Identification of implants that have been inserted previously by other dentists is only possible from radiographs. The following are a few descriptions of the radiographic image of a number of dental implant fixtures (**Table 31.5**).

BIBLIOGRAPHY

1. Avrahami R, Watemberg S, Danish Philips E, et al. Hiss J Endoscopic Autopsy. Am J Forensic Med Patho.1995;(1)16. AEW, Miles. Dentition in Age Estimation, J Dent Res. Supplement to 1963;42(1):255-63.
2. Birguil Azral et al. Usefulness of combining clinical and radiological dental findings for a more accurate noninvasive age estimation. J Forensic Science. 2007;52:(1).
3. Brodgon BG, Forensic radiology, Boca Raton, FL: CRC Press 1998;98.
4. Brown KA, Hollanmb C, Clarke BJ, et al. A video technique of raniofacial photo super imposition.Proceeding of 8th international meet of IAFS kasas abstract. 1978;199:59.
5. Cameron JM, Sims BG. Dental identifications forensic dentistry. Churchill livingstone publication, Edinburg Page 46-59.
6. Chandra Sakharam P. Electronics skull identification device. J Foren Sci Soc. 1985;1(1):169-74.
7. Dahl, Solheim. Computer aided dental identification. Odontostomatol. 1985;3:7.
8. Demirjian A, Goldstein H, Tanner JM. A new system of dental age assessment. Hum Bioi. 1973;45:211.
9. Dental clinics of North America - Forensic Odontology. 2001;45(2):237-49.
10. Dental clinics of North America Forensic. Odontology. 2001; 45(2):316-24.
11. De-Saucey MJ, et al. Postmortem dental radiography a useful innovation. J Odontostomatol. 1991;9(1):24-8.
12. Donald R, Morse, et al. Comparision of clinical and statistical models in age estimation using dental periapical radiographic parameters, Compend Contin Edu Dent, Vol. XIV, No 6.
13. Donald R. Morse, et al. Age estimation using dental radiographs. Am J Forensic Med Pathol. 1994;15:4.
14. Evans KT, Knight B. As cited in "Forensic Radiology". Backwell Scientific Publication, Oxford London Edinburg, Boston, Melbourn; 1981.
15. Funtz L. History of forensic dentistry. Dent Clin North America. 1977;21:3.
16. Griffin JH, Malan D. Age determination of children from radiographic analysis of eight stages in the mineralization of the lower left permanent dentition, excluding the third molar. Dissertation for diploma in forensic odontology, London hospital medical college, 1987.
17. Gustafson G. Age determination of teeth. J Am Dent Assoc. 1950;41:45.
18. Gustafson G. Microscopic examination of teeth as a means of identification in Forensic Medicine. J Am Dent Ass. 1947;7:35:720.
19. Haglund. The NCIC missing and unidentified persons system revisited. J Forens Sci. 1993;38:365.
20. Hagmeier H. "Identification electronic superimposition I images". Int Crim Pol Rer. 1983;373:286-90.
21. Hame SDH. Identification in man disasters from dental prosthesis. Int J Forens Dent. 1973;1:11.
22. Happonen RP, et al. Use of orthopantomographs in forensic identification. Am J For Med Pathol. 1991;12(1): 59-63.
23. Harrey W. Dental identification and forensic odontology. Henry Kimpton Publishers, London; 1976.pp.101.
24. Harvey OW. Identity by teeth and the marking of dentures. Brit Dent J. 1966;121:334.
25. Hawey W. Dental identification and F O London, 1976;104.
26. Heriting, et al. Role of dental panaroma in identification procedure. J Radiol. 1990;72(10):489-90.
27. Isaque S, et al. As cited in "Determination of sex from necrotic human dental pulp and its utility in forensic odontology". Dissertation submitted to Bombay University. 1987.
28. Kalender W, Klotz E, Vock P, et al. Spiral volumetric CT with single breath hold technique transport and continuous scanner rotation. Radiology. 1990;176:181-91.
29. Kalra. As cited in "Age Evaluation from Lower Right Permanent Molar Teeth". Dissertation submitted to Bombay University, 1976.

30. Karjodar FR, Maideo A. Identification from dental implants, medico-legal update. 2012;12.

31. Karjodkar FR, Anuradha Maideo Identification from Dental Implants, Medico-legal update. 2012;12:1.

32. Karjodkar FR, Saxena SV. Fractals in Forensic, J Indo Pacific Acad For Odont. 2011;2(2):16-21.

33. Kasat V, Karjodkar FR Vaz W. Age estimation in 25-45 years old females by physical and radiological methods. J Forens Dent Sci. 2010;2:(2).

34. Keiser-Nielsen. Dental identifications: Certainty vs probability. Forens Sci. 1977;9:87.

35. Lorton, Rethman, Friedman. The CAPMI system. J Forens Sci. 1988;33:977.

36. Mincer HH, Harris EF, Berryman HE. The ABFO study of third-molar development and its use as an estimator of chronological age. J Forens Sci. 1993;38:379.

37. Moorees CFA, Fanning EA, Hunt EE. Age variation of formation stages for ten permanent teeth. J Dental Res 1963;42:264-73.

38. Oliver WR, Boxwala A, Rosenman J, Cullip T, Symon J. Wag nor G. Three-dimensional visualization and image processing in the evaluation of patterned injuries: the AFIP/UNC experience in the Rodney King case. Am J forensic med pathol. 1997;18:1-10.

39. Patil N, Karjodkar RF, Sontakke S, Kaustubh Sansare, Rohini Salvi, Uniqueness of radiographic patterns of the frontal sinus for personal identification; Imaging Sci Dent. 2012;42(4):213-217. English. Published online 2012 December http://dx.doi.org/10.5624/isd.2012.42.4.213.

40. Reichs KJ, Demirjian A. A multimedia tool for the assessment of age in immature remains: The electronic encyclopedia for maxillofacial, dental and skeletal development. In Reichs KJ (Ed): Forensic Osteology, Ed 2. Springfield, IL, Charles C Thomas 1998 .

41. Roberto Cameriere, et al. Age estimation by pulp/tooth ratio in canines by periapical X-rays. J Forensic Science. 2007;52:(1).

42. Role of Dental Radiology in Forensic Odontology 963

43. Sarode V. As cited from "Simple methods for age determination and sex identification from permanent teeth: Their application in forensic odontology". Dissertation submitted to Bombay University, 1992.

44. Sekharan C. The problems of positioning skulls for video superimposition technique. J Cad Soc Foren Sci 1989;22:21-4.

45. Serwin Ib. Identification of dental implants on radiographs. Quintessence International. 1992;23:9.

46. Shendarkar A. Dissertation submited to Mumbai University. Estimation of age in the living in the age group 25-45 years in Municipal employees by Physical and Radiological examination. 2005;32.

47. Shendarkar AT, Kharat R, Vaz WF, et al. Estimation of Age in Living Municipal Employees in Age Group of 24–45 years by physical and radiological examination. J Indian Acad. Forens Med. 32(2)113-9.

48. Shirodkar RP. As cited from "Ascertaining the attainment of 18 years, age in Indian subject by morphometric study of the third molar's". Dissertation submitted to Bombay University, 1984.

49. Siegel. Sperber. 10 through the computerization of dental records. J Forens Sci. 1977;22:434.

50. Smith BC. Reconstruction of root morphology in skeletonized remains with postmortem dental loss. J For Sci. 1992;37(1):176-84.

51. Southard, Pierce. Applications of digitized image transmission to forensic dentistry. Milit Med. 1986;150:413.

52. Sweet O, DiZinno JA. Personal identification through dental evidence: Tooth fragments to DNA. Calif Dent Assoc J. 1996;24:35.

53. T Harley W (1966), Butler O, Furness J and Laird R (1968). Value of keeping accurate dental records, 1968.

54. Tanner JM, Whitehouse RM, Marshall WA, et al. (Eds). Assessment of Skeletal Maturity and Prediction of Adult Height TW2 Method. London, Academic Press, 1975.

55. The dental clinics of North America—forensic odontology. 2001;45(2):217-19.

56. Udupa JK. Three-dimensional visualization and analysis methodologies; a current perspective. Radiographic. 1999; 19:789-806.

57. Vale GL. Forensic odontology. Jou Soc Calif Dent Assoc. 1969;37:248.

58. Vikrant Kasat. Disseration submitted to Mumbai University, estimation of age in the living in the age group of 25-45 years in female volunteers by physical and radiological examination, 2006.

59. Willems G, Van Olman A, Spiessens B, et al. Dental age estimation in Belgian children: Demirjian's technique revisited. J Forens Sci. 2001;46(4). In press.

Index

Page numbers followed by *f* refer to figure and *t* refer to table